# *The Esophagus*

## *Third Edition*

# The Esophagus

## Third Edition

### Editor

**Donald O. Castell, M.D.**
*Kimbel Professor and Chairman*
*Department of Medicine*
*Graduate Hospital*
*Philadelphia, Pennsylvania*

### Associate Editor

**Joel E. Richter, M.D.**
*Chairman*
*Center for Swallowing and Esophageal Disorders*
*Department of Gastroenterology*
*The Cleveland Clinic Foundation*
*Professor*
*Department of Medicine*
*The Cleveland Clinic Foundation Health Science*
*Center of the Ohio State University*
*Cleveland, Ohio*

LIPPINCOTT WILLIAMS & WILKINS
PHILADELPHIA · NEW YORK · BALTIMORE

Acquisitions Editor: Beth Barry
Developmental Editor: Anne Snyder
Manufacturing Manager: Tim Reynolds
Production Manager: Liane Carita
Production Editor: Robin E. Cook
Cover Designer: Sandy Mohindru
Indexer: Pam Edwards
Compositor: Maryland Composition
Printer: Maple-Vail

**Library of Congress Cataloging-in-Publication Data**

The esophagus / edited by Donald O. Castell and Joel E. Richter.—
  3rd ed.
     p.     cm.
  Includes bibliographical references and index.
  ISBN 0-7817-1535-0
  1. Esophagus—Diseases.   I. Castell, Donald O.   II. Richter, Joel
E.
  [DNLM:  1. Esophagus Diseases.    WI 250E792   1999]
  RC815.7.E763   1999
  616.3′2—dc21
  DNLM/DLC
  for Library of Congress                          98-42497
                                                       CIP

To the loves of my life—Marci, Nicole, Mandy, and Jason.

*Joel E. Richter*

To those in my family who share my excitement for intellectual activity: June Anne, Daniel, Kathleen, Celine, Mary, Karen, Steve, Cynthia, Richard, Marianna, Jessica, and David. Hopefully, this same spirit will naturally be transmitted to Fiona and Sophia. Deep appreciation for the immeasurable support and encouragement by Debra Bruestle and to the ''Esophageal Team''—Matt Gideon, Nicole Bracy, Vera Paoletti, Phil Katz, and David Katzka.

*Donald O. Castell*

# Contents

Color plate sections appear in Chapters 15 and 36

# Contributors

**Edgar Achkar, M.D.**
*Department of Gastroenterology*
*The Cleveland Clinic Foundation*
*9500 Euclid Avenue NE*
*Cleveland, Ohio 44195*

**John R. Bennett, M.D.**
*Treasurer*
*Royal College of Physicians*
*11 St. Andrews Place*
*London NW1 4LE*
*United Kingdom*

**Michelle L. Bennett, M.D.**
*Resident*
*Department of Dermatology*
*Wake Forest University School of Medicine*
*Medical Center Boulevard*
*Winston-Salem, North Carolina 27157–1071*

**Susan A. Branton, M.D.**
*Department of Surgery*
*Mayo Clinic Jacksonville*
*4500 San Pablo Road*
*Jacksonville, Florida 32224*

**Alan J. Cameron, M.D.**
*Department of Gastroenterology*
  *and Hepatology*
*Mayo Clinic*
*200 First Street SW*
*Rochester, Minnesota 55905*

**Donald O. Castell, M.D.**
*Department of Medicine*
*Graduate Hospital*
*One Graduate Plaza*
*1800 Lombard Street*
*Pepper Pavilion, Suite 501*
*Philadelphia, Pennsylvania 19146*

**June A. Castell, M.S.**
*Director*
*Clinical Research*
*Department of Medicine*
*Graduate Hospital*
*1800 Lombard Street*
*Suite 501, Pepper Pavilion*
*Philadelphia, Pennsylvania 19146*

**Ian J. Cook, M.D., F.R.A.C.P.**
*Associate Professor*
*Faculty of Medicine*
*University of New South Wales*
*Kensington*
*New South Wales 2052, and*
*Director*
*Department of Gastroenterology*
*St. George Hospital*
*Kogarah*
*New South Wales 2217*
*Australia*

**Tom R. DeMeester, M.D.**
*Chief of Surgery*
*Department of Surgery*
*University of Southern California Medical Center*
*1510 San Pablo, Suite 514*
*Los Angeles, California 90033*

**Kenneth R. DeVault, M.D.**
*Associate Professor*
*Department of Medicine*
*Mayo Medical School*
*200 First Street SW*
*Rochester, Minnesota 55905, and*
*Consultant*
*Department of Medicine*
*Mayo Cliic Jacksonville*
*4500 San Pablo Road*
*Jacksonville, Florida 32224*

**Steven A. Edmundowicz, M.D.**
*Associate Professor*
*Department of Medicine*
*Graduate Hospital*
*1800 Lombard Street*
*Suite 1101, Pepper Pavilion*
*Philadelphia, Pennsylvania 19146*

**Thomas R. Eubanks, D.O.**
*Acting Assistant Professor*
*Department of Surgery*
*University of Washington*
*Box 356410*
*1959 NE Pacific Street*
*Seattle, Washington 98195-6410*

**David E. Fleischer, M.D.**
*Chief, Endoscopy*
*Professor of Medicine*
*Division of Gastroenterology*
*Georgetown University Medical Center*
*Room 2122*
*3800 Reservoir Road, NW*
*Washington, D.C. 20007*

**Neil R. Floch, M.D.**
*Laparoscopic Surgery Fellow*
*Department of Surgery*
*Mayo Clinic Jacksonville*
*4500 San Pablo Road*
*Jacksonville, Florida 32224*

**Lawrence S. Friedman, M.D.**
*Associate Professor*
*Department of Medicine*
*Harvard Medical School, and*
*Physician*
*Gastrointestinal Unit (Medical Services)*
*Massachusetts General Hospital*
*55 Fruit Street, Blake 456D*
*Boston, Massachusetts 02114*

**Kim R. Geisinger, M.D.**
*Director, Surgical Pathology and Cytopathology*
*North Carolina Baptist Hospital, and*
*Professor*
*Department of Pathology*
*Wake Forest University School of Medicine*
*Medical Center Boulevard*
*Winston-Salem, North Carolina 27157-1072*

**R. Matthew Gideon**
*Director*
*Esophageal Function Laboratory*
*Graduate Hospital*
*Philadelphia, Pennsylvania 19146*

**Raj K. Goyal, M.D.**
*Mallinckrodt Professor of Medicine*
*Center for Swallowing and Motility Disorders*
*Brockton/West Roxbury VA Medical Center*
*Department of Veterans Affairs*
*Research Service 151*
*1400 VFW Parkway*
*West Roxbury, Massachusetts 02132, and*
*Harvard Medical School*
*Boston, Massachusetts 02115*

**Nadim G. Haddad, M.D.**
*Trad Hospital*
*Klemenceau*
*Beruit, Lebanon*

**Susan M. Harding, M.D.**
*Associate Professor of Medicine*
*Medical Director*
*Department of Medicine*
*UAB Sleep/Wake Disorders Center*
*Division of Pulmonary, Allergy, and Critical*
*   Care Medicine*
*University of Alabama at Birmingham*
*Tinsley-Harrison Tower, Room 215*
*Birmingham, Alabama 35294*

**Ronald A. Hinder, M.D., PhD**
*Professor and Chairman*
*Department of Surgery*
*Mayo Clinic Jacksonville*
*4500 San Pablo Road*
*Jacksonville, Florida 32224*

**Anthony Infantolino, M.D., FACP**
*Assistant Clinical Professor of Medicine*
*Division of Gastroenterology and Hepatology*
*Thomas Jefferson Medical College, and*
*Clinical Director of Endoscopic Ultrasound*
*Division of Gastroenterology and Hepatology*
*Thomas Jefferson University Medical Center*
*132 South 10th Street, 480 Main Building*
*Philadelphia, Pennsylvania 19107*

**Jozef Janssens, M.D., PhD**
*Professor of Medicine*
*Department of Gastroenterology*
*University of Leuven (Kul), and*
*Head*
*Department of Gastroenterology*
*University Hospital Gasthuisberg*
*Herestraat*
*3000 Leuven*
*Belgium*

**David A. Johnson, M.D., F.A.C.P., F.A.C.G.**
*Professor*
*Department of Gastroenterology*
*Eastern Virginia School of Medicine, and*
*Digestive and Liver Disease Specialists, Ltd.*
*844 Kempsville Road, Suite 106*
*Norfolk, Virginia 23502*

**Joseph L. Jorizzo, M.D.**
*Professor and Chair*
*Department of Dermatology*
*Wake Forest University School of Medicine*
*Medical Center Boulevard*
*Winston-Salem, North Carolina 27157-1071*

**Peter J. Kahrilas, M.D.**
*Professor of Medicine*
*Departments of Medicine and Communication*
  *Sciences and Disorders*
*Northwestern University Medical School, and*
*Medical Director*
*Division of Gastroenterology and Hepatology*
*Northwestern University Hospital*
*Passavant Pavilion, Suite 746*
*303 East Superior Street*
*Chicago, Illinois 60611*

**Philip O. Katz, M.D.**
*Vice Chairman*
*Department of Medicine*
*Chest Pain and Swallowing Center*
*Graduate Hospital*
*Suite 501, Pepper Pavilion*
*1800 Lombard Street*
*Philadelphia, Pennsylvania 19146*

**David A. Katzka, M.D.**
*Chief*
*Division of Gastroenterology*
*Graduate Hospital*
*1800 Lombard Street*
*Philadelphia, Pennsylvania 19146*

**James Walter Kikendall, M.D.**
*Gastroenterology Service*
*Walter Reed Army Medical Center*
*6900 Georgia Avenue, NW, Room 7F*
*Washington, D.C. 20307-5001*

**Paul J. Klingler, M.D.**
*Department of General Surgery*
*University Hospital of Innsbruck*
*Annichstrasse 35*
*A-6020 Innsbruck, Austria*

**Elizabeth Klinkenberg-Knol, M.D., Ph.D.**
*Department of Gastroenterology*
*Free University Hospital*
*P.O. Box 7057*
*1007 MB Amsterdam*
*The Netherlands*

**Corinne L. Maydonovitch, M.D.**
*Gastroenterology Service*
*Walter Reed Army Medical Center*
*Building 2, Room 7F*
*Washington, D.C. 20307-5001*

**Ravinder K. Mittal, M.D.**
*Professor of Medicine*
*Department of Gastroenterology*
*University of California, San Diego*
*4028 Basic Science Building*
*9500 Gilman Drive*
*La Jolla, California 92093-0688, and*
*Chief*
*Gastroenterology Section*
*Department of Veterans Affairs Medical Center*
*3350 La Jolla Village Drive*
*La Jolla, California 92123*

**J. Barry O'Connor, M.D.**
*Center for Swallowing and Esophageal Disorders*
*Department of Gastroenterology*
*The Cleveland Clinic Foundation*
*9500 Euclid Avenue*
*Cleveland, Ohio 44195*

**Roy C. Orlando, M.D.**
*Professor of Medicine and Physiology*
*Chief, Gastroenterology and Hepatology*
*Tulane University Medical Center*
*1430 Tulane Avenue*
*New Orleans, Louisiana 70112-2699*

**David J. Ott, M.D.**
*Professor of Radiology*
*Department of Radiology*
*Wake Forest University School of Medicine*
*Wake Forest University Baptist Medical Center*
*Medical Center Boulevard*
*Winston-Salem, North Carolina 27157*

**Carlos Pellegrini, M.D.**
*The Henry N. Harkins Professor and Chairman*
*Department of Surgery*
*University of Washington, and*
*Attending Surgeon*
*University of Washington Medical Center*
*1959 NE Pacific Street*
*Box 356410*
*Seattle, Washington 98195*

**Jeffrey H. Peters, M.D.**
*Associate Professor*
*Department of Surgery*
*University of Southern California School of*
  *Medicine*
*Chief, Section of General Surgery*
*University of Southern California University*
  *Hospital, and*
*University of Southern California Healthcare*
  *Consultation Center*
*1510 San Pablo Street, Suite 514*
*Los Angeles, California 90033*

**David A. Peura, M.D.**
*Professor of Medicine*
*Associate Chief*
*Division of Gastroenterology and Hepatology*
*University of Virginia Health Sciences Center*
*Hospital West GI Division*
*P.O. Box 10013*
*Charlottesville, Virginia 22906*

**Joel E. Richter, M.D.**
*Chairman*
*Center for Swallowing and Esophageal Disorders*
*Department of Gastroenterology*
*The Cleveland Clinic Foundation, and*
*Professor*
*Department of Medicine*
*The Cleveland Clinic Foundation Health Science*
  *Center of The Ohio State University*
*9500 Euclid Avenue*
*Cleveland, Ohio 44195*

**Malcolm Robinson, M.D., F.A.C.G., F.A.C.P.**
*Clinical Professor of Medicine*
*Division of Gastroenterology*
*Department of Medicine*
*University of Oklahoma Teaching Hospitals*
*Oklahoma City, Oklahoma 73104*

**Robert Thayer Sataloff, M.D., D.M.A.**
*Chairman*
*Department of Ortolaryngology—Head and Neck*
  *Surgery*
*Graduate Hospital*
*1800 Lombard Street #608*
*Philadelphia, Pennsylvania 19146, and*
*Professor*
*Department of Otolaryngology—Head and Neck*
  *Surgery*
*Thomas Jefferson University*
*1020 Walnut Street*
*Philadelphia, Pennsylvania 19107*

**Matthias H. Seelig, M.D.**
*Chief Resident*
*Department of Surgery*
*General Hospital Ludwigshafen*
*Bremserstrasse 79*
*D-67063 Ludwigshafen/Rhein*
*Germany*

**Steven S. Shay, M.D.**
*Department of Gastroenterology*
*The Cleveland Clinic Foundation*
*9500 Euclid Avenue*
*Cleveland, Ohio 44195*

**Elizabeth F. Sherertz, M.D.**
*Professor and Vice Chair*
*Department of Dermatology*
*Wake Forest University School of Medicine*
*Medical Center Boulevard*
*Winston-Salem, North Carolina 27157-1071*

**D. V. Sivarao, Ph.D.**
*Center for Swallowing and Motility Disorders*
*Brockton/West Roxbury VA Medical Center*
*Department of Veterans Affairs*
*Research Service 151*
*1400 VFW Parkway*
*West Roxbury, Massachusetts 02132, and*
*Harvard Medical School*
*Boston, Massachusetts 02115*

**André J. P. M. Smout, M.D., Ph.D.**
*Professor of Gastroenterology*
*Gastrointestinal Research Unit*
*Departments of Gastroenterology and Surgery*
*University Hospital Utrecht*
*P.O. Box 85500*
*3508 GA Utrecht*
*The Netherlands*

**Joseph R. Spiegel, M.D., F.A.C.S.**
*Chairman*
*Department of Otolaryngology—Head and Neck*
  *Surgery*
*Graduate Hospital*
*1800 Lombard Street*
*Philadelphia, Pennsylvania 19146, and*
*Associate Professor*
*Department of Otolaryngology—Head and Neck*
  *Surgery*
*Thomas Jefferson University*
*1020 Walnut Street*
*Philadelphia, Pennsylvania 19107*


**Anita E. Spiess, M.D.**
*Department of Gastroenterology*
*Northwestern University School of Medicine*
*33 West Higgins, Suite 5000*
*Chicago, Illinois 60610*


**Jan Tack, M.D., Ph.D.**
*Associate Professor*
*Center for Gastrointestinal Research, and*
*University of Leuven*
*Staff Member*
*Division of Internal Medicine*
*University Hospital Gasthuisberg*
*Herestratt 49*
*B-3000 Leuven, Belgium*


**Lisa A. Teot, M.D.**
*Associate Professor of Pathology*
*Director, Department of Cytopathology*
*University of Rochester Medical Center*
*601 Elmwood Avenue, Box 626*
*Rochester, New York 14642*


**Roland B. Ter, M.D.**
*Fellow in Gastroenterology*
*Division of Gastroenterology*
*Graduate Hospital*
*1800 Lombard St.*
*Philadelphia, Pennsylvania 19146*


**Richard W. Tobin, M.D.**
*Assistant Professor*
*Department of Medicine*
*Division of Gastroenterology*
*University of Washington School of Medicine*
*1959 NE Pacific Street*
*Seattle, Washington 98195*


**Michael F. Vaezi, M.D., Ph.D.**
*Department of Gastroenterology*
*The Cleveland Clinic Foundation*
*9500 Euclid Avenue*
*Cleveland, Ohio 44195*


**C. Mel Wilcox, M.D.**
*Associate Professor*
*Department of Medicine*
*University of Alabama at Birmingham, and*
*Director of Clinical Research*
*Chief of Endoscopy*
*Division of Gastroenterology*
*University Hospital*
*703 South 19th Street*
*633 Zeigler*
*Birmingham, Alabama 35294-0007*


**Roy K.H. Wong, M.D.**
*Gastroenterology Service*
*Walter Reed Army Medical Center*
*6825 Georgia Avenue, NW*
*Building 2, Room 7F*
*Washington, D.C. 20307-5001*


**Joseph Carl Yarze, M.D., F.A.C.P., F.A.C.G.**
*Attending Gastroenterologist*
*Division of Gastroenterology*
*Department of Medicine*
*Glens Falls Hospital, and*
*Gastroenterology Associates of Northern*
  *New York*
*5 Irongate Center*
*Glens Falls, New York 12801*


**Paul Yeaton, M.D.**
*Digestive Health Center*
*University of Virginia Health Science Center*
*Box 10013*
*Charlottesville, Virginia 22906-0013*

# Preface

This third edition of *The Esophagus* not only brings changes in chapters and authors, but also a new publisher and associate editor. I am extremely pleased that my respected colleague of many years, Dr. Joel E. Richter, has agreed to work with me to maintain the high level of clinical utility and new information that was achieved in the first two editions. In the process of planning the third edition, Dr. Richter and I have made a conscious attempt to revise old chapters, to provide current and clinically relevant information, and to add new chapters where appropriate. Thus, the chapters on anatomy and physiology, endoscopy, oropharyngeal dysphagia, rings and webs, diverticula, hiatal hernia, motility factors in gastroesophageal reflux disease (GERD), Barrett's esophagus, pulmonary complications of GERD, infectious esophagitis, non-cardiac chest pain, and perforation have undergone considerable revision; and new chapters on bile reflux and esophageal strictures appear for the first time in this edition. We have also invited new authors, including many of international stature, to write chapters in the hope of continuing to provide a fresh and up-to-date discussion of each area of esophagology contained within this text. This is particularly true with esophageal surgery, where Drs. Hinder and Pellegrini have joined the list of authors. Dr. Richter and I are delighted to have the opportunity to continue to develop this textbook with a respected, reputable publishing company such as Lippincott Williams & Wilkins. We anticipate that this collaboration will allow us to disseminate important information on esophageal function and disease more widely throughout the world. The preparation of the text material for *The Esophagus* remains a labor of love and an honest attempt to provide information that we believe is of clinical importance to those internists, gastroenterologists, and surgeons who frequently care for patients with esophageal disorders and often seek direction for diagnosis and treatment of perplexing clinical scenarios. It is our hope that you will find the material in this third edition as helpful and exciting as we do.

*Donald O. Castell*
*Joel E. Richter*

*The Esophagus*, Third Edition,
edited by D. O. Castell and J. E. Richter.
Lippincott Williams & Wilkins, Philadelphia © 1999.

CHAPTER 1

# Functional Anatomy and Physiology of Swallowing and Esophageal Motility

Raj K. Goyal and D. V. Sivarao

The oral cavity, pharynx, and esophagus constitute the swallowing passage that transports food into the stomach. The oropharyngeal part of the swallowing passage is not a simple conduit as it is a crossroad that is shared by a variety of vital functions, including respiration and swallowing. Oropharyngeal muscles make precise and split-second adjustments to allow its use by respiratory or swallowing functions as mixing of swallowing and respiration can be fatal. The swallowing passage also serves as a conduit for the backflow of digestive contents that may occur during vomiting and belching. During these activities, an abrupt conversion of the pharynx from a respiratory to a digestive conduit is required. The pharynx is also well armed to handle any mishaps that might occur if timely movement of food does not take place in the pharyngeal passage, by means of special local reflexes. The passage of food through the esophagus is less demanding than that through the pharynx. The upper esophageal sphincter (UES) also has an important task of stopping the backflow of gastric contents into the pharynx and larynx. The lower esophageal sphincter (LES) has to constantly guard against gastric acid moving up into the esophagus, opening only transiently to allow passage of the swallowed food into the stomach. Clearly, swallowing is one of the very demanding reflex activities. The details of this reflex are still not fully understood. Many general and more focused reviewers have summarized past research advances that we now take for granted [51, 52, 80, 105, 108, 111, 133, 141, 172, 218, 237, 282, 299]. There are also some excellent recent reviews that describe aspects of oropharyngeal and esophageal motility in detail [13, 22, 31, 114, 116, 162, 173, 175, 177, 238]. This chapter provides a general review of the physiology of swallowing and oropharyngeal and esophageal motility.

## SWALLOWING REFLEX

The act of swallowing can be divided into voluntary and involuntary phases. The voluntary component of the oral stage of swallowing involves mastication and mixing of a food bolus with saliva and positioning of an appropriate-sized food bolus on the dorsum of the tongue. The involuntary component of the oral stage includes opening of the glossopalatal gate, which separates the oral cavity from the pharynx, and a wave-like contraction starting from the anterior part of the tongue and working backward to squeeze the bolus against the hard palate and propel it into the pharynx. Movement of the bolus through the pharynx and the UES constitutes the pharyngeal stage. After entering the esophagus, the food bolus is carried across the esophagus and LES into the stomach, and this constitutes the esophageal stage. Oral, pharyngeal, and esophageal stages are the motor expression of the swallowing reflex. Normal human subjects swallow about 500 times during a 24-hour period [157]. The onset of the swallowing reflex is marked by contraction of the mylohyoid muscle. The muscles involved in swallowing are shared by other complex reflexes, including mastication, gagging, retching, vomiting, belching, respiration, and speech [80].

### Initiation

Stimulation of receptors at the base of the tongue, tonsils, anterior and posterior pillars of the fauces, soft palate, uvula, posterior pharyngeal wall, epiglottis, and larynx can elicit the swallowing reflex [3, 80, 246]. Even though the nature of these receptors is unclear, they are apparently very superficial in that when fluids of different chemical composition

R. K. Goyal and D. V. Sivarao: Center for Swallowing and Motility Disorders, Brockton/West Roxbury VA Medical Center, Department of Veterans Affairs, West Roxbury, Massachusetts 02132, and Harvard Medical School, Boston, Massachusetts 02115.

are applied to sensitive regions, the deglutition reflex is quickly activated [246]. There are significant interspecies differences in the relative sensitivity of these areas in initiating deglutition. In humans, the anterior and posterior tonsillar pillars and posterior wall of the pharynx appear to be the most sensitive areas for initiating the reflex. The afferents initiating the deglutitive reflex are carried in the maxillary branch of the trigeminal nerve (cranial nerve V), the glossopharyngeal nerve (cranial nerve IX), and the superior laryngeal branch of the vagus nerve (cranial nerve X) [80, 140].

Swallowing can also be initiated voluntarily from the cerebral cortex [142, 162], but this requires some additional sensory input from the pharynx because voluntary deglutition is very difficult when the pharynx is anesthetized or if there is no bolus present. Esophageal distention may also induce swallowing in humans, as does perfusion of the esophagus with a fluid of low pH and reflux of gastric acid [68, 188].

Electrical stimulation of the superior laryngeal nerve (SLN) is a popular method of inducing swallowing in experimental animals [21, 100, 156]. However, SLN stimulation elicits other reflexes as well, and a specific pattern and intensity of stimuli are necessary for eliciting swallowing. For example, higher intensities of electrical SLN stimulation elicit gagging, whereas lower intensities produce swallowing and even lower intensities produce only LES relaxation [10, 79]. In the opossum, contraction of the cricopharyngeus, which resembles gagging, is elicited after the onset of SLN stimulation. However, with continued stimulation, cricopharyngeal inhibition associated with the swallowing reflex is induced [10].

**Central Organization**

Peripheral afferent and cortical inputs activate swallowing-center neurons to elicit the swallowing reflex [73, 172, 173, 218, 237]. *Swallowing center* is an operational term that describes a complex of organizing and follower excitatory and inhibitory interneurons which produce a patterned sequence of inhibitory and excitatory discharges for the motor neurons that innervate the muscles participating in the swallowing reflex. The complex of interneurons involved in the swallowing reflex is also called the swallowing pattern generator (SPG) because, once activated, it carries out the entire sequence of swallowing without additional sensory input.

Electrical recording of medullary neurons during swallowing, by Jean [140, 141] and others [172, 173], has established that the swallowing-center neurons are located in two main brainstem areas, namely, the nucleus tractus solitarius (NTS) and the adjacent reticular formation and the nucleus ambiguus (NA) and the adjacent reticular formation. The areas in and around the NTS and NA are called dorsal and ventral regions of the swallowing center, respectively. Organization of swallowing has been reviewed by Miller [173].

The earliest neurons of the SPG are the organizing neurons that orchestrate the activities of other interneurons and the premotor neurons that provide sequential activation of motor neurons innervating the muscles involved in swallowing. Within the NTS, the organizing neurons for the oropharyngeal phase of swallowing are located in the intermediate part (NTSint) and those for the esophageal phase in the central part (NTSc) [32]. The organizing neurons for the oropharyngeal phase are closely connected with those for the esophageal phase, thereby linking oropharyngeal and esophageal phases of swallowing. Stimulation of oropharyngeal swallowing inhibits the esophageal phase and provides central contribution to the phenomenon of "deglutitive inhibition" [32].

The organizing neurons for oropharyngeal swallowing project onto a pool of excitatory and inhibitory interneurons located within the dorsal region and orchestrate sequential and patterned discharges from these interneurons. Output from these dorsal interneurons projects onto a second set of interneurons, which are located in the ventral region. These neurons have been called switch neurons because they relay patterned inhibitory and excitatory discharges to motor neurons involved in oropharyngeal swallowing. These premotor switch neurons for oropharyngeal swallowing project onto the motor nuclei of trigeminal (V), the facial (VII), the hypoglossal (XII), and the loose formation of the NA of glossopharyngeal (IX) and vagus (X) nerves [33, 152, 155].

The organizing neurons for the esophageal phase of swallowing project from the NTSc in the dorsal complex to a group of inhibitory and excitatory interneurons in the ventral complex. The fiber tracts that connect the neurons in the NTSc in the dorsal complex to the ventral complex neurons for the esophageal phase of swallowing pass through an area between the NTS and dorsal motor nucleus of vagus (DMNV). This is supported by the observation that while stimulation of the dorsal swallowing complex elicits both pharyngeal and esophageal phases of swallowing, lesion in the area between the NTS and DMNV abolishes the esophageal phase, leaving only pharyngeal swallow activity upon stimulation of the dorsal swallowing complex in the NTS. The premotor neurons from the ventral complex project onto the compact formation of the NA, which contains cell bodies of lower motor neurons carried in cranial nerves IX and X to the striated muscle portion of the esophagus [33]. The DMNV contains cell bodies of vagal preganglionic motor neurons that provide innervation to excitatory cholinergic myenteric neurons in the smooth muscle portion of the esophagus. The DMNV also appears to contain preganglionic neurons for the myenteric inhibitory neurons innervating the esophageal smooth muscle [100, 219]. Recent studies using neural fiber tract tracing techniques lead to somewhat different conclusions regarding locations of the premotor neurons [14, 16, 36]. Further studies will help to reveal the complex neuronal network that the swallowing center is.

The chemical mediators and neurotransmitters of the swallowing center are not well understood. Bieger [31, 32] has shown that glutamatergic afferent fibers activate the SPG for the oropharyngeal phase of swallowing via *N*-methyl-D-aspartate (NMDA) receptors, while cholinergic afferent fibers activate the esophageal phase of swallowing via muscarinic receptors. Moreover, thyrotropin-releasing hormone, substance P, oxytocin, and antidiuretic hormone also activate the swallowing center. However, their physiological importance is not known. On the other hand, γ-aminobutyric acid (GABA), released by GABAergic interneurons, exerts a tonic inhibitory action on the swallowing center so that inhibitors of GABAergic neurotransmitters stimulate the swallowing center. Dopamine, norepinephrine, enkephalin, and somatostatin also inhibit the swallowing center [31, 32]. Some esophageal premotor neurons have nitric oxide synthase (NOS), suggesting their inhibitory influence on the lower motor neurons [292].

The activity of the swallowing center is intimately linked with that of other medullary centers, such as respiratory and cardiovascular centers, allowing for close integration of swallowing with other reflex activities [241, 264]. The swallowing centers in each half of the medulla are also well connected so that in the event of destruction of the swallowing center on one side, the contralateral half of the center can execute the entire swallowing sequence [172].

The pattern of output by the swallowing center is programmed to be reproducible; however, it is not rigid and is modifiable. The pattern of swallowing reflex can be modified in several different ways. First, as mentioned above, oropharyngeal and esophageal stages can be dissociated so that either oropharyngeal or esophageal stages alone are expressed. Similarly, pharyngeal swallowing can occur without the oral phase [243]. Moreover, there is evidence to suggest that the esophageal vagal inhibitory pathway can be activated alone without the excitatory pathway, leading to deglutitive inhibition without esophageal peristaltic contraction. Second, the pattern of efferent swallowing discharge can be modified by the extensive sensory input from the pharynx and the esophagus [3, 21]. Finally, a variety of vagovagal reflexes that involve individual swallowing muscles can occur independent of the swallowing reflex. Some examples of these reflexes include transient LES relaxation, belching and vomiting reflexes, and UES and airway protective reflexes elicited by esophageal stimulation [177, 244].

### Cortical Influence

Although swallows can be elicited by cortical stimulation in experimental animals, recent studies show that transcranial magnetic stimulation of the motor cortex in humans does not initiate swallowing, probably because of the weakness of the applied stimulus [13]. However, it evokes two distinct electromyographic (EMG) responses in the oropharyngeal and esophageal striated muscles [13, 118]. The nerve fibers mediating these cortical responses may pass through the SPG, but this is uncertain [12]. Cortical topographic representation of muscles involved in the oropharyngeal and esophageal phases of swallowing with three-dimensional magnetic resonance imaging (MRI) scans using transcranial magnetic stimulation are now available [13, 118, 256]. The swallowing muscles are bilaterally represented with somatotopic organization on the motor cortex. Responses of swallowing muscles to cortical stimulation are facilitated by stimulation of afferents that evoke swallowing. Cortical ischemic lesions that involve the dominant hemisphere for swallowing lead to dysphagia and reorganization of the contralateral hemisphere; this plasticity underlies the improvement in swallowing seen after cortical stroke [118].

## OROPHARYNGEAL STAGE

### General Description

The oral stage includes both voluntary and involuntary phases of swallowing. The voluntary stage includes components such as oral filling, chewing, mixing with saliva, loading of food bolus on the tongue, and voluntary shift of food toward the posterior part of the tongue. The involuntary phase involves glossopalatal expulsion and clearing of the food bolus. A food bolus loaded on the tongue is contained in a cavity that is closed on all sides by the peripheral edges of the tongue contracting against the hard palate, and the glossopalatal gate remains closed. As the glossopalatal gate opens, bulk volume of the food bolus is expulsed into the pharyngeal cavity. This forceful expulsion of bulk volume is followed by clearing of residue by an anterior–posterior glossopalatal occluding contraction wave [148]. Kahrilas and co-workers [147, 148] have investigated the effect of bolus volume on the oral phase of swallowing. Larger-volume boluses require greater loading times than smaller-volume ones [148]. The size of the bolus chamber on the dorsum of the tongue varies with the size of the ingested bolus. However, in general, the period of expulsion and oral clearance of a barium bolus is similar regardless of the volume, being around 0.5 seconds. Larger volumes are associated with a larger opening of the posterior glossopalatal gate as well as a faster change in volume of the bolus chamber on the dorsum of the tongue. Thus, the overall pattern of lingual motion is similar among bolus volumes; however, larger-volume boluses are expulsed into the pharynx more rapidly and more vigorously than smaller-volume ones [148], but the clearance of residues of large- and small-volume boluses is similar. The oral phase of swallowing is generally investigated by videofluoroscopy, and disturbances in tongue contour have been investigated by sonography [286].

Just prior to the involuntary oral stage, in anticipation of the arrival of a food bolus, respiration is temporarily suppressed and the pharynx is converted from a respiratory to a swallowing pathway. Conversion of the pharynx to a swallowing pathway requires (a) closure of openings of the pharynx to nasal passages, oral cavity, and laryngeal vestibule [83]; (b) opening of the UES; and (c) shortening and widening of the pharyngeal chamber.

A food bolus enters the pharynx close to the onset of swallowing, and as soon as the food enters the pharynx, pharyngeal emptying starts. Most of the pharyngeal emptying into the esophagus occurs prior to the start of the pharyngeal peristaltic contraction. Ergun et al. [88], using ultrafast computerized tomography, reported that, during filling, the pharyngeal chamber volume was estimated to be 4.6 cm$^2$ after 0.36 seconds and 1 cm$^2$ after 0.42 seconds following the onset of swallowing, around which time the pharyngeal contraction started. The pharyngeal propulsive peristaltic contraction begins by apposition of the soft palate and the contracting posterior pharyngeal wall (Passavant's ridge). It then proceeds toward the esophagus by sequential appositions of the posterior pharyngeal wall with the posterior surface of the tongue, epiglottis, laryngeal, arytenoid and interarytenoid muscles, and finally the posterior surface of the cricoid cartilage [52, 149]. The anatomy of the pharynx, the epiglottis and cricoid cartilage effectively occlude the medial part of the swallowing chamber, splitting the bolus into two lateral halves before complete occlusion.

Pharyngeal clearance is also highly reproducible in timing and does not appear to vary much by the size of the bolus. Larger-volume boluses exit earlier and move with a greater velocity than smaller-volume swallows. Kahrilas et al. [149] reported velocity of propagation to be 50 cm per second for a 10-mL swallow and only 15 cm per second for a 1-mL swallow. However, the craniocaudal velocity of propagation of the tail end of the bolus representing the velocity of propagation of pharyngeal contraction does not vary with the bolus volume. So that the early and rapid movement of large-volume boluses through the pharynx can be properly handled, the UES opens much earlier than the onset of pharyngeal contraction [149].

The pharyngeal stage of swallowing is usually investigated by videofluoroscopy. Pharyngeal pressures reveal marked radial and axial asymmetry because of the anatomy of the pharynx [40, 230]. Moreover, head position markedly affects the dynamics of the pharynx [39]. Therefore, results of manometric studies of the pharynx are not reproducible and may not be helpful in clinical practice. Measurement of intrabolus pressure using swallowing videofluoroscopy and manometry is sometimes performed to evaluate resistance to the distal flow of a barium bolus.

**Neuromuscular Control**

Almost two dozen individual muscles innervated by branches of six cranial nerves (V, VII, IX, X, XI, and XII) with their motor neurons in the nucleus of cranial nerves V, VII, and XII and the NA (loose formation) participate to accomplish the wonder of oropharyngeal swallowing [116]. EMG of individual key muscles during swallowing provides information regarding inhibition and excitation [81].

The hyoid bone is critically located at the posterior part of the base of the oral cavity and the upper part of the fibrocartilaginous anterior wall of the pharynx. Movement of the hyoid bone with its attached muscle therefore controls the critical junction where a swallowed food bolus takes a 90-degree downward turn as it flows from the oral to the pharyngeal cavity. Hyoid muscles are active throughout the oropharyngeal phase of swallowing. In the first half of oropharyngeal swallowing (about 0.5 seconds), which includes the entire oral stage and filling and free flow of bolus through the pharynx, the hyoid bone moves up by 10 to 12 mm and forward also by 10 to 12 mm [135]. In the second half of the pharyngeal phase (also lasting about 0.5 seconds), the hyoid bone descends to its resting place (Fig. 1–1). The ascent of the hyoid bone is associated with raising of the floor of the mouth, which is important in accomplishing the oral phase. Elevation of the hyoid bone also brings the epiglottis from its vertical orientation to a horizontal one, which can provide a cover for the laryngeal opening during the passage of the food bolus, and shortens the length of the pharyngeal passage by over 1 cm. Forward displacement of the hyoid bone is essential for opening up the angle where the food bolus makes a turn into the pharynx, widening the pharyngeal passage and the opening of the UES. The descent of the hyoid bone corresponds with the pharyngeal peristaltic contraction wave. Jacob et al. [135] have shown that movement of the hyoid during its ascent and descent does not follow the same path but describes an ellipse so that its path of descent is up to 5 mm anterior to its path of ascent. It rises rapidly to reach a maximum height in about 0.4 seconds. It then moves forward for only 0.2 seconds, descends for ~0.4 seconds, and finally moves back to its original position (Fig. 1–1).

The main muscles that cause elevation and forward movement of the hyoid include the mylohyoid, the anterior belly of the digastric (innervated by V), the stylopharnyngeus (IX), and the geniohyoid (XII) muscles. Inhibition of activity in these muscles and contractions of infrahyoid muscles ensure orderly descent of the hyoid. The hyoid bone finally moves posteriorly to its natural resting position. The suprahyoid and infrahyoid muscles provide for a well-balanced movement of the hyoid bone during swallowing.

Just prior to the onset of the oral stage of swallowing, closure of the glossopalatal passage is ensured by elevation of the posterior surface of the tongue by styloglossus (innervated by XII) and palatoglossus (IX, X, and XI cranial nerve branches) muscles. The palatoglossus muscles play a particularly important role in the closure of this passage (Fig. 1–2). At the onset of the oral stage of swallowing, opening of the palatoglossal passage is facilitated by suppression of activities of the styloglossus and palatoglossus muscles and anterior pull on the hyoid bone and the posterior part of the tongue by geniohyoid muscle, supplied by cranial nerve XII. Elevation of the soft palate and uvula by levator veli palatini and uvular muscles, both innervated by cranial nerves X and XI, plays an important role in the opening of this passage.

A sequential anterior–posterior wave of apposition between the tongue and the palate move food residues from the oral cavity into the pharynx. This is brought about by activities of the hypoglossus and genioglossus muscles supplied by cranial nerve XII. As the contraction wave reaches the palatoglossal sphincter area, the palatoglossus, styloglos-

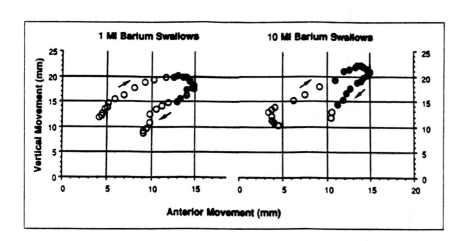

**FIG. 1–1.** Movement patterns of the hyoid bone during 1-mL and 10-mL swallows. Each circle represents the hyoid position during a single video frame of the recorded fluoroscopic sequence (0.03-second interval). *Arrows* indicate the direction of movement. *Open circles* denote frames during which the sphincter was closed; *solid circles* indicate times at which the sphincter was open; *hatched circles* indicate times that it was variably open, depending on the subject. Sphincter opening and closing occurred at nearly identical hyoid coordinates among subjects and among volumes. Larger-volume swallows were associated with persistence of the hyoid superior to and anterior to the opening coordinates. (From ref. 135, with permission.)

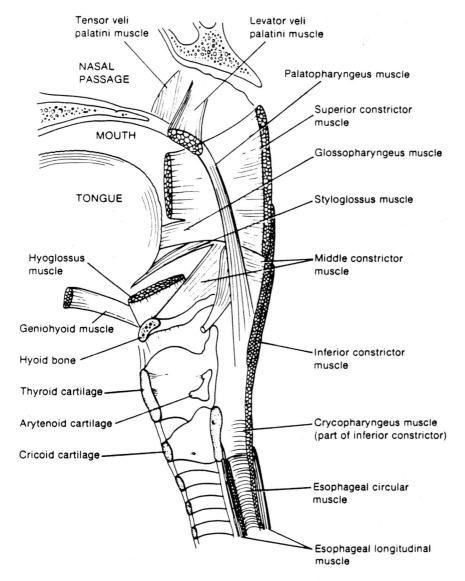

**FIG. 1–2.** Schematic of pharyngeal musculature. The pharynx, bridging the nose and mouth on one end to the esophagus and trachea on the other, is responsible for separating food and air as they pass through this area. The exquisite motor control required for this task is reflected by the complexity of its structure. The pharynx consists of several distinct muscle groups and, in its lower portion, is supported anteriorly by arytenoid, cuneiform, corniculate, and cricoid cartilages. Traditionally, the pharynx has been divided into the nasopharynx, oropharynx, and hypopharynx. The nasopharynx, extending from the base of the skull behind the soft palate to the distal edge of the soft palate, is not part of the alimentary tract. Muscles in the nasopharynx, such as the tensor veli palatini, levator veli palatini, and others, contribute to elevating the soft palate and closing the nasopharyngeal passage during swallowing, preventing bolus entry into the nasal passage. The oropharynx extends from the soft palate above to the base of the tongue and the level of the hyoid bone below and contains the upper border of the epiglottis, called the vallecula. In this area, the respiratory and gastrointestinal tracts cross. Muscles in the oropharynx are responsible for bolus propulsion (e.g., middle constrictor) and for elevation (e.g., palatopharyngeus) and forward displacement (e.g., geniohyoid) of the pharynx. The hypopharynx extends from the vallecula at the base of the tongue to the lower border of the cricoid cartilage and contains the inferior constrictor muscle and the upper esophageal sphincter. (From ref. 22, with permission.)

sus, and posterior belly of digastric muscles contract to close the oral cavity from the pharynx once more.

The pharyngeal phase of swallowing consists of conversion of the pharynx from a respiratory to a swallowing passage, pharyngeal filling, passive transport, and active pharyngeal peristalsis. One of the important components of conversion of the pharynx from a respiratory passage to a food passage is closure of the nasopharynx, which is accomplished by muscles attached to the soft palate (Fig. 1–3).

These are levator veli palatini, tensor veli palatini, uvular, and palatopharyngeus muscles. These muscles, except tensor veli palatini, are innervated by motor fibers carried in the vagus and accessory nerves with cell bodies in the NA. Tensor veli palatini is innervated by motor fibers in the trigeminal (V) nerve.

Another important component of the pharyngeal phase is closure of the larynx. Elevation of the hyoid causes the epiglottis to assume a horizontal position, to direct the food

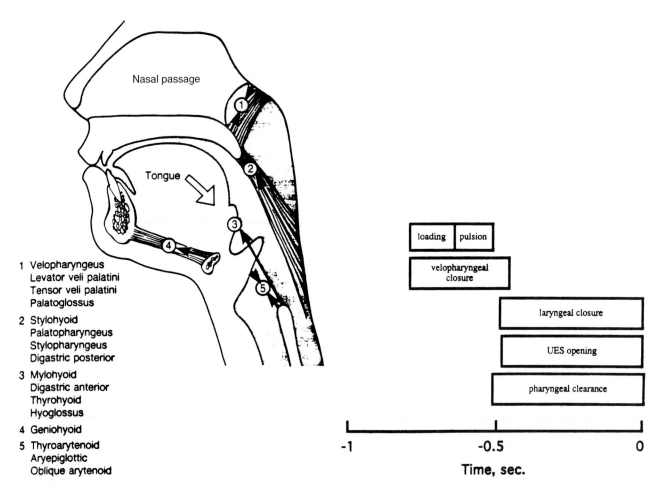

1 Velopharyngeus
  Levator veli palatini
  Tensor veli palatini
  Palatoglossus
2 Stylohyoid
  Palatopharyngeus
  Stylopharyngeus
  Digastric posterior
3 Mylohyoid
  Digastric anterior
  Thyrohyoid
  Hyoglossus
4 Geniohyoid
5 Thyroarytenoid
  Aryepiglottic
  Oblique arytenoid

**FIG. 1–3.** **Left:** List of extrinsic muscles, which are responsible for altering the shape of the pharynx and closing the airways, and intrinsic muscles, which are responsible for collapsing the lumen of the pharynx and propelling the bolus. The extrinsic muscles, including the levator veli palatini, tensor veli palatini, and palatoglossus, are located in the nasopharynx; they raise and tense the soft palate and uvula and close the nasal passage, preventing pressure generated in the mouth from being dissipated through the nose. The stylohyoid, palatopharyngeus, stylopharyngeus, digastric posterior, and other muscles located posteriorly cause elevation; and the geniohyoid, mylohyoid, digastric anterior, thyrohyoid, and other muscles located anteriorly cause forward displacement of the larynx and pharynx and contribute to opening the upper esophageal sphincter (UES). The thyroarytenoid, aryepiglottic, and oblique arytenoid muscles and others close the larynx to prevent food from entering the trachea. **Right:** Time course of events during swallowing of a 1-mL liquid bolus: closure of the velopharyngeus to prevent reflux into the nose, closure of the larynx to prevent aspiration, pharyngeal peristalsis to clear the bolus out of the pharynx, laryngeal upward and forward displacement to move the larynx out of the path of the bolus and to force open the cricopharyngeal region, and opening of the UES. Time zero represents the end of the swallow, determined by the occurrence of UES closure. Velopharyngeal closure occurs as the bolus is gathered on the tongue (i.e., loading) and propelled forward (i.e., pulsion). Laryngeal closure and UES opening occur later, during the phase of pharyngeal clearance. (From ref. 22, with permission.)

bolus from entering the larynx. The laryngeal opening during swallowing is further protected by adduction of three tiers of thyroarytenoid muscle [160, 226]. The first level involves approximation of aryepiglottic folds to allow coverage of the superior inlet of the larynx by the epiglottic tubule anteriorly and the arytenoid cartilages posteriorly. This is brought about by contraction of the most superior division of the thyroarytenoid muscle. A second tier of protection occurs at the level of the false vocal folds that form the roof of the laryngeal ventricle. Adduction of these folds is due to contraction of fibers of the thyroarytenoid muscles present in these folds. The third tier of protection occurs at the level of the true vocal cords. This is the most effective of the three barriers against aspiration. Adduction of the true vocal cords is brought about by contraction of the thyroarytenoid muscle. Thyroarytenoid receives its motor innervation from the recurrent laryngeal branch of the vagus. Other muscles of the larynx, namely, lateral and posterior cricoarytenoids, thyroarytenoid, and interarytenoid muscles (all innervated by the recurrent laryngeal nerve) and cricothyroid muscle (innervated by the external branch of the SLN), also help in adduction and closure of the vocal cords.

Apart from swallowing, a variety of protective reflexes against aspiration in response to afferent stimulation from the pharynx and esophagus have been identified [239, 242, 244, 245]. These reflexes are important in avoiding respiratory complications of gastroesophageal reflux disease [240].

Elevation of the hyoid bone by the suprahyoid muscle raises and shortens the anterior wall of the pharynx. The posterior and lateral muscular pharynx is shortened and elevated by the inner longitudinal muscles in the pharyngeal wall, i.e., the stylopharyngeus and salpingopharyngeus muscles. Motor neurons innervating these muscles are located in the NA, and the motor fibers are carried along the vagus (for salpingopharyngeus) and glossopharyngeal (for stylopharyngeus) nerves. The duration of elevation of the hyoid bone during swallowing can be voluntarily augmented (as in the Mendelsohn maneuver) so as to increase the period of pharyngeal swallowing. This allows for behavioral modification by biofeedback therapy for oropharyngeal dysphagia [116].

The craniocaudal sequential contraction (peristaltic wave) begins at the level of the superior pharyngeal constrictor and the palatopharyngeus muscle and travels down the overlapping middle and inferior pharyngeal constrictor muscles (Fig. 1–2). The pharyngeal constrictors are also innervated by large motor neurons in the semicompact formation of the NA, and the lower motor neurons are carried in the pharyngeal branches of the vagus nerve [155].

## Upper Esophageal Sphincter: Inferior Pharyngeal Sphincter

### General Description

The UES refers to a zone of intraluminal high pressure that exists between the pharynx and the upper esophagus.

Although it is generally called UES, it may be more justifiably called the inferior pharyngeal sphincter. Anatomically, the UES is comprised of the muscular cartilaginous hypopharynx along with the cricoid cartilage ventrally and the cricopharyngeus muscle both dorsally and laterally. The cricopharyngeus muscle has oblique and horizontal components. It is generally agreed that the horizontal portion of the cricopharyngeus is part of the UES. This muscle, however, is only 1 cm wide and therefore cannot itself account for the entire high-pressure zone, which measures between 2 and 4 cm [107]. The inferior pharyngeal constrictor joins with the cricopharyngeus in forming the UES [107].

The cricopharyngeus muscle is structurally, biochemically, and mechanically different from the surrounding pharyngeal muscles [156]. It is composed of striated muscle fibers of small average diameter (25 to 35 $\mu$m), which are not oriented in strict parallel fashion [34, 37], and a large amount of connective tissue and no muscle spindles [34]. The cricopharyngeus has both slow-twitch (type I) and fast-twitch (type II) muscle fibers; however, the predominant fiber is the slow-twitch type, which is more oxidative [75]. Mechanically, the length at which the cricopharyngeus develops maximum tension is larger than usual [166]. Innervation is also distinctive. Glycogen depletion studies have shown that it is innervated by both the pharyngeal nerve and the SLN [155]. The cell bodies of lower motor neurons carried in these nerves are located in the NA and additional neurons are located outside this nucleus [155].

### Basal Pressure

The closing pressure of the UES varies somewhat with the circumstances under which the measurements are made [39, 41, 57, 296]. The pressure profile of the UES shows axial asymmetry with a sharp ascent in its upper part and a more gradual decline in its lower part, as well as marked radial asymmetry [39, 291]. Welch et al. [291] constructed a three-dimensional pressure profile of the UES. The pressures are higher in the anterior–posterior than in the lateral orientation, but there is also a dissociation of peak pressures along the anterior and posterior aspects. Peak pressure occurs 1 cm below the upper border of the high-pressure zone anteriorly and 2 cm below the upper portion of the high-pressure zone posteriorly (Fig. 1–4). The radial and axial asymmetry is not observed after laryngectomy, indicating that the rigid cartilages of the larynx forming the anterior wall of the UES are responsible for the asymmetry [291]. Reported resting UES pressures in normal subjects with low-compliance recording systems have ranged from 35 to 200 mm Hg [39, 291, 296]. Pressure recorded with a laterally oriented manometric device is 33% of the magnitude of pressures recorded when the device is oriented in the anterior or posterior direction. Resting UES pressures may be lower in infancy, in the aged, and during sleep [144]. The UES opens with each swallow to permit passage of the bolus into the esophagus. Pressure recordings demonstrate a fall

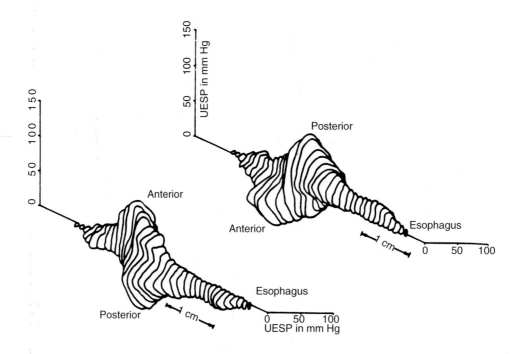

**FIG. 1–4.** Three-dimensional pressure profiles of the upper esophageal sphincter. Note that pressures are higher in the anteroposterior orientation than on the sides. (From ref. 291, with permission.)

in UES pressure immediately after the onset of deglutition. Pressures at the nadir of relaxation may reach subatmospheric levels [52] but do not usually reach intraesophageal levels.

Several studies have demonstrated continuous electrical spike activity in the cricopharyngeus muscle (Fig. 1–5) [10, 84, 85, 247, 281]. The significance of this activity, however, is a subject of debate. Doty [80] concluded that resting UES pressure is entirely due to passive forces caused by elasticity of the tissues and that tonic electrical spike activity is caused by reflex stimulation by the intraluminal manometry tube or other reflexes [156, 166]. Asoh and Goyal [10], in contrast, suggest that continuous electrical spike activity in both the cricopharyngeus and the caudal-most fibers of the inferior pharyngeal constrictor muscle combined with passive forces

are responsible for the resting UES pressure. The activity of the UES muscles is depressed during deep sleep and during anesthesia and shows a phasic change in activity with inspiration [10, 247].

Reflex increases in UES pressure occur with pharyngeal stimulation [167, 244], esophageal distention [87], and intraesophageal acid infusion [96]. The reflex increase in UES pressure induced by acid infusion or balloon distention is less marked when the more distal, rather than the more proximal, esophageal segments are stimulated [156]. The reflex increase in UES pressure caused by esophageal distention or acid infusion is largely mediated by vagal afferent pathways [92]. Bilateral cervical vagosympathetic cooling does not change the resting UES pressure but partially antagonizes the increase in pressure caused by distention or acid infusion.

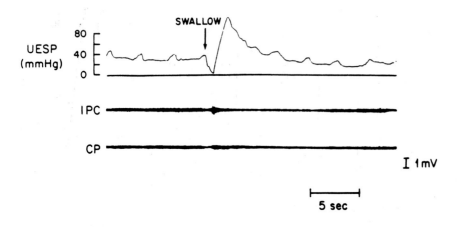

**FIG. 1–5.** Simultaneous manometric and electromyographic recordings from opossum upper esophageal sphincter (UES). Sphincter pressure (*UESP*) falls abruptly on swallowing, and this is associated with cessation of tonic electrical spike activity in cricopharyngeus (*CP*) and inferior pharyngeal constrictor (*IPC*) muscles. UESP then recovers and actually rises to well above baseline (postrelaxation contraction). This corresponds to increased spike-burst activity in CP and IPC. (From ref. 104, with permission.)

UES pressure also increases with inspiration, glossopharyngeal breathing, and gagging and during the Valsalva maneuver when it is performed against a closed mouth and nose as opposed to a closed glottis [108].

### Relaxation

Relaxation and opening of the UES occur during deglutition, rumination, vomiting, regurgitation, and belching [156, 242]. During swallow-induced relaxation of the UES, the continuous spike activity of the cricopharyngeus muscle ceases (Fig. 1-5) [9, 247]. This is due to inhibition of lower motor neurons in the brainstem that innervate the UES. The inhibition of tonic muscle activity is in itself not sufficient to open the UES because its closure due to passive factors persists even after cessation of all cricopharyngeal electrical activity. Elevation and anterior displacement of the larynx by the suprahyoid muscles, such as the geniohyoid muscle, are required to abolish this residual pressure and open the sphincter, though in experimental settings contraction of the geniohyoid muscle may obliterate the UES high-pressure zone even when the cricopharyngeus continues to be active (Figs. 6 and 7) [10]. Under normal circumstances, the cessation of activity in the cricopharyngeus and the contraction of the suprahyoid muscles are coordinated to ensure efficient opening of the UES [58, 145]. Paralysis of suprahyoid muscles, such as the geniohyoid, significantly impairs UES opening even when the cricopharyngeus functions normally [10]. On the other hand, contraction of the suprahyoid muscles may cause considerable opening of the UES despite impaired cricopharyngeal relaxation. Because UES opening is related to two factors, it is best to distinguish between cricopharyngeal relaxation and UES opening. The relaxation component is due to the cessation of tonic activity in the cricopharyngeal and inferior pharyngeal constrictor muscles,

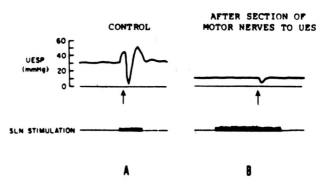

**FIG. 1-7.** Effect of transecting motor nerves to the upper esophageal sphincter (*UES*) on resting pressures and deglutitive responses as evoked by superior laryngeal muscle (*SLN*) stimulation. During control period **(A)**, resting UES pressure (*UESP*) is ~30 mm Hg. Stimulation of SLN causes initial transient UES contraction, followed by relaxation upon activation of deglutition reflex (*arrow*). After sectioning motor nerves to the UES **(B)**, resting UESP falls to ~10 mm Hg and deglutition, which is induced by SLN stimulation, causes a further drop in pressure, due to opening of the UES by contraction of the suprahyoid muscles. (From ref. 10, with permission.)

whereas the opening is due to contraction of the suprahyoid muscles. Impaired relaxation of the cricopharyngeus muscle or loss of its compliance by fibrosis is responsible for the prominent cricopharyngeal bar or cricopharyngeal achalasia [3, 58, 267]. In contrast, paralysis of the suprahyoid muscle and lack of opening of the UES are responsible for paralytic upper sphincter achalasia [107]. Simultaneous EMG and manometric studies are useful for investigating dysfunction of the UES [85].

## ESOPHAGEAL STAGE

### General Description

In adults, the body of the esophagus, exclusive of the sphincters, is 18 to 22 cm long [282]. The upper level of the esophageal body begins ~18 cm from the incisors and ends at 40 cm (range 26 to 50 cm) in men and at 37 cm (range 22 to 41 cm) in women. The esophageal wall, like other regions of the gut, consists of mucosa, submucosa, and muscularis propria; however, unlike the other regions, it has no serosal covering. The outer esophageal wall is bounded by a thin, poorly defined layer of connective tissue. The mucosa consists of stratified squamous epithelium in all regions except the LES, where esophageal squamous epithelium joins gastric columnar epithelium. Relatively few glands are present in the esophageal mucosa; hence, its secretory function is rather limited. The muscularis propria consists of inner circular and outer longitudinal muscle layers, in addition to a longitudinally oriented muscle layer called the muscularis mucosa located between the muscle layers and the mucosa.

During swallowing of liquid food, the food bolus enters

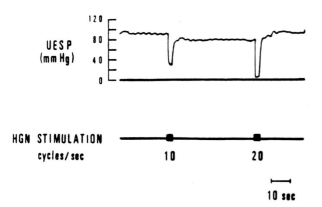

**FIG. 1-6.** Effect of geniohyoid muscle contraction on upper esophageal sphincter pressure (*UESP*) in opossum. Electrical stimulation of a branch of the hypoglossal nerve (*HGN*) to the geniohyoid muscle causes contraction of the muscle and a precipitous fall in UESP. This indicates that the suprahyoid muscles function to open UES independent of relaxation of the intrinsic UES muscles. (From ref. 10, with permission.)

the esophagus very early, soon after it enters the pharynx. In the upright position, the head of the liquid barium bolus traverses the esophagus and enters the stomach within a few seconds from the onset of swallowing. The tail of the bolus is propelled by the esophageal peristaltic contraction. Thus, in the upright position, because of gravity, the head of the liquid bolus moves faster than its tail. On the other hand, when the effect of gravity is removed, as in the recumbent position, the head and tail of the bolus move closely together. Normally, the esophagus is completely cleared of the ingested food bolus in 8 to 10 seconds (Fig. 1–8).

The esophageal peristaltic wave associated with swallowing is called primary peristalsis and is recognized by its association with pharyngeal peristaltic contraction and UES relaxation and activity in the mylohyoid muscle. The peristaltic wave is produced by a lumen-occluding contraction of the esophageal muscle. The characteristics of this

wave vary with the segment of esophagus in which it is measured [211]. The duration of the pressure wave varies from 2 to 7 seconds and increases in an aboral direction. Recording peak pressures with an intraesophageal transducer system reveals values of 53.4 ± 9.0 mm Hg (mean ± SE) in the upper esophagus, 35.0 ± 6.4 mm Hg in the middle portion, and 69.5 ± 12.1 mm Hg in the lower esophagus. The lower pressures in the midesophagus correspond to the junction of striated and smooth muscle. The average peristaltic speed is ~4 cm per second; it is ~3 cm per second in the upper esophagus, accelerates to ~5 cm per second in the midregion, and then slows again to ~2.5 cm per second just above the LES (Fig. 1–9). Several factors may influence the amplitude, duration, and propagation velocity of the peristaltic wave. Within the same individual and with the same technique, peristaltic amplitude remains reasonably constant when examined serially and is unaffected by age [127]. Am-

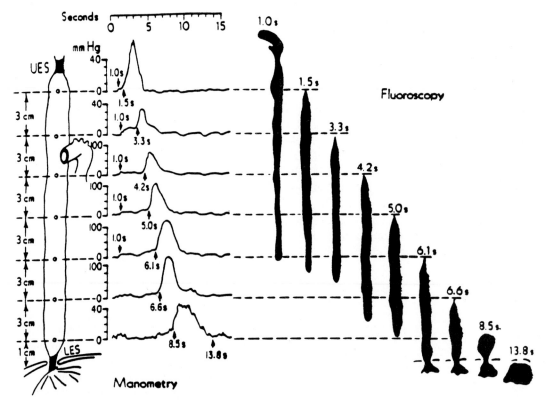

**FIG. 1–8.** Concurrent manometric and video recording of a 5-mL barium swallow. Tracings from the video images of the fluoroscopic sequence on the **right** show the distribution of the barium column at the times indicated above the individual tracings and by *arrows* on the manometric record. In this example, a single peristaltic sequence completely cleared the barium bolus from the esophagus. Pharyngeal injection of barium into the esophagus occurs at the 1.0-second mark. The entry of barium causes distension and a slightly increased intraluminal pressure, indicated by the *downward pointing arrows* marked "1.0 s." Shortly thereafter, esophageal peristalsis is initiated. During esophageal peristalsis, luminal closure and, hence, the tail of the barium bolus passed each recording site concurrent with the onset of the manometric pressure wave. Thus, at 1.5 seconds, the peristaltic contraction had just reached the proximal recording site and barium had been stripped from the esophagus proximal to that point. Similarly, at 4.2 seconds, the peristaltic contraction was beginning at the third recording site and, correspondingly, the tail was located at the third recording site. Finally, after completion of the peristaltic contraction (time 13.8 seconds), all of the barium was cleared into the stomach. (From ref. 145, with permission.)

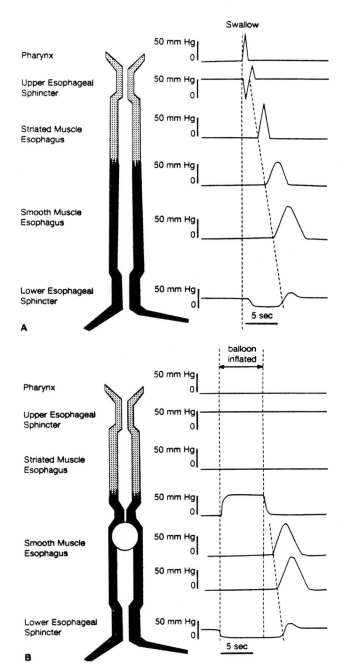

**FIG. 1–9. A:** Manometric profile of a primary peristalsis. At rest, the normal esophagus is quiescent and the sphincters are tonically contracted. Swallow triggers relaxation of the upper and lower esophageal sphincters (LES) and gives rise to a peristaltic contraction traveling smoothly through the striated and then the smooth muscle portion of the esophagus. Each location along the esophageal axis contracts with a latency that increases gradually from the upper esophagus to the LES. The latencies are site-dependent and reproducible. In the upper third of the esophagus, contraction occurs within 1 to 2 seconds after swallowing; in the middle third, within 3 to 5 seconds; and in the lower third, between 5 and 8 seconds. The velocity of the peristaltic wave is slower in the striated muscle and faster in the smooth muscle segments of the esophagus. Contractions reach the smooth muscle segment within 2 seconds after the onset of the swallow, traveling at a speed of about 3 cm per second; in the smooth muscle segment, the velocity of propagation may be as fast as 5 cm per second. The contractions in the striated muscle segment are shorter (1 to 2 seconds), and in the smooth muscle segment, they are longer (4 to 7 seconds). Contractions in the distal one-third of the esophagus are usually stronger (50 to 150 mm Hg) than those in the upper third (40 to 120 mm Hg), and both are stronger than those in the middle third (20 to 80 mm Hg), where they are relatively weak, probably occurring at the transition between the striated and smooth muscle esophagus. **B:** Manometric profile of a secondary peristalsis. Secondary peristalsis results when a bolus remains in the esophagus after an ineffective primary peristalsis or when gastric contents reflux into the esophagus. It is thought to be caused by distension and can be demonstrated by inflating a balloon in the esophagus. Upon inflation, the esophagus contracts proximal to and relaxes distal to the balloon, including the LES. When the balloon is deflated, peristalsis proceeds down the esophagus. (From ref. 22, with permission.)

plitudes of esophageal contractions are less when recorded in the upright position, with velocity greater in the upper esophagus and decreasing in the mid- to lower esophagus [229]. Also, the duration and amplitude are increased and the velocity is decreased when a fluid bolus is swallowed as opposed to a dry bolus, i.e., gulping air [128]. Moreover, larger bolus volumes elicit stronger peristaltic contractions [138, 139]. Increases in intraabdominal pressure or outflow obstruction slow the speed of peristalsis. Warm boluses augment and cold boluses inhibit peristaltic contraction, but bolus osmolality is without significant effect [86, 297]. The esophageal peristaltic mechanism is not well developed in premature infants [187].

The amplitude (force) of peristalsis ensures that it completely sweeps the bolus without leaving any residue behind. However, weaker contractions can leave some residue behind. Moreover, if the bolus pressure is increased due to distal obstruction or reduced compliance of the lumen, the liquid bolus may appear to flow back through the ineffective peristaltic wave. Nonperistaltic contractions do not propel the food bolus but break it up into segments. On barium swallow examination, nonperistaltic contractions are responsible for a corkscrew or beaded appearance of the esophagus.

Food residue left behind in the esophagus by ineffective primary peristalsis is removed by the so-called secondary peristalsis. Secondary peristalsis is distinguished from primary peristalsis by the fact that it is localized to the esophagus and not accompanied by pharyngeal peristalsis or UES relaxation. Experimentally, secondary peristalsis is elicited by transient esophageal distention and deflation of an intraluminal balloon (Fig. 1–9) [194]. Esophageal distention may also induce primary peristalsis. Air and water boluses can also trigger a peristaltic response. However, slow infusion of fluids into the esophagus elicits either peristaltic or simultaneous contractions. Patients with reflux esophagitis have higher thresholds for eliciting a secondary peristalsis and reduced frequency of peristalsis [227]. The amplitude and velocity of secondary peristaltic contractions resemble those of primary peristalsis [91], but there are some differences in the sensitivity to atropine [191].

Winship and Zboralske [298] reported that if a balloon is inflated in the human esophageal body and prevented from moving distally, an aborally directed steady force of up to 200 g is exerted on the balloon, called the esophageal propulsive force. The esophageal propulsive force appears to increase with increasing bolus size and is greatest in the distal esophagus. During the period of fixed balloon distention, no contractions occur in the esophagus distal to the balloon; however, when restraints are removed from the balloon, the contraction producing the localized propulsive force is converted to a peristaltic sequence that progresses distally, pushing the balloon ahead of it [298]. Williams et al. [293] have shown that this propulsive force is produced by phasic and tonic contractions of the circular and longitudinal muscles at and just above the balloon. These consist of simultaneous contractions that become multipeaked, repetitive, and associated with a sustained rise in the basal pressure with increasing distention volumes [196, 293]. Generation of the esophageal propulsive force appears to be reflexly mediated, involving both central and local, afferent and efferent pathways [193].

Normally, the esophagus responds on a one-to-one basis to each pharyngeal swallow. However, the time required for the pharyngeal stage of swallowing is much shorter than that for the esophageal stage (1 second versus 8 seconds). Moreover, during rapid drinking, successive oropharyngeal swallows are performed up to every 2 seconds. During the period of rapid successive swallowing, the esophageal activity is inhibited and only the last swallow of the swallowing train is associated with esophageal peristaltic contraction (Fig. 1–10) [8, 171]. This phenomenon of deglutitive inhibition has been quantified by investigating responses to paired swallows made at different time intervals [171, 248, 280]. During normal food ingestion, when swallows are performed in rapid succession but irregularly, fewer peristaltic waves than swallows are observed. Moreover, the amplitudes are variable, presumably due to deglutitive inhibition [169]. Mayrand et al. [164] measured esophageal resting tone *in vivo* and Sifrim et al. [249, 250] have demonstrated a wave of inhibition prior to peristaltic contraction motility. Deglutitive inhibition is critically important for the passage of swallowed food through the esophagus, and failing deglutitive

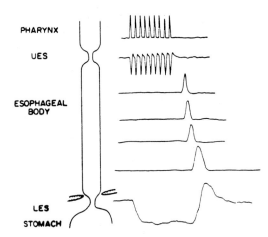

**FIG. 1–10.** Diagrammatic representation of deglutitive inhibition. Swallows taken in rapid succession are marked by repeated phasic pressure changes recorded in the pharynx. The upper esophageal sphincter relaxes and recovers with each swallow on a one-to-one basis. However, peristalsis in the esophageal body does not ensue until after the last swallow. Also, the lower esophageal sphincter relaxes to first swallow and does not recover until after the peristaltic wave initiated by the last swallow has traversed the esophagus. (From ref. 108, with permission.)

inhibition is associated with esophageal motility disorders [250].

### Striated Muscle (Cervical Esophagus)

The human cervical esophagus is composed of striated muscle in both the inner circular and outer longitudinal muscle layers. The longitudinal muscle fibers arise from the superior aspect of the median ridge on the dorsal surface of the cricoid cartilage and are joined by muscle bundles from the cricopharyngeus and posteriolateral cricoid cartilage on each lateral aspect. Fibers course dorsally and caudally to join ~3 cm below the cricoid cartilage posteriorly. This arrangement leaves a triangular area devoid of longitudinal muscle that is called Laimer's triangle. Esophageal striated muscle develops from esophageal smooth muscle by a process of transdifferentiation [190]. Approximately ~4 cm (2 to 6 cm) of the proximal end of the esophageal body is constituted by striated muscle [170, 282]. Smooth and striated muscles are present in nearly equal amounts between 4 and 8 cm from the upper end. This mixture of striated and smooth muscle extends to a point 10 to 13 cm from the lower border of the cricopharyngeus. From that point distally, it is exclusively smooth muscle, so the distal one-half to one-third of the esophagus is entirely smooth muscle in both the inner circular and outer longitudinal coats. There have been rare reports of striated muscle extending the length of the entire esophagus in humans [133].

The somatic motor fibers to the striated muscles of the esophagus arise from lower motor neurons located in the nucleus retrofacialis and the compact formation of the NA

[33] and contain choline acetyltransferase and calcitonin gene-related peptide (CGRP). Axons of the lower motor neurons projecting to the esophagus are carried in the vagus nerve. Nerve fibers to the striated muscle portion of the esophagus depart from the vagus in the upper part of the neck as the recurrent laryngeal nerve. Therefore, electrical stimulation of the vagus nerve in the midportion of the neck produces no response in the striated muscle segment of the esophagus. The lower motoneurons are myelinated and make direct contact with individual striated muscle fibers, which contain choline acetyltransferase and CGRP, via the motor end plate. Acetylcholine is the excitatory neurotransmitter involved at the motor end plate, exerting its effects through stimulation of nicotinic cholinergic receptors [277]. The role of CGRP is not known. The striated muscle portion of the esophagus also has a myenteric plexus with a large number of neurons that are NOS-positive [186, 225, 255]. These neurons provide nitrergic innervation to the motor end plates that is unique to the esophageal striated muscle. These nitrergic neurons may receive preganglionic input from the DMNV; however, this remains to be documented.

Peristalsis in the striated muscle portion of the esophagus is mediated by the lower motoneurons, the fibers of which are carried in the vagus nerve, as evidenced by the fact that bilateral cervical vagotomy above the origin of the pharyngoesophageal branches abolishes peristalsis in the striated muscle esophagus [137, 282]. Andrew [7] suggested that sequential discharge of the motoneurons destined for progressively more distal levels was responsible for peristalsis. Roman and Gonella [218] performed experiments in which the central portion of a sectioned vagus (containing nerve fibers from lower motor neurons to the striated muscle portion of the esophagus) was sutured to the distal end of the motor nerve innervating the sternocleidomastoid and trapezius muscles, allowing vagal motor fibers to reinnervate these muscles. They then recorded EMG activity in muscle units in the neck in response to swallowing. It was found that activation of deglutition induced sequential contraction of the reinnervated muscles and that this coincided with esophageal peristaltic contractions. This observation further supported the view that sequential activation of vagal motoneurons elicited peristaltic activity. The esophageal sensory afferent input can quantitatively affect the peristaltic amplitude and velocity by modulating the central vagal efferent discharge.

Distention-induced peristalsis in the striated muscle segment of the dog and sheep esophagus is also entirely dependent on central vagal pathways. Thus, there is no difference between primary and secondary peristalsis in the striated muscle segments other than in the method of initiation and in the fact that the occurrence of the latter is independent of the oropharyngeal component. In humans, esophageal balloon distention has been reported to induce pharyngeal peristalsis that passes through the striated muscle segment and into the smooth muscle segment [248]. The distention-induced secondary peristalsis and esophageal propulsion in the

striated muscle portion are mediated by central reflexes. The deglutitive inhibition of the striated muscle esophagus is thought to be centrally mediated by inhibiting lower motoneurons in the compact formation of the NA [31]. Whether the intramural NOS-positive neurons in the myenteric plexus within the striated muscle play a role in peristalsis and deglutitive inhibition is not known.

### Smooth Muscle (Thoracic Esophagus)

The thoracic esophagus in humans is mostly composed of smooth muscle fibers that receive innervation from preganglionic neurons in the DMNV via the vagus [54]. These fibers then branch to form the esophageal plexus and finally enter the esophagus at different levels. The preganglionic fibers travel within the esophageal wall for several centimeters before reaching the postganglionic neurons in the intramural plexuses. The smooth muscle portion of the esophagus also receives a sympathetic nerve supply that arises from the cell bodies in the intermediolateral cell columns of spinal segments T1–T10. Preganglionic fibers enter the cervical sympathetic ganglia, ganglia in the thoracic sympathetic chain, and possibly the celiac ganglia. Most fibers to the lower esophagus travel in the greater splanchnic nerves to enter the celiac ganglia, where they synapse with postganglionic neurons [17]. Postganglionic branches accompany the blood vessels, and a few fibers join the vagus to reach the esophagus. Most of the postganglionic axons terminate in the myenteric plexus [17, 136] and submucosal plexus. Very few terminate directly on the muscle cells. The density of the adrenergic innervation is less in the lower sphincter than in the more proximal esophagus [17].

Intramural neural ganglia in the esophagus, like in other parts of the gut, are located in the myenteric and submucous plexuses. In the esophagus, the intramural neurons are fewer in number and more haphazard in arrangement than elsewhere in the gut [48, 233]. The esophageal neurons contain many different peptide and nonpeptide chemical markers [231, 254, 255, 285]. However, there are two predominant types of motor neuron: those staining for NOS and vasoactive intestinal polypeptide (VIP) and those that stain for substance P and choline acetyltransferase. Although indirect studies suggest that there are two populations of neurons that receive separate preganglionic projections, this has not yet been documented by morphological studies.

The neurophysiology of primary peristalsis and other motor activities in the smooth muscle portion of the esophagus is more complicated. It is clear, however, that swallow-induced primary peristalsis in the smooth muscle portion of the esophagus is also dependent on activation of the swallowing center and the vagal pathways to the esophagus since bilateral cervical vagotomy or vagal cooling abolishes primary peristalsis in the esophagus [171, 209, 220, 271]. However, unlike the striated muscle, sequential firing of vagal efferent neurons destined for progressively more caudal smooth muscle esophageal segments is not essential to activate peristalsis. This is demonstrated experimentally by simultaneously stimulating all vagal efferent fibers with an electric current and observing that peristalsis is still induced [98, 99, 101].

It was initially proposed that esophageal peristalsis in the smooth muscle portion of the esophagus was also due to sequential cholinergic excitation. Tieffenbach and Roman [271], using recordings from baboon skeletal muscle that had been reinnervated by vagal preganglionic efferent fibers, detected a vagal efferent discharge that coincided with peristaltic activity in the smooth muscle esophagus. The pattern of this discharge was sequential, indicating that vagal preganglionic fibers destined for the smooth muscle esophagus are activated by a central sequencing mechanism in the same manner as is seen with the vagal lower motoneurons that supply the striated muscle esophagus. Tieffenbach and Roman [271] suggested that these preganglionic efferent fibers synapse with postganglionic cholinergic fibers in the smooth muscle esophageal wall, which in turn produce the peristaltic contractions. This was consistent with the demonstration of atropine sensitivity of esophageal circular muscle contractions elicited by intramural nerve stimulation *in vitro*. According to this model, during swallowing, the esophageal circular muscle remains in its resting, quiescent state, responsible for the latency period, which is followed by contraction due to sequential activation of excitatory cholinergic neurons [218].

The above model of sequential activation of the cholinergic pathway leading to peristalsis was called into question when it was found that simultaneous electrical stimulation of vagal efferents elicits peristalsis rather than simultaneous contraction at all levels of the esophagus. These studies raised the possibility that vagal efferents to all levels of the smooth muscle portion of the esophagus may be activated simultaneously and pointed to a peripheral mechanism for peristalsis. Moreover, Rattan et al. [199] and others have reported that vagal efferent stimulation as well as swallowing cause a sequence of inhibition followed by contraction of the esophageal circular muscle. The sequence of mechanical inhibition (latency) and contraction correlated with the membrane potential changes of hyperpolarization followed by depolarization of esophageal circular smooth muscle (Fig. 1–11). Weisbrodt and Christensen [287] made the original observation that transmural stimulation of esophageal circular muscle strips produces a contraction after a period of latency and well after the end of the stimulus. They called it the ''off'' contraction. They also found that this contraction was not cholinergically mediated but was due to a nonadrenergic and noncholinergic inhibitory neurotransmitter. Electrophysiological studies have shown that transmural stimulation elicits membrane hyperpolarization followed by depolarization, which correlate with the latency period and ''off'' contractions, respectively, in mechanical studies [199]. Both of these responses are noncholinergic and are now thought to be mediated by the gaseous neurotransmitter nitric oxide (NO) [303]. Furthermore, Weisbrodt and Chris-

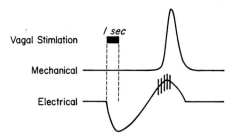

**FIG. 1–11.** Schematic illustrating simultaneous mechanical and electrical potential changes recorded from opossum esophageal circular smooth muscle. Note that vagal stimulation elicited hyperpolarization ([inhibitory junction potential (IJP), trough] followed by a rebound depolarization [excitatory junctional potential (EJP), crest] with superimposed spikes in the electrical activity trace. Mechanical trace shows a period of latency after vagal stimulation, followed by a contraction. The latency corresponds to the IJP and the contraction to EJP and spike activity. The neurotransmitter nitric oxide (NO) seems to be responsible for the hyperpolarization and associated latency of the smooth muscle, while the EJP and smooth muscle contraction seem to be due to a blend of NO-associated rebound and cholinergic excitation.

tensen [287] reported that the latency of circular muscle contraction increased progressively in caudal segments of the esophageal circular smooth muscle and suggested that esophageal peristalsis was due to noncholinergic inhibitory nerves and that a gradient in their influence or a regional difference in smooth muscle was responsible for swallow-induced peristalsis [108]. This model, however, could not explain the fact that the latency gradient elicited by vagal efferent stimulation did not match the slower velocity of swallow-induced peristalsis. Moreover, this model also could not explain the observed effect of atropine on primary peristalsis [74, 77].

More recent studies suggest that both noncholinergic inhibitory and sequential cholinergic excitatory pathways are involved in esophageal peristalsis. The presence of two parallel pathways in the vagal efferents was suggested by studies of Gidda and Buyniski [97]. They recorded swallow-evoked potentials from single cervical vagal efferent fibers of the opossum (Fig. 1–12) and found two types of preganglionic efferent fiber destined for the smooth muscle esophagus based on electrophysiological characteristics and latency distributions [100]. Short-latency fibers began firing within 1 second of the onset of swallowing, as recorded by mylohyoid activity. Long-latency fibers had latencies to onset of discharge that ranged between 1 and 5 seconds. The respective latency distributions indicate that short-latency discharges correlate with deglutitive inhibition and long-latency fibers correlate with peristaltic contractions. The swallow-evoked efferent discharge in each fiber lasts ~1 second with four to six spikes per discharge. These results were consistent with sequential activation of excitatory nerves during swallowing, as proposed by Roman and Gonella [218]. However, Gidda and Buyniski [97] suggested the ex-

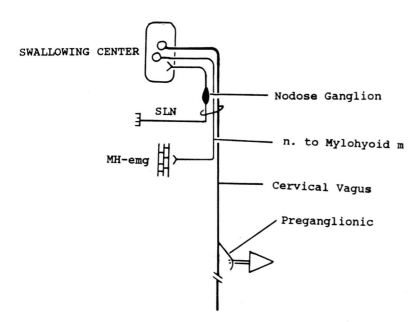

SWALLOWING CENTER

SLN

MH-emg

Nodose Ganglion

n. to Mylohyoid m

Cervical Vagus

Preganglionic

**FIG. 1–12.** Schematic illustrating the setup used for recording swallow-evoked responses from single-unit efferent vagal fibers of opossums. The superior laryngeal nerve (SLN) was stimulated to evoke swallowing, while mylohyoid muscle activity (EMG) was monitored as an index of swallowing.

istence of a parallel inhibitory vagal pathway that is also activated during swallowing.

Evidence for both cholinergic and noncholinergic peripheral pathways was first furnished by Dodds et al. [78], who showed that, depending on the intensity of stimulus used, vagal efferent stimulation can elicit either a cholinergic or a noncholinergic contraction in the esophageal circular muscle, as evidenced by sensitivity to atropine. They also showed that with long trains of vagal stimulation, the cholinergic contraction occurred with the onset ("on" contraction) and the noncholinergic contraction occurred after the end ("off," or rebound, contraction) of the stimulus. Careful *in vitro* studies of circular smooth muscle strips also showed that, depending on the stimulus used, either cholinergic or noncholinergic contractions can be elicited. Moreover, long-train electrical stimuli also produced a cholinergic ("on") contraction near the onset and a noncholinergic ("off") contraction after the end of the stimulus (Fig. 1–13). Recent studies have shown that "off" contractions are blocked by chemical inhibitors of the enzyme NOS [55, 184, 304].

The above observations are consistent with the view that during short train electrical vagal efferent or transmural stimulations, the contraction waves may be a blend of overlapping cholinergic and noncholinergic contractions. However, they do not explain the roles of cholinergic and noncholinergic nerves in esophageal peristalsis, i.e., the latency gradient along the esophagus. It appears that peristalsis in the smooth muscle portion of the esophagus is due to the latency gradient that is determined both by noncholinergic inhibitory as well as cholinergic excitatory nerves.

Weisbrodt and Christensen [287] were the first to demonstrate a latency gradient along the esophagus due to noncholinergic inhibitory nerves. Studies of membrane potential recording also show that, on transmural stimulation of noncholinergic nerves, the duration of the inhibitory junction

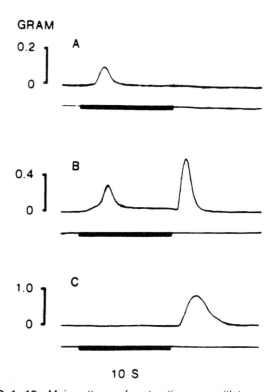

GRAM

0.2 — A

0 —

0.4 — B

0 —

1.0 — C

0 —

10 S

**FIG. 1–13.** Main patterns of contraction seen with transmural electrical stimulation of opossum esophageal circular smooth muscle strips. Stimulus train duration and pulse width were constant at 10 seconds and 1 millisecond, respectively. **A:** Stimulus of 60 V and 40 Hz resulted in only an "on" contraction, occurring shortly after onset of stimulus. **C:** Stimulus of 80 V and 10 Hz evoked only an "off" contraction, occurring after termination of stimulus. **B:** Stimulus 80 V and 20 Hz produced both "on" and "off" contractions. "On" contractions were sensitive to cholinergic blockade with atropine, whereas "off" contractions were not sensitive to cholinergic or adrenergic blockade. (From ref. 60, with permission.)

potential (IJP) is shorter in circular smooth muscle from proximal rather than distal sites [63, 65]. This may be due to increasing noncholinergic influence distally along the esophagus.

The cholinergic influence has been shown to decrease the latency of contraction [61]. A craniocaudally decreasing cholinergic influence would have the effect of slowing the velocity of peristalsis, as seen during swallowing. Crist et al. [61] have reported that cholinergic motor influence was maximal in the proximal portion of the esophagus and decreased distally. This was evidenced by greater sensitivity to atropine of the contraction amplitude and latency elicited by transmural stimulation of the circular muscle strips from proximal than from distal esophageal segments. Studies of membrane potential recordings more clearly showed a greater expression of cholinergic influence in reducing the duration of the IJP at proximal rather than distal esophageal sites [65] (Fig. 1–14). These and other observations led Crist et al. [61] to suggest a model showing gradients of decreasing cholinergic and increasing noncholinergic influences distally along the esophagus. These gradients explain, at

least in part, how vagal efferent or transmural nerve stimulation elicits the peristaltic sequence of esophageal contractions and how changing the intensity of electrical stimulation of the vagus nerve could change the velocity of esophageal peristalsis by altering the cholinergic and noncholinergic components in the peristaltic contractions [98]. In addition to the peripheral mechanism of peristalsis explained by the regional gradients of noncholinergic and cholinergic nerves, central sequential activation of the cholinergic pathway during swallowing would further aid in the normal slow speed of primary peristalsis (Fig. 1–15). During swallowing, there is immediate, near simultaneous activation of the inhibitory pathway but a delayed and sequential activation of the cholinergic excitatory neural pathway in the vagus. The early and more prominent cholinergic activation in the proximal esophageal site would cause greater shortening of latencies of contraction at the more proximal sites, resulting in increased velocity of esophageal peristalsis.

Successive vagal stimulation has been used to study whether the phenomenon of deglutitive inhibition in the esophageal circular muscle is also due to active peripheral inhibition by the noncholinergic inhibitory nerves [99]. These studies show that, similar to successive swallows, vagal stimulation exerts an inhibitory effect on the esophagus and that a peripheral mechanism for inhibition exists in the smooth muscle esophagus. Studies also show that the duration of deglutitive inhibition increases distally along the esophagus; explain the phenomenon of rebound contraction, which is due to ongoing active inhibition throughout the

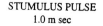

STUMULUS PULSE
1.0 m sec

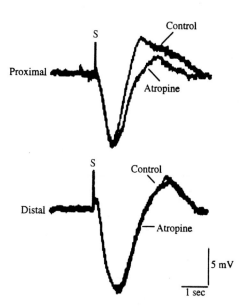

FIG. 1–14. Intracellular recording from opossum esophageal smooth muscle taken from proximal and distal esophageal sites. Note that transmural stimulation (at S) caused a hyperpolarization response in the smooth muscle cells from both sites. The control trace from the proximal site shows a shorter duration of hyperpolarization (inhibitory junctional potential [IJP]). However, following atropine treatment, the duration of IJP increased, suggesting cholinergic mediation in shortened duration of IJP. At the distal site, atropine had no marked effect, suggesting minimal cholinergic mediation. These observations illustrate that there is a gradient of cholinergic activity along the esophagus with the greatest influence at the proximal sites.

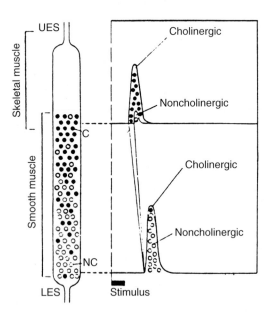

FIG. 1–15. Schematic drawing illustrating gradients of cholinergic (C) and noncholinergic (NC) nerve influence along the smooth muscle portion of the esophagus. Cholinergic influence is most prominent proximally and progressively decreases distally, whereas noncholinergic influence is most prominent distally and progressively decreases proximally. (From ref. 61, with permission.)

period of vagal stimulation; and reveal that esophageal peristaltic contractions are followed by a period of refractoriness [101].

The esophageal body circular muscle is a phasic muscle; i.e., it contracts transiently and does not develop sustained tone upon stimulation. This phasic property may be related to the composition of its contractile proteins, which revealed a greater proportion of a unique seven amino acid–inserted myosin isoform, acidic essential light chain (LC17a), caldesmon, and less $\alpha$-actin in the phasic esophageal muscle than the tonic sphincter muscle [266]. A variety of ion channels (potassium, chloride, nonselective cations, and calcium) have been identified in the esophagus. These channels modulate the membrane potential and influence calcium entry into the smooth muscle cells, thereby modifying contractility [1, 2, 283].

NO and acetylcholine (ACh) have been shown to be the major inhibitory and excitatory neurotransmitters, respectively. The redox form of NO involved in inhibitory neurotransmission has been shown to be the nitric oxide gas (NO$^\bullet$) [106], and its inhibitory effect has been shown to be due to a wide variety of signaling pathways that lead to a fall in intracellular $Ca^{2+}$ and inhibition of contractile activity. One of the important actions of NO$^\bullet$ is to produce membrane hyperpolarization, thereby causing inhibition of voltage-dependent calcium entry in smooth muscle cells. Goyal and co-workers [64, 106, 306] have shown that this hyperpolarization is due to cyclic guanosine monophosphate (cGMP)-dependent inhibition of a resting chloride conductance. Others have suggested that nitrergic IJP is due to opening of potassium channels [143].

ACh affects many ionic currents in esophageal circular muscle [121, 283]. Carbachol activates a $Ca^{2+}$-sensitive chloride and nonselective cation currents [283]. These currents appear to be activated by the release of $Ca^{2+}$ from intracellular stores. Activation of the chloride currents would cause depolarization of the smooth muscle membrane, leading to $Ca^{2+}$ entry into the cells via voltage-sensitive $Ca^{2+}$ channels. The nonselective cation channels are also permeable to $Ca^{2+}$ and to other cations but not anions. The nonselective cation channels have a large conductance but are sparsely distributed on the smooth muscle membrane; therefore, single channel currents can be observed. Their activation is not associated with significant depolarization. These channels may serve as a source for nonvoltage-dependent $Ca^{2+}$ entry [120]. ACh also inhibits a variety of potassium channels. These effects on potassium channels are most likely involved in the enhancement of the excitatory effect of ACh [121]. The signaling cascade for ACh-induced contraction of the esophageal circular muscle is different from that in the LES [26, 27, 260]. In the esophageal circular muscle, ACh acts on $M_2$ muscarinic receptors to activate phospholipase D (PLD), phosphotidyl-specific phospholipase C (PLC) via guanosine triphosphate (GTP)-binding protein ($G_{i3}$), and phospholipase $A_2$ (PLA$_2$) via an as yet unknown GTP-binding protein [258, 259]. Activation of

these enzymes requires influx of extracellular $Ca^{2+}$ [260]. These phospholipases produce diacylglycerol (DAG) and arachadonic acid (AA). DAG and AA act synergistically to stimulate protein kinase C$_\Sigma$ (PKC$_\Sigma$) [260]. Activated PKC$_\Sigma$ appears to act via mitogen-associated protein (MAP) kinase to inactivate actin-based inhibitory proteins such as caldesmon to cause muscle contraction. In experimental esophagitis, ACh-elicited contraction is not significantly affected [24]. Inflammatory mediators may suppress esophageal contraction in vivo by inhibiting the release or action of ACh.

Muscarinic antagonists such as atropine suppress the amplitude of esophageal contractions and prolong the latency of contractions in the smooth muscle but have no effect on the striated muscle. This effect is more marked in proximal than in distal parts of the esophagus [61, 77]. Moreover, peristaltic contractions in certain species, such as cats, are more sensitive to atropine than those in opossums [97]. Chemical blockers of NOS reduce the latency of contractions, particularly in the most distal parts of the esophagus, leading to simultaneous-onset contractions in response to swallowing [302, 303]. A combination of atropine and NOS blockers eliminates peristaltic contractions. Stroma-free hemoglobin solution binds and thereby scavenges released NO, resulting in effects on the esophageal peristalsis that are similar to those of NOS blockers used in animals [43, 56]. Esophageal peristalsis is also affected by agents that act centrally, at neuronal synapses of esophageal neurons and at smooth muscle directly.

The above discussion has focused on the esophageal circular muscle. However, the esophageal longitudinal muscle, by causing esophageal shortening, also plays an important role in various reflex activities [150]. Swallowing causes sequential activation of longitudinal muscle segments and is associated with inhibition and excitation, as seen in the esophageal circular muscle. The esophageal longitudinal muscle has prominent cholinergic and substance P innervation [62], and its pharmacology differs in some respects from that of the esophageal circular muscle. For example, NO donors and cGMP cause contraction (in addition to transient relaxation), and this contraction is mediated by a tyrosine kinase-signaling pathway [125].

## LOWER ESOPHAGEAL SPHINCTER

### General Description

The LES can be readily identified by intraluminal manometry as a 2 to 4 cm zone of high pressure at the gastroesophageal junction. The manometrically defined LES is marked by a ring of thickened circular muscle [29, 232]. Ultrastructural studies of the sphincter muscle in the opossum suggest that muscle cells from the LES are of larger diameter and form fewer gap junctions than do those of the esophageal body. These sphincter muscle cells also have irregular surfaces and evaginations that are not seen in the esophageal body. The evaginations may be related to the tonically contracted state of the sphincter muscle [232]. The LES can also be distinguished from the esophageal body, by the presence of more numerous intermuscular spaces containing blood vessels and connective tissue [232]. Mitochondria and the smooth endoplasmic reticulum mass are greater in the LES than in the esophageal body [47].

The LES is innervated by vagal preganglionic and sympathetic postganglionic efferents [20]. These efferents largely innervate neurons in the myenteric plexus. The myenteric neurons contain many chemical markers [254, 255, 285]; however, two prominent populations of motor neurons are noteworthy: those that contain NOS and VIP are inhibitory motor neurons and those that contain choline acetyltransferase and substance P are excitatory motor neurons. The motor neurons supply innervation to the muscle layers, including the interstitial cells of Cajal (ICC) that may serve as intermediary to amplify actions of neurotransmitters on the smooth muscle cells [46, 67, 89].

## Basal Pressure

The high-pressure zone caused by the LES shows axial as well as radial asymmetry [261]. Axially, the LES pressure has a bell-shaped configuration with a total length of between 2 and 4 cm. Pressures tend to be higher in the more distal segment of the LES. The LES is radially symmetrical in its oral half, but in the aboral half, it shows higher pressures on the left side [210, 289, 290]. The diaphragm makes an impression on the left side of the terminal esophagus. Thus, both diaphragmatic and gastric sling fibers that buttress the left side of the LES may help to create higher pressures in this region.

In humans, the pressures in the upper and lower halves of the LES are usually affected by respiration in opposite ways. In the lower part, inspiration causes a rise in LES pressure, whereas the opposite occurs in the upper part [290]. This is thought to represent abdominal and thoracic influences at the distal and proximal locations, respectively. The point at which the respiratory pressure transition occurs is called the point of respiratory reversal or the pressure inversion point. This often occurs over a wide region that shows biphasic pressure changes with respiration. This zone is ~0.5 cm wide and is usually located in the middle of the high-pressure zone, but its precise location is variable. The point of respiratory reversal may be related to the crura of the diaphragm, which separates thoracic from abdominal cavities and provides opposing pressure environments during respiration. It may also be related to the LES itself as it separates intraesophageal from intragastric pressure or axial movement of the esophagus relative to the recording device. In addition, because of the position of the LES, within the diaphragmatic hiatus, the sphincter pressure may be influenced by the respiratory contractions of the crural diaphragm [35, 123, 158, 290, 299]. Slow phasic contractions in phase with the gastric component of the migrating myoelectrical

complex (MMC) have been described in humans and animals [70, 130, 131, 134].

The basal LES pressure is due to myogenic tone, which is normally modulated by excitatory and inhibitory neurohormonal influences. The hallmark of the sphincter muscle is its propensity to maintain tonic contraction [45]. This ability distinguishes the LES from the esophageal body muscle. The cellular mechanisms involved in stress or tone maintenance in the LES are not fully understood. The tonic behavior of the LES muscle has been attributed to a depolarized state and the presence of spikes that cause influx of $Ca^{2+}$ in the resting state of the muscle. Papasova et al. [189] found that the sphincter muscle exhibited tone in the absence of spike activity and that this spike-independent tone varied directly with the resting membrane potential. A relatively depolarized resting state of the sphincter muscle, which would result in increased tone, has been reported in studies with direct intracellular recordings. Zelcer and Weisbrodt [305] reported that resting membrane potential of the sphincter smooth muscle was approximately $-40$ mV, in contrast to the resting membrane potential of esophageal body circular muscle, which is $-50$ mV. Asoh and Goyal [9] showed that the opossum LES *in vivo* shows continuous spike activity. Moreover, increases in spike activity are associated with an increase in the maintained sphincter tone and abolition of the spike activity is associated with a decrease (Fig. 1–16). Continuous spike activity has also been shown to be present in the cat LES [208]. The depolarized state of the sphincter smooth muscle has been suggested to be due to resting chloride conductance [224]. Studies have also shown that sphincter muscles have higher resting intracellular $Ca^{2+}$ levels than nonsphincteric muscles. Biancani et al. [26] have proposed that high levels of intracellular $Ca^{2+}$ in the LES are supported by spontaneously active PLC, leading to elevated inositol 1,4,5-triphosphate ($IP_3$). The mildly elevated intracellular $Ca^{2+}$ levels are insufficient to activate calmodulin and myosin light-chain kinase (MLCK), leading to myosin light-chain phosphorylation and contraction. However, these $[Ca^{2+}]_i$ levels are sufficient to interact with DAG to generate tone through a PKC-dependent pathway [26, 124].

Weisbrodt and Murphy [288] studied the phosphorylation of myosin during force development and maintenance in the opossum LES. They found that the phosphorylation rate was ~4% of maximum during the relaxed state of the sphincter, increased to 33% during tone development, and then fell to 16% during tone maintenance, supporting the role of the latch phenomenon in LES tone. Szymanski et al. [266] have reported that LES has a different contractile protein composition than the esophageal circular muscle. The LES muscle has proportionally more $\alpha$-actin and basic essential light chains LC17b and less of a seven amino acid–inserted myosin isoform and caldesmon than esophageal body circular muscle. These differences in the contractile protein may determine the tonic phenotype of the LES muscle. The energy required to maintain sphincter tone is evidenced by its marked sensitivity to anoxia compared to that of esophageal body muscle [44, 228]. It has been reported that the LES

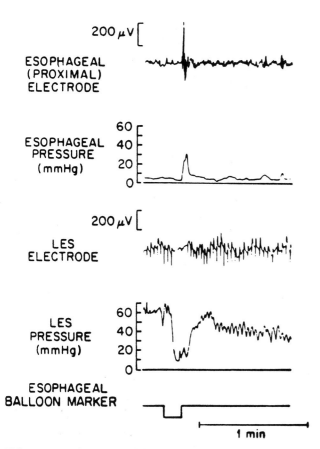

200 μV [

ESOPHAGEAL
(PROXIMAL)
ELECTRODE

ESOPHAGEAL
PRESSURE
(mmHg)

60
40
20
0

200 μV [

LES
ELECTRODE

LES
PRESSURE
(mmHg)

60
40
20
0

ESOPHAGEAL
BALLOON MARKER

1 min

**FIG. 1–16.** Influence of inflation of an intraluminal esophageal balloon on electrical activity and pressures of distal esophageal body and lower esophageal sphincter (LES). Balloon inflation causes cessation of tonic LES spike activity and simultaneous fall in LES pressure. Balloon deflation causes spike activity that precedes contraction in the esophageal body; in LES, tonic spike activity reappears as LES pressure returns toward baseline. (From ref. 9, with permission.)

has lower levels of cytochrome *c* oxidase activity than does the esophageal body [212]. This may help to explain why the LES is more dependent on exogenous $O_2$.

The mechanical advantage afforded by the Laplace law to the tonic sphincter muscle *in vivo* explains the ability of the LES to stay closed at rest with a small tension requirement and to generate fairly stable pressures over a wide range of luminal diameters [25, 29]. Excitatory and inhibitory nerve activity on the myogenic tone of the sphincter can influence its resting pressure. However, it is now clear that the major component of the resting basal pressure of the sphincter *in vivo* is not due to tonic excitatory nerve activity [110].

### Relaxation

Deglutition causes relaxation of the LES, which may start with the onset of the deglutition. Usually, LES relaxation onsets less than 2 seconds after the initiation of swallowing. At this time, the swallowed bolus is in the esophagus and

the peristaltic contraction is oral to the bolus in the cervical esophagus. In the upright position, the swallowed bolus may reach the LES very quickly due to gravity, and when this happens, it may be transiently delayed at the sphincter before passage into the stomach. The LES normally relaxes to a pressure equal to or very close to intragastric pressure. Relaxation of the LES may last for a total of 8 to 10 seconds and is followed in the oral part of the sphincter by an aftercontraction, which is in continuity with the peristaltic contraction in the esophageal body. The aftercontraction lasts for 7 to 10 seconds. The lower part of the LES does not show aftercontractions, and the sphincter pressure simply returns to the resting level. Electrical recordings show that swallow-induced LES relaxation is associated with cessation of spike activity when present [9].

Relaxation of the LES is the most sensitive component of the swallowing reflex. Thus, it is possible to have LES relaxation without any other motor evidence of the swallowing reflex (Fig. 1–17). Isolated LES relaxation can be induced experimentally by applying pharyngeal tactile stimulation, which is subthreshold for producing a full swallowing response. Similarly, electrical stimulation of the SLN with stimulus frequencies that fail to produce esophageal peristalsis causes isolated LES relaxation. Low-intensity stimulation of the swallowing center can also cause isolated LES relaxation [15]. When repeated swallows are made in succession, as during rapid drinking, the LES remains relaxed and returns to the baseline state of tone after the last swallow [51]. The LES relaxation associated with primary peristalsis, as well as the isolated LES relaxation due to pharyngeal or SLN stimulation, is mediated by vagal efferent nerves and abolished by bilateral cervical vagal section or cooling [209, 220].

Distention of either the striated or smooth muscle portion of the esophagus produces a reflex relaxation of the LES that is associated with secondary peristalsis in the esophageal body. During prolonged, localized esophageal distention, the LES may recover from relaxation despite ongoing distention [191, 194]. The sphincter relaxation due to distention in the striated muscle is centrally mediated and abolished by vagotomy, whereas the relaxation due to distention in the smooth muscle portion is mediated by intramural nerves and remains after bilateral vagotomy. However, recent studies have shown that the vagus nerves may exert a facilitative influence on LES relaxation evoked by balloon distention of the smooth muscle portion of the esophagus [194, 209]. As with primary peristalsis, LES relaxation is also the most sensitive component of secondary peristalsis. Thus, isolated LES relaxation without esophageal contraction occurs with distentions that are subthreshold for activation of full secondary peristalsis.

### Transient Lower Esophageal Sphincter Relaxation

Apart from primary and secondary peristalsis, relaxation of the LES also occurs during belching, retching, vomiting,

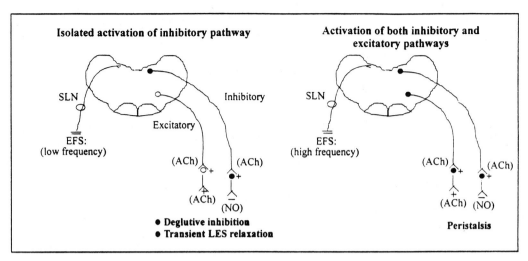

**FIG. 1–17.** Model depicts the activation of neurons in the medulla responsible for peristalsis. Low-frequency stimulation of the superior laryngeal nerve activates only the inhibitory pathway, while high-frequency stimulation activates both the inhibitory and excitatory pathways.

and rumination [51, 165, 257, 282]. During belching and vomiting, there is no esophageal contraction in association with LES relaxation [301]. With rumination, LES relaxation is associated with reverse peristalsis. Dent and colleagues [68] performed long-term recording of LES pressure using a sleeve device and observed that normal volunteers showed esophageal reflux episodes that were related to transient relaxations of the LES which were not associated with swallows [see also 132]. These relaxation episodes are also called inappropriate relaxations. These transient relaxations cause a significant number of reflux episodes in normal subjects as well as in patients with reflux esophagitis. Transient LES (tLES) relaxations are frequently associated with reflux of gas and are a component of the belch reflex. However, not all tLES relaxations are accompanied by reflux episodes. The percentage of tLES relaxations accompanied by reflux varies, depending on experimental circumstances, from as few as 10% to 15% [178] to as many as 93% [68]. The tLES relaxation is a vagally mediated reflex. The efferent arm of this reflex appears to involve vagal efferents that synapse on nitrergic postganglionic neurons, the same pathway that is involved in swallow-induced relaxation. The tLES relaxations are facilitated by gastric distention with gas or after a meal. They are also facilitated by the presence of a nasogastric tube [177, 180].

The neurotransmitters involved in the vagal inhibitory pathway to the LES have been investigated in some detail [109, 201]. This pathway consists of a chain of at least two neurons consisting of pre- and postganglionic neurons. The preganglionic neurons are carried in the vagus and synapse on postganglionic inhibitory neurons present intramurally in the LES.

The preganglionic neurons release predominantly ACh, which activates the postganglionic inhibitory neurons by stimulating both nicotinic and $M_1$ muscarinic receptors

[109]. There is also evidence that serotonin participates to a lesser degree in this synaptic transmission [202]. However, the combination of $M_1$ and serotonergic antagonists does not modify LES relaxation due to electrical stimulation of intramural inhibitory nerves. These observations show that the effect of the antagonists is exerted at the synaptic site between pre- and postganglionic neurons [205]. The intramural neural pathway involved in distention-induced LES relaxation is not known. Transient LES relaxation is also mediated via the vagal pathway as it is blocked by vagotomy or vagal cooling [177].

The inhibitory neurotransmitter released by the intramural inhibitory neurons remains unknown but is clearly not cholinergic or adrenergic in nature. Hence, this neurotransmitter is called noncholinergic, nonadrenergic [109, 274]. However, there is now strong evidence to suggest that NO gas is the major inhibitory neurotransmitter for relaxation induced by swallowing, esophageal distention, or tLES relaxation [55, 177, 192, 275, 304]. Chemical blockers of NO block transmurally stimulated relaxation of the LES *in vitro* [275] (Fig. 1–18) and swallow-induced relaxation in anesthetized animals [304] (Fig. 1–19). There is also evidence for the involvement of VIP in inhibitory neurotransmission [113, 265]. In some systems, VIP serves as an intermediary agent to release NO upon nerve stimulation [122, 161, 163]. VIP may also act in parallel to NO to participate in inhibitory neurotransmission.

The cellular basis of reflex LES relaxation is not fully understood. However, it is clear that it is an active process. It is associated with inhibition of continuous spike activity and hyperpolarization of the muscle cell membrane, which may be due to suppression of a resting chloride conductance by NO or activation of a potassium conductance. Smooth muscle hyperpolarization would cause muscle relaxation (electromechanical coupling) due to suppression of $Ca^{2+}$ in-

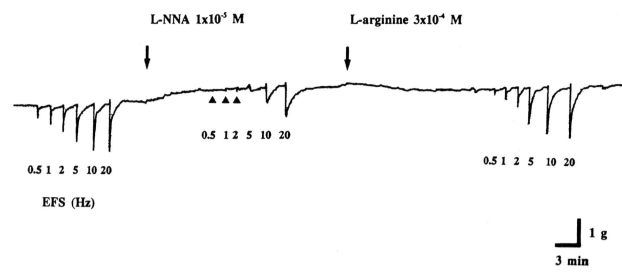

**FIG. 1–18.** Nitric oxide (NO) mediates lower esophageal sphincter (LES) relaxation. Electrical field stimulation (EFS) causes frequency-dependent relaxation in the opossum LES circular smooth muscle. Pretreatment with the NO synthase inhibitor $N^W$ nitro-L-arginine (L-NNA) inhibits this response. Pretreatment with L-arginine, a competitive substrate to the enzyme and a precursor of NO, restores relaxatory responses to EFS.

flux, leading to cessation of myosin phosphorylation. Both cyclic adenosine monophosphate (cAMP) and cGMP mediate LES relaxation [174, 207, 273] by activating protein kinases A and G, respectively. These signaling molecules can cause smooth muscle relaxation without causing membrane hyperpolarization (pharmacomechanical coupling). These kinases may lower the free intracellular $Ca^{2+}$ for the enzyme MLCK.

### Contraction

The upper part of the LES displays reflex contraction immediately after the peristalsis-related relaxation. This

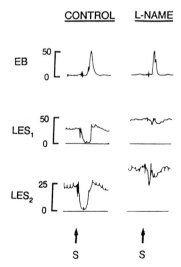

**FIG. 1–19.** Effect of nitric oxide synthase blocker on swallow (*S*)-induced relaxation in the lower esophageal sphincter (LES). Note that nitro-L-arginine methyl ester (L-NAME) (20 mg/kg) markedly antagonized relaxation in both LES leads.

contraction occurs in continuity with the peristaltic wave of the esophageal body and may represent the response of esophageal body type: circular muscle mixed with the sphincter muscle. A similar behavior is seen in muscle strips *in vitro*. This aftercontraction is somehow related to the level of baseline tone. Human LES circular muscle strips show prominent aftercontractions when basal tone is low, but as the tone increases, the aftercontraction is abolished.

Short-lived increases in LES pressure also occur secondary to increases in intraabdominal pressure. Considerable controversy exists as to whether this rise in LES pressure is due to reflex contraction or merely to a passive transmission of the increased intraabdominal pressure [159, 183]. The studies that show this to be a true reflex also suggest that it is vagally mediated and dependent on cholinergic neurons. The LES also contracts transiently, in phase with stomach contractions. This is closely tied to the phasic antral contractions that occur during different stages of the MMC [70, 130, 131]. During the first phase of the MMC, the LES pressure is stable, whereas during late phase II and throughout phase III, large-amplitude phasic contractions occur without there being a major change in the basal pressure. These MMC-related contractions are abolished by atropine and anesthesia [129, 130]. Studies suggest that they are initiated by the circulating hormone motilin [131]. The effect of infused motilin is abolished by hexamethonium and markedly inhibited by atropine and the selective $M_3$ antagonist 4-DAMP. This indicates that motilin may stimulate preganglionic cholinergic fibers, which in turn activate nicotinic receptors on postganglionic cholinergic excitatory fibers. These latter neurons then release ACh.

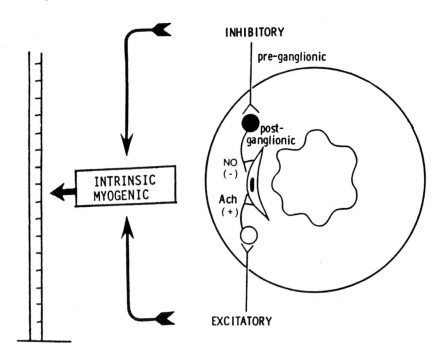

**FIG. 1–20.** Diagram explaining the origin of tone in the lower esophageal sphincter (LES) as a function of neurogenic and myogenic factors. Neurally mediated LES tone (shown as a sliding scale) is a summation of inhibitory (dilatory) and excitatory (contractile) neurotransmitter influences. Diminution or blockade in one (e.g., inhibitory) leads to an unbridled opposite effect (e.g., contraction). Total ablation of all neural influences will still leave the LES with some tone, which is attributed to the intrinsic, myogenic nature of the sphincteric smooth muscle.

The signaling pathway for ACh-induced contraction has been examined in detail by Biancani and colleagues [28]. In the LES smooth muscle of cat, ACh stimulates $M_3$ muscarinic receptors that activate PLC via the GTP-binding protein $(G_q)$ to produce $IP_3$. $IP_3$ causes release of $Ca^{2+}$ from the sarcolemmal store. The released $Ca^{2+}$ activates calmodulin, and $Ca^2_{\pm}$ calmodulin activates MLCK, which phosphorylates myosin light chains (MLCs), causing contraction. In experimental esophagitis, there is a change in the signaling cascade in that ACh causes contraction via the PKC-dependent pathway [24]. Infusion of acid into the esophageal lumen also causes a neurally mediated reflex contraction of the LES. This reflex contraction involves substance P-containing nerves [208].

**Pharmacology**

Figure 1–20 represents three major factors that influence sphincter pressure. These are the myogenic tone [110] of the LES and the inhibitory [NO (6, 154, 276)] and excitatory [ACh (95, 103, 119, 129)] influences. A multitude of endogenous compounds, hormones [76, 268, 269, 278], and classical [102, 103, 119, 205, 270] and putative [23, 43, 151, 195, 222, 223] neurotransmitters affect LES pressure in pharmacological experiments by affecting one or more of these three mechanisms. The physiological significance of their effect is, however, not clear. Additionally, lifestyle and dietary habits affect LES activity [146, 300]. Table 1–1 summarizes the effect of some endogenous chemicals on LES function.

## EXTERNAL LOWER ESOPHAGEAL SPHINCTER: DIAPHRAGMATIC CRURA

Mittal et al. [175, 179] and others [35, 153] have provided overwhelming evidence to suggest that the diaphragmatic crura of the esophageal hiatus acts on the external LES (Fig. 1–21). Manometric recordings of LES pressure are characterized by inspiratory spike-like increases in pressure that result from inspiratory contractions of the diaphragmatic crura that encircle the LES [35, 175]. The crural diaphragm acts independently of the costal diaphragm under certain gastrointestinal functions. For example, during vomiting and eructation, when the costal diaphragm shows marked electrical activity consistent with its contractile state, the esophageal crural diaphragm is inactive, consistent with its relaxation [272]. Similarly, during esophageal distention, the crural diaphragm becomes inactive when the costal diaphragm is contracting. These observations indicate that the esophageal crural diaphragm relaxes during reflex relaxation of the smooth muscle LES [5]. The crural diaphragm has also been shown to be inhibited during other reflex activities that cause LES relaxation, such as swallowing and LES relaxation [176, 178].

The crural diaphragm is composed of striated muscle, and it receives excitatory motor innervation by the phrenic nerve, similar to the costal diaphragm. Its inhibitory reflex activity could be mediated by unique, selective inhibition of lower motor neurons in the brainstem during such reflexes. It has been shown that vagotomy abolishes the reflex inhibition of the crural diaphragm, indicating a role for the vagus in this reflex [71]. This could represent a vagophrenic inhibitory

**TABLE 1–1.** *Effects of some hormones and putative neurotransmitters on the lower esophageal sphincter (LES)*

| Agent | Effect | Circular smooth muscle | Inhibitory neurons | Excitatory neurons | Comments | Reference |
|---|---|---|---|---|---|---|
| Bombesin | Contraction | √ | — | √ | Releases norepinephrine from adrenergic neurons | 59, 111 |
| Calcitonin gene-related peptide | Relaxation | √ | √ | — | | 200, 279 |
| Cholecystokinin | Biphasic | √ | √ | — | Inhibition overrides excitation, causes paradoxical excitation in achalasia patients | 18, 69 |
| Dopamine | Relaxation ($D_2$) | √ | — | — | | 111 |
| | Contraction ($D_1$) | √ | — | — | | 252 |
| Galanin | Contraction | √ | — | — | | 206 |
| Gastric inhibitory polypeptide | Relaxation | ? | ? | ? | | 253 |
| Gastrin | Contraction | √ | — | — | | 198 |
| Glucagon | Relaxation | √ | — | — | Releases catecholamines from adrenal medulla | 19 |
| Histamine | Contraction | √ ($H_1$) | — | — | | 22 |
| Motilin | Contraction | √ | — | √ | | 117 |
| Neurotensin | Contraction | √ | — | — | | 22 |
| Nitric oxide | Relaxation | √ | — | — | | 6, 56, 82, 112, 154, 275, 276, 303 |
| Pancreatic polypeptide | Contraction | √ | — | √ | | 203 |
| $PGF_{2\alpha}$ | Contraction | √ | — | — | | 66, 204 |
| $PGE_{1,2}$ | Relaxation | √ | — | — | | 204 |
| Progesterone | Relaxation | | — | — | | 90, 185 |
| Secretin | Relaxation | √ | — | — | | 19 |
| Serotonin | Contraction | √ | — | — | | 22 |
| Somatostatin | Contraction | ? | ? | ? | | 115 |
| Substance P | Contraction | √ | — | √ | | 181 |
| VIP | Relaxation | √ | — | — | | 19 |

PGF, prostaglandin F; PGE, prostaglandin E; VIP, vasoactive intestinal peptide.

reflex in which the afferent arc of the reflex is in the vagal afferents. It is also possible that vagal efferents provide inhibitory input to the crural striated muscle. Recent studies have shown that motor endplates of the crural striated muscle are innervated by nitrergic fibers. These nitrergic fibers may represent postganglionic fibers in the vagal inhibitory pathway. The nitrergic inhibitory vagal pathway may mediate reflex inhibition of the crural fibers. It has recently been shown that NO suppresses the excitatory potentials at the crural end plates [175]. A part of the esophageal crural diaphragm develops from esophageal mesenchyma. It is possible that, like esophageal striated muscle, a part of the esophageal crural diaphragm develops from smooth muscle transdifferentiation.

The amplitude of inspiratory pressure increases with increased inspiratory effort, and the pressure augmentation observed during sustained inspiration corresponds with augmentation of the crural EMG activity both temporally and quantitatively. The inspiratory augmentations in pressure may play an important role in gastroesophageal reflux dis-

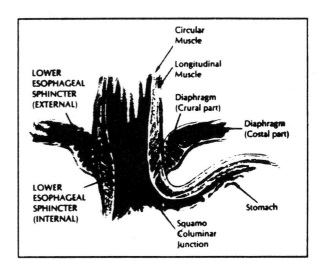

**FIG. 1–21.** The anatomy at the region of the esophagogastric junction, showing the innermost fibers of the diaphragm around the esophageal hiatus. These fibers behave like a sphincter. (From ref. 175, with permission.)

## ESOPHAGEAL TENSION RECEPTORS

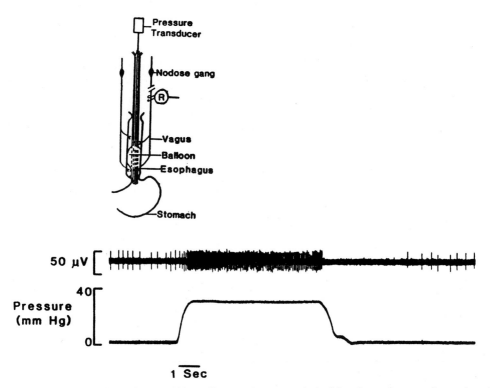

**FIG. 1–22.** Esophageal tension-sensitive afferents increase their firing frequency to distension. The vagal fibers showed three broad phases in response to the esophageal distension (stimulus): a rapid increase in firing at the onset of distension; an adaptation to sustained distension by a decrease in frequency that was still far greater than the resting frequency; and finally, following withdrawal of distension, a decrease in frequency to a lower than resting level. The schematic diagram at the **top** represents the setup employed in this study.

ease. The crural diaphragmatic contractions are involved only in inspiratory augmentation, and therefore, end-expiratory pressure measurements reflect the intrinsic pressure of the LES [35, 175].

## ESOPHAGEAL SENSATIONS

Afferent fibers from the esophagus course along the vagal and splanchnic nerves. The vagal afferent fibers have their cell bodies in the nodose ganglion and project to the nucleus solitarius [94]. Sympathetic afferents travel via dorsal root ganglia into the spinal cord at T1–L2 [53].

Ultrastructural studies by Rodrigo et al. [213–217] reveal the presence of perivascular and free nerve endings in the esophageal submucosa of cats, as well as free intraepithelial nerve endings and peculiar tape-like nerve endings within the myenteric ganglia. The latter have been termed intraganglionic laminar endings [215] and are thought to be ideally located to serve as mechanoreceptors. The afferent nature of these endings has been confirmed by studies that show their degeneration after extirpation of the nodose ganglion [213, 217]. The intraepithelial nerve endings may serve as mechanoreceptors and as thermo-, osmo-, and chemorecep-

tors in the esophagus [49, 50, 86]. The afferent receptors appear to be concentrated at the upper and the lower portions of the thoracic esophagus [215].

Esophageal mechanoceptors also transduce painful sensations [42]. Esophageal distention with a compliant balloon in awake persons elicited three types of response depending on the degree of balloon distention. At small distention pressures, secondary esophageal peristalsis is produced without any sensory perception. At moderate distention pressures, the subjects experience pressure sensation only; but at high distention pressures, they experience chest discomfort and pain. According to the intensity theory of pain, all of these sensory responses were transduced by the same mechanoreceptor-afferent fiber so that the intensity of its stimulation determined whether discomfort or pain sensations were transduced. Sengupta and colleagues [234–236] showed that esophageal distention elicits spike activity in single vagal and splanchnic afferent fibers (units) (Fig. 1–22). They studied the quantitative stimulus intensity response relationship of single afferent units. Based on their findings, these units were classified as low-threshold mechanoreceptors (LTMs), wide dynamic range mechanonociceptors (WDR-MNs), and high-threshold mechanonocioceptors (HTMNs) (Fig. 1–23)

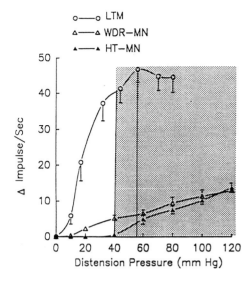

**FIG. 1–23.** Stimulus-response relationships in the three types of esophageal, distension-sensitive unit. The esophageal distension-sensitive afferents were classified into three types based on the threshold pressure for activation and saturation pressure. Note that low-threshold mechanoceptors (*LTMs*) saturated near the noxious threshold pressures. Wide dynamic range mechanonociceptors (*WDR-MNs*) had an intermediate activation threshold and showed no evidence of saturation. They were active in both innocuous and noxious stimulus ranges and had low discharge rates. On the other hand, high-threshold mechanoceptors (*HTMNs*) had a very high threshold pressure that was in the noxious range and showed no sign of saturation with very low discharge rates. *Shaded area* indicates noxious range of stimuli. (From ref. 114, with permission.)

[234, 235]. These observations suggested that all afferent units were not homogenous and that distinct afferent units transduced different sensations and, therefore, supported the specificity theory of pain [42]. Furthermore, it was shown that HTMNs were highly sensitive to the autacoid bradykinin [236]. Properties of the three types of afferent unit are summarized in Table 1–2 [114].

These studies also showed that LTM units were present only in the vagus nerve, whereas WDR-MN and HTMN units were present in the splanchnic nerves. These observations are consistent with the view that the esophageal vagal afferents are involved in physiological reflexes that occur without sensory perception, whereas the spinal splanchnic afferents transduce esophageal sensations and nociception. However, nociceptive pathways from the lower esophagus are not affected in patients with C-6 or C-7 spinal cord injury [72]. These conclusions do not exclude a role for vagal afferents in the modulation of esophageal nociception as they have been shown to suppress signal nociceptive mechanisms.

The vagal sensory units have their cell bodies in the nodose ganglia lying just below the jugular foramen. The nodose ganglia display rostrocaudal organization of the gut, with some neurons from the oropharynx and esophagus located superiorly [4]. The central projections of the nodose ganglion cells terminate in the medial division of the NTS, where they also display rostrocaudal viscerotropic organization within the subnuclei [4]. The NTS neurons project to different levels, including (a) neurons in the DMN and NA (containing swallowing neurons); (b) antero-mediolateral cell column of the spinal cord (containing sympathetic pathway nerves); (c) neurons in the thalamus, hypothalamus, and limbic and insular cortical regions (which are concerned with autonomic, neuroendocrine, and behavioral functions); and (d) parabrachial nuclei, which are in turn connected to higher brain centers (Fig. 1–24) [13].

The splanchnic sensory units have the cell bodies in the dorsal root ganglia. They contain substance P and CGRP. The central projections of these neurons terminate in the spinal column and in the nucleus gracilis and cuneatus in

**TABLE 1–2.** *Esophageal mechanosensitive receptors*

| Characteristics | Low-threshold mechanoreceptors | Wide dynamic range mechanonociceptors | High-threshold mechanonociceptors |
|---|---|---|---|
| Fiber type | A$\delta$, C | A$\delta$, C | A$\delta$, C |
| Mean threshold pressure for activation (mm Hg) | 3 | 10 | 40 |
| Mean saturation pressure (mm Hg) | 50 | >120 | >120 |
| Max. discharge rate | 60 | 17 | 10 |
| Resting activity | 100% | 73% | 42% |
| Activity rate (impulses/sec) | ~10 | <1 | <0.5 |
| Response to physiological peristalsis | | | |
| % responding | 100% | 100% | 0% |
| Response rate as % maximum | 100% | 25% | 0% |
| Activation by algogenic bradykinin | No | Yes | Yes (highly sensitive) |
| Anatomic course | Vagus | Splanchnic | Splanchnic |
| Physiological role | Nonnoxious information | Nonnoxious to noxious information | Nociceptive information |

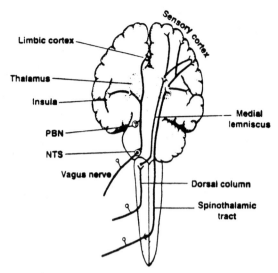

**FIG. 1–24.** The bulbar and suprabulbar projections of vagal and spinal afferent pathways. Vagal afferents terminate in the nucleus tractus solitarius (*NTS*), from which projections ascend via the parabronchial nucleus (*PBN*) to the thalamus and the limbic and insular cortices. Spinal afferents ascend in the spinothalamic tract and the dorsal columns. The spinothalamic tracts ascend to the thalamus, and the dorsal columns ascend to the nuclei gracilus and cuneatus in the rostral medulla, from which they project to the thalamus via the medial lemniscus. From the thalamus, projections ascend to the primary somatosensory and insular cortices. (From ref. 13, with permission.)

the brainstem and then ascend to terminate in the thalamus. From the thalamus, projections ascend to primary somatosensory and insular cortical areas (Fig. 1–24) [13]. Sensitization of nociceptors may play an important role in esophageal sensation [168].

Aziz and Thompson [13] have reviewed recent information on the projection of nerves conveying esophageal sensations to the brain in humans by studying cortical evoked potentials (CEPs), magnetoencephalography, positron emission tomography (PET), and functional magnetic resonance imaging (fMRI) following esophageal distention or electrical stimulation.

PET scan studies suggest that esophageal sensation, like somatic sensation, is processed in the primary somatosensory cortex (for sensoridiscriminative aspects) and the anterior cingulate cortex (for affective motivational aspects) and inhibits the medial prefrontal cortex (a region known for cognitive-evaluation aspects of sensation) [11]. fMRI studies have found that parieto-occipital and midparietal cortices were activated by distention of the distal and proximal esophagus, respectively. Moreover, esophageal distention and acid perfusion induces spatially and temporally distinct cortical activation. Painful stimuli induce activation in the same cortical area as nonpainful stimuli and cause activation of anterior cingulate gyri [13].

Mechanical and electrical stimuli of the esophagus also produce CEPs [93]. Sensory perception is usually necessary

to evoke CEPs, and there is a progressive increase in CEP magnitude with increasing perception scores. The magnitude of cortical response to esophageal electrical stimulation is intensity-dependent [126], and it has been suggested that CEPs might be mediated by stimulation of wide dynamic range mechanosensitive afferents that are carried in the splanchnic nerves [13]. CEPs have been used to determine the integrity of esophageal afferents [13, 197].

## REFERENCES

1. Akbarali HI, Goyal RK. Effect of sodium nitroprusside on $Ca^{2+}$ currents in opossum esophageal circular muscle cells. Am J Physiol 1994; 266:G1036
2. Akbarali HI, et al. Transient outward current in opossum esophageal circular muscle. Am J Physiol 1995;268:G979
3. Ali GN, et al. Influence of mucosal receptors on deglutitive regulation of pharyngeal and upper esophageal sphincter function. Am J Physiol 1994;267:G644
4. Altschuler SM, et al. Viscerotopic representation of the upper alimentary tract in the rat: sensory ganglia and nuclei of the solitary and spinal trigeminal tracts. J Comp Neurol 1989;283:248
5. Altschuler SM, et al. Simultaneous reflex inhibition of lower esophageal sphincter and crural diaphragm in cats. Am J Physiol 1985;249: G586
6. Anand N, Paterson WG. Role of nitric oxide in esophageal peristalsis. Am J Physiol 1994;266:G123
7. Andrew BL. The nervous control of the cervical oesophagus of the rat during swallowing. J Physiol 1956;134:729–740
8. Ask P, Tibbling L. Effect of time interval between swallows on esophageal peristalsis. Am J Physiol 1980;238:G485
9. Asoh R, Goyal RK. Electrical activity of the opossum lower esophageal sphincter in vivo. Its role in the basal sphincter pressure. Gastroenterology 1978;74:835
10. Asoh R, Goyal RK. Manometry and electromyography of the upper esophageal sphincter in the opossum. Gastroenterology 1978;74:514
11. Aziz Q, et al. Identification of human brain loci processing esophageal sensation using positron emission tomography. Gastroenterology 1997;113:50
12. Aziz Q, et al. The topographic representation of esophageal motor function on the human cerebral cortex. Gastroenterology 1996;111: 855
13. Aziz Q, Thompson DG. Brain–gut axis in health and disease. Gastroenterology 1998;114:559
14. Bao X, Wiedner EB, Altschuler SM. Transsynaptic localization of pharyngeal premotor neurons in rat. Brain Res 1995;696:246
15. Barone FC, Lombard DM, Ormsbee HS, III. Effects of hindbrain stimulation on lower esophageal sphincter pressure in the cat. Am J Physiol 1984;247:G70
16. Barrett RT, et al. Brain stem localization of rodent esophageal premotor neurons revealed by transneuronal passage of pseudorabies virus. Gastroenterology 1994;107:728
17. Baumgarten HG, Lange W. Adrenergic innervation of the esophagus in the cat (*Felis domestica*) and rhesus monkey (*Macacus rhesus*). Z Zellorsch Mikrosk Anat 1969;95:529
18. Behar J, Biancani P. Effect of cholecystokinin-octapeptide on lower esophageal sphincter. Gastroenterology 1977;73:57
19. Behar J, Biancani P. Effect of glucagon, secretin, and vasoactive intestinal polypeptide on the feline lower esophageal sphincter. Mechanism of action. Gastroenterology 1979;77:1001
20. Behar J, Kerstein M, Biancani P. Neural control of the lower esophageal sphincter in the cat: studies on the excitatory pathways to the lower esophageal sphincter. Gastroenterology 1982;82:680
21. Beyak MJ, et al. Superior laryngeal nerve stimulation in the cat: effect on oropharyngeal swallowing, oesophageal motility and lower oesophageal sphincter activity. Neurogastroenterol Motil 1997;9:117
22. Biancani P, Behar J. Esophageal motor function. In Yamada T, ed, Textbook of Gastroenterology. Philadelphia: JB Lippincott Co, 1995: 158
23. Biancani P, et al. Role of peptide histidine isoleucine in relaxation of cat lower esophageal sphincter. Gastroenterology 1989;97:1083

24. Biancani P, et al. Acute experimental esophagitis impairs signal transduction in cat lower esophageal sphincter circular muscle. Gastroenterology 1992;103:1199

25. Biancani P, et al. Mechanics of sphincter action. Studies on the lower esophageal sphincter. J Clin Invest 1973;52:2973

26. Biancani P, et al. Differential signal transduction pathways in cat lower esophageal sphincter tone and response to ACh. Am J Physiol 1994;266:G767

27. Biancani P, et al. Contraction mediated by $Ca^{2+}$ influx in esophageal muscle and by $Ca^{2+}$ release in the LES. Am J Physiol 1987;253:G760

28. Biancani P, et al. Signal transduction pathways in esophageal and lower esophageal sphincter circular muscle. Am J Med 1997;103:23S

29. Biancani P, Zabinski MP, Behar J. Pressure, tension, and force of closure of the human lower esophageal sphincter and esophagus. J Clin Invest 1975;56:476

30. Biancani P, et al. Lower esophageal sphincter mechanics: anatomic and physiologic relationships of the esophagogastric junction of cat. Gastroenterology 1982;82:468

31. Bieger D. Neuropharmacologic correlates of deglutition: lessons from fictive swallowing. Dysphagia 1991;6:147

32. Bieger D. The brainstem esophagomotor network pattern generator: a rodent model. Dysphagia 1993;8:203

33. Bieger D, Hopkins DA. Viscerotopic representation of the upper alimentary tract in the medulla oblongata in the rat: the nucleus ambiguus. J Comp Neurol 1987;262:546

34. Bonington A, Mahon M, Whitmore I. A histological and histochemical study of the cricopharyngeus muscle in man. J Anat 1988;156:27

35. Boyle JT, et al. Role of the diaphragm in the genesis of lower esophageal sphincter pressure in the cat. Gastroenterology 1985;88:723

36. Broussard DL, et al. Solatarial premotor neuron projections to the rat esophagus and pharynx: implications for control of swallowing. Gastroenterology 1998;114:1268.

37. Brownlow H, Whitmore I, Willan PL. A quantitative study of the histochemical and morphometric characteristics of the human cricopharyngeus muscle. J Anat 1989;166:67

38. Castell DO, et al. Cerebral electrical potentials evoked by balloon distention of the human esophagus. Gastroenterology 1990;98:662

39. Castell JA, et al. Effect of head position on the dynamics of the upper esophageal sphincter and pharynx. Dysphagia 1993;8:1

40. Castell JA, Dalton CB, Castell DO. Effects of body position and bolus consistency on the manometric parameters and coordination of the upper esophageal sphincter and pharynx. Dysphagia 1990;5:179

41. Castell JA, Dalton CB, Castell DO. Pharyngeal and upper esophageal sphincter manometry in humans. Am J Physiol 1990;258:G173

42. Cervero F, Janig W. Visceral nociceptors: a new world order? Trends Neurosci 1992;15:374

43. Chakder S, Rosenthal GJ, Rattan S. In vivo and in vitro influence of human recombinant hemoglobin on esophageal function. Am J Physiol 1995;268:G443

44. Christensen J. Oxygen dependence of contractions in esophageal and gastric pyloric and ileocecal muscle of opossums. Proc Soc Exp Biol Med 1982;170:194

45. Christensen J, Conklin JL, Freeman BW. Physiologic specialization at esophagogastric junction in three species. Am J Physiol 1973;225:1265

46. Christensen J, Rick GA, Soll DJ. Intramural nerves and interstitial cells revealed by the Champy-Maillet stain in the opossum esophagus. J Auton Nerv Syst 1987;19:137

47. Christensen J, Roberts RL. Differences between esophageal body and lower esophageal sphincter in mitochondria of smooth muscle in opossum. Gastroenterology 1983;85:650

48. Christensen J, Robison BA. Anatomy of the myenteric plexus of the opossum esophagus. Gastroenterology 1982;83:1033

49. Clerc N, Mei N. Thoracic esophageal mechanoreceptors connected with fibers following sympathetic pathways. Brain Res Bull 1983;10:1

50. Clerc N, Mei N. Vagal mechanoreceptors located in the lower oesophageal sphincter of the cat. J Physiol 1983;336:487

51. Code CF, Schlegel JF. Motor action of the esophagus and its sphincters. In Code CF, ed, Handbook of Physiology. Washington DC: Am Physiol Soc, 1968;1821

52. Cohen BR, Wolf BS. Cineradiographic and intraluminal correlations in the pharynx and esophagus. In Code CF, ed, Handbook of Physiology. Washington DC: Am Physiol Soc, 1968;1841

53. Collman PI, Tremblay L, Diamant NE. The distribution of spinal and vagal sensory neurons that innervate the esophagus of the cat. Gastroenterology 1992;103:817

54. Collman PI, Tremblay L, Diamant NE. The central vagal efferent supply to the esophagus and lower esophageal sphincter of the cat. Gastroenterology 1993;104:1430

55. Conklin JL, et al. Characterization and mediation of inhibitory junction potentials from opossum lower esophageal sphincter. Gastroenterology 1993;104:1439

56. Conklin JL, et al. Effects of recombinant human hemoglobin on motor functions of the opossum esophagus. J Pharmacol Exp Ther 1995;273:762

57. Cook IJ, Dent J, Shannon S, Collins SM. Measurement of upper esophageal sphincter pressure. Effect of acute emotional stress. Gastroenterology 1987;93:526

58. Cook IJ, et al. Opening mechanisms of the human upper esophageal sphincter. Am J Physiol 1989;257:G748

59. Corazziari E, et al. Effect of bombesin on lower esophageal sphincter pressure in humans. Gastroenterology 1982;83:10

60. Crist J, Gidda JS, Goyal RK. Characteristics of ''on'' and ''off'' contractions in esophageal circular muscle in vitro. Am J Physiol 1984;246:G137

61. Crist J, Gidda JS, Goyal RK. Intramural mechanism of esophageal peristalsis: roles of cholinergic and noncholinergic nerves. Proc Natl Acad Sci USA 1984;81:3595

62. Crist J, Gidda J, Goyal RK. Role of substance P nerves in longitudinal smooth muscle contractions of the esophagus. Am J Physiol 1986;250:G336

63. Crist J, Surprenant A, Goyal RK. Intracellular studies of electrical membrane properties of opossum esophageal circular smooth muscle. Gastroenterology 1987;92:987

64. Crist JR, He XD, Goyal RK. Chloride-mediated inhibitory junction potentials in opossum esophageal circular smooth muscle. Am J Physiol 1991;261:G752

65. Crist JR, Kauvar D, Goyal RK. Gradient of cholinergic innervation in opossum esophageal circular smooth muscle. Gullet 1991;1:92

66. Daniel EE, Crankshaw J, Sarna S. Prostaglandins and tetrodotoxin-insensitive relaxation of opossum lower esophageal sphincter. Am J Physiol 1979;236:E153

67. Daniel EE, Posey-Daniel V. Neuromuscular structures in opossum esophagus: role of interstitial cells of Cajal. Am J Physiol 1984;246:G305

68. Dent J, et al. Mechanism of gastroesophageal reflux in recumbent asymptomatic human subjects. J Clin Invest 1980;65:256

69. Dent J, et al. Effect of cholecystokinin-octapeptide on opossum lower esophageal sphincter. Am J Physiol 1980;239:G230

70. Dent J, et al. Interdigestive phasic contractions of the human lower esophageal sphincter. Gastroenterology 1983;84:453

71. De Troyer A, Rosso J. Reflex inhibition of the diaphragm by esophageal afferents. Neurosci Lett 1982;30:43

72. DeVault KR, et al. Esophageal sensation in spinal cord-injured patients: balloon distension and cerebral evoked potential recording. Am J Physiol 1996;271:G937

73. Diamant NE. A glimpse at the central mechanism for swallowing? Gastroenterology 1995;109:1700

74. Diamant NE, El-Sharkawy TY. Neural control of esophageal peristalsis. A conceptual analysis. Gastroenterology 1977;72:546

75. Dick TE, van Lunteren E. Fiber subtype distribution of pharyngeal dilator muscles and diaphragm in the cat. J Appl Physiol 1990;68:2237

76. Dilawari JB, et al. Response of the human cardia sphincter to circulating prostaglandins F2$\alpha$ and E2 and to antiinflammatory drugs. Gut 1975;16:137

77. Dodds WJ, et al. Pharmacologic investigation of primary peristalsis in smooth muscle portion of opossum esophagus. Am J Physiol 1979;237:E561

78. Dodds WJ, et al. Esophageal contractions induced by vagal stimulation in the opossum. Am J Physiol 1978;235:E392

79. Doty RW. Influence of stimulus pattern on reflex deglutition. Am J Physiol 1951;166:142

80. Doty RW. Neural organization of deglutition. In Code CF, ed, Handbook of Physiology. Washington DC: Am Physiol Soc, 1968;1861

81. Doty RW, Bosma JF. An electromyographic analysis of reflex deglutition. J Neurophysiol 1956;19:44

82. Du C, et al. Nitric oxide: mediator of NANC hyperpolarization of opossum esophageal smooth muscle. Am J Physiol 1991;261:G1012

83. Dua KS, et al. Coordination of deglutitive glottal function and pharyngeal bolus transit during normal eating. Gastroenterology 1997;112:73

84. Elidan J, et al. Manometry and electromyography of the pharyngeal muscles in patients with dysphagia. Arch Otolaryngol Head Neck Surg 1990;116:910

85. Elidan J, et al. Electromyography of the inferior constrictor and cricopharyngeal muscles during swallowing. Ann Otol Rhinol Laryngol 1990;99:466

86. El Ouazzani T, Mei N. Electrophysiologic properties and role of the vagal thermoreceptors of lower esophagus and stomach of cat. Gastroenterology 1982;83:995

87. Enzmann DR, Harell GS, Zboralske FF. Upper esophageal responses to intraluminal distention in man. Gastroenterology 1977;72:1292

88. Ergun GA, et al. Shape, volume, and content of the deglutitive pharyngeal chamber imaged by ultrafast computerized tomography. Gastroenterology 1993;105:1396

89. Faussone-Pellegrini MS, Cortesini C. Ultrastructural features and localization of the interstitial cells of Cajal in the smooth muscle coat of human esophagus. J Submicrosc Cytol 1985;17:187

90. Fisher RS, et al. Inhibition of lower esophageal sphincter circular muscle by female sex hormones. Am J Physiol 1978;234:E243

91. Fleshler B, et al. The characteristics and similarity of primary and secondary peristalsis in the esophagus. J Clin Invest 1959;38:110

92. Freiman JM, El-Sharkawy TY, Diamant NE. Effect of bilateral vagosympathetic nerve blockade on response of the dog upper esophageal sphincter (UES) to intraesophageal distention and acid. Gastroenterology 1981;81:78

93. Frieling T, Enck P, Wienbeck M. Cerebral responses evoked by electrical stimulation of the esophagus in normal subjects. Gastroenterology 1989;97:475

94. Fryscak T, Zenker W, Kantner D. Afferent and efferent innervation of the rat esophagus. A tracing study with horseradish peroxidase and nuclear yellow. Anat Embryol 1984;170:63

95. Gaumnitz EA, et al. Electrophysiological and pharmacological responses of chronically denervated lower esophageal sphincter of the opossum. Gastroenterology 1995;109:789

96. Gerhardt DC, et al. Human upper esophageal sphincter. Response to volume, osmotic, and acid stimuli. Gastroenterology 1978;75:268

97. Gidda JS, Buyniski JP. Swallow-evoked peristalsis in opossum esophagus: role of cholinergic mechanisms. Am J Physiol 1986;251:G779

98. Gidda JS, Cobb BW, Goyal RK. Modulation of esophageal peristalsis by vagal efferent stimulation in opossum. J Clin Invest 1981;68:1411

99. Gidda JS, Goyal RK. Influence of successive vagal stimulations on contractions in esophageal smooth muscle of opossum. J Clin Invest 1983;71:1095

100. Gidda JS, Goyal RK. Swallow-evoked action potentials in vagal preganglionic efferents. J Neurophysiol 1984;52:1169

101. Gidda JS, Goyal RK. Regional gradient of initial inhibition and refractoriness in esophageal smooth muscle. Gastroenterology 1985;89:843

102. Gilbert R, Rattan S, Goyal RK. Pharmacologic identification, activation and antagonism of two muscarine receptor subtypes in the lower esophageal sphincter. J Pharmacol Exp Ther 1984;230:284

103. Gilbert RJ, Dodds WJ. Effect of selective muscarinic antagonists on peristaltic contractions in opossum smooth muscle. Am J Physiol 1986;250:G50

104. Goyal RK, Cobb BW. Motility of the pharynx, esophagus, and esophageal sphincter. In Johnson LR, ed, Physiology of the Gastrointestinal Tract. New York: Raven Press, 1981:359

105. Goyal RK, Gidda JS. Evidence for NO redox form of nitric oxide as nitrergic inhibitor neurotransmitter in gut. Am J Physiol 1981;240:G305

106. Goyal RK, He XD. Different mechanisms of ileal smooth muscle hyperpolarization based on redox forms of nitric oxide: NO as the nitrergic neurotransmitter. Am J Physiol 1998;275

107. Goyal RK, et al. The role of cricopharyngeus muscle in pharyngoesophageal disorders. Dysphagia 1993;8:252

108. Goyal RK, Paterson WG. Esophageal motility. In Wood JD, Schultz SG, eds, Handbook of Physiology. The Gastrointestinal System. Washington DC: Am Physiol Soc, 1987:865

109. Goyal RK, Rattan S. Nature of the vagal inhibitory innervation to the lower esophageal sphincter. J Clin Invest 1975;55:1119

110. Goyal RK, Rattan S. Genesis of basal sphincter pressure: effect of tetrodotoxin on lower esophageal sphincter pressure in opossum in vivo. Gastroenterology 1976;71:62

111. Goyal RK, Rattan S. Neurohumoral, hormonal, and drug receptors for the lower esophageal sphincter. Gastroenterology 1978;74:598

112. Goyal RK, Rattan S. Effects of sodium nitroprusside and verapamil on lower esophageal sphincter. Am J Physiol 1980;238:G40

113. Goyal RK, Rattan S, Said SI. VIP as a possible neurotransmitter of non-cholinergic non-adrenergic inhibitory neurones. Nature 1980;288:378

114. Goyal RK, Sengupta JN, Saha JK. Properties of esophageal mechano-sensitive receptors. In Holle GE, ed, Advances in the Innervation of the Gastrointestinal Tract. New York: Elsevier Science, 1992

115. Greco AV, et al. Effect of somatostatin on lower esophageal sphincter (LES) pressure and serum gastrin in normal and achalasic subjects. Horm Metab Res 1982;14:26

116. Groher ME. Dysphagia: Diagnosis and Management. Boston: Butterworth-Heineman, 1997

117. Gutierrez JG, et al. Effect of motilin on the lower esophageal sphincter of the opossum. Am J Dig Dis 1977;22:402

118. Hamdy S, et al. The cortical topography of human swallowing musculature in health and disease. Nat Med 1996;2:1217

119. Harris LD, Ashworth WD, Ingelfinger FJ. Esophageal aperistalsis and achalasia produced in dogs by prolonged cholinesterase inhibition. J Clin Invest 1960;39:1744

120. Hatakeyama N, et al. Tyrosine kinase-dependent modulation of calcium entry in rabbit colonic muscularis mucosae. Am J Physiol 1996;270:C1780

121. Hatakeyama N, et al. Muscarinic suppression of ATP-sensitive $K^+$ channel in rabbit esophageal smooth muscle. Am J Physiol 1995;268:C877

122. He XD, Goyal RK. Nitric oxide involvement in the peptide VIP-associated inhibitory junction potential in the guinea-pig ileum. J Physiol 1993;461:485

123. Heitmann P, et al. Simultaneous cineradiographic-manometric study of the distal esophagus: small hiatal hernias and rings. Gastroenterology 1966;50:737

124. Hillemeier C, et al. Protein kinase C mediates spontaneous tone in the cat lower esophageal sphincter. J Pharmacol Exp Ther 1996;277:144

125. Hirano I, et al. Tyrosine phosphorylation in contraction of opossum esophageal longitudinal muscle in response to SNP. Am J Physiol 1997;273:G247

126. Hollerbach S, et al. The magnitude of the central response to esophageal electrical stimulation is intensity dependent. Gastroenterology 1997;112:1137

127. Hollis JB, Castell DO. Esophageal function in elderly man. A new look at ''presbyesophagus.'' Ann Intern Med 1974;80:371

128. Hollis JB, Castell DO. Effect of dry swallows and wet swallows of different volumes on esophageal peristalsis. J Appl Physiol 1975;38:1161

129. Holloway RH, et al. Electrical control activity of the lower esophageal sphincter in unanesthetized opossums. Am J Physiol 1987;252:G511

130. Holloway RH, et al. Variability of lower esophageal sphincter pressure in the fasted unanesthetized opossum. Am J Physiol 1985;248:G398

131. Holloway RH, et al. Motilin: a mechanism incorporating the opossum lower esophageal sphincter into the migrating motor complex. Gastroenterology 1985;89:507

132. Holloway RH, Penagini R, Ireland AC. Criteria for objective definition of transient lower esophageal sphincter relaxation. Am J Physiol 1995;268:G128

133. Ingelfinger FJ. Esophageal motility. Physiol Rev 1958;38:533

134. Itoh I, et al. Control of lower esophageal sphincter contractile activity by motilin in conscious dogs. Am J Dig Dis 1978;23:341

135. Jacob P, et al. Upper esophageal sphincter opening and modulation during swallowing. Gastroenterology 1989;97:1469

136. Jacobowitz D, Nemir P Jr. The autonomic innervation of the esophagus of the dog. J Thorac Cardiovasc Surg 1969;58:678

137. Janssens J, et al. Peristalsis in smooth muscle esophagus after transection and bolus deviation. Gastroenterology 1976;71:1004

138. Janssens J, et al. Studies on the necessity of a bolus for the progression of secondary peristalsis in the canine esophagus. Gastroenterology 1974;67:245

139. Janssens J, et al. Is the primary peristaltic contraction of the canine esophagus bolus-dependent? Gastroenterology 1973;65:750

140. Jean A. Control of the central swallowing program by inputs from the peripheral receptors. A review. J Auton Nerv Syst 1984;10:225

141. Jean A. Brainstem control of swallowing: localization and organiza-

tion of the central pattern generator for swallowing. In Taylor A, ed, Neurophysiology of the Jaws and Teeth. London: MacMillan Press, 1990

142. Jean A, Car A. Inputs to the swallowing medullary neurons from the peripheral afferent fibers and the swallowing cortical area. Brain Res 1979;178:567

143. Jury J, Jager LP, Daniel EE. Unusual potassium channels mediate nonadrenergic noncholinergic nerve-mediated inhibition in opossum esophagus. Can J Physiol Pharmacol 1985;63:107

144. Kahrilas PJ, et al. Effect of sleep, spontaneous gastroesophageal reflux, and a meal on upper esophageal sphincter pressure in normal human volunteers. Gastroenterology 1987;92:466

145. Kahrilas PJ, et al. Upper esophageal sphincter function during deglutition. Gastroenterology 1988;95:52

146. Kahrilas PJ, Gupta RR. Mechanisms of acid reflux associated with cigarette smoking. Gut 1990;31:4

147. Kahrilas PJ, et al. Oropharyngeal accommodation to swallow volume. Gastroenterology 1996;111:297

148. Kahrilas PJ, et al. Deglutitive tongue action: volume accommodation and bolus propulsion. Gastroenterology 1993;104:152

149. Kahrilas PJ, Logemann JA, Lin S, Ergun GA. Pharyngeal clearance during swallowing: a combined manometric and videofluoroscopic study. Gastroenterology 1992;103:128

150. Kahrilas PJ, et al. Attenuation of esophageal shortening during peristalsis with hiatus hernia. Gastroenterology 1995;109:1818

151. Kim N, et al. Leukotrienes in acetylcholine-induced contraction of esophageal circular smooth muscle in experimental esophagitis. Gastroenterology 1997;112:1548

152. Kitamura S, et al. Location of the motoneurons supplying the rabbit pharyngeal constrictor muscles and the peripheral course of their axons: a study using the retrograde HRP or fluorescent labeling technique. Anat Rec 1991;229:399

153. Klein WA, et al. Sphincterlike thoracoabdominal high pressure zone after esophagogastrectomy. Gastroenterology 1993;105:1362

154. Knudsen MA, Svane D, Tottrup A. Action profiles of nitric oxide, S-nitroso-L-cysteine, SNP, and NANC responses in opossum lower esophageal sphincter. Am J Physiol 1992;262:G840

155. Kobler JB, et al. Innervation of the larynx, pharynx, and upper esophageal sphincter of the rat. J Comp Neurol 1994;349:129

156. Lang IM, Shaker R. Anatomy and physiology of the upper esophageal sphincter. Am J Med 1997;103:50S

157. Lear CS, Flanagan JB, Moorrees CF. The frequency of deglutition in man. Arch Oral Biol 1965;10:83

158. Lind JF, et al. Effect of thoracic displacement and vagotomy on the canine gastresophageal junctional zone. Gastroenterology 1969;56:1078

159. Lind JF, Warrian WG, Wankling WJ. Responses of the gastroesophageal junctional zone to increases in abdominal pressure. Can J Surg 1966;9:32

160. Logemann JA, et al. Closure mechanisms of laryngeal vestibule during swallow. Am J Physiol 1992;262:G338

161. Mao YK, Wang YF, Daniel EE. Distribution and characterization of vasoactive intestinal polypeptide binding in canine lower esophageal sphincter. Gastroenterology 1993;105:1370

162. Martin RE, Sessie BJ. The role of the cerebral cortex in swallowing. Dysphagia 1993;8:195

163. Mashimo H, et al. Neuronal constitutive nitric oxide synthase is involved in murine enteric inhibitory neurotransmission. J Clin Invest 1996;98:8

164. Mayrand S, Tremblay L, Diamant N. In vivo measurement of feline esophageal tone. Am J Physiol 1994;267:G914

165. McNally EF, Kelly JE, Ingelfinger FJ. Mechanism of belching: effects of gastric distention with air. Gastroenterology 1964;46:254

166. Medda BK, et al. Correlation of electrical and contractile activities of the cricopharyngeus muscle in the cat. Am J Physiol 1997;273:G470

167. Medda BK, et al. Characterization and quantification of a pharyngo-UES contractile reflex in cats. Am J Physiol 1994;267:G972

168. Mehta AJ, et al. Sensitization to painful distention and abnormal sensory perception in the esophagus. Gastroenterology 1995;108:311

169. Mellow MH. Esophageal motility during food ingestion: a physiologic test of esophageal motor function. Gastroenterology 1983;85:570

170. Meyer GW, et al. Muscle anatomy of the human esophagus. J Clin Gastroenterol 1986;8:131

171. Meyer GW, Castell DO. Human esophageal response during chest pain induced by swallowing cold liquids. JAMA 1981;246:2057

172. Miller AJ. Deglutition. Physiol Rev 1982;62:129

173. Miller AJ. The search for the central swallowing pathway: the quest for clarity. Dysphagia 1993;8:185

174. Miller CA, et al. Cyclic nucleotide-dependent protein kinases in the lower esophageal sphincter. Am J Physiol 1986;251:G794

175. Mittal RK, Balaban DH. The esophagogastric junction. N Engl J Med 1997;336:924

176. Mittal RK, Fisher MJ. Electrical and mechanical inhibition of the crural diaphragm during transient relaxation of the lower esophageal sphincter. Gastroenterology 1990;99:1265

177. Mittal RK, et al. Transient lower esophageal sphincter relaxation. Gastroenterology 1995;109:601

178. Mittal RK, McCallum RW. Characteristics of transient lower esophageal sphincter relaxation in humans. Am J Physiol 1987;252:G636

179. Mittal RK, Rochester DF, McCallum RW. Electrical and mechanical activity in the human lower esophageal sphincter during diaphragmatic contraction. J Clin Invest 1988;81:1182

180. Mittal RK, Stewart WR, Schirmer BD. Effect of a catheter in the pharynx on the frequency of transient lower esophageal sphincter relaxations. Gastroenterology 1992;103:1236

181. Mukhopadhyay AK. Effect of substance P on the lower esophageal sphincter of the opossum. Gastroenterology 1978;75:278

182. Mukhopadhyay A, Rattan S, Goyal RK. Effect of prostaglandin $E_2$ on esophageal motility in man. J Appl Physiol 1975;39:479

183. Muller-Lissner SA, Blum AL. Fundic pressure rise lowers lower esophageal sphincter pressure in man. Hepatogastroenterology 1982;29:151

184. Murray J, et al. Nitric oxide: mediator of nonadrenergic noncholinergic responses of opossum esophageal muscle. Am J Physiol 1991;261:G401

185. Nelson JL III, et al. Esophageal contraction pressures are not affected by normal menstrual cycles. Gastroenterology 1984;87:867

186. Neuhuber WL, et al. NADPH-diaphorase-positive nerve fibers associated with motor endplates in the rat esophagus: new evidence for co-innervation of striated muscle by enteric neurons. Cell Tissue Res 1994;276:23

187. Omari TI, et al. Esophageal body and lower esophageal sphincter function in healthy premature infants. Gastroenterology 1995;109:1757

188. Orr WC, Johnson LF, Robinson MG. Effect of sleep on swallowing, esophageal peristalsis, and acid clearance. Gastroenterology 1984;86:814

189. Papasova M, et al. On the changes in the membrane potential and the contractile activity of the smooth muscle of the lower esophageal and ileo-caecal sphincters upon increased K in the nutrient solution. Acta Physiol Pharmacol Bulg 1980;6:41

190. Patapoutian A, Wold BJ, Wagner RA. Evidence for developmentally programmed transdifferentiation in mouse esophageal muscle. Science 1995;270:1818

191. Paterson WG. Neuromuscular mechanisms of esophageal responses at and proximal to a distending balloon. Am J Physiol 1991;260:G148

192. Paterson WG, Anderson MA, Anand N. Pharmacological characterization of lower esophageal sphincter relaxation induced by swallowing, vagal efferent nerve stimulation, and esophageal distention. Can J Physiol Pharmacol 1992;70:1011

193. Paterson WG, Hynna-Liepert TT, Selucky M. Comparison of primary and secondary esophageal peristalsis in humans: effect of atropine. Am J Physiol 1991;260:G52

194. Paterson WG, Rattan S, Goyal RK. Esophageal responses to transient and sustained esophageal distension. Am J Physiol 1988;255:G587

195. Penagini R, Bianchi PA. Effect of morphine on gastroesophageal reflux and transient lower esophageal sphincter relaxation. Gastroenterology 1997;113:409

196. Pouderoux P, Lin S, Kahrilas PJ. Timing, propagation, coordination, and effect of esophageal shortening during peristalsis. Gastroenterology 1997;112:1147

197. Rathmann W, et al. Visceral afferent neuropathy in diabetic gastroparesis. Diabetes Care 1991;14:1086

198. Rattan S, Colin D, Goyal RK. The mechanisms of action of gastrin on the lower esophageal sphincter. Gastroenterology 1976;70:828

199. Rattan S, Gidda JS, Goyal RK. Membrane potential and mechanical responses of the opossum esophagus to vagal stimulation and swallowing. Gastroenterology 1983;85:922

200. Rattan S, Gonella P, Goyal RK. Inhibitory effect of calcitonin gene-related peptide and calcitonin on opossum esophageal smooth muscle. Gastroenterology 1988;94:284

201. Rattan S, Goyal RK. Neural control of the lower esophageal sphincter: influence of the vagus nerves. J Clin Invest 1974;54:899

202. Rattan S, Goyal RK. Evidence of possible 5-HT participation in the vagal inhibitory pathway to the opossum LES. Am J Physiol 1978; 234:E273

203. Rattan S, Goyal RK. Effect of bovine pancreatic polypeptide on the opossum lower esophageal sphincter. Gastroenterology 1979;77:672

204. Rattan S, Goyal RK. Role of prostaglandins in the regulation of lower esophageal sphincter. In Christensen JM, ed, Gastrointestinal Motility. New York: Raven Press, 1980

205. Rattan S, Goyal RK. Identification of $M_1$ and $M_2$ muscarinic receptor subtypes in the control of the lower esophageal sphincter in the opossum. Trends Pharmacol Sci 1984;(suppl):78

206. Rattan S, Goyal RK. Effect of galanin on the opossum lower esophageal sphincter. Life Sci 1987;41:2783

207. Rattan S, Moummi C. Influence of stimulators and inhibitors of cyclic nucleotides on lower esophageal sphincter. J Pharmacol Exp Ther 1989;248:703

208. Reynolds JC, Ouyang A, Cohen S. A lower esophageal sphincter reflex involving substance P. Am J Physiol 1984;246:G346

209. Reynolds RP, El-Sharkawy TY, Diamant NE. Lower esophageal sphincter function in the cat: role of central innervation assessed by transient vagal blockade. Am J Physiol 1984;246:G666

210. Richardson BJ, Welch RW. Differential effect of atropine on rightward and leftward lower esophageal sphincter pressure. Gastroenterology 1981;81:85

211. Richter JE, et al. Esophageal manometry in 95 healthy adult volunteers. Variability of pressures with age and frequency of "abnormal" contractions. Dig Dis Sci 1987;32:583

212. Robison BA, Percy WH, Christensen J. Differences in cytochrome c oxidase capacity in smooth muscle of opossum esophagus and lower esophageal sphincter. Gastroenterology 1984;87:1009

213. Rodrigo J, et al. Sensory vagal nature and anatomical access paths to esophagus laminar nerve endings in myenteric ganglia. Determination by surgical degeneration methods. Acta Anat (Basel) 1982;112:47

214. Rodrigo J, et al. Vegetative innervation of the esophagus. III. Intraepithelial endings. Acta Anat (Basel) 1975;92:242

215. Rodrigo J, et al. Vegetative innervation of the esophagus. II. Intraganglionic laminar endings. Acta Anat (Basel) 1975;92:79

216. Rodrigo J, et al. Calcitonin gene-related peptide immunoreactive sensory and motor nerves of the rat, cat, and monkey esophagus. Gastroenterology 1985;88:444

217. Rodrigo J, et al. Sensorivagal nature of oesophageal submucous layer nerve endings. Determination of surgical degeneration methods. Acta Anat (Basel) 1980;108:540

218. Roman C, Gonella J. Extrinsic control of digestive tract motility. In Johnson LR, ed, Physiology of the Gastrointestinal Tract. New York: Raven Press, 1987:289

219. Rossiter CD, et al. Control of lower esophageal sphincter pressure by two sites in dorsal motor nucleus of the vagus. Am J Physiol 1990; 259:G899

220. Ryan JP, Snape WJ Jr, Cohen S. Influence of vagal cooling on esophageal function. Am J Physiol 1977;232:E159

221. Saha JK, Hirano I, Goyal RK. Biphasic effect of SNP on opossum esophageal longitudinal muscle: involvement of cGMP and eicosanoids. Am J Physiol 1993;265:G403

222. Saha JK, Sengupta JN, Goyal RK. Effect of bradykinin on opossum esophageal longitudinal smooth muscle: evidence for novel bradykinin receptors. J Pharmacol Exp Ther 1990;252:1012

223. Saha JK, Sengupta JN, Goyal RK. Effects of bradykinin and bradykinin analogs on the opossum lower esophageal sphincter: characterization of an inhibitory bradykinin receptor. J Pharmacol Exp Ther 1991; 259:265

224. Saha JK, Sengupta JN, Goyal RK. Role of chloride ions in lower esophageal sphincter tone and relaxation. Am J Physiol 1992;263: G115

225. Sang Q, Young HM. Development of nicotinic receptor clusters and innervation accompanying the change in muscle phenotype in the mouse esophagus. J Comp Neurol 1997;386:119

226. Sasaki CT, Weaven EM. Physiology of the larynx. Am J Med 1997; 103:9S

227. Schoeman MN, Holloway RH. Stimulation and characteristics of secondary oesophageal peristalsis in normal subjects. Gut 1994;35:152

228. Schulze-Delrieu K, Crane SA. Oxygen uptake and mechanical tension in esophageal smooth muscle from opossums and cats. Am J Physiol 1982;242:G258

229. Sears VW Jr, Castell JA, Castell DO. Comparison of effects of upright versus supine body position and liquid versus solid bolus on esophageal pressures in normal humans. Dig Dis Sci 1990;35:857

230. Sears VW Jr, Castell JA, Castell DO. Radial and longitudinal asymmetry of human pharyngeal pressures during swallowing. Gastroenterology 1991;101:1559

231. Seelig LL Jr, et al. Acetylcholinesterase and choline acetyltransferase staining of neurons in the opossum esophagus. Anat Rec 1984;209: 125

232. Seelig LL Jr, Goyal RK. Morphological evaluation of opossum lower esophageal sphincter. Gastroenterology 1978;75:51

233. Sengupta A, Paterson WG, Goyal RK. Atypical localization of myenteric neurons in the opossum lower esophageal sphincter. Am J Anat 1987;180:342

234. Sengupta JN, Kauvar D, Goyal RK. Characteristics of vagal esophageal tension-sensitive afferent fibers in the opossum. J Neurophysiol 1989;61:1001

235. Sengupta JN, Saha JK, Goyal RK. Stimulus-response function studies of esophageal mechanosensitive nociceptors in sympathetic afferents of opossum. J Neurophysiol 1990;64:796

236. Sengupta JN, Saha JK, Goyal RK. Differential sensitivity to bradykinin of esophageal distension-sensitive mechanoreceptors in vagal and sympathetic afferents of the opossum. J Neurophysiol 1992;68:1053

237. Sessle BJ, Henry JL. Neural mechanisms of swallowing: neurophysiological and neurochemical studies on brain stem neurons in the solitary tract region. Dysphagia 1989;4:61

238. Shaker R. First Multi-Disciplinary International Symposium on Supraesophageal Complications of Reflux Disease (abstract). Am J Med 1997;103:1s

239. Shaker R, et al. Esophagoglottal closure reflex: a mechanism of airway protection. Gastroenterology 1992;102:857

240. Shaker R, Lang IM. Reflex mediated airway protective mechanisms against retrograde aspiration. Am J Med 1997;103:64S

241. Shaker R, et al. Coordination of deglutition and phases of respiration: effect of aging, tachypnea, bolus volume, and chronic obstructive pulmonary disease. Am J Physiol 1992;263:G750

242. Shaker R, et al. Mechanisms of airway protection and upper esophageal sphincter opening during belching. Am J Physiol 1992;262:G621

243. Shaker R, et al. Identification and characterization of the esophagoglottal closure reflex in a feline model. Am J Physiol 1994;266:G147

244. Shaker R, et al. Characterization of the pharyngo-UES contractile reflex in humans. Am J Physiol 1997;273:G854

245. Shaker R, et al. Effect of aging, position, and temperature on the threshold volume triggering pharyngeal swallows. Gastroenterology 1994;107:396

246. Shingai T, Shimada K. Reflex swallowing elicited by water and chemical substances applied in the oral cavity, pharynx, and larynx of the rabbit. J J Physiol 1976;26:455

247. Shipp T, Deatsch WW, Robertson K. Pharyngoesophageal muscle activity during swallowing in man. Laryngoscope 1970;80:1

248. Siegel CI, Hendrix TR. Evidence for the central mediation of secondary peristalsis in the esophagus. Bull Johns Hopkins Hosp 1961;108: 297

249. Sifrim D, Janssens J. Secondary peristaltic contractions, like primary peristalsis, are preceded by inhibition in the human esophageal body. Digestion 1996;57:73

250. Sifrim D, Janssens J, Vantrappen G. A wave of inhibition precedes primary peristaltic contractions in the human esophagus. Gastroenterology 1992;103:876

251. Sifrim D, Janssens J, Vantrappen G. Failing deglutitive inhibition in primary esophageal motility disorders. Gastroenterology 1994;106: 875

252. Sigala S, et al. Different neurotransmitter systems involved in the development of esophageal achalasia. Life Sci. 1995;56:1311–1320

253. Sinar DR, et al. Effect of gastric inhibitory polypeptide on lower esophageal sphincter pressure in cats. Gastroenterology 1978;75:263

254. Singaram C, et al. Peptidergic innervation of the human esophageal smooth muscle. Gastroenterology 1991;101:1256

255. Singaram C, et al. Nitrinergic and peptidergic innervation of the human oesophagus. Gut 1994;35:1690

256. Singh KD, et al. Topographic mapping of transcranial magnetic stimulation data on surface rendered MR images of the brain. Electroencephalog Clin Neurophysiol 1997;105:345

257. Smith CC, Brizzee KR. Cineradiographic analysis of vomiting in the cat. Gastroenterology 1960;40:654

258. Sohn UD, et al. Agonist-independent, muscle-type-specific signal transduction pathways in cat esophageal and lower esophageal sphincter circular smooth muscle. J Pharmacol Exp Ther 1995;273:482

259. Sohn UD, et al. Distinct muscarinic receptors, G proteins and phospholipases in esophageal and lower esophageal sphincter circular muscle. J Pharmacol Exp Ther 1993;267:1205

260. Sohn UD, et al. Role of 100-kDa cytosolic PLA2 in ACh-induced contraction of cat esophageal circular muscle. Am J Physiol 1994; 267:G433

261. Stein HJ, et al. Three-dimensional pressure image and muscular structure of the human lower esophageal sphincter. Surgery 1995;117:692

262. Sugarbaker DJ, Rattan S, Goyal RK. Mechanical and electrical activity of esophageal smooth muscle during peristalsis. Am J Physiol 1984;246:G145

263. Sugarbaker DJ, Rattan S, Goyal RK. Swallowing induces sequential activation of esophageal longitudinal smooth muscle. Am J Physiol 1984;247:G515

264. Sumi T. The activity of brain stem respiratory neurons and spinal respiratory motoneuron during swallowing. J Neurophysiol 1963;26:466

265. Szewczak SM, et al. VIP-induced alterations in cAMP and inositol phosphates in the lower esophageal sphincter. Am J Physiol 1990;259:G239

266. Szymanski PT, et al. Differences in contractile protein content and isoforms in phasic and tonic smooth muscles. Am J Physiol 1998;275:C684

267. Templeton FE, Kredel RH. The cricopharyngeal sphincter: a roentgenologic study. Laryngoscope 1943;53:1

268. Terenghi G, et al. Calcitonin gene-related peptide-immunoreactive nerves in the tongue, epiglottis and pharynx of the rat: occurrence, distribution and origin. Brain Res 1986;365:1

269. Thor K, Rokaeus A. Studies on the mechanisms by which (Gin4)-neurotensin reduces lower esophageal sphincter (LES) pressure in man. Acta Physiol Scand 1983;118:373

270. Thorpe JA. Effect of propranolol on the lower oesophageal sphincter in man. Curr Med Res Opin 1980;7:91

271. Tieffenbach L, Roman C. The role of extrinsic vagal innervation in the motility of the smooth-musculed portion of the esophagus: electromyographic study in the cat and the baboon. (in French). J Physiol (Paris) 1972;64:193

272. Titchen DA. Diaphragmatic and oesophageal activity in regurgitation in sheep: an electromyographic study. J Physiol 1979;292:381

273. Torphy TJ, et al. Lower esophageal sphincter relaxation is associated with increased cyclic nucleotide content. Am J Physiol 1986;251:G786

274. Tottrup A, et al. Effects of transmural field stimulation in isolated muscle strips from human esophagus. Am J Physiol 1990;258:G344

275. Tottrup A, Knudsen MA, Gregersen H. The role of the L-arginine–nitric oxide pathway in relaxation of the opossum lower oesophageal sphincter. Br J Pharmacol 1991;104:113

276. Tottrup A, Svane D, Forman A. Nitric oxide mediating NANC inhibition in opossum lower esophageal sphincter. Am J Physiol 1991;260:G385

277. Toyama T, Yokoyama I, Nishi K. Effects of hexamethonium and other ganglionic blocking agents on electrical activity of the esophagus induced by vagal stimulation in the dog. Eur J Pharmacol 1975;31:63

278. Tuma SN, Mukhopadhyay A. The effect of parathyroid hormone on the esophageal smooth muscle of the opossum. Am J Gastroenterol 1980;74:415

279. Uc A, Murray JA, Conklin JL. Effects of calcitonin gene-related peptide on opossum esophageal smooth muscle. Gastroenterology 1997; 113:514

280. Vanek AW, Diamant NE. Responses of the human esophagus to paired swallows. Gastroenterology 1987;92:643

281. van Overbeek JJ, et al. Simultaneous manometry and electromyography in the pharyngoesophageal segment. Laryngoscope 1985;95:582

282. Vantrappen G, Hellemans J. Diseases of the Esophagus. New York: Springer-Verlag, 1974

283. Wang Q, et al. Caffeine- and carbachol-induced $Cl^-$ and cation currents in single opossum esophageal circular muscle cells. Am J Physiol 1996;271:C1725

284. Wang YT, Bieger D. Role of solitarial GABAergic mechanisms in control of swallowing. Am J Physiol 1991;261:R639

285. Wattchow DA, Furness JB, Costa M. Distribution and coexistence of peptides in nerve fibers of the external muscle of the human gastrointestinal tract. Gastroenterology 1988;95:32

286. Wein B, Bockler R, Klajman S. Temporal reconstruction of sonographic imaging of disturbed tongue movements. Dysphagia 1991;6:135

287. Weisbrodt NW, Christensen J. Gradients of contractions in the opossum esophagus. Gastroenterology 1972;62:1159

288. Weisbrodt NW, Murphy RA. Myosin phosphorylation and contraction of feline esophageal smooth muscle. Am J Physiol 1985;249:C9

289. Welch RW, Drake ST. Normal lower esophageal sphincter pressure: a comparison of rapid vs. slow pull-through techniques. Gastroenterology 1980;78:1446

290. Welch RW, Gray JE. Influence of respiration on recordings of lower esophageal sphincter pressure in humans. Gastroenterology 1982;83:590

291. Welch RW, et al. Manometry of the normal upper esophageal sphincter and its alterations in laryngectomy. J Clin Invest 1979;63:1036

292. Wiedner EB, Bao X, Altschuler SM. Localization of nitric oxide synthase in the brain stem neural circuit controlling esophageal peristalsis in rats. Gastroenterology 1995;108:367

293. Williams D, et al. Responses of the human esophagus to experimental intraluminal distension. Am J Physiol 1993;265:G196

294. Williams D, et al. Esophageal clearance function following treatment of esophagitis. Gastroenterology 1994;106:108

295. Williams D, et al. Identification of an abnormal esophageal clearance response to intraluminal distention in patients with esophagitis. Gastroenterology 1992;103:943

296. Wilson JA, et al. Normal pharyngoesophageal motility. A study of 50 healthy subjects. Dig Dis Sci 1989;34:1590

297. Winship DH, Viegas de Andrade SR, Zboralske FF. Influence of bolus temperature on human esophageal motor function. J Clin Invest 1970;49:243

298. Winship DH, Zboralske FF. The esophageal propulsive force: esophageal response to acute obstruction. J Clin Invest 1967;46:1391

299. Wolf BS. The inferior esophageal sphincter—anatomic, roentgenologic and manometric correlation, contradictions, and terminology. Am J Roentgenol Radium Ther Nucl Med 1970;110:260

300. Wright LE, Castell DO. The adverse effect of chocolate on lower esophageal sphincter pressure. Am J Dig Dis 1975;20:703

301. Wyman JB, et al. Control of belching by the lower oesophageal sphincter. Gut 1990;31:639

302. Xue S, Valdez D, Collman PI, Diamant NE. Effects of nitric oxide synthase blockade on esophageal peristalsis and the lower esophageal sphincter in the cat. Can J Physiol Pharmacol 1996;74:1249

303. Yamato S, Saha JK, Goyal RK. Role of nitric oxide in lower esophageal sphincter relaxation to swallowing. Life Sci 1992;50:1263

304. Yamato S, Spechler SJ, Goyal RK. Role of nitric oxide in esophageal peristalsis in the opossum. Gastroenterology 1992;103:197

305. Zelcer E, Weisbrodt NW. Electrical and mechanical activity in the lower esophageal sphincter of the cat. Am J Physiol 1984;246:G243

306. Zhang Y, Vogalis F, Goyal RK. Nitric oxide suppresses a $Ca^{2+}$-stimulated $Cl^-$ current in smooth muscle cells of opossum esophagus. Am J Physiol 1998;274:G886

*The Esophagus*, Third Edition,
edited by D. O. Castell and J. E. Richter.
Lippincott Williams & Wilkins, Philadelphia © 1999.

CHAPTER 2

# Overview and Symptom Assessment

John R. Bennett and Donald O. Castell

Traditional teaching in medicine has stressed the importance of careful evaluation of the patient's clinical history as a major component of the diagnostic evaluation. This dictum is particularly applicable in the approach to a patient with possible esophageal disease. Although often considered little more than a conduit to assist the passage of food from mouth to stomach, the esophagus has been the subject of many clinical and physiological studies that clarified the relevance of specific symptoms and the mechanisms by which they occur. So while it is tempting to leap from main symptom to special investigation, omission of the intermediate steps of detailed, sympathetic patient interrogation and the deductive process which should accompany it is always an error. At worst, the diagnostic scheme may set off in entirely the wrong direction; at best, the clinician may reach the "correct" diagnosis, in anatomical or physiological terms, but will not have learned other aspects of the patient's story which assist in subsequent management.

There are essentially three clinical presentations of esophageal disorders—*heartburn, dysphagia,* and *chest pain.* Each of these may vary in detail and may be associated with other minor symptoms, but they should all suggest the possible presence of an underlying esophageal abnormality to the clinician. In subsequent chapters of this text, the specific esophageal defects to be considered are discussed in detail.

## HEARTBURN

It has been estimated that a symptom identified as heartburn (or possibly indigestion or dyspepsia) occurs daily in approximately 10% of persons in Western society and at least weekly in 20%, with an overall prevalence of 40% [24, 25, 30], and that intermittent symptoms are present in more than one-third of the population in the United States, Europe, and Australia. The majority of these patients will treat their symptoms with over-the-counter medication and not consult a physician for this particular problem, and it has been shown that more than 80% of the antacid preparations purchased over the counter are being used for symptoms of heartburn and regurgitation [21]. Patients who do seek a physician's help for their reflux symptoms or who mention them during evaluation of other clinical problems are often seen by a primary-care physician. The subspecialist in gastroenterology or gastrointestinal surgery is likely to see only the "tip of the iceberg" from this patient group when the symptoms have become particularly severe and persistent or unresponsive to standard therapy or when complications have developed. It becomes important, therefore, that physicians in all specialties who see such patients become familiar with the meaning of these symptoms and develop a reasonable clinical approach to them. In addition to heartburn, there are a variety of other symptoms, both esophageal and extraesophageal, that may occur secondary to gastroesophageal (GE) reflux. The term *GE reflux disease* (GERD) is particularly useful for describing the whole spectrum of manifestations of chronic reflux. Thus, this term should include the patient who has recurring heartburn without objective disease (esophagitis) as well as the person who presents with severe esophageal injury with or without the common symptoms. In addition, GERD encompasses patients with other manifestations of reflux often missed by the clinician, including unexplained chest pain, chronic hoarseness, nonallergic asthma, and chronic cough. The concept of the GERD spectrum is discussed further in Chapter 19.

How does the patient describe the esophageal symptoms? Classic heartburn is a substernal burning sensation with a tendency to radiate toward the mouth. It may be associated with an acid or bitter taste, usually occurs within 30 minutes to 2 hours after meals, and is made worse when the patient lies down or bends over. It may waken patients from sleep. A large meal, especially if it contains fat, chocolate, coffee, or alcohol, is particularly likely to precipitate heartburn. The

J. R. Bennett: Royal College of Physicians, London NW1 4LE, United Kingdom.

D. O. Castell: Department of Medicine, Graduate Hospital, Philadelphia, Pennsylvania 19146.

discomfort often disappears quickly on drinking water or milk or after taking an antacid. If heartburn occurs frequently, it can interfere with the patient's way of life, particularly work or pleasure involving lying or bending, including gardening and sexual intercourse.

Heartburn is considered always to be the consequence of contact of an irritant substance (most commonly acid) with the esophageal mucosa. Most patients with regular heartburn can be shown, by intraesophageal pH monitoring, to have episodes of acid reflux more frequently, or for longer periods, than the normal, symptomless population [27, 43]. There is, nevertheless, a substantial proportion of patients with characteristic heartburn who have normal levels of acid reflux [40, 47], though in many of these the "symptom index" [52] (the correlation between acid reflux and an episode of heartburn) is positive.

Although recurrent heartburn, as an isolated symptom, strongly suggests GERD as the diagnosis, there are other possibilities [17, 37]. Peptic ulceration, of the duodenum or stomach, sometimes causes heartburn rather than epigastric pain as its predominant symptom. Delayed gastric emptying, whether functional (as in diabetic gastroparesis) or organic (as in carcinoma of the gastric antrum), may cause heartburn.

Sudden, unprecedented heartburn may indicate acute esophagitis or esophageal erosion caused by a corrosive, especially a drug.

## ODYNOPHAGIA

The term *odynophagia* is used to describe the symptom of pain caused by swallowing. This important symptom is clearly indicative of a pharyngeal or esophageal problem but is not always volunteered by patients, who should be specifically asked about it. A sensation of burning or pain soon after swallowing hot, spicy, or acidic food or drink is characteristic of "esophagitis." It occurs in up to 50% of patients with GERD, though will often need to be elicited by direct questioning. It is common in infective esophagitis and, in one study, was reported in 31% of acquired immunodeficiency syndrome (AIDS) patients [8].

In corrosive esophagitis (particularly "pill"-induced injury), odynophagia may be severe enough to cause complete cessation of swallowing.

## REGURGITATION

Heartburn is often associated with the symptom of regurgitation, best described as the effortless appearance of an acid or bitter taste in the mouth or awakening from sleep because of coughing or choking and sometimes finding secretions on the pillow. Regurgitation is particularly severe at night or when bending over and may occur with or independently from heartburn. Apart from GERD, regurgitation may be a symptom of a pharyngeal pouch, esophageal obstruction, or gastric outlet obstruction.

### Water Brash

This term *water brash,* which is frequently misused, is intended to describe the sudden filling of the mouth with clear, slightly salty fluid. The fluid is not regurgitated gastric contents but, rather, secretions from the salivary glands occurring by reflex stimulation secondary to acid irritation in the distal esophagus [22].

### Vomiting

An esophageal problem alone does not cause true vomiting. Patients, however, may complain of "vomiting" when, in fact, they are experiencing some form of regurgitation.

## HICCUP

The easily recognized hiccup (hiccough, singultus) is caused by an abrupt, involuntary lowering of the diaphragm and closure of the glottis, producing a characteristic sound. Although most doctors are aware that various systemic disorders, notably uremia, may cause hiccup, almost all sporadic hiccuping is of unclear origin [26]. Undoubtedly, esophageal disease can be a cause [15], e.g., GE reflux [19, 41]. The fact that sporadic hiccup particularly occurs after a large meal is compatible with the view that reflux is frequently the cause. Esophageal obstruction may also cause hiccup, sometimes without dysphagia, and is sometimes reported by patients with achalasia or with benign or malignant strictures [15].

## RESPIRATORY SYMPTOMS

Certain respiratory symptoms are associated with and possibly caused by GE reflux and may be considered symptoms of esophageal disease. A higher than expected incidence of detectable reflux in patients with respiratory problems, such as asthma [20, 44] and bronchitis [13], has been repeatedly observed in recent years.

The suggestion that extraesophageal manifestations of chronic GERD may bring patients to various specialists is not a new concept. Otolaryngologists have been aware for many years that hoarseness might be a manifestation of GERD secondary to reflux laryngitis (the so-called Cherry-Donner syndrome) [5, 53]. Respiratory and laryngeal associations with GERD are discussed in Chapters 28 and 29.

## DYSPHAGIA

The word *dysphagia,* which is derived from the Greek *phagia* (to eat) and *dys* (with difficulty), is the symptom most specifically indicating an esophageal disorder. It refers to the sensation of food being hindered in its normal passage from the mouth to the stomach. Patients with dysphagia most frequently complain that food "sticks," "hangs up," "gets caught," or "just won't go down right." They may occasionally note some associated pain, but the symptom of dysphagia should not be used interchangeably with odynophagia (see above). It is not uncommon, and 10% of people over 50 years old report troublesome dysphagia [29]. The importance of the clinical history in suggesting the specific etiology of dysphagia cannot be overstated. When Schatzki [38] described the lower esophageal ring that bears his name, he asserted that a careful history should give the physician a strong suspicion of the correct diagnosis in 80% to 85% of patients with dysphagia. Although Schatzki was referring to what we now classify as *esophageal dysphagia,* that statement helps to emphasize the critical importance of the medical history in clarifying the cause of this symptom.

## Globus

A generally accepted clinical truth is that dysphagia almost always indicates the presence of organic dysfunction. It is important, therefore, that one should not confuse dysphagia with globus sensation, the feeling of a lump, fullness, or "tickle" in the throat. Globus is usually a more constant symptom that does not interfere with swallowing and, in fact, may be relieved during deglutition. Globus has often been considered a symptom occurring in patients having hysterical personality traits, leading to the outdated term *globus hystericus.* This is not an appropriate indictment since psychological evaluations have revealed an increase in depression [35] and obsessive-compulsive tendencies [36] in patients with globus but little evidence of hysteria. Thus, the term *globus,* or *globus sensation,* is preferable. It is also important to recognize that symptoms consistent with the diagnosis of globus might also occur in patients with organic esophageal disease. The diagnosis of globus should never be made without a thorough investigation for a lesion in the pharynx, larynx, or neck. Reports of various manometric abnormalities in the cricopharyngeal sphincter or of increased acid reflux have not been confirmed, and the symptom is probably entirely psychological [10]. Recent observations from our laboratory have found a surprising association of hypertensive upper esophageal sphincter (UES) pressure with globus sensation (Fig. 2–1). This finding was gender-

related in that almost all male subjects with globus had elevated UES pressures, whereas female subjects were equally likely to have a UES pressure in the normal range. These observations suggested that increased visceral afferent sensation might play a greater role in the genesis of globus sensation in women. In addition, ambulatory pH monitoring failed to confirm a relationship between abnormal GE reflux and globus in either men or women [11].

## Classification of Dysphagia

Dysphagia can usually be divided into two distinct syndromes, that produced by abnormalities affecting the finely tuned neuromuscular mechanism of the striated muscle of the mouth, pharynx, and UES (oropharyngeal dysphagia) and that due to any one of the variety of disorders affecting the smooth muscle esophagus (esophageal dysphagia).

*Oropharyngeal dysphagia* is usually described as a problem with the initiation of swallowing. It is a transfer problem, due to impaired ability to transfer food from mouth to upper esophagus or due to an impaired oral preparatory phase. These patients present with a variety of complaints, including food sticking in the throat, nasal regurgitation, and coughing during swallowing. They may also complain of dysarthria or display nasal speech because of associated muscle weakness. Many local, neurological, and muscular diseases can produce oropharyngeal dysphagia (see Chapter 9). Usually, the dysphagia is only one of the manifestations of a relatively obvious disease and does not pose a diagnostic problem, but careful radiological and manometric investigation may be required to make a specific diagnosis and to assist in planning therapy.

*Esophageal dysphagia* can result from a variety of structural or neuromuscular defects in the smooth muscle portion of the esophagus and the lower esophageal sphincter (LES), causing difficult *transport* of ingested material down the esophagus (Table 2–1). Conceptually, dysphagia is likely with either of two generic mechanisms: the first is due to any condition producing obstruction to luminal flow, including rings, strictures, carcinoma, extrinsic masses, or muscular contractions in the esophageal body (diffuse spasm) or LES (achalasia), and the second is failure of peristalsis (achalasia, scleroderma) or disruption of the normal peristaltic progression (diffuse spasm). In some patients, both elements are present and additive, for example, the modest extrinsic pressure of a dilated aorta combined with feeble peristalsis, producing the syndrome of dysphagia aortica (see Chapter 39). Further details of pathophysiology are discussed with specific conditions.

## History and Physical Examination

As noted previously, the patient with oropharyngeal dysphagia usually describes trouble initiating a swallow. Other features which may provide important diagnostic clues include the presence of a speech disorder or evidence of cranial

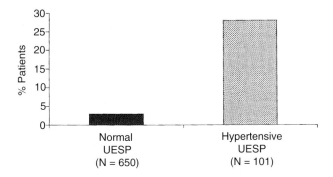

**FIG. 2–1.** Globus sensation was the presenting symptom in only 3% of 650 patients with normal upper esophageal sphincter pressure (UESP) versus 28% of 101 patients with hypertensive (greater than 118 mm Hg) UESP (*p* < 0.01).

**TABLE 2–1.** *Etiologies of esophageal dysphagia*

Neuromuscular (motility) disorders
  Primary
    Achalasia
    Other primary motility abnormalities
      Diffuse esophageal spasm
      Nutcracker esophagus (hypertensive peristalsis)
      Hypertensive lower esophagus
      Ineffective esophageal motility
  Secondary
    Scleroderma
    Other collagen disorders
    Chagas' disease
Mechanical lesions—intrinsic
  Most common
    Peptic stricture
    Lower esophageal (Schatzki's) ring
    Carcinoma
  Other
    Esophageal webs
    Esophageal diverticula
    Benign tumors
    Foreign bodies
    Medication-induced injury
Mechanical lesions—extrinsic
  Vascular compression
  Mediastinal abnormalities
  Cervical osteoarthritis

nerve deficits, limb weakness, or changes in sleep pattern, including sleep apnea or the recent onset of snoring; the recent onset of a stroke; or the development of weakness due to a muscular disease. This is in contrast to esophageal dysphagia, wherein the dysphagia is usually the prominent manifestation.

Any patient presenting with oropharyngeal dysphagia deserves a careful neurological examination and evaluation of the pharynx and larynx, including direct laryngoscopy. In patients with Zenker's diverticula, the earliest symptoms may be transient oropharyngeal dysphagia. When the pharyngeal sac becomes large enough to retain food, the more classic symptoms of persistent cough, fullness in the neck, gurgling in the throat, postprandial regurgitation, and aspiration develop. Some diverticula become so large that patients perform various maneuvers, such as applying pressure on the neck and repeatedly coughing, to empty them. These sacs can become large enough to produce a visible mass in the neck or to obstruct the esophagus by compression (see Chapter 15 for further details).

When approaching the patient with apparent esophageal dysphagia, a careful evaluation of the history is equally important. Three questions are crucial: (a) What kind of food (liquid or solid) produces the symptom? [For research purposes, this can be scored quantitatively (12)]. (b) Is the dysphagia intermittent or progressive? (c) Is there associated heartburn? On the basis of the answers to these questions, it is often possible not only to identify the etiology as either a mechanical or a neuromuscular defect, but also to postulate which of the three major causes in each of these two subdivi-

sions is the more likely. An algorithm for the historical aspects of the common causes of esophageal dysphagia is shown in Figure 2–2. Additional helpful features to ascertain are duration, onset (sudden or gradual), frequency (occasional or invariable), associated pain, weight loss, associated coughing or choking, drug history [especially nonsteroidal antiinflammatory drugs (NSAIDs), antibiotics].

Patients with esophageal motility disorders usually complain of slowly progressive dysphagia for both liquids and solids from the onset. Conversely, patients with mechanical obstruction usually have dysphagia initially for solids only and more progressive symptoms, although the onset is occasionally sudden [33]. The exception is the lower esophageal ring, in which intermittent dysphagia is the rule.

The site at which the patient localizes his or her dysphagia is of limited value. Although dysphagia in the epigastric or retrosternal areas frequently corresponds to the site of obstruction, dysphagia localized by the patient to the neck is frequently referred from below. The term *cervical dysphagia* should be avoided since localization of sensation in the suprasternal area can occur with either oropharyngeal or esophageal dysphagia.

Physical examination usually is not revealing in patients with esophageal dysphagia, with the exception of scleroderma, in which other manifestations of CREST syndrome (*c*alcinosis, *R*aynaud's phenomenon, *e*sophagus, *s*clerodactyly, *t*elangiectasia) may be present.

## Clinical Presentations

The clinical presentation of patients with oropharyngeal dysphagia is discussed above. Details of some conditions causing esophageal dysphagia are discussed below.

### Rings and Webs

Patients who have only *intermittent dysphagia for solids* most frequently are noted to have either rings or webs (see also Chapter 14). A mucosal ring at the junction of the esophageal and gastric mucosa is commonly referred to as a *Schatzki's ring* or a *B ring*. Although the prevalence of B rings noted on barium x-ray studies is reported to be up to 14%, the majority are asymptomatic. Symptoms generally occur only when the intraluminal diameter is less than 13 mm [39]. Dysphagia that occurs every day is not likely to be caused by a lower esophageal ring. The diagnosis can essentially be made by this history, although barium studies are needed to confirm this impression (see Chapter 3).

The other ring of the lower esophagus is called a *muscular, contractile,* or *A ring*. This type occurs less frequently than B rings and is rarely symptomatic. When present, symptoms are identical to those of B rings. In contrast to mucosal rings, muscular rings appear on barium esophagograms as broad constrictions a few centimeters above the squamocolumnar junction.

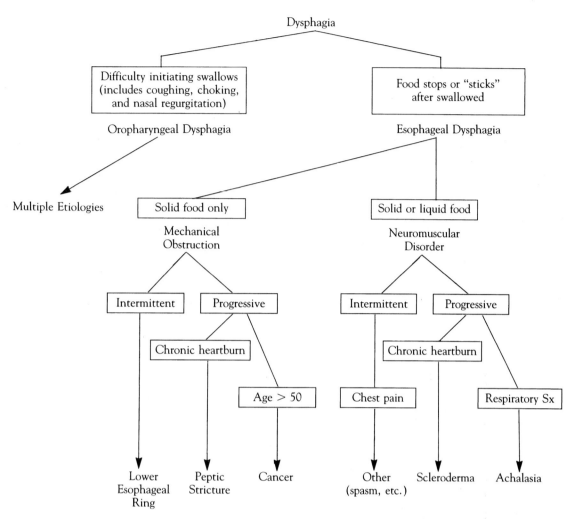

**FIG. 2–2.** Algorithm for diagnostic symptom analysis of patients with dysphagia. *Sx,* symptoms.

### Peptic Stricture

If the solid-food dysphagia is clearly progressive, then the major considerations in the differential diagnosis are peptic esophageal stricture and carcinoma. Patients with peptic stricture are usually middle-aged or elderly and typically have a long antecedent history of heartburn and chronic antacid use. They have often taken NSAIDs. Radiographically, these strictures are smooth, vary in length, and usually are in the lower third of the esophagus. Evaluation should always include endoscopy with biopsy and cytology to exclude carcinoma. A peptic stricture located more proximally in the esophagus strongly suggests a diagnosis of Barrett's esophagus (see also Chapter 27).

### Esophageal Carcinoma

Patients with carcinoma of the esophagus are more likely to present with a history of rapidly progressive dysphagia. They frequently do not have a long history of heartburn, but the chance association of reflux may occur. The exception to this rule is the patient with Barrett's esophagus secondary to chronic reflux disease who develops an adenocarcinoma in the metaplastic epithelium. Patients with esophageal cancer frequently have anorexia and greater weight loss than the severity or duration of their dysphagia would support. Heavy alcohol and tobacco use are associated with esophageal squamous carcinoma. The diagnosis of esophageal carcinoma can be strongly suggested by the history alone, but radiology and/or endoscopy are the methods of initial diagnosis. All patients should undergo endoscopy with biopsy and cytology to confirm the diagnosis (see Chapter 12 for details on esophageal cancer).

### Vascular Anomalies

Several vascular anomalies may produce dysphagia by compression of the esophagus. The most common complete vascular rings reported to cause dysphagia are, in order of frequency, (a) double aortic arch, (b) right aortic arch with retroesophageal left subclavian artery and left ligamentum arteriosum, and (c) right aortic arch with mirror-image branching and left ligamentum arteriosum. The most com-

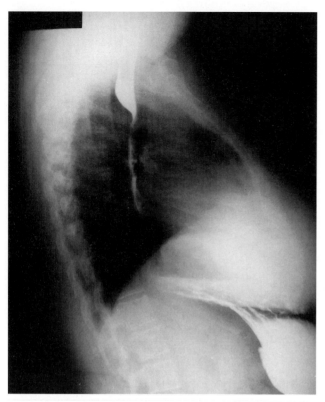

**FIG. 2–3.** Barium swallow revealing posterior esophageal compression at the level of the aortic arch. (From ref. 34, with permission.)

mon incomplete rings are retroesophageal right aberrant subclavian artery (arteria lusoria) and anomalous left pulmonary artery. The dysphagia associated with these lesions (so-called dysphagia lusoria, from *lusus naturae,* meaning "a freak of nature") usually begins early in childhood. Occasionally, symptoms may present in the adult, after increasing atherosclerosis or aneurysmal changes.

The incidence of arteria lusoria is approximately 0.75%, but clinically important obstructive manifestations are unusual. When present, the dysphagia is usually a constant, daily problem, described as a temporary arrest of a solid bolus beneath the manubrium.

Barium swallow may show compression of the esophagus posteriorly (Fig. 2–3), and manometry may reveal a zone of increased pressure with arterial pulsations at the level of vascular compression (Fig. 2–4) [45]. Computed tomography (Fig. 2–5A) or magnetic resonance imaging may help to establish the specific vascular anomaly (Fig. 2–5B).

### Dysphagia Aortica

A diagnosis of dysphagia aortica includes impingement on the thoracic esophagus by a massive thoracic aortic aneurysm or compression of the anatomically restricted distal esophagus between a rigid atherosclerotic aorta posteriorly and the heart or the ventral margin of the esophageal hiatus anteriorly. As expected, this is a disorder of the elderly, the average age at diagnosis being in the seventies.

### Cervical Hypertrophic Osteoarthropathy

Although hypertrophic spurs on the anterior surface of the cervical vertebrae occur in 20% to 30% of the elderly population, dysphagia secondary to compression of the esophagus by them is unusual. Since the esophagus is anchored at the cricoid cartilage, an osteophyte at the fourth through seventh cervical vertebrae may produce this symptom [14]. The most common complaint is difficulty swallowing solid foods, but patients also complain of odynophagia, a foreign-body sensation, cough, hoarseness, or an urge to clear the throat. Diagnosis can be made by barium esophagogram (lateral view), although careful endoscopy should be performed to exclude intraluminal pathology.

### Mediastinal Abnormalities

Dysphagia may be caused by a variety of pathological processes resulting in mediastinal adenopathy, including bronchial carcinoma and sarcoidosis.

### Achalasia

Idiopathic achalasia is an esophageal motility disorder characterized clinically by slowly progressive dysphagia and regurgitation of ingested foods (see also Chapter 10). There are two main defects in achalasia: obstruction of the esophagogastric junction and abnormal esophageal peristalsis.

The majority of patients present between the ages of 20 and 40, although the disease occurs in children and in the elderly. The most common initial complaint is progressive dysphagia for either liquids or solids. Regurgitation of undigested food that had been eaten many hours previously is a common complaint, particularly at night, when it may result in aspiration and nocturnal coughing.

The diagnosis of achalasia is sometimes apparent on a routine chest x-ray. Possible findings include absence of a gastric air bubble, mediastinal widening with a double shadow created by the dilated esophagus, and evidence of aspiration pneumonia. Characteristic features on barium esophagogram include esophageal dilatation with a smoothly tapered narrowing at the distal end and the presence of a fluid level in the upper portion due to the retention of esophageal secretions and ingested material. The beaklike, symmetric narrowing of the distal end of the esophagus helps to differentiate achalasia from the more ragged appearance of carcinoma.

Manometry is the preferred method to make the diagnosis of achalasia and reveals absent peristalsis and incomplete LES relaxation.

The diagnosis of idiopathic achalasia should not be considered conclusive until a thorough endoscopic evaluation of the esophagogastric junction has been made, including a

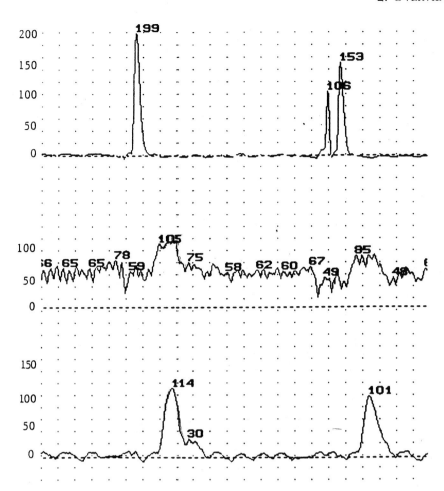

**FIG. 2–4.** Esophageal manometry showing zone of high pressure in the **middle tracing** (at 25 cm from the nares) with small, regular spikes synchronous with the heart rate. There is a failure of relaxation of this pressure zone with swallows. Recording sites are at 20, 25, and 30 cm from the nares (**top** to **bottom tracings**). Pressure on the vertical axis is in millimeters of mercury. (From ref. 34, with permission.)

retroflexed view from within the stomach. The ability of the endoscope easily to "pop through" the tight LES and the absence of nodularity or mucosal defects are important findings to help exclude cancer in this area, which may mimic achalasia [48].

### Progressive Systemic Sclerosis

The other major motility disorder that may present with slowly progressive dysphagia for liquids and solids is that seen with progressive systemic sclerosis (PSS) or scleroderma (see also Chapter 16). Esophageal involvement occurs in more than 80% of patients with PSS and correlates best with the presence of Raynaud's phenomenon [7, 46]. A similar association of Raynaud's phenomenon and esophageal dysfunction is seen in mixed connective tissue disease.

The motility defects are marked diminution of peristalsis in the lower two-thirds (smooth muscle) of the esophagus and hypotension of the LES but with normal contraction pressures in the upper one-third (striated muscle) and a normal UES. Dysphagia may be a major complaint, but heartburn is a more prevalent symptom, separating these patients from those with achalasia. Severe reflux has been reported to result in strictures in up to 40% of these patients [54],

though long-term acid-suppressive therapy may prevent this complication [23].

### Diffuse Esophageal Spasm and Related Syndromes

Symptomatic diffuse esophageal spasm (DES) is a disorder of esophageal motility associated clinically with dysphagia or chest pain (see also Chapter 11). It is important to stress that this diagnosis must not be made without clinical symptoms since the radiographic and manometric findings can be seen in asymptomatic individuals. The cause of the disorder is unknown, although the functional abnormalities of the esophagus suggest both muscular and neural defects.

The dysphagia of DES may occur with liquids or solid food and is usually highly variable. It is generally intermittent and nonprogressive and occasionally is associated with pain, features that separate it from the other motility disorders. Patients may report that a variety of factors might precipitate dysphagia or chest pain, including ingestion of hot or cold foods or carbonated beverages or being exposed to stress.

The barium esophagogram reveals simultaneous, nonperistaltic contractions with resultant segmentation of the barium column. This has led to a variety of descriptive terms that

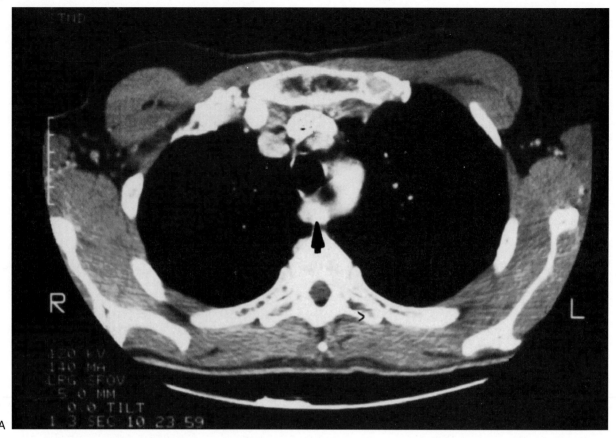

**FIG. 2–5. A:** Chest computed tomography scan showing an aberrant right subclavian artery (*arrow*) posterior to the esophagus and trachea. **B:** Chest magnetic resonance image showing the double aortic arch (*arrows*). (From ref. 34, with permission.)

attempt to depict the spectrum of findings, from mild serration of the margin of the esophagus (*tertiary contractions*) to frank subdivision of the esophageal outline (*rosary bead esophagus*) to marked tortuosity of the esophagus (*corkscrew esophagus*).

The manometric findings typically found in DES and related dysmotility patterns are discussed in Chapter 11.

### Miscellaneous Disorders

A number of other abnormalities of esophageal motility have been identified in patients presenting with dysphagia or chest pain. The symptom patterns in these patients—intermittent dysphagia or chest pain—are similar to those in patients with DES. Like DES, their relation to abnormal physiology or to a specific disease entity remains to be clarified.

### Hypercontractile Esophagus

Code and co-workers [6] described the manometric finding of a *hypertensive* LES in patients with chest pain or dysphagia. It is characterized by resting LES pressure exceeding the upper limit of normal (usually higher than 45

mm Hg) with normal peristalsis in the body of the esophagus. The majority of these patients will also demonstrate the high-amplitude peristaltic contractions (average greater than 180 mm Hg) seen in the *nutcracker esophagus.* Radiographic and scintigraphic studies usually have found normal esophageal function without bolus retardation at the level of the LES. Manometric studies using a more quantitative assessment of sphincter relaxation have revealed some degree of abnormality of relaxation of the LES in these patients, with a residual pressure of 5 to 10 mm Hg at the nadir of relaxation [16, 51].

### Assessment

The preferred diagnostic test in patients with dysphagia is a barium swallow. Because of the rapid sequence of pressure changes and movement of anatomic structures in the oropharynx, special techniques must be employed for adequate study. Video recording of a series of swallows with radiographic projections in the anteroposterior and lateral directions will provide imaging information that can be replayed at slower speed to identify abnormalities of movement of the various anatomic structures and muscle

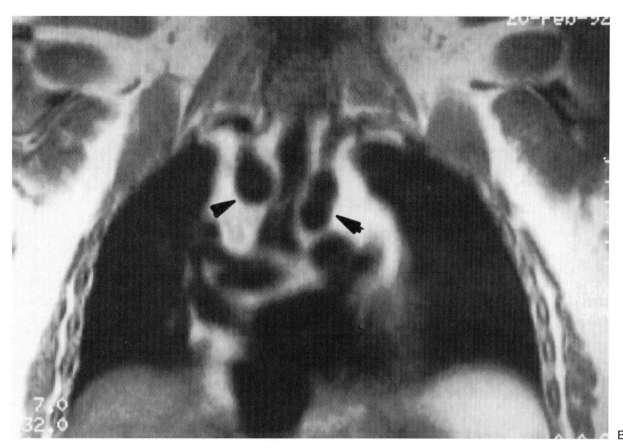

**FIG. 2–5.** *(continued)*

activities in the mouth, pharynx, and UES. A modified barium swallow can be performed with the addition of thick barium and a solid bolus (small cookie, marshmallow, or barium tablet) [50]. These techniques improve the overall assessment of the ability of the patient to transfer food from mouth to esophagus.

Endoscopy should always be done in patients with dysphagia, and if the history suggests an obstructive lesion, this may be the first investigation. If the radiological study suggests obstruction, endoscopy with biopsy and cytology is necessary to confirm or elucidate the lesion.

The development of improved techniques for measuring pharyngeal and UES pressures and pressure dynamics during swallowing has allowed more quantitative assessment of these functions in health and disease [4]. By the use of solid-state transducer systems or the combination of solid-state pharyngeal transducers and sleeve recording sensors spanning the UES, more accurate pressure and coordination sequences during swallowing are obtainable. With the development of on-line computer analysis of the rapid pressure changes occurring in this area with swallowing, the technology has advanced to a stage where subtle changes in pressure dynamics can be identified and categorized (see Chapter 5).

If the x-ray findings are negative or suggest a motility disorder, an esophageal motility study should be performed. These concepts are summarized in Figure 2–6.

## CHEST PAIN OF UNCERTAIN ORIGIN

Many patients (e.g., up to one-third of patients admitted urgently because of chest pain) with angina-like chest pain are found to have no evidence of ischemic heart disease, and many of these may have an esophageal disorder.

Initial interest in the significant proportion who could be shown to have abnormalities of esophageal motility waned when it became apparent that most patients, "reassured" that the problem had been identified, continued complaining of the pain [32]. More recently, interest has moved in two directions: the frequent relationship between GE reflux and chest pain and consideration of the network of pain perception.

The relationship between pain and abnormal esophageal events has been clarified by the development of a symptom index, intended to show whether episodes of pain are significantly linked in time to abnormal esophageal events (pH drops or motility change) or occur by chance [52]. By this means, patients in whom there is a statistical relationship, can be clearly identified. Some patients have pain during pH-

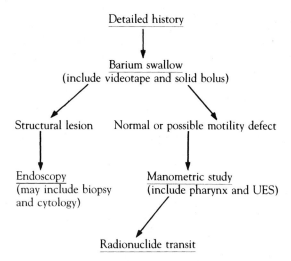

Detailed history

↓

Barium swallow
(include videotape and solid bolus)

Structural lesion ← → Normal or possible motility defect

↓ ↓

Endoscopy
(may include biopsy
and cytology)

Manometric study
(include pharynx and UES)

↓

Radionuclide transit

**FIG. 2–6.** Suggested diagnostic testing sequence for the evaluation of patients with dysphagia. *UES,* upper esophageal sphincter.

recorded episodes of reflux, even though the total amount of reflux is not necessarily "abnormal" [42, 52].

For some time, it has been recognized that some patients with "chest pain of uncertain origin" had an esophagus which could more readily be stimulated to cause pain than could normals [49]. This may also be likely in individuals whose UES relaxes less easily in response to esophageal distention ("high-threshold belcher") [18]. This phenomenon is not confined to patients with obscure chest pain, for the esophageal pain threshold is lower in patients with irritable bowel, too [9].

Anxiety, even panic disorder [3], is well recognized to be a feature of these patients' personalities [28], and this notably alters the patient's pain perception [2].

It seems increasingly likely that these chest pain-experiencing individuals have abnormal visceral perception, localized to the chest because the "sensitive" viscus may be heart, esophagus, or other thoracic structure. The abnormality rendering them "sensitive" may be local nociceptors in the viscera, higher processing centers, or cortical connections and possibly other factors (including anxiety) [1, 31].

These problems are discussed further in Chapter 36.

## REFERENCES

1. Bass C. Chest pain and breathlessness: relationship to psychiatric illness. Am J Med 1992;92(suppl 1A):125
2. Bass C, Wade W, Gardner WN, et al. Unexplained breathlessness and psychiatric morbidity in patients with normal and abnormal coronary arteries. Lancet 1983;i:605
3. Barsky AJ. Palpitation, cardiac awareness and panic disorder. Am J Med 1992;92(suppl 1A):315
4. Castell JA, Dalton CB, Castell DO. Pharyngeal and upper esophageal sphincter manometry in humans. Am J Physiol 1990;258:G173
5. Cherry J, Siegel C, Margulies S, Donner M. Pharyngeal localization of symptoms of gastroesophageal reflux. Ann Otol Rhinol Laryngol 1970;79:912
6. Code CF, Schlegel JF, Kelley ML, et al. Hypertensive gastroesophageal sphincter. Mayo Clin Proc 1986;35:391
7. Cohen S, Laufer I, Snape WJ, et al. The gastrointestinal manifestations of scleroderma. Gastroenterology 1980;79:155
8. Connolly GM. Oesophageal symptoms, their causes, treatment and prognosis in patients with the acquired immunodeficiency syndrome. Gut 1989;30:1033
9. Constantini M, Sturniolo GC, Zaninotto G, et al. Altered esophageal pain threshold in irritable bowel syndrome. Dig Dis Sci 1993;38:206
10. Cook IJ. Globus—real or imagined? Gullet 1991;1:68
11. Corso M, Pursnani K, Mohiuddin M, Gideon R, Castell J, Katzka D, Kate P, Castell D. Globus sensation is associated with hypertensive upper esophageal sphincter but not with gastroesophageal reflux. Dig Dis Sci 1998; (in press)
12. Dakkak M, Bennett JR. A new dysphagia score with objective validation. J Clin Gastroenterol 1992;14:99
13. Duclone A, Vendevenne A, Jovin H, et al. Gastro-esophageal reflux in patients with asthma and chronic bronchitis. Am Rev Respir Dis 1987;135:327
14. Eviatar E, Harell M. Diffuse idiopathic skeletal hyperostosis with dysphagia. J Laryngol Otol 1987;101:627
15. Fass R, Higa L, Kodner A, Mayer EA. Stimulus and site specific induction of hiccups in the oesophagus of normal subjects. Gut 1997;41:590
16. Friedin N, Mittal RK, Traube M, McCallum R. Hypertensive lower esophageal sphincter: a definable motility disorder. Am J Gastroenterol 1987;82:927A
17. Gibson MAR, Varghese A, Clarke KE, et al. Heartburn for the patient—heartache for the doctor? BMJ 1983;287:465
18. Gignoux C, Bost R, Hostein J, et al. Role of upper esophageal reflex and belch reflex dysfunctions in non-cardiac chest pain. Dig Dis Sci 1993;38:1909
19. Gluck M, Pope CE. Chronic hiccups and gastroesophageal reflux disease: the acid perfusion test as a provocative maneuver. Ann Intern Med 1986;605:219
20. Goldman J, Bennett JR. Gastro-oesophageal reflux respiratory disorders in adults. Lancet 1988;ii:493
21. Graham DY, Smith JL, Patterson DJ. Why do apparently healthy people use antacid tablets? Am J Gastroenterol 1983;78:257
22. Helm JF, Dodds WJ, Hogan WJ. Salivary responses to esophageal acid in normal subjects and patients with reflux esophagitis. Gastroenterology 1982;93:1393
23. Hendel L. Esophageal and small intestinal manifestations of progressive systemic sclerosis: a clinical and experimental study. MD thesis. University of Copenhagen, 1994
24. Johnson R, Bernersen B, Staume B, et al. Prevalence of endoscopic and histologic findings in subjects with and without dyspepsia. BMJ 1991;302:749
25. Jones RH, Lydeard SE, Hobbs FD, et al. Dyspepsia in England and Scotland. Gut 1990;31:401
26. Kahrilas PJ, Shi G. Why do we hiccup? Gut 1997;41:712
27. Kruse-Andersen S, Wallin L, Madsen T. Reflux patterns and related oesophageal motor activity in gastro-oesophageal reflux disease. Gut 1990;31:633
28. Lantinga LJ, Spratkin RD, McCroskery, et al. One year psychosocial follow-up of patients with chest pain and angiographically normal coronary arteries. Am J Cardiol 1988;62:209
29. Lindgren S, Janzon L. Prevalence of swallowing complaints and clinical findings among 50–79 year old men and women. Dysphagia 1991;6:187
30. Locke GR, Talley NJ, Fett SL, et al. Prevalence and clinical spectrum of gastroesophageal reflux: a population-based study in Olmsted County, Minnesota. Gastroenterology 1997;112:1448
31. Malagelada J-R. Disturbed upper gastrointestinal sensation: an important abnormality? Aliment Pharmacol Ther 1997;11(suppl 2):51
32. Mayou RA. Patients' fear of illness: chest pain and palpitations in patients with medically unexplained physical symptoms. In Creed F, Mayou R, Hopkins A, eds, Medical symptoms not explored by organic disease. London: Royal College of Physicians and Royal College of Psychiatrists, 1991
33. Nebel OT, Fornes MF, Castell DO. Symptomatic gastroesophageal reflux: incidence and precipitating factors. Dig Dis Sci 1976;21:955
34. Nguyen P, Gideon RM, Castell DO. Dysphagia lusoria in the adult. Am J Gastroenterol 1994;89:620
35. Pratt LW, Tobin WH, Gallagher R. Globus hystericus—office evaluation by psychological testing with the MMPI. Laryngoscope 1976;86:1540

36. Puhakka H, Lehtenen V, Aalto T. Globus hystericus—a psychosomatic disease? J Laryngol Otol 1976;90:1021
37. Rune SJ. Heartburn and dyspepsia: the utility of symptom analysis. Aliment Pharmacol Ther 1997;11(suppl 2):9
38. Schatzki R. Panel discussion on diseases of the esophagus. Am J Gastroenterol 1959;31:117
39. Schatzki R. The lower esophageal ring. Am J Radiol 1963;90:805
40. Schofield PM, Bennett DH, Whorwell PJ, et al. Exertional gastro-oesophageal reflux: a mechanism for symptoms in patients with angina pectoris and normal coronary angiograms. BMJ 1987;294:1459
41. Shay SS, Myers RL, Johnson LF. Hiccups associated with reflux esophagitis. Gastroenterology 1984;87:204
42. Singh S, Richter JE, Bradley LA, et al. The symptom index: differential usefulness in suspected acid-related complaints of heartburn and chest pain. Dig Dis Sci 1993;38:1402
43. Smout AJPM, Breedijk M, van der Zouw C, Akkermans LM. Physiological gastroesophageal reflux and esophageal motor activity studied with a new system for 24-hour recording and automated analysis. Dig Dis Sci 1989;34:372
44. Sontag SJ, Schnell TG, Miller TQ, et al. Prevalence of oesophagitis in asthmatics. Gut 1992;33:872
45. Stagias JG, Ciarolla D, Campo S, Burrell MI, Traube M. Vascular compression of the esophagus. Dig Dis Sci 1994;39:782
46. Treacy WL, Baggenstoss AH, Slocumub CH, Code CF. Scleroderma of the esophagus. Ann Intern Med 1963;59:351
47. Trimble KC, Douglas S, Pryde A, et al. Clinical characteristics and natural history of symptomatic but not excess gastroesophageal reflux. Dig Dis Sci 1995;40:1098
48. Tucker HJ, Snape WJ, Cohen S. Achalasia secondary to carcinoma: manometric and clinical features. Ann Intern Med 1978;89:315
49. Vantrappen G, Janssens J. What is irritable esophagus? Another point of view. Gastroenterology 1988;94:1092
50. van Westen D, Ekberg O. Solid bolus swallowing in the radiologic evaluation of dysphagia. Acta Radiol 1993;34:372
51. Waterman DC, Dalton CB, Ott D. The hypertensive lower esophageal sphincter: what does it mean? J Clin Gastroenterol 1989;11:139
52. Wiener GJ, Richter JE, Copper JB, Wu WC, Castell DO. The symptom index: a clinically important parameter of ambulatory 24-hour esophageal pH monitoring. Am J Gastroenterol 1988;38:358
53. Wilson TA. Reflux and the larynx. Gullet 1992;2:11
54. Zamost BJ, Hirschberg J, Ippoliti AF, et al. Esophagitis in scleroderma. Gastroenterology 1987;92:421

*The Esophagus*, Third Edition,
edited by D. O. Castell and J. E. Richter.
Lippincott Williams & Wilkins, Philadelphia © 1999.

CHAPTER 3

# Radiology of the Oropharynx and Esophagus

David J. Ott

Radiologic imaging of the oropharynx and esophagus has improved considerably in recent years. These improvements have resulted from better understanding of oropharyngeal and esophageal structure and function and the introduction of new techniques, including computed tomography (CT), radionuclide imaging, and endoscopic ultrasonography (EUS). In this chapter, the various imaging techniques used to evaluate the oropharynx and esophagus are discussed briefly, emphasizing the barium examination. This is followed by separate sections on the oropharynx and esophagus. Normal radiographic anatomy and structural and functional abnormalities of these anatomic regions are covered.

## IMAGING TECHNIQUES

### Oropharyngeal Techniques

Radiographic examination of the oropharynx is often neglected because the area is easily inspected visually. However, visual examination may not adequately evaluate certain structural abnormalities and does not assess functional disturbances. The oropharynx is usually studied as part of the radiographic examination of the esophagus or upper gastrointestinal tract. In patients with major swallowing difficulty who are at substantial risk of aspiration, a more limited examination of the oropharynx using small amounts of various materials is often needed.

#### Standard Techniques

Plain films of the neck, particularly in the lateral position, assess for radiopaque foreign bodies, soft tissue masses, and adjacent bony or cartilaginous abnormalities. Barium exami-

D. J. Ott: Department of Radiology, Wake Forest University School of Medicine, Wake Forest University Baptist Medical Center, Winston-Salem, North Carolina 27157.

nation should combine static filming with motion-recording techniques to evaluate properly structural and functional abnormalities of the oropharynx and cervical esophagus [43, 83, 111]. Videotaping is the most convenient motion-recording technique available, although cineradiography can also be used. The examination starts with the patient upright in the frontal position. Motion recording of one or several swallows is done. A spot film is taken after the swallow (Fig. 3–1). Then the sequence is repeated with the patient in the lateral position.

#### Oropharyngeal Function Study

The oropharyngeal function study (or modified barium swallow) is used in patients with major oropharyngeal transport problems who are at risk for aspiration [83, 100]. These patients usually are recovering from strokes or closed head injuries, are being studied after neck surgery, or have neurologic diseases. The patient is first evaluated sitting in the lateral position. The examination is primarily performed using motion recording. Small amounts (3 to 5 mL) of different materials are used, including a low- and high-viscosity barium suspension, a barium paste, and a paste-coated cookie. The patient may be turned to the frontal position and the examination repeated, usually using only several of the materials mentioned.

### Esophageal Techniques

Radiographic examination of the esophagus may be done separately, often combined with oropharyngeal evaluation or as part of an upper gastrointestinal series. Effective radiology of the esophagus requires a thorough understanding of a variety of radiographic techniques. The multiphasic examination of the esophagus combining different techniques is most effective [34, 76, 78, 83]. Each technique has advantages and limitations, and no one method optimally examines

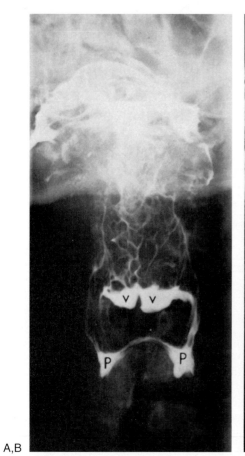
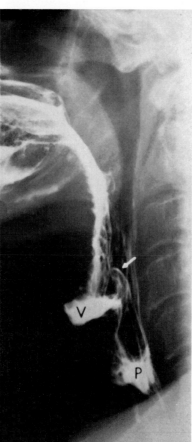

FIG. 3–1. Frontal **(A)** and lateral **(B)** spot films of the hypopharynx with residual barium in the valleculae (*v*) and piriform (*P*) sinuses. The epiglottis (*arrow*) is well shown on the lateral view.

A,B

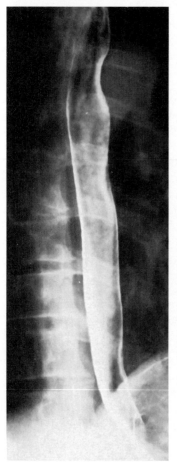
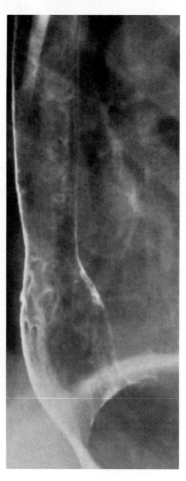

A,B

FIG. 3–2. **A:** Normal double-contrast view of the esophagus. **B:** Mucosal irregularity and ulceration of the lower esophagus due to reflux esophagitis and hiatal hernia. (From ref. 77A, with permission.)

the esophagus. In addition to the standard methods, supplemental techniques may be needed occasionally.

### Standard Techniques

The following techniques are used for the routine multiphasic examination of the esophagus: (a) double-contrast, (b) full-column, (c) mucosal relief, and (d) fluoroscopic observation and motion recording [34, 76, 78, 83]. Double-contrast films are obtained by coating the esophagus with dense barium suspension and distending the organ with gas (Fig. 3–2). The main advantage of this method is simultaneous visualization of the distended esophagus and its mucosal surface. Small neoplasms and various types of esophagitis are well shown on double-contrast films (Fig. 3–2). In about one-third of patients, however, the esophagogastric region is not adequately distended and small hiatal hernias, lower esophageal mucosal rings, and peptic strictures may not be detected [11, 78, 83].

The full-column technique requires rapid filling of the esophagus with barium and is done with the patient prone. Esophageal motility is best assessed fluoroscopically in this position by observing multiple single swallows of barium. Hiatal hernias, lower esophageal mucosal rings, and peptic strictures are optimally shown (Fig. 3–3). Circumferential lesions, contour deformity, and more severe forms of esophagitis also can be seen. Conversely, small and eccentric neoplasms, milder forms of esophagitis, and esophageal varices may not be detected.

Mucosal relief films are taken with the esophagus collapsed and coated with a dense barium suspension. The smooth, longitudinal folds are well seen (Fig. 3–4). Irregularity or thickening of these folds suggests abnormality. Small neoplasms, various types of esophagitis, and esophageal varices can be detected. Indeed, varices are best shown by this technique [15]. Lesions requiring maximal distention of the esophagus are not well seen.

Fluoroscopic observation is integral to the radiographic

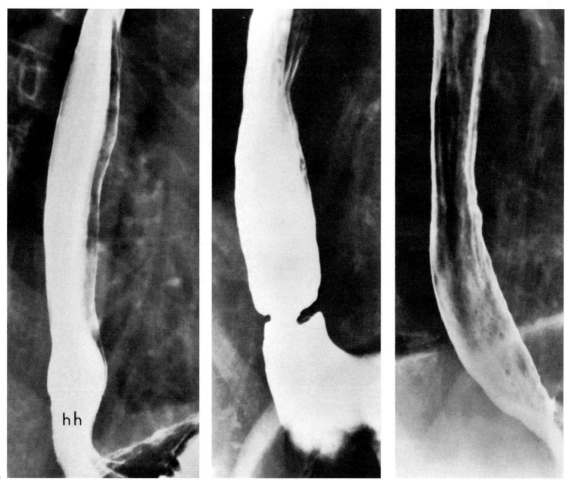

A B,C

**FIG. 3–3. A:** Normal full-column film of the esophagus with a small hiatal hernia (*hh*) that shows serration from areae gastricae of the stomach. **B:** Prone full-column view of an 8-mm mucosal ring in a patient with dysphagia. **C:** Normal upright double-contrast view in the same patient. (Parts **B** and **C** From ref. 93, with permission.)

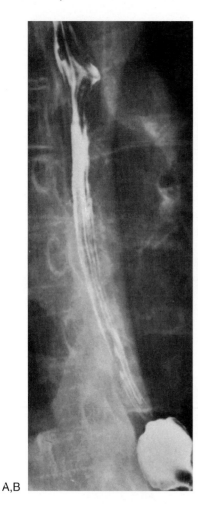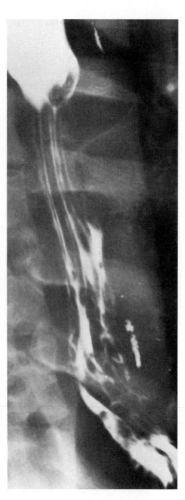

A,B

**FIG. 3–4. A:** Normal mucosal relief film showing thin, smooth longitudinal folds of the collapsed esophagus. **B:** Thickened and irregular folds from reflux esophagitis. (From ref. 106, with permission.)

examination of the esophagus. Permanent motion-recording techniques supplement fluoroscopy and include videotape recording, cineradiography, and spot-film cameras. Digital fluoroscopy and videodisc recording are newer innovations. Motion-recording techniques aid in evaluating functional disorders of the oropharynx and esophagus. The rapidity of events, especially in the oropharynx, makes static filming of transient abnormalities difficult.

### Supplemental Techniques

A variety of supplemental examining techniques may further aid in evaluating the esophagus, especially when the results from the standard methods are unsatisfactory. Inadequate distention of the esophagus may be a problem if the patient cannot ingest barium rapidly. The relaxant effect of iced barium on the esophagus often promotes better distention, especially in the esophagogastric region [92]. Use of solid boluses, such as marshmallows, is important in patients with dysphagia, to show abnormalities or reproduce symptoms better [78, 83, 97, 98]. Occasionally, a solid bolus will bring out a lesion not seen on the examination with liquid

barium (Fig. 3–5). Esophageal intubation and pharmacologic aids are used for specific indications.

### Computed Tomography

CT of the neck and thorax is useful to evaluate bowel wall thickening, extent of neoplastic spread, adjacent adenopathy, and intramural or extrinsic processes. Barium examination and endoscopy are limited to assessment of the mucosal surface, caliber of the bowel, and contour of the lumen but provide little information regarding intramural lesions and extrinsic abnormalities. Detailed discussion of CT for evaluating the neck and esophagus has been reported [49, 127].

### Radionuclide Imaging

Nuclear medicine techniques have been used for studying functional disorders of the oropharynx, esophagus, and stomach [18, 81]. Advantages of radioisotopes include incorporation into foodstuff with minimal change in the nature of the material, ready detection of the ingested radiolabeled material, generation of temporal images, and quantification

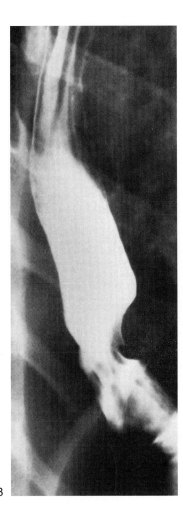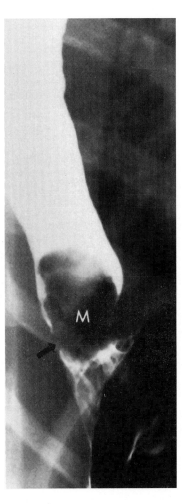

A,B

FIG. 3–5. **A:** Prone full-column view shows a small hiatal hernia in a patient with dysphagia. **B:** Marshmallow (*M*) bolus impacted at a 10-mm mucosal ring (*arrow*), producing dysphagia. Endoscopy confirmed the presence of a ring.

of information, especially with the use of computers. Such procedures have been used to evaluate oropharyngeal transport, to demonstrate and quantitate gastroesophageal reflux, and to study esophageal transit and emptying (Fig. 3–6).

### Endoscopic Ultrasonography

EUS is a newer technology uniting flexible endoscopy and ultrasonic imaging. The instrument permits intraluminal placement of a real-time ultrasonic probe in the esophagus, stomach, duodenum, rectum, or colon. EUS is useful in the esophagus for evaluating both mucosal and intramural abnormalities [4, 108, 112, 121, 128]. Extramucosal processes can be characterized and their anatomic location in the esophageal wall determined. Extrinsic and intrinsic compression can be differentiated. Most importantly, preoperative staging of esophageal carcinoma by EUS has proved effective in assessing the depth of malignant infiltration [4, 108, 112, 128].

A variety of EUS systems are available which use real-time transducers attached to the end of the endoscope that produce a radial sector or linear scan depending on the de-

sign of the instrument. Optimal ultrasound transmission is obtained in the esophagus by a water-filled balloon. Ultrasonic anatomy of the esophageal wall shows five discrete and alternating echogenic and echolucent layers [48, 128]. These ultrasonic layers have histologic equivalents, and their identification is useful in evaluating the presence and location of extramucosal lesions, extent of malignant invasion, and extrinsic compression (Fig. 3–7).

### Magnetic Resonance Imaging

Magnetic resonance imaging (MRI) is the newest technique that produces thin tomographic depictions of anatomy. In contrast to CT, MRI does not involve radiation but is based on interaction between radio waves and atomic nuclei in the presence of a strong magnetic field. The application of MRI in the neck and thorax is similar to that of CT [49, 108, 127]. The main uses have been in the staging of malignancies involving the larynx, pharynx, and esophagus. Although MRI offers more options than CT for planar imaging of the esophagus, both methods are comparable in their anatomic evaluation [108].

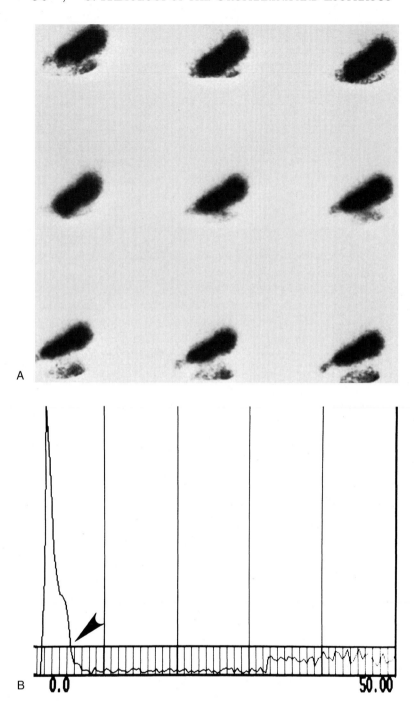

**FIG. 3–6. A:** Normal radionuclide gastroesophageal reflux study showing no esophageal activity and prominent gastric activity in sequential images. **B:** Computer-generated normal single-bolus esophageal transit curve, with the *arrowhead* indicating the 90% clearance line. Total recording time, 50 seconds.

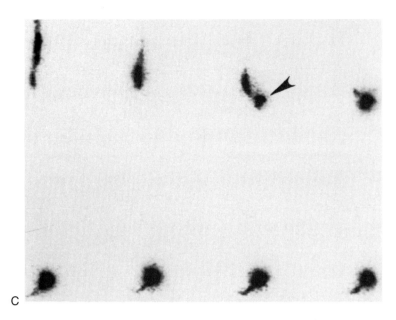

C

**FIG. 3–6.** (*continued*) **C:** Two-second serial anterior images of a normal single-swallow transit study show rapid progression through the esophagus and entry into the stomach (*arrowhead*). (From ref. 18, with permission.)

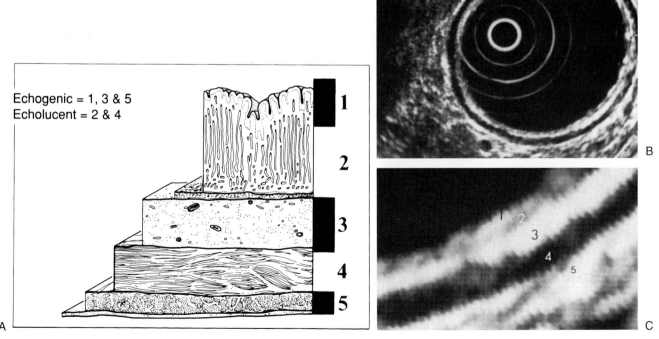

**FIG. 3–7. A:** Correspondence between endoscopic ultrasonography (EUS) and anatomic layers of normal gastrointestinal wall. *1,* luminal and mucosal interface; *2,* remainder of mucosa and muscularis mucosae; *3,* submucosa and interface with muscularis propria; *4,* muscularis propria; *5,* serosal interface and adjacent tissues. (From ref. 6a, with permission.) **B:** EUS of the water-filled gastric antrum showing the typical alternating echogenic and echolucent layers **(top).** The *lower* view is magnified and is keyed similarly to the diagram in **A.**

## OROPHARYNX

### Normal Radiographic Anatomy

#### Normal Anatomy

The pharynx consists of the nasopharynx, oropharynx, and hypopharynx. The hypopharynx extends from the epiglottis to the esophageal inlet [34, 43, 83, 111]. On the frontal view, the epiglottis is seen as a smooth arcuate shadow projecting just above the paired valleculae. The hypopharynx extends inferiorly as the piriform sinuses, which surround much of the laryngeal vestibule. Superimposition of structures of the hypopharynx complicates the lateral view. The epiglottis is located just posterior to the valleculae at the level of the hyoid bone (Fig. 3–1). The aryepiglottic folds slant posteriorly downward to the arytenoid cartilages. The posterior pharyngeal wall is well shown. The cricopharyngeal muscle may cause an indentation posteriorly at the pharyngoesophageal level.

#### Anatomic Variants

The valleculae often contain small filling defects representing lymphoid tissue. The laryngeal cartilages and their membranous attachments may produce smooth compressions on the hypopharynx. Just below the cricoid cartilage impression, a small indentation may be seen as a normal variant called the postcricoid impression [33, 83, 111]. This is ascribed to redundant mucosa and has a variety of appearances that may mimic a web or neoplasm (Fig. 3–8).

### Structural Abnormalities

#### Congenital Anomalies

Hypopharyngeal anomalies are rare. Congenital diverticula may occur laterally from remnants of the third or fourth pharyngeal pouches. Communicating branchial cleft cysts or sinuses opening on the neck also occur.

#### Webs

Hypopharyngeal and cervical esophageal webs arise from the anterior wall, often extending laterally and rarely circumferentially. Webs appear as thin, smooth structures and must be distinguished from the posterior indentation of the cricopharyngeal muscle or the normal postcricoid impression anteriorly (Fig. 3–9). Webs are best shown by motion recording and have been reported in 1% to 5% of asymptomatic people and in up to 15% of patients with dysphagia

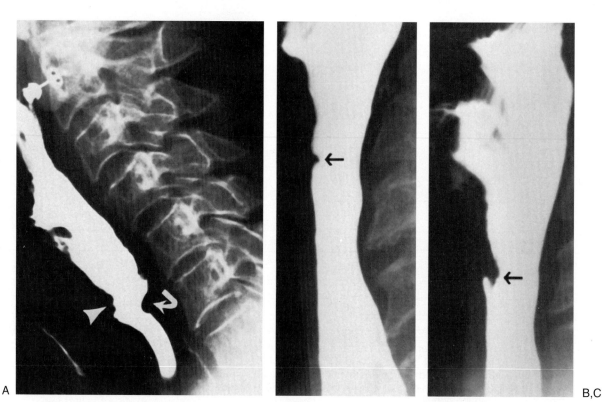

**FIG. 3–8.** **A:** Cricopharyngeus muscle seen as a posterior indentation (*curved arrow*) at the pharyngoesophageal junction. Anteriorly, a broad postcricoid impression (*arrowhead*) is evident. **B:** Postcricoid impression (*arrows*) in two different patients.

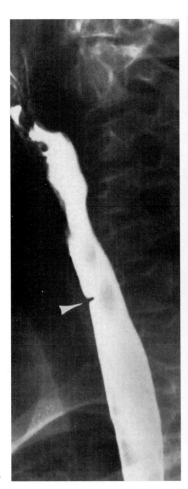 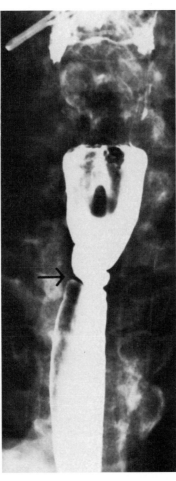

**FIG. 3–9. A:** Upper cervical esophageal web (*arrowhead*) near the pharyngoesophageal junction. **B:** Circumferential web (*arrow*) at the pharyngoesophageal junction.

[74, 111]. The relationship between esophageal webs and iron-deficiency anemia, the so-called Plummer-Vinson (or Paterson-Kelly) syndrome, is disputed [74, 111].

### Diverticular Disease

Pharyngeal diverticula may be classified by origin, as congenital or acquired, or by location [44, 111]. Zenker's diverticulum, an acquired posterior pouch, is most common. Lateral pharyngeal diverticula are rare, and the terms used for them are confusing. Lateral bulging of the distended pharynx due to anatomic weakness of the thyrohyoid membrane is often seen on frontal views. These pouches are more common with age and have been called *hypopharyngeal ears* and *pharyngoceles*. Lateral bulges may also occur in the tonsillar fossae. Zenker's diverticulum protrudes through the midline of the posterior hypopharyngeal wall in an area of muscular thinning called Killian's dehiscence. This point of anatomic weakness results from the divergence of the oblique fibers of the inferior pharyngeal constrictor and the cricopharyngeus muscles inferiorly. It is an acquired pulsion diverticulum of uncertain etiology. Although cricopharyn-

geal dysfunction has previously been considered a cause of Zenker's diverticulum, more recent studies have questioned this association [17, 107, 124].

Zenker's diverticula have a variety of radiographic appearances (Fig. 3–10). Small diverticula may be transient, have a spiculated shape, and are best seen on motion recording [107]. Larger diverticula have a more permanent, clubbed appearance and arise posteriorly just above the cricopharyngeus muscle, which is often seen as a smooth impression. Larger diverticula are saccular and extend inferiorly, often compressing the esophagus. Retention of food, secretions, and barium is seen in larger diverticula.

### Neoplasms

Epithelial malignancies comprise most tumors arising from the pharynx [44, 111]. Many are detected by visual inspection, although their exact anatomic origin and extent of spread are usually better shown radiographically. Since squamous cell carcinomas of the oropharynx and esophagus may be synchronous, evaluation of the esophagus is also important. Malignant neoplasms of the pharynx present as

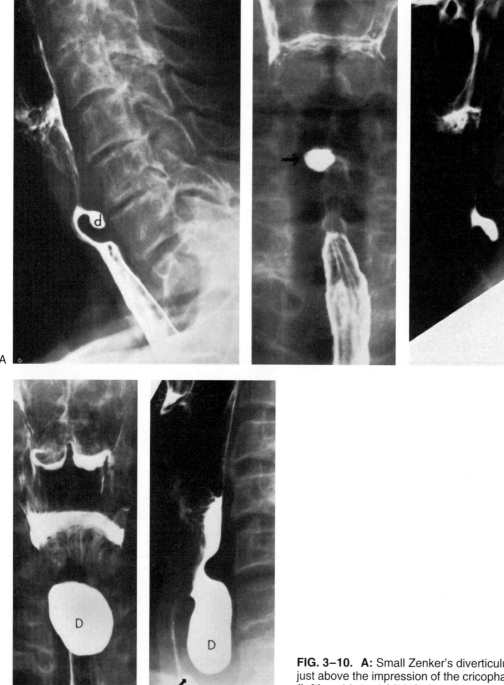

**FIG. 3–10.  A:** Small Zenker's diverticulum (*d*) protrudes posteriorly just above the impression of the cricopharyngeus muscle. **B:** Frontal **(left)** and lateral **(right)** views of a small Zenker's diverticulum (*arrows*). **C:** Frontal **(left)** and lateral **(right)** views of a larger Zenker's diverticulum (*D*) compressing the upper cervical esophagus (*arrows*).

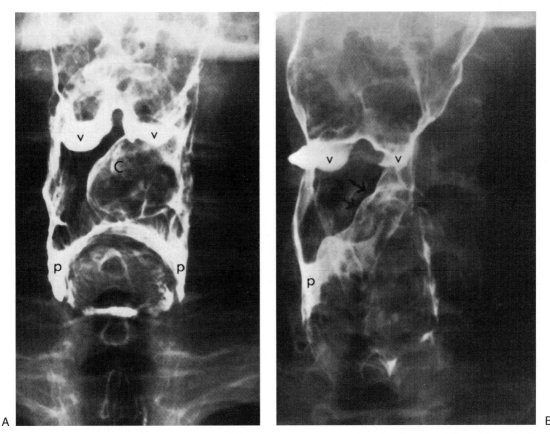

**FIG. 3–11. A:** Polypoid carcinoma *(C)* of the left hypopharynx. *v*, valleculae; *p*, piriform sinuses. **B:** Infiltrative carcinoma (*arrows*) of the left piriform sinus causing hypopharyngeal asymmetry. *p*, right piriform sinus.

a polypoid mass or deformity from tumor infiltration causing focal pharyngeal deformity (Fig. 3–11). Small malignancies produce minimal mucosal changes and may be difficult to show or differentiate from normal anatomic variants.

### Postoperative Appearances

Surgery for pharyngeal or laryngeal carcinoma is the usual reason for postoperative changes [44, 111]. Both functional and structural alterations affect the operated pharynx, including aspiration potential if a tracheostomy is not made. Alterations include absence of portions of the pharyngeal recesses, pharyngeal deformity, and focal or diffuse narrowing. The latter may be caused by scarring, radiation, or tumor recurrence. More recent surgical advances, including placement of voice prostheses and jejunal grafts, have their own unique radiographic appearances [123, 126].

### Extrinsic Effects

Adjacent diseases may secondarily involve the hypopharynx, causing extrinsic deformity. The larynx, thyroid and parathyroid glands, cervical lymph nodes, and spine are the main considerations. Cervical spondylosis can encroach on the hypopharynx posteriorly and be a rare cause of dysphagia. However, degenerative spondylosis is common in the elderly, and other reasons for dysphagia must be excluded [130].

### Functional Abnormalities

Swallowing difficulty is the major reason for radiographic examination of the oropharynx, and functional disorders are an important cause of oropharyngeal dysphagia. Normal swallowing is divided into oral, pharyngeal, and esophageal stages, which involve rapid and complex events, beginning as a voluntary act and ending with an involuntary initiation of esophageal peristalsis [19, 26, 43, 44, 100].

### General Abnormalities

The oral stage of swallowing involves the voluntary transport of a bolus from the oral cavity to the pharynx. Labial and nasopharyngeal closure direct the bolus posteriorly into the oropharynx. As the material enters the pharynx, the reflex pharyngeal stage of swallowing is initiated. The hyoid bone and larynx elevate and the epiglottis inverts. The upper

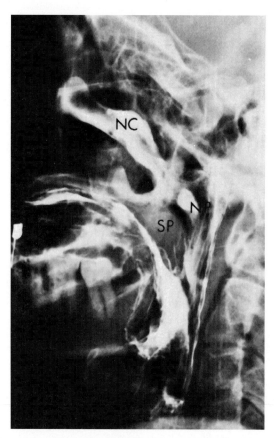

**FIG. 3–12.** Swallowing dysfunction due to brain metastases with misdirection of barium above the soft palate (*SP*) into the nasopharynx (*NP*) and nasal cavity (*NC*).

esophageal sphincter relaxes as the bolus is rapidly transported through the hypopharynx into the esophagus. The upper esophageal sphincter quickly returns to its resting state as esophageal peristalsis begins.

A wide variety of heterogeneous disorders can alter oropharyngeal function, but the types of abnormalities seen are limited and often not specific [24, 43, 44, 100]. Oral transport difficulty appears as poor control of the bolus in the oral cavity, discoordinated movement of the material posteriorly, and misdirection into the nasopharynx or out of the mouth (Fig. 3–12). The pharyngeal stage may be disrupted by a delayed or absent swallowing reflex, with spillover of material and early aspiration. Pharyngeal paresis reduces laryngeal motion and may cause aspiration with swallowing and stasis in the hypopharyngeal recesses after swallowing, the so-called vallecular sign (Fig. 3–13). A persistent cricopharyngeal impression, along with other signs of oropharyngeal abnormality, may indicate upper esophageal sphincter dysfunction.

### Specific Disorders

Oropharyngeal dysphagia may result from a variety of neuromuscular causes (Table 3–1), many of which produce similar functional disturbances in the oropharynx necessitating clinical correlation. The major role of radiographic evaluation in these patients is to identify the types and severity of functional disturbances and risk of aspiration, particularly with different types of materials. Also, structural diseases of the oropharynx may mimic functional abnormalities and must be excluded. Unilateral pharyngeal paresis, for example, can cause asymmetry of the hypopharynx and may be confused with neoplastic involvement.

Since the radiographic findings in many of these neuromuscular disorders are similar, only a few specific comments are made. Cerebrovascular accidents, a common cause of swallowing difficulty, can present uncommonly as unilateral pharyngeal paresis. Myasthenia gravis typically shows diffuse functional abnormalities with progressive worsening on repeated swallows but improvement after parenteral injection of neostigmine. Myotonic dystrophy appears as a continuous column of barium extending from the pharynx into the cervical esophagus with an open cricopharyngeal segment.

### Cricopharyngeal Dysfunction

The cricopharyngeus muscle is the main contributor to the resting high-pressure zone known as the upper esophageal sphincter [39, 43]. This sphincter normally relaxes before the arrival of the bolus, and its relaxation is seen indirectly as opening of the pharyngoesophageal segment by the distending bolus. Possible functional abnormalities of the cricopharyngeus muscle include (a) elevated or low resting pressure, the latter typically seen in myotonic dystrophy; (b) delayed opening, as in familial dysautonomia; (c) premature closure, a debatable cause of Zenker's diverticulum; and (d)

**TABLE 3–1.** *Neuromuscular disorders causing functional abnormalities of the oropharynx*

Central nervous system
  Cerebrovascular accident
  Parkinson's disease
  Huntington's chorea
  Demyelinating disease
  Amyotrophic lateral sclerosis
  Tumors (primary, metastatic)
  Congenital disorders
  Miscellaneous degenerations

Peripheral nervous system
  Bulbar poliomyelitis
  Peripheral neuropathies

Myoneural junction
  Myasthenia gravis

Skeletal muscle
  Polymyositis
  Dermatomyositis
  Muscular dystrophies
  Metabolic myopathy

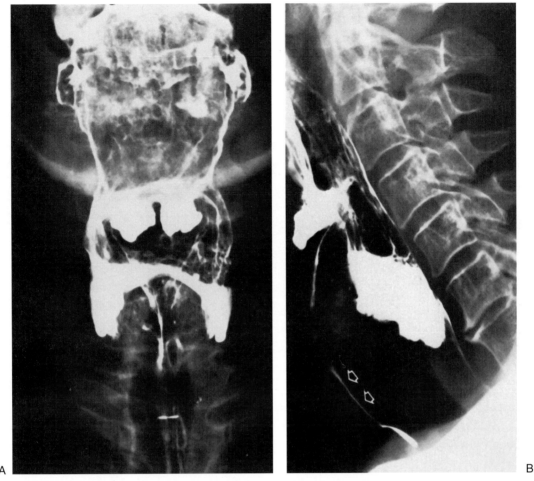

**FIG. 3–13.** Frontal **(A)** and lateral **(B)** views of the pharynx showing barium stasis and aspiration (*arrows*) in a patient with amyotrophic lateral sclerosis. Repetitive swallowing failed to clear barium from the hypopharyngeal recesses.

failure of relaxation, so-called cricopharyngeal achalasia [20, 39, 43].

Cricopharyngeal achalasia has been described radiographically as a persistent or transient posterior indentation (or cricopharyngeal bar) at the pharyngoesophageal junction (Fig. 3–14) [20, 44, 100]. The clinical significance of this indentation, however, has been controversial [20, 32, 75, 100]. Approximately 5% to 15% of individuals without oropharyngeal dysphagia show a minor cricopharyngeal impression, using motion recording [28, 32]. Normal manometric relaxation of the upper esophageal sphincter occurs in many of these asymptomatic patients with minor cricopharyngeal impressions, calling into question the validity of the term *cricopharyngeal achalasia*. Thus, minimal cricopharyngeal impression in asymptomatic people with no other oropharyngeal abnormalities is of debatable importance [32]. About 20% of patients with oropharyngeal dysphagia show a cricopharyngeal impression, which is often found with other swallowing abnormalities [29]. Consequently, *cricopharyngeal dysfunction* is the pre-

ferred term to describe these upper esophageal sphincter abnormalities [32, 39].

## ESOPHAGUS

### Normal Radiographic Anatomy

#### Normal Anatomy

The cervical esophagus begins at the pharyngoesophageal junction and continues into the chest as the thoracic esophagus. The cervical and thoracic parts of the esophagus have a smooth appearance when distended and are indistinguishable (Fig. 3–2). Several smooth, longitudinal folds course the length of the normal collapsed esophagus (Fig. 3–4). The cervical and thoracic portions together are called the *tubular esophagus*. Important structures lie adjacent to the esophagus and may normally cause extrinsic impressions, especially at the levels of the aortic arch, left main stem bronchus, and heart.

The anatomic transition between the lower end of the tho-

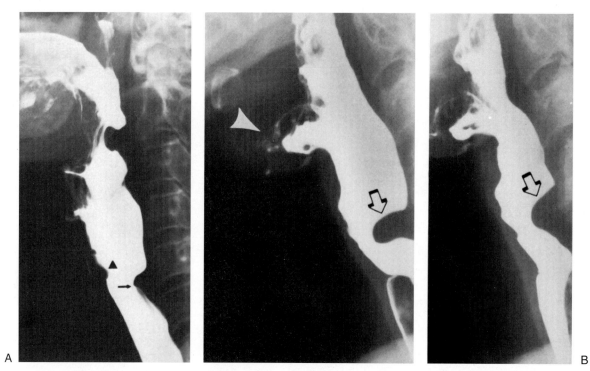

**FIG. 3–14. A:** Mild persistent cricopharyngeal bar (*arrow*) in a patient with dysphagia. A postcricoid impression is seen anteriorly (*arrowhead*). Nasopharyngeal reflux and aspiration also are present. **B:** Two views of a more prominent but persistent cricopharyngeal bar (*arrows*) in a patient with oropharyngeal dysphagia. Laryngeal penetration (*arrowhead*) also is seen.

racic esophagus and stomach is complex (Fig. 3–15). The tubular esophagus terminates as a bell-shaped structure called the *esophageal vestibule* [76, 78, 93]. The tubular esophagus and vestibule unite at the tubulovestibular junction, or *A level*. A portion of the esophageal vestibule is intraabdominal under normal resting conditions. The esophagogastric junction is the union of the vestibule with the stomach. The squamocolumnar mucosal transition is often called the *B level* and lies at the lower margin of the vestibule. The lower esophageal sphincter is a manometric high-pressure zone coinciding in position to the esophageal vestibule, although a distinct anatomic structure representing the sphincter has not been clearly identified.

### Anatomic Variants

Structural and physiologic variants may affect the esophagus and mimic disease. The aorticobronchial triangle is a potential space that exists between the aortic arch and left main stem bronchus. The esophagus may focally protrude into this space and resemble a diverticulum [34, 83]. A fine nodular appearance of the esophageal mucosa due to glycogen acanthosis is occasionally seen, particularly in older individuals [36]. These glycogen deposits are typically less than 5 mm and of no clinical significance except for confu-

sion with disease, such as esophagitis. Transient esophageal motility patterns, especially tertiary contractions, may momentarily alter the smooth contour of the esophagus and must be distinguished from fixed deformity. Fleeting transverse folds, often called *esophageal rimpling,* may be seen [37]. These are probably due to muscularis mucosae contractions and may be more prevalent in gastroesophageal reflux disease.

### Congenital Anomalies

Congenital esophageal anomalies include atresia, stenosis and webs, and duplications [5]. Esophageal atresia, usually accompanied by a tracheoesophageal fistula, is the most common anomaly. Classification of esophageal atresia usually includes five types, with approximately 85% being associated with a fistula to the lower esophageal segment. Isolated atresia and the H-type fistula account for most of the rest. Focal stricture usually occurs after surgical repair, and abnormal esophageal motility is present in many patients. Congenital stenosis and webs are rare. The esophagus is a common site for duplication in the gastrointestinal tract (Fig. 3–16). Duplications resemble a cyst and compress the esophagus but rarely communicate with the lumen.

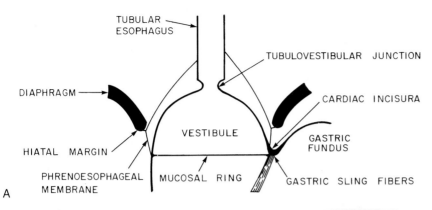

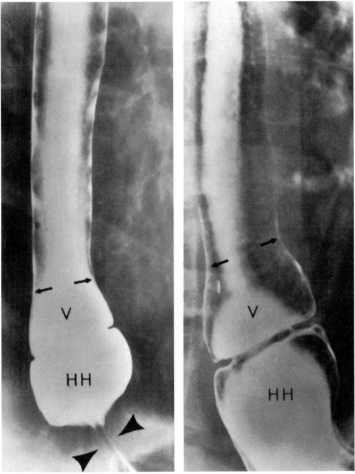

FIG. 3–15. **A:** Diagram of lower esophageal anatomy with simplification of terminology. The esophageal vestibule is defined by the tubulovestibular junction superiorly and the upper margin of the gastric sling fibers inferiorly. When present, the mucosal ring occurs at a lower level of the esophageal vestibule. (From ref. 129a, with permission.) **B:** A widely patent mucosal ring projects 3 cm above the pinchcock effect of the diaphragmatic hiatus (*arrowheads*). **C:** A smooth, symmetric mucosal ring in another patient with a patulous esophageal hiatus. *HH,* hiatal hernia; *V,* vestibule; *arrows* indicate tubulovestibular junction. (Parts **B** and **C** from ref. 93, with permission. Copyright by American Roentgen Ray Society.)

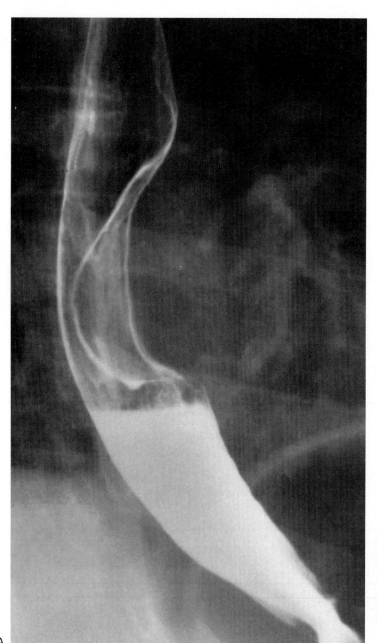

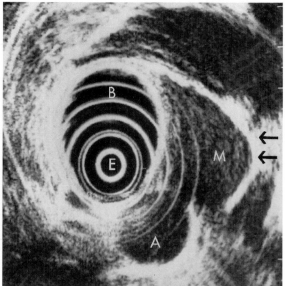

**FIG. 3–16. A:** A lower esophageal mass with a smooth impression measuring 5 cm in length. **B:** An intramural esophageal mass (*M*) with fine homogeneous echotexture and far-wall acoustic enhancement (*arrows*). Compared to the adjacent aorta (*A*), the lesion shows more internal echoes. *E,* echoendoscope; *B,* balloon. At surgery, an esophageal duplication cyst was found and contained tenacious, thick mucus. (From ref. 98a, with permission.)

A

B

## Hiatal Hernia and Rings

### Hiatal Hernia

Hiatal hernia is upward protrusion of part of the stomach through the esophageal hiatus and is the most common diaphragmatic hernia. It is classified into three types: (a) sliding, or axial; (b) paraesophageal; and (c) mixed. Most hiatal hernias are of the sliding type, in which the esophagogastric junction is the most orad portion of the herniated stomach [53, 79, 93]. Axial hernias are usually small and generally slide relative to the esophageal hiatus. Hiatal hernias are best shown on the full-column examination, and radiographic diagnosis depends on showing landmarks of the esophagogas-

tric junction extending above the esophageal hiatus (Fig. 3–17). The most important landmarks include the lower esophageal mucosal ring, the notch from the gastric sling fibers, and the orad level of the areae gastricae of the stomach.

Although hiatal hernia is often used as a predictor of reflux esophagitis, a direct causal relationship between hernia and gastroesophageal reflux disease has not been established [72, 94, 96, 117]. Lower esophageal sphincter dysfunction is believed to be the primary cause of abnormal gastroesophageal reflux [23, 72]. Hiatal hernia is found radiographically in nearly half of adults, but only a minority will have reflux esophagitis endoscopically [106]. Conversely, about 90% of

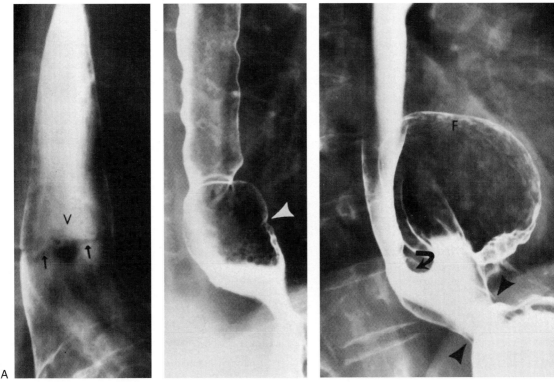

A

B,C

**FIG. 3–17. A:** Widened esophageal hiatus with sliding hernia. The esophagogastric junction is identified by the lower end of the vestibule (*V*) and squamocolumnar mucosal transition (*arrows*). **B:** Sliding hiatal hernia with the notch from the gastric sling fibers (*arrowhead*) seen clearly. There is a reticulated pattern of areae gastricae in the herniated stomach. **C:** Large, mixed hiatal hernia with the esophagogastric junction (*curved arrow*) above the level of the esophageal hiatus (*arrowheads*) but with the fundus (*F*) of the stomach more orad.

those with reflux disease will be seen to have hiatal hernias if appropriate radiographic techniques and criteria are used. Patients without hiatal hernia are furthermore unlikely to have the more severe forms of endoscopic esophagitis. Thus, hiatal hernia is not likely the primary cause of abnormal gastroesophageal reflux but may be permissive in some patients by enhancing lower esophageal sphincter dysfunction or impeding esophageal emptying [23, 72, 79, 81].

Paraesophageal hernias are rare, accounting for a small percent of hiatal hernias [53, 79]. The esophagogastric junction remains below the hiatus, but part of the gastric fundus herniates into the chest alongside the lower esophagus. The herniated stomach may be small or large and may twist. Mechanical complications can occur, such as volvulus and strangulation, which require surgical repair. The mixed hernia is a large sliding type with the fundus more orad; it is usually large, with much of the stomach being intrathoracic [35, 53, 79]. Patients are often asymptomatic, but gastric rotation and inversion can cause mechanical complications.

### Esophageal Rings

Thin constrictions have been found at locations throughout the esophagus. *Web* and *ring* are most commonly used to describe these constrictions, and the varying uses of these terms have been confusing [53, 79, 93]. For descriptive purposes, *esophageal web* is limited to constrictions covered by squamous epithelium only and located above the tubulovestibular junction. Esophageal webs are not common and usually occur in the cervical region. Webs appear as thin, transverse folds and are best detected with the esophagus distended. *Esophageal ring* is limited to annular narrowings situated at the upper and lower borders of the esophageal vestibule. These are most commonly classified as muscular or mucosal rings. The muscular ring occurs at the tubulovestibular junction and appears as a broad, smooth narrowing. Its caliber varies, and the ring may disappear completely on maximal distention of the esophagus (Fig. 3–18). Muscular rings rarely cause dysphagia.

The lower esophageal mucosal ring, or Schatzki's ring, encircles the lower border of the vestibule and appears as a thin, transverse structure with a fixed caliber [53, 79, 93, 114]. Its margins are typically smooth and symmetric (Fig. 3–19). The full-column technique best shows mucosal rings and requires distention of the esophagogastric region above the caliber of the ring. Occasionally, use of a solid bolus will show a mucosal ring not seen on the examination with liquid barium and often reproduces symptoms [78, 93, 97, 98]. Radiology is more sensitive than endoscopy in detecting

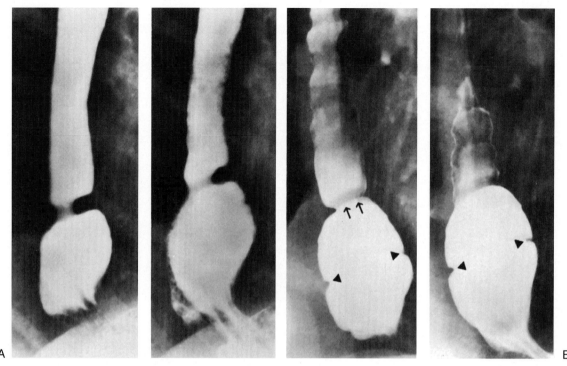

**FIG. 3–18. A:** Broad, smooth narrowing of muscular ring at the tubulovestibular junction on two views. The caliber of the ring changes from 6 mm **(left)** to 12 mm **(right). B:** Muscular ring (*arrows*) at the tubulovestibular junction **(left)** disappears moments later **(right).** A mucosal ring (*arrowheads*) remains static in appearance. (From ref. 93, with permission. Copyright by American Roentgen Ray Society.)

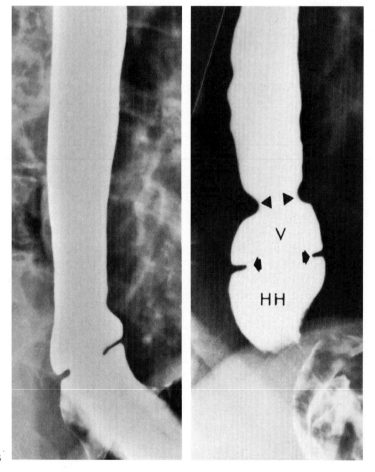

**FIG. 3–19. A:** Smooth, symmetric lower esophageal mucosal ring demarcating the junction of the vestibule and hiatal hernia. **B:** Widely patent mucosal ring (*arrows*) at the esophagogastric junction and muscular ring (*arrowheads*) at the tubulovestibular junction *V,* vestibule; *HH,* hiatal hernia.

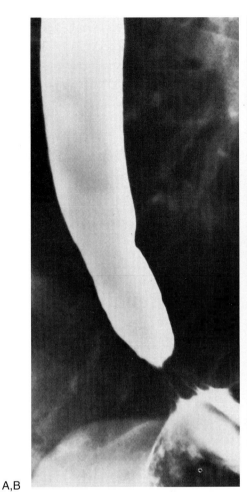
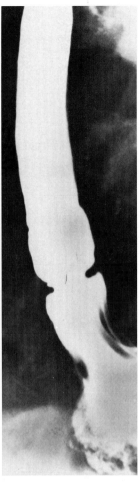

A,B

**FIG. 3–20. A:** Initial barium esophagogram in a patient with intermittent dysphagia and normal findings on endoscopy. **B:** Repeat esophagogram supplemented by use of a marshmallow bolus showed a 12-mm mucosal ring. (From ref. 93, with permission. Copyright by American Roentgen Ray Society.)

mucosal rings, especially if smaller-caliber endoscopes are used (Fig. 3–20) [87]. The lower esophageal mucosal ring is an important cause of solid-food dysphagia. The prevalence of dysphagia is related to the caliber of the ring and is rarely present in rings larger than 20 mm [113]. Conversely, rings of less than 13 mm nearly always cause dysphagia, whereas 13- to 20-mm rings are symptomatic in approximately half of the patients.

## Reflux Esophagitis

Reflux esophagitis is the most common esophageal inflammation (Table 3–2). Patients with symptomatic gastroesophageal reflux may have a normal-appearing esophageal mucosa, histologic abnormalities only, or gross morphologic changes of reflux esophagitis [77, 81]. The term *gastroesophageal reflux disease* (GERD) has been used to include all of these patients. The following are believed important to the development of GERD: (a) inadequate antireflux mechanism, (b) volume and potency of reflux material, (c) esophageal mucosal resistance, and (d) efficacy of esophageal clearance and gastric emptying [23]. The barium esophagram and radionuclide methods can assess several of

**TABLE 3–2.** *Causes of esophagitis*

Common causes
  Reflux esophagitis
  Infectious esophagitis
    *Candida* esophagitis
    Herpetic esophagitis
    Cytomegalovirus
  Acquired immunodeficiency syndrome
  Caustic esophagitis
  Radiation esophagitis
  Medication-induced injury

Rare causes
  Crohn's disease
  Pemphigoid
  Epidermolysis bullosa
  Ulcerative colitis
  Behçet's syndrome
  Graft-versus-host disease
  Zollinger-Ellison syndrome
  Eosinophilic esophagitis
  Thermal injury
  Trauma

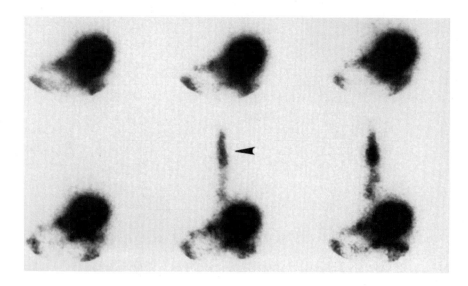

**FIG. 3–21.** Radionuclide gastroesophageal reflux study showing spontaneous reflux (*arrow*). (From ref. 18, with permission.)

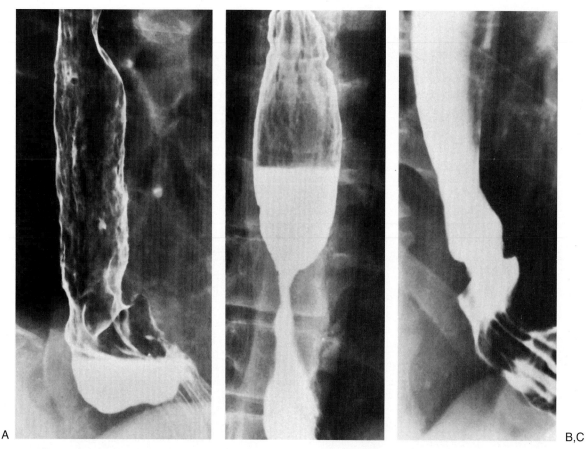

A

B,C

**FIG. 3–22. A:** Double-contrast view of severe reflux esophagitis showing mucosal irregularity, marginal serration, erosions, and ulceration. (From ref. 34, with permission.) **B:** Tapered, slightly irregular peptic stricture of the lower esophagus. (From ref. 106, with permission.) **C:** Slightly irregular annular stricture measuring 6 mm long. The thickness of the narrowing favors a peptic stricture rather than a mucosal ring.

these pathogenetic factors and the resultant gross morphologic changes of reflux esophagitis [18, 23, 77, 81].

## Morphologic Findings

Nearly 60% of patients with GERD have endoscopic abnormalities [77, 81, 82]. The remaining 40% may show mild epithelial erosions or histologic inflammation on biopsy examination. Endoscopy has been the benchmark for judging the presence and severity of the gross morphologic changes of reflux esophagitis. Endoscopic signs include erythema, friability, exudation, erosions, ulceration, and stricture. Erythema alone is not reliable unless accompanied by other findings, such as exudation [82, 85]. Various endoscopic criteria have classified the severity of reflux esophagitis for radiologic correlation, usually into three categories: (a) mild, erythema with exudation or friability; (b) moderate, erosions or ulcerations, and (c) severe, marked ulceration or stricture [77, 81, 85, 106].

## Radiologic Findings

In evaluating GERD, the barium esophagram best detects reflux esophagitis and its complications [77, 81, 85]. Abnor-

malities of esophageal motility and clearance are common in GERD and may also be assessed by radiologic imaging. However, abnormal gastroesophageal reflux is most effectively evaluated by 24-hour pH monitoring using ambulatory devices [13, 99, 119, 125]. The barium esophagram is much less sensitive than prolonged pH monitoring for identifying reflux. Barium reflux may occur spontaneously or during various provocative tests, such as the water siphon test, but is observed in only 35% or so of symptomatic patients [77, 81, 82]. Provocative maneuvers improve the radiographic demonstration of gastroesophageal reflux, but the specificity in many studies is less [82, 119]. Despite initial enthusiasm, the radionuclide reflux study has shown only approximately a 60% average detection rate of gastroesophageal reflux (Fig. 3–21) [18, 77, 81, 82].

The more common radiographic abnormalities seen in reflux esophagitis include contour irregularity, fold thickening, erosions, ulcers, wall thickening, and segmental narrowing, particularly from stricture (Figs. 3–2B, 3–4B, 3–22) [54, 77, 81, 85, 106]. Pseudodiverticula, inflammatory polyps, and esophagogastric fistula are seen less often. Radiographic detection of reflux esophagitis depends most impor-

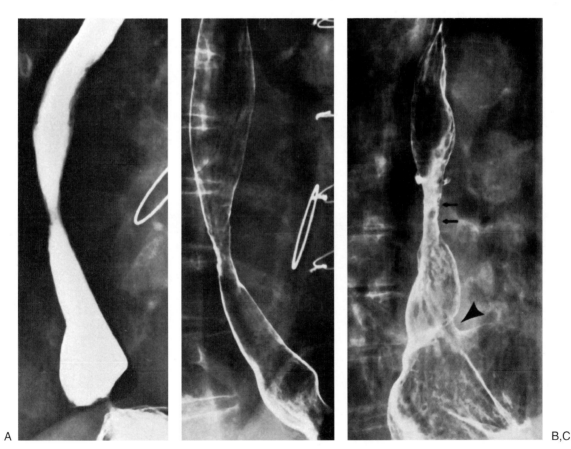

A                                                                                          B,C

**FIG. 3–23. A:** Full-column **(left)** and double-contrast **(right)** views in a patient with Barrett's esophagus showing a midesophageal stricture. (From ref. 77, with permission.) **B:** Large hiatal hernia with peptic stricture (*arrows*) well above the level of the esophagogastric junction (*arrowhead*) in a patient with Barrett's esophagus. Pseudodiverticula are present at the upper level of the stricture. (From ref. 77a, with permission.)

tantly on its endoscopic severity, as well as on the quality of the examination. A multiphasic esophagram is needed for optimal evaluation [77, 81, 85, 106]. Radiographic detection is poor in mild esophagitis. However, the combined sensitivity for diagnosing moderate and severe reflux esophagitis has averaged 90%, with 95% detection of peptic stricture [77, 81, 85, 91, 106]. Endoscopic detection of peptic stricture is somewhat less effective with the use of smaller-caliber endoscopes [86].

### Barrett's Esophagus

Barrett's esophagus represents progressive columnar metaplasia of the lower esophagus caused by chronic reflux esophagitis [2, 9, 51, 54]. The overall prevalence of Barrett's esophagus is approximately 10% in patients with reflux disease. Barrett's esophagus is a premalignant condition with an increased risk of adenocarcinoma [2, 51, 64]. Barrett's esophagus is suggested radiographically when focal esophagitis, ulcer, or stricture is separated from an accompanying hiatal hernia by a normal segment of esophagus (Fig. 3–23). A reticular mucosal pattern has been described as being more specific for columnar-lined esophagus, but its prevalence and specificity have been debated [9, 54, 65].

### Nonreflux Esophagitis

Nonreflux esophagitis results from numerous causes (Table 3–2). The rarer causes require clinical correlation since the radiographic findings mimic those seen in other forms of esophagitis.

### Infectious Esophagitis

Infectious esophagitis results from a wide variety of fungal, viral, or bacterial agents. *Candida albicans* is the most common cause, usually of an opportunistic infection [55]. Dysphagia and odynophagia are the usual presenting complaints, and importantly, oral lesions are absent in approximately 50% of patients [55, 89]. *Candida* esophagitis has various radiologic features depending on its severity (Fig. 3–24). Fine ulcers and a cobblestone pattern are early findings. Abnormal motility, severe ulceration, and pseudomem-

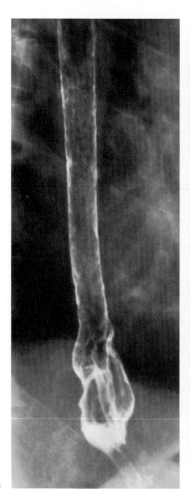
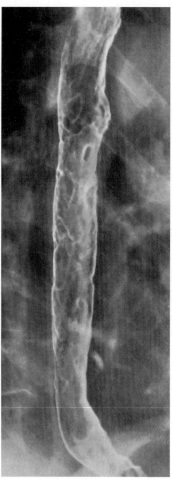

A,B

**FIG. 3–24. A:** Extensive mucosal irregularity from *Candida* esophagitis. **B:** Severe, diffuse esophagitis from candidiasis with larger plaques. (From ref. 77a, with permission.)

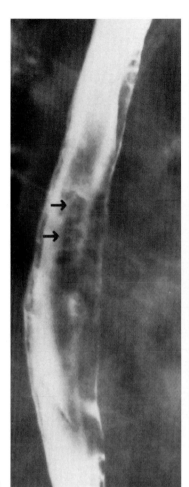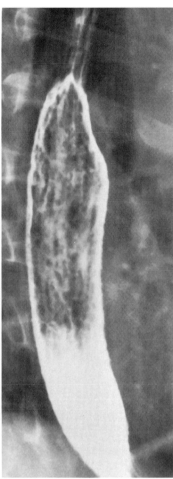

A,B

**FIG. 3–25. A:** Discrete ulcers (*arrows*) in a patient with herpetic esophagitis. **B:** Diffuse herpetic esophagitis indistinguishable from *Candida* infection. (From ref. 77A, with permission.)

brane formation are later features. Stricture, fungal masses, and fistula with abscess are rare [55, 89]. Radiographic detection of *Candida* esophagitis has varied from 80% to 92% [68, 122].

Herpes simplex and cytomegalovirus most often cause viral esophagitis [55]. Although usually opportunistic and causing symptoms similar to *Candida* esophagitis, herpetic infection has occurred in healthy individuals [116]. Discrete ulceration may be a suggestive finding in early viral infection, but histologic examination is needed for definitive diagnosis (Fig. 3–25). Severe viral disease shows appearances indistinguishable from fungal esophagitis. Radiographic detection of viral esophagitis has been 90% or more, although a specific diagnosis is suggested in only about half of patients [55, 67, 122].

Acquired immunodeficiency syndrome (AIDS) is associated with unusual malignancies and opportunistic infections of the gastrointestinal tract. Infectious esophagitis secondary to AIDS may result from numerous causes, including the usual fungal and more common viral agents [55, 70]. Also, unusual infections due to various mycobacterial or-

ganisms, *Cryptosporidium,* and other rare types can occur [38, 55]. More recently, human immunodeficiency virus (HIV)-related giant esophageal ulcers have been described and may mimic specific viral infections (Fig. 3–26) [55, 66].

### Caustic Esophagitis

The severity of caustic esophagitis depends on the type, quantity, and concentration of material ingested and on the duration of mucosal contact [14, 57]. Esophageal dilatation, atony, and poor distensibility with segmental contractions are early functional disturbances. Mucosal injury can be graded endoscopically depending on the depth of tissue damage. Radiographic findings in patients with more severe caustic esophagitis include exudates, pseudomembranes, erosions, and ulcers. Intramural dissection and even perforation with mediastinitis can occur acutely. Strictures may result and usually develop several weeks or more after the initial caustic insult (Fig. 3–27).

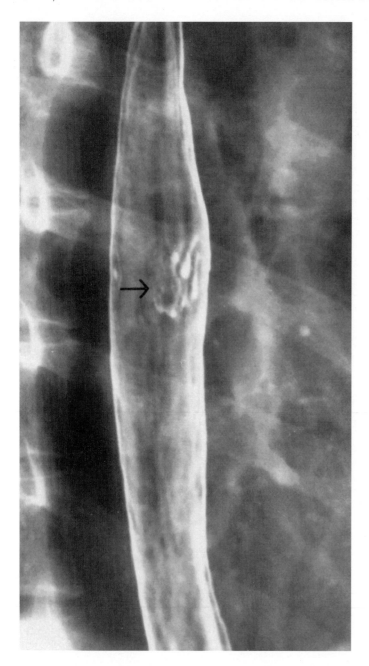

**FIG. 3–26.** Oval ulcers (*arrow*) in a patient with acquired immunodeficiency syndrome (AIDS) and dysphagia. Endoscopic examination recovered no specific infectious agents, and the patient did not respond symptomatically to antiviral or antifungal drugs.

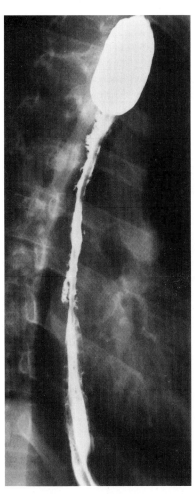

**FIG. 3–27.** Long, irregular stricture of the midesophagus due to caustic injury from lye ingestion.

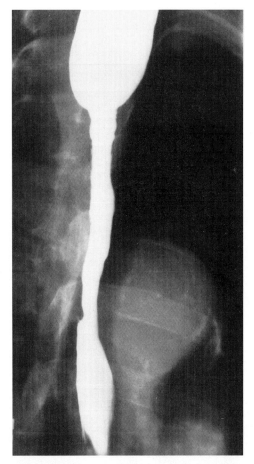

**FIG. 3–28.** Stricture located at and above the level of the aortic arch (*A*) in an elderly man taking numerous cardiac medications. Endoscopic examination showed erosive esophagitis but no malignancy or Barrett's epithelium.

### Radiation Esophagitis

Esophageal radiation injury is seen mainly in treated esophageal carcinoma but can occur after mediastinal radiation for other malignancies. Acute and chronic radiation effects of the esophagus generally occur after 4,500 to 6,000 rads given over 6 to 8 weeks [16, 50, 57]. Chemotherapy and radiation combined enhance the chance of esophageal damage [3]. Radiologic abnormalities include abnormal esophageal motility, mucosal irregularity, ulceration, stricture, pseudodiverticula, and fistula. The occurrence and temporal appearance of these abnormalities depend on the dosage and schedule, field size, use of chemotherapy, and individual susceptibility. Motility disturbances usually occur within 1 to 3 months following radiotherapy and stricture, generally at 6 to 8 months [16, 50, 57].

### Medication-induced Injury

A wide variety of medications can cause focal esophagitis [1, 57]. The most common have been emepronium, tetracy-cline, and slow-releasing potassium chloride. Slow esophageal clearance of the medication or abnormal motility may prolong contact between the ingested material and the esophageal mucosa. The usual site involved has been the midesophagus near the aortic arch. Superficial erosions and ulcerations are the typical endoscopic abnormalities, which may be shown radiographically. Focal esophageal narrowing, often caused by spasm, edema, or (rarely) stricture, may be present (Fig. 3–28). The findings usually resolve quickly on withdrawal of the medication.

### Neoplastic Disease

A diversity of neoplasms and tumor-like lesions may involve the esophagus (Table 3–3). Benign and malignant primary neoplasms, secondary neoplasms, and an assortment of nonneoplastic conditions have been described. Only the more common lesions are discussed.

**TABLE 3–3.** *Neoplasms and tumor-like lesions of the esophagus*

Benign neoplasm
  Leiomyoma
  Squamous papilloma[a]
  Myoblastoma[a]
  Vascular tumors[a]
  Adenoma[a]
  Lipoma[a]
Malignant neoplasms
  Squamous cell carcinoma
  Adenocarcinoma
  Barrett's carcinoma
  Carcinosarcoma[a]
  Lymphoma[a]
  Leiomyosarcoma[a]
Secondary neoplasms
  Contiguous spread
  Lymph node metastases
  Hematogenous metastases[a]
Tumor-like lesions
  Inflammatory reflux polyp
  Inflammatory fibroid polyp[a]
  Fibrovascular polyp[a]
  Congenital or acquired cysts[a]
  Intramural hematoma[a]

[a] Extremely rare.

### Benign Neoplasms

Leiomyoma is the most common benign esophageal tumor but is rare [30, 31, 52]. Many patients are asymptomatic, and the leiomyoma is found incidentally. The lesion is generally solitary, most often found in the lower esophagus, and usually 2 to 6 cm in size (Fig. 3–29). Leiomyoma typically presents as a smooth, eccentric contour defect due to its intramural location, which may be identified by EUS (Fig. 3–30) [121]. Ulceration and calcification are rare. Larger leiomyomas show an adjacent mass effect and may be apparent on chest films.

### Malignant Neoplasms

Squamous cell carcinoma and adenocarcinoma are the most common primary esophageal neoplasms [30, 58, 63]. Squamous cell carcinomas show a wide spectrum of morphologic and, thus, radiologic appearances, including superficial, polypoid or fungating, ulcerative, and infiltrative forms (Fig. 3–31). Small, superficial carcinomas may appear as focal mucosal irregularity or nodular protrusion. Polypoid malignancies vary from small, eccentric defects to large, intraluminal tumors. Ulceration may accompany the other morphologic types or be a predominant finding surrounded

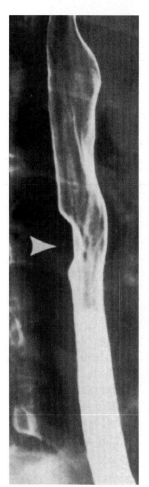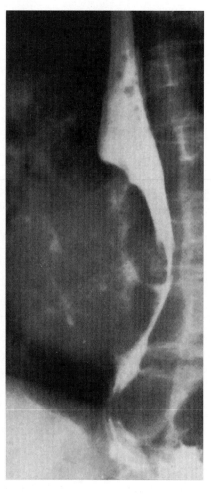

A,B

**FIG. 3–29. A:** Leiomyoma measuring 1.5 cm (*arrowhead*) found incidentally in a patient without esophageal symptoms. **B:** Large (6.5 × 7.5 cm) leiomyoma with mass effect in a patient with dysphagia. (From ref. 77a, with permission.)

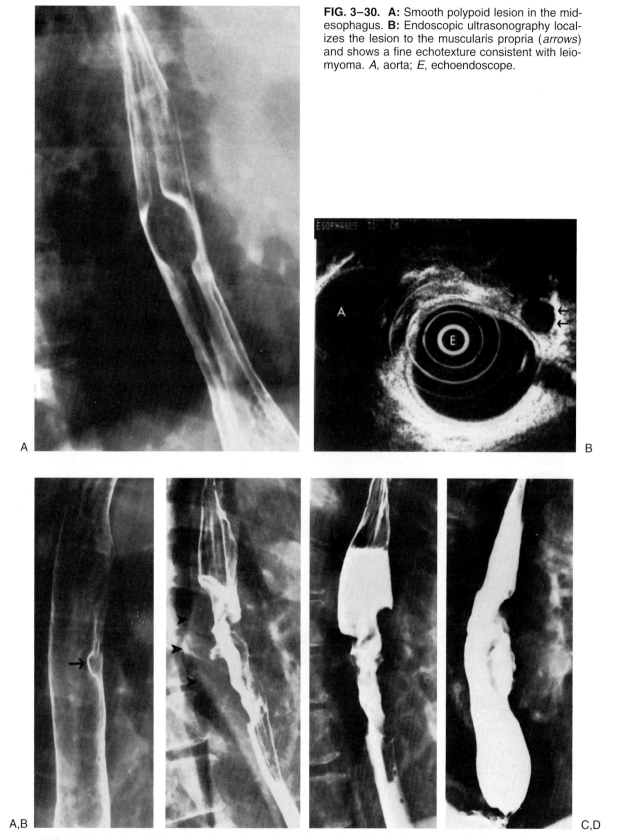

**FIG. 3–30. A:** Smooth polypoid lesion in the mid-esophagus. **B:** Endoscopic ultrasonography local-izes the lesion to the muscularis propria (*arrows*) and shows a fine echotexture consistent with leio-myoma. *A,* aorta; *E,* echoendoscope.

A

B

A,B

C,D

**FIG. 3–31. A:** Small (6 × 8 mm) esophageal carcinoma (*arrow*) clearly seen on double-contrast view. (From ref. 77a, with permission.) **B:** Circumferential squamous cell carcinoma with ulceration and wall thickening (*arrowheads*). **C:** Irregular annular carcinoma of the midesophagus. **D:** Ulcerative squamous cell carcinoma.

by tumor mass. Infiltrative carcinoma often causes eccentric or annular constriction with a typically irregular, ulcerated contour. Malignant infiltration with a smooth contour is rare, except after radiotherapy, but may mimic a benign stricture.

Radiologic detection of esophageal squamous cell carcinoma depends on its size and the techniques used [61–63]. Large circumferential or polypoid malignancies are easily shown. Using a multiphasic radiographic examination, virtually all symptomatic esophageal carcinomas are detected [21, 41, 105]. Early diagnosis of esophageal carcinoma por-

tends longer survival since size of the lesion and extent of invasion are related. Infiltration by small carcinomas may be limited to the submucosa, whereas more advanced types often have invaded adjacent structures and are not resectable [4, 108, 112, 128].

CT and EUS have become important in evaluating patients with esophageal carcinoma, for assessing extraluminal extent of disease and staging of malignancy [4, 49, 108, 112, 128]. CT evaluates transmural extension of esophageal carcinoma, regional lymphadenopathy, direct invasion into the

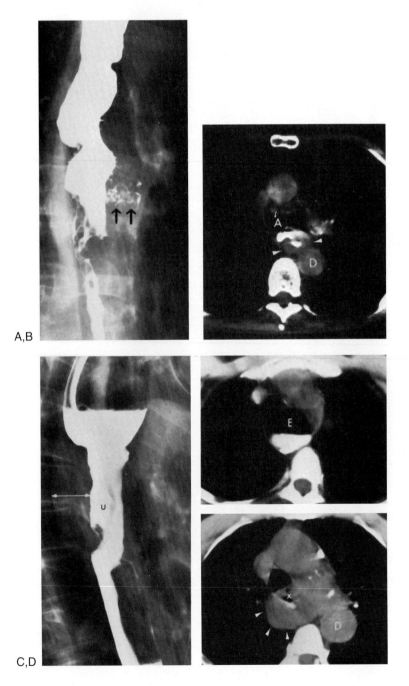

A,B

C,D

FIG. 3–32. **A:** Carcinoma of the midesophagus with a sinus tract (*arrows*). **B:** Computed tomography (CT) scan in the same patient as in **A,** showing a thickened esophageal wall (*arrowheads*) and contrast material adjacent to the airway (*A*). *D,* descending aorta. (Courtesy Robert E. Bechtold, Winston-Salem, NC.) **C:** Annular carcinoma of the midesophagus with orad dilatation, ulceration (*U*), and wall thickening (*connected arrow*). **D:** Two CT scans 3 cm apart. The orad view **(top)** shows dilatation of the esophagus (*E*) with air-contrast level. The lower view **(bottom)** shows narrowing of the esophageal lumen with ulceration (*x*) and marked wall thickening (*arrowheads*). *D,* descending aorta. (Courtesy Robert E. Bechtold, Winston-Salem, NC.)

aorta and airway, and distant metastases, especially to the liver. EUS is superior to CT in evaluating the depth of malignant infiltration, particularly in the early stages, and in assessing regional lymph node metastases [4, 108, 112, 128]. EUS also shows invasion into adjacent organs but is limited by severe esophageal stenosis and does not detect distant metastases (Figs. 3–32, 3–33, 3–34). At present, MRI is less accurate than CT or EUS in staging esophageal carcinoma [49, 108].

Adenocarcinoma is increasing in prevalence and accounts for 10% or more of primary esophageal malignancies [10, 30, 63]. Adenocarcinoma originates mainly in the lower esophagus and may arise from the esophageal glands, heterotopic gastric mucosa, or metaplastic columnar epithelium, so-called Barrett's carcinoma. Indeed, the most common origin is believed to be dysplastic Barrett's epithelium [10, 30, 54, 63]. Barrett-type adenocarcinoma is often superimposed on changes of chronic reflux esophagitis, especially long stricturing [54, 63, 64]. Radiologic appearances of Barrett's carcinoma overlap features of squamous cell carcinoma and secondarily invading gastric carcinoma and include infiltra-tive, varicoid, polypoid, ulcerative, and mixed forms (Fig. 3–35).

### Secondary Neoplasms

Secondary neoplasms may involve the esophagus by contiguous spread, lymph node metastases, or hematogenous metastases [58]. Hematogenous metastasis is least common, resulting most often from melanoma and carcinomas of the breast and lung. Mediastinal lymph node metastases are the second most common source of secondary esophageal neoplasms. Lung and breast are the usual sources of metastatic mediastinal tumor invading the esophagus. Contiguous tumor extension from carcinomas of adjacent organs is the most frequent route. Malignancies of the larynx, thyroid, lung, and gastric cardia predominate. Invasion of gastric carcinoma into the esophagus is well known and may mimic achalasia.

### Tumor-like Lesions

A diversity of nonneoplastic lesions that may simulate esophageal neoplasms have been described. Since most

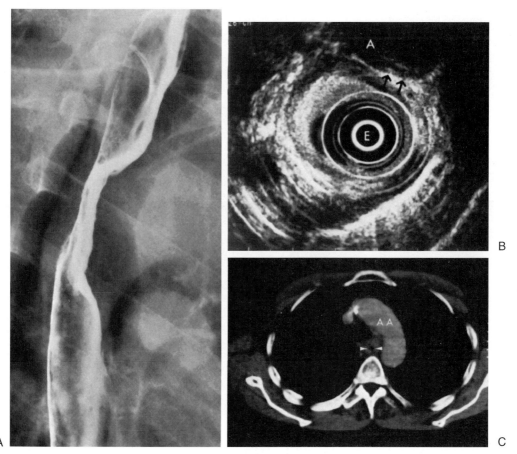

**FIG. 3–33. A:** Annular carcinoma of the esophagus at the level of the aortic arch. **B:** Endoscopic ultrasonography shows wall thickening and obliteration of the typical ultrasonic layers. Interface (*arrows*) with the aorta (*A*) is preserved. *E,* echoendoscope. **C:** Computed tomography scan at the level of the aortic arch (*AA*) shows luminal narrowing (*arrowheads*) and esophageal wall thickening.

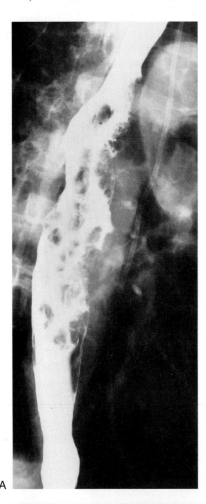

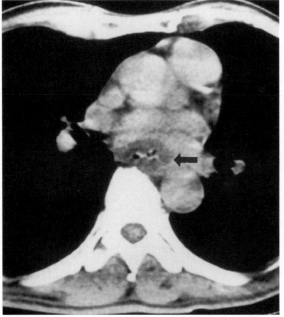

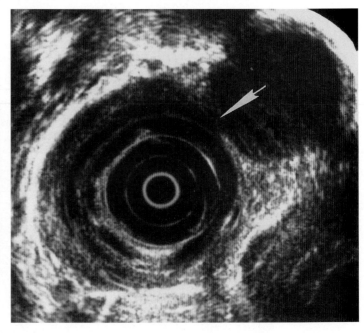

**FIG. 3–34. A:** Circumferential, irregular carcinoma of the esophagus. **B:** Computed tomography scan at a level below the aortic arch shows thickening of the esophageal wall and possible aortic invasion (*arrow*). **C:** Endoscopic ultrasonography at a similar level also shows diffuse esophageal wall thickening, extension of malignancy into the periesophageal tissues, and invasion of the aorta (*arrow*).

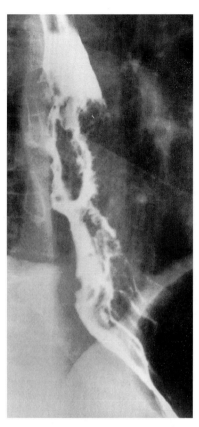

**FIG. 3–35.** Adenocarcinoma of the lower esophagus arising from Barrett's epithelium.

are rare, only the inflammatory reflux polyp is discussed. An uncommon endoscopic finding in reflux esophagitis, it is an enlarged, inflamed gastric fold near the squamocolumnar junction [54, 118]. The reflux polyp is also called the sentinel fold and is seen as a polypoid defect radiographically. The inflammatory polyp must be differentiated from a true neoplasm or may appear compressible and resemble an esophageal varix. Endoscopy is needed for differentiation.

## Diverticular Disease

Esophageal diverticula are acquired abnormalities, usually of the pulsion variety [6, 31, 56]. They may be classified by cause, location, or appearance. Diverticula increase in prevalence with age, are often incidental, and rarely cause symptoms. Pulsion diverticula are mucosal herniations through the esophageal muscularis and may relate to motility disorders, mechanical obstruction, or chronic wear-and-tear forces. The latter is likely the main mechanism in the formation of Zenker's diverticulum and the underlying cause, along with motility disturbances, of most esophageal diverticula.

### Midesophageal Diverticula

Midesophageal diverticula are most often of the pulsion type (Fig. 3–36). However, traction diverticula due to extrinsic inflammatory involvement of the esophagus also occur at this site. Fibrotic healing of adjacent infected lymph nodes exerts traction and initiates a focal outpouching of the esophageal wall. Local pulsion forces within the esophagus may also contribute. Traction diverticula are generally small, have a conical or triangular shape, and often show changeable deformity during esophageal peristalsis.

### Epiphrenic Diverticula

Epiphrenic diverticula occur in the lower esophagus just above the diaphragm, usually accompanied by hiatal hernia [6]. Nearly all are pulsion diverticula (Fig. 3–37). Most are larger than those in the midesophagus and vary in size from 1 to 7 cm. The shape of epiphrenic diverticula depends on their size, position, and phase of esophageal peristalsis. Typical small pulsion diverticula have a smooth, rounded appearance. Larger diverticula have well-defined necks with a dependent portion acting as a passive reservoir, trapping food and secretions and compressing the adjacent esophagus. A large esophageal diverticulum may be seen on chest films, often containing an air-fluid level.

### Intramural Pseudodiverticulosis

Intramural pseudodiverticulosis is unusual and may involve the esophagus segmentally or diffusely [31, 57, 69]. Multiple small outpouchings seen in the esophageal wall are believed to represent dilated submucosal glands, possibly related to chronic mucosal inflammation (Figs. 3–23B, 3–38). This cause is likely in segmental pseudodiverticulosis, which typically is associated with esophageal stricture, usually from reflux esophagitis. Diffuse pseudodiverticulosis may also occur with stricture, *Candida* esophagitis, herpetic esophagitis, or even esophageal carcinoma.

## Esophageal Motility Disorders

Esophageal motility disorders are an important cause of esophageal complaints, especially when symptoms are not readily explained by a structural abnormality [41, 78]. Evaluation of esophageal function is integral to radiographic examination of the esophagus. An understanding of esophageal physiology is needed to assess functional disorders properly. This section discusses radiographic evaluation of esophageal motility and its abnormalities, with the more common primary motility disorders emphasized.

### General Principles

Radiographic evaluation of esophageal motility includes examination of the esophageal body and the upper and

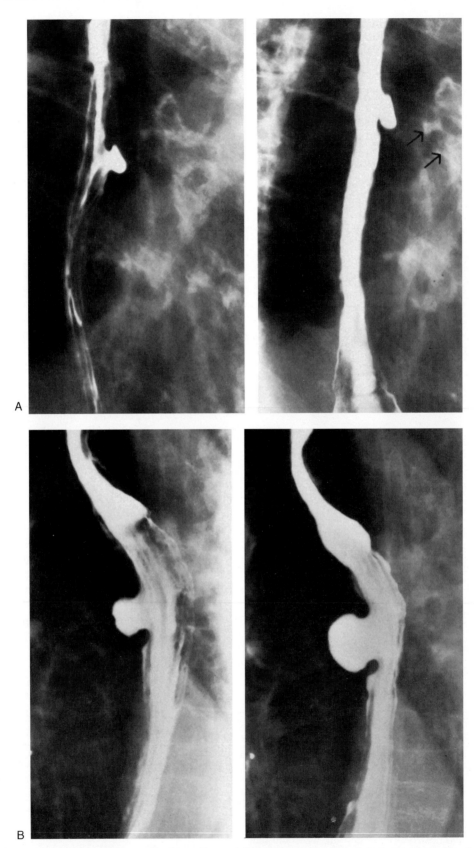

**FIG. 3–36. A:** Two views of a small midesophageal diverticulum. The angulated appearance and adjacent calcifications (*arrows*) suggest a traction origin. **B:** Two views of a larger midesophageal diverticulum. The changeable spherical shape suggests a pulsion origin. A nonspecific esophageal motility disorder was present fluoroscopically and manometrically.

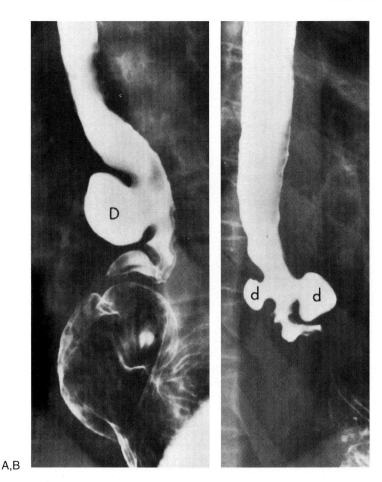

A,B

FIG. 3–37. A: Epiphrenic diverticulum (*D*) in a patient with a nonspecific esophageal motility disorder. A hiatal hernia also is present. B: Multiple epiphrenic diverticula (*d*).

lower esophageal sphincters [22, 78, 80]. Fluoroscopic observation is usually adequate for functional study of the esophagus and lower esophageal sphincter. The patient is examined in the prone oblique position to eliminate the effect of gravity on bolus transport. Single swallows of barium are observed because rapid multiple swallows inhibit primary peristalsis and may be mistaken for functional abnormality. Repetitive swallowing distends the esophagus for structural evaluation.

A normal primary peristaltic sequence is seen as an aboral contraction wave that obliterates the esophageal lumen (Fig. 3–39). The peristaltic wave imparts an inverted V configuration to the top of the barium column and normally strips all of the barium from the esophagus. Occasionally, some proximal escape of barium occurs at the level of the aortic arch because of the lower-amplitude pressure trough normally present at the transition from striated to smooth muscle of the esophagus. Proximal escape is more common with increasing age and may be misinterpreted as abnormal [40].

Esophageal motility disorders are usually classified as primary or secondary (Table 3–4) [80, 115]. Primary motility disorders involve the esophagus predominantly, whereas secondary motility disorders result from local disease (such as esophagitis) or from a variety of systemic, neurologic, and other types of disorders. The classification of primary esophageal motility disorders is still evolving.

TABLE 3–4. *Esophageal motility disorders*

| |
| --- |
| Primary motility disorders |
|     Achalasia and variants |
|     Diffuse esophageal spasm |
|     Nonspecific motility disorder |
|     Nutcracker esophagus |
|     Presbyesophagus? |
| Secondary motility disorders |
|     Collagen vascular disease |
|     Reflux esophagitis |
|     Caustic esophagitis |
|     Radiation injury |
|     Medication-induced injury |
|     Infectious esophagitis |
|     Alcoholism |
|     Diabetes mellitus |
|     Thyroid disease |
|     Neuromuscular disorders[a] |

[a] See Table 3–1 (similar causes).

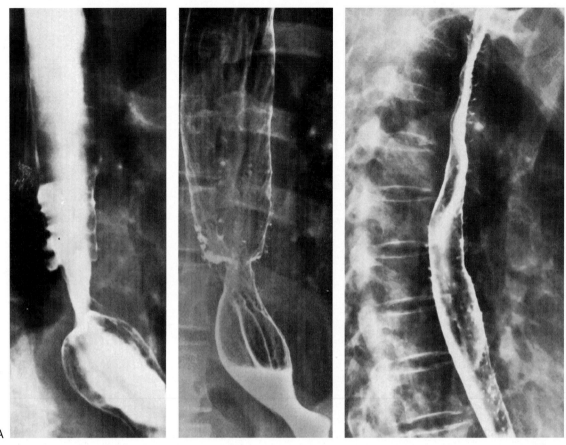

A                                                                                B,C

**FIG. 3–38. A:** Peptic stricture associated with multiple smooth outpouchings representing pseudodiverticula endoscopically. **B:** Peptic stricture with numerous small collections of barium. Ulcers and pseudodiverticula were found at endoscopy. (Parts **A** and **B** From ref. 77, with permission.) **C:** Intramural pseudodiverticulosis involving the esophagus diffusely.

### Primary Motility Disorders

Achalasia is characterized by esophageal aperistalsis and lower esophageal sphincter dysfunction [46, 78, 80]. Primary peristalsis is absent on all swallows, and the lower end of the esophagus is smoothly tapered, reflecting failure of the barium bolus to distend the dysfunctional sphincter (Fig. 3–40). Repetitive nonperistaltic contractions may occasionally be seen, a variant called *vigorous achalasia.* Another variant may be early achalasia, in which there is aperistalsis but sphincter relaxation [102]. Radiographic findings in this entity have been similar to classic achalasia except for less esophageal dilatation. In more severe disease, the esophagus is markedly dilated and retains food, secretions, and barium.

Other causes of lower esophageal narrowing and dysfunction, such as intrinsic and extrinsic neoplasms, peptic stricture, and complicated scleroderma, may mimic achalasia. Carcinoma of the lower esophagus or stomach must be excluded, especially in older patients [25, 58, 80]. Uncommonly, gastric carcinoma or an extrinsic neoplasm involving the lower esophagus causes smooth tapering with abnormal peristalsis and may resemble achalasia (Fig. 3–41). Hiatal hernia is uncommon in achalasia but usually accompanies peptic stricture [95]. Scleroderma typically shows a widened esophageal hiatus but may be complicated by peptic stricture.

Radiographic imaging may aid management and treatment of patients with achalasia. Radionuclide transit and emptying studies can quantitate esophageal retention before and following therapy (Fig. 3–42) [18, 102]. Achalasia is treated surgically with a Heller myotomy or by pneumatic dilatation. Radiographic evaluation of the esophagus immediately following pneumatic dilatation is most useful for detecting serious complications, such as perforation (Fig. 3–43) [88, 103]. Following a Heller myotomy, a diverticulum-like outpouching is typically present at the lower end of the esophagus.

Diffuse esophageal spasm is not common. Manometric criteria are intermittent normal peristalsis with simultaneous

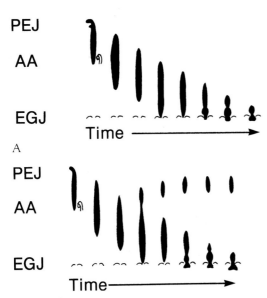

PEJ

AA

EGJ

Time ⟶

A

PEJ

AA

EGJ

Time ⟶

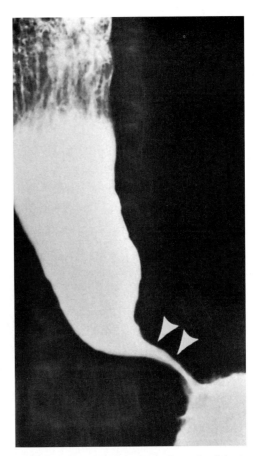

**FIG. 3–39. A:** Schematic representation of normal primary peristalsis with the lumen-obliterating contraction wave stripping all of the barium from the esophagus. **B:** Normal primary peristalsis with proximal escape because the contraction wave fails to obliterate the esophageal lumen completely at the level of the aortic arch. Note that the peristaltic sequence continues aborally. *PEJ,* pharyngoesophageal junction; *AA,* aortic arch; *EGI,* esophagogastric junction. (From ref. 77a, with permission.)

**FIG. 3–40.** Esophageal dilatation and aperistalsis shown fluoroscopically in achalasia. The smooth tapering at the lower end of the esophagus (*arrowheads*) represents the dysfunctional lower esophageal sphincter.

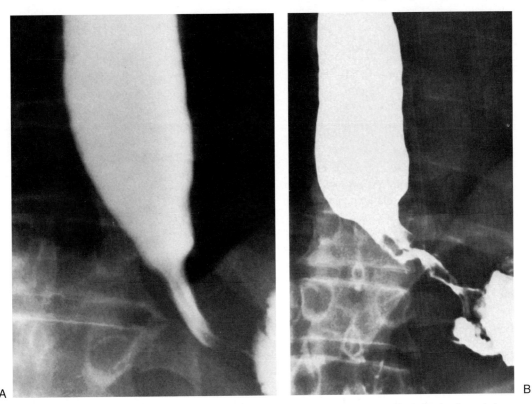

A

B

**FIG. 3–41. A:** Smooth narrowing of the esophagogastric junction simulating achalasia. Pathologically, scirrhous carcinoma of the stomach is infiltrating the esophagus. (From ref. 77a, with permission.) **B:** Fluoroscopically evident aperistalsis, esophageal dilation, and irregular tapering of the esophagogastric region due to carcinoma of the adjacent stomach.

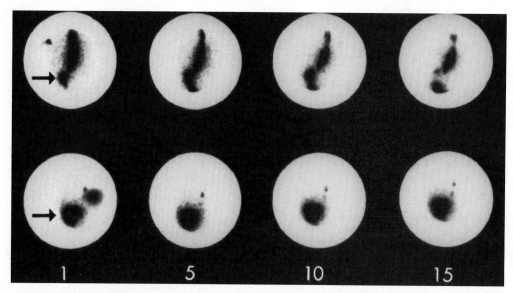

**FIG. 3–42.** Radionuclide emptying studies before **(top)** and after **(bottom)** pneumatic dilatation in a patient with achalasia. Selective images at 1, 5, 10, and 15 minutes. There is delayed retention in the esophagus before treatment and normal emptying following dilatation. The *arrows* indicate gastric activity. (From ref. 102, with permission.)

contractions and usually normal lower esophageal sphincter function [80, 109]. Radiographically, esophageal peristalsis is disrupted periodically in the smooth muscle segment and replaced by nonperistaltic contractions (Fig. 3–44) [12, 78, 80]. Spontaneous, obliterating contractions may segment the esophageal lumen, creating the corkscrew or rosary-bead appearance. The esophageal musculature may be thickened in diffuse esophageal spasm, although radiographic and EUS studies have shown that most patients have normal esophageal wall thickness [12, 80].

*Nonspecific esophageal motility disorder* has become a catchall term to describe symptomatic patients with motility abnormalities that defy specific classification [8, 80]. The natural history and clinical significance of this disorder are not clear. Manometric findings include intermittent absence of peristalsis, low-amplitude peristalsis, repetitive contractions, or incomplete lower esophageal sphincter relaxation. Radiographically, primary peristaltic disturbances and tertiary contractions suggest an indeterminant motility disorder.

Nutcracker esophagus is a controversial motility disorder associated with chest pain. Manometrically, primary peristalsis is intact, but lower esophageal peristaltic contractions have abnormally high amplitude and prolonged duration [8, 80]. The radiographic findings are normal in most patients, although nonspecific tertiary contractions may be present [80, 104]. Nutcracker esophagus is, thus, a manometric diagnosis.

Presbyesophagus has become a questionable entity; as described originally, it referred to esophageal dysmotility associated with aging [42, 129]. The major manometric criteria included decreased incidence of peristalsis, increased tertiary contractions, and occasional lower esophageal sphincter dysfunction. Radiographic abnormalities reflected the manometric findings. However, many patients from earlier reports of this entity had neurologic disorders or diabetes mellitus, which may have produced esophageal dysmotility. Other studies in healthy older people have shown only minor changes in esophageal function [40, 42, 47, 110].

Radiologic efficacy for evaluating esophageal motility depends on the quality of the examination. Radiographic specificities for identifying normal primary peristalsis have been 91% to 95% using multiple single barium swallows [22, 71, 84, 101]. Radiographic sensitivities vary with the motility disorder being evaluated. Detection rates of approximately 95% for achalasia, 75% for diffuse esophageal spasm, and 50% for nonspecific esophageal motility disorders have been reported [12, 101]. Nutcracker esophagus is not specifically diagnosed radiographically [104]. The use of five single barium swallows has shown excellent correlation with manometry and would likely improve radiographic detection of diffuse spasm and nonspecific dysmotility [71, 84].

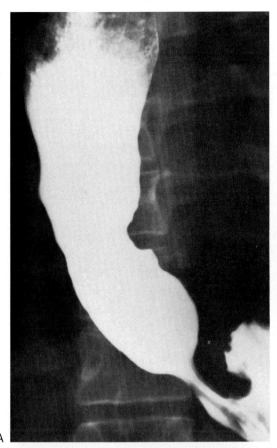

A

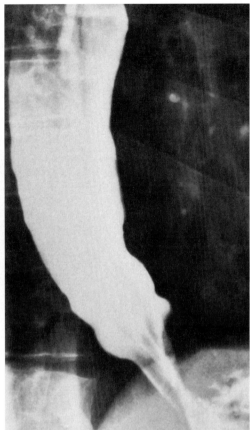

B

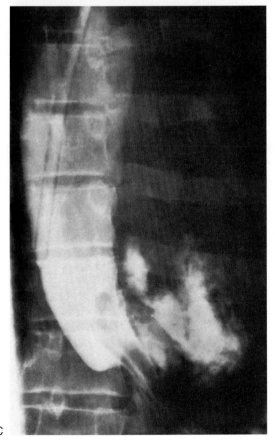

C

FIG. 3–43. **A:** Esophagogram before pneumatic dilatation of achalasia. The luminal diameter of the esophagogastric junction is 6 mm. **B:** Intubated examination of the esophagus after dilatation in the same patient as in **A.** The esophagogastric caliber is 10 mm, and the contour is smooth. **C:** Free perforation immediately following pneumatic dilatation shown with water-soluble contrast material. (From ref. 103, with permission.)

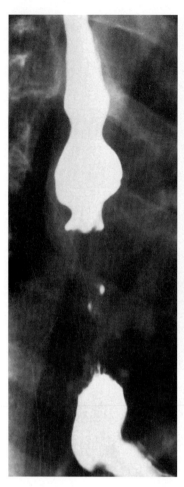 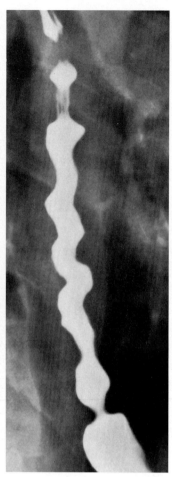

A,B

**FIG. 3–44. A:** Diffuse esophageal spasm with intermittent disruption of primary peristalsis at fluoroscopy and focally obliterative simultaneous contractions. (From ref. 77a, with permission.) **B:** Diffuse esophageal spasm with typical curling or corkscrew appearance.

### Secondary Motility Disorders

Radiographic diagnosis of secondary motility disorders is based on showing nonspecific functional disturbances combined with clinical correlation. Scleroderma is the most important and is characterized by peristaltic abnormalities in the smooth muscle segment and lower esophageal sphincter hypotension, which predisposes to reflux esophagitis [115]. Radiographically, primary peristalsis is disordered or absent in the lower two-thirds of the esophagus, the organ is often dilated, and hiatal hernia is typically present. Peptic stricture may complicate scleroderma.

### Miscellaneous Esophageal Disorders

### Esophageal Varices

Esophageal varices are most commonly of the ''uphill'' variety due to portal hypertension from cirrhosis of the liver [60]. Other causes include thrombosis of the splenic, portal, or hepatic veins and compression by tumors or congenital stenosis of the same venous structures. Varices are best shown by the mucosal relief technique and appear as change-

able fold thickening or as serpiginous and polypoid defects in the lower esophagus (Fig. 3–45). EUS can detect esophageal varices and evaluate portal hypertension and may monitor patients following various types of treatment [7]. A variety of esophageal changes have been described after sclerotherapy, including the development of stricture [120].

### Traumatic Effects

Esophageal trauma may result from foreign body, surgery, endoscopic and therapeutic procedures, blunt or penetrating injury, and postemetic trauma [56]. Esophageal perforation is the most serious consequence and is often due to endoscopy, dilatation procedures, or surgery. Postemetic trauma related to severe vomiting shows a spectrum of injury that includes the Mallory-Weiss tear, intramural hematoma, and spontaneous Boerhaave rupture. Water-soluble contrast material is used for initial examination of the esophagus for suspected trauma. If perforation is not present, examination with barium should follow for detection of more subtle abnormalities [27, 56, 90].

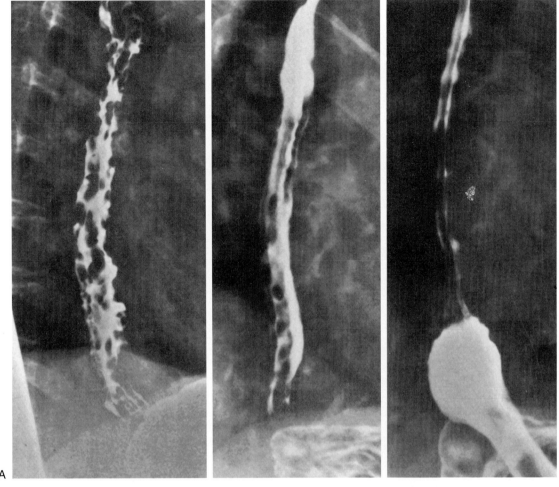

A                                                                                                                                    B,C

**FIG. 3–45.** **A:** Esophageal varices well shown by the mucosal relief technique. **B:** Nodular filling defects due to esophageal varices. **C:** Disappearance of varices in the same patient as in **B,** following a peristaltic contraction.

### Foreign Bodies

A wide variety of foreign objects may be swallowed purposely by infants, children, or psychiatric patients and unintentionally by adults [56]. The most common foreign body found in adults is a meat bolus that lodges at an area of anatomic or pathologic narrowing. A lower esophageal mucosal ring or peptic stricture is the usual pathologic cause of narrowing. An impacted meat bolus may be dislodged by the use of glucagon and a gas-producing agent or may be removed endoscopically (Fig. 3–46) [45]. Proteolytic enzyme digestion of a food impaction is no longer recommended owing to the risk of esophageal perforation.

### Postprocedural Effects

Surgery or therapeutic endoscopy of the esophagus includes a variety of procedures (Table 3–5), many of which produce characteristic changes, such as the Nissen fundoplication,

or may be associated with a variety of complications. An understanding of the procedure performed, its typical normal radiographic appearances, and the possible complications is required to evaluate these patients properly [59].

### Extrinsic Effects

Extrinsic structural lesions are easily detected if the abnormality encroaches on the esophagus [56]. In the neck, thyroid enlargement can compress and displace the cervical esophagus. Neoplastic or inflammatory disease of the mediastinum and cardiac enlargement are causes of extrinsic involvement. Symptomatic compression of the esophagus by the aorta or by aberrant vessels can also occur. Dysphagia lusoria results from a symptomatic impression on the upper thoracic esophagus from an aberrant right subclavian artery, which produces an oblique posterior defect. Most patients with this anomaly, however, do not have dysphagia. Dysphagia aor-

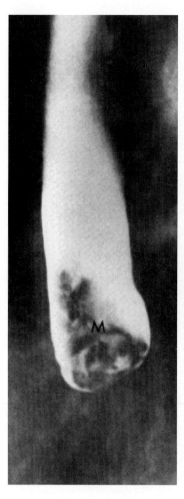
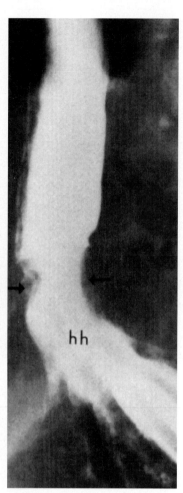

A,B

**FIG. 3–46. A:** Impacted meat (*M*) bolus at the lower end of the esophagus. Glucagon and a gas-producing agent were given and dislodged the obstruction. **B:** Repeat esophagogram shows an irregular peptic stricture (*arrows*) at the level of previous impaction and a hiatal hernia (*hh*).

tica describes symptomatic compression of the lower esophagus by a tortuous descending thoracic aorta [73]. Although displacement and compression of the lower esophagus by an atherosclerotic aorta are often seen in the elderly, most patients will not have dysphagia. Cardiac enlargement and kyphosis of the thoracic spine may aggravate the symptoms.

**TABLE 3–5.** *Surgical and therapeutic endoscopic procedures*

| | |
|---|---|
| Antireflux surgery | Other surgical procedures |
|   Nissen fundoplication |   Congenital anomalies |
|   Other procedures |   Esophageal varices |
|   Angelchik device |   Trauma or foreign bodies |
|   Peptic stricture repairs |   Nonpeptic stricture |
| Motility disorders | Therapeutic endoscopy |
|   Cricopharyngeal myotomy |   Foreign-body removal |
|   Heller myotomy |   Endoscopic pneumatic |
|     (achalasia) |     dilatation |
|   Long myotomy (diffuse |   Peptic stricture dilatation |
|     spasm) |   Sclerotherapy (varices) |
|   Diverticular surgery |   Endoprosthesis placement |
| Carcinoma surgery | |
|   Esophagogastrostomy | |
|   Bowel interposition | |

## REFERENCES

1. Agha FP, Wilson JA, Nostrand TT. Medication-induced esophagitis. Gastrointest Radiol 1986;11:7
2. Armstrong D. Reflux disease and Barrett's oesophagus. Endoscopy 1994;26:9
3. Boal DKB, Newburger PE, Teele RL. Esophagitis induced by combined radiation and adriamycin. Am J Roentgenol 1979;132:567
4. Botet JF, Lightdale CJ, Zauber AG, Gerdes H, Urmacher C, Brennan MF. Preoperative staging of esophageal cancer: comparison of endoscopic US and dynamic CT. Radiology 1991;181:419
5. Boyle BT. Congenital disorders of the esophagus. In Cohen S, Soloway RD, eds, Diseases of the Esophagus. New York: Churchill-Livingstone, 1982:97
6. Bruggeman LL, Seaman WB. Epiphrenic diverticula—an analysis of 80 cases. Am J Roentgenol 1973;119:266
6a.Caletti G. The normal gastrointestinal tract wall: problems and variations. Syllabus from International Symposium on Endoscopic Ultrasonography, Cleveland, OH, March 2–3, 1989
7. Caletti G, Brocchi E, Baraldini M, Ferrari A, Gibilaro M, Barbara L. Assessment of portal hypertension by endoscopic ultrasonography. Gastrointest Endosc 1990;36:S21
8. Castell DO. The nutcracker esophagus and other primary esophageal motility disorders. In Castell DO, Richter JE, Dalton CB, eds, Esophageal Motility Testing. New York: Elsevier Science, 1987:130
9. Chen YM, Gelfand DW, Ott DJ, Wu WC. Barrett esophagus as an extension of severe esophagitis: analysis of radiologic signs in 29 cases. Am J Roentgenol 1985;145:275
10. Chen MYM, Ott DJ, Gelfand DW. More evidence for the increasing prevalence of adenocarcinoma of the esophagus over an 18-year period. J Clin Gastroenterol 1995;21:254

11. Chen YM, Ott DJ, Gelfand DW, Munitz HA. Multiphasic examination of the esophagogastric region for strictures, rings, and hiatal hernia: evaluation of the individual techniques. Gastrointest Radiol 1985;10: 311

12. Chen YM, et al. Diffuse esophageal spasm: radiographic and manometric correlation. Radiology 1989;170:807

13. Chen MYM, Ott DJ, Sinclair JW, Wu WC, Gelfand DW. Gastroesophageal reflux disease: correlation of esophageal pH testing and radiographic findings. Radiology 1992;185:483

14. Chen YM, Ott DJ, Thompson JN, Gelfand DW. Progressive roentgenographic appearance of caustic esophagitis. South Med J 1988;81:724

15. Cockerill EM, Miller RE, Chernish SM, McLaughlin GC III, Rodda BE. Optimal visualization of esophageal varices. Am J Roentgenol 1976;126:512

16. Collazzo LA, Levine MS, Rubesin SE, Laufer I. Acute radiation esophagitis: radiographic findings. Am J Roentgenol 1997;169:1067

17. Cook IJ, et al. Pharyngeal (Zenker's) diverticulum is a disorder of upper esophageal sphincter opening. Gastroenterology 1992;103:1229

18. Cowan RJ. Radionuclide evaluation of the esophagus in patients with dysphagia. In Gelfand DW, Richter JE, eds, Dysphagia—Diagnosis and Treatment. New York: Igaku-Shoin Medical Publishers, 1989: 127

19. Curtis DJ. Radiologic evaluation of oropharyngeal swallowing. In Gelfand DW, Richter JE, eds, Dysphagia—Diagnosis and Treatment. New York: Igaku-Shoin Medical Publishers, 1989:161

20. Dantas RO, Cook IJ, Dodds WJ, Kern MK, Lang IM, Brasseur JG. Biomechanics of cricopharyngeal bars. Gastroenterology 1990;99: 1269

21. DiPalma JA, Prechter GC, Brady CE III. X-ray negative dysphagia: is endoscopy necessary? J Clin Gastroenterol 1984;6:409

22. Dodds WJ. Current concepts of esophageal motor function: clinical implications for radiology. Am J Roentgenol 1977;128:549

23. Dodds WJ. The pathogenesis of gastroesophageal reflux disease. Am J Roentgenol 1988;151:49

24. Dodds WJ, Logemann JA, Stewart ET. Radiologic assessment of abnormal oral and pharyngeal phases of swallowing. Am J Roentgenol 1990;154:965

25. Dodds WJ, Stewart ET Kishk SM, Kahrilas PJ, Hogan WJ. Radiologic amyl nitrite test for distinguishing pseudoachalasia from idiopathic achalasia. Am J Roentgenol 1986;146:21

26. Dodds WJ, Stewart ET, Logemann JA. Physiology and radiology of the normal oral and pharyngeal phases of swallowing. Am J Roentgenol 1990;154:953

27. Dodds WJ, Stewart ET, Vlymen WJ. Appropriate contrast media for evaluation of esophageal disruption. Radiology 1982;144:439

28. Ekberg O, Nylander G. Cineradiography of the pharyngeal stage of deglutition in 150 individuals without dysphagia. Br J Radiol 1982; 55:253

29. Ekberg O, Nylander G. Dysfunction of the cricopharyngeal muscle. Radiology 1982;143:481

30. Fenoglio-Preiser CM, Lantz PE, Listrom MB, Davis M, Rilke FO. The neoplastic esophagus. In Gastrointestinal Pathology—An Atlas and Text. New York: Raven Press, 1989:85

31. Fenoglio-Preiser CM, Lantz PE, Listrom MB, Davis M, Rilke FO. The non-neoplastic esophagus. In Gastrointestinal Pathology—An Atlas and Text. New York: Raven Press 1989:33

32. Frederick MG, Ott DJ, Grishaw EK, Gelfand DW, Chen MYM. Functional abnormalities of the pharynx: a prospective analysis of radiographic abnormalities relative to age and symptoms. Am J Roentgenol 1996;166:353

33. Friedland GW, Filly R. The postcricoid impression masquerading as an esophageal tumor. Am J Dig Dis 1975;20:287

34. Gelfand DW, Ott DJ. Anatomy and technique in evaluating the esophagus. Semin Roentgenol 1981;16:168

35. Gerson DE, Lewicki AM. Intrathoracic stomach—when does it obstruct? Radiology 1976;119:257

36. Ghahremani GG, Rushovich AM. Glycogenic acanthosis of the esophagus: radiographic and pathologic features. Gastrointest Radiol 1984; 9:93

37. Gohel VK, Edell SL, Laufer I, Rhodes WH. Transverse folds in the human esophagus. Radiology 1978;128:303

38. Goodman P, Pinero SS, Rance RM, Mansell PW, Uribe-Botero G. Mycobacterial esophagitis in AIDS. Gastrointest Radiol 1989;14:103

39. Green WE, Castell DO. The upper esophageal sphincter. In Castell DO, Richter JE, Dalton CB, eds, Esophageal Motility Testing. New York: Elsevier Science 1987:183

40. Grishaw EK, Ott DJ, Frederick MG, Gelfand DW, Chen MYM. Functional abnormalities of the esophagus: a prospective analysis of radiographic findings relative to age and symptoms. Am J Roentgenol 1996;167:719

41. Halpert RD, Feczko PJ, Spickler EM, Ackerman LV. Radiological assessment of dysphagia with endoscopic correlation. Radiology 1985;157:599

42. Hollis JB, Castell DO. Esophageal function in elderly men—a new look at ''presbyesophagus.'' Ann Intem Med 1974;80:371

43. Jones B. The pharynx—disorders of function. Radiol Clin North Am 1994;32:1103

44. Jones B, Gayler BW, Donner MW. Pharynx and cervical esophagus. In Levine MS, ed, Radiology of the Esophagus. Philadelphia: WB Saunders, 1989:311

45. Kaszar-Seibert DJ, Korn WT, Bindman DJ, Shortsleeve MJ. Treatment of acute esophageal food impaction with a combination of glucagon, effervescent agent, and water. Am J Roentgenol 1990;154:533

46. Katz PO. Achalasia. In Castell DO, Richter JE, Dalton CB, eds, Esophageal Motility Testing. New York: Elsevier Science, 1987:107

47. Khan TA, Shragge BW, Crispin JS, Lind JE. Esophageal motility in the elderly. Dig Dis Sci 1977;22:1049

48. Kimmey MB, Martin RW, Haggitt RC, Wang KY, Franklin DW, Silverstein FE. Histologic correlates of gastrointestinal ultrasound images. Gastroenterology 1989;96:433

49. Koehler RE, Memel DS, Stanley RJ. Gastrointestinal tract. In Lee JK, Sagel SS, Stanley RJ, Heiken JP, eds, Computed Body Tomography with MRI Correlation (3rd ed). New York: Lippincott-Raven, 1998:637

50. Lepke RA, Libshitz HI. Radiation-induced injury of the esophagus. Radiology 1983;148:375

51. Levine MS. Barrett's esophagus: a radiologic diagnosis? Am J Roentgenol 1988;151:433

52. Levine MS. Benign tumors. In Gore RM, Levine MS, Laufer I, eds, Textbook of Gastrointestinal Radiology, vol 1. Philadelphia: WB Saunders, 1994:431

53. Levine MS. Gastroesophageal junction. In Gore RM, Levine MS, Laufer I, eds, Textbook of Gastrointestinal Radiology, vol 1. Philadelphia: WB Saunders, 1994:531

54. Levine MS. Gastroesophageal reflux disease. In Gore RM, Levine MS, Laufer I, eds, Textbook of Gastrointestinal Radiology, vol 1. Philadelphia: WB Saunders, 1994:360

55. Levine MS. Infectious esophagitis. In Gore RM, Levine MS, Laufer I, eds, Textbook of Gastrointestinal Radiology, vol 1. Philadelphia: WB Saunders, 1994:385

56. Levine MS. Miscellaneous abnormalities. In Gore RM, Levine MS, Laufer I, eds, Textbook of Gastrointestinal Radiology, vol 1. Philadelphia: WB Saunders, 1994:512

57. Levine MS. Other esophagitides. In Gore RM, Levine MS, Laufer I, eds, Textbook of Gastrointestinal Radiology, vol 1. Philadelphia: WB Saunders, 1994:403

58. Levine MS. Other malignant tumors. In Gore RM, Levine MS, Laufer I, eds, Textbook of Gastrointestinal Radiology, vol 1. Philadelphia: WB Saunders, 1994:479

59. Levine MS. Postoperative esophagus. In Gore RM, Levine MS, Laufer I, eds, Textbook of Gastrointestinal Radiology, vol 1. Philadelphia: WB Saunders, 1994:542

60. Levine MS. Varices. In Gore RM, Levine MS, Laufer I, eds, Textbook of Gastrointestinal Radiology, vol 1. Philadelphia: WB Saunders, 1994:499

61. Levine MS, Chu P, Furth EE, Rubesin SE, Laufer I, Herlinger H. Carcinoma of the esophagus and esophagogastric junction: sensitivity of radiographic diagnosis. Am J Roentgenol 1997;168:1423

62. Levine MS, Dillon EC, Saul SH, Laufer I. Early esophageal cancer. Am J Roentgenol 1986;146:507

63. Levine MS, Halvorsen RA. Esophageal carcinoma. In Gore RM, Levine MS, Laufer I, eds, Textbook of Gastrointestinal Radiology, vol 1. Philadelphia: WB Saunders, 1994:446

64. Levine MS, Herman JB, Furth EE. Barrett's esophagus and esophageal adenocarcinoma: the scope of the problem. Abdom Imaging 1995;20:291

65. Levine MS, Kressel HY, Caroline DF, Laufer I, Herlinger H, Thompson JJ. Barrett esophagus: reticular pattern of the mucosa. Radiology 1983;147:663

66. Levine MS, Loercher G, Katzka DA, Herlinger H, Rubesin SE, Laufer I. Giant, human immunodeficiency virus-related ulcers in the esophagus. Radiology 1991;180:323

67. Levine MS, Loevner LA, Saul SH, Rubesin SE, Herlinger H, Laufer I. Herpes esophagitis: sensitivity of double-contrast esophagography. Am J Roentgenol 1988;151:57

68. Levine MS, Macones AJ Jr, Laufer I. Candida esophagitis: accuracy of radiographic diagnosis. Radiology 1985;154:581

69. Levine MS, Moolten DN, Herlinger H, Laufer I. Esophageal intramural pseudodiverticulosis: a reevaluation. Am J Roentgenol 1986; 146:1165

70. Levine MS, Woldenberg R, Herlinger H, Laufer I. Opportunistic esophagitis in AIDS: radiographic diagnosis. Radiology 1987;165: 815

71. Massey BT, et al. Abnormal esophageal motility—an analysis of concurrent radiographic and manometric findings. Gastroenterology 1991;101:344

72. Mittal RK, Balaban DH. The esophagogastric junction. N Engl J Med 1997;336:924

73. Mittal RK, Siskind BN, Hongo M, Flye MW, McCallum RW. Dysphagia aortica—clinical, radiological, and manometric findings. Dig Dis Sci 1986;31:379

74. Nosher JL, Campbell WL, Seaman WB. The clinical significance of cervical esophageal and hypopharyngeal webs. Radiology 1975;117: 45

75. Olsson R, Ekberg O. Videomanometry of the pharynx in dysphagic patients with a posterior cricopharyngeal indentation. Acad Radiol 1995;2:597

76. Ott DJ. Radiologic evaluation of the esophagus. In Castell DO, Johnson LF, eds, Esophageal Function in Health and Disease. New York: Elsevier Science 1983:211

77. Ott DJ. Barium esophagram. In Castell DO, Wu WC, Ott DJ, eds, Gastroesophageal Reflux Disease. Mt Kisco: Futura, 1985:109

77A. Ott DJ. Radiologic evaluation of esophageal dysphagia. Curr Probl Diagn Radiol 1988;17:1

78. Ott DJ. Radiographic techniques and efficacy in evaluating esophageal dysphagia. Dysphagia 1990;5:192

79. Ott DJ. The esophagus: diaphragmatic hernias. In Taveras JM, Ferrucci JT, eds, Radiology: Diagnosis, Imaging, Intervention, vol 4. Philadelphia: JB Lippincott Co, 1993:1

80. Ott DJ. Motility disorders of the esophagus. Radiol Clin North Am 1994;32:1117

81. Ott DJ. Gastroesophageal reflux disease. Radiol Clin North Am 1994; 32:1147

82. Ott DJ. Gastroesophageal reflux: what is the role of barium studies? Am J Roentgenol 1994;162:627

83. Ott DJ. Pharynx and esophagus. In Ott DJ, Gelfand DW, Chen MYM, eds, Manual of Gastrointestinal Fluoroscopy. Springfield, IL: Charles C. Thomas Publisher, 1996:24

84. Ott DJ, et al. Esophageal motility: assessment with synchronous videotape fluoroscopy and manometry. Radiology 1989;173:419

85. Ott DJ, Chen YM, Gelfand DW, Munitz HA, Wu WC. Analysis of a multiphasic, radiographic examination for detecting reflux esophagitis. Gastrointest Radiol 1986;11:1

86. Ott DJ, Chen YM, Wu WC, Gelfand DW. Endoscopic sensitivity in the detection of esophageal strictures. J Clin Gastroenterol 1985;7: 121

87. Ott DJ, Chen YM, Wu WC, Gelfand DW, Munitz HA. Radiographic and endoscopic sensitivity in detecting lower esophageal mucosal ring. Am J Roentgenol 1986;147:261

88. Ott DJ, Donati D, Wu WC, Chen MYM, Gelfand DW. Radiographic evaluation of achalasia immediately after pneumatic dilatation with the Rigiflex dilator. Gastrointest Radiol 1991;16:279

89. Ott DJ, Gelfand DW. Esophageal stricture secondary to candidiasis. Gastrointest Radiol 1978;2:323

90. Ott DJ, Gelfand DW. Gastrointestinal contrast agents indications, uses, and risks. JAMA 1983;249:2380

91. Ott DJ, Gelfand DW, Lane TG, Wu WC. Radiologic detection and spectrum of appearances of peptic esophageal stricture. J Clin Gastroenterol 1982;4:11

92. Ott DJ, Gelfand DW, Munitz HA, Chen YM. Cold barium suspensions in the clinical evaluation of the esophagus. Gastrointest Radiol 1984; 9:193

93. Ott DJ, Gelfand DW, Wu WC, Castell DO. Esophagogastric region and its rings. Am J Roentgenol 1984;142:281

94. Ott DJ, Glauser SJ, Ledbetter MS, Chen MYM, Koufman JA, Gelfand DW. Association of hiatal hernia and gastroesophageal reflux: correlation between presence and size of hiatal hernia and 24-hour pH monitoring of the esophagus. Am J Roentgenol 1995;165:557

95. Ott DJ, Hodge RG, Chen MYM, Wu WC, Gelfand DW. Achalasia associated with hiatal hernia: prevalence and potential implications. Abdom Imaging 1993;18:7

96. Ott DJ, Katz PO, Wu WC. Anti-reflux barrier. In Castell DO, Wu WC, Ott DJ, eds, Gastroesophageal Reflux Disease. Mt Kisco: Futura, 1985:35

97. Ott DJ, Kelley TF, Chen MYM, Gelfand DW. Evaluation of the esophagus with a marshmallow bolus: clarifying the cause of dysphagia. Gastrointest Radiol 1991;16:1

98. Ott DJ, Kelley TF, Chen MYM, Gelfand DW, Wu WC. Use of a marshmallow bolus for evaluating lower esophageal mucosal rings. Am J Gastroenterol 1991;86:817

98a. Ott DJ, et al. Endoscopic ultrasonography of benign esophageal cyst simulating leiomyoma. J Clin Gastroenterol 1992;15:85

99. Ott DJ, McManus CM, Ledbetter MS, Chen MYM, Gelfand DW. Heartburn correlated to 24-hour pH monitoring and radiographic examination of the esophagus. Am J Gastroenterol 1997;92:1827

100. Ott DJ, Pikna LA. Clinical and videofluoroscopic evaluation of swallowing disorders. Am J Roentgenol 1993;161:507

101. Ott DJ, Richter JE, Chen YM, Wu WC, Gelfand DW, Castell DO. Esophageal radiography and manometry: correlation in 172 patients with dysphagia. Am J Roentgenol 1987;149:307

102. Ott DJ, Richter JE, Chen YM, Wu WC, Gelfand DW, Castell DO. Radiographic and manometric correlation in achalasia with apparent relaxation of the lower esophageal sphincter. Gastrointest Radiol 1989;14:1

103. Ott DJ, Richter JE, Wu WC, Chen YM, Castell DO, Gelfand DW. Radiographic evaluation of esophagus immediately after pneumatic dilatation for achalasia. Dig Dis Sci 1987;32:962

104. Ott DJ, Richter JE, Wu WC, Chen YM, Gelfand DW, Castell DO. Radiologic and manometric correlation in "nutcracker esophagus." Am J Roentgenol 1986;147:692

105. Ott DJ, Wu WC, Gelfand DW. Efficacy of radiology of the esophagus for evaluation of dysphagia. Gastrointest Radiol 1981;6:109

106. Ott DJ, Wu WC, Gelfand DW. Reflux esophagitis revisited: prospective analysis of radiologic accuracy. Gastrointest Radiol 1981;6:1

107. Ponette E, Coolen J. Radiological aspects of Zenker's diverticulum. Hepatogastroenterology 1992;39:115

108. Reeders JW, Bartelsman JF. Radiological diagnosis and preoperative staging of oesophageal malignancies. Endoscopy 1993;25:10

109. Richter JE. Diffuse esophageal spasm. In Castell DO, Richter JE, Dalton CB, eds, Esophageal Motility Testing. New York: Elsevier Science, 1987:118

110. Richter JE, et al. Esophageal manometry in 95 healthy adult volunteers. Dig Dis Sci 1987;32:583

111. Rubesin SE. The pharynx—structural disorders. Radiol Clin North Am 1994;32:1083

112. Saunders HS, Wolfman NT, Ott DJ. Esophageal cancer—radiologic staging. Radiol Clin North Am 1997;35:281

113. Schatzki R. The lower esophageal ring—long term follow-up of symptomatic and asymptomatic rings. Am J Roentgenol 1963;90:805

114. Schatzki R, Gary JE. Dysphagia due to a diaphragm-like localized narrowing in the lower esophagus ("lower esophageal ring"). Am J Roentgenol 1953;70:911

115. Scobey MW. Secondary motility disorders. In Castell DO, Richter JE, Dalton CB, eds, Esophageal Motility Testing. New York: Elsevier Science, 1987:163

116. Shortsleeve MJ, Levine MS. Herpes esophagitis in otherwise healthy patients: clinical and radiographic findings. Radiology 1992;182:859

117. Sloan S, Kahrilas PJ. Impairment of esophageal emptying with hiatal hernia. Gastroenterology 1991;100:596

118. Styles RA, Gibb SP, Tarshis A, Silverman ML, Scholz FJ. Esophagogastric polyps: radiographic and endoscopic findings. Radiology 1985;154:307

119. Thompson JK, Koehler RE, Richter JE. Detection of gastroesophageal reflux: value of barium studies compared with 24-hr pH monitoring. Am J Roentgenol 1994;162:621

120. Tihansky DP, Reilly JJ, Schade RR, Van Thiel DH. The esophagus after injection sclerotherapy of varices. Radiology 1984;153:43

121. Tio TL, Tytgat GNJ, den Hartog Jager FC. Endoscopic ultrasonogra-

phy for the evaluation of smooth muscle tumors in the upper gastrointestinal tract: an experience with 42 cases. Gastrointest Endosc 1990; 36:342

122. Vahey TN, Maglinte DDT, Chemish SM. State-of-the-art barium examination in opportunistic esophagitis. Dig Dis Sci 1986;31:1192

123. Vincent ME, Robbins AH, Walsh M, Vaughan C. Evaluation of Blom-Singer voice prosthesis. Am J Roentgenol 1984;143:745

124. Watemberg S, Landau O, Avrahami R. Zenker's diverticulum: reappraisal. Am J Gastroenterol 1996;91:1494

125. Wiener GJ, et al. Ambulatory 24-hour esophageal pH monitoring—reproducibility and variability of pH parameters. Dig Dis Sci 1988;33:1127

126. Williford ME, Rice RP, Kelvin FM, Fisher SR, Meyers WC, Thompson WM. Revascularized jejunal graft replacing the cervical esophagus: radiographic evaluation. Am J Roentgenol 1985;145:533

127. Wippold FJ II. Neck. In Lee JK, Sagel SS, Stanley RJ, Heiken JP, eds, Computed Body Tomography with MRI Correlation (3rd ed). New York: Lippincott-Raven, 1998:107

128. Wolfman NT, Scharling ES, Chen MYM. Esophageal squamous carcinoma. Radiol Clin North Am 1994;32:1183

129. Zboralske FF, Amberg JR, Soergel KH. Presbyesophagus: cineradiographic manifestations. Radiology 1964;82:463

129a. Zboralske FF, Friedland GW. Diseases of the esophagus—present concepts. West J Med 1970;112:33

130. Zerhouni EA, Bosma JF, Donner MW. Relationship of cervical spine disorders to dysphagia. Dysphagia 1987;1:129

*The Esophagus*, Third Edition,
edited by D. O. Castell and J. E. Richter.
Lippincott Williams & Wilkins, Philadelphia © 1999.

# CHAPTER 4

# Endoscopy

Steven A. Edmundowicz

Endoscopic evaluation of the esophagus has evolved from a rarely used, invasive procedure to a standard outpatient diagnostic test. As an extension of the physical examination, it has become the gold standard for the detection of all mucosal and most structural disorders of the esophagus. Endoscopy has become so prominent in the diagnosis and management of esophageal disease that it is difficult to imagine patient care without this technology. In the last decade, exciting new developments in endoscopy-related technologies have allowed us to imagine beyond the mucosa of the esophagus. At the same time, the evolution of flexible endoscopic therapeutic techniques has led to the development of significant new, minimally invasive treatment alternatives for patients with esophageal disorders.

This evolution of the diagnostic and therapeutic capabilities of modern endoscopy has been the cumulative result of the work of many innovative individuals who have furthered endoscopic development over the past 150 years. Their combined efforts are described in historical works that delineate the development of the modern videoendoscope from the steel tube that was first introduced in 1868 to visualize the esophagus and stomach [15, 55]. Current upper endoscopes are sophisticated instruments that provide high-quality video images, improved flexibility, and smaller-diameter insertion tubes [12, 63] (Figs. 4–1, 4–2). These changes allow for improved diagnostic abilities, more extensive options for image documentation and transmission, and easier delivery of endoscopic therapies. In addition, endoscopes have been specifically modified to incorporate ultrasound transducers and adapted to allow for band ligation, suturing, and mucosal resections. The current armamentarium of endoscopic devices is extensive and growing rapidly as modifications of new technologies that can be applied to the esophagus continue to evolve [67].

## THE TECHNIQUE OF ENDOSCOPY OF THE ESOPHAGUS

The technique of diagnostic upper endoscopy has not changed significantly in the past decade. Most patients can easily undergo upper endoscopy with minimal effort and preparation. Relative contraindications to upper endoscopy are listed in Table 4–1. While patient preparation, facilities, and certain aspects of endoscopy may vary by region, the procedure is essentially performed in the same manner at all locations. A number of different endoscope manufacturers provide instruments, which vary slightly in design and characteristics. In general, they appear to be well suited for diagnostic upper endoscopy. For those not familiar with the procedure, diagnostic upper endoscopy has been described in detail by several authors [1, 13].

Examination of the esophagus by endoscopy begins with insertion of the endoscope into the posterior pharynx. The posterior pharynx and larynx are examined for abnormalities (see Chapter 28). The endoscope is advanced under direct vision into the upper esophageal sphincter, and the patient is instructed to swallow. With relaxation of the sphincter, the endoscope is advanced into the upper esophagus and the mucosa is carefully examined. The esophageal mucosa is continuously examined for abnormalities as the endoscope is slowly advanced. Extrinsic compression of the esophagus by the aortic arch, right atrium, or right ventricle may be noted. The area of the gastroesophageal junction is carefully examined to document the location of the Z line or ora serrata. This is the transition point between squamous (esophageal) and columnar (gastric) mucosa. This area should be examined for irregularities of the Z line that might signify Barrett's esophagus. The endoscope should then be advanced into the stomach and the cardia examined in retroflexion to visualize a hiatal hernia or other abnormality of the cardia.

Several situations require special consideration when endoscopy is employed to evaluate patients with suspected spe-

S. A. Edmundowicz: Department of Medicine, Graduate Hospital, Philadelphia, Pennsylvania 19146.

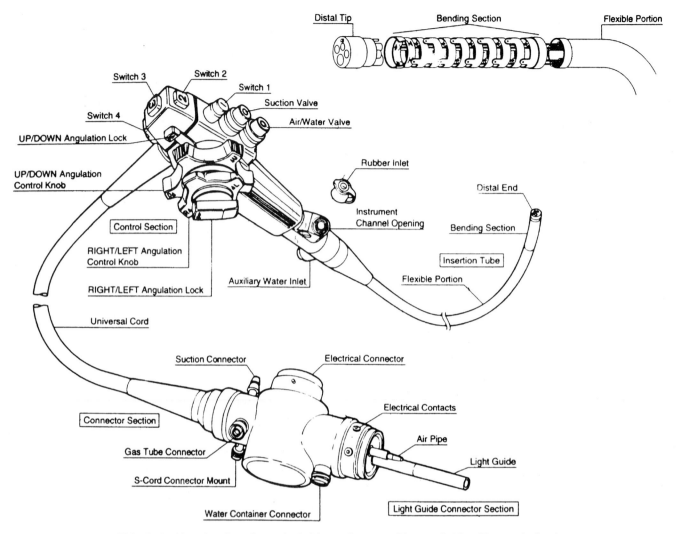

Distal Tip    Bending Section    Flexible Portion

Switch 3    Switch 2    Switch 1
Switch 4    Suction Valve
UP/DOWN Angulation Lock    Air/Water Valve
UP/DOWN Angulation Control Knob    Rubber Inlet    Distal End
Control Section    Instrument Channel Opening    Bending Section
RIGHT/LEFT Angulation Control Knob    Insertion Tube
RIGHT/LEFT Angulation Lock    Auxiliary Water Inlet    Flexible Portion
Universal Cord
Suction Connector    Electrical Connector
Connector Section    Electrical Contacts
Gas Tube Connector    Air Pipe
S-Cord Connector Mount    Light Guide
Water Container Connector    Light Guide Connector Section

**FIG. 4–1.** Line drawing of a typical videoendoscope. (From ref. 12, with permission.)

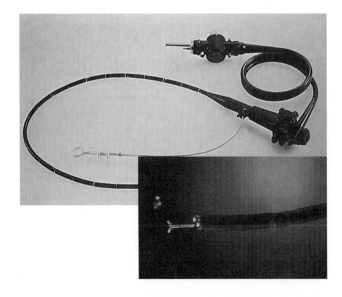

**FIG. 4–2.** Photograph of a videoendoscope for upper endoscopy. Inset: Biopsy forceps in position through the biopsy channel. (Courtesy Olympus Corporation, Tokyo, Japan.)

**TABLE 4–1.** *Relative contraindications to upper endoscopy*

Medically unstable patient (i.e., marked hypotension, acute myocardial infarction, respiratory distress)
Unstable cervical spine
Coagulopathy, unresponsive to therapy
Known or suspected perforation of the gastrointestinal tract

cific esophageal disorders. Patients with suspected achalasia should have a prolonged fast preceded by a clear liquid diet for 24 to 48 hours to allow any food matter to pass into the stomach prior to endoscopy (see Chapter 10). Large-bore tube lavage may be required to remove semisolid material that does not pass spontaneously into the stomach. The staff assisting with the endoscopy should be prepared to suction the oropharynx and prevent aspiration. Similar precautions should be used in patients with significant dysphagia. They may have structural abnormalities of the upper esophagus that could increase the risk of perforation and/or aspiration. If a recent barium study is not available, caution should be used in passing the endoscope. If patients have severe dysphagia for solids, it may be advantageous to schedule the procedure with the availability of fluoroscopy to assist in dilatation if a significant stricture is encountered. Patients with a known or suspected Zenker's diverticulum should also be endoscoped with caution as the lumen of the esophagus may be difficult to identify and follow. Forceful manipulation of the endoscope inside the diverticulum could lead to perforation (see Chapter 15).

## DIAGNOSTIC UPPER ENDOSCOPY

The refinement of the endoscope and ancillary diagnostic techniques has led to an increased ability to diagnose and treat patients with diseases of the esophagus. The ability to inspect the mucosa of the esophagus alone is extremely useful in characterizing and classifying many of the disorders discussed in this text. The addition of biopsy and brush cytology techniques further augments this ability. The use of absorptive stains that are sprayed on the mucosa during endoscopy has been described by several groups and can assist in the detection and definition of abnormalities. Endoscopic ultrasonography has expanded the diagnostic capabilities of endoscopists by imaging the wall layers of the esophagus as well as the surrounding structures. Additional techniques that appear to have endoscopic applications include molecular biologic investigation of specimens obtained at endoscopy, tissue autofluorescence, and magnetic resonance imaging during endoscopy.

Imaging of the esophageal mucosa during endoscopy is extremely useful in clarifying symptoms. Fiberoptic technology allows the endoscopist to view the mucosa of the esophagus with excellent detail and resolution. High-resolution video images allow the endoscopist and others in the endoscopy suite to view mucosal irregularities with great conve-

nience and excellent image quality. While the appearance of some abnormalities may be unique enough to lead to a specific diagnosis, most abnormalities will require histologic or cytologic confirmation. This can be easily accomplished with standard biopsy techniques or brush cytology.

Biopsy forceps are utilized to obtain tissue at endoscopy. Forceps vary by size, style, and design. Adequate mucosal sampling can be obtained with most standard biopsy forceps. Certain endoscopic maneuvers, such as the "turn and suction" technique [38], may be used to increase the biopsy size. Jumbo, or large-capacity, forceps are available from several manufacturers. Jumbo forceps require an endoscope with a 3.2-mm diameter biopsy channel. These accessories also allow the endoscopist to obtain larger (but not necessarily deeper) samples of mucosa and submucosa for histologic evaluation [3].

Brush cytology is routinely performed in all areas of the gastrointestinal (GI) tract with specially designed disposable brushes [6]. The sheathed cytology brush is advanced through the biopsy channel of the endoscope and placed in contact with the mucosa to be examined. Vigorous motion of the brush against the mucosa allows cells to be captured on the bristles of the brush. The brush is then retracted into its sheath and removed from the endoscope. The brush is then placed in contact with a glass slide, and the captured cells are transferred to its surface. The slide is treated with a fixative and submitted to the cytologist for staining. Malignancy [6], infections, dysplasia, and even *Helicobacter pylori* [43] can be detected by brush cytology (see Chapter 8).

Submucosal lesions may be identified at endoscopy and confirmed with endoscopic ultrasound. Ultrasound confirmation of the submucosal and nonvascular nature of the lesion is essential, especially if aggressive biopsy techniques are contemplated. Fine needle aspiration [66] or deep biopsy of these lesions may reveal a specific diagnosis with minimal additional risk. "Core" biopsies (repeated biopsy of the same site to obtain a deeper specimen) may be utilized to obtain tissue from submucosal lesions when standard techniques fail [66].

Chromoscopy has been useful during endoscopy of the esophagus. The use of two absorptive stains in the evaluation of esophageal disorders has recently been reviewed [17]. Lugol's solution will stain normal esophageal mucosa containing glycogen dark green-brown. Any abnormality of the squamous epithelium that does not contain glycogen (carcinoma, intestinal metaplasia, and inflammation) will appear unstained when the dye is sprayed throughout the mucosa [17]. Up to 50 mL of a 1% solution can be sprayed onto the mucosa during endoscopy to detect subtle areas of abnormality. Lugol's iodine has been used to detect early carcinoma of the esophagus and areas of dysplasia [17] (see Chapter 12, Fig. 12–12). Methylene blue is another stain that will be taken up by actively absorbing epithelial cells. While normal esophageal epithelium will not absorb methylene blue, areas of intestinal metaplasia will. Canto et al. [7] have recently described the use of methylene blue dye sprayed during endoscopy to help delineate areas of intestinal metaplasia in patients with Barrett's esophagus. The mucosa is prepared by applying a mucolytic, 20 mL of 10% *N*-acetylcysteine (Mucomyst). Methylene blue in a 0.5% to 1.0% solution is then sprayed on the mucosa to highlight areas of intestinal metaplasia [7]. Dye spraying is a quick, easy technique to employ and may provide additional diagnostic information with minimal cost or time requirements.

Endoscopic ultrasonography has added another diagnostic dimension to endoscopy of the esophagus. This technology allows placement of a specialized ultrasound transducer in close proximity to the abnormality to be studied. This results in high-resolution images of the esophageal wall and adjacent structures (see Chapter 3). Currently available ultrasound technologies include dedicated endoscope systems and through-the-scope miniprobes (Figs. 4–3, 4–4, Color Plate 1). These devices are attached to an ultrasound processor that includes a control panel to manipulate the ultrasound image on a high-resolution monitor. The oldest and most commonly used system for the evaluation of esophageal disease is the Olympus (Tokyo, Japan) 360-degree sector-scanning instrument operating at 7.5 and 12 MHz. This system provides excellent images of the esophageal wall and adjacent structures. A modified sector-scanning endoscope has recently been made available for ultrasound-guided needle biopsies [58]. This device uses the same ultrasound processor as the other Olympus sector scanners, with an acoustic mirror to alter the ultrasound orientation to allow guided

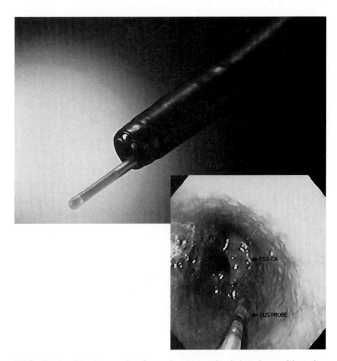

**FIG. 4–4.** Photograph of an ultrasound miniprobe exiting the biopsy channel of a therapeutic upper endoscope. Inset: Endoscopic ultrasound miniprobe in position in the esophagus for staging of a malignant stricture.

needle aspiration. Its clinical utility has been reported in one series [58]. Miniprobes are available in 7 French 360-degree sector-scanning catheters imaging at 12 and 20 MHz. These devices are passed through a therapeutic endoscope or advanced blindly into the esophagus. They can be utilized with the same image processor as the previously mentioned Olympus sector-scanning instruments. The miniprobes provide excellent resolution of the esophageal wall but have a limited depth of penetration [10]. They are best utilized for imaging mucosal and small submucosal abnormalities involving the esophageal wall. They can be used to investigate the lower esophageal sphincter, varices, and Barrett's epithelium, in addition to other superficial processes.

Two dedicated endoscope systems with curved linear array transducers are currently available. Both systems require the purchase of a dedicated ultrasound processor that may have Doppler capabilities. The Pentax endoscope (see Chapter 12) has been widely used and allows ultrasound-guided fine needle aspiration of submucosal masses and adjacent lesions [68]. The Olympus system has recently been released and should offer similar capabilities with the advantage of a larger biopsy channel [5]. Both devices are designed primarily for ultrasound guidance during fine needle aspiration procedures. The Pentax device has been used to identify and sample periesophageal lymph nodes in patients with lung cancer [68]. These devices can be used to identify and target lymph nodes or lesions in the tissues adjacent to the upper GI tract.

Endoscopic ultrasonography has many applications in the

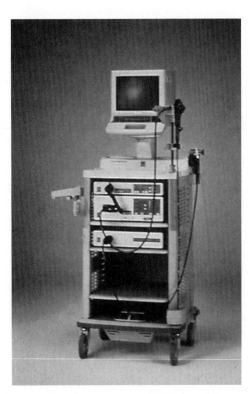

**FIG. 4–3.** Photograph of the Olympus EUM-30 endoscopic ultrasound system. (Courtesy Olympus Corporation, Tokyo, Japan.)

evaluation of esophageal disorders [11, 65]. This technique has been demonstrated to be particularly useful in the evaluation of esophageal malignancy and potentially metastatic lymph nodes in the periesophageal and celiac axis regions [52]. Preoperative staging of esophageal malignancies can be accomplished with these technologies with superior accuracy when compared to other imaging modalities [52]. Endoscopic ultrasonography also has a role in the evaluation of patients after radiation and chemotherapy if surgery is contemplated [26]. It may also be a sensitive modality to detect recurrent cancer in patients who have undergone resection [39].

## OTHER DIAGNOSTIC MODALITIES

Tissue spectroscopy is a technology that is in the early stages of clinical development [47]. One may use the specific characteristics of autofluorescence of tissue when exposed to a frequency of laser light to identify dysplastic mucosa. This technology has been used in patients with Barrett's esophagus to identify those individuals with high-grade dysplasia [49]. If the modifications of this technique prove to be effective and are confirmed by others, one would be able to obtain an ''optical biopsy'' of a region at the time of endoscopy. This technique may be used to direct endoscopic biopsy or other therapies.

A magnetic resonance endoscope has been used in animals and humans to image the GI wall [16, 35]. The technology appears to be capable of imaging the wall layers of the GI tract as well as adjacent structures. Further study is needed to determine the clinical utility of magnetic resonance endoscopy.

Molecular biologic testing has also influenced the way in which we perform diagnostic endoscopy. Endoscopists may now sample the mucosa of the esophagus to obtain DNA for analysis. This type of analysis is being used in Barrett's esophagus and other disorders [53]. Esophageal specimens can also be analyzed in the molecular biology lab for evidence of viral or fungal infections.

## ENDOSCOPIC FINDINGS IN COMMON ESOPHAGEAL DISORDERS

### Gastroesophageal Reflux Disease

Patients with symptoms of gastroesophageal reflux disease (GERD) are often evaluated with endoscopy to document the presence and extent of reflux disease and to exclude other diagnoses. The endoscopic findings in GERD can range from normal-appearing mucosa to severe esophagitis with ulcerations or stricture formation. The inflammatory changes in GERD should always involve the Z line and distal esophagus. Isolated inflammatory changes in other areas of the esophagus without involvement of the esophageal mucosa that is adjacent to the Z line should suggest other etiologies, such as medication-induced or infectious esophagitis.

Several classification systems have been devised to more accurately define or grade reflux changes by using characteristics seen at endoscopy [51]. Each classification scheme has specific advantages and disadvantages. By their nature, they all have some inter- and intra-observer variability. Two of the more commonly used classification systems are the Savary-Miller New Endoscopic Grading System [48], listed in Table 4–2, and that used by Hetzel et al. [25], listed in Table 4–3. Examples of the different grades of GERD are demonstrated in Color Plates 2 and 3. Mucosal biopsy at endoscopy may detect changes of reflux esophagitis even when the endoscopic appearance of the esophagus is normal (see Chapter 8).

### Barrett's Esophagus

In general terms, Barrett's esophagus is a condition in which a gastric-type columnar epithelium replaces the normal squamous epithelial lining of the esophagus. This is recognized endoscopically as the presence of salmon pink-appearing gastric mucosa in the distal esophagus (Color Plate 4). The ectopic mucosa may have one of several appearances in the distal esophagus, including a confluent and circumferential pattern, irregular finger-like extensions, or isolated islands of gastric-type mucosa surrounded by squamous epithelium (Color Plates 5 and 6). The diagnosis of this ectopic gastric mucosa is made at endoscopy and is dependent on the endoscopist's ability to identify the anatomic gastroesophageal junction and the squamocolumnar–mucosal junction. The anatomic gastroesophageal junction is clinically defined at the location of the proximal margin of the gastric folds. This can be accurately localized in most patients. The anatomic gastroesophageal junction can be difficult to localize in patients with hiatal hernia. Alternatively, the histologic confirmation of specialized columnar epithelium (intestinal metaplasia with goblet cells) at any location in the esophagus is diagnostic of Barrett's. An area of isolated ectopic gastric mucosa in the upper esophagus at the level of the upper esophageal sphincter is known as an inlet patch (Color Plate 7). This is identified in almost 4% of patients undergoing diagnostic endoscopy when the mucosa of the upper esophageal sphincter is care-

TABLE 4–2. *Savary-Miller New Endoscopic Grading System*

| Grade I | Single, erosive, or exudative lesion; oval or linear; taking only one longitudinal fold |
|---|---|
| Grade II | Noncircular, multiple erosion or exudative lesion taking more than one longitudinal fold, with or without confluence |
| Grade III | Circular erosive or exudative lesion |
| Grade IV | Chronic lesions: ulcers, strictures, or short esophagus, isolated or associated with lesion grades I–III |
| Grade V | Barrett's epithelium isolated or associated with lesion grades I–III |

**TABLE 4–3.** *Classification system of Hetzel et al. [25]*

| | |
|---|---|
| Grade 0 | Normal-appearing mucosal endoscopy |
| Grade 1 | Mucosal edema, hyperemia, and/or friability of mucosa |
| Grade 2 | Superficial erosions involving <10% of mucosal surface of last 5 cm of esophageal squamous mucosa |
| Grade 3 | Superficial erosions/ulcerations involving 10% to 50% of distal esophagus |
| Grade 4 | Deep peptic ulceration anywhere in the esophagus or confluent erosion of >50% of the distal esophageal squamous mucosa |

fully examined [28]. The inlet patch is usually an incidental finding; however, rare complications of focal ulceration, stricture, and even adenocarcinoma have been reported [8, 59]. Figure 4–10 demonstrates the typical appearance of an inlet patch. The endoscopic aspects of Barrett's esophagus are discussed in detail in Chapter 26.

## Esophageal Infections

Endoscopic examination of the esophagus with tissue sampling by cytology or biopsy is the primary diagnostic modality for esophageal infections. The pathogens that lead to infectious esophagitis, their pathophysiology, and therapy are discussed in detail in Chapter 33. The endoscopic characteristics of candidiasis (Color Plate 8) and herpes simplex virus (Color Plate 9) are also discussed in Chapter 33.

## Pill-induced Esophageal Injury

Medication-induced esophageal injury has become increasingly identified as a major cause of focal esophagitis and esophageal ulceration. Pill-induced esophagitis is discussed in detail in Chapter 32. Color Plate 10 demonstrates a pill-induced ulceration with stricture formation.

## Esophageal Rings and Webs

Esophageal rings and webs are discussed in detail in Chapter 14. The endoscopic appearance of an esophageal web is shown in Color Plate 11. A Schatzki ring is demonstrated in Color Plate 12.

## Mallory-Weiss Tear

The Mallory-Weiss tear is a fissure-like mucosal tear located at the gastroesophageal junction. It is the third most common cause of upper GI bleeding, following peptic ulcer and varices [40]. The classic history of vomiting followed by hematemesis is reported in only one-third to one-half of patients presenting with bleeding Mallory-Weiss tears [40]. The typical appearance of a Mallory-Weiss tear is shown in Color Plate 13.

Additional endoscopic findings of many of the esophageal

disorders discussed in this textbook are reviewed in their respective chapters.

## THERAPEUTIC ENDOSCOPY OF THE ESOPHAGUS

### Esophageal Hemorrhage

Endoscopy has become the primary method for evaluation and treatment of GI bleeding. Early endoscopic examination of the esophagus in patients with suspected hemorrhage could identify the site as well as the status of GI bleeding. In addition, extremely effective hemostatic therapy can be initiated during the same session. Distinguishing vericeal from nonvariceal sources of bleeding is of prime importance as specific therapies directed toward portal hypertension will be utilized if esophageal varices are identified.

### Hemostasis of Nonvariceal Hemorrhage

Advances in endoscopic hemostatic modalities allow endoscopists to approach and control most causes of GI bleeding in the esophagus. Nonvariceal hemorrhage from the esophagus may originate from a number of lesions, as listed in Table 4–4. While most upper GI bleeding stops spontaneously prior to endoscopy, endoscopic control of recent or active bleeding from these lesions is possible in most cases, using one or more of the techniques listed below.

#### *Injection Therapy*

Injection of submucosal epinephrine or sclerosants can be an extremely effective modality to control nonvariceal hemorrhage from a number of lesions [37]. Using a commercially available injection needle passed through the biopsy channel of a standard endoscope, a 1 : 10,000 epinephrine to saline mixture is injected into the submucosa around the bleeding site. This results in a prompt blanching of the mucosa, followed by a slowing or cessation of bleeding. Injection therapy can be used alone or in combination with thermal therapies to control bleeding. Up to 10 cc of the 1 : 10,000 solution can be injected to control hemorrhage. Some authors prefer to add a sclerosant to the mixture, while others use the epinephrine solution alone. Reported results are similar with either approach [37]. Some investigators

**TABLE 4–4.** *Nonvariceal sources of bleeding in the esophagus*

Esophagitis, infectious or acid reflux
Esophageal ulceration
Malignancy, primary and metastatic disease
Mallory-Weiss tear
Dieulafoy's lesion
Arteriovenous malformation
Crohn's disease
Vascular enteric fistula

and clinicians are now combining injection therapy with a thermal therapy as preliminary reports in ulcer therapy demonstrate improvement in hemostasis rates with combination therapy. Complications of injection therapy are uncommon but may include precipitation of an arrhythmia or myocardial ischemia, esophageal perforation, or bacteremia [37].

### Thermal Therapies

Thermal therapies revolutionized the approach to hemorrhage in the GI tract [36]. Monopolar electrocautery was initially used to treat bleeding in the upper GI tract with some utility. Difficulties with tissue adherence and depth of injury prompted a search for other technologies.

Laser therapy was initially used to control bleeding from peptic ulcers [61]. It became readily apparent that this technology was useful and effective in treating upper GI bleeding. With the development of portable, less expensive thermal devices, such as the BICAP unit and the heater probe, laser therapy has fallen out of favor as the primary method to treat active GI bleeding. It is still used in some clinical situations, such as tumor bleeding and treatment of areas with extensive vascular malformation.

### Coaptation with BICAP or Heater Probe

Coaptive technology with the heater probe or BICAP device has become the primary endoscopic treatment of GI bleeding at most institutions [36]. These devices allow for extremely effective, safe therapy of bleeding lesions in the esophagus. Portability and low cost have allowed them to become the standard of care for GI bleeding in most centers in the world. These devices convert electrical energy to heat. When applied to a bleeding lesion with pressure, they create a coaptive coagulation of the bleeding site, leading to hemostasis (Color Plate 14). In animal experiments, arterial vessels up to 2.5 mm in diameter can be occluded with these techniques [32].

### Argon Plasma Coagulator

The argon plasma coagulator (APC) is a unique device that allows monopolar electrocautery to be applied to the mucosa of the GI tract by way of an ionized plasma of argon gas (Fig. 4–5). This form of delivery allows for a uniform

and safe dispersion of electrical energy to the surface mucosa in a noncontact mode. While there is limited experience with the device, it has been demonstrated to be useful in the treatment of vascular malformations and active bleeding from other mucosal sites. It has the advantage of being able to treat large areas of mucosa in a single setting by using the selective properties of the argon plasma for conduction. Comparison trials of argon plasma coagulation and other thermal modalities are ongoing.

### Mechanical Therapies

#### Hemoclip

A recent review listed several reports demonstrating the effectiveness of the hemoclip device in the control of active GI bleeding [57]. This device is passed through the biopsy channel of the endoscope and allows the endoscopist to place a metallic clip directly on a bleeding site in the GI mucosa. Multiple clips can be placed with the reusable applicator. Preliminary comparison studies with other hemostatic modalities demonstrate similar efficacy [22].

#### Variceal Ligators

Standard variceal ligation devices have occasionally been used with success to treat nonvariceal bleeding sources. Matsui et al. [42] reported use of the variceal ligator to treat a bleeding Dieulafoy's lesion. Bleeding sites in the esophagus could potentially be treated in this manner.

### Hemostasis of Variceal Hemorrhage

Endoscopy plays an essential role in the diagnosis and management of variceal hemorrhage. Urgent endoscopy is extremely useful in patients with upper GI bleeding and suspected varices to document the site of bleeding and exclude other etiologies. Specific treatment options for patients with variceal hemorrhage can then be employed with confidence. The pathophysiology of esophageal varices and endoscopic therapies of sclerotherapy and variceal ligation are discussed in recent reviews [4, 9].

### TREATMENT OF ESOPHAGEAL LESIONS

#### Endoscopic Mucosal Resection

Several authors [44, 56, 62] have described the technique of endoscopic resection of mucosal lesions of the esophagus. Esophageal lesions can be safely resected in a manner similar to mucosal resection techniques used in early gastric cancer. The lesion is first confirmed to be limited to the mucosa or superficial submucosal layer of the esophagus by endoscopic ultrasound examination. Submucosal saline infiltration is often used to elevate the lesion from the muscularis propria. Using one of several mechanical techniques described in the

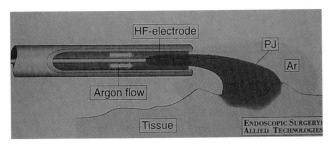

**FIG. 4–5.** Argon plasma coagulation catheter with coaxial argon gas flow. Ionized argon gas conducts electrical coagulation energy to the tissue in a noncontact mode. (From ref. 15A with permission.)

above references, the lesion is removed from the esophageal wall using electrocautery and a snare.

## Ablation of Mucosal Lesions of the Esophagus

Superficial lesions of the esophagus can be identified and treated without resection. This technique does not allow complete pathologic examination of the lesion that is treated; therefore, its use is usually limited to those lesions known to be mucosally based and not invasive. Follow-up endoscopies with biopsy can be completed to document superficial destruction of the lesion. Endoscopic ablation of mucosal lesions of the esophagus can be accomplished using one of several available techniques. Ablation techniques allow the mucosal and superficial submucosal layers of the esophagus to be destroyed. The depth of injury is purposely limited to these layers to avoid perforation of the esophageal wall. As with endoscopic mucosal resection, pretreatment endoscopic ultrasound examination should be used to investigate the depth of lesion penetration into the esophageal wall. A number of modalities can be used to ablate superficial lesions, including BICAP, heater probe, APC, laser, and photodynamic therapy (PDT).

The depth of injury to the esophageal mucosa is dependent on a number of factors at the time of treatment. In general, the depth of injury is also related to the modality used to create the injury. PDT and the neodymium-yttrium-aluminum-garnet (Nd:YAG) laser cause the deepest injuries, followed by heater probe, APC, BICAP, and the argon laser [23, 54]. It is important to recognize that the operator can vary the actual depth of injury and that any of the techniques can lead to perforation if applied excessively. Clinical trials are needed to establish the safety and efficacy of these modalities used in mucosal ablation.

## Ablation of Barrett's Mucosa

Endoscopic ablation of Barrett's mucosa is possible using the modalities listed above [54]. The complexities involved in assessing the usefulness of this approach and other therapeutic options are discussed in Chapter 26.

## Endoscopic Therapy of Esophageal Stricture

Stricture, or narrowing, of the esophagus is a common finding during diagnostic endoscopy in patients with complaints of dysphagia. Benign and malignant strictures of the esophagus occur from a number of possible etiologies. In this setting, without a prior barium study of the esophagus, the endoscopist (and patient) should be prepared to dilate an esophageal stricture for symptom relief if one is encountered. Regardless of the etiology of the luminal narrowing, the endoscopist has a number of treatment options available to attempt to relieve the dysphagia. While attempts to classify the narrowing as malignant or benign are useful and

essential, often cytologic and pathologic examination of specimens obtained at endoscopy will be required to secure the diagnosis.

If the endoscope cannot be advanced beyond the stricture, through-the-scope balloons or a savory guide wire can be advanced into and through the stricture for dilatation. If there is any difficulty in advancing the device beyond the stricture, one should consider fluoroscopic guidance for the dilatation. Usually, the balloon or guide wire can be easily advanced into the stomach. Either device can then be utilized to dilate the narrowing to a size to allow endoscope passage. For benign strictures, the relative advantages and disadvantages of the different dilator systems are discussed in Chapter 27.

Some esophageal strictures that have been resistant to standard dilatation therapy have been managed with intra-stricture corticosteroid injection. This has seemed to benefit some patients; however, randomized and controlled studies have not been completed. Little is known about stricture characteristics that would predict difficulty in dilatation. With some perseverance, most strictures can be safely dilated and maintained open.

## Endoscopic Treatment of Malignant Obstruction of the Esophagus

Malignant obstruction of the esophagus is commonly managed with endoscopic therapy. Palliative therapy to allow oral intake of nutrients and medication includes stricture dilatation, tumor ablation, or stent placement. In addition, complications of esophageal malignancies, such as tracheoesophageal fistulas and esophageal perforation, can be managed conservatively in the nonoperative candidate with covered metallic stent placement.

The initial management of a malignant stricture or obstruction of the esophagus is identical to that of a benign stricture. A tissue diagnosis is confirmed and the stricture is dilated to allow passage of the endoscope. Treatment is then individualized to meet the needs of the patient and match the predicted clinical course.

Serial dilatation of the esophagus can be effective in managing some forms of malignancy. Usually, the lesion initially responds but rapidly returns to its predilatation lumen and symptoms recur. As the interval between dilatations becomes progressively shorter, alternative approaches should be considered.

Tumor ablation can be accomplished endoscopically with injection of ethanol, BICAP probe, APC, lasers, or PDT. All of the ablative modalities increase luminal diameter by destroying the malignant tissue that is obstructing the esophagus.

Injection therapy has been advocated as an inexpensive, effective method to ablate exophytic malignant lesions of the esophagus [50]. The exophytic portion of the tumor is injected with a sclerosing agent [50] or chemotherapy [69], which leads to tumor necrosis and sloughing of tissue. The technique is limited by the inability to control the depth of tumor destruction. While used by some centers, it has not received widespread acceptance.

The BICAP tumor probe was developed as a thermal modality to treat circumferential, partially obstructing neoplasms in a single session. The device consists of bipolar electrodes oriented around metal olive dilators ranging in size from 6 to 15 mm [31]. The device has been used by some centers and in trials compared favorably with laser photoablation [18, 29]. It has largely been replaced by other ablative modalities.

The APC utilizes an ionized argon gas plasma to conduct monopolar electrocautery to the esophageal wall [64]. This noncontact mode of electrocautery has been used to coagulate and ablate esophageal cancers with good result [30]. This technique has a limited depth of penetration due to the unique characteristics of electrical conduction with the argon plasma. This should reduce or eliminate transmural injury and reduce the incidence of perforation due to ablative treatment [30]. Unlike laser therapies, APC cannot vaporize tumor. Neoplasms treated with APC will usually require more frequent treatments when compared to ND:YAG therapy. Argon plasma coagulation has been used to treat tumor ingrowth of metallic stents with good result and no perceivable damage to the stents [20].

Laser photoablation of obstructing esophageal neoplasm has been the mainstay of palliative endoscopic therapy for this disorder since the early 1980s [19]. The Nd:YAG laser has been the most widely used laser for this purpose. The use of laser therapy for esophageal cancer has been recently reviewed [21]. Essentially, the technique involves application of laser energy to the esophageal cancer either with a coaxial noncontact fiber or with sapphire contact tips. This thermally destroys or, at higher energy levels, vaporizes the tumor. Once a lumen has been established, the patient may be retreated to improve dysphagia at regular intervals or only when symptoms recur.

PDT currently involves utilizing an injected photosensitizing agent that is selectively taken up in malignant cells. It is activated by exposure to laser energy at 630 nm, releasing free oxygen radicals and causing cell death. Injection of the photosensitizing agent is followed by laser activation 48 to 72 hours later. Endoscopy is completed to identify the lesion, and a fiberoptic diffusing catheter is positioned to illuminate the lesion with laser light. The duration of therapy and output wattage of the laser determine the depth of injury. Retreatment is possible within 7 days. Treatment causes significant mucosal sloughing and edema. Treated individuals often require intravenous hydration and pain control. Comparison with Nd:YAG laser therapy for palliation of esophageal carcinoma revealed that PDT resulted in a similar relief of dysphagia, improved performance status at 1 month, and longer duration of response [24]. Additional photosensitizing agents under development will hopefully be better tolerated and have fewer side effects.

Endoscopic stent placement for malignant obstruction of the esophagus has evolved as a very effective approach for the palliation of malignant dysphagia. The development of expandable metallic stents has furthered the endoscopist's ability to provide palliation in this setting [34]. Large-diameter plastic stents are effective in relieving dysphagia in selected patients [60]. Their placement requires extensive dilatation of the malignant stricture, the need for general anesthesia, and a relatively high incidence of complications [14]. Once in place, the large-diameter plastic stents are often effective. Stent migration, tumor overgrowth, and stent obstruction have occurred but can usually be managed with additional endoscopic therapy [14].

Expandable metallic stents provide an alternative approach to malignant dysphagia that offers several advantages. The stent introducers are now of a smaller diameter, therefore limiting the need for excessive dilatation of the malignant stricture before stent deployment. The stents have designs that incorporate radial dilatation forces that slowly increase the lumen diameter until the stents are fully expanded. Coated stents are available that prevent tumor ingrowth through the metallic mesh as well as allow for closure of fistulas and perforations of the esophagus [46]. The advantages of the expandable metallic stents are balanced by their increased cost, difficulties with stent migration, and the potential for tumor overgrowth. Coated expandable metallic stents are particularly useful in the management of tracheoesophageal fistulas. With adequate stent placement, the fistula can be closed and resumption of an oral diet instituted rapidly [46] (Fig. 4–6).

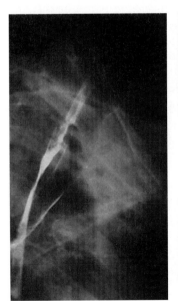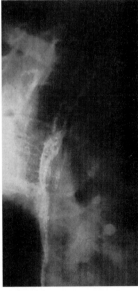

A,B

**FIG. 4–6.** Radiographs of a coated metallic stent placement to close a tracheoesophageal fistula. **A:** Tracheoesophageal fistula that occurred following radiation therapy for primary lung cancer. **B:** Same patient following placement of a coated nitinol metallic stent with closure of the fistula tract. Patient could tolerate a regular diet following stent placement.

## Endoscopic Treatment of Miscellaneous Conditions

Zenker's diverticulum is an uncommon condition that is discussed in detail in Chapter 15. Flexible endoscopic management of this condition has been reported [27, 45]. With this technique, the bridge of tissue between the esophageal wall and diverticulum is incised during endoscopy with electrocautery or laser. This creates a wide-mouthed diverticulum that reduces symptoms. The procedure has been accomplished with minimal morbidity [27, 45] (see also Chapter 15).

For years, individuals have hoped to develop an endoscopic therapy for GERD. Techniques such as submucosal collagen injection and laser scarring of the gastroesophageal junction have been attempted in animal models with variable success. Endoscopic techniques that show promise involve manipulation of the gastroesophageal junction with suture or staples. These techniques augment or elongate the gastroesophageal junction and in preliminary reports appear to reduce or eliminate gastroesophageal reflux [41]. One technique utilizes a specially modified endoscope to suture the cardia of the stomach, creating an elongated sphincter zone that apparently reduces reflux [33]. The procedure is accomplished in other outpatient examinations or therapy in a standard endoscopy facility. Reports of larger human trials with various techniques are anticipated soon. The lasting effect of these procedures and their effect on esophageal function require clarification by long-term outcome studies.

Submucosal lesions of the esophagus can be readily identified by endoscopy. Endoscopic ultrasound examination can be used to identify the wall layer of origin of the lesion. It can also provide useful information to further classify the lesion. Biopsy techniques to obtain tissue confirmation of the lesion include "jumbo bite" forceps, "core" biopsies, and needle aspiration with or without ultrasound guidance. Some authors have reported successful endoscopic resection of submucosal esophageal lesions [2]. Most physicians still recommend surgical resection of symptomatic, large (>4 cm), or histologically uncharacterized masses.

## REFERENCES

1. Baillie J. Gastrointestinal Endoscopy: Basic Principles and Practice. Boston: Butterworth-Heinemann, 1992
2. Bennedetti G, et al. Fiberoptic endoscopic resection of symptomatic leiomyoma of the upper esophagus. Acta Chir Scand 1990;156:807
3. Bernstein D, et al. Standard biopsy forceps versus large-capacity forceps with and without needle. Gastrointest Endosc 1995;41:573
4. Binmoeller KF, Soehendra N. Non-surgical treatment of variceal bleeding: new modalities. Am J Gastroenterol 1995;90:1923
5. Binmoeller KF, et al. Endoscopic ultrasound-guided, 18-gauge, fine needle aspiration biopsy of the pancreas using a 2.8mm channel convex array echoendoscope. Gastrointest Endosc 1998;47:121
6. Camp R, et al. A prospective, randomized, blinded trial of cytological yield with disposable cytology brushes in upper gastrointestinal tract. Am J Gastroenterol 1992;87:1439
7. Canto MI, et al. Methylene blue selectively stains intestinal metaplasia in Barrett's esophagus. Gastrointest Endosc 1996;44:1
8. Carrie A. Adenocarcinoma of the upper end of the esophagus arising from ectopic gastric epithelium. Br J Surg 1950;37:474
9. Cello JP. Endoscopic management of esophageal variceal hemorrhage: injection, banding, glue, octreotide, or a combination? Semin Gastrointest Dis 1997;8:179
10. Chak A, et al. Clinical applications of a new through-the-scope ultrasound probe: prospective comparison with an ultrasound endoscope. Gastrointest Endosc 1997;45:291
11. Chak A, et al. Endosonographic differentiation of benign and malignant stromal cell tumors. Gastrointest Endosc 1997;45:468
12. Chen YK, Kovacs BJ. The structure and function of the endoscope. In DiMarino AJ, Benjamin SB, eds, Gastrointestinal Disease: An Endoscopic Approach. Malden: Blackwell Science, 1997:25
13. Cotton PB, Williams CB (eds). Practical Gastrointestinal Endoscopy (3rd ed.) Cambridge: Blackwell Science, 1990
14. De Palma GD, et al. Plastic prosthesis versus expandable metal stents for palliation of inoperable esophageal thoracic carcinoma: a controlled prospective study. Gastrointest Endosc 1996;43:478
15. Edmonson JM. History of the instruments for gastrointestinal endoscopy. Gastrointest Endosc 1991;37:S27
15A. Favin G, Grund KE. Technology of argon plasma coagulation with particular regard to endoscopic applications. End Surg 1994;2:71
16. Feldman DR, et al. MR endoscopy: preliminary experience in human trials. Radiology 1997;202:868
17. Fennerty MB. Tissue staining. Gastrointest Endosc Clin N Am 1994;4:297
18. Fleischer D. A comparison of endoscopic laser therapy and BICAP tumor probe therapy for esophageal cancer. Am J Gastroenterol 1987;82:608
19. Fleischer D, Kessler F. Endoscopic Nd:YAG laser therapy for carcinoma of the esophagus: a new form of palliative treatment. Gastroenterology 1983;85:600
20. Grund KE, Storek D, Becker HD. Highly flexible self-expanding meshed metal stents for palliation of malignant esophagogastric obstruction. Endoscopy 1995;7:486
21. Haddad N, Fleischer D. Endoscopic laser therapy for esophageal cancer. Gastrointest Endosc Clin N Am 1994;4:863
22. Handa K, Takahashi K, Fujita R. Endoscopic hemostasis for GI bleeding. Endoscopy 1996;28:S66
23. Heier SK, et al. Argon plasma coagulation: comparison to other candidate therapies for Barrett's ablation using the canine esophagus. Gastrointest Endosc 1997;45:A27
24. Heier SK, et al. Photodynamic therapy for obstructing esophageal cancer: light dosimetry and randomized comparison with Nd:YAG laser therapy. Gastroenterology 1995;109:63
25. Hetzel DJ, et al. Healing and relapse of severe peptic esophagitis after treatment with omeprazole. Gastroenterology 1988;95:903
26. Hordijk ML. Restaging after radiotherapy and chemotherapy: value of endoscopic ultrasonography. Gastrointest Endosc Clin N Am 1995;5:601
27. Ishioka S, et al. Endoscopic incision of Zenker's diverticula. Endoscopy 1995;27:433
28. Jabbari M, et al. The inlet patch: heterotopic gastric mucosa in the upper esophagus. Gastroenterology 1985;89:352
29. Jensen DM, et al. Comparison of low-power YAG laser and BICAP tumor probe for palliation of esophageal cancer strictures. Gastroenterology 1988;94:1263
30. Johanns W, et al. Argon plasma coagulation (APC) in gastroenterology: experimental and clinical experiences. Eur J Gastroenterol Hepatol 1997;9:581
31. Johnston JH, et al. Palliative bipolar electrocoagulation therapy of obstructing esophageal cancer. Gastrointest Endosc 1987;33:349
32. Johnston JR, Jensen DM, Auth R. Experimental comparison of endoscopic yttrium-aluminum-garnet laser electrosurgery, and heater probe for canine gut arterial coagulation. Importance of compression and avoidance of erosion. Gastroenterology 1987;92:1101
33. Kadirkamanathan SS, et al. Antireflux operations at flexible endoscopy using endoluminal stitching techniques: an experimental study. Gastrointest Endosc 1996;44:133
34. Knyrim K, et al. A controlled trial of an expansile metal stent for palliation of esophageal obstruction due to inoperable cancer. N Engl J Med 1993;329:1302
35. Kulling D, et al. Histological correlates to pig gastrointestinal wall layers imaged in vitro with the magnetic resonance endoscope. Gastroenterology 1997;112:1568
36. Kumar P, Fleischer DE. Thermal therapy for gastrointestinal bleeding. Gastrointest Endosc Clin N Am 1997;4:593

37. Lau JY, Leung JW. Injection therapy for bleeding peptic ulcers. Gastrointest Endosc Clin N Am 1997;4:575

38. Levine DS, Reid BJ. Endoscopic biopsy technique for acquiring larger mucosal samples. Gastrointest Endosc 1991;37:332

39. Lightdale CJ. Detection of anastomotic recurrence by endoscopic ultrasonography. Gastrointest Endosc Clin N Am 1995;5:595

40. Lum DF, et al. Endoscopic hemostasis of nonvariceal, non-peptic ulcer hemorrhage. Gastrointest Endosc Clin N Am 1997;7:657

41. Mason RJ, et al. A new intraluminal antigastroesophageal reflux procedure in baboons. Gastrointest Endosc 1997;45:283

42. Matsui S, et al. Endoscopic band ligation for hemostasis of non-variceal upper gastrointestinal bleeding. Endoscopy 1996;28:S67

43. Mendoza ML, et al. *H. pylori* infection: rapid diagnosis with brush cytology. Acta Cytol 1993;37:181

44. Moreira LF, et al. Endoscopic mucosal resection for superficial carcinoma and high-grade dysplasia of the esophagus. Surg Laparosc Endosc 1995;5:171

45. Mulder CJ, et al. Flexible endoscopic treatment of Zenker's diverticulum: a new approach. Endoscopy 1995;27:438

46. Nelson DB, et al. Silicone-covered Wallstent prototypes for palliation of malignant esophageal obstruction and digestive-respiratory fistulas. Gastrointest Endosc 1997;45:31

47. Nishioka NS. Laser-induced fluorescence spectroscopy. Gastrointest Endosc Clin N Am 1994;4:313

48. Ollyo JB, et al. Savary's new endoscopic grading of reflux oesophagitis: a simple, reproducible, logical, complete and useful classification. Gastroenterology 1990;89:A100

49. Panjehpour M, et al. Endoscopic fluorescence detection of high-grade dysplasia in Barrett's esophagus. Gastroenterology 1996;111:93

50. Payne-James JJ, et al. Use of ethanol-induced tumor necrosis to palliate dysphagia in patients with esophagogastric cancer. Gastrointest Endosc 1990;36:43

51. Richter JE. Severe reflux esophagitis. Gastrointest Endosc Clin N Am 1994;4:677

52. Rosch T. Endosonographic staging of esophageal cancer: a review of the literature results. Gastrointest Endosc Clin N Am 1995;5:537

53. Rustgi AK. Biomarkers for malignancy in the columnar-lined esophagus. Gastroenterol Clin North Am 1997;26:599

54. Sampliner RE. Ablative therapies for the columnar-lined esophagus. Gastroenterol Clin North Am 1997;26:685

55. Schuman B. The development of the endoscope. In DiMarino AJ, Benjamin SB, eds, Gastrointestinal Disease: An Endoscopic Approach. Malden: Blackwell Science, 1997:9

56. Soehendra N, et al. Endoscopic snare mucosectomy in the esophagus without any additional equipment: a simple technique for resection of flat early cancer. Endoscopy 1997;29:380

57. Soehendra N, Bohnacker S, Binmoeller KF. New and alternative hemostatic techniques. Gastrointest Endosc Clin N Am 1997;7:641

58. Soetikno RM, et al. Is the linear-oriented radial scanning echoendoscope (GF-UM30-P) adequate for performing endoscopic ultrasound (EUS) guided fine needle aspiration (FNA)? Gastrointest Endosc 1998;47:AB39

59. Steadman C, et al. High esophageal stricture. A complication of "inlet patch" mucosa. Gastroenterology 1988;94:521

60. Stemerman DH, et al. Nonexpandable silicone esophageal stents for treatment of malignant tracheoesophageal fistulas: complications and radiographic appearances. Abdom Imaging 1997;22:14

61. Swain CP. Laser therapy for gastrointestinal bleeding. Gastrointest Endosc Clin N Am 1997;4:611

62. Takeshita K, et al. Endoscopic treatment of early oesophageal or gastric cancer. Gut 1997;40:123

63. Vakil N, Knyrim K. Endoscopic imaging technology. Gastrointest Endosc Clin N Am 1994;4:463

64. Wahab PJ, et al. Argon plasma coagulation in flexible gastrointestinal endoscopy: pilot experiences. Endoscopy 1997;29:176

65. Waxman I. Endosonography in the columnar lined esophagus. Gastroenterol Clin N Am 1997;26:607

66. Wegener M, Adamek R. Puncture of submucosal and extrinsic tumors: is there a clinical need? Puncture techniques and their accuracy. Gastrointest Endosc Clin N Am 1995;5:615

67. Wiersema MJ (ed). Emerging technologies in gastrointestinal endoscopy. Gastrointest Clin N Am 1997;7:191

68. Wiersema MJ, et al. Endosonography-guided real-time fine-needle aspiration. Gastrointest Endosc 1994;40:700

69. Wright RA, O'Conner KW. A pilot study of endoscopic injection chemo/sclerotherapy of esophageal carcinoma. Gastrointest Endosc 1990;36:47

*The Esophagus*, Third Edition,
edited by D. O. Castell and J. E. Richter.
Lippincott Williams & Wilkins, Philadelphia © 1999.

CHAPTER 5

# Esophageal Manometry

## June A. Castell and R. Matthew Gideon

Esophageal manometry is a diagnostic test that measures intraluminal pressures and coordination of pressure activity of the muscles of the esophagus (Fig. 5–1). It provides both qualitative and quantitative assessment of esophageal pressures, coordination, and motility. During the 1970s, there was a remarkable resurgence of interest in studies of esophageal function, due in large part to improvements in methodology for accurate measurement of intraluminal pressures. Although primitive manometric studies were first performed more than 100 years ago [35, 39], it was not until the development of a low-compliance perfusion system in the last 20 years that accurate measurements of esophageal pressures were made possible. The studies of Pope [44] and Winans and Harris [56] led to the replacement of static water-filled catheters within the esophagus by systems employing a constant infusion of minute quantities of water. Further studies, using solid-state intraluminal transducers as the standard measure of actual esophageal peristaltic pressures, determined the effect of infusion rates [27, 50] and led to refinements in technology that allowed accurate measurement of transient changes in intraesophageal pressure without the necessity of high infusion rates [2]. These developments led to extensive use of manometry in clinical research laboratories studying the esophagus—its normal function and alterations of its function, both through pharmacologic agents and in various disease states. More recently, refinement of intraluminal transducers that can measure the very rapid pressure changes in the pharynx and the development of a transducer that averages circumferential pressures and can thus be used to measure sphincters generating asymmetric pressures have allowed manometric investigation of the upper esophageal sphincter and pharynx [13]. The advent of computer technology and its application to esophageal manometry has added a new level to the understanding, versatility, and accuracy of this technique [6, 8, 9, 11, 12].

Esophageal manometric testing has proved to be a useful tool in both the clinical and the basic research laboratory [10]. Studies performed in a variety of species, including humans, primates, cats, dogs, and opossum, have provided much new information on both normal esophageal function and disease states. Esophageal manometric testing has made possible more precise and quantitative measurements of abnormal esophageal pressures and has gained greater clinical utility [7]. Manometric studies are used in the assessment of patients with symptoms suggestive of esophageal origin such as dysphagia, odynophagia, and noncardiac chest pain. A manometric study is also indicated prior to antireflux surgery and in assessing possible esophageal involvement in systemic disorders such as scleroderma and chronic idiopathic pseudoobstruction (Table 5–1).

## MATERIALS AND EQUIPMENT

The materials and equipment necessary to perform an esophageal manometry study consist of two general groups. The primary equipment is comprised of a group of relatively expensive, interconnected, and essentially permanent pieces. The group of secondary materials and equipment consists mainly of relatively inexpensive, consumable items used during the performance of the study.

### Primary Equipment

The function of the primary equipment is to sense the pressure activity of the muscles of the esophagus and to transmit and convert this to a permanent record that is easily read, measured, and stored. This equipment includes the manometry catheter system, transducers, and the physiograph or computer.

The manometry catheter is inserted into the esophagus and measures the pressures of the esophageal contractions. It is a specially designed long, flexible tube. There are

J. A. Castell: Department of Medicine, Graduate Hospital, Philadelphia, Pennsylvania 19146.
R. M. Gideon: Esophageal Function Laboratory, Graduate Hospital, Philadelphia, Pennsylvania 19146.

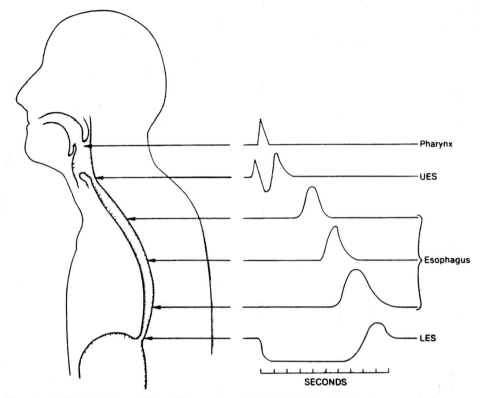

**FIG. 5–1.** A schematic representation of the intraluminal pressure activity of the muscles of the esophagus. At the onset of the swallow, both the upper and lower esophageal sphincters relax. A peristaltic contraction begins at the pharynx and continues through the esophagus. UES, Upper esophageal sphincter; LES, lower esophageal sphincter.

two main types of manometry catheter systems. The water infusion system consists of a catheter composed of small capillary tubes, a low-compliance hydraulic capillary infusion pump, and external transducers (Fig. 5–2). The small capillary tubes that make up the manometry catheter have an internal diameter of approximately 0.8 mm and an

**TABLE 5–1.** *Suggested clinical indications for manometric testing*

Evaluation of patients with dysphagia
  Pharyngeal or upper esophageal sphincter abnormalities
  Primary esophageal motility disorders (e.g., achalasia)
  Secondary esophageal motility disorders (e.g., scleroderma)
Evaluation of patients with possible gastroesophageal reflux disease
  Assist in placement of pH probe
  Evaluate lower esophageal sphincter pressure (e.g., poor treatment response)
  Evaluate defective peristalsis (particularly prior to fundoplication)
Evaluation of patients with noncardiac chest pain
  Primary esophageal motility disorders
  Pain response to provocative testing
Exclude generalized gastrointestinal tract disease
  Scleroderma
  Chronic idiopathic intestinal pseudo-obstruction
Exclude esophageal etiology for suspected anorexia nervosa

opening or port at a known point along the length of the catheter. One commonly used catheter has eight capillary tubes around a larger central tube with an overall diameter of 4.5 mm (Fig. 5–3). The eight orifices, or ports, of this catheter are arranged so that the four distal ports have a radial orientation of 90 degrees and are either 1 cm apart or at the same level. The four proximal ports are 5 cm apart and are also radially oriented. Each lumen is connected to an external transducer. The infusion pump perfuses the capillary tubes with water at a constant rate of 0.5 mL/min. When a catheter port is occluded (e.g., by a muscular contraction), the water pressure builds within the catheter exerting a force which is transmitted to the external transducer (see Fig. 5–2).

The *Dent sleeve manometry catheter* is a water infusion catheter with a specially constructed tip. One side of a 6-cm segment at the distal end is covered with a thin, flexible membrane. A constant infusion of water occurs under this membrane, which produces a pressure-sensitive area along the entire length. This catheter is especially useful for long-term monitoring of esophageal sphincters, as it is not affected by small displacements of the sensor relative to the high-pressure zone of resting sphincters. It is used extensively in research. Original studies showed good correlation between measurements of resting lower esophageal sphincter (LES) pressure made with the sleeve device and with

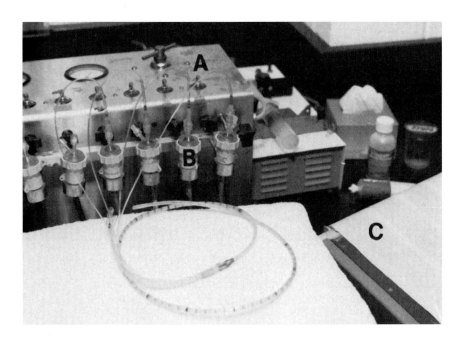

**FIG. 5–2.** Primary equipment for esophageal manometry using the water infusion system. Shown are (**A**) pneumohydraulic capillary infusion pump, (**B**) external transducers, and (**C**) physiograph.

the more common side-hole sensor [19]. Other studies also demonstrated comparable resting LES pressures, but showed significant differences in the measured duration of LES relaxation, with the sleeve consistently measuring a shorter duration of relaxation [12]. This apparent foreclosure of the relaxation seen with the Dent sleeve is an artifact caused when the oncoming peristaltic contraction reaches the proximal tip of the sleeve.

Water infusion systems have two inherent shortcomings. First, the equipment is difficult to move from the laboratory, and, second, because the pressure measurement is relative to the height of a column of water, studies are best performed with the patient supine so as to ensure that the external transducers are at the same level as the esophagus.

The *solid-state esophageal manometry catheter* is a soft, flexible catheter in which microtransducers are contained. These microtransducers directly measure the esophageal contractions. The diameter of this catheter is comparable to that of the eight-lumen water infusion catheter, which is an important consideration since catheters of different diameters will measure pressures differently [37]. Solid-state catheters have the advantage that, unlike the water infusion system, pressures are measured directly and are unrelated to the relative position of the subject and the equipment; therefore,

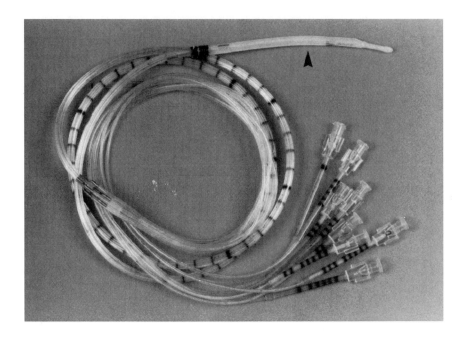

**FIG. 5–3.** Eight-lumen esophageal manometry catheter showing the location of the ports (*arrowhead*). The overall diameter of the pressure-sensing portion of this catheter is 4.5 mm.

studies may be performed with the subject in the upright position. This, and the fact that no continuous source of water is required, make studies such as long-term ambulatory monitoring possible. In addition, the response time of solid-state catheters is much faster than that of the water infusion system, making possible more accurate measurements of the striated-muscle response in the cricopharyngeal region.

A specialized solid-state transducer that senses pressures circumferentially over 360 degrees has also been developed (Fig. 5–4). The ability to sense pressures in more than one direction is accomplished through the use of a Silastic circumferential annulus filled with a viscous fluid such as glycerine or cod liver oil that surrounds a single miniature titanium strain gauge. The oil-filled chamber surrounding the transducer produces an extremely noncompliant system. Studies by the manufacturer (Konigsberg Instruments, Pasadena, CA) reveal low hysteresis (0% to 40% of full scale) and low volumetric compliance ($7 \times 10^{-6}$ mm$^3$/mm Hg). In our laboratory, this transducer has a pressure rise rate in excess of 2,000 mm Hg/sec. The pressure-sensing portion has an active length of 3.1 mm and a diameter ranging from 4 to 5.6 mm. The transducer's pressure-sensing diaphragm is exposed to the fluid-filled annulus, whose silicon rubber membrane makes contact directly with the sphincter wall. The pressure exerted by the sphincter is transmitted through the contained fluid to the transducer [14]. This assembly provides a measure of circumferential squeeze that is especially useful for pressure measurements in areas where pressure is not exerted symmetrically, such as the upper esophageal sphincter (UES). Pursnani and colleagues [45] compared LES pressure and length measurements between a circumferential transducer and the mean of four unidirectional transducers oriented at 90 degrees and found no differences. In our laboratory, we use a catheter with two circumferential transducers (diameter 4.6 mm) spaced 3 cm apart at the distal end, and two unidirectional solid-state transducers at 2 and 5 cm proximal to the second

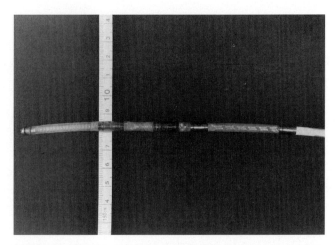

**FIG. 5–5.** A solid-state esophageal manometry catheter with four microtransducers. The two most distal transducers are circumferential sphincter transducers; the other two are unidirectional transducers. The transducers, starting at the distal end, are separated by 3, 2, and 5 cm, respectively.

circumferential transducer (Fig. 5–5). Knowing the exact length of the catheter, distance of the distal transducer (or port) from the tip of the catheter, and spacing between the transducers (or ports) and orientation is essential to accurate esophageal measurement.

The physiograph or computer receives the electrical signal from the transducers and produces a graphic record that is easy to read, measure, and interpret. A physiograph or chart recorder produces the pressure tracing on special graph paper, whereas the computer displays the pressure wave on a monitor and stores the data on computer disks. It is possible to use both a chart recorder and a computer, with the chart recorder producing a paper analog record of the study and the computer collecting, digitizing, and analyzing the data. Technological advances have resulted in specialized equipment that not only produces a high-quality pressure tracing, if desired, but also can store digitized records of the study for later review on a computer monitor and can automatically analyze pressure parameters.

### Secondary Equipment

In addition to the primary equipment, there are pieces of smaller equipment and consumable supplies that are needed for esophageal manometry. A mercury manometer attached to a calibration chamber (stoppered flask or test tube) should be available for use in calibrating the equipment. Viscous lidocaine, lubricating jelly, tissues, an emesis basin, a straw with a container of water at room temperature, a penlight, and a tongue blade should be available for the insertion of the tube. Surgical tape is used to secure the catheter at the desired level. A 20-mL syringe is useful for giving measured wet swallows during the study. After the study, a mild germicidal solution such as 2% glutaraldehyde (Cidex) is used to

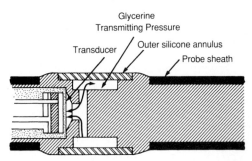

**FIG. 5–4.** Cross section of the circumferential pressure-sensing sphincter transducer showing the strain gauge surrounded by a glycerine-filled chamber through which the pressure is transmitted.

clean the catheter. Materials needed for provocative testing may include 0.1 N hydrochloric acid solution, normal saline solution, edrophonium chloride (1 ml, 10-mg vial), and 1-ml syringes. Atropine should be available to counteract the rare adverse response to edrophonium.

## STUDY TECHNIQUE

Careful attention to details is essential for a successful manometric study. The esophageal manometry study is performed while the patient is awake and alert; therefore, the cooperation and comfort of the patient are very important for a good study.

### Patient Preparation

The patient should have fasted for at least 6 hours. Medications that might alter normal esophageal function should be discontinued at least 24 hours before the study. These include nitrates, calcium channel blockers, anticholinergics, promotility agents, and sedatives. Patients who must take one or more of these medications for a serious, chronic medical condition may be studied while on medication. All medications prescribed ''as needed'' (PRN) should be discontinued.

### Intubation and Patient Calibration

Intubation with the manometry catheter is, in general, the most uncomfortable part of the entire study. It is essential to do this gently and carefully. Begin by lubricating the tube. Viscous lidocaine or a similar topical anesthetic can be applied to the tip of the catheter if necessary, unless it is believed that this might hinder swallowing function. The patient should be seated comfortably and should remove eyeglasses. Gently insert the tip of the catheter into the nose and slowly move it straight back, angling the tip so as to traverse the floor of the sinus cavity. When the patient can feel the catheter in back of the throat, stop advancing the catheter and reassure the patient. Having the patient sip some water and bend the neck forward (chin down) will facilitate passage of the catheter into the esophagus. Once it is in the esophagus, advance to the 60-cm level and tape it in place. At this point, in most patients, the recording sites are in the stomach. The patient is then placed in a supine position and a ''patient calibration'' is performed. This procedure simply zeros all recording sites, regardless of the pressure exerted against them. This allows gastric pressure to be used as a zero baseline when measuring LES pressures. The patient remains supine during evaluation of the LES and esophageal body. There are two reasons for this: first,

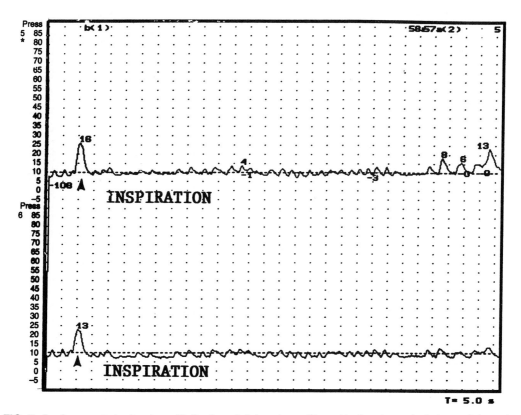

**FIG. 5–6.** A manometry tracing with the two distal ports positioned in the stomach during quiet respiration. Note the rise in pressure with inspiration (*arrowheads*).

all published normal values for stationary manometry are from supine studies, and second, this removes gravity as a compounding factor.

## Lower Esophageal Sphincter

Manometric assessment of the LES is aimed at measuring the resting pressure of the sphincter and assessing relaxation of the sphincter during swallowing. In our laboratory we begin the study with the two distal transducers (the circumferential transducers) in the stomach. A relatively flat, smooth tracing with a small pressure rise with inspiration indicates gastric placement (Fig. 5–6). This can be confirmed by having the patient take a deep breath and noting a rise in pressure with full inspiration. The station pullthrough technique for determining LES pressure involves a slow, stepwise withdrawal of the catheter through the LES. The catheter is moved in 0.5-cm increments and should remain at each "station" long enough to assess a stable resting pressure of the sphincter, usually three to five respirations. The LES is first identified in the proximal channel by an increase in the respiratory variation, followed by the bottom of the pressure tracing rising above the baseline (Fig. 5–7).

As the catheter is withdrawn, the pressure will increase, and at the point where the transducer moves from the abdominal portion of the sphincter to the thoracic portion, the tracing will show a marked change in configuration, with a fall in pressure during inspiration instead of a rise in pressure (Fig. 5–8). This is called the *pressure inversion point* (PIP). It is important to note that the PIP is not the end of the sphincter, but rather a landmark within the sphincter that is used to calculate the ratio of intraabdominal to intrathoracic LES length. This ratio and total LES length are used as important parameters in the assessment of the LES as a competent reflux barrier in some laboratories [4, 42]. As the catheter is further withdrawn, the pressure tracing will drop and flatten until a point is reached where there is no more change. At the point where the transducer has left the LES, the pressure drops below gastric baseline pressure, indicating that the transducer is now measuring esophageal baseline pressure (see Fig. 5–7). Accurate recording of the location of the LES and the UES will allow for a determination of esophageal length [36].

Measurement of the resting pressure of the LES (LESP) must take into account the added influence of respirations. Two popular ways to measure the LESP are from gastric

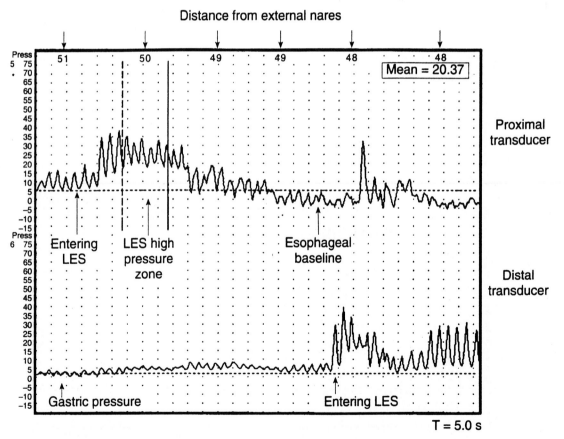

**FIG. 5–7.** Station pullthrough of the lower esophageal sphincter (LES). As the catheter is advanced, there is a rise in respiratory variations as the proximal transducer enters the LES, followed by the identification of the high-pressure zone. Note that the esophageal baseline pressure is *below* gastric baseline pressure. (From ref. 15, with permission.)

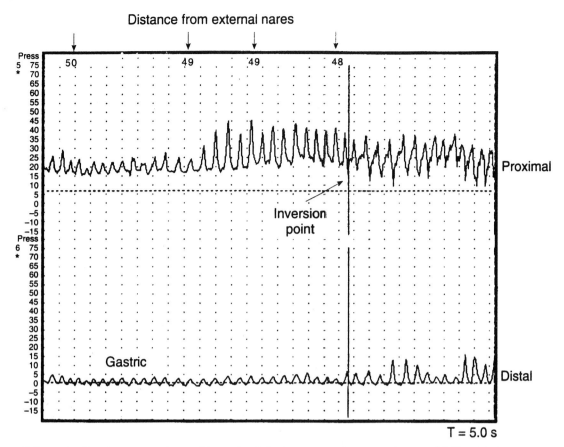

**FIG. 5–8.** Esophageal station pullthrough of the lower esophageal sphincter (LES) with the cursor positioned at the pressure inversion point in the proximal channel. It is at this point in the sphincter pullthrough that the transducer moves from the abdomen into the chest. (From ref. 15, with permission.)

baseline to either midexpiration or end-expiration pressure at the station with the highest overall pressures (Fig. 5–9). Some controversy exists concerning which of these methods is the most accurate way to measure the sphincter pressure. One study suggested that end-expiratory pressures are more indicative of the true LESP, as at this point in the respiratory cycle the diaphragmatic contribution to the observed pressure is at a minimum [5]. While this is true, other investigators have shown that the midexpiratory pressure provides a LESP measurement that most reliably distinguishes patients with normal amounts of gastroesophageal reflux from those with abnormal amounts [34]. Thus the pressure contributed by the diaphragm during respiration may be an important component of the antireflux mechanism of the LES and should be included in the assessment of overall resting pressure.

Whichever method is chosen, it is necessary to compare the results to a cohort of age-matched normal subjects measured with the same technique. The most comprehensive study of normal esophageal manometric parameters [47] established the following normal values (relative to gastric pressure) in 95 healthy adult volunteers (mean age, 43 years; range, 22 to 79 years): end inspiration, 39.7 ± 13.2 mm Hg; midexpiration, 24.4 ± 10.1 mm Hg; end expiration,

15.2 ± 10.7 mm Hg. All values are expressed as the mean plus or minus 1 standard deviation.

Once the resting LES pressure has been measured with the proximal transducer, the distal transducer is placed in the high-pressure zone to evaluate sphincter relaxation during deglutition. Dry swallows often do not induce complete relaxation of the sphincter; therefore, in our laboratory we use a 5-ml water bolus. Following a swallow, the pressure should drop to approximately the level of the gastric baseline (Fig. 5–10). Parameters normally evaluated include the duration of the relaxation and either the percent relaxation or the residual pressure. The residual pressure is defined as the difference between the lowest pressure achieved during relaxation and the gastric baseline pressure, and since this residual pressure is independent of the resting LES baseline pressure, it is a better indicator of function than is percent relaxation [12] (Fig. 5–11).

Manual interpretation of LES parameters, particularly the relaxation parameters, is highly subjective and often qualitative. Attempts to provide a more subjective and quantitative measure of these parameters have resulted in computer algorithms for an automated analysis [8, 12]. In addition to improved objectivity in the measurement of LES parameters, computer technology has also been used to identify and

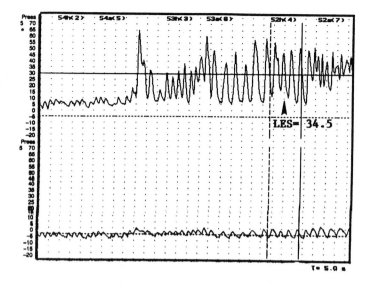

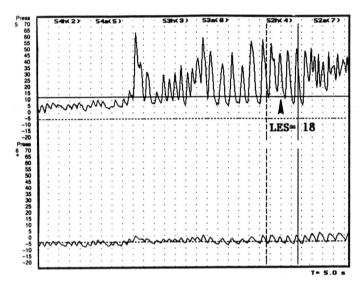

**FIG. 5–9.** Two different ways to measure lower esophageal sphincter (LES) pressure. The tracing on the top has the LES calculated as the *midrespiratory* pressure, while the same tracing on the bottom has the LES calculated as the *end-expiratory* pressure. Before values from different laboratories are compared, it is necessary to know the method used to calculate this pressure.

evaluate parameters that would be impossible to evaluate manually. One such parameter is the LES vector volume (LESVV), which is the volume of an inverse polygon used as a three-dimensional graphic representation of the LES pressure profile, considered by Bombeck and co-workers [3] to be a parameter for measuring LES mechanical integrity. More recently, Stein et al. [51] used this three-dimensional technique to correlate radial muscular thickness with manometric pressures at the gastroesophageal junction. Most of these computer algorithms for LES evaluation have been adapted by manufacturers of motility equipment and are commercially available.

Low LES pressures can be associated with gastroesophageal reflux disease, whereas abnormally high LES pressures are often associated with symptoms of dysphagia or noncardiac chest pain. Failure of the sphincter to relax adequately contributes to symptoms of dysphagia and is usually associated with diffuse esophageal spasm and achalasia.

**Esophageal Body**

Manometric studies of the esophageal body are used to assess the strength and duration of the muscular contractions, to evaluate peristaltic activity, and to detect any motility abnormalities. A complete evaluation should include measurements of both the smooth muscle of the distal esophagus and the striated muscle of the proximal esophagus. The distal esophagus is evaluated by locating the distal transducer 3 cm above the upper border of the LES, with two more proximal transducers at 5-cm intervals. Ten wet swallows are given at 30-second intervals, and the response of the esophagus to the swallows is closely monitored. The proximal esophagus is evaluated in a like manner with the proximal transducer located 1 cm below the lower border of the upper esophageal sphincter and two more distal transducers at 5-cm intervals. Figure 5–12 illustrates the catheter placement used in our laboratory for a complete esophageal manometric evaluation.

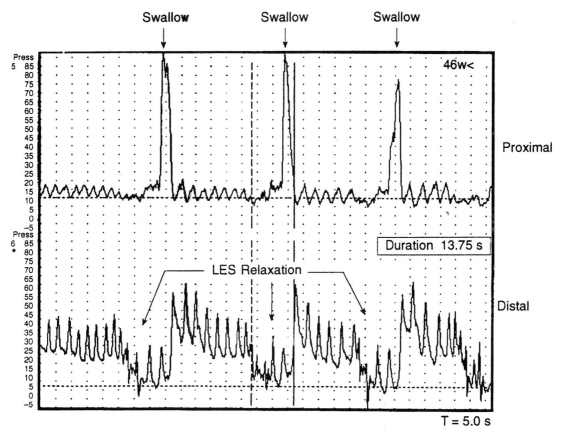

**FIG. 5-10.** A normal relaxation of the lower esophageal sphincter (LES) during deglutition. The proximal channel is recording in the esophagus and the distal channel is recording in the high-pressure zone of the LES. The cursors have marked the relaxation for the second wet swallow and show a relaxation to gastric baseline (zero residual pressure) and a relaxation duration of 13.75 seconds. (From ref. 15, with permission.)

Measures are made of at least the following peristaltic parameters: amplitude, duration, and velocity. Amplitude is a measure of the strength of the contraction and is expressed in millimeters of mercury (mm Hg). Duration of the contraction is expressed in seconds. Velocity is the rate of progression of the contraction down the esophagus and is expressed in centimeters per second (Fig. 5-13). Usually ten wet swallows are assessed, and parameters are based on the mean.

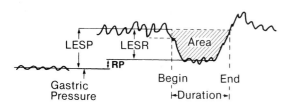

**FIG. 5-11.** Schematic representation of pressure parameters measurable during lower esophageal sphincter (LES) relaxation. Resting LES pressure (LESP) is the pressure rise measured from gastric pressure; residual pressure (RP) is the difference between the pressure at the nadir of the relaxation and gastric pressure; LES relaxation (LESR) is the difference between LESP and RP, expressed as a percentage. Duration and area of the relaxation phase are also shown.

A study from our laboratory evaluated the reproducibility of swallow parameters and concluded that the mean values from five to eight swallows would reliably characterize an individual's esophageal peristalsis [20]. Analysis of these parameters, especially those involving the identification of the onset of the peristaltic wave, can be very subjective and time-consuming. In attempts to obtain more objective and quantitative data, several laboratories have developed or evaluated computer systems that collect, digitize, and automatically analyze esophageal body pressure data [8, 52, 54]. Most manufacturers of manometric equipment have adapted and improved upon these programs for general use and they are commercially available.

Initially, esophageal peristalsis was evaluated with dry swallows. However, it soon became apparent that afferent stimulation by a liquid bolus (a so-called wet swallow) was important for reproducible and accurate quantitative assessment of the peristaltic sequence [21, 28]. Studies traditionally are done with the patient in the supine position. Increased use of intraluminal transducers and the advent of long-term ambulatory pressure monitoring have promoted interest in studies performed in the more physiologic upright position [14, 32, 48]. In addition, some investigators are

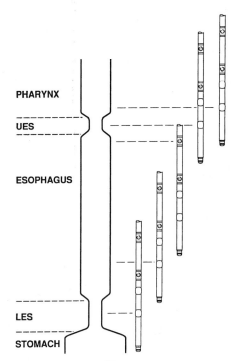

**FIG. 5–12.** Schematic representation of sequential catheter positions showing the locations of the four transducers for a complete manometric assessment of the esophagus. UES, Upper esophageal sphincter; LES, lower esophageal sphincter.

evaluating the effects of bolus size and composition [14, 23, 48] and the effects of food ingestion [1, 38] on esophageal peristalsis.

Normal peristalsis in the distal esophagus is an orderly, sequential contraction down the esophagus, with amplitude,

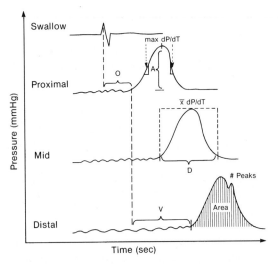

**FIG. 5–13.** Schematic representation of esophageal peristaltic parameters: A, wave amplitude; D, wave duration; V, propagation velocity; x̄ dP/dT, mean rate of pressure change per unit time; max dP/dT, maximum pressure change per unit time.

duration, and velocity in the normal range (Fig. 5–14). Wet swallows in the proximal esophagus produce a somewhat different appearance (Fig. 5–15). The contraction in the striated-muscle segment is usually sharper, with a shorter duration. If a transducer is placed in the transition zone between the striated and smooth-muscle portions of the esophagus (generally about 6 cm below the UES), no, or at best very low, contractions (''pressure trough'') may be seen. The presence of a midesophageal pressure trough was confirmed by Clouse et al. [16–18], who recorded esophageal pressures at 1-cm intervals and generated isobaric contour plots for a detailed analysis of intraesophageal pressures. They also showed a difference in shape and peristaltic velocity between the distal and proximal esophagus. A recent study by Peghini et al. [43] determined, however, that the striated muscle of the esophagus has manometric characteristics much closer to those of the esophageal smooth muscle of the esophagus than to those of the striated muscle in the pharynx. They also confirmed the presence of a pressure trough in the middle esophagus, although they found it in less than one-third of the subjects studied.

The definition of normal range comes from measurements of these parameters in a large number of asymptomatic or ''normal'' volunteer subjects. The largest such study to date is the one by Richter and colleagues [47] in 1987. This study presents normal values in 95 healthy adults. The values from that study are given in Table 5–2, and are considered to be standard for wet swallows in the distal esophagus. In addition, the effect of age on the measured parameters is shown (Fig. 5–16). When comparing studies done in patients to this or any other group of normal values, it is necessary to remember that these measurements are affected by the age of the subject, body position, size of the bolus, size of the catheter, and location of the transducer.

Examples of abnormal contractions include simultaneous, nontransmitted, triple-peaked, and retrograde (Fig. 5–17). An excellent compendium of the interpretation of both normal and abnormal esophageal motility tracings can be found in the Atlas of GI Motility in Health and Disease [15]. Peristaltic contractions where the overall mean amplitude is either very weak (30 mm Hg or less) or very strong (180 mm Hg or greater) are also abnormal. Simultaneous comparisons of manometry with radiography [26] and scintigraphy [46] have shown that contractions with an amplitude of less than 30 mm Hg lack the necessary force to move a bolus through the esophagus. Mean distal contraction amplitudes in excess of 180 mm Hg are more than 2 standard deviations above normal and, while found in less than 2.5% of the normal population, occur in 48% of patients with a possible esophageal cause of noncardiac chest pain [31].

## Upper Esophageal Sphincter and Pharynx

A manometric evaluation of the UES and pharynx includes a determination of the resting pressure of the UES, the relaxation of the UES, pharyngeal contraction and peri-

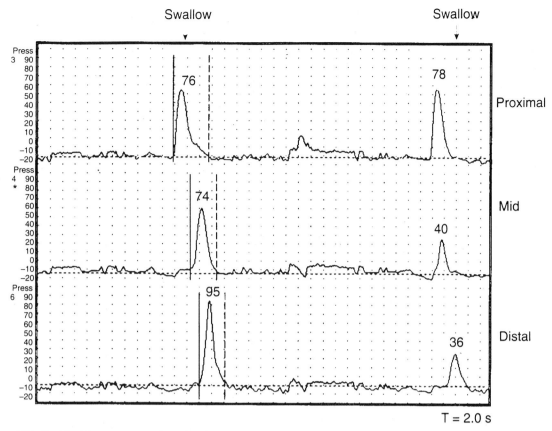

**FIG. 5–14.** Manometry tracing showing three pressure transducers in the body of the distal esophagus (distal transducer 3 cm above the proximal margin of the lower esophageal sphincter), illustrating a normal peristaltic sequence in response to a wet swallow. (From ref. 15, with permission.)

stalsis, and an assessment of the coordination between UES relaxation and the pharyngeal contraction [10]. This study is best performed with the patient in a sitting position.

The UES and pharyngeal region differs from the body of the esophagus in several ways that markedly affect the manner in which manometry must be performed. First, the UES and pharynx are composed of striated muscle; therefore, the muscular contractions and responses are much more rapid than those in the smooth-muscle distal esophagus. The more rapid rate of contraction of the striated muscle far exceeds the response time of low-compliance infusion systems, which will substantially misrecord pharyngeal waveforms [22]. Intraluminal transducers, however, do have a frequency response time within the range required. In addition to limitations imposed by the response of the transducer system, an analog recording system has a recording frequency that will impact on the interpretation of the signal from the transducers. The mechanical recording pens of the polygraph generally record faithfully only to a frequency of 20 to 40 Hz [50]. A computerized manometry system allows more flexibility in recording frequencies. Though it is possible to collect data at much higher rates, practical considerations of memory and disk space utilization have kept those computer systems currently in use to a recording frequency of 100 to 128 Hz [9], which allows for a resolution of ± 10 msec.

The second difference that affects UES–pharyngeal manometry is inherent in the anatomy of the UES, which is discussed extensively in Chapter 1. The asymmetry of the UES pressure profile has been confirmed in humans by the use of an eight-lumen perfused manometry catheter where the orientation of each orifice was known [53, 55]. The highest pressures are recorded from the anterior and posterior directions, and the lowest from the lateral direction. One possible solution to this dilemma which has been tried is to use an oval catheter that ensures proper orientation within the sphincter and records only maximum and minimum pressures [24, 33]. Use of such a catheter instead of the round tube routinely used for esophageal manometry would present, some practical problems. Green and colleagues [25] reported on a comparison between a round and an oval catheter each with four orifices spaced radially at 90 degrees. They found that mean values for the oval and round catheters were not significantly different. Therefore, the recording of average sphincter pressures over 360 degrees is independent of catheter shape. The development of a circumferential sphincter transducer has allowed for accurate sphincter measurements without the need to control catheter orientation [14].

The high-pressure zone of the UES is usually found by the slow or station pullthrough method. The UES is quite

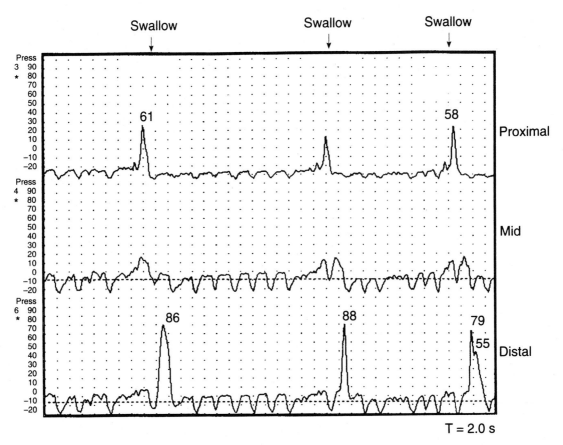

**FIG. 5–15.** Manometry tracing showing three pressure transducers in the body of the proximal esophagus (proximal transducer 1 cm below the distal margin of the upper esophageal sphincter), illustrating a normal sequence in response to a wet swallow. The middle channel is located in the transition zone between the striated and smooth muscle where a "pressure trough" or area of low pressure exists. (From ref. 15, with permission.)

**TABLE 5–2.** *Normal esophageal pressure data: wet swallows (95 subjects)[a]*

| Parameter measured at given recording site | Value |
|---|---|
| Amplitude (mm Hg) | |
| At 18 cm above LES | 62 ± 29 |
| At 13 cm above LES | 70 ± 32 |
| At 8 cm above LES | 90 ± 41 |
| At 3 cm above LES | 109 ± 45 |
| ⅜ (DEA) | 99 ± 40 |
| Duration (sec) | |
| At 18 cm above LES | 2.8 ± 0.8 |
| At 13 cm above LES | 3.5 ± 0.7 |
| At 8 cm above LES | 3.9 ± 0.9 |
| At 3 cm above LES | 4.0 ± 1.1 |
| ⅜ DED | 3.9 ± 0.9 |
| Velocity (cm/sec) | |
| Proximal | 3.0 ± 0.6 |
| Distal | 3.5 ± 0.9 |

[a] LES, Lower esophageal sphincter; DEA, distal esophageal amplitude; DED, distal esophageal duration. All values are mean values ±1 standard deviation.

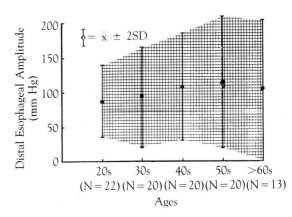

**FIG. 5–16.** Values for mean ±2 standard deviations (SD) for distal esophageal contractile amplitudes analyzed by decade. The observed linear increase of normal pressures with age should be considered when evaluating older patients.

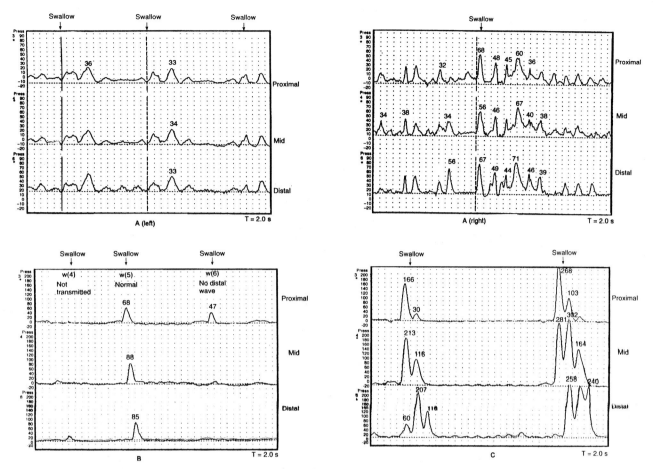

**FIG. 5–17. (A)** Two manometry tracings that illustrate simultaneous contractions. The onsets (marked by the cursors) of all waves for each swallow occur at the same time. The left tracing shows isobaric waveforms typical of achalasia, while the right tracing shows multiple simultaneous contractions more typical of diffuse esophageal spasm. **(B)** This tracing illustrates nontransmitted contractions. There is no peristaltic response to the first swallow, the second swallow is normal, and the third swallow elicits a response in the proximal transducer, but the contraction is not transmitted distally. **(C)** This tracing shows abnormal multiple peaks (more than two) in the distal contractions. In addition, these contractions have higher amplitudes and longer durations than do normal contractions. (From ref. 15, with permission.)

reactive to catheter movement, so it is necessary to allow the recording device to remain in the high-pressure zone for 15 to 20 seconds before measuring the pressure (Fig. 5–18). This allows the pressures to stabilize, and a man pressure over about a 5-second period can be measured.

In addition to measuring the resting UES pressure, a manometric evaluation must also include an analysis of UES relaxation during swallowing (Fig. 5–19). This analysis has been confounded by swallow-related movements of the sphincter [29]. Kahrilas and co-workers [30] have shown that a measuring device positioned in the high-pressure zone of the UES records a duration of UES relaxation considerably longer than the period of UES opening radiographically. They concluded that this is an artifact caused by the sensor falling distal to the sphincter (i.e., into the body of the esophagus) as the UES moves orad. This artifact can be avoided by placing the sensor proximal to the high-pressure zone of

the sphincter. If the sensor is properly positioned, the tracing seen during a swallow will describe an M configuration, as shown in Fig. 5–20. Initially, the pressure will be well below that of the UES high-pressure zone. However, as the UES moves orad with the initiation of the swallow, the pressure increases, corresponding to the movement of the high-pressure zone onto the sensor. The pressure then drops and again increases as the sphincter relaxes and regains its resting tone. There is finally a slow drop in pressure as the high-pressure zone returns to its original position distal to the sensor.

Once the sensor is properly positioned, it is possible to study both the UES function during swallowing and the coordination between the relaxation of the UES and the contraction of the pharynx. The pharynx, like the UES, is asymmetric both circumferentially and longitudinally. A study using a special catheter with four solid-state transducers separated by 3 cm and oriented circumferentially at 90 degrees mea-

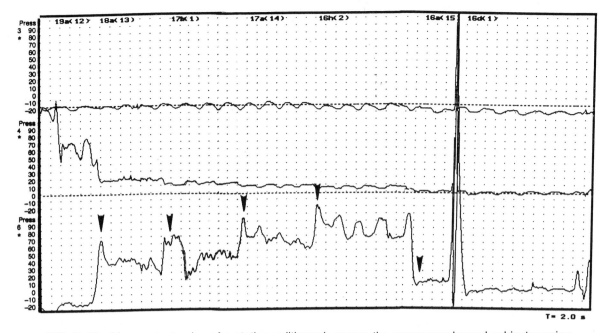

**FIG. 5–18.** Manometry tracing of a station pullthrough across the upper esophageal sphincter using the sphincter transducer. Movement of the catheter through the sphincter creates an initial pressure rise that equilibrates in approximately 10 seconds.

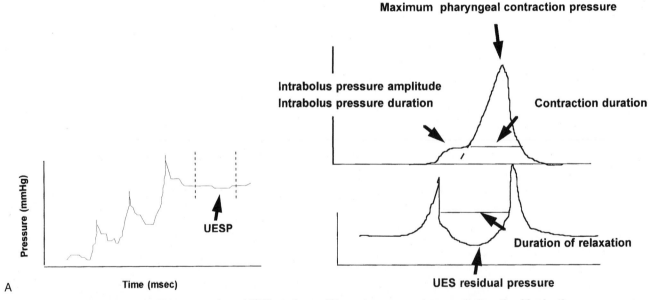

**FIG. 5–19.** (A) Representation of UES station pullthrough pressure is recorded on the *Y* axis, time on the *X* axis. Resting UES pressure (UESP) is measured as a mean of pressures over 4 to 6 seconds in the high-pressure zone after stabilization. (B) Parameters of UES relaxation and pharyngeal contraction. Pressure is recorded on the *Y* axis, time on the *X* axis. Coordination is measured in milliseconds from the beginning of the pharyngeal contractions (extension of major upstroke to the baseline) to the beginning of the UES relaxation. The UES residual pressure is measured relative to the esophageal baseline.

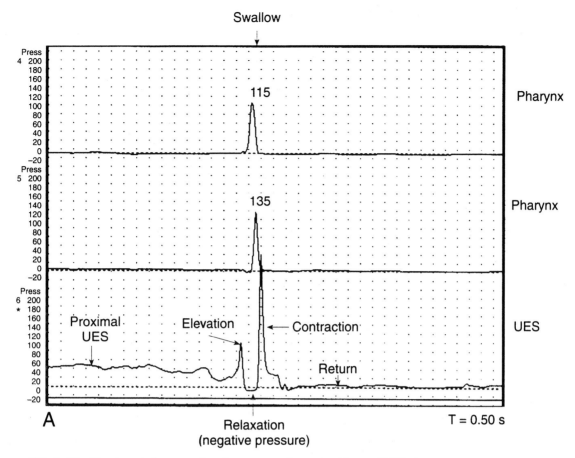

**FIG. 5–20.** Tracing of pharyngeal and upper esophageal sphincter (UES) dynamics during deglutition. The two distal transducers are circumferential, so that orientation is not critical. The proximal transducer is used only to record the onset of the pharyngeal contraction so that peristaltic velocity can be measured. The sphincter transducer is positioned in the most proximal segment of the UES. During the swallow, the sphincter moves upward onto the transducer, relaxes, closes, and moves downward to the resting state, producing the M configuration seen here. The residual pressure (pressure at the nadir of the relaxation) in a normal subject is a negative value. (From ref. 15, with permission.)

sured pharyngeal pressures in four directions from the proximal edge of the UES through the hypopharynx and oropharynx [49]. The results are shown in Figure 5–21. There was statistically significant asymmetry in both the longitudinal and radial directions. Pressures varied from 365 ± 29 to 86 ± 13 mm Hg (mean plus or minus 1 standard error of the mean). In our laboratory we use the second circumferential transducer to measure mean pharyngeal pressures 3 cm proximal to the UES and a unidirectional transducer 2 cm proximal to the pharyngeal circumferential transducer to measure the onset of the pharyngeal contraction wave (see Fig. 5–20). If a second circumferential transducer is not used in the pharynx, then close attention must be paid to the orientation of the catheter to obtain maximum pharyngeal pressures during swallow studies. Maintaining a known orientation is quite difficult, as the catheter is flexible, with a certain amount of torque produced during intubation.

The accurate evaluation of pharyngeal peristalsis and UES–pharyngeal coordination requires computer analysis. The sequence of events is so rapid (usually less than 1 sec-

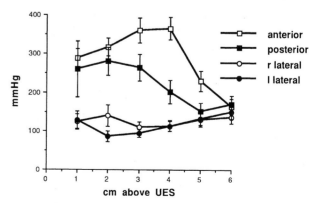

**FIG. 5–21.** Mean pharyngeal contraction pressures during wet swallows in 90-degree orientation at 1 to 6 cm above the upper esophageal sphincter (UES). Vertical lines indicate ± 1 standard error of the mean.

**TABLE 5–3.** *Normal values for upper esophageal sphincter (UES)–pharyngeal manometry: 5-mL water swallows*[a]

| | |
|---|---|
| **UES** | |
| Resting pressure | 73 ± 29 mm Hg |
| Residual pressure | −0.7 ± 3.7 mm Hg |
| Relaxation time (from beginning of relaxation to nadir) | 174 ± 46 msec |
| Duration (time from beginning of relaxation to end) | 561 ± 74 msec |
| Recovery (time from nadir of relaxation to end) | 387 ± 64 msec |
| **Pharynx** | |
| Peak pressure | 122 ± 36 mm Hg |
| dP/dT (rate of pressure change from beginning to peak) | 443 ± 182 mm Hg/sec |
| Contraction (time from beginning of contraction to peak) | 327 ± 138 msec |
| Duration (time from beginning of contraction to end) | 627 ± 168 msec |
| Recovery (time from peak of contraction to end) | 300 ± 82 msec |
| **Coordination** | |
| Beginning of pharyngeal contraction to: | |
|     Beginning of UES relaxation | −53 ± 146 msec |
|     Nadir of UES relaxation | 121 ± 150 msec |
|     End of UES relaxation | 508 ± 127 msec |
| Peak of pharyngeal contraction to: | |
|     Beginning of UES relaxation | −380 ± 86 msec |
|     Nadir of UES relaxation | −206 ± 92 msec |
|     End of UES relaxation | 181 ± 58 msec |
| End of pharyngeal contraction to: | |
|     Beginning of UES relaxation | −681 ± 122 msec |
|     Nadir of UES relaxation | −506 ± 121 msec |
|     End of UES relaxation | −119 ± 106 msec |

[a] Data are means ± standard deviations.

ond) that the higher resolution of computer-recorded data is necessary. Figure 5–19 shows the parameters of UES–pharyngeal coordination that are most commonly analyzed in our laboratory. Studies in our laboratory to determine normal values for these parameters are ongoing. Preliminary normal values obtained by this method are shown in Table 5–3.

Until very recently, it was believed that the barium examination was the only useful technique for assessing patients with pharyngeal dysphagia, since it provides the opportunity to assess actual bolus transfer and the possible presence of aspiration. However, using the technology described, manometric studies can also provide important information on the swallowing mechanism of the pharynx and the UES. In particular, such studies can provide details of the force of the pharyngeal contraction and specific timing of this contraction and the relaxation of the UES. A manometric evaluation allows quantitation of the forces of the pharyngeal propulsive wave, the squeezing tone of the UES, and the timing of the coordination between the pharyngeal contraction and the UES relaxation to an accuracy of 1/100 second. We believe that this information will augment that provided by the barium swallow and allow for a more complete assessment of the dysphagia patient. An example of this is shown in Fig. 5–22. This study was performed on a 42-year-old man with an acute onset of dysphagia and muscle weakness considered to be due to neurotrophic virus infection. Barium swallow with videotaping revealed mildly dilated hypopharynx and inability of barium to pass into the upper esophagus. A diagnosis of cricopharyngeal achalasia was made. The UES–pharyngeal manometric study shown in Fig. 5–22 doc-

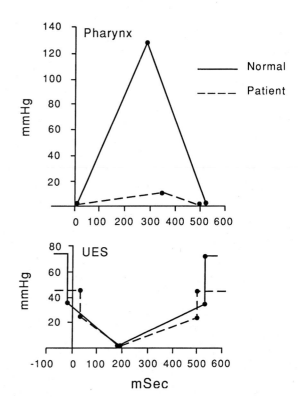

**FIG. 5–22.** Schematic representation of pharyngeal–upper esophageal sphincter (UES) coordination in a patient with a diagnosis of cricopharyngeal achalasia, superimposed on a diagram representing the mean values for 12 normal volunteers. Note the normal UES function and absence of pharyngeal pressure.

umented normal UES relaxation, but marked weakness of the pharynx and only questionable peristalsis, thus identifying the correct pathophysiologic basis for the patient's dysphagia. More recently, combined videomanometric studies such as those done by Olsson and colleagues [40, 41] are beginning to describe pressure abnormalities in dysphagic patients that are not found in barium studies alone.

## REFERENCES

1. Allen ML, et al. Water swallows versus food ingestion as manometric tests for esophageal dysfunction. Gastroenterology 1988;95:831
2. Arndorfer RC, et al. Improved infusion system for intraluminal esophageal manometry. Gastroenterology 1977;73:23
3. Bombeck CT, et al. Computerized axial manometry of the esophagus. Ann Surg 1987;206:465
4. Bonavina L, Evander A, DeMeester TR. Length of the distal esophageal sphincter and competency of the cardia. Am J Surg 1986;151:25
5. Boyle JT, et al. Role of the diaphragm in the genesis of lower esophageal sphincter pressure in the cat. Gastroenterology 1985;88:723
6. Brasseur JG, Dodds WJ. Interpretation of intraluminal manometric measurements in terms of swallowing mechanics. Dysphagia 1991;6:100
7. Castell DO. Clinical applications of esophageal manometry. Dig Dis Sci 1982;27:769
8. Castell JA, Castell DO. Computer analysis of human esophageal peristalsis and lower esophageal sphincter pressure: 11. An interactive system for online data collection and analysis. Dig Dis Sci 1986;31:121
9. Castell JA, Castell DO. Modern solid state computerized manometry of the pharyngoesophageal segment. Dysphagia 1993;8:270
10. Castell JA, Castell DO. Stationary esophageal manometry. In Scarpignato C, Galmiche JP, eds, Functional Investigation in Esophageal Disease (1st ed). Basel: Karger, 1994:109–129
11. Castell DO, et al. Computer-aided analysis of human esophageal peristalsis. Dig Dis Sci 1984;29:65
12. Castell JA, Dalton CB, Castell DO. On-line computer analysis of human lower esophageal sphincter relaxation. Am J Physiol 1988;255:G794
13. Castell JA, Dalton CB, Castell DO. Pharyngeal and upper esophageal sphincter manometry in humans. Am J Physiol 1990;258:G173
14. Castell JA, Dalton CB, Castell DO. Effects of body position and bolus consistency on the manometric parameters and coordination of the upper esophageal sphincter and pharynx. Dysphagia 1990;5:179
15. Castell JA, Gideon RM, Castell DO. Esophagus. In Schuster MM, ed, Atlas of GI Motility in Health and Disease (1st ed). Baltimore: Williams & Wilkins, 1993:134–157
16. Clouse RE, Staiano A. Topography of normal and high-amplitude esophageal peristalsis. Am J Physiol 1993;268:G1098
17. Clouse RE, Staiano A. Topography of the esophageal peristaltic pressure wave. Am J Physiol 1991;261:G677
18. Clouse RE, et al. Characteristics of the propagating pressure wave in the esophagus. Dig Dis Sci 1996;41:2369
19. Dent J, Chir B. A new technique for continuous sphincter pressure measurement. Gastroenterology 1976;71:263
20. DeVault K, Castell JA, Castell DO. How many swallows are required to establish reliable esophageal peristaltic parameters in normal subjects? An on-line computer analysis. Am J Gastroenterol 1987;82:754
21. Dodds WJ, et al. A comparison between primary esophageal peristalsis following wet and dry swallows. J Appl Physiol 1973;35:851
22. Dodds WJ, et al. Considerations about pharyngeal manometry. Dysphagia 1987;1:209
23. Dooley CF, Schlossmacher B, Valenzuela JE. Effects of alterations in bolus viscosity on esophageal peristalsis in humans. Am J Physiol 1988;254:G8
24. Gergardt DC, et al. Esophageal dysfunction in esophagopharyngeal regurgitation. Gastroenterology 1980;78:893
25. Green WER, Castell JA, Castell DO. Upper esophageal sphincter pressure recording: is an oval manometry catheter necessary? Dysphagia 1988;2:162
26. Hogan WJ, Dodds WJ, Stewart ET. Comparison of roentgenology and

intraluminal manometry for evaluating oesophageal peristalsis. Rend Gastroenterol 1973;5:28
27. Hollis JB, Castell DO. Amplitude of esophageal peristalsis as determined by rapid infusion. Gastroenterology 1972;63:417
28. Hollis JB, Castell DO. Effect of dry swallows and wet swallows of different volumes on esophageal peristalsis. J Appl Physiol 1975;38:1161
29. Isberg A, Nilsson ME, Schiaratzki H. Movement of the upper esophageal sphincter and a manometric device during deglutition, a cineradiographic investigation. Acta Radiol [Diagn] (Stockh) 1985;26:381
30. Kahrilas P, et al. Upper esophageal sphincter function during deglutition. Gastroenterology 1988;95:52
31. Katz PO, et al. Esophageal testing of patients with noncardiac chest pain and/or dysphagia. Results of a three year experience with 1161 patients. Ann Intern Med 1987;106:593
32. Kaye MD, Wexler RM. Alteration of esophageal peristalsis by body position. Dig Dis Sci 1981;26:897
33. Knuff TE, Benjamin SB, Castell DO. Pharyngoesophageal (Zenker's) diverticulum, a reappraisal. Gastroenterology 1982;82:734
34. Kraus BB, Wu WC, Castell DO. Comparison of lower esophageal sphincter manometrics and gastroesophageal reflux measured by 24-hour pH recording. Am J Gastroenterol 1990;85:692
35. Kronecker H, Meltzer SJ. Der Schluckmechanismus, seine Erregung und seine Hummung. Arch Ges Anat Physiol (Suppl) 1983;7:328
36. Li Q, Castell JA, Castell DO. Manometric determination of esophageal length. Am J Gastroenterol 1994;89:722
37. Lydon SB, et al. The effect of manometric assembly diameter on intraluminal esophageal pressure recording. Dig Dis Sci 1975;20:968
38. Mellow MH. Esophageal motility during food ingestion: a physiologic test of esophageal motor function. Gastroenterology 1983;85:570
39. Meltzer SJ. Recent experimental contributions to the physiology of deglutition. NY State J Med 1984;59:389
40. Olsson R, Castell JA, Castell DO, Ekberg O. Solid-state computerized manometry improves diagnostic yield in pharyngeal dysphagia: simultaneous videoradiography and manometry in dysphagia patients with normal barium swallows. Abdom Imaging 1995;20:230
41. Olsson R, et al. Combined videomanometric identification of abnormalities related to pharyngeal retention. Acad Radiol 1997;4:349
42. O'Sullivan GC, DeMeester TR, Joelsson BE. Interaction of lower esophageal sphincter pressure and length of sphincter in the abdomen as determinants of gastroesophageal competence. Am J Surg 1982;143:40
43. Peghini PL, et al. Proximal and distal esophageal contractions have similar manometric features. Am J Physiol 1998;37:G325
44. Pope CE. A dynamic test of sphincter strength: its application to the lower esophageal sphincter. Gastroenterology 1967;52:770
45. Pursnani KG, Oeffner C, Gideon RM, Castell DO. Comparison of lower oesophageal sphincter pressure measurement using circumferential vs unidirectional transducers. Neurogastroenterol Motil 1997;9:177
46. Richter JE, et al. Relationship of radionuclide liquid bolus transport and esophageal manometry. J Lab Clin Med 1987;109:217
47. Richter JE, et al. Esophageal manometry in 95 healthy adult volunteers. Dig Dis Sci 1987;32:583
48. Sears VW, Castell JA, Castell DO. Comparison of effects of upright versus supine body position and liquid versus solid bolus on esophageal pressures in normal humans. Dig Dis Sci 1990;35:857
49. Sears VW, Castell JA, Castell DO. Radial and longitudinal asymmetry of the human pharynx. Gastroenterology 1991;101:1559
50. Stef JJ, et al. Intraluminal esophageal manometry: an analysis of variables affecting recording fidelity of peristaltic pressures. Gastroenterology 1974;67:221
51. Stein HJ, et al. Three dimensional pressure image and muscular structure of the human lower esophageal sphincter. Surgery 1995;117:692
52. Tijskens G, et al. Validation of a fully automated analysis of esophageal body contractility and lower esophageal sphincter function: a study on the effect of the PGE₂ analogue Rioprostil on human esophageal motility. J Gastrointest Motil 1989;1:21
53. Welch RW, et al. Manometry of the normal upper esophageal sphincter and its alteration in laryngectomy. J Clin Invest 1979;63:1036
54. Wilson JA, et al. Computerized manometric recording: an evaluation. Gullet 1991;1:87
55. Winans CS. The pharyngoesophageal closure mechanism. A manometric study. Gastroenterology 1972;63:768
56. Winans CS, Harris LD. Quantitation of lower esophageal sphincter competence. Gastroenterology 1966;52:754

*The Esophagus*, Third Edition,
edited by D. O. Castell and J. E. Richter.
Lippincott Williams & Wilkins, Philadelphia © 1999.

# CHAPTER 6

# Ambulatory Monitoring of Esophageal pH and Pressure

André J. P. M. Smout

During the last decade, both researchers and clinicians have learned to appreciate the relevance of prolonged recording of esophageal functions in ambulatory subjects. The first report on prolonged recording of esophageal pH dates from 1969 [56]. This pioneering work was done with stationary equipment in hospitalized patients. Esophageal pH monitoring in truly ambulatory subjects was first described in 1980 [17]. The first report on ambulatory 24-hour esophageal pressure recording dates from 1982 [62]. Since the early 1980s, the development in this field has been very rapid and numerous reports on ambulatory monitoring of esophageal function have been published. In this chapter, information on ambulatory esophageal pH and pressure monitoring in health and disease is reviewed. Because ambulatory pH recording has found and will find more widespread clinical application than ambulatory pressure recording, emphasis is placed on the former technique.

## pH RECORDING

### Recording Techniques and Conditions

Some of the technical details of intraesophageal pH recording greatly influence the outcome of the procedure and are thus relevant to the clinician. In this chapter, technical details are discussed only when considered of clinical relevance.

### pH Electrodes

Several types of small pH electrodes suitable for intraesophageal use are commercially available. Important differences exist between monopolar electrodes, requiring an external reference electrode, and combination electrodes with

A. J. P. M. Smout: Gastrointestinal Research Unit, Departments of Gastroenterology and Surgery, University Hospital Utrecht, 3508 GA Utrecht, The Netherlands.

a built-in reference. The former recording technique is more liable to artifacts than the latter. The cutaneous reference electrode may be the source of totally unreadable tracings due to loose contact, and inaccurate readings may be caused by perspiration-induced changes of the ionic composition of the electrolyte solution surrounding the electrode [15, 19, 36]. However, pH electrodes with built-in reference are currently available only as glass electrodes. They have a larger diameter (up to 4.5 mm) than monopolar electrodes, making transnasal insertion somewhat more difficult.

Monocrystalline antimony electrodes are less expensive than glass electrodes, but have a much shorter life. Furthermore, their performance is clearly inferior to that of glass electrodes. *In vitro* studies have shown that antimony electrodes respond more slowly to sudden pH changes, drift more, and have a far less linear response than glass electrodes [19, 36]. In addition, the response curves of antimony electrodes show considerable hysteresis [36]. From the standpoint of a basic scientist, these shortcomings of antimony electrodes render them inadequate for accurate measurement of intraesophageal pH. In clinical esophageal pH studies, however, both types of electrodes appear to provide similar results [19, 68].

Recently, the ion-sensitive field effect (ISFET) pH electrode was developed. ISFET pH sensors appear to be comparable to glass electrodes with respect to linearity and drift, but have the ability to respond more rapidly to sudden pH changes [14, 33]. They offer the advantage of miniaturization, which makes it feasible to incorporate up to six sensors into one catheter. Currently available ISFET pH electrodes are monopolar.

Prior to each 24-hour pH study, a two-point calibration of the pH electrode must be performed using a neutral buffer and an acidic buffer. At return of the patient after the 24-hour recording period, the calibration should be repeated to rule out pH electrode failure and to allow for correction for slow pH drift. When glass electrodes are used, any type of pH buffer will suffice. With antimony electrodes, only the buffer solutions provided by the manufacturer should be used, since antimony electrodes are also sensitive to agents other than the hydrogen ion.

## Data Loggers

Various types of portable data loggers are commercially available. The analog recording systems initially used have generally been replaced by digital data loggers. A sampling rate of eight per minute and a resolution of 0.1 pH unit are sufficient for clinical purposes [15]. The minimal amount of memory required for 24-hour recording of one pH signal is 11.5 kbytes, the storage of which in a portable housing is technically comfortable. All available systems contain one or more event markers that allow the patient to indicate when symptoms occur (Fig. 6–1). Although the availability of a larger number of event markers seems to be advantageous at first sight, most users of this equipment have become disappointed by the capability of the average patient to use these multiple event markers appropriately.

## Electrode Positioning

Global consensus has been reached that the pH electrode should be positioned at 5 cm above the upper border of the lower esophageal sphincter. For accurate positioning, an esophageal manometric study should be performed prior to the 24-hour pH study, in order to determine the distance from the lower sphincter to the nares. Because esophageal manometry is not as widely available as 24-hour pH recording, other techniques for electrode placement have been used. Measurement based on the pH profile recorded on withdrawal of the electrode from the stomach has been found to be inferior to placement on manometric guidance [38]. Measurement of the distance from the sphincter to the mouth at endoscopic examination, fluoroscopic placement, and use of certain formulas in which body height is employed to calculate sphincter depth are other alternatives, with obvious disadvantages. Fluoroscopic placement carries the risk that the pH electrode will be inadvertently positioned in a hiatal hernia. The endoscopic placement technique suffers from the disadvantage that sphincter-to-mouth and sphincter-to-nose distances vary from patient to patient.

## Patient's Food Intake and Exercise Level

The acidity and buffering capacity of meals and beverages consumed during the 24-hour study period can vary considerably. Therefore, standardization of food intake during pH monitoring has been recommended. Acidic foods, such as carbonated beverages, fruit-based products, pickles, and yogurt, are usually forbidden. It should be realized, however, that the intake of these products has a rather short-lived effect on esophageal pH, so that the quantitative effect of their consumption on reflux variables is minimal. Hence, the use of acid-restricted or nonacidic diets probably is not required for a routine clinical study. Exclusion of the actual eating period from the overall analysis eliminates the artifact introduced by meal constituents having pH below 4.0 (coffee, tea, citrus, carbonated drinks) and improves the separation of normal and abnormal total times for which pH is less than 4 [76]. In some institutions, the use of coffee or cigarettes is routinely prohibited to patients undergoing 24-hour pH monitoring. Apart from the fact that it is doubtful whether all patients are able and willing to adhere to these regulations, the evidence for a substantial influence of these factors on esophageal acid exposure is poor. It has been shown that alcohol and chocolate consumption have a significant reflux-promoting effect [41, 65]. It is likely that other, as-yet-unexplored food constituents also have demonstrable effects on gastroesophageal reflux. Clearly, for research purposes the ideal pH study would be one during which the patient ingests standardized meals at standardized times. In clinical practice, however, such an approach would be unfeasible, and

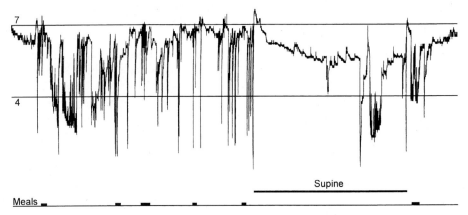

**FIG. 6–1.** Twenty-four-hour overview plot of esophageal pH recorded in an ambulatory subject with gastroesophageal reflux disease. Periods of eating and drinking are indicated by *horizontal bars*. Supine position is indicated by *horizontal line*.

perhaps even undesirable: Information on esophageal pH profile and symptoms during a period in which the patient adheres to his or her own dietary habits is probably more relevant. Other factors of considerable influence are the level of physical exercise displayed by the patient during 24-hour recording [10] and the time spent in a supine position [12].

### Data Reproducibility

The intrasubject reproducibility of 24-hour recording of esophageal pH was studied by several groups of investigators. In some studies, subjects (patients and healthy controls) underwent two ambulatory pH studies on separate days [67, 74]. In another, reflux patients were studied for 48 hours, that is, during 2 consecutive days [27]. Consecutive-day testing was also performed in infants and children [61]. Reproducibility was found to be most consistent for the parameters of percent of time with a pH of less than 4. Total percent of time with a pH of less than 4 showed 85% reproducibility (i.e., 85% of the tested subjects retained a normal or abnormal test result on both study days) [74]. The degree of concordance for this parameter was 77% [27]. Whereas most groups concluded that the reproducibility was ''good'' or ''satisfactory'' [27, 61, 67], others stressed the fact that the total percent of time with a pH of less than 4 may vary between tests by a factor of 3.2-fold (218% higher to 69% lower) [74]. This latter interpretation was supported by the results of a study in which two antimony pH electrodes were positioned at the same level in the esophagus. Discrepancies between the readings from the two electrodes were such that a change in clinical diagnosis (normal versus abnormal) occurred for 2 of the 10 patients studied [42].

### Duration of pH Monitoring

There has been some debate on the optimal duration of a prolonged ambulatory pH monitoring study. Some investigators have made a case for short-term postprandial recording rather than a 24-hour study [21, 29]. However, evidence for the superiority of 24-hour over shorter interval pH monitoring has been produced; the sensitivity of a 24-hour test is significantly higher than that of a 12-hour test [2]. Furthermore, in outpatients a 24-hour recording period usually is more practical than a shorter test and the reproducibility of 24-hour recordings is significantly better than that of 4-hour or 8-hour recordings [27]. Although most clinicians and investigators would now agree that 24-hour recording is the method of choice, a 16-hour study from 1600 to 0800 hours can provide accurate information and improve patient tolerance [13].

### INTERPRETATION

#### Criteria for Reflux

In the analysis of esophageal pH recordings, pH drops below 4 are usually taken as evidence of acid gastroesopha-

geal reflux. The cutoff limit of pH 4 has been chosen arbitrarily, but there seems to be some rationale for this choice; first, because the proteolytic enzyme pepsin is inactive above pH 4.0 and, second, because patients with symptomatic reflux usually report heartburn at an intraesophageal pH below 4 [59]. Different cutoff limits have been formally compared in a number of studies. In an early study in nonambulatory subjects, the discriminatory power of pH cutoff levels 3, 4, and 5 was calculated and the best discrimination between healthy controls and patients with reflux symptoms was found to be obtained with pH 5 [58]. Others compared cutoff levels of pH 3, 4, 5, and 6 using an ambulatory technique. The best discrimination between healthy subjects and reflux patients occurred within the full range from pH 3 to 6 rather than at any single pH [64]. Yet another group reported cutoff limits of pH 3, 4, and 5 to be superior to pH 2 with respect to the discrimination of patients with endoscopic evidence of grade II or III esophagitis from normal subjects [28]. A combination of cutoff limits was not found to be superior in the latter group's data. Consequently, the authors suggested that pH 4 should be used to define reflux episodes [28].

In a recent study in which we used pH distribution curves to identify the point of separation between ''reflux'' and ''nonreflux'' pH values, optimal pH thresholds from 5.0 to 6.4 (upright) and from 4.5 to 5.7 (supine) were found [73]. On the basis of the results it can be concluded that use of the conventional threshold of pH 4 leads to underestimation of the severity of gastroesophageal reflux. Nevertheless, given the widespread acceptance of the pH 4 threshold, it would be unwise to advocate the use of any other threshold in clinical practice. In the analysis of the association between symptoms and reflux, however, we advocate taking rapid pH falls of more than 1 pH unit into account, even when the threshold of 4 is not reached (see section on Association between Symptoms and Reflux).

The proportion of time that the pH is below the cutoff level of 4, called *reflux time* or *acid exposure time,* is the most widely used reflux variable. It can be expressed either in minutes or in percentage of time. It has the often-underestimated advantage that its calculation is straightforward. In contrast, the number of reflux episodes counted during a 24-hour study period depends highly on the algorithm used for identification of a reflux episode. With some algorithms, oscillations of the pH around the threshold value lead to a spuriously high number of reflux episodes counted (Fig. 6–2) [15, 23]. It is obvious that the results from different centers cannot be compared as far as the numbers of reflux episodes are concerned. The number of reflux episodes shows a much poorer correlation with the grade of esophagitis than does reflux time. In addition, the parameter of number of episodes was found to be less reproducible than the parameter of percent of time with a pH less than 4 [74]. These limitations of the number-of-episodes parameter have made some investigators abandon its use completely.

The mean duration of a reflux episode can be calculated

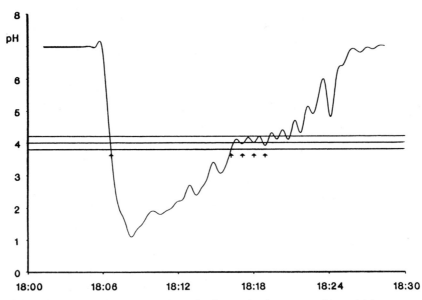

**FIG. 6–2.** Figure illustrating that the number of reflux episodes counted in a 24-hour esophageal pH study depends on the algorithm used for determination of onset and end of a reflux episode. Small oscillations around the threshold level of pH 4 may lead to a spuriously high number of reflux episodes. (From ref. 23, with permission.)

by dividing the reflux time by the number of reflux episodes. The variable has been called the acid clearance time since it is dependent on the clearance capacity of the esophagus. It should be realized that this variable is as algorithm dependent as is the number of reflux episodes.

The number of reflux episodes longer than 5 minutes, a variable introduced in 1974 [25], is still popular. Whereas one should be aware that the choice of a 5-minute period is arbitrary, many clinicians have learned to appreciate this variable as a measure of esophageal clearance capacity. Three or more reflux episodes longer than 5 minutes occurring in a 24-hour study is considered abnormal.

Mean and median pH in certain time intervals have been used as variables by some investigators in this field, but have not gained much popularity.

More complex reflux parameters composed of a number of different variables have been advocated by some users of the 24-hour recording technique. The frequency–duration index (FDI), e.g., is defined as the mean number of reflux episodes per hour multiplied by the mean cumulative duration of reflux episodes per hour [4]. Johnson and DeMeester [25, 26] advocated the use of a pH score that takes into account the six different variables listed in Table 6–1. It is questionable whether such composite scores have sufficient advantages over simpler variables. Studies that compared composite scores with reflux time (time with a pH less than 4) showed that the latter discriminates at least as well as the former between health and disease [28, 49].

The patterns of reflux in healthy subjects are very different during the day and during the night. At night, reflux episodes are rare, although their incidence increases with age [20, 33, 70]. When nighttime gastroesophageal reflux occurs, it

appears to be related to the interdigestive migrating motor complex [20]. During the day, up to 50 reflux episodes may be observed in health. These observations necessitate the separate analysis of daytime (upright) and nighttime (supine) portions of the recordings.

DeMeester and colleagues [12] described three patterns of abnormal gastroesophageal reflux: reflux in the upright position only, in the supine position only, and in both positions. Of the 100 symptomatic patients studied, 9 were upright refluxers, 37 were supine refluxers, and 54 were combined refluxers. In patients with an upright reflux pattern reflux occurred predominantly in the postprandial period. Supine refluxers differed from upright refluxers by having a higher incidence of esophagitis. Combined refluxers had an even higher incidence of esophagitis than supine refluxers [12]. Others were unable to confirm that three distinct patterns of reflux occur [11]. Also, acid exposure during the 3 hours following the evening meal was more closely corre-

**TABLE 6–1.** *Normal values in 24-hour esophageal pH recording as derived from the pioneering study by Johnson and DeMeester [25]*[a]

| Variable | Normal value |
|---|---|
| Percent of time pH <4 | |
|   Total period | <4.2% |
|   Upright period | <6.3% |
|   Supine period | <1.2% |
| Number of episodes | |
|   Total | <50 |
|   Longer than 5 min | <3 |
| Duration of longest episode | <9.2 min |

[a] From ref. 25, with permission.

lated with esophagitis than was nighttime exposure [11]. Others reported that although the increase in nighttime reflux in esophagitis patients was proportionally greater than the increase in postprandial reflux, the latter still formed the greatest contribution to the acid contact time [32].

Reflux of alkaline duodenal contents into the esophagus has been put forward as a putative factor in the pathogenesis of reflux esophagitis, and it has been claimed that episodes of alkaline gastroesophageal reflux can be detected as rises of esophageal pH in excess of 7. However, in a patient with an intact and acid-secreting stomach the gastric pH seldomly exceeds 7. It has been shown that esophageal pH values of greater than 7 may also occur as a result of increased secretion of saliva [52]. Furthermore, recent studies have shown that the esophageal mucosa can also be a source of bicarbonate in the esophageal lumen [39]. Using an esophageal aspiration technique, Mittal and colleagues found that in patients with gastroesophageal reflux disease, bile acids do not reflux into the esophagus in potentially harmful quantities [40]. In a study using a bilirubin-sensitive probe, significant correlations were found between esophageal acid and bilirubin exposure values, but not between alkaline and bilirubin exposures. This observation suggests that bilirubin exposure of the esophagus mainly runs parallel with acid exposure and that duodenogastroesophageal reflux cannot be recorded reliably by esophageal pH monitoring [9]. Therefore there is no rationale for quantifying the number of episodes or percentages of time with an esophageal pH greater than 7 in a clinical 24-hour esophageal pH study.

## Normal Values

A prerequisite for any diagnostic test aimed at detecting disease is that the limits of normal for that test have been well defined. This is usually done by subjecting a sufficiently large group of healthy subjects to the test. When the values found in these normal subjects are normally distributed, the mean plus or minus 2 standard deviations can be used to determine the upper and lower limits of normal. Many investigators have indeed used the mean plus or minus 2 standard deviations in calculating the upper limit of normal of ambulatory esophageal pH variables. It has been shown, however, that most variables measured in ambulatory 24-hour esophageal recording do not fit the assumption of Gaussian distribution [28, 54]. Nonparametric methods, such as estimation of the 5th and 95th percentiles (or the 2.5th and 97.5th percentiles), must therefore be used in the determination of normal values in ambulatory 24-hour esophageal pH recording. Another approach is to study a group of healthy control subjects and a group of patients with reflux disease and to determine the values that provide optimal separation between the groups. This can be done with discriminant analysis or with receiver-operating characteristics analysis [49]. The threshold values found with such an approach should be evaluated prospectively in a new group of patients and controls before statements about the sensitivity and specificity of the test are made.

As shown in Table 6–2, the normal values for ambulatory esophageal pH recording in adults reported in the literature vary widely [3, 11, 19, 20, 25, 28, 47, 49, 64, 68, 70] due to differences in the age distribution of the control subjects studied and in the algorithms used for calculation of the parameters, as well as to the method used for determination of the upper limit of normal.

Controversial data have been published on the relation between age and pH variables in normal subjects. Whereas some investigators found no significant relation with age [57], others reported an increase in some reflux variables with age [47, 54].

In a study of 285 infants, the esophageal exposure time was found to be relatively low in the first months of life (1.20 ± 0.91% to 2.52 ± 2.25%) [60]. At 4 months, the reflux index had increased significantly (to 4.18 ± 2.6%). At 15 months, the reflux index had decreased again, to 2.65 ± 1.90%. The low values of the reflux variables found in newborns have been attributed to a low level of body movements and the hyposecretion of gastric acid.

**TABLE 6–2.** *Reported limits of normal values as found in ambulatory esophageal pH recording in adults*

| Study | Ref. | Percent of time esophageal pH <4 | | Analytic method used[a] |
|---|---|---|---|---|
| | | Upright | Supine | |
| Johnson and DeMeester 1974 | 25 | 6.3 | 1.2 | Mean ± 2 SD |
| Weiser et al. 1982 | 70 | 5.9 | 2.1 | Mean ± 2 SD |
| Vitale et al. 1985 | 64 | 5.9 | 4.6 | Mean ± 2 SD |
| Ward et al. 1986 | 68 | 5.9 | 1.8 | Mean ± 2 SD |
| Bonavina et al. 1986 | 3 | 6.3 | 4.6 | Mean ± 2 SD |
| De Caestecker 1989 | 11 | 9.1 | 11.2 | 95th percentile |
| Gignoux et al. 1987 | 19 | 14.2 | 3.6 | Mean ± 2 SD |
| Schindlbeck et al. 1987 | 49 | 10.5 | 6.0 | ROC |
| Johnsson et al. 1987 | 28 | 4.6 | 3.2 | 95th percentile |
| Smout et al. 1989 | 54 | | | |
|    <45 yr | | 7.3 | 3.6 | 95th percentile |
|    >45 yr | | 16.0 | 6.7 | 95th percentile |
| Richter et al. 1992 | 47 | 8.15 | 3.45 | 95th percentile |

[a] SD, Standard deviation; ROC, receiver-operating characteristic analysis.

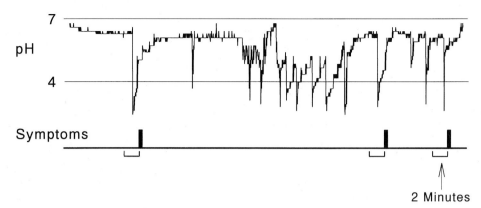

**FIG. 6–3.** Association between reflux symptoms and esophageal pH drops in a patient with pyrosis and regurgitation, but without esophagitis. The three vertical bars mark the onset of reflux symptoms, as indicated by the patient by pressing the symptom marker button on the pH recorder. Each of the three symptom episodes is preceded by reflux.

### Association between Symptoms and Reflux

As discussed in more detail later, the importance of determining whether a patient's reflux is pathologic or is still within physiologic limits is probably overstressed. Rather, the most important piece of information to be obtained from a 24-hour pH study is whether and to what extent the symptoms reported by the patient are related to gastroesophageal reflux. The temporal correlation between symptoms and reflux can be convincing on inspection of the pH–time curves (Fig. 6–3), but a quantitative measure of such a relationship is desirable. In the (automated) analysis of the relationship between symptoms and reflux a 2-minute time window beginning at 2 minutes before the onset of the symptoms appears to be optimal [35].

In 1988, Wiener and colleagues [75] proposed a parameter to express the relationship between symptoms and reflux episodes which they labeled the symptom index (SI). It is defined as the percentage of the symptom episodes that are related to reflux,

$$\frac{\text{Number of reflux-related symptom episodes}}{\text{Total number of symptom episodes}} \times 100\%$$

There is evidence, based on receiver operating characteristic analysis, that 50% is the optimal threshold for the SI [53].

The distribution of symptom indices in a population of patients with reflux disease is bimodal (i.e., high and low values occur more often than intermediate values; Fig. 6–4). It is important to note that the correlation between the severity of esophageal acid exposure and the symptom index is rather poor (Fig. 6–4), indicating that acid exposure and acid sensitivity are different phenomena.

The disadvantage of the symptom index is that it does not take into account the number of reflux episodes. Obviously, the significance of a symptom index of 100% in a patient with only a single reflux episode per 24 hours is different from that in a patient with more than 100 reflux episodes per 24 hours. For this reason, Breumelhof and colleagues

proposed the additional use of another index, which they called the symptom sensitivity index (SSI) [6], defined as

$$\frac{\text{Number of symptom-associated reflux episodes}}{\text{Total number of reflux episodes}} \times 100\%$$

SSI values of 10% or higher are considered to be positive [6]. Calculation of both SI and SSI for one and the same pH monitoring test may yield discordant results. From discordant test results, conclusions can be drawn as to the cause of the patient's symptoms. When the SSI is high and the SI is low, e.g., this would indicate that the patient's esophagus is sensitive to reflux, but that other causes than acid reflux are likely to contribute to the symptoms as well.

Both the SI and the SSI suffer from the disadvantage that they do not integrate all factors determining the relationship between symptoms and reflux. Weusten and colleagues therefore developed another parameter that expresses the

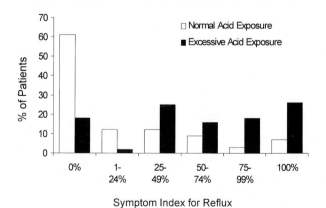

**FIG. 6–4.** Distribution of symptom indices (SI) for the symptom heartburn or chest pain in 125 patients who experienced one or more symptom episodes during a 24-hour esophageal pH study. Note that many patients with a low SI have excessive esophageal acid exposure and that some patients with a high SI have normal acid exposure. (From ref. 71, with permission.)

likelihood that a patient's symptoms are related to reflux [7]. This parameter, labeled the symptom association probability (SAP), is calculated by dividing the 24-hour pH data into 2-minute segments. Then for each of these 2-minute segments it is determined whether reflux occurred in it and whether a symptom was reported. A $2 \times 2$ contingency table is then made in which the number of 2-minute segments with and without reflux and with and without symptom are tabulated. A modified chi-square test is used to calculate the probability that the observed distribution could have been brought about by chance. The SAP is calculated as $(1 - P) \times 100\%$. By statistical convention SAP values greater than 95% are positive.

In the analysis of the association between symptoms and reflux, rigorous adherence to the criterion that a threshold of pH 4 should be passed may lead to underestimation of the reflux-related origin of the symptoms. In patients using acid secretion inhibitors, in patients with atrophic gastritis, and during postprandial periods the intragastric pH may be above 4. In our laboratory any decrease in pH of more than one pH unit that occurs within 8 seconds is considered as indicative of gastroesophageal reflux. It has been shown that these episodes may be responsible for up to one-third of reflux-related symptom episodes [31].

### Clinical Relevance of Ambulatory pH Recording

#### pH Monitoring in Patients with Reflux Esophagitis

It will come as no surprise to learn that patients with reflux esophagitis have more reflux episodes and a higher esophageal acid exposure time than do normal controls [18, 32, 37, 45, 48] and that the severity of reflux esophagitis is significantly correlated with the extent of gastroesophageal reflux (reflux time) (Fig. 6–5) [37]. Given the accuracy with which the diagnosis of reflux esophagitis can be made endoscopically, however, it is amazing to witness how much effort has been made to determine the sensitivity and specificity of 24-hour pH recording in making this diagnosis. Sensitivities between 84% and 96% and specificities ranging from 91% to 98% have been reported [2, 18, 28, 49, 50, 64]. The gold standard in the above referenced reports was variable; hence, the results of the various studies cannot be compared directly. Furthermore, the design of some of the studies was insufficient in that determination of the optimally discriminating pH values and the calculation of specificity and sensitivity were done in the same patient group and control group. This may result in spuriously high sensitivity and specificity values. More importantly, however, it is incorrect to view esophageal pH monitoring as an alternative to endoscopy in the diagnosis of reflux esophagitis, and therefore calculation of sensitivity and specificity with esophagitis as the gold standard is useless.

Once the diagnosis of reflux has been made endoscopically, there is generally no indication for 24-hour monitoring. Only when the esophagitis fails to respond to medical treatment should 24-hour pH recording be considered. Ideally, the pH study should then be performed repetitively with the patient using increasingly high doses of an acid secretion-inhibiting drug. With this approach, one should be able to find the dose that adequately reduces esophageal acid exposure. It has been argued, however, that the large intrasubject variability in 24-hour acid exposure may limit this test's usefulness as a measurement of therapeutic improvement [74]. Dual pH monitoring with one electrode in the esophagus and one in the stomach may be helpful in the management of these therapy-resistant patients [30].

#### pH Monitoring in Patients with Reflux Symptoms

The symptoms of heartburn and regurgitation are commonly held to be reliable indicators of gastroesophageal reflux. However, heartburn may also be the principal complaint of patients with peptic ulcer disease, cholelithiasis, and nonulcer dyspepsia. On the other hand, patients with severe reflux disease (resulting in severe esophagitis) may deny all typical reflux symptoms. Not infrequently, atypical symptoms—in particular, anginalike chest pain and pulmonary symptoms—are the only manifestations of reflux disease. Therefore, ambulatory pH monitoring is the preferred method to document abnormal reflux and its association with specific symptoms. The correlation between typical reflux symptoms and 24-hour esophageal acid exposure, as measured by 24-hour monitoring, has been found to be rather weak (Fig. 6–6) [37, 71]. This finding should not be interpreted as indicative of a limited value of 24-hour esophageal pH monitoring, but rather as a result of the large individual variability in the perception of reflux. Esophageal pH monitoring is the most appropriate technique to prove (or disprove) that the symptoms (typical or not) are reflux related [22]. For quantitative analysis of the temporal relation between symptoms and reflux, the symptom index, the symptom sensitivity index, and the symptom association probability can be used [6, 72, 75], as discussed previously. The indications for ambulatory 24-hour esophageal pH recording are summarized in Table 6–3.

### PRESSURE RECORDING

#### Recording Technique

Since the early 1980s, esophageal pressure signals have been recorded in ambulatory subjects, using intraesophageal microtransducers. All groups that have evaluated 24-hour esophageal pressure recording have combined this technique with 24-hour esophageal pH recording. The pioneering work in this field was done with analog recording systems, using Holter types of tape recorders and audiocassettes [22, 24, 43, 44, 55, 63]. With the advent of digital recording systems with large memory capacity many of the technical problems of ambulatory esophageal pressure recording have been overcome [5, 8, 16]. One of the advantages of digital record-

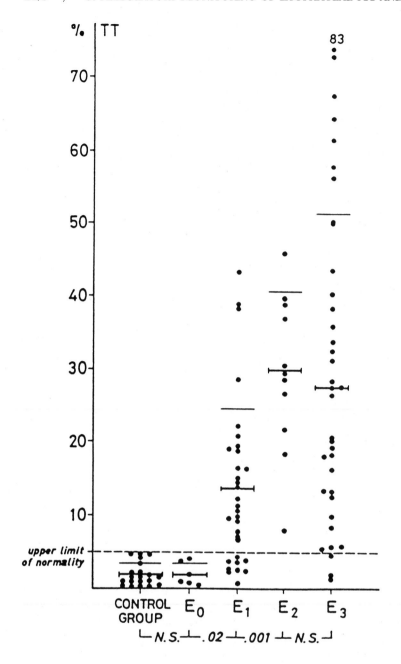

**FIG. 6–5.** Relationship between percent total time (%TT) with esophageal pH of less than 4 and grade of esophagitis. $E_0$, No esophagitis; $E_1$, microscopic esophagitis; $E_2$, nonconfluent erosions; $E_3$, confluent erosions, ulcer, stenosis, or Barrett's esophagus; N.S., not significant. (From ref. 37, with permission.)

ing is that the digitized data can easily be displayed graphically at any desired time base and amplitude scale, without excessive paper consumption. When a digital system is used to store 24-hour esophageal pressure data, the sampling rate must be 4 Hz or higher to prevent unacceptable waveform distortion and underestimation of contraction amplitude.

Since esophageal contractile activity is different during meals and between meals and different during sleep and during the day (see Fig. 6–7), it is imperative that records be kept of these activities. These records must be precise to the minute. Use of a marker button to indicate accurately the beginning and end of a meal and supine episodes is helpful.

At present, 24-hour recording of esophageal pH and pressure no longer is a research technique. Clinical application of this technique in the noncardiac chest pain syndrome has been shown to be worthwhile [24, 34, 43, 55]. Unfortunately, standardization of recording and analysis techniques has not yet been achieved.

**Analysis Techniques**

The problems encountered in the analysis of 24-hour esophageal pressure data are far more complex than those encountered in the analysis of 24-hour pH data. As mentioned earlier, esophageal motility and its relation to symptoms cannot be adequately assessed by simply looking at a 24-hour plot. It can be estimated that complete manual analysis of a 24-hour pressure recording, comprising categoriza-

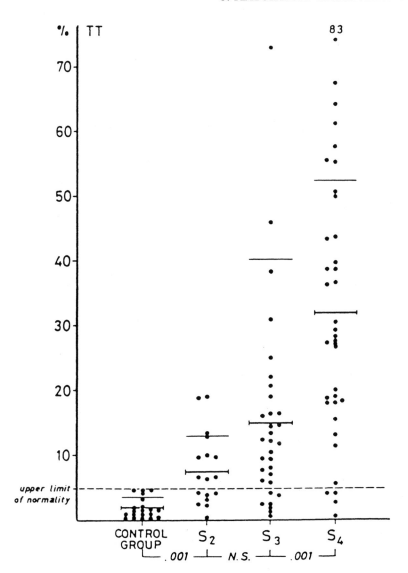

**FIG. 6-6.** Relationship between percent of total time (%TT) with esophageal pH of less than 4 and severity of reflux symptoms. $S_2$, Postural heartburn or pain once or twice daily; $S_3$, postural or spontaneous heartburn or pain up to four times daily; $S_4$, spontaneous or postural heartburn or pain more than four times per day; N.S., not significant. (From ref. 37, with permission.)

tion of each contraction and measurement of its amplitude, duration, and propagation velocity, would take one person approximately 2 weeks. Even in a research environment, this is an unacceptable investment of time and money. Solutions to this problem are to just browse through the data and analyze only certain proportions (e.g., the episodes during which the patient reported presence of a symptom) or to rely on computer algorithms for fully automated analysis of the data.

**TABLE 6-3.** *Indications for ambulatory 24-hour esophageal pH recording*

Assessment of relationships between symptoms and (acid) reflux
   Typical reflux symptoms in the absence of esophagitis
   Atypical symptoms with or without esophagitis
   When antireflux surgery is considered
Evaluation of the effect of symptomatically or endoscopically unsuccessful treatment (conservative or surgical) on esophageal acid exposure

Even when commercially developed computer software can be used, the clinician relying on it must be sure that he or she fully understands what the program does. Ambulatory esophageal pressure recording is certainly an area in medicine wherein the danger of incorrect decisions being made on the basis of insufficiently understood computer-generated figures is real.

In the automated analysis of ambulatorily recorded esophageal pressure, criteria have been developed to differentiate contractions from artifacts (e.g., respiration artifacts) and to categorize contractions as peristaltic, simultaneous, or nontransmitted (nonpropagated). It should be realized that the majority of contractions recorded in a 24-hour study are not initiated by wet swallows and that these have a considerably lower amplitude than those recorded in a conventional manometric study. Even in healthy controls, the smallest esophageal contractions are indistinguishable from respiratory pressure variations and other artifacts. A threshold of approximately 15 mm Hg above baseline is usually em-

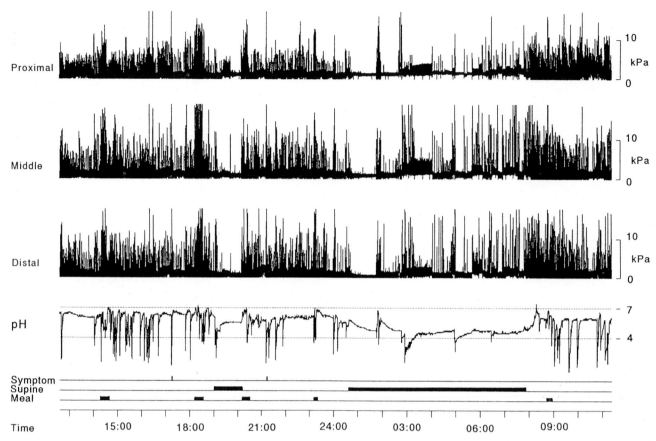

**FIG. 6–7.** Twenty-four-hour overview plot of esophageal pH signal (lower panel) and three esophageal pressure signals (upper three panels) recorded in an ambulatory patient with chest pain. The proximal, middle, and distal pressure transducers were positioned 15, 10, and 5 cm proximal to the upper border of the lower esophageal sphincter, respectively. 10 kPA equals 77 mm Hg.

ployed to distinguish contractions from artifacts [5, 16]. The criteria to differentiate peristaltic contractions from simultaneous and nontransmitted contractions are summarized in Table 6–4 [5, 16, 64]. Results of automated pressure data analysis have been validated by comparing the results of computer analysis with those of manual analysis by a panel of experts [8, 54].

In a study in 32 healthy volunteers ranging in age from 20 to 73 years, it was found that contractions recorded during meal consumption (perprandial contractions) had a signifi-

**TABLE 6–4.** *Propagation velocities used as criteria in computerized classification of esophageal contractions in ambulatory 24-hour studies*

| Contraction type | Velocity (cm/sec) | |
|---|---|---|
| | Breedijk et al. 1989 [5][a] Smout et al. 1989 [54][a] | Emde et al. 1990 [16][b] |
| Peristaltic | ≥1.8 and ≤12.5 | >1 and <10 |
| Simultaneous | >12.5 or <−25.0 | >10 |
| Nontransmitted | <1.8 and ≥−25.0 | <1 |

[a] Reference point: passing of 15-mm Hg threshold.
[b] Reference point: maximal slope during upstroke.

cantly ($p$ less than 0.001) higher amplitude (66 ± 5.3 mm Hg) than the interprandial contractions recorded at daytime (49.6 ± 3.8 mm Hg). Only 50.9 ± 2.0% of the 2,141 ± 163 contractions recorded in the 24-hour period were peristaltic, 10.4 ± 1.2% were simultaneous, and the remaining portion was nontransmitted (segmental). Repetitive contractions, defined as having more than two peaks, were rare [54]. Upper and lower limits of normal are listed in Table 6–5.

As in the analysis of pH data, the analysis of the temporal association between symptoms and abnormalities in tracings is of more importance than the overall analysis. This symptom-oriented analysis is rather complex, since the pressure tracings must be analyzed for abnormal contraction amplitude, abnormal contraction duration, abnormal contraction configuration (repetitive contractions), and abnormal contraction type (increased number of simultaneous waves). The optimal approach appears to be to use the patient as his or her own control (i.e., to use the motor activity in symptom-free episodes to determine what is normal for that patient). It has been shown that an analysis that uses asymptomatic baseline periods throughout the entire 24-hour period leads to more reliable results than an analysis in which only 10-minute periods before each chest pain episode are used [46].

**TABLE 6–5.** *Normal values in 24-hour ambulatory esophageal manometry (2.5th and 97.5th percentiles) as derived from a study in 32 healthy subjects [54]*[a]

| | 15 cm from LES | 5 cm from LES |
|---|---|---|
| Mean amplitude (kPa) | | |
| Peristaltic contractions | | |
|     Interprandial, day-time | 3.71–9.31 | 3.84–10.39 |
|     Interprandial, night-time | 3.38–12.63 | 3.26–13.97 |
|     Perprandial | 3.50–11.42 | 3.60–15.09 |
| Simultaneous contractions | | |
|     Interprandial, day-time | 3.63–7.65 | 3.84–8.13 |
|     Interprandial, night-time | 3.11–9.73 | 3.68–15.41 |
|     Perprandial | 3.43–7.59 | 3.48–7.51 |
| Nontransmitted contractions | | |
|     Interprandial, day-time | 3.43–7.24 | 3.56–6.86 |
|     Interprandial, night-time | 2.91–6.93 | 3.59–8.08 |
|     Perprandial | 3.60–9.29 | 3.54–10.85 |
| Mean duration (sec) | | |
| Peristaltic contractions | | |
|     Interprandial, day-time | 1.3–2.9 | 1.3–3.5 |
|     Interprandial, night-time | 1.3–3.7 | 1.8–4.9 |
|     Perprandial | 1.5–3.7 | 1.4–3.7 |
| Simultaneous contractions | | |
|     Interprandial, day-time | 1.0–2.2 | 1.2–2.9 |
|     Interprandial, night-time | 1.2–3.3 | 1.4–6.3 |
|     Perprandial | 0.9–2.4 | 1.1–2.8 |
| Nontransmitted contractions | | |
|     Interprandial, day-time | 1.1–2.2 | 1.1–2.4 |
|     Interprandial, night-time | 1.2–2.3 | 1.4–3.4 |
|     Perprandial | 1.2–4.0 | 1.2–2.9 |
| Percent peristaltic contractions | 30.4–71.1 | |
| Percent simultaneous contractions | 2.65–29.8 | |
| Percent nontransmitted contractions | 19.6–59.4 | |

[a] LES, Lower esophageal sphincter. 1 kPa equals 7.5 mm Hg.

Algorithms for fully automated computer analysis according to this principle have been developed and applied and are now commercially available [46]. In this symptom association analysis, different time windows have been used arbitrarily by various groups. A recent study has indicated, however, that a window beginning at 2 minutes before the onset of pain and ending at the onset of pain yields optimal results [35]. This is the same window that is also optimal for the analysis of reflux-related symptoms.

## Clinical Relevance of Ambulatory Pressure Recording

The development of systems for ambulatory recording of esophageal motor acitivity was prompted by the frequency with which diagnostic problems are encountered in patients with noncardiac chest pain. Since some of the esophageal

motor abnormalities that may lead to esophageal chest pain occur intermittently, they can easily be missed during a brief conventional study. The aim of 24-hour pressure monitoring is to increase the chance of catching these abnormalities. Second, the demonstration of a continuously present esophageal motor abnormality, such as the nutcracker esophagus, does not yet prove that the patient's intermittent symptoms are caused by that abnormality. Much more convincing evidence of the causal role of such an abnormality is obtained when a temporal relationship between symptoms and abnormal motor events is found.

It is not likely that 24-hour esophageal pressure monitoring will prove to be very useful in the diagnosis of continuously present (i.e., nonintermittent) esophageal motor disorders. It may be argued that prolonged monitoring is slightly more sensitive and specific in the diagnosis of nutcracker esophagus, since the diagnosis of this condition depends on the quantitative evaluation of contraction amplitude, but it is doubtful whether this diagnostic yield outweighs the costs and efforts associated with ambulatory pressure monitoring.

The first report on 24-hour ambulatory pressure monitoring in noncardiac chest pain was published in 1986 [24]. In that year, the Louvain group reported that in a group of 60 patients with chest pain of unexplained origin, combined 24-hour monitoring of esophageal pH and pressure increased from 16 to 29 the number of patients in whom an esophageal origin of the pain could be proved [24]. The authors described their findings in a rather positive way, by stating that the combination of all conventional examinations and the 24-hour test made an esophageal origin of the pain likely in 48% of the patients (29 of 60 patients) [18]. However, a correlation between chest pain and abnormal motility alone was demonstrated in only 8 of the 60 patients, 6 of whom also showed abnormalities during the conventional manometric study. Therefore, the most pessimistic interpretation of the data would be that in only 2 of the 60 patients studied did the ambulatory pressure study provide new evidence of the esophageal origin of the symptoms.

One year later, the same group of investigators described a group of 33 patients with anginalike chest pain in whom a positive correlation between chest pain and reflux or an esophageal motor disorder was found on 24-hour monitoring [63]. An intriguing finding was that in 10 of these patients, some of the episodes of chest pain were associated with reflux and other episodes with motor abnormalities. The increased tendency to perceive esophageal stimuli of various types as pain was designated "irritable esophagus."

In a U.S. study in 24 patients with daily noncardiac chest pain in which quantitative criteria were used to determine whether a patient's esophageal motility was (more) abnormal during symptom episodes than during asymptomatic periods, the majority of the symptom episodes (64%) were found to have no associations with abnormal motility or reflux, 20% were reflux-related, 18% were dysmotility-related, and 4% of the episodes were related to both abnormalities [43]. Overall, 13 patients (59%) had at least one chest pain episode correlating with abnormal motility or pH. The authors concluded that ambulatory monitoring of esophageal motility and pH is useful in the evaluation of noncardiac chest pain. However, their individual patient data show that some association between chest pain and abnormal motility alone was found in only 4 patients (14%), only 1 of whom had a symptom index higher than 50% (for motor abnormality).

In a study from the United Kingdom of 20 patients with noncardiac chest pain, ambulatory pH and pressure recording were reported to have a low diagnostic yield. The ambulatory pH study helped to establish the esophagus as the likely source of pain in 1 patient, and the ambulatory pressure recording did the same in another [55].

Our first experiences with 24-hour pH and pressure monitoring in unexplained chest pain were published in 1990 [46]. Breumelhof and colleagues studied 44 consecutive tertiary referral patients with daily chest pain without making a selection of the basis of the frequency of their pain attacks. As could have been expected, 19 of the patients did not experience chest pain during the 24-hour study period. Using computerized analysis of the association between chest pain and reflux or abnormal motility and using the rather stringent criterion of SI greater than 75% proof of an esophageal origin of the symptoms was found in 8 of the remaining 25 patients (reflux in 2, dysmotility in 2, both reflux and dysmotility in 4 patients). Thus, it had to be concluded that combined esophageal monitoring provided a diagnosis in 8 of the 44 patients (18%) only.

Later we learned that the yield of ambulatory 24-hour pH and pressure monitoring in noncardiac chest pain depends largely on patient selection. Whereas the test was positive in only 18% of tertiary referral patients, much higher yields were found in patients acutely referred to a general hospital. Lam and colleagues studied 41 patients admitted to the coronary care unit as soon as it was considered unlikely that their pain was of cardiac origin [34]. Using the same techniques for recording and data analysis as in Breumelhof's study [46], they found pain episodes to be related to reflux in 14 patients (34%) and to abnormal motility in 12 patients (29%) [34]. In another general hospital, a 24-hour monitoring study was carried out in 28 patients who were newly referred to a cardiac outpatient clinic because of chest pain. Symptomatic gastroesophageal reflux disease was identified as the cause of the pain in 36% of the patients. In none of the patients was evidence of a esophageal motility disorder found [66].

Hewson and colleagues compared the yield of conventional tests, such as short-term esophageal manometry, the acid perfusion test, and the edrophonium test, with that of 24-hour pH and pressure monitoring in 45 patients with noncardiac chest pain [22]. All patients experienced chest pain during ambulatory monitoring. Patients with normal manometry were significantly more likely to have acid reflux chest pain than did nutcracker esophagus patients. A positive result on the acid perfusion test was significantly associated with abnormal motility during pain, whereas a positive result

on the edrophonium test predicted acid reflux-associated pain. The authors concluded that conventional tests may point to the esophagus as the likely source of the chest pain, but that ambulatory monitoring is required to prove the association between symptoms and reflux or dysmotility. However, an association between pain and abnormal motility alone (i.e., in the absence of an association with reflux) occurred in only 4 of the 45 patients (9%) [22].

The general conclusion to be drawn from these studies is that, in tertiary referral patients, the addition of 24-hour pressure recording to 24-hour pH recording does not lead to a substantial increase in the number of cases in which evidence for an esophageal origin of the symptoms can be obtained. On the basis of currently available information, it can be estimated that the additional diagnostic yield in these patients is less than 10%. One of the problems encountered is that only a minority of the noncardiac chest pain patients have their pain every day. The diagnostic yield of the technique appears to be higher, however, when it is applied to patients in an early phase of the diagnostic workup or to patients with frequent pain attacks.

However, even though the yield of combined pH and pressure monitoring in unselected patients with chest pain is limited, we consider it worthwhile to perform the test because a positive result may greatly influence the patient's quality of life. It has been reported that an affirmative diagnosis of esophageal chest pain reduces the number of coronary care unit admissions, the consumption of drugs, and even the incidence of chest pain episodes [69].

## Ambulatory Lower Esophageal Sphincter Pressure Monitoring

Recent technological developments have made it possible to record lower esophageal sphincter (LES) pressure during prolonged periods of time in ambulatory subjects. Basically, two types of devices can be used to measure LES pressure continuously. Both employ a sensor of several centimeters length that is positioned across the LES. With such a sensor small longitudinal movements of the sphincter with respect to the sensor (caused by respiration, body movements, or swallowing) do not influence the LES pressure readings. One of these devices is a so-called sphinctometer, consisting of a nonperfused chamber filled with a viscous fluid [1]. The other is a modification of the water-perfused sleeve sensor, requiring a portable perfusion pump and transducer assembly [51]. A disadvantage of the latter system is that it is rather bulky and heavy. These technical obstacles, and the fact that the additional value of LES pressure monitoring for clinical decision making has not yet been established, presently limit the application of the technique to the research domain. Important new observations on the mechanisms of gastroesophageal reflux have been made with this technique [51]. In particular, the important role of transient LES relaxations in the pathogenesis of gastroesophageal re-

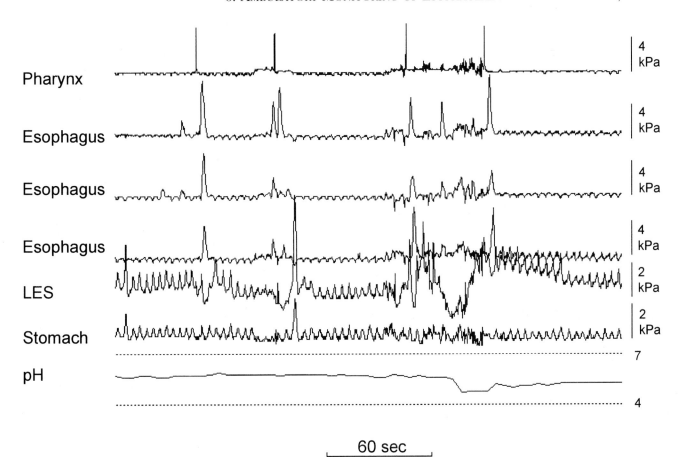

**FIG. 6–8.** Detail of a 24-hour study in which pharyngeal, esophageal, lower esophageal sphincter (LES), and gastric pressures were recorded in a patient with (endoscopy-negative) reflux disease. A reflux episode can be seen during which the esophageal pH falls from 5.8 to 4.7. This reflux episode is caused by a transient LES relaxation.

flux has been elucidated with the aid of ambulatory LES pressure monitoring (Fig. 6–8).

## REFERENCES

1. Barham CP, Gotley DC, Mills A, Alderson D. Oesophageal acid clearance in patients with severe reflux oesophagitis. Br J Surg 1995;82:333–337
2. Bianchi Porro G, Pace F. Comparison of three methods of intra-esophageal pH recording in the diagnosis of gastroesophageal reflux. Scand J Gastroenterol 1988;23:743–750
3. Bonavina L, DeMeester TR. Prolonged esophageal pH monitoring. In Sigel B, ed, Diagnostic Patient Studies in Surgery. Philadelphia: Lea & Febiger, 1986:353–363
4. Branicki FJ, Evans DF, Jones JA, Ogilvie AL, Atkinson M, Hardcastle JD. A frequency-duration index (FDI) for the evaluation of ambulatory recordings of gastro-oesophageal reflux. Br J Surg 1984;71:425–430
5. Breedijk M, Smout AJPM, Van der Zouw C, Verwey H, Akkermans LMA. Microcomputer based system for 24-hour recording of oesophageal motility and pH profile with automated analysis. Med Biol Eng Comput 1989;27:41–46
6. Breumelhof R, Smout AJPM. The symptom sensitivity index: a valuable additional parameter in 24-hour esophageal pH recording. Am J Gastroenterol 1991;86:160–164
7. Breumelhof R, Nadorp JHSM, Akkermans LMA, Smout AJPM. Analysis of 24-hour esophageal pressure and pH data in unselected patients with noncardiac chest pain. Gastroenterology 1990;99:1257–1264
8. Bumm R, Emde C, Armstrong D, Bauerfeind P, Blum AL. Ambulatory esophageal manometry: comparison of expert and computer-aided manometry analyses. J Gastrointest Motil 1990;2:216–223
9. Champion G, Richter JE, Vaezi MF, Singh S, Alexander R. Duodeno-gastroesophageal reflux: relationship to pH and importance in Barrett's esophagus. Gastroenterology 1994;107:747–754
10. Clark CS, Kraus BB, Sinclair J, Castell DO. Gastroesophageal reflux induced by exercise in healthy volunteers. JAMA 1989;261:3599–3601
11. De Caestecker JS. Twenty-four-hour oesophageal pH monitoring: advances and controversies. Neth J Med 1989;34:S20–S39
12. DeMeester TR, Johnson LF, Joseph GJ, Toscano MS, Hall AW, Skinner DB. Patterns of gastroesophageal reflux in health and disease. Ann Surg 1976;184:459–469
13. Dobhan R, Castell DO. Prolonged intraesophageal pH monitoring with 16-hour overnight recording. Dig Dis Sci 1992;37:857–864
14. Duroux P, et al. The ion sensitive field effect transistor (ISFFT) pH electrode: a new sensor for long term ambulatory pH monitoring. Gut 1991;32:240–245
15. Emde C, Garner A, Blum A. Technical aspects of intraluminal pH-metry in man: current status and recommendations. Gut 1987;28:1177–1188
16. Emde C, Armstrong D, Bumm R, Kaufhold HJ, Riecken EO, Blum AL. Twenty-four-hour continuous ambulatory measurement of oesophageal pH and pressure: a digital recording system and computer-aided manometry analysis. J Ambul Monit 1990;3:47–62
17. Falor WH, Hansell JR, Chang B, Kraus FC, White HA. Outpatient 24-hour esophageal monitoring by pH telemetry. Gastroenterology 1980;78:1163–1168
18. Fuchs KH, DeMeester TR, Albertucci M. Specificity and sensitivity of objective diagnosis of gastroesophageal reflux disease. Surgery 1987;102:575–580

19. Gignoux C, Bonnet-Eymard DO, Holstein J, Fournet J. Enregistrement ambulatoire du pH oesophagien pendant 24 heures dans une population de 27 témoins: analyse des facteurs techniques et methodologiques influençant les resultats. Gastroenterol Clin Biol 1987;11:17–23

20. Gill RC, Kellow JE, Wingate DI. Gastro-oesophageal reflux and the migrating motor complex. Gut 1987;28:929–934

21. Grande L, et al. Intraesophageal pH monitoring after breakfast and lunch in gastroesophageal reflux. J Clin Gastroenterol 1988;10:373–376

22. Hewson LG, Dalton CB, Richter JE. Comparison of esophageal manometry, provocative testing, and ambulatory monitoring in patients with unexplained chest pain. Dig Dis Sci 1990;35:302–309

23. Hopert R, Emde C, Riecken EO. Recommendations for long-term oesophageal pH monitoring. Neth J Med 1989;34:S55–S61

24. Janssens J, Vantrappen G, Ghillebert G. 24-hour recording of esophageal pressure and pH in patients with noncardiac chest pain. Gastroenterology 1986;90:1978–1984

25. Johnson LF, DeMeester TR. Twenty-four-hour pH monitoring of the distal esophagus. Am J Gastroenterol 1974;62:323–332

26. Johnson LF, DeMeester TR. Development of the 24-hour intraesophageal pH monitoring composite scoring system. J Clin Gastroenterol 1986;8(Suppl 1):52–58

27. Johnsson F, Joelsson B. Reproducibility of ambulatory oesophageal pH monitoring in the diagnosis of gastroesophageal pH monitoring. Gut 1988;29:886–889

28. Johnsson F, Joelsson B, Isberg PE. Ambulatory 24 hour intraesophageal pH monitoring in the diagnosis of gastroesophageal reflux disease. Gut 1987;28:1145–1150

29. Jörgensen F, Elsborg L, Hesse B. The diagnostic value of computerized short term esophageal pH monitoring in suspected gastroesophageal reflux. Scand J Gastroenterol 1988;23:363–367

30. Katzka DA, Paoletti V, Lelte L, Castell DO. Prolonged ambulatory pH monitoring in patients with persistent gastroesophageal reflux symptoms: testing while on therapy identifies the need for more aggressive anti-reflux therapy. Am J Gastroenterol 1996;91:2110–2113

31. Klauser AG, Schindlbeck HC, Müller-Lissner SA. Is long-term esophageal pH monitoring of clinical value? Am J Gastroenterol 1989;84:362–366

32. Kruse-Andersen S, Wallin L, Madsen T. Acid gastro-oesophageal reflux and oesophageal pressure activity during postprandial and nocturnal periods. Scand J Gastroenterol 1987;22:926–930

33. Kuit JA, Schepel SJ, Bijleveld CMA, Kloibouker JH. Evaluation of a new catheter for esophageal pH monitoring. Hepatogastroenterology 1991;38:78–80

34. Lam HGT, Dekker W, Kan G, Breedijk M, Smout AJPM. Acute noncardiac chest pain in a coronary care unit: evaluation by 24-hour pressure and pH monitoring of the esophagus. Gastroenterology 1992;102:453–460

35. Lam HGT, Breumelhof R, Roelofs JMM, van Berge Henegouwen GP, Smout AJPM. What is the optimal time window in symptom analysis of 24-hour esophageal pressure and pH data? Dig Dis Sci 1994;39:402–409

36. McLauchlan G, Rawlings JM, Lucas ML, McCloy RT, Crean GP, McColl KEL. Electrodes for 24-hour pH monitoring: a comparative study. Gut 1987;28:935–939

37. Mattioli S, Pilotti V, Spangaro M, et al. Reliability of 24-hour home esophageal pH monitoring in diagnosis of gastroesophageal reflux. Dig Dis Sci 1989;34:71–78

38. Mattox HE, Richter JE, Sinclair JW, Price JP, Case LD. Gastroesophageal pH step-up inaccurately locates proximal border of lower esophageal sphincter. Dig Dis Sci 1992;37:1185–1195

39. Meyers RL, Orlando RC. In vivo bicarbonate secretion by the human esophagus. Gastroenterology 1992;103:1174–1178

40. Mittal RK, Reuben A, Whitney JO, McCallum RW. Do bile acids reflux into the esophagus? Gastroenterology 1987;92:371–375

41. Murphy DW, Castell DO. Chocolate and heartburn: evidence of increased esophageal acid exposure after chocolate ingestion. Am J Gastroenterol 1988;83:633–636

42. Murphy DW, Yuan Y, Castell DO. Does the intraesophageal pH probe accurately detect acid reflux? Simultaneous recording with two pH probes in humans. Dig Dis Sci 1989;34:649–656

43. Peters L, et al. Spontaneous noncardiac chest pain. Gastroenterology 1988;94:878–886

44. Pfister CJ, Harrison MA, Hamilton JW, Tompkins WJ, Webster JG. Development of a three-channel, 24-h ambulatory esophageal pressure monitor. IEEE Trans Biomed Eng 1989;36:487–490

45. Pujol A, Grande L, Ros F, Pera C. Utility of inpatient 24-hour intraesophageal pH monitoring in diagnosis of gastroesophageal reflux. Dig Dis Sci 1988;33:1134–1140

46. Richter JF, Castell DO. 24-hour ambulatory oesophageal motility monitoring: how should motility data be analyzed? Gut 1989;30:1040–1047

47. Richter JE, Bradley LA, DeMeester TR, Wu WC. Normal 24-hour ambulatory esophageal pH values. Influences of study center, pH electrode, age and gender. Dig Dis Sci 1992;37:849–856

48. Rokkas T, Sladen GE. Ambulatory esophageal pH recording in gastroesophageal reflux. Relevance to the development of esophagitis. Am J Gastroenterol 1988;83:629–632

49. Schindlbeck NE, Heinrich C, König A, Dendorfer A, Pace F, Müller-Lissner SA. Optimal thresholds, sensitivity, and specificity of long-term pH-metry for the detection of gastroesophageal reflux disease. Gastroenterology 1987;93:85–90

50. Schlesinger PK, Donahue PE, Schmid B, Layden TJ. Limitations of 24-hour intraesophageal pH monitoring in the hospital setting. Gastroenterology 1985;98:797–804

51. Schoeman MN, Tippett M, Akkermans LMA, Dent J, Holloway RH. Mechanisms of gastroesophageal reflux in ambulant healthy human subjects. Gastroenterology 1995;108:83–91

52. Singh S, Bradley LA, Richter JE. Determinants of oesophageal "alkaline" pH environment in controls and patients with gastro-oesophageal reflux disease. Gut 1993;34:309–316

53. Singh S, Richter JE, Bradley LA, Haile JM. The symptom index. Differential usefulness in suspected acid-related complaints of heartburn and chest pain. Dig Dis Sci 1993;38:1402–1408

54. Smout AJPM, Breedijk M, Van der Zouw C, Akkermans LMA. Physiological gastroesophageal reflux and esophageal motor activity studied with a new system for 24-hour recording and automated analysis. Dig Dis Sci 1989;34:372–378

55. Soffer EE, Scalabrini P, Wingate DL. Spontaneous noncardiac chest pain: value of ambulatory esophageal pH and motility monitoring. Dig Dis Sci 1989;34:1651–1655

56. Spencer J. Prolonged pH recording in the study of gastro-oesophageal reflux. Br J Surg 1969;56:912–914

57. Sponce RAJ, Collins BJ, Parks TG, Love AHG. Does age influence normal gastroesophageal reflux? Gut 1985;26:799–801

58. Stanciu R, Hoarc RC, Bennett JR. Correlations between manometric and pH tests for gastro-oesophageal reflux. Gut 1977;18:536–540

59. Tuttle SG, Rufin F, Bettarello A. The physiology of heartburn. Ann Intern Med 1961;55:292–300

60. Vandenplas Y, Sacre L. Continuous 24-hour esophageal pH monitoring in 285 asymptomatic infants (from 0 to 15 months old). J Pediatr Gastroenterol Nutr 1987;6:220–224

61. Vandenplas Y, Helven R, Goyvaerts H, Sacré L. Reproducibility of continuous 24 hour oesophageal pH monitoring in infants and children. Gut 1990;31:374–377

62. Vantrappen G, Servaes J, Janssens J, Peeters T. Twenty-four hour esophageal pH- and pressure recording in outpatients. In Wienbeck M, ed, Motility of the digestive tract. New York: Raven Press, 1982:293–297

63. Vantrappen G, Janssens J, Ghillebert G. The irritable oesophagus: a frequent cause of angina-like pain. Lancet 1987;2:1232–1234

64. Vitale GC, et al. Computerized 24-hour ambulatory esophageal pH monitoring and esophagogastroduodenoscopy in the reflux patient. J Lab Clin Med 1985;105:686–693

65. Vitale GC, Cheddle WG, Patel B, Sadek SA, Michel M, Cusschieri A. The effect of alcohol on nocturnal gastroesophageal reflux. JAMA 1987;258:2077–2079

66. Voskuil JH, Cramer MJ, Broumelhof R, Timmer R, Smout AJPM. Prevalence of esophageal disorders in patients with chest pain newly referred to the cardiologist. Chest 1996;109:1210–1214

67. Wang H, Beck IT, Paterson WG. Reproducibility and physiological characteristics of 24-hour ambulatory esophageal manometry/pH-metry. Am J Gastroenterol 1996;91:492–497

68. Ward BW, et al. Ambulatory 24-hour esophageal pH monitoring: technology searching for a clinical application. J Clin Gastroenterol 1986;8:59–67

69. Ward BW, Wallace C, Wu WC, Richter JE, Hacksaw BT, Castell DO. Longterm follow-up of symptomatic status of patients with noncardiac chest pain: is diagnosis of esophageal etiology helpful? Am J Gastroenterol 1987;82:215–218

70. Weiser HF, Pace F, Lepsien C, Müller-Lissner SA, Blum AL, Siewert

JR. Gastroösophagealer Reflux—was ist physiologisch? Dtsch Med Wochenschr 1982;107:366–370

71. Weusten BLAM, Akkermans LMA, van Berge Henegouwen GP, Smout AJPM. Ambulatory combined oesophageal pressure and pH monitoring: relationships between pathological reflux, oesophageal dysmotility and symptoms of oesophageal dysfunction. Eur J Gastroenterol Hepatol 1993;5:1055–1060

72. Weusten BLAM, Roelofs JMM, Akkermans LMA, van Berge Henegouwon GP, Smout AJPM. The symptom association probability: an improved method for symptom analysis of 24-hour esophageal pH data. Gastroenterology 1994;107:1741–1745

73. Weusten BLAM, Roelofs JMM, Akkermans LMA, Van Berge Hene-

gouwen GP, Smout AJPM. Objective determination of pH thresholds in the analysis of 24 h ambulatory oesophageal pH monitoring. Eur J Clin Invest 1996;26:151–158

74. Wiener GJ, et al. Ambulatory 24-hour esophageal pH monitoring. Reproducibility and variability of pH parameters. Dig Dis Sci 1988;33:1127–1133

75. Wiener GJ, Richter JE, Copper JB, Wu WC, Castell DO. The symptom index: a clinically important parameter of ambulatory 24-hour esophageal pH monitoring. Am J Gastroenterol 1988;83:358–361

76. Wo JM, Castell DO. Exclusion of meal periods from ambulatory pH monitoring may improve diagnosis of esophageal acid reflux. Dig Dis Sci 1994;39:1601–1607

*The Esophagus*, Third Edition,
edited by D. O. Castell and J. E. Richter.
Lippincott Williams & Wilkins, Philadelphia © 1999.

CHAPTER 7

# Provocative Tests for Pain of Esophageal Origin

## Applied Sensory Physiology

Kenneth R. DeVault

Recurrent chest pain in patients with negative findings on cardiac evaluation is a common and important clinical challenge. Although these patients have a low cardiac morbidity and mortality, they continue to consume large amounts of medical resources with frequent emergency room and physician office visits despite knowledge of their normal coronary anatomy [76, 106]. It has been suggested that by providing a firm, noncardiac diagnosis, peace of mind can be increased, allowing a return to normal activity and a decrease in health care-seeking behavior [105]. To overcome the anxiety produced by fear of a potentially fatal cardiac condition in the substantial proportion of patients who have an esophageal etiology for their chest pain, strong and reasonably unequivocal esophageal data must be presented and reinforced.

Possible esophageal causes for chest pain include mucosal irritation secondary to gastroesophageal reflux, abnormal contractions (e.g., nutcracker esophagus or diffuse spasm), and an abnormal sensory response to normal contractions. When 910 patients with noncardiac chest pain were referred for esophageal testing, only 28% had abnormal manometry findings [53]. A significant proportion of patients with negative results on esophageal motility studies may have undiagnosed esophageal pain. This has led to a search for specific and sensitive provocation tests to increase the diagnostic yield of esophageal testing.

### PHYSIOLOGY OF ESOPHAGEAL PAIN

The mechanisms of gastrointestinal pain in general and esophageal pain in particular are incompletely understood. It

has been traditionally held that pain from the gastrointestinal tract is carried in the spinal nerves to the spinal cord and then to the brain via the spinothalamic tracts. The understanding that a majority of fibers in the vagus nerve are sensory in nature has challenged this concept. To study pain, there must be a method to provoke pain in normal control subjects and patients that is both safe and reproducible. Pain can be provoked from the gastrointestinal tract using several stimulus modalities. Receptors sensitive to mucosal stimulation have been isolated in the gastrointestinal tract [66]. Theoretically, these receptors underlie the pain produced with esophageal acid, both in gastroesophageal reflux and with acid infusion in the Bernstein test. While these receptors produce a brief burst of impulses with mechanical stimulation of the gastrointestinal tract, there is another set of receptors which respond to mechanical changes in the esophageal wall [48]. These receptors are located deeper in the muscle layers and are activated by tension in the wall produced by distention, contraction, or compression of the viscus [42, 62]. Most visceral organs, including the esophagus, are compliant within physiologic pressure ranges, while further increases in distention beyond this physiologic range may result in sharp increases in both pressure and mechanoreceptor discharge [48]. Intraganglionic laminar nerve endings found in the myenteric plexus may function as the receptor organ for this type of sensation. To provoke painful esophageal sensation, these various types of receptors have been stimulated with both acid and pharmacologic agents designed to increase the amplitude and duration of esophageal contractions (ergonovine, edrophonium, bethanechol). Direct mechanical or electrical stimulation of the esophagus may also provide a physiologic and specific form of afferent sensory stimulation.

K. R. DeVault: Department of Medicine, Mayo Medical School, Rochester, Minnesota 55905, and Division of Gastroenterology, Mayo Clinic Jacksonville, Jacksonville, Florida 32224.

## ESOPHAGEAL PROVOCATION TESTS

### The Acid Perfusion Test (Bernstein Test)

Bernstein and Baker [9] introduced the acid perfusion test as an objective method to reproduce symptoms. After a 15- to 30-minute control period of intraesophageal saline infusion at a rate of 6 to 8 mL/min, 0.1 N hydrochloric acid (HCl) is administered at the same rate for a period of 30 minutes or until symptoms occur. If the acid perfusion provokes the familiar anginalike chest pain and saline solution does not induce the pain, the test suggests an esophageal origin of the pain. Some have additionally required that for a result to be positive, the acid-induced symptoms should quickly disappear by the reinfusion of saline or bicarbonate [8]. Although the test appears to be highly specific [90], its sensitivity is relatively low, with figures ranging from 6% to almost 60% [25, 39, 47, 73, 82, 98, 104]. A negative test result has little clinical value and does not exclude an esophageal origin of the chest pain. Patients with Barrett's esophagus have been noted to have a decrease in their sensitivity to acid, resulting in even more false negatives [51]. Interestingly, a recent study found that the acid sensitivity in Barrett's patients returned after their squamous epithelium was reestablished using ablative and acid suppressant therapy [35]. It is important to follow closely a protocol when doing the acid perfusion test since many factors can influence the results. For example, a prior acid infusion decreases the amount of acid required to produce symptoms in normal controls [93].

Because of low sensitivity compared to 24-hour pH monitoring with symptom assessment, some authors have considered the acid perfusion test to be obsolete [46, 89]. The test is easy to perform and has almost no side effects, and therefore it is reasonable to include in the diagnostic evaluation of patients with noncardiac chest pain. The test has little to offer in the patient with typical reflux symptoms, which are highly specific for reflux [56], or in the patient with esophagitis on endoscopy, in which case the diagnosis has been established.

It has been debated whether the contact of acid with the mucosa on its own, or acid-induced motility disorders [12, 87], or a combination of both are involved in the pain production. Smith and colleagues [94] showed that symptom production is clearly pH dependent, which strongly suggests that acid and not the associated motility disorder is responsible for the symptoms.

### The Edrophonium Test

Provocation tests have been developed to pharmacologically induce esophageal motility disorders and chest pain. The parasympathomimetic agents bethanechol and edrophonium, the sympathomimetic agent ergonovine, and pentagastrin have all been used, but edrophonium offers the best results with the lowest level of side effects.

Intravenous injection of 80 μg per mg of edrophonium reproduces esophageal manometric changes and chest pain in 20% to 30% of noncardiac chest pain patients [22, 86]. Larger doses of 10 mg have been used as well, but without apparent gain in sensitivity [61]. The pain occurs on swallowing, within 5 minutes after the administration of the drug, and disappears quickly as the drug is rapidly metabolized. Edrophonium has shown no effect on coronary artery diameter and actually decreases cardiac workload [86]. The side effects are minimal and the antidote atropine is almost never required. As with the acid perfusion test, figures for the sensitivity of the edrophonium test widely vary in the literature from as high as 55% to as low as 0% [25, 39, 73, 82, 98, 104]. The correct sensitivity is unknown because of the lack of a gold standard. Although edrophonium is known to increase esophageal contraction amplitude and duration as well as the number of repetitive contractions after swallowing, some studies showed that this increase is not greater in chest pain patients with a positive (pain) response as compared with patients in whom the test did not induce pain. The changes in contractions observed in chest pain patients are similar to those in healthy control subjects who never experience pain during the test [86]. This indicates that we do not clearly understand the mechanism by which edrophonium induces pain in the positive-response patient unless we accept that these patients have a lower threshold for pain induced by increased contractility. It also means that if a subjective parameter such as pain is the endpoint for a positive test result, a placebo control is necessary to interpret the test correctly.

Other motility-stimulating agents have been used as a provocation test. They have no higher sensitivity as compared to edrophonium and they are less specific or have more side effects. Bethanechol, 40 to 50 μg per kg, induced chest pain in 12% to 33% of noncardiac chest pain patients [8, 70, 75]. When the dose of bethanechol was increased to two injections of 50 μg per kg, with an interval of 15 minutes, as many as 77% of the patients had their chest pain reproduced, but at the cost of severe side effects [75]. Ergonovine is a sympathomimetic agent of the ergoalkaloid group and is used by cardiologists to diagnose vasospastic angina in chest pain patients with normal coronary arteries. The drug reportedly is as sensitive as edrophonium in the provocation of esophageal chest pain in patients without changes in the ST-T segment on electrocardiogram (ECG) or coronary artery spasm on angiography [23, 33, 57, 65]. However, as side effects are common and serious cardiac effects and even death have been reported, the drug should not used for esophageal provocation [13]. Pentagastrin directly stimulates esophageal smooth muscle, especially in patients with primary esophageal motility. Its sensitivity to induce pain in patients with noncardiac chest pain is low and the drug is no longer used for a provocation test.

### Balloon Provocation

Balloon distention of the gastrointestinal tract has been used to stimulate mechanoreceptors involved in various re-

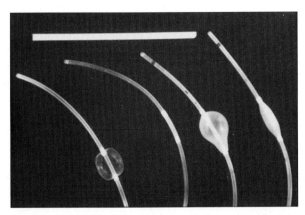

**FIG. 7–1.** Commercially available balloon distention catheters with either silicone (right) or latex (left) balloons attached to a manometry catheter (Wilson-Cooke, Winston-Salem, NC). Both balloon types are shown deflated and inflated with 20 ml of air.

flex and pain pathways in health and disease. Subjects with the diagnosis of the irritable bowel syndrome and with chronic idiopathic dyspepsia have a lowered pain threshold to distention of the colon and stomach, respectively [63, 91].

Studies in the opossum esophagus demonstrated tension-sensitive mechanoreceptors associated with vagal afferents that are activated by both normal peristalsis and balloon distention. These mechanoreceptors appear to be associated with both the longitudinal and circular muscle layers [92]. Over 40 years ago, intraesophageal balloon distention in humans was reported to produce pain referred to the chest [58]. Early data indicated that in patients with documented ischemic heart disease, balloon distention of the esophagus produced pain indistinguishable from anginal pain, but without ECG changes [64]. This may be explained by convergence of sensory pathways at the level of the spinal cord or in the midbrain. Despite this similarity in pain, it appears that esophageal balloon distention itself has no effect on

coronary function or blood flow [109]. Intraesophageal balloon distention also has a high degree of intrasubject reproducibility in both normal controls and patients [45, 59] (Fig. 7–1).

Several painful clinical syndromes are associated with esophageal distention. These include esophageal dilation and aperistalsis induced by the ingestion of cold liquids [72], acute food impaction, the drinking of carbonated beverages [55], and dysfunction of the belch reflex [52]. It has also been suggested that esophageal pain is at times due to esophageal dilation secondary to a lack of coordination between the esophageal body and the lower esophageal sphincter (LES) [54]. These findings led to increased interest in balloon distention as a provocation test for esophageal pain. When air was injected in 1-mL increments to a maximum of 10 mL into a latex balloon attached to a manometry catheter, patients with noncardiac chest pain were more likely to experience pain (18 of 30) than normal control subjects (6 of 30) [88] (Fig. 7–2). Concurrent ECG monitoring showed no ischemic changes. In this seminal study the intraesophageal volume at the onset of pain also distinguished patients from control subjects, with chest-pain patients experiencing pain at balloon volumes of less than 8 mL and the few control subjects experiencing pain at volumes of 9 mL or more. A second report evaluating 50 patients with noncardiac chest pain found that 28 (56%) had their ''typical'' chest pain during balloon inflation. Again, the majority of these patients (24 of 28) had their pain at volumes less than 8 mL [7]. Abnormal motility did not predict a positive test result. When intraballoon pressures were used as a measure of esophageal wall tone, no difference between control subjects and noncardiac chest pain patients was noted. The response appears to be fairly specific since only 1 patient had a negative response on the balloon study and a positive result on the edrophonium test and no patient had a negative response on the balloon study and a positive result on the acid perfusion test.

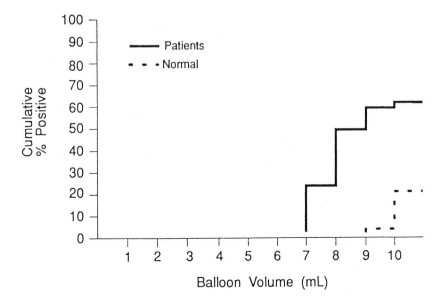

**FIG. 7–2.** Esophageal pain with balloon distention. Sixty percent of chest pain patients (solid line) experienced pain, compared to only 20% of normal subjects (broken line) ($p < 0.005$). Not only did pain develop more frequently in the patients, but the pain occurred at smaller balloon volumes, suggesting a lower pain threshold to esophageal distention.

Further reports have clarified this response. In a study where 29 (45%) of 77 patients referred for esophageal testing had a positive result on the balloon distention test, the only manometric finding associated with a positive result was an increased number of multipeaked contraction waves [17]. Interestingly, patients with dysphagia tended to have pain at lower volumes, while those with abnormal psychologic profiles did not have increased positive responses. A clinical correlation between sensitivity to balloon distention and an abnormal belch reflex has also been suggested [40]. Balloon distention was more likely to yield a positive response in those who were less likely to belch with intraesophageal air infusion (64%) than in those who belched easily. Furthermore, patients with the irritable bowel syndrome and with fibromyalgia have a lower pain threshold to esophageal distention, suggesting a common alteration in visceral receptor sensitivity or modulation [20, 43]. Interestingly, women, who are more likely to experience ''functional'' gastrointestinal pain, also have a lower esophageal pain threshold than do men, independent of body size [74]. Caution must be used in the interpretation of balloon distention testing in older patients, since both visceral sensation from the esophagus and the ability of an inflated balloon to induce secondary peristalsis seem to diminish with aging in normal subjects [60, 85].

While it seems likely that intraesophageal balloon distention produces pain secondary to activation of esophageal mechanoreceptors, there is some evidence to suggest that the balloon may initiate either ''normal'' or ''abnormal'' secondary peristalsis that could contribute to the pain response. Esophageal balloon distention has been shown to produce increased motility proximal to the balloon and inhibition distally and to initiate secondary peristalsis in normal subjects [21, 34]. Sustained balloon distention produces a strong, proximal, aboral contraction force referred to as the duration response or the esophageal propulsive force [107]. In the opossum this contraction proximal to a distending balloon is abolished with cervical vagotomy, while contractions distal to the balloon are retained and believed to be mediated by an intramural nonadrenergic noncholinergic (NANC) system [78]. Human studies showed that atropine inhibits proximal contraction when balloon distention is carried out in the distal, but not proximal esophagus, indirectly indicating some difference in the innervation of these two regions [79]. In addition to the above-mentioned effects in the body of the esophagus, balloon distention produces increases in upper esophageal sphincter (UES) and decreases in LES pressure [1]. In studies performed on a group of dysphagia patients, both patients and control subjects experienced a sustained increase in pressure proximal to the balloon. In 21 (70%) of 30 patients, but in no control subjects, there was evidence of repeated simultaneous contractions (spasm) distal to the balloon [26]. Similar findings of distal esophageal ''spasm'' with balloon distention were noted in 38 (61%) of 62 chest pain patients, but in no control subjects [27].

The use of balloon distention as a tool to test the pharmacologic response to various agents being considered for use in patients with chest pain is evolving. Imipramine has been demonstrated to improve symptoms in patients with noncardiac chest pain [14] and also has been shown to increase pain, but not sensation, threshold to balloon distention in a group of normal controls [81]. A preliminary report found octreotide to improve both sensory and pain thresholds in a group of chest pain patients [44]. Nifedipine has been studied using both standard balloon distention and with barostat testing and has not been found to change reliably sensory thresholds or esophageal wall tone [28, 96].

Electrical stimulation has been suggested as an alternative to balloon distention. It has the advantage of being able to deliver a precise stimulus, which has been exploited in the evoked potential studies discussed below. A recent report found electrical stimulation to reproduce chest pain in 43% of patients with unexplained chest pain, although an additional preliminary report showed no advantage of electrical over balloon testing [10, 110]. The risk of possible induction of cardiac dysrhythmias makes this technique less desirable than balloon distention.

## Esophageal Evoked Potentials

Esophageal balloon distention is a potent and specific stimulus for esophageal pain. Whereas the ability to reproduce ''typical'' symptoms is a strength of this technique, the subjective endpoint of pain can be a source of confusion in interpretation. Pain is mediated by personal experience, cultural values, and other life events, making it difficult to compare pain responses between subjects and even within the same subject on different days [108]. Some evidence indicates that fluctuating levels of endogenous enkephalins may lead to variable intrasubject pain thresholds [68]. This variability is especially bothersome in the evaluation of therapeutic changes, which are often difficult to blind to the patient and investigator. What is needed is an objective measure of the subjective sensation of esophageal pain.

Cerebral evoked potentials are recorded as a reflection of the electrical activity of the brain in response to stimuli applied in the periphery (Fig. 7–3). Visual evoked potentials (secondary to a flashing light) and auditory evoked potentials (secondary to repetitive clicks) have found clinical applicability. In addition, somatosensory evoked potentials (secondary to repetitive electrical stimulation) have been used to evaluate peripheral nerves. The recording of cerebral evoked potentials in response to visceral stimulation is a recently described technique providing objective information in response to the provocation of visceral pain. Electrical stimulation of the bladder and urethra evokes cerebral potentials and is being used clinically [5, 6]. The technique of electrical stimulation has been applied to the rectum and the esophagus to evoke reproducible cerebral potentials [37, 38]. While electrical stimulation may be appropriate for the study of nerve function in the peripheral nervous system, the gastro-

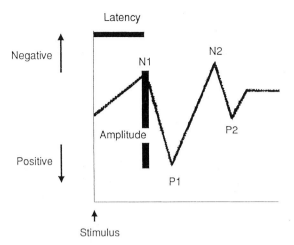

**FIG. 7–3.** Schematic illustration of a hypothetical evoked potential. By convention, negative is up and positive is down. The peaks are numbered consecutively as negative (N1, N2) or positive (P1, P2). Amplitude is expressed on the vertical axis as a difference between peaks (N1 to P1, P1 to N2, etc.). Latency is on the horizontal axis and is measured from the stimulus to a given peak.

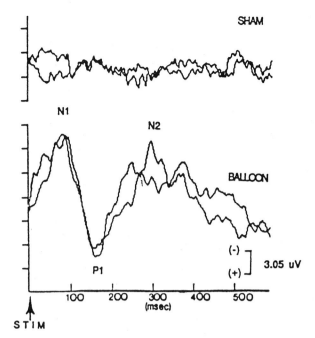

**FIG. 7–4.** Evoked potential recorded after esophageal balloon distention (50 repetitions). Amplitude is expressed in microvolts on the vertical axis, while latency from stimulus (Stim) to peak in milliseconds is on the horizontal axis. The typical configuration of two negative peaks (N1, N2) and one positive peak (P1) is demonstrated. Note the close similarity of the two studies in this subject and the lack of evoked potential with sham distention.

intestinal tract has multiple sensory modalities (chemoreceptive, thermoreceptive, and mechanoreceptive) that are likely to be nonspecifically stimulated with electrical discharge. More recent studies evaluated balloon distention as the stimulus modality.

Evoked potential recording after mechanical distention of a visceral organ was first reported for the rectum [18]. This led to initial studies of cerebral potentials evoked by esophageal balloon distention [15]. In this study a latex balloon was placed in the distal esophagus and inflated repeatedly at the level of pain threshold by a mechanical pump that also triggered the evoked potential recorder. A characteristic triphasic evoked potential was obtained (Fig. 7–4). Considerable intersubject, but minimal intrasubject variability was noted. In a follow-up study, Smout and colleagues [95] clarified this response. A rapid inflation rate (170 mL/min) was found to be superior to a slower rate (30 mL/min) in the production of evoked potentials. No improvement in potentials was noted with 100 repetitions compared to 50, nor was a random time interval between inflations important. Perhaps most importantly, evoked potential quality and amplitude were found to be dependent on the level of sensation provided by the stimulus. The specificity and reproducibility of esophageal evoked potential recordings have been confirmed [31]. Balloon distention with cerebral evoked potential recording was sequentially carried out in the distal and proximal esophageal body. The latencies were significantly shorter with balloon distention in the proximal esophagus (Fig. 7–5). This change in latency is similar whether electrical or mechanical stimulation is used [37].

Evoked potential recording has been performed in patients with esophageal disease [97]. Ten patients with noncardiac chest pain having either nutcracker esophagus or diffuse

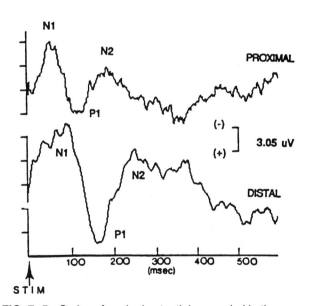

**FIG. 7–5.** Series of evoked potentials recorded in the same subject after distal and proximal esophageal stimulation (50 repetitions each). A recognizable evoked potential was noted after distal and proximal stimulation. In this example the latencies with proximal stimulation (N1 = 75 msec, P1 = 120 msec, N2 = 210 msec) were shorter than those with distal stimulation (N1 = 105 msec, P1 = 160 msec, N2 = 256 msec).

esophageal spasm (DES) experienced chest pain at lower balloon volumes than did control subjects. Both amplitude and quality of the evoked potential increased with increasing sensation while the latencies remained stable. Interestingly, the amplitude and quality of the evoked potentials were lower in patients than control subjects, with similar levels of sensation produced by lower balloon volumes in the patients. The authors concluded that these data suggest an abnormality in central processing of visceral sensory information in noncardiac chest pain patients and not an abnormality at the peripheral receptor. An interesting correlate to this was provided by a recent report of increased evoked potentials produced with auditory stimulation in patients with somatization disorder, which may indicate an increase in general central nervous system sensitivity [49], and by the finding of abnormal pain thresholds in multiple areas in patients with nonulcer dyspepsia and irritable bowel syndrome [101].

Esophageal balloon distention and cerebral evoked potential recording may help define the pathway and type of nerves involved in esophageal nociception in the human. In a recent report, both esophageal pain perception and esophageal evoked potentials were found to be normal in patients with C5 to C6 sensory spinal cord lesions [32]. This appears to indicate pain conveyance by the vagus nerve, although spinal esophageal afferents have been suggested to have cell bodies as high as the C5 dorsal root ganglion [19], raising the possibility that some nociceptive data may travel up the spinal cord in these patients. Two comparisons of evoked potentials obtained with balloon and electrical stimulation concluded that sensation evoked by balloon distention was carried by unmyelinated C fibers, while electrical stimulation more likely activated myelinated A delta fibers [99, 100]. Conversely, Aziz and co-workers [2] found a decrease in evoked potential amplitude, but an increase in sensation with increasing frequency of stimulation. They suggested that the evoked potential may therefore be dependent on slowly adapting fibers, although an alternative explanation would hold that their higher frequency stimulation may have initiated motor or other activity too diffuse to be measured with evoked potential recording. The above studies emphasize the utility of esophageal evoked potential recording in examining the innervation of the human esophagus.

Evoked potential recording is beginning to provide evidence that a specific portion of the brain is the source of esophageal pain. A small study used source modeling to suggest that the scalp evoked potential was coming from cortical sources located in the cingulate gyri and insular cortex [36]. An additional study supported the role of the insular cortex and suggested that there was some evidence for hemispheric dominance that was independent of handedness [3].

The application of newer imaging technologies to the study of esophageal sensation is an exciting area of study. Positron emission tomography has been used to record brain activity after balloon distention [4]. This study suggested that esophageal sensation activated the insula, primary so-

matosensory cortex, and operculum, while pain stimulated the right anterior insular cortex and anterior cingulate gyrus.

## NEW TECHNIQUES IN THE EVALUATION OF ESOPHAGEAL SENSATION AND COMPLIANCE

Barostat testing is another form of balloon distention that has been used to measure wall tone in several visceral organs. In these studies, the volume of intraballoon air is varied to maintain a set pressure. The balloon or bag attached to the barostat is large enough essentially to allow infinite distensibility at the volume required to fill the given viscera. This results in a change in volume needed to maintain the set pressure even with quite small changes in wall tone. The use of this technology is well described in both the stomach and colon, but has only recently been applied to the esophagus [67]. Esophageal barostat experiments were able to measure a difference in tone between the smooth and striated esophagus and record changes in tone after application of the smooth muscle relaxant amyl nitrite. A recent study used a barostat device to find a reduction, but not loss of esophageal wall tone in patients with achalasia [41]. A similar technique has been used to both measure esophageal tone and document a fall in esophageal tone which commenced with deglutition and persisted until passage of the peristaltic wave [30].

Impedance planimetry is another new method of measurement of esophageal tone [77, 83]. This method is able to estimate the cross-sectional area of the esophagus using changes in the impedance within a balloon as it enlarges [77]. This is similar to reporting the volume of a balloon needed to produce a given pressure with the barostat technique, and compliance in the wall of the esophagus can then be calculated. This technique has also been applied to a group of patients with unexplained chest pain [84]. A 50% reduction in compliance and 50% lower thresholds for both pain and secondary peristalsis were noted in the patients with chest pain and normal coronary arteries compared to normal controls.

## PROVOCATION TESTS VERSUS 24-HOUR pH AND PRESSURE MONITORING

The best (if not only) way to ascribe noncardiac chest pain to the esophagus is to correlate in time the pain attack with an abnormal esophageal event. As this is only rarely the case during conventional esophageal testing, prolonged 24-hour pH and pressure monitoring has been developed to increase the chance of documenting a spontaneous chest pain attack. The sensitivity of the technique varies in the literature from 47% to 10%, according to the population studied and according to the method of analysis [11, 39, 47, 50, 82]. It is evident that patients with few pain episodes will benefit less from the technique than patients with daily pain.

Ghillebert and co-workers [39] compared provocation tests and ambulatory monitoring in a group of 50 consecutive patients with noncardiac chest pain who all underwent 24-hour pH and pressure recordings as well as a number of provocation tests, including the acid perfusion test, the edrophonium test, the balloon distention test, and the vasopressin test. They found that 24-hour pH and pressure recording, the acid perfusion test, and the edrophonium test were almost equally sensitive in establishing the esophageal origin of the pain, the test results being positive in 38%, 36%, and 32% of the patients, respectively. The balloon distention test and the vasopressin test were less sensitive. More importantly, the combined use of provocation tests (especially the acid perfusion test and the edrophonium test) made it possible to establish the esophageal origin of the pain in 52% of the patients, as compared to 38% for the 24-hour pH and pressure recording. Moreover, the gain in establishing the esophageal origin of the chest pain by performing 24-hour recordings on patients who had already undergone provocation tests was only 10%, as 90% of the patients with a positive 24-hour recording also had at least one positive provocation test result.

## WHAT IS THE MEANING OF A POSITIVE RESULT ON A PROVOCATION TEST?

Most authors accept that a positive response on a provocation test in a patient with noncardiac chest pain indicates that the esophagus is the source of the chest pain. Although very reasonable, this conclusion should nevertheless be taken with some caution. Acid perfusion in the esophagus may induce chest pain by producing myocardial ischemia in susceptible patients, a phenomenon referred to as linked angina. Mellow and colleagues [71] instilled HCl into the esophagi of 15 subjects with coronary artery stenosis. In 3 of the subjects, pain and ECG changes developed when the rate–pressure product exceeded the figure at which ischemic pain had previously occurred during exercise. The authors suggested that the sympathetic response to esophageal pain had increased myocardial oxygen demand beyond a critical point. Instillation of acid into the esophagus of patients with coronary artery disease lowers the exertional angina threshold. In 10 of 12 patients studied by Davies and co-workers [24], the angina point was reached after the patient walked a significantly shorter distance on the treadmill when acid was instilled than when saline was infused. Chauhan and associates [16] showed that in patients with microvascular angina (syndrome X), gastroesophageal reflux disease can indeed cause a decreased myocardial oxygen supply. These studies suggest that acid in the esophagus may, in a way that is not fully understood, affect the heart so as to cause cardiac ischemia and angina. It is of course possible for a patient to have both angina pectoris and chest pain from esophageal causes.

Problems may also arise when several provocation tests are performed on the same patient during the same diagnostic session. In normal controls, infused acid has no effect on pain threshold and a nonspecific effect on sensory threshold [29]. There have been two studies that evaluated this issue in patients. In the first, a lower volume to pain threshold to balloon distention (11.7 versus 9.1 mL, p less than 0.02) was noted after acid infusion, although a nonsignificant drop was also

noted with a saline infusion (11.7 to 10.6 mL) [68]. In an additional study, a subgroup of patients with mucosal sensitivity to acid were noted to have a lower threshold for balloon distention after acid infusion [80]. The interaction between acid exposure and the balloon response was recently examined further. A group of patients with symptomatic, but not excessive gastroesophageal reflux (by ambulatory pH monitoring) were found to have lower balloon thresholds than either normal controls or patients with esophagitis or Barrett's esophagus [102].

The most important point in the interpretation of esophageal provocation tests is related to the finding that although provocation tests may indicate the esophageal origin of the noncardiac chest pain, they do not identify the nature of the underlying esophageal abnormality that causes the spontaneous chest pain. Acid perfusion may induce the familiar chest pain in a patient whose spontaneous pain during 24-hour recording seems exclusively related to motor disturbances. Edrophonium may induce the customary anginalike chest pain in a patient having reflux without motor disorders at the time of spontaneous pain. Results of the acid perfusion, edrophonium, and balloon distention tests may be positive in the same patient and produce identical chest pain [103]. Only 24-hour pH and pressure recording is able to identify the underlying esophageal event occurring at the time of the spontaneous pain attacks. Thus, while sensory provocation of the esophagus may not provide a diagnosis in all patients, it is clear that these tests add to the understanding of symptoms in individual patients and to our understanding of both the physiology and the pathophysiology of esophageal pain.

## REFERENCES

1. Andreollo NA, Thompson DG, Kendall GP, Earlam RJ. Functional relationships between cricopharyngeal sphincter and oesophageal body in response to graded intraluminal distention. Gut 1988;29:161–166
2. Aziz Q, et al. Effect of stimulation frequency on sensory perception and cortical evoked potentials in the human esophagus. Gastroenterology 1993;104:A810
3. Aziz Q, et al. Topographic mapping of cortical potentials evoked by distension of the human proximal and distal esophagus. Electroencephal Clin Neurophysiol 1995;96:219–228
4. Aziz Q, et al. Identification of human brain loci processing esophageal sensation using positron emission tomography. Gastroenterology 1997;113:50–59
5. Badr G, Carlsson CA, Fall M, Friberg S, Lindstrom L, Ohlsson B. Cortical evoked potentials following stimulation of the urinary bladder in man. Electroencephal Clin Neurophysiol 1982;54:494–498
6. Badr GG, Fall M, Carlsson CA, Lindstrom L, Friberg S, Ohlsson B. Cortical evoked potentials obtained after stimulation of the lower urinary tract. J Uro 1984;131:L306–L309
7. Barish CF, Castell DO, Richter JE. Graded esophageal balloon distention. A new provocative test for noncardiac chest pain. Dig Dis Sci 1986;31:292–298
8. Benjamin SB, Richter JE, Cordova CM, Knuff TE, Castell DO. Prospective manometric evaluation with pharmacologic provocation of patients with suspected esophageal motility dysfunction. Gastroenterology 1983;84:893–901
9. Bernstein LM, Baker LA. A clinical test for esophagitis. Gastroenterology 1958;34:760
10. Bovero E, De Iaco F, Poletti M, Torre F. New provocative tests in the diagnosis of esophageal pain. Rev Esp Enferm Dig 1993;83:183–186
11. Breumelhof R, Nadorp JH, Akkermans LM, Smout AJ. Analysis of

24-hour esophageal pressure and pH data in unselected patients with noncardiac chest pain. Gastroenterology 1990;99:1257–1264

12. Burns TW, Venturates SG. Esophageal motor function and response to acid perfusion in patients with symptomatic reflux esophagitis. Dig Dis Sci 1985;30:529–535

13. Buxton A, et al. Refractory ergonovine-induced coronary vasospasm: importance of intracoronary nitroglycerin. Am J Cardiol 1980;46: 329–334

14. Cannon RO, et al. Imipramine in patients with chest pain despite normal coronary angiograms. N Engl J Med 1994;330:1411–1417

15. Castell DO, Wood JD, Frieling T, Wright FS, Vieth RF. Cerebral electrical potentials evoked by balloon distention of the human esophagus. Gastroenterology 1990;98:662–666

16. Chauhan A, Petch MC, Schofield PM. Effect of esophageal acid instillation on coronary blood flow. Lancet 1993;341:1309–1310

17. Clouse RE, McCord GS, Lustman PJ, Edmundowicz SA. Clinical correlates of abnormal sensitivity to intraesophageal balloon distention. Dig Dis Sci 1991;36:1040–1045

18. Collet L, Meunier P, Duclaux R, Chery-Croze S, Falipou P. Cerebral evoked potentials after endorectal mechanical stimulation in humans. Am J Physiol 1988;254:G477–G482

19. Collman PI, Tremblay L, Diamant NE. The distribution of spinal and vagal sensory neurons that innervate the esophagus of the cat. Gastroenterology 1992;103:817–822

20. Costantini M, et al. Altered esophageal pain threshold in irritable bowel syndrome. Dig Dis Sci 1993;38:206–212

21. Creamer B, Schlegel J. Motor responses of the esophagus to distention. J Appl Physiol 1957;100:498

22. Dalton CB, Hewson EG, Castell DO, Richter JE. Edrophonium provocation test in noncardiac chest pain. Dig Dis Sci 1990;35:1445–1451

23. Davies HA, Kaye MD, Rhodes J, Dart AM, Herderson AH. Diagnosis of esophageal spasm by ergometrine provocation. Gut 1982;23:89–97

24. Davies HA, Page Z, Rush EM, Brown AL, Lewis MJ, Petch MC. Oesophageal stimulation lowers exertional angina threshold. Lancet 1985;1:1101–1104

25. De Caestecker JS, Pryde A, Heading RC. Comparison of intravenous edrophonium and esophageal acid perfusion during esophageal manometry in patients with non-cardiac chest pain. Gut 1988;29: 1029–1034

26. Deschner WK, Maher KA, Cattau EL, Benjamin SB. Manometric responses to balloon distention in patients with nonobstructive dysphagia. Gastroenterology 1989;97:1181–1185

27. Deschner WK, Maher KA, Cattau EL, Benjamin SB. Intraesophageal balloon distention versus drug provocation in the evaluation of noncardiac chest pain. Am J Gastroenterol 1990;85:938–943

28. DeVault KR. Nifedipine does not alter barostat determined esophageal smooth muscle tone. Gastroenterology 1995;108:A591

29. DeVault KR. Acid infusion does not affect intraesophageal balloon distention-induced sensory and pain thresholds. Am J Gasoenterol 1997;92:947–949

30. DeVault KR. Effects of Nifedipine and swallowing on esophageal smooth muscle tone. Am J Gastroenterol 1995;90:1557

31. DeVault KR, Beacham S, Streletz LJ, Castell DO. Cerebral evoked potentials: a method of quantification of the central nervous system response to esophageal pain. Dig Dis Sci 1993;38:2241–2246

32. DeVault KR, Beacham S, Castell DO, Streletz LJ, Ditunno JF. Esophageal sensation in spinal cord-injured patients: balloon distension and cerbral evoked potential recording. Am J Physiol 1996;271: G937–G941

33. Eastwood GL, et al. Use of ergonovine to identify esophageal spasm in patients with chest pain. Ann Intern Med 1981;94:768–771

34. Enzmann DR, Harell GS, Zburalske EF. Upper esophageal responses to intraluminal distention in man. Gastroenterology 1977;72: 1292–1298

35. Fass R, Yalam JM, Camargo L, Johnson C, Garewal HS, Sampliner RE. Increased esophageal chemoreceptor sensitivity to acid in patients after successful reversal of Barrett's esophagus. Dig Dis Sci 1997; 42:1853–1858

36. Franssen H, Weusten BL, Wieneke GH, Smout AJ. Source modeling of esophageal evoked potentials. Electroencephal Clin Neurophysiol 1996;100:85–95

37. Frieling T, Enck P, Wienbeck M. Cerebral responses evoked by electrical stimulation of the rectosigmoid in normal subjects. Dig Dis Sci 1989;34:202–205

38. Frieling T, Enck P, Wienbeck M. Cerebral responses evoked by elec-

trical stimulation of the esophagus in normal subjects. Gastroenterology 1989;97:475–478

39. Ghillebert G, Janssens J, Vantrappen G, Nevens F, Piessens J. Ambulatory 24-hour intraesophageal pH and pressure recordings v. provocation tests in the diagnosis of chest pain of esophageal origin. Gut 1990;31:738–744

40. Gignoux C, et al. Role of upper esophageal reflex and belch reflex dysfunctions in noncardiac chest pain. Dig Dis Sci 1993;38: 1909–1914

41. Gonzalez M, Mearin F, Vasconez C, Armengol JR, Malagelada JR. Oesophageal tone in patients with achalasia. Gut 1997;41:291–296

42. Grundy D, Scratcher T. Sensory afferents from the gastrointestinal tract. In Schultz SG, Wood JD, Rauner BB, eds, Handbook of Physiology, sec 6, vol 1. New York: Oxford University Press, 1989

43. Gupta PK, Clauw DJ, Maher KA, Blank CA, Benjamin SB. Patients with fibromyalgia have lowered thresholds of visceral nociception. Am J Gastroenterol 1993;88:1488 (abstract)

44. Hazan S, Buckley E, Castell DO, Achem SR. Octreotide improves sensory and pain thresholds in patients with noncardiac chest pain. Gastroenterology 1996;110:A132

45. Hazan S, Steinberg A, Morris N, Affronti J, Achem SR. Long-term reproducibility of intraesophageal balloon distention studies in patients with unexplained chest pain. Gastroenterology 1997;112:A145

46. Hewson EG, Sinclair JW, Dalton CB, Wu WC, Castell DO, Richter JE. Acid perfusion test: does it have a role in the assessment of non cardiac chest pain. Gut 1989;30:305–310

47. Hewson EG, Dalton CB, Richter JE. Comparison of esophageal manometry, provocative testing, and ambulatory monitoring in patients with unexplained chest pain. Dig Dis Sci 1990;35:302–309

48. Iaenig W, Morrison JFB. Functional properties of spinal visceral afferents supplying abdominal and pelvic organs, with special emphasis on visceral nociception. In Cervero F, Morrison JFB, eds, Progress in Brain Research, vol 67. New York: Elsevier, 1986

49. James L, Gordon E, Kraiuhin C, Howson A, Meares R. Augmentation of auditory evoked potentials in somatization disorder. J Psychiatr Res 1990;24:155–163

50. Janssens J, Vantrappen G, Ghillebert G. 24-hour recording of esophageal pressure and pH in patients with noncardiac chest pain. Gastroenterology 1986;90:1978–1984

51. Johnson DA, Winters C, Spurling TJ, Chobanian SJ, Cattau EL. Esophageal acid sensitivity in Barrett's esophagus. J Clin Gastroenterol 1987;9:23–27

52. Kahrilas PJ, Dodds WJ, Hogan WJ. Dysfunction of the belch reflex. Gastroenterology 1987;93:818–822

53. Katz PO, Dalton CB, Richter JE, Wu WC, Castell DO. Esophageal testing in patients with noncardiac chest pain or dysphagia: results of three years' experience with 1161 patients. Ann Intern Med 1987; 106:593–597

54. Kaye MD. Anomalies of peristalsis in idiopathic diffuse esophageal spasm. Gut 1981;22:217–222

55. Kaye MD, Kilby AE, Harper PC. Changes in distal esophageal function in response to cooling. Dig Dis Sci 1987;32:22–27

56. Klauser AG, Schindbeck NE, Muller-Lissner SA. Symptoms in gastro-esophageal reflux disease. Lancet 1990;335:205–208

57. Koch KL, Curry RC, Feldman RL, Pepine CJ, Long A, Mathias JR. Ergonovine-induced esophageal spasm in patients with chest pain resembling angina pectoris. Dig Dis Sci 1982;27:1073–1080

58. Kramer P, Hollander W. Comparison of experimental esophageal pain with clinical pain of angina pectoris and esophageal disease. Gastroenterology 1955;29:719

59. Lasch H, Devault KR, Castell DO. Intraesophageal balloon distention in the evaluation of sensory thresholds: studies on reproducibility and comparison of balloon composition. Am J Gastroenterol 1994; 89:1185–1190

60. Lasch H, Castell DO, Castell JA. Evidence for diminished visceral pain with aging: studies using graded intraesophageal balloon distention. Am J Physiol 1997;272:G1–G3

61. Lee CA, Reynolds JC, Ouyang A, Baker L, Cohen S. Esophageal chest pain: value of high dose provocative testing with edrophonium chloride in patients with normal manometrics. Dig Dis Sci 1987;32: 682–688

62. Leek BF. Abdominal and pelvic visceral receptors. Br Med Bull 1977; 33:163–168

63. Lemann M, Dederding JP, Flourie B, Franchisseur C, Rambaud JC, Jian R. Abnormal perception of visceral pain in response to gastric

distention in chronic idiopathic dyspepsia. The irritable stomach syndrome. Dig Dis Sci 1991;36:1249–1254

64. Lipkin M, Sleisenger MH. Studies of visceral pain: measurements of stimulus intensity and duration associated with the onset of pain in esophagus, ileum and colon. J Clin Invest 1958;37:28

65. London RL, Ouyang A, Snape MJ, Goldberg S, Hirshfeld JW, Cohen S. Provocation of esophageal pain by ergonovine or edrophonium. Gastroenterology 1981;81:10–14

66. Mayer EA, Raybould HE. Role of visceral afferent mechanisms in functional bowel disorders. Gastroenterology 1990;99:1688–1704

67. Mayrand S, Diamant NE. Measurement of human esophageal tone *in vivo*. Gastroenterology 1993;105:1411–1420

68. McGivern RF, Berntson GG. Mediation of diurnal fluctuations in pain sensitivity in the rat by food intake patterns: reversal by naloxone. Science 1980;210–211

69. Mehta AJ, De Caestecker JS, Camm AJ, Northfield JC. Sensitization to painful distention and abnormal sensory perception in the esophagus. Gastroenterology 1995;108:311–319

70. Mellow M. Symptomatic diffuse esophageal spasm. Manometric follow-up and response to cholinergic stimulation and cholinesterase inhibition. Gastroenterology 1977;73:237– 240

71. Mellow MH, Simpson AG, Watt L, Schoolmeester L, Haye OL. Esophageal acid perfusion in coronary artery disease. Gastroenterology 1983;85:306–312

72. Meyer GW, Castell DO. Human esophageal response during chest pain induced by swallowing cold liquids. JAMA 1981;246:2057–2059

73. Nevens F, Janssens J, Piessens J, Ghillebert G, De Geest H, Vantrappen G. Prospective study on prevalence of esophageal chest pain in patients referred on an elective basis to a cardiac unit for suspected myocardial ischemia. Dig Dis Sci 1991;36:229–235

74. Nguyen P, Castell D. Evidence of gender differences in esophageal pain threshold. Am J Gastroenterol 1995;90:901–905

75. Nostrant TT, Saves J, Haber T. Bethanechol increases the diagnostic yield in patients with esophageal chest pain. Gastroenterology 1986;91:1141–1146

76. Ockene IS, Shay MJ, Alpert JS, Weiner BH, Dalen JE. Unexplained chest pain in patients with normal coronary arteriograms: a follow-up study of functional status. N Engl J Med 1980;303:1249–1252

77. Orvar KB, Gregersen H, Christensen J. Biomechanical characteristics of the human esophagus. Dig Dis Sci 1993;38:197–205

78. Paterson WG. Neuromuscular mechanisms of esophageal responses at and proximal to a istending balloon. Am J Physiol 1991;260:G148–G55

79. Paterson WG, Selucky M, Hynna-Liepert TT. Effect of intra-esophageal location and muscarinic blockade on balloon-distention-induced chest pain. Dig Dis Sci 1991;36:282–288

80. Peghini PL, Johnston BT, Leite HP, Castell DO. Mucosal acid exposure sensitized a subset of normal subjects to intra-oesophageal balloon distention. Eur J Gastroenterol Hepatol 1996;8:979–983

81. Peghini P, Katz P, Castell D. Imipramine decreases oesophageal pain perception in human male volunteers. Gut 1998 (in press)

82. Peters L, et al. Spontaneous noncardiac chest pain: evaluation by 24-hour ambulatory esophageal motility and pH monitoring. Gastroenterology 1988;94:878–886

83. Rao SS, Hayek B, Summers RW. Impedance planimetry: an integrated approach for assessing sensory, active and passive biomechanical properties of the human esophagus. Am J Gastroenterol 1995;90:431–438

84. Rao SS, Gregersen H, Hayedk B, Summers RW, Christensen J. Unexplained chest pain: the hypersensitive, hyperreactive and poorly compliant esophagus. Ann Intern Med 1996;124:950–958

85. Ren J, et al. Effect of aging on the secondary esophageal peristalsis: presbyesophagus revisited. Am J Physiol 1995;268:G772–G779

86. Richter JE, Hackshaw BT, Wu WC, Castell DO. Edrophonium: a useful provocative test for esophageal chest pain. Ann Intern Med 1985;103:14–21

87. Richter JE Johns DN, Wu WC, Castell DO. Are esophageal motility abnormalities produced during the intraesophageal acid perfusion test? JAMA 1985;253:1914–1917

88. Richter JE, Barish CF, Castell DO. Abnormal esophageal perception in patients with esophageal pain. Gastroenterology 1986;91:845–852

89. Richter JE, Hewson EG, Sinclair JW, Dalton CB. Acid perfusion test and 24-hour esophageal pH monitoring with symptom index: comparison of tests for esophageal acid sensitivity. Dig Dis Sci 1991;36:565–571

90. Richter JE. Provocative tests in esophageal diseases. In Scarpignato C, Galmiche JP, eds, Functional Evaluation in Esophageal Disease. Basel: Karger, 1994

91. Ritchie J. Pain from distention of the pelvic colon by inflating a balloon in the irritable colon syndrome. Gut 1973;14:125–132

92. Sengupta JN, Kauvar D, Royal RK. Characteristics of vagal esophageal tension-sensitive afferent fibers in the opossum. J Neurophysiol 1989;61:1001–1010

93. Siddiqui MA, Johnston BT, Leite LP, Katzka DA, Castell DO. Sensitization of esophageal mucosa by prior acid infusion: effect of decreasing intervals between infusions. Am J Gastroenterol 1996;91:1745–1748

94. Smith JL, Opekun AR, Larkai E, Graham DY. Sensitivity of the esophageal mucosa to pH in gastroesophageal reflux disease. Gastroenterology 1989;96:683–689

95. Smout AJ, Devore MS, Castell DO. Cerebral potentials evoked by esophageal distention in humans. Am J Physiol 1990;259:G955–G959

96. Smout AJ, Devore MS, Dalton CB, Castell DO. Effects of nifedipine on esophageal tone and perception of esophageal distention. Dig Dis Sci 1992;37:598–602

97. Smout AJ, DeVore MS, Dalton CB, Castell DO. Cerebral potentials evoked by esophageal distention in patients with noncardiac chest pain. Gut 1992;33:298–302

98. Soffer EE, Scalabrini P, Wingate DL. Spontaneous noncardiac chest pain: value of ambulatory esophageal pH and motility monitoring. Dig Dis Sci 1989;34:1651–1655

99. Sollenbohmer C, Enck P, Haussinger D, Frieling T. Electrically evoked cerebral potentials during esophageal distension at perception and pain threshold. Am J Gastroenterol 1996;91:970–975

100. Tougas G, Fitzpatrick D, Upton ARM, Hunt RH. The cortical evoked responses produced by balloon distention and electrical stimulation of the esophagus involve different vagal fibers. Gastroenterology 1993;104:A592

101. Trimble KC, Farouk A, Pryde A, Douglas S, Heading RC. Heightened visceral sensation in functional gastrointestinal disease is not site-specific. Evidence for a generalized disorder of gut sensitivity. Dig Dis Sci 1995;40:1607–1613

102. Trimble KC, Pryde A, Heading RC. Lowered oesophageal sensory thresholds in patients with symptomatic but not excess gastro-oesophageal reflux: evidence for a spectrum of visceral sensitivity in GORD. Gut 1995;37:7

103. Vantrappen G, Janssens J. What is irritable esophagus? Another point of view. Gastroenterology 1988;94:1092–1094

104. Vantrappen G, Janssens J, Ghillebert G. The irritable esophagus: a frequent cause of angina-like chest pain. Lancet 1987;1:1232–1234

105. Ward BW, Wu WC, Richter JE, Hackshay BT, Castell DO. Long term follow-up of symptomatic status of patients with noncardiac chest pain: is diagnosis of esophageal etiology helpful? Am J Gastroenterol 1987;82:215–218

106. Wielgosz AT, et al. Unimproved chest pain in patients with minimal or no coronary disease: a behavioral phenomenon. Am Heart J 1984;108:67–72

107. Winship DH, Zboralske FF. The esophageal propulsive force: esophageal response to acute obstruction. J Clin Invest 1967;46:1391–1401

108. Wolff BB. Behavioral measurements of human pain. In Steinbach RA, ed, The Psychology of Pain. New York: Raven Press, 1978:129–168

109. Yakshe PN, et al. Does provocative esophageal testing influence coronary blood flow or coronary flow reserve? Preliminary results of concurrent esophageal and cardiac testing. Gastroenterology 1993;104:A227

110. Zacchi P, Freiling T, Kuhlbusch R, Wilhelm K, Enck P, Lubke HJ. What is more physiological: electrical or mechanical stimulation of the human esophagus? Gastroenterology 1992;102:A538

*The Esophagus*, Third Edition,
edited by D. O. Castell and J. E. Richter.
Lippincott Williams & Wilkins, Philadelphia © 1999.

CHAPTER 8

# Role of Histology and Cytology in Esophageal Disease

Kim R. Geisinger and Lisa A. Teot

In many individuals with esophageal disorders, the diagnosis rests completely with the clinical symptomatic picture. That is, patients are not examined radiographically or endoscopically. An even greater proportion of patients with diseases of this organ do not undergo a pathologic examination of their esophageal tissues. However, in some patients morphologic confirmation of the clinical and endoscopic picture is needed and requires the gastroenterologist to obtain endoscopic biopsies and cytologic brushings. Such morphologic evaluation, furthermore, may provide the initial consideration of a specific diagnosis. Both of these scenarios apply to tumors and nonneoplastic abnormalities.

It is our impression that endoscopically obtained biopsies and brushings are diagnostically complementary [38, 40, 41]. Although this may be especially valid for the diagnosis of neoplastic lesions, this also is true for other conditions, especially infections. This recurrent theme will be emphasized at multiple points throughout this chapter.

## NORMAL HISTOLOGY AND CYTOLOGY

In order to attain a complete appreciation of many aspects of the morphologic pathology of the esophagus, it is important to have a firm grasp on the appearance of the normal esophagus in histologic sections [25]. Furthermore, the histologic architecture and cytomorphologic structure of the esophagus form the substrate for cytopathologic specimens [40]. Thus, an understanding of normal anatomy, including cytomorphologic features, is a prerequisite to recognizing and identifying pathologic abnormalities in patients with dis-

ease. As with other organs of the gastrointestinal tract, the esophagus has four concentric layers: mucosa, submucosa, muscularis propria, and adventitial tissue.

The esophageal mucosa is lined by stratified nonkeratinizing squamous epithelium which possesses basal, intermediate, and superficial layers. The basal cell compartment is composed normally of two or three cellular layers and comprises no more than 15% of the full thickness of the epithelium. Mitotic figures are uncommon and occur only in the basal cell zone. As these cells mature within the epithelium, the cytoplasm increases, the nuclear-to-cytoplasmic (N/C) ratios decline, and the space between neighboring nuclei increases. Keratohyaline granules are generally absent. The lamina propria is composed of loose fibrovascular tissue which is richly endowed with lymphatic vessels. Papillae in the lamina propria normally project no further than two-thirds of the way through the overlying epithelium. The muscularis mucosae consists of thin slips of smooth muscle. The distalmost 1 to 2 cm may be lined by a simple columnar cell epithelium with or without mucus production [25]. Throughout the entire length of the esophagus, the lamina propria contains glandular structures which histologically resemble those present in the gastric cardia. Normally, goblet cells are not present in the esophagus [49].

Accordingly, cytologic smears are dominated by squamous epithelial cells of the superficial and intermediate types [40]. The former are characterized by polygonal contours, delicate voluminous eosinophilic cytoplasm, and a single, centrally positioned pyknotic nucleus. According to Shen et al. [113], the majority of the cells have an intermediate level of maturation. Thus, the nuclei are larger and have finely granular chromatin and small chromocenters. Nucleoli are generally not present. In smears, both types of squamous cells are present in large, flat sheets, small clusters, concentric arrangements (pearls), and as single cells. Rarely, cytologic preparations may also contain parabasal cells, presum-

K. R. Geisinger: Surgical Pathology and Cytopathology, North Carolina Baptist Hospital, and Department of Pathology, Wake Forest University School of Medicine, Winston-Salem, North Carolina 27157-1072.

L. A. Teot: Department of Cytopathology, University of Rochester Medical Center, Rochester, New York 14642.

ably the consequence of very vigorous sampling. These will typically present as solitary cells with round contours with dense cyanophilic cytoplasm and relatively high N/C ratios.

Normal esophageal brushings may also contain glandular cells, the consequence of either inadvertent sampling of the stomach and/or procurement of columnar cells that may normally be present in the distalmost portion of this organ. These cells are present in small to large, generally flat sheets with sharply delineated edges, well-defined cellular borders, and small, round nuclei with finely granular, pale chromatin and inconspicuous nucleoli. Cytoplasm is delicate and finely granular; vacuoles are generally not evident. In addition, normal cytologic specimens may contain a variety of contaminants. These may include ciliated respiratory cells, alveolar macrophages, plant cells, and talc crystals.

Histologically, the submucosa is composed of relatively hypocellular, denser collagenous and elastic connective tissue through which blood vessels, lymphatic vessels, and nerves are evident. The muscularis propria consists of skeletal muscle in the upper third and smooth muscle in the lower third of the organ; the middle portion shows a mixture of cell types. Ganglia of the myenteric plexus are located between the inner and outer muscle layers. The adventia is composed of loose connective tissue which blends with the surrounding mediastinal soft tissues.

## ESOPHAGITIS

Inflammation represents the common final pathway by which tissues respond to a wide variety of noxious stimuli. Although clinical and radiologic findings may suggest a specific etiology and diagnosis, the histologic and cytologic alterations in the esophagitides are, for the most part, nonspecific. The major exceptions are the infectious conditions in which the presence of fungal elements, viral inclusions, or rarely, pathogenic bacteria may permit a specific diagnosis.

### *CANDIDA* ESOPHAGITIS

By far, *Candida albicans* is the most frequent cause of clinically significant infectious esophagitis. Most individuals with this infection are immunosuppressed or at least receiving antibiotics. In our experience, it is commonly identified in patients with leukemia or lymphoma, those who have received systemic chemotherapy and/or radiation for the treatment of cancer, and individuals infected by the human immunodeficiency virus. Obstruction due to achalasia, stricture, or neoplasm also predisposes to a *Candida* infection [37, 77].

The gross appearance of *Candida* esophagitis varies from small, slightly raised plaques on a background of an erythematous mucosa to large nodules associated with ulcers. *Candida* infection typically results in a pseudomembrane that covers and is attached to the underlying squamous mucosa.

Histologically, this pseudomembrane consists of a mix-

ture of fungal organisms (pseudohyphae), fibrinopurulent exudate, and, at times, dead squamous epithelial cells (Color Plate 15). The fungal organisms, both yeast and pseudohyphae, are present within the epithelium and are often associated with a neutrophilic infiltrate (Color Plate 16). The epithelium may show erosions and ulcers which are associated with degenerative and regenerative alterations within the adjacent squamous epithelium.

The cytopathologic diagnosis of *Candida* esophagitis is usually straightforward [40]. In Papanicolaou-stained preparations, characteristic pseudohyphae and yeast cells appear brightly eosinophilic or magenta and are often conspicuous, even at low magnifications (Color Plate 17). The pseudohyphae are delicate and do not show true septation; rather, indentations along their long axes are usually apparent. The smaller round or ovoid budding yeast are more difficult to identify, but can usually be found. In addition to lying free within the smear, the fungi may be trapped within an acute inflammatory exudate and/or appear to infiltrate the squamous epithelium. Degenerative and necrotic alterations within the squamous epithelium may be present in such smears. The squamous epithelial cells may manifest marked reparative atypia.

Reparative alterations occur within epithelium in response to a significant inflammatory infiltrate and/or a mucosal defect [40]. In repair, the body attempts to heal the injury through regeneration of the adjacent mucosa. The histologic appearance of this mending process is distinctive (Color Plate 18). The regenerating epithelial cells have nuclei which are larger than normal and often somewhat more ovoid, having pale-stained chromatin and prominent nucleoli. The cytoplasm in regenerating squamous cells may appear less dense and homogeneous than in the normal resting state. Repair is the cytomorphologic picture seen in cytologic preparations in this healing phase (Color Plate 19). The cytomorphologic features of repair include the presence of cohesive, generally flat sheets of enlarged epithelial cells. These aggregates vary from small to large. This preservation of intercellular cohesion is a major hallmark of this benign atypia. In fact, only rarely do the smears contain individually dispersed atypical cells with intact cytoplasm. Within the aggregates, normal polarity is relatively well maintained. In addition, there may be a streaming effect in which the cells and their nuclei all appear to be traveling in the same direction. The squamous nuclei will have round to oval, smooth contours with finely granular, uniformly distributed, and often pale chromatin. The distinctive nuclear membranes are thin and uniform. Characteristically, huge nucleoli are present within the vesicular chromatin. The N/C ratios may be elevated. Finally, mitotic figures may be evident within the squamous epithelium.

*Candida albicans* frequently inhabits the oropharynx and the gastrointestinal tract in healthy individuals. Accordingly, the presence of characteristic yeast alone in a cytologic preparation should not be misinterpreted as definite esophageal infection. Rather, the identification of pseudohyphae in the background of necrotic debris and inflammatory cells is essential to a correct cytologic diagnosis of *Candida* esophagitis.

In our experience, brushings have a higher level of diagnostic sensitivity for *Candida* esophagitis than do biopsies [38]. In large part, this may be related to two factors, namely, greater sampling of the mucosal surface by the brush than the forceps and the proclivity for this fungus to proliferate on and near the luminal surface. However, biopsies and brushings are diagnostically complementary in this situation.

It has also been our experience that endoscopy is not always able to predict with a high level of accuracy the presence of *Candida* esophagitis. Biopsies and brushings may be able to provide a more definitive diagnosis. Isaac et al. [60] demonstrated that biopsies were important in the initiation of specific antimicrobial therapy in pediatric patients with cancer. Brushings may be a diagnostic procedure which may be pursued rather than biopsies in patients who harbor malignancies and are severely thrombocytopenic.

## HERPES ESOPHAGITIS

Herpes simplex virus (HSV) is the most frequently recognized cause of viral esophagitis. Predisposing conditions include mucosal trauma, cancer, chemotherapy, radiotherapy, immunosuppressive therapy, and other immunodeficiency states [17, 90, 105]. Furthermore, herpetic esophagitis also occurs in apparently immunocompetent patients of all ages [6, 26, 95, 122]. Herpetic esophagitis often resolves spontaneously, even in immunocompromised patients.

The actual incidence of herpetic esophagitis remains unknown due at least in part to the often asymptomatic nature of the infection and in part to probable underdiagnosis in patients with symptoms. In the past, diagnosis was most frequently made at postmortem examination. In a review of nearly 7,000 autopsies at a cancer hospital, Rosen and Hajdu [105] found histologic changes consistent with a herpes virus infection in the esophagi of 25 individuals. Only 1 of their patients had an antemortem diagnosis of esophagitis. In their review of nearly 4,000 autopsies in a general hospital, Buss and Scharyj [17] discovered herpes esophagitis in 50 patients. In the vast majority of these individuals, an antemortem diagnosis was not suspected. Nash and Ross [90], in their review of 3,000 autopsies, identified 14 instances of herpes esophageal infection. In not a single patient had herpetic esophagitis been suspected clinically.

The classic endoscopic appearance of herpetic esophagitis is that of multiple shallow, small ulcers with sharply delineated borders, generally in the distal third of the esophagus. In other patients, more extensive mucosal sloughing or a nonspecific inflammatory picture may be evident. It is important for the endoscopist to sample the edges of ulcers in an attempt to diagnose HSV infections.

Squamous epithelium is the prime target of HSV, and thus the major alterations are evident within these cells [74, 133]. Basically, two types of viral cytopathic alterations may be

evident in biopsies and brushings (Color Plate 20). In one, classic Cowdry type A inclusion bodies are present. These eosinophilic structures are round, dense, and uniform in structure, and are separated from a thickened nuclear membrane by a clear zone or halo. The other type of virocyte is characterized by homogeneous, faintly basophilic chromatin. The latter is often referred to as having a "ground glass" appearance. In both types of virocytes, the nuclei and the cytoplasm are increased in volume, but the N/C ratios are not always elevated. In addition, multinucleation of the infected squamous cells is characteristically seen. Within these cells, the nuclei are typically compressed against one another: this is referred to as molding. The large inclusions need to be distinguished from prominent nucleoli, especially those in malignant cells. In HSV-infected squamous epithelial cells, a definite agranular clear zone separates the central inclusion from the peripheral chromatin rim. In contrast, nuclei with large nucleoli usually have variably sized and shaped granulated chromatin within the surrounding nucleoplasm. Cytoplasmic inclusions are not present within HSV virocytes.

Histologically, the earliest alterations are nonspecific cytopathic effects in infected superficial squamous cells. These include ballooning degeneration and bland necrosis. Small and at times multiple intranuclear inclusions, easily confused with chromocenters, may also be present. Separation of the infected, devitalized superficial epithelium results in an intraepithelial vesicle containing an inflammatory exudate. Subsequent sloughing of the necrotic epithelium results in erosion or ulcer. The bases of ulcers are composed of necrotic cellular debris, fibrin, inflammatory cells, and granulation tissue. The characteristic virocytes are present predominantly at the ulcer margins (Color Plate 20). Thus, it is important for the endoscopist to sample the edges of ulcers, as this will provide the highest diagnostic yield. Recently, Singh and Odze [110] called attention to the presence of multinucleated squamous epithelial giant cells in patients with nonherpetic esophagitis. These cells were most frequently located next to an ulcer or areas of prominent epithelial injury. The nuclei in these cells demonstrated a very finely granulated chromatin and often a solitary large eosinophilic nucleolus. Thus, such cells need to be distinguished from herpetic virocytes. However, the nuclei in these giant cells did not have inclusion bodies or the chromatin smudging typical of virally infected cells. Furthermore, these cells tended to be concentrated in the deeper portion of the epithelium, in contrast to the more superficial location in herpes infection.

The cytologic diagnosis of esophageal HSV infection is often straightforward [40]. As in biopsies, the cytopathologic diagnosis depends on the identification of squamous epithelial cells with the characteristic alterations of HSV infection [40, 79, 80, 111]. In smears, virocytes appear as enlarged squamous epithelial cells, both singly and in flat sheets (Color Plate 21). The enlarged nuclei may contain inclusion bodies which vary from round to irregular and are centrally positioned. The inclusions are separated from the nuclear envelope by a clear agranular zone. The nuclear membrane is variably thickened and may appear beaded, probably due to degeneration. In our experience, the ground glass appearance is more frequent. In smears, it is characterized as a chromatin with a smooth or homogeneous pale basophilic appearance (Color Plates 21 and 22). At times, it has an almost refractile presentation. Multinucleated squamous cells are usually present in the smears and show characteristic molding of the enlarged nuclei. In such cases the already thickened membranes are further accentuated. Cytoplasm of the infected cells may appear scanty, dense, and cyanophilic. As ulcers are frequently present, reparative atypia, neutrophils, and granular necrotic debris are also present. A potential pitfall in the interpretation of brushings from herpetic esophagitis is confusing the intranuclear inclusion bodies with the macronucleoli of cancer cells. Combined with the presence of bizarre, reparative epithelial cells, this could lead to a false-positive diagnosis of squamous cell carcinoma.

Although not universally agreed upon, most authors believe that endoscopic brushing samples have a higher level of diagnostic sensitivity than do biopsies for herpetic esophagitis [38, 40]. In any case, brushings and biopsies are complementary for the diagnosis of this infection.

## CYTOMEGALOVIRUS ESOPHAGITIS

Cytomegalovirus (CMV) is second to HSV as a cause of viral esophagitis and, as with HSV, tends to affect immunocompromised patients [108]. In contrast to HSV, CMV involves the esophagus much less frequently than the glandular lined mucosa of the stomach and intestines.

The radiographic and endoscopic attributes are totally nonspecific. Grossly, alterations vary from a mild, nonspecific inflammatory picture to one of irregularly contoured ulcers. In general, CMV does not infect squamous epithelial cells, in contrast to HSV. Rather, this virus infects fibroblasts within granulation tissue, capillary endothelial cells, neurons, and the epithelium of submucosal glands. Accordingly, in biopsies, the characteristic cytopathic changes are noted not within the epithelial cells, but rather within the cells in the base of ulcers (Color Plate 23). If the endoscopist does not sample an ulcer bed, then the infection may very well be missed. The CMV virocytes are characterized, as their name suggests, by a marked enlargement of both nuclear and cytoplasmic volumes [108]. The nucleomegaly and cytomegaly are greater than one typically expects in HSV infections. The enlarged nucleus possesses a huge homogeneous basophilic inclusion body which is separated from a thickened nuclear membrane by a clear halo. Some virocytes may contain minute cytoplasmic inclusions which are generally eosinophilic. Unlike HSV, CMV virocytes almost never show multinucleation or ground glass chromatin patterns.

Greenson [47] recently reported that clusters of macrophages in granulation tissue and inflammatory exudates were a characteristic reaction to the virus; 86% of the examined biopsies showed macrophage aggregates. He claimed that the aggregates may show a peculiar perivascular distribution strongly suggestive of CMV esophagitis.

In esophageal brushing smears, only rare CMV virocytes are scattered against a background of reparative epithelial cells, acute inflammation, necrotic debris, and granulation tissue [40, 124]. The infected cells present as single elements, that is, they are unassociated with other cells (Color Plate 24). The diagnostic cells demonstrate both prominent nucleomegaly and cytomegaly, thick, marginated chromatin, and huge, round to reniform basophilic inclusion bodies within the nucleus. The latter are surrounded by huge, clear halo, the consequence of chromatin clearing. Granular eosinophilic inclusions may be seen in the cytoplasm of some virocytes.

It is important for the endoscopist to biopsy and brush the base of esophageal ulcers to sample CMV virocytes. A diligent search is necessary for the identification in smears, as the number of infected cells in the given specimen is generally quite low. Although biopsies are more sensitive for the diagnosis of this esophageal infection, histologic and cytologic examinations are diagnostically complementary [38, 130].

The major entity in the differential diagnosis with CMV esophagitis is infection by HSV [40]. As stated earlier, HSV typically infects squamous epithelium, whereas CMV infects both glandular and mesenchymal elements. Multinucleation and ground glass chromatin are common in herpes infections, but are almost never seen with CMV. Conversely, cytoplasmic inclusions occur only within CMV viroctyes. In brushings, HSV virocytes are typically present in much greater numbers than in CMV virocytes.

## OTHER INFECTIONS OF THE ESOPHAGUS

Esophagitis due primarily to bacterial infection is an apparently uncommon clinical problem. Affected patients are usually immunocompromised, have a history of prolonged antibiotic therapy, or both. The causative agents are often normal flora or saprophytes [85, 128].

Grossly and microscopically, primary bacterial infections may present as ulcerative or pseudomembranous esophagitis or simply as a nonspecific inflammatory picture. In biopsies, the bacteria may be seen within the epithelium or deeper tissues. When inflammation and necrosis are pronounced, Gram's staining of tissue may be needed to demonstrate the organisms. Evidence of cancer or infection with viral or fungal agents precludes the diagnosis of primary bacterial esophagitis, as superinfection is a common occurrence in these settings.

In cytologic smears, the presence of morphologically uniform bacteria, acute inflammatory cells, necrotic debris, and reactive epithelium, as well as the absence of other specific findings, may suggest primary bacterial esophagitis. Whether these bacteria are contaminants or are contributing to the pathogenesis of disease is often uncertain. However, it is prudent to mention in the cytology report that bacteria are present in the smears.

*Aspergillus, Mucor, Histoplasma,* and *Cryptococcus* species have been implicated as rare causes of esophagitis [64, 68, 86, 87]. To the best of our knowledge, the cytologic diagnosis of these diseases has not been reported. We have seen a single example of *Aspergillus* esophagitis in brushings from a patient with acute myeloblastic leukemia (Color Plate 25). The smears were poorly cellular with scattered benign squamous epithelial cells and abundant granular debris. In addition, throughout the specimen were three-dimensional aggregates of fungal hyphae. They were deeply cyanophilic and composed of moderately thick, uniform, septated structures. Inflammatory cells were extremely sparse, as the patient was severely leukopenic. Biopsies were not obtained from this patient due to a profound thrombocytopenia. In histologic material, we have seen a single example of esophageal infection by *Histoplasma.* Both the lamina propria and submucosa were extensively infiltrated by budding yeasts, which grew in nodular aggregates and sheets. The host inflammatory reaction was nonexistent. The patient had the acquired immunodeficiency syndrome. Cytologic smears were not performed in this patient.

## RADIATION- AND CHEMOTHERAPY-ASSOCIATED ESOPHAGITIS

Esophagitis is an unfortunate but well-recognized complication of radiotherapy to the chest and mediastinum. In general, the severity of injury appears to be related to several factors, including the total dose of the radiation received, the fraction delivered per treatment, and the time period over which the therapy is administered [10, 67, 92]. Irreversible damage to the tissues of the esophagus is believed to occur at doses of 60 Gy (6,000 rad) or more [10]. A number of cytotoxic chemotherapeutic agents may also cause injury to the esophagus in a similar manner [94]. Indeed, the effects of chemotherapy and radiation may potentiate each other, lowering the threshold for injury [45, 94, 98, 112].

Endoscopically, radiation- and chemotherapy-associated esophagitis may be characterized by mucosal erythema, edema, and friability which may progress to erosions and ulcers. With extreme damage, extensive mucosal sloughing occurs and may be accompanied by life-threatening hemorrhage. Radiation-induced fibrosis is a chronic process which often develops silently.

Histologically, radiation esophagitis is distinguished from other inflammatory processes, with which it shares nonspecific features such as neutrophilic infiltrates, by the presence of bizarre-appearing epithelial and mesenchymal cells, including fibroblasts and capillary angioblasts [10]. The enlarged squamous epithelial cells are characterized by increased volumes of both cytoplasm and nucleoplasm with retention of a relatively normal N/C ratio; in practice, however, this ratio may be increased to the point that it resembles malignant cells. With radiation, the chromatin typically appears pale or washed out rather than hyperchromatic. In addition, nucleoli are not usually prominent. Multinucleation of squamous cells is a constant feature, but, in contrast to HSV virocytes, the nuclei are not necessarily centrally concentrated or compressed against one another. Within the epithelial layer, mitoses are increased, may show abnormal configurations, and are present at levels higher than the basal cell zone. In the subacute and chronic phases, parakeratosis and acanthosis are common, and superficial blood vessels within the lamina propria may appear hyalinized and thick walled. Furthermore, highly atypical mesenchymal elements may be present within the lamina propria and muscle layers. These cells are characterized by enlarged, irregularly shaped, and hyperchromatic nuclei, at times with well-developed nucleoli.

In cytologic preparations, as in tissue sections, the hallmark of radiation esophagitis is the presence of highly atypical epithelial cells [40]. Characteristic morphologic features include marked but proportionate nucleomegaly and cytomegaly, multinucleation, and vacuolization of the cytoplasm and occasionally the nucleus. Irregular infolding, wrinkling, and focal thickening of the nuclear membrane are common attributes. Chromatin is usually pale stained and coarsely granular, although occasional nuclei exhibit hyperchromatism. As in tissue sections, the multinucleated squamous epithelial cells can usually be distinguished from HSV virocytes. Rarely, individually dispersed huge and bizarre stromal cells are also noted in the smears. These cells may have very high N/C ratios and indistinct cellular borders.

The histopathologic features of chemotherapy-associated esophagitis are similar to those induced by radiation. For example, markedly enlarged cells with huge nuclei and multinucleation are common. Compared to the radiation case, however, the chromatin may be much more darkly stained and nucleoli may be more prominent. Mitotic figures may be numerous.

The cytologic findings in esophageal brushings from 19 patients who had neither esophageal nor gastric carcinoma, but who had received a variety of cytotoxic chemotherapeutic agents, either alone or with radiotherapy, were reported by O'Morchoe and colleagues [94]. Cytomorphologic features observed in the specimens from 3 of the 10 patients who had received only chemotherapy included increased N/C ratios, crowded and overlapped nuclei, nuclear pleomorphism, nuclear membrane irregularities, chromatin clumping, and hyperchromatism which was marked in some nuclei; prominent, often multiple and irregularly shaped nucleoli were evident. In addition, cytologic changes similar to those seen with radiotherapy were present, although none of these patients had been irradiated. Curiously, these attributes were not identified in brushings from any of the 9 patients who had received both chemotherapy and radiation, although mild epithelial atypia was diagnosed in 4. This study suggests that chemotherapy-induced cytologic alterations may mimic those of cancer cells more closely than do radiation-induced changes and thus create a potentially serious diagnostic dilemma for the morphologist [94]. However, in practice there should only be a major problem if the patient had been treated for carcinoma of the esophagus.

In fact, a major diagnostic challenge may be posed by the distinction between therapy-induced cytologic abnormalities and malignant transformation. Relative preservation of the N/C ratio, relatively uniform alterations among the sampled cells, and an absence of diffuse hyperchromatism are major features that serve to separate neoplastic cells from the benign but bizarre atypia that may be induced in epithelial elements by radiation or chemotherapy [40]. Admittedly, differentiation between these two is not always possible. Furthermore, these two diagnoses are not mutually exclusive and radiation atypia may also be induced in truly malignant cells. In these situations, having both biopsies and cytologic brushings may prove very useful in achieving the correct diagnosis [38].

## REFLUX ESOPHAGITIS

The most common cause of inflammation of the esophagus is damage secondary to reflux of gastric and possibly duodenal contents into the esophageal lumen through a relatively incompetent lower esophageal sphincter [39]. Accordingly, reflux esophagitis is a common clinical problem and it accounts for significant morbidity in a sizable proportion of the population. Often, the diagnosis rests solely on the basis of classic symptoms. This is often supplemented with an endoscopic examination of the esophageal mucosa, especially in patients with apparently severe disease and with atypical clinical presentations. Other clinical tests may also be performed, such as pH monitoring. As a result, several investigators have claimed that there is little need for mucosal biopsies [2, 28]. However, other investigators, including us, believe that biopsy is warranted and increases both the diagnostic sensitivity and specificity for the identification of gastroesophageal reflux disease [32, 39]. Furthermore, biopsy aids in excluding other causes of inflammation and in diagnosing and confirming major complications of reflux, especially Barrett's esophagus.

These arguments in support of esophageal biopsy must be tempered with the knowledge that the pathologic findings needed to make a diagnosis of reflux esophagitis are not agreed upon unanimously [12, 16, 20, 32, 39, 62, 126]. Arguments have revolved about the histopathologic criteria necessary in this setting. For the most part, controversy has weighed the value of inflammatory cell infiltrates against the merits of reactive epithelial hyperplasia as markers of acid-induced esophagitis. Lack of total agreement about the diagnostic criteria stems from a number of factors. The clinical parameters used to determine whether patients have reflux esophagitis have varied among published series, the spectrum ranging from symptoms of heartburn [62, 76] to the use of intraesophageal 24-hour pH monitoring [70]. The histologic findings in some studies have relied on well-oriented suction-type biopsies, whereas others utilize generally smaller pinch-type biopsy specimens. The methods by which quantitative characteristics were evaluated has also differed among the investigations. In some, quantitation via an ocular micrometer was utilized [12, 70, 109], whereas others relied on visual estimation of the alterations [8, 61, 62]. Finally, the location and numbers of biopsies per patient have shown considerable heterogeneity.

## INFLAMMATORY CELLS

Almost all investigators agree that the presence of inflammatory cells in the esophagus is a major criterion to identify esophagitis. Yet, a lack of uniformity exists in defining distribution and type(s) of inflammatory cells that are important in diagnosing reflux esophagitis. Essentially everyone agrees that the presence of neutrophilic leukocytes is diagnostic (Color Plate 26). However, as stated by Yardley [136], this specific histologic marker occurs in only a minority of biopsy specimens from patients with clinically well-defined reflux disease. The fact that the neutrophil was a specific, but insensitive indicator was confirmed by Behar and Sheahan [8], who studied biopsy specimens from 40 patients and 15 controls. Neutrophils were identified in 5% and 40% of patients with mild and severe clinical reflux esophagitis, respectively, but they were not recognized in any of the specimens from the normal controls. However, neither report stated specifically whether the leukocytic infiltrates were present within the squamous epithelium, the lamina propria, or both. Mitros [88] also stated the high specificity and low sensitivity of the neutrophils in either the epithelium or the lamina propria.

The report of Collins et al. [20] is interesting in that they did not find the presence of segmented leukocytes to be a statistically significant discriminator between patients with esophagitis and controls. Several other authors reported similar findings [31, 109, 126]. For example, Seefeld and colleagues [109] looked for the presence of segmented leukocytes, both neutrophils and eosinophils, in the lamina propria of biopsies and found them in 62% of the patients with definite reflux esophagitis as well as 10% of the control subjects. They claimed that the neutrophil was more specific than the eosinophil, yet both were claimed to be insensitive for this diagnosis. Fink et al. [31] studied 18 normal subjects and found rare neutrophils in 1 (5.5%), but did not specify whether they were present in the squamous epithelium or the lamina propria. Although Black and co-workers [12] did not find intraepithelial neutrophils within the esophageal mucosa of autopsied infants, Shub et al. [116] did identify slightly more than one neutrophilic leukocyte per high-powered microscopic field in a similar study population. Unfortunately, several good investigations apparently did not study the diagnostic role of neutrophils or other inflammatory cells [36, 70, 76].

We believe that the presence of neutrophilic leukocytes, at least within the squamous epithelium, is a rather specific histologic marker for esophagitis, despite reservations that one might have from reviewing the literature [44]. It has been recognized that neutrophils are often present in association with morphologic damage to the squamous epithelial cells [8, 88]. In this setting, their presence is usually easy to identify (Color Plate 26). Conversely, in the presence of morphologically unremarkable epithelium, it may be more difficult to identify these cells specifically when they are present in extremely low numbers. In part, this is due to the pale staining of the cytoplasmic granules, which do not contrast sharply with the cytoplasm of adjacent squamous epithelial cells. In addition, it may be difficult to differentiate between a neutrophilic leukocyte and an intraepithelial lymphocyte. This challenge is especially evident in deeper portions of the epithelium.

A more recent focus of interest has centered on the importance of the intraepithelial eosinophil. Brown, Goldman, and Winter and their colleagues [16, 44, 135] have championed the eosinophilic leukocyte as a very sensitive and specific histologic marker of reflux esophagitis (Color Plate 27). Winter and associates [135] studied 113 esophageal biopsy specimens from 46 children with chronic reflux esophagitis, all of whom underwent continuous overnight intraesophageal pH monitoring; the majority of the biopsies were the suction type, and up to 36 sections were prepared per specimen. The authors found that the presence of eosinophils within the epithelium correlated well with abnormal acid clearance. Overall, of the 46 patients, eosinophils, usually in small numbers, were identified in 18 children, 17 of whom had abnormal clearances. Eosinophils were found in a single patient who had a normal acid clearance. Several relationships to patient age were noted by Winter et al. [135]. First, the number of eosinophils was greater in the specimens from older children than in the younger ones; Chadwick et al. [18] also noticed that in infants, eosinophils were not a reliable marker of esophagitis in patients 4 months of age or younger. More importantly, in the Winter study [135] eosinophils occurred in the absence of epithelial hyperplasia in patients younger than 2 years. The presence of intraepithelial eosinophils in biopsies from more proximal sites in the esophagus corresponded to more severe disease. Eosinophils could be identified equally well in pinch- and suction-type biopsy specimens. Other authors also found intraepithelial eosinophils to be a sensitive indicator of esophagitis in young children [12, 58, 116]. Friesen et al. [33] found that suction biopsies were preferable to pinch biopsies for the histologic diagnosis of esophagitis in infants 6 months of age or younger.

Subsequently, Brown and co-workers [16] examined pinch biopsy specimens from 50 consecutive adult patients. Whereas the evaluation of epithelial hyperplasia was feasible in only 14%, the majority of patients (62%) had intraepithelial segmented leukocytes or squamous cell necrosis. Of these, the eosinophil was the most common abnormality, being noted in 52% of the patients and being the sole histologic marker of esophagitis in 23%. The number of intraepithelial eosinophils was variable from case to case, but they were generally scanty and required that up to 24 sections be examined to discover them. Their concentrations did not correspond to the degree of severity of esophagitis. However, Mitros [88] claimed that eosinophils became more numerous with increasing severity. When present in very large numbers within the epithelium, however, eosinophils may not be related specifically to reflux esophagitis [73]. Rather, they may be a marker of an allergic phenomenon similar to asthma.

Palmer [96] stated that eosinophils were always present, although usually in small quantities; he did not specifically relate whether they were in the epithelium, lamina propria, or both. Similarly, Behar and Sheahan [8] and Fink and co-workers [31] failed to designate a specific site for the residence of the cells. The latter authors found eosinophils in one of their 18 controls [31]. According to Black et al. [12], eosinophils within the lamina propria are a rather specific marker for reflux esophagitis in infants. Their presence in this location possessed a greater level of diagnostic sensitivity than did intraepithelial eosinophils. Furthermore, in this specific site, eosinophils correlated with the other histologic parameters of inflammation. Collins and colleagues [20] found intraepithelial eosinophils in one-fourth of their controls and believed that eosinophils and neutrophils were too nonspecific to be of diagnostic value. Tummala et al. [126] examined 103 suction biopsy specimens from 73 adult patients with well-documented reflux esophagitis for both intraepithelial leukocytes and epithelial hyperplasia, and reported that high levels of sensitivity and specificity were lacking for the intraepithelial eosinophil. More precisely, one-third of their patients and their normal controls had this histologic finding. In contrast to most other reported investigations, their controls were examined for and were found to have normal results during pH monitoring.

Although we have not specifically examined biopsy specimens from normal, asymptomatic volunteers, it is our opinion that intraepithelial eosinophils are a sensitive tissue marker for esophagitis in both pediatric and adult patients with clinical and endoscopic evidence supportive of reflux esophagitis (Color Plate 27). We are unaware of any data that adequately explain the greater sensitivity of the eosinophil versus the neutrophil in this setting; at least in part, it may be related to the relative ease with which the eosinophil is observed in tissue sections. Neutrophil granules do not stain intensely with hematoxylin and eosin. On the other hand, the eosinophil's cytoplasm is packed with round granules of intensely reddish, at times almost refractile, hyaline quality that often permits their recognition at low magnification, even when present in scanty numbers. It is necessary to separate eosinophils from erythrocytes within the epithelium; the latter are larger and generally do not pose a diagnostic challenge. One may identify eosinophils within tissue sections without recognizing their typically bilobate nucleus; not infrequently, only thin strands of cytoplasm containing their characteristic granules can be seen extending between squamous cells at all levels of the stratified epithelium. As suggested by Brown et al. [16], eosinophilic migration may be stimulated by specific inflammatory mediators or it may be only a part, albeit prominent, of a nonspecific chronic inflammatory reaction. Unfortunately, the intraepithelial eosinophil may not be an extremely sensitive diagnostic marker, being absent in a significant minority of patients, even with the examination of a large number of histologic sections and levels. If the presence of either the neutrophil or the eosinophil within the epithelium is considered as diagnostic, then increased sensitivity, and probably specificity, are the result. Unlike the neutrophil, the eosinophil is found more often than not within epithelium which does not manifest any morphologic evidence of damage.

Goldman and Antonioli [44] wrote that the only diagnostically important exudative finding on biopsy is the presence of the segmented leukocyte within the squamous epithelium. Thus, defining neutrophils or eosinophils within the lamina propria would be construed as lacking diagnostic significance. This, however, is not proved, and it may be that segmented white cells within the lamina propria also have merit in confirming reflux esophagitis by biopsy. It stands to reason that intraepithelial leukocytes migrate from the small blood vessels in the underlying connective tissue and thus must be present in the lamina propria at some point before reaching the epithelium. A major advantage of relying on intraepithelial segmented leukocytes over epithelial hyperplasia is that one is not handicapped by relatively small and poorly oriented biopsy specimens. As long as the inflammatory cells are present among the squamous elements, a diagnosis can be rendered with a high level of certainty [39]. Consequently, pinch biopsies are adequate.

Palmer [96] reported on the biopsy findings from 61 patients with endoscopic erosive esophagitis; all specimens included the muscularis mucosae. In 19 patients, inflammatory cells were present within the epithelium, predominantly in the deeper portions. The majority of these inflammatory infiltrates were composed of mononuclear cells, especially lymphocytes. In all 61 specimens, the inflammatory reaction was greater in the lamina propria, especially just beneath the basal cell layer. Lymphocytes and plasma cells were the major components. Ballem and co-workers [7] also diagnosed esophagitis on the basis of subepithelial infiltrates of mononuclear elements.

The consensus is the simple presence of lymphocytes within the squamous epithelium is not diagnostic of esophagitis, as lymphocytes can be found in control esophagi [8, 16, 20, 44, 62, 88, 135, 136]. We believe that intraepithelial lymphocytes can be found in specimens without any other abnormalities, but agree with other authors that they may very well be more numerous in patients with reflux esophagitis [35, 83, 88]. A major reason for identifying these cells within the epithelium is to distinguish them from pathologic cells, namely the segmented leukocytes. In most tissue infiltrates, the nuclei of lymphocytes have a rounded configuration with little or no visible surrounding cytoplasm. However, when they percolate between squamous cells, their

contours may become contorted, and their nuclei may appear elongated and wavy. This needs to be separated from true nuclear segmentation. Furthermore, lymphocytes do not have visible cytoplasmic granules. Recently, Chadwick et al. [18] evaluated the earliest ages at which histologic alterations can be utilized to diagnose esophagitis. They studied 113 infants between the ages of 2 and 18 months with clinically significant reflux esophagitis. Intraepithelial lymphocytes were the earliest histologic attribute noted and were found earlier than 4 months of age. The numbers of intraepithelial eosinophils and lymphocytes and the presence of papillomatosis all increased with age. These authors also concluded that endoscopy was highly specific, but had poor sensitivity for predicting esophagitis in this age group; they felt that biopsy was an essential part of the diagnostic evaluation in infants [18].

## EPITHELIAL HYPERPLASIA AND PAPILLOMATOSIS

By publishing the histologic results of the investigation of suction biopsy specimens, Ismail-Beigi and co-workers [62] created a landmark article that has generated controversy for more than two decades. They studied specimens taken 2 cm above the gastroesophageal junction of 33 patients with reflux esophagitis and 21 control subjects. Basically, they claimed that by measuring two parameters of the squamous epithelium, namely basal cell zone thickness and papillary height, a diagnosis of reflux esophagitis could be rendered in the absence of inflammatory cell infiltrates (Color Plates 28–30). According to these authors, in the normal esophageal mucosa, the basal cell layer comprised less than 15% of the full epithelial thickness, with a mean of 10% [62].

In patients with esophagitis, the mean thickness of this deep zone was 30% with a range of 16% to 80% (Color Plate 28). In controls, the vascularized connective tissue of the underlying lamina propria extended upward to no greater than two-thirds of the full thickness of the epithelium. With reflux esophagitis, papillae appear longer, so that the lamina propria approaches to within a few epithelial cell layers of the lumen (papillomatosis) (Color Plate 29). The combination of these two alterations was present in 85% of the reflux patients, but in one-fourth of the patients, these alterations were present in only one of the two biopsy specimens, demonstrating the patchiness of the lesions.

Ismail-Beigi et al. [62] hypothesized that noxious agents in refluxed gastric juice accelerate the rate of cellular desquamation. Thus, the papillae are actually closer to the luminal surface, and hyperplasia occurs in the germinative zone from the need for enhanced cellular replacement. When neutrophils were present (in the lamina propria), the hyperplastic changes were always developed, supporting their sensitivity for diagnosing esophagitis. However, the reactive epithelial changes were also noted in one of the two biopsies from each of two controls, reducing their diagnostic specificity.

Using molecular biologic and immunohistochemical tools, Katada et al. [71] recently demonstrated that apoptosis is greatly enhanced in the squamous epithelium of patients with reflux esophagitis; the authors suggested that this enhanced cell death may be a protective mechanism to counteract the accelerated proliferation of squamous epithelium.

Ismail-Beigi and associates [62] did not believe that the number of papillae was increased, only their relative lengths. However, we and others are impressed that capillaries and their associated connective tissue within the lamina propria proliferate in response to reflux, increasing their numbers [76, 88, 136]. This led Kobayashi and Kasugai [76] to examine nonoriented pinch biopsy specimens, which revealed this ingrowth of new blood vessels as increased numbers of capillary profiles (Color Plate 30). Their system called for constructing imaginary lines perpendicular to the basement membrane of the epithelium; overlapping of the papillae on any of these lines was construed as evidence of esophagitis (papillomatosis). Without providing much detail, Komorowski and Leinicke [78] were unable to reproduce these results. We are unaware of other published studies of this exact approach, but believe it is one that should be repeated.

In their subsequent investigation, Ismail-Beigi and Pope [61] reviewed multiple biopsy specimens of the distal 8 cm of the esophagus in 34 patients with clinical reflux and 10 controls. Based on their own histologic criteria, 29 (85%) of their patients had two or more abnormal biopsy specimens, and 31 (91%) had at least one specimen consistent with reflux esophagitis. Yet, 2 of their controls (20%) also had a single abnormal specimen; thus they recommended four or more biopsy specimens from patients suspected of having reflux. Such findings in two or more specimens was considered diagnostic of esophagitis. They claimed a random distribution of reflux changes in the distal esophagus without any tendency for the hyperplastic alterations to be concentrated just above the junction. However, this report was quickly followed by the work of Weinstein and his colleagues [134]. Using the criteria of Ismail-Beigi and associates [62], they examined 95 suction biopsy specimens systematically obtained from the distal 10 cm of the esophagus from 19 asymptomatic volunteers. Fourteen of their subjects had at least one abnormal specimen, and 7 (37%) had three or more hyperplastic specimens. Thirty-eight percent of all of the biopsy specimens and more than half of those from the distal 2.5 cm were considered altered secondary to what they termed physiologic reflux. Thus, they stated that the criteria of Ismail-Beigi could not be applied at least to biopsy specimens from the distal most part of this organ [134]. However, in turn, their study was criticized by Fink and associates [31] in that Weinstein's subjects did not undergo pH reflux tests or other functional testing to confirm that they were truly normal and not just asymptomatic refluxers. Furthermore, 2 of their patients did have positive Bernstein tests and 3 had abnormal manometry results.

Fink and colleagues [31] examined multiple biopsy specimens taken at 2 cm intervals from the distal 10 cm of the esophagi of 18 asymptomatic subjects with normal results in pH reflux tests. These authors developed a histologic scoring system to rank the severity of changes seen in specimens, with grade 0 for those of normal appearance and grade 5 for Barrett's metaplasia. Their grade 1 specimens met both of Ismail-Beigi's criteria, namely, basal cell hyperplasia and papillomatosis exceeding 15% and 66%, respectively, of the epithelial thickness. When segmented leukocytes were present in the lamina propria or epithelium, a grade 2 score was provided. Grades 3 and 4 resulted from the presence of erosions and ulcers, respectively. Only grade 0 biopsies were found in 17 of their subjects. As one of their subjects (6%) had four abnormal specimens (grades 1 and 2), they proclaimed that although not perfect, these criteria do have a high level of diagnostic specificity.

Several other good clinical studies critically examined the ability of reactive epithelial hyperplasia to diagnose and confirm reflux esophagitis [8, 12, 58, 70, 76, 109]. Unfortunately, the manner in which the pathologic changes, especially papillomatosis, were defined has varied from study to study. For example, thresholds for abnormal height have been set at 50%, 55%, and 60% of the epithelial thickness. Behar and Sheahan assayed multiple suction biopsy specimens from 40 reflux patients and 15 controls [8]. Both basal cell hyperplasia and papillomatosis were found in two or more specimens in 95% of the patients and in none of the controls. These authors [8] proclaimed squamous hyperplasia to be sensitive, as it was noted in their patients with mild symptoms and endoscopically normal-appearing esophageal mucosa. They also believed that multiple specimens with a normal appearance excluded reflux disease. One of the largest and most meticulous studies is that of Johnson and coworkers. They evaluated biopsy specimens from 100 individuals who underwent 24-hour intraesophageal pH monitoring [70]. Although up to 54 sections per biopsy were required in some subjects, all patients' specimens were considered adequate for study. The basal cell zone thickness was measured from the basement membrane to the point at which the epithelial nuclei were separated by a distance equal to the nuclear diameter. This is the criterion we use in practice, as we believe it is highly reproducible. For papillary height, Johnston and colleagues [70] measured all of the papillae with perpendicular orientations and calculated a mean height for each specimen. Relative and absolute papillary heights correlated well with the degree of acid exposure, as did the extent of basal cell hyperplasia. They found that both of these epithelial parameters declined following successful antireflux surgery.

However, using the same threshold as Johnson's group, Seefeld and colleagues [109] concluded that there was no correlation between these measurements of hyperplasia and any clinical function test. Their study included 24 patients with proved reflux esophagitis and 20 controls; they could not demonstrate significant differences between the two groups. In acknowledging the difficulty in accurately and precisely measuring the thickness of the basal cell layer, two separate distances from the basement membrane were made at each point of interest and then averaged. The authors suggested that in the normal esophagus, there is an inverse relationship between the length of the connective tissue papillae and the total thickness of the epithelium. Most other studies did not find major differences in the latter measurement.

Collins and associates [20] compared biopsy specimens from 12 controls, 20 patients with symptomatic reflux, but no endoscopic abnormalities, and 24 patients with both appropriate symptoms and mucosal friability and erosions. Very wide ranges of values for both papillary height and basal cell zone thickness were recorded, with extensive overlapping among the three study groups. In fact, the longest papillary lengths occurred in a control subject. Yet, when the authors applied the criteria of both Ismail-Beigi [62] and of Behar and Sheahan [8] for the subgroup of patients with more than one biopsy specimen, statistically significant differences were noted between those with erosive esophagitis and their controls. It is of interest that for all comparisons, the reactive epithelial values of the symptomatic group with normal endoscopic findings more closely approached the control values than those with endoscopic abnormalities.

Based mostly on a pinch biopsy experience, it is our opinion that basal cell hyperplasia and papillomatosis are reliable histologic markers of esophagitis. When the biopsy specimens can be evaluated adequately, these two parameters are often present in patients with other nonhistologic evidence of reflux esophagitis. However, this raises one of the most serious objections to depending on these markers, namely the need for adequately oriented and sufficiently large biopsy specimens so that these measurements can be made objectively. Too often, pinch biopsy specimens are too small in that they include little or no lamina propria and muscularis mucosae. In turn, this makes optimal orientation of a specimen difficult or impossible, and thus tangential histologic sections result. All published studies that compared suction and pinch biopsies found the former to be preferable [4, 18, 31, 58, 75, 76, 78, 135]. For example, Knuff and co-workers [75] reported that 59% of the pinch biopsy specimens in patients with mild esophagitis were uninterpretable with regard to hyperplasia; somewhat surprisingly, 23% of the suction biopsies were also less than optimal. It should be noted, however, that the data of Johnson and associates [70] were generated from pinch biopsy specimens, all 100 of which were assessed as adequate for interpretation. As stated earlier, the goal of Kobayashi's study [76] was to create diagnostic criteria that would be more reproducible and applicable to specimens obtained through the fiberoptic endoscope.

Several authors have also found it difficult to define the basal cell layer or basal zone even in well-oriented specimens [70, 109]. The basal cells are primitive elements with regenerative activity as their major purpose and are characterized by a thin rim of basophilic cytoplasm surrounding the oval, dark-staining nucleus, the long axis of which appears at right angles to the surface of the epithelium. With the criteria of Johnson [70], the upper boundary of this layer is defined as ending when the internuclear distance exceeds the diameter of the nuclei. This occurs as the cell matures and produces greater volumes of cytoplasm. Basal cells have little in the way of cytoplasmic glycogen, but it is well represented in the more superficial and mature squamous elements. Thus, the periodic acid-Schiff (PAS) histochemical reaction for glycogen has been suggested as an aid in defining the exact cutoff between the basal zone and the intermediate squamous zone. For example, Mitros [88] claimed that the PAS stain assists in accentuating the point of maturation. However, Collins and associates [20], Jarvis and colleagues [65], and we do not find it to be a consistent value. Perhaps the acid injury to the epithelial cells or the resultant inflammation-related damage reduces the amount of glycogen produced or increases its utilization by the cells. In any event, this demarcation line can still be somewhat blurry and irregular. It has been pointed out that using the PAS reaction will tend to reduce the perceived thickness of the basal cell layer [88].

A potentially important caveat in the evaluation of these reactive hyperplastic changes is the variation and interpretation among microscopists and even by the same observer [2, 20, 62, 88, 89]. Although details were not provided, the initial report of Ismail-Beigi and co-workers [62] stated that the biopsy specimens were independently assessed by three reviewers and that agreement by all three occurred 80% of the time; this, of course, means that one-fifth of the specimens prompted an interpretative disagreement. This problem was specifically addressed by Adami and associates [2], who sectioned 11 esophagi obtained from autopsies as if they were biopsies. The sections were examined twice independently by two people for basal zone thickness and papillary height. When the sections were graded simply as either normal or abnormal, interobserver differences occurred 26% of the time. Intraobserver variation was found 12.5% and 20% of the time. Similar results emerged from Mitros's laboratory [88]. In their evaluation of intraepithelial inflammatory infiltrates, Shub and co-workers found interobserver variation in less than 20% of all cases [116].

Although not as well studied, the histopathologic changes associated with long-standing and severe reflux esophagitis are widely recognized [39, 88, 89, 96]. Denudation of the mucosa may occur to varying depths. An erosion exists when only the more superficial layers of the squamous cells are destroyed. The squamous elements at the base of the erosion range from normal in appearance to irreversibly degenerated. Although Palmer [96] stated that an inflammatory reaction was absent at the eroded surface, we have seen cells, predominantly neutrophils, in and immediately about an erosion. The same is true of an ulcer which is present when the full thickness of the mucosa including muscularis mucosae is destroyed. The epithelium adjacent to an ulcer may manifest cytologic atypia with enlarged nuclei and nucleoli. This should not be mistaken for malignant change. This is the histologic counterpart to cytologic repair which can be seen in smears of such epithelium [40]. It is not rare to find bacterial colonies and *Candida* organisms in the exudate overlying these epithelial defects, presumably as secondary pathogens. The granulation tissue in the base of an ulcer develops into a scar, which may occupy broad zones of the submucosa. Although the overlying epithelium is capable of regenerating and covering over the defects, the submucosal fibrotic reaction persists. In esophageal resection specimens, both Palmer [96] and Moersch and colleagues [89] found that peptic ulcers did not penetrate as deeply as might be expected. Usually, the muscularis propria remained intact and rather unaffected.

Jessurun and co-workers [69] described a distinctive epithelial alteration, the balloon cell, which they claimed is a very sensitive indicator of early injury to the esophageal mucosa. Although it is not specific for reflux esophagitis, it is not present in the normal esophagus (Color Plate 31). The balloon cell is an enlarged, rounded squamous cell with pale-stained cytoplasm, often with marked degenerative changes in the nucleus. In reflux esophagitis, they occur mostly in the middle of the epithelial layer and often aggregate in clusters. The presence of the balloon cells did not correlate with endoscopic appearances or with any other known histologic feature [69]. Apparently, these cells result from pathologic swelling, as both albumin and immunoglobulin light chains were accentuated in their cytoplasm immunohistochemically. More recently, Singh and Odze [110] described the presence of benign multinucleated giant squamous epithelial cells in biopsies from 14 patients with esophagitis. Although not specific as to etiology, the most common cause of inflammation was reflux. These giant cells tended to be concentrated in the depths of the mucosa and possessed two to nine regular nuclei with distinct nucleoli. The authors [110] suggest that this represents a nonspecific regenerative reaction to injury.

In 1972, Yardley [136] noted changes in the microvasculature of the connective tissue papillae of the lamina propria. He stated that the vessels could be greatly dilated and appeared to have lost their collar of basal epithelial cells. Vascular alterations were emphasized by Geboes and associates [36] as a very early histologic feature of reflux esophagitis. The small blood vessels in the superficial portion of the mucosa were greatly distended, and, at times, associated with extravasation of erythrocytes in 83% of reflux patients; in more than one-fourth of these individuals, the vascular alterations were the only histologic abnormality present on biopsy (Color Plate 32). The epithelial cells immediately surrounding the vessels frequently appeared degenerated. Goldman and Antonioli [44] confirmed this distention and congestion of vessels in the elongated papillae, especially near the luminal surface, as an early change in esophagitis. These authors warned that the trauma of endoscopy and biopsy can itself induce dilatation of vessels, although it is limited to the deeper layers of the mucosa. Thus, as with epithelial hyperplasia, proper orientation of biopsies is important in evaluating this change. Mitros [88] stated that the usefulness of this criterion remains unknown, but suggested that it may be too sensitive. Collins and associates [20] did

not find it helpful in discriminating between controls and reflux patients.

Within the last several years, several investigative groups have attempted to define new diagnostic criteria for reflux esophagitis in biopsies by morphometric assessments of individual cells and components, especially the nuclei [21, 65]. Jarvis et al. [65] evaluated biopsies from 6 patients before and after drug therapy for 13 nuclear and nucleolar features in cells of both the basal and intermediate zones of the squamous epithelium. In pretherapy specimens, the mean number of nuclei per unit area in both intermediate and basal zones was increased relative to the subsequent specimens (after omprezole), supportive of increased proliferative activity in injured, but nonuclerated squamous epithelium. One advantage of this assay is that specimen orientation was not essential. However, the amount of time and work per specimen is relatively enormous. Collins and associates [21] reported the results of two investigations in which nucleolar dimensions, nuclear area, and nuclear concentrations were studied. None of the evaluated parameters corresponded to the results of pH monitoring; also, none of them could distinguish between biopsy specimens from normal controls and those of patients with symptomatic and endoscopic esophagitis. As stated by Collins and co-workers [21] morphometry cannot be recommended as a diagnostic tool in cases of suspected reflux esophagitis. It is also unlikely that ultrastructural studies have any diagnostic role [55].

Cytologic brushings do not offer any positive diagnostic assistance in patients with reflux esophagitis [40]. The major value of cytologic examination in such individuals is to exclude other cytologically recognizable causes of esophageal inflammation such as fungal or viral infections. Within brushings, acute and inflammatory cells, parabasal cells, and regenerative epithelial alterations are constant features. As in other proliferative conditions, reactive epithelial cells are characterized by enlarged nuclei with vesicular or very finely granular chromatin and distinct, but delicate, uniform nuclear membranes. Solitary large nucleoli are typically present. Key features to note are the preservation of intercellular cohesion and the absence of both diffuse hyperchromasia and distinct irregularities of the nuclear membrane. Degenerative changes may also be evident within the squamous epithelium including marked enlargement of the nuclei with loss of internal structure, pyknosis, and karyorrhexis. Cytoplasmic vacuolization may be evident, and unusually prominent cytoplasmic eosinophilia may be noted in some intermediate squamous cells. In the presence of an erosion or ulcer, necrotic debris and fibrin are present, providing the smear background a dirty appearance.

## BARRETT'S ESOPHAGUS

It is well recognized that Barrett's esophagus represents a benign metaplastic change in which the normal stratified squamous epithelium of the esophagus is variably replaced by glandular epithelium [49]. Histologically, this glandular epithelium may resemble gastric and/or intestinal mucosa. Although somewhat variable from study to study, the prevalence of this complication is probably approximately 10% of all patients with long-standing reflux disease [23, 44, 125]. The various morphologic types of columnar epithelium that may occur were well characterized by Paull and colleagues [97]. These authors defined three histologic and cytologic patterns in their biopsy series of 11 adult patients. One pattern, termed the junctional type, morphologically resembles the cardiac mucosa of the stomach. The surface and underlying glands are composed of cells resembling gastric mucus surface and glandular cells. The second type resembles gastric fundic mucosa, complete with parietal and chief cells. Usually, this is modified by atrophic changes and thus somewhat resembles atrophic gastritis. The third and most distinctive pattern, termed the specialized variant, was their most common finding. It was characterized by a villous architecture, goblet cells, and mucus glands (Color Plate 33). Some authors claim that Barrett's metaplasia does not exist unless one identifies intestinal metaplasia, generally in the form of goblet cells [8]. The majority of the patients had more than one of these types of glandular arrangements, and, in this situation, distinct topographic order or zonation was found. The specialized type was always in the most proximal locations and the fundic type assumed the most distal position. Similar findings were reported in two biopsy series of children [23, 53].

The exhaustive study of Thompson et al. [125], however, dispelled some of these concepts. They extensively examined esophagogastrectomy specimens from eight patients with Barrett's esophagus plus an adenocarcinoma, and established that metaplasia was a complex mosaic of cellular and architectural types. Essentially, all cell types in the stomach and intestine, including neuroendocrine cells and Paneth cells, are present to varying degrees. In contrast to the previously cited biopsy studies, the architectural patterns created a continuous spectrum, with hybrid forms intimately mixed with one another in an apparent random fashion. Except for a tendency for fundic-type elements to occur distally, no distinct zonation could be demonstrated. They agreed with Paull et al. [97] that the finding of goblet, mucus, and absorptive cells in a villous arrangement, reminiscent of the small intestine, was diagnostic of Barrett's esophagus. The authors also described a common association of atrophic alterations affecting all of the glandular patterns [125]. At times, squamous epithelium can overlie the columnar elements of Barrett's esophagus, with or without preceding therapy [11, 106]. It should be mentioned that not all "ectopic" glandular tissue seen in biopsies of the esophagus is Barrett's metaplasia. Congenital abnormalities such as the inlet patch do occur and may be responsible for symptoms indistinguishable from those of reflux esophagitis [63, 100, 127].

In cytologic brushings from patients with benign Barrett's esophagus, the smears generally contain abundant glandular epithelium [40]. These specimens are dominated by large, flat sheets of cohesive, uniform-appearing glandular epithelial cells (Color Plate 34). The sheets and aggregates have sharp, smooth borders; that is, they do not appear frayed and irregular. This reflects the retention of a normal level of intercellular cohesion among the glandular cells. Normal polarity is also well maintained. Thus, within the sheets, the nuclei appear equidistant from one another, and intercellular borders are distinct. This creates the classic honeycomb appearance. In the presence of reparative atypia in benign Barrett's epithelium, as may occur with well-developed inflammation or ulcer, there may be a streaming effect in which the cells and their nuclei all appear to flow in the same direction [40, 129, 131]. The metaplastic nuclei are, in general, uniform from cell to cell, having round or slightly ovoid contours, delicate, smooth nuclear membranes, and very finely granular, pale-stained chromatin. In general, nucleoli are inconspicuous, but in some cases of atypia they may be quite enlarged. When viewed on end, the cardiac-type mucus cells have a hexagonal configuration and a granular, somewhat bluish-gray appearance, whereas the goblet cells of intestinal metaplasia have a more rounded contour and optically clear cytoplasm (Color Plate 34). Typically, the smear background is clean, although a few inflammatory elements are often scattered about.

## SQUAMOUS CELL CARCINOMA

Squamous cell carcinoma comprises the vast majority of esophageal cancers worldwide. These are insidious neoplasms that usually become symptomatic only at an advanced stage and are typically highly invasive or metastatic at initial diagnosis. Regardless of the therapeutic modalities employed, prognosis is grim, unless the tumor is diagnosed in an early stage. In one series, the mean survival time from initial diagnosis was less than 6 months with invasive carcinoma and less than 3 months when metastases were identified [3].

Histologically, squamous cell carcinoma of the esophagus has the same appearance as these lesions occurring in other body sites. Tumors are classified as well, moderately, or poorly differentiated, and as keratinizing or nonkeratinizing. Well-differentiated squamous cell carcinoma is characterized by architectural and cytomorphologic features that allow the immediate recognition of its squamous origin (Color Plate 35). Prominent features include stratification, intercellular bridges (desmosomes), and cytoplasmic keratinization. Compared to benign squamous epithelium, the N/C ratios are increased. However, relative to the less-differentiated carcinomas, these ratios are relatively low. Nuclei are much larger than normal and often have irregular contours; frequently, the nuclei show squared-off or angulated shapes. The chromatin is often very darkly stained and may have a structureless pattern; nucleoli are relatively inconspicuous. In tissue sections, "pearls" may be seen; these represent concentric whorling of the malignant cells, often with central keratinization. Moderately differentiated carcinoma, although recognizable as squamous in type, lacks some of the distinct architectural and cytologic features of the better differentiated lesions (Color Plate 36). In well-differentiated carcinoma, nests of invasive tumor often broach the underlying connective tissue in relatively smooth, broad interfaces. In the less-differentiated neoplasms, more irregular and thinner cords of neoplastic cells invade the stroma. Overall, the component cells are smaller, and more pleomorphic, and have higher N/C ratios. Poorly differentiated squamous cell carcinoma is characterized by the near absence of cytomorphologic and histologic features indicative of a squamous origin. Specifically, the malignant cells are relatively small, possess relatively high N/C ratios, and lack keratinization and intercellular bridges. In some cases, the neoplastic cells are quite uniform in appearance, but in others pleomorphism is striking, including bizarre-appearing tumor giant cells. Relative to the better differentiated carcinomas, the nuclear chromatin may be more finely granular and nucleoli may be much more prominent.

In resection specimens, several different histologic parameters may carry prognostic significance. These include the histologic grade of the neoplasm, which is based on the most poorly differentiated portion of the neoplasm. If any of the surgical resection margins are involved by tumor, then the likelihood of local recurrence is increased and the overall prognosis is worse. Probably the single most important histologic factor as relating to the patient's outcome is the depth of invasion by the tumor into the wall of the esophagus. In general, the deeper the invasion, the worse the prognosis. Early squamous cell carcinomas are defined as those in which invasion is limited to the mucosa or submucosa [93]. In the more superficial invasive neoplasms, the presence of tumor cells within vascular lumens also portends a worse prognosis.

Overall, the cytologic appearance of invasive squamous cell carcinoma in brushings is variable, reflecting the degree of histologic differentiation of the tumor [40]. In well-differentiated carcinomas, intercellular cohesion is relatively well maintained and thus smears tend to contain relatively large aggregates of large neoplastic cells (Color Plate 37). The latter possess abundant dense cytoplasm. With the Papanicolau stain, many of the neoplastic cells may have orangeophilic cytoplasm. Nuclei characteristically are centrally positioned and have sharply angulated shapes. Their chromatin is characteristically very darkly stained and coarsely granular or almost structureless (pyknotic) in quality. Although the nuclei are much larger than in normal epithelial cells, the N/C ratios are relatively low compared to less-differentiated carcinomas. In smears, keratin pearls, elongated cellular shapes (tadpole cells), and many enucleated squames may be present. Nucleoli tend to be inconspicuous. A dirty background composed of necrotic cellular debris and inflammatory cells is common.

Moderately differentiated squamous cell carcinoma is characterized in smears by round to oval cells with cyanophilic cytoplasm and moderately enlarged, irregular nuclei (Color Plate 38). The neoplastic cells vary in size, but are typically smaller than those of well-differentiated carcinomas. Nuclei are hyperchromatic with finely to coarsely granular chromatin and often distinct nucleoli. The N/C ratios are further increased. Identification of malignant cells with orangeophilic cytoplasm and cell-in-cell arrangements are helpful in establishing the squamous origin of the cancerous elements. Although rarely seen, intercellular bridges are also diagnostically helpful. In the smears, the malignant cells occur singly and in sheets. Again, the smear background is dirty.

Poorly differentiated squamous cell carcinoma is characterized in smears by large or small cells with relatively scanty basophilic cytoplasm and irregular, markedly enlarged nuclei (Color Plate 39). Cells may show considerable variation in size and shape and often have relatively indistinct cellular borders. Nucleoli may be quite prominent, being large and/or multiple. In smears, the cells occur singly or as small, irregular aggregates. The latter are often referred to as syncytia, as their malignant nuclei are crowded and overlapped, and cytoplasmic borders are inapparent. Evidence of squamous differentiation is scanty and in some cases the cell of origin may be unclear.

In the vast majority of instances, the histologic and cytologic diagnosis of invasive squamous cell carcinoma is straightforward. Most commonly, differential diagnosis involves markedly atypical, but benign regenerative and degenerative cells obtained from mucosa adjacent to benign ulcers and striking inflammation. Overall, the benign cells are more homogeneous in appearance, have relatively low N/C ratios, and lack true hyperchromatism. In biopsies, when invasion of connective tissue is apparent, then the diagnosis is clinched. In cytologic smears, distinct loss of cohesion and disruption of normal polarity are very helpful in rendering a malignant diagnosis. In our experience, biopsies and brushings are diagnostically complementary for squamous cell carcinoma of the esophagus [38].

## INTRAEPITHELIAL NEOPLASIA (DYSPLASIA AND CARCINOMA-IN-SITU)

Histologically, intraepithelial neoplasia is characterized by a broad spectrum of architectural and especially cytologic abnormalities that include loss of epithelial maturation and polarity, nuclear aberrations, and increased mitotic activity [114, 115]. At the lower end of the spectrum are changes which may be so subtle that the distinction between dysplasia and reactive atypia is difficult. At the upper end, the malignant nature of the epithelium is readily apparent. Between these extremes lies a continuum of quantitative and qualitative abnormalities that reflect progressive involvement of the epithelium by neoplastic transformation.

Dysplasia may be classified as mild or low grade, moderate or intermediate grade, or severe or high grade based on the extent to which immature cells replace the normal epithelium. Abnormalities in polarity, nuclear attributes, and mitotic activity tend to parallel the loss of maturation, although variation exists between lesions of the same histologic grade.

In mild squamous dysplasia, immature cells occupy approximately the lower one-third of the epithelium. Thus, the lower portion of the epithelium consists of uniform-appearing small cells with high N/C ratios with solitary hyperchromatic nuclei. As the cells approach the luminal surface, they acquire progressively greater quantities of dense cytoplasm. Mitotic figures may be seen above the normal basal cell layer. In moderate dysplasia, the dysplastic cells involve the lower and middle thirds of the epithelial thickness. Cellular density is increased and loss of polarity may be prominent. Dyskeratotic cells may be encountered. In severe squamous dysplasia, the primitive cells extend through all but the most superficial layers of the epithelium. The neoplastic epithelium is characterized by a high degree of cellularity, dyspolarity, and nuclear crowding. Nuclear pleomorphism may be striking, although a relatively monotonous population of abnormal nuclei is found in some lesions. Nuclei with irregular contours and thickened membranes accompany coarsely granular, darkly stained chromatin. Nucleoli tend to be rare. Abnormal appearing mitotic figures may be seen at essentially all levels of the epithelium. Carcinoma-in-situ may be distinguished from severe dysplasia by the full-thickness involvement of the epithelium by the primitive neoplastic cells. However, this distinction is not always clear-cut and certainly is subjective.

In our opinion, the cytologic criteria for diagnosing esophageal squamous dysplasia and carcinoma-in-situ are analogous to those used for the evaluation of these lesions in cervical epithelium. However, not all authors [115] would be totally in agreement with this statement. Mild dysplasia may be characterized by superficial and intermediate-type cells within large hyperchromatic nuclei. The abnormal cells contain voluminous cytoplasm and are as large as or even slightly larger than their normal counterparts. Cytoplasmic maturation is rather well maintained and in addition may progress to keratinization as witnessed by deeply orangeophilic cytoplasm. Nuclei are relatively uniform, round to oval to slightly irregular, and bordered by relatively smooth nuclear membranes. Compared to normal, the N/C ratios are increased.

In moderate squamous dysplasia, a more heterogeneous population of abnormal cells is present, at least some of which have higher N/C ratios than in the mild category. Generally, this is due to reduced cytoplasmic volumes, whereas the nuclei maintain relatively similar diameters. Occasional elongated or bizarre cellular forms may be encountered. Nuclear pleomorphism is typical and in addition nuclei may exhibit irregular notching or indentation.

Severe squamous dysplasia is characterized by cells with very high N/C ratios, hyperchromatic nuclei with coarse chromatin granules, and generally cyanophilic cytoplasm. They are variably mixed with cells with lesser degrees of dysplastic alterations. In some instances, large keratinized cells with bizarre, very darkly stained nuclei are present and

may even dominate the picture. In clusters of dysplastic cells, intercellular borders remain relatively well defined. By contrast, in aggregates of cells derived from squamous carcinoma-in-situ, these borders are blurred (formation of syncytia).

It may be stated that the majority of pathologists in the United States do not have a vast experience with the histopathology and cytopathology of preinvasive squamous cell abnormalities of the esophagus [27, 46]. In part at least, this is related to the relatively low frequency of invasive squamous cell carcinoma in this country. On the other hand, in countries such as China in which squamous cell carcinoma is so common, morphologists are much more familiar with these cytologic and histologic alterations [9, 24, 113–115].

## SURVEILLANCE FOR SQUAMOUS CELL CARCINOMA

In some portions of the world, especially China, large-scale surveillance programs exist to detect early squamous cell carcinoma and preferably its precursors [9, 24, 113–115]. Early detection is crucial for good survival, as the most important prognostic attribute is the depth of invasion by tumor into the esophageal wall. For screening programs to be technically and financially feasible in these nations, nonendoscopic or blinded sampling methodologies using different types of abrasive instruments have evolved. Most commonly, an inflatable balloon-tipped catheter with an abrasive, absorbent surface is used in an attempt to sample the entire esophageal mucosal surface. Patients with abnormal cytologic findings subsequently undergo endoscopy with directed biopsy or, in the absence of grossly identifiable lesions, multiple random biopsies.

In his review of cytologic screening conducted in various Chinese provinces from 1963 to 1978, Shu reported overall accuracy rates of 95% and 98% for the diagnosis of cancerous and noncancerous lesions, respectively [114, 115]. Of the malignant lesions detected in mass screenings, 56% to 89% were either carcinoma-in-situ or minimally invasive carcinoma. In their study of 500 high-risk South African patients, Berry and co-workers [9] identified 26 examples of dysplasia and 15 squamous cell carcinomas, 10 of which were carcinoma-in-situ or only minimally invasive. In each of these cases, the cytologic diagnosis was subsequently confirmed by histology. Within the last few years, several large studies have been published by the investigative group which includes Liu, Shen, and Dawsey [24, 82, 113]. In one large screening study, the initial balloon cytologic diagnosis was invasive cancer in 3% and squamous dysplasia above a mild level in another 6%. The prevalence of these abnormalities increased with patient age at the time of initial surveillance procedure. Liu et al. [82] reported the results of screening of over 10,000 individuals from a high-risk region of China in 1983 in which the individuals were followed for a mean period of 7.5 years. During this period, 747 cancers developed, which accounted for 322 cancer-related deaths. The authors found that higher levels of abnormalities in the initial cytologic sampling correlated strongly with progressively increased risk of developing carcinoma during the follow-up period. However, 16% of the malignant neoplasms developed in individuals whose initial balloon sampling was interpreted as normal.

## ADENOCARCINOMA AND GLANDULAR DYSPLASIA

In the United States and other portions of the developed world, the incidence of adenocarcinoma of the esophagus is rising in epidemic proportions [48]. For example, 20 years ago, adenocarcinoma constituted no more than 10% of all primary cancers of this organ. Today, it represents nearly one-half. Essentially, all adenocarcinomas of the esophagus arise on a background of preexisting benign Barrett's metaplasia and thus are related to chronic reflux disease [19, 49]. These carcinomas almost always originate and present in the distal one-third of the organ and often appear to straddle the gastroesophageal junction [49].

Although adenocarcinomas of the esophagus are histologically classified into three categories—well, moderately, or poorly differentiated—based on architectural and cytomorphologic features, the vast majority are well to moderately differentiated [49]. Well-differentiated adenocarcinomas are composed predominantly of gland-forming structures with central lumens (Color Plate 40). Nuclear stratification, crowding, and overlapping are prominent. Nuclei are typically elongated, but may be round or oval and have irregular contours. Additional nuclear attributes include enlargement, hyperchromatism, and the presence of one or more large nucleoli. Cytoplasmic mucin vacuoles are present in some cells and may compress the nucleus, creating a sharply angulated nuclear contour. In moderately differentiated adenocarcinomas, the neoplastic cells are arranged in solid aggregates as well as within lumen-containing glands. In addition, there may be a greater degree of nuclear and cellular pleomorphism and more prominent nucleoli. In poorly differentiated neoplasms, the malignant cells are arranged singly and in solid sheets with infrequent and often incomplete glandular structures identified. Pleomorphism and hyperchromasia are often striking, and anaplastic cells with bizarre giant or multiple nuclei may be encountered. In contrast to the stomach, signet-ring carcinomas are quite uncommon.

In cytologic preparations, adenocarcinomas characteristically appear as single malignant cells mixed with irregular, often three-dimensional cellular aggregates that have irregular or frayed borders, with individual tumor cells seeming to fall away from the main cluster [22, 40, 42, 52, 81, 104, 117]. Within these cellular aggregates, cytoplasmic borders are indistinct and polarity is disrupted as evidenced by the haphazard arrangement of crowded, overlapped nuclei (Color Plate 41). Compared to normal, the malignant nuclei are much larger. They may maintain a round or ovoid configuration with only relatively subtle irregularities in their

membranes, which are often variably thickened. Chromatin is finely to coarsely clumped, and one or more often irregular nucleoli are present. Nuclear pleomorphism and hyperchromatism vary with the histologic grade of the neoplasm. Variable numbers of malignant cells will contain mucin vacuoles that appear as punched-out holes in their cytoplasm, often indenting the nucleus and creating sharply angulated nuclear shapes. However, the majority of the malignant cells in most cases do not show evidence of cytoplasmic mucin production. Cytoplasm is cyanophilic and more delicate than typically seen in squamous cell carcinoma. The smear background is usually dirty, due to the presence of necrotic cellular debris and inflammatory cells (the classic tumor diathesis).

It is generally agreed that adenocarcinoma can be reliably diagnosed by cytology [40, 117]. More importantly, esophageal cytologic brushings may contain cellular material diagnostic of adenocarcinoma when concurrently obtained biopsy specimens do not, that is, we believe that biopsies and brushings are diagnostically complementary in the evaluation of patients with Barrett's esophagus [38, 40]. We emphatically recommend the inclusion of both diagnostic modalities in surveillance programs.

As might be expected, glandular dysplasia shares many of the histologic and cytologic attributes of adenocarcinoma (Color Plates 42 and 43). Endoscopically, glandular dysplasia is generally indistinguishable from the surrounding benign Barrett's epithelium [43, 49, 118–120]. Rarely, obvious nodular or polypoid lesions are encountered, and may be termed adenomas [84, 121].

Although Hamilton and Smith [51] recognized three histologic grades of glandular dysplasia, other investigators have generally employed a system in which dysplasia is classified as either low grade or high grade [5, 42, 49, 50, 101, 102, 107]. This two-tier system provides histologic distinctions that are clinically useful and furthermore circumvent overuse of the intermediate category. Unfortunately, interobserver variation in interpretation is greater than optimal, especially for the low-grade lesions [102].

In low-grade dysplasia, architectural distortion, as evidence by irregularities in size, shape, and distribution of the glands and by papillary infolding of the glandular epithelium, is relatively minimal [49]. Individual glands are composed of enlarged cells with round, oval, or elongated nuclei that exhibit moderate enlargement, hyperchromatism, and mild pleomorphism. Chromatin is finely granular, and one or more often small nucleoli are evident. Subtle irregularities in the nuclear membrane may be encountered. Maintenance of normal polarity, as evidence by nuclear stratification, is relatively well preserved, with the abnormally enlarged nuclei persisting in the basal or lower half of the cells. Mitotic figures may be increased in number, but are generally confined to the deeper portions of the glands as well. Some leading authorities claim that it may be impossible to distinguish reliably between benign regenerative glandular epithelium and true low-grade dysplasia [49, 102].

In high-grade glandular dysplasia, the mucosal architecture is clearly distorted by irregularly distributed and often crowded glands of various sizes and shapes [49]. The glands may be so densely arrayed that there appears to be no intervening stroma; this results in a typical cribriform pattern (Color Plate 42). Papillary infolding of the glandular epithelium may be prominent, and loss of polarity is often striking, with the abnormal nuclei residing toward the apical ends of the cells. Nuclear enlargement, hyperchromatism, and pleomorphism may be marked, although on a cell-for-cell basis it may be impossible to distinguish reliably between low- and high-grade cellular elements. Increased numbers of mitotic figures are present throughout the entire length of the dysplastic glands.

As might be expected, many of the cytologic criteria for dysplasia are the same as those for adenocarcinoma [40]. Although the criteria for the cytologic diagnosis of dysplasia in Barrett's epithelium are not well established, two groups independently have described similar diagnostic criteria of this entity in cytologic brushings [42, 129]. The dysplastic cells are characteristically arranged in irregularly shaped, three-dimensional aggregates with frayed edges, with individual cells appearing to fall away from the cluster (Color Plate 43). In addition, infrequent solitary dispersed abnormal intact cells are also encountered, that is, in comparison with normal glandular epithelium, intercellular cohesion is reduced. Within the cellular aggregates, polarity is also disrupted as evidenced by haphazard arrangements of crowded, overlapped enlarged nuclei and indistinct cytoplasmic borders. Similar to adenocarcinoma, the nuclei are darkly stained and somewhat pleomorphic, and the cells manifest increased N/C ratios. The nuclei are characteristically ovoid or almost elongated in contour with finely to coarsely granular chromatin and one or more nucleoli. Aberrations in the nuclear membrane are frequent, but are often subtle. In the absence of active esophagitis, the smear background is clean, as true tissue invasion is not evident (lack of a tumor diathesis).

The distinction between high-grade dysplasia and adenocarcinoma is difficult and in some cases impossible. The two major features that serve to distinguish these entities are the presence of poorly differentiated or pleomorphic malignant cells in adenocarcinoma and the number of individually dispersed abnormal glandular cells [42, 129]. In adenocarcinoma, single cells are typically moderate to abundant in number, whereas in dysplasia, cohesion is much better preserved and only occasional individual cells are encountered. Although nuclear pleomorphism, hyperchromatism, and nuclear membrane irregularities are also greater in adenocarcinoma than in dysplasia, these features are difficult to assess objectively.

## SURVEILLANCE OF PATIENTS WITH BARRETT'S ESOPHAGUS

It is now widely recognized that there is an intermediate morphologic stage between benign Barrett's metaplasia and adenocarcinoma, namely glandular dysplasia. This knowledge has led to the development of surveillance programs in patients known to have this benign metaplastic process [5, 49, 101, 103, 118, 119]. In general, these involve obtaining numerous endoscopic biopsies systematically procured circumferencially throughout the entire length of the metaplastic esophageal segment. A minority of programs have also included brushing cytology into their evaluations [29, 57, 132]. As in essentially all other situations, it is preferable to obtain the brushing specimen prior to the endoscopic biopsies. It has been demonstrated that obtaining the biopsies first may result in less than optimal cytologic preparations; on the other hand, the reverse appears not to be true [72, 137]. Overall, the surveillance programs have been successful in detecting patients with early invasive adenocarcinoma and glandular dysplasia. Still, the diagnostic yields from these programs, while still not well defined, are considered by some to be inadequate based purely on classic histopathology (and cytopathology). In addition, these endoscopic surveillance programs are relatively expensive when the combined costs of endoscopic examination, preparation, and interpretation of histologic and cytologic specimens and time away from work by the patients are considered [1, 43, 99].

The latter considerations and the success of nonendoscopic sampling by the Chinese for squamous cell carcinoma have prompted several investigative groups to consider nonendoscopic sampling with a balloon in patients with documented Barrett's esophagus. Fennerty and colleagues [30] published a small series in which balloon samples were compared with endoscopic biopsies. Overall, the biopsies were much more sensitive for the detection of the specialized or intestinal variant of Barrett's mucosa. These authors claimed that the balloon was also less sensitive for the detection of glandular dysplasia than were biopsies. However, review of their data does not support, we believe, this last conclusion. A much larger series of patients was published recently by Falk and colleagues [29]. This investigation included endoscopic biopsies and balloon sampling in 63 adult patients. The majority also had endoscopic brushings obtained. Glandular epithelium was noted in only 83% of the balloon samples and 97% of the brushings. These cytologic specimens were independently reviewed by two investigators who were blinded to both the endoscopic and histologic results. Using the biopsy diagnoses as the gold standards, brushing cytology was positive in all cases of carcinoma and high-grade glandular dysplasia. However, it had a much lower sensitivity in individuals with histologically documented low-grade dysplasia. The levels of diagnostic sensitivity by the balloon samples for high-grade dysplasia and adenocarcinoma combined and for low-grade dysplasia were 80% and 25%, respectively. It appears as if the balloon utilized in that study did not retrieve proportionately large numbers of glandular elements. Although these data are quite promising, they may be improved by modification of the balloon's surface to procure greater numbers of glandular cells.

## SMALL-CELL CARCINOMA

Neuroendocrine neoplasms of the esophagus are very uncommon, constituting far less than 5% of all malignancies of this organ [14]. In contrast to the rest of the gastrointestinal tract, carcinoids are not the most frequent tumor type in this category. Rather, it is the highly lethal small-cell carcinoma [59]. With now more than 100 reported examples of this malignancy, the literature suggests that this neoplasm accounts for 2% of all esophageal cancers.

Although young adults may be affected, this tumor typically occurs in the middle or distal portions of the esophagus in middle-aged or older individuals. Histologically, these highly cellular tumors are composed of small, uniform-appearing malignant cells [14]. Each possesses a solitary ovoid to somewhat elongated nucleus, very darkly stained, coarsely granular chromatin, and exceedingly high N/C ratios.

Cytologic brushings are dominated by small, homogeneous neoplastic cells [54, 56]. Each tumor cell possesses a single round, ovoid, or fusiform nucleus with inconspicuous nucleoli. Other characteristic features include very hyperchromatic, finely to especially coarsely granular and evenly distributed chromatin and very high N/C ratios. Both individually dispersed and aggregated neoplastic cells may be present in the smears. The latter may include chains, densely packed nests, and even rarely rosettelike structures. Within the cohesive aggregates, the nuclei are crowded and often appear to overlap one another with indistinct cell borders. Compression or molding of adjacent nuclei may be evident as well.

The histologic and cytologic differential diagnosis of small-cell carcinoma includes metastases from elsewhere in the body, high-grade squamous cell carcinomas of the small-cell type, and malignant lymphoreticular neoplasms [40]. If a small-cell cancer is known or suspected of having originated in a different organ, then an esophageal origin should not ascribed. However, the cytologic picture could be indistinguishable. Lymphoma cells should have more discernible nucleoli, but do not manifest any evidence of intercellular cohesion or nuclear molding. In very poorly differentiated squamous cell carcinomas, at least a small fraction of the neoplastic elements are larger, having greater volumes of cytoplasm, better developed nucleoli, and more pleomorphism than is expected in a pure small-cell carcinoma. When features of small-cell carcinoma and poorly differentiated squamous cell carcinoma are present, the possibility of a small-cell carcinoma with squamous differentiation should be entertained. For example, three of the seven cases of primary esophageal small-cell carcinoma reported by Horai et al. [56] exhibited cytologic features that led to misdiagnosis as poorly differentiated squamous cell carcinoma. In these cases, histologic sections revealed foci of squamous differentiation.

## MELANOMA

Malignant melanoma, whether of primary esophageal origin or metastatic to this site, is rare [15, 66, 91, 123]. Primary melanoma characteristically exhibits an exophytic growth pattern, producing an intraluminal polypoid mass, often with a thick pedicle. Ulcers are common, but tend to be superficial. Although metastases may produce a similar appearance, they more typically occur as submucosal nodules with deep central ulcers. In both primary and metastatic lesions, pigmentation is variable.

The histologic appearance of esophageal melanoma is diverse, but generally leaves little doubt as to the highly aggressive nature of the neoplasm. Junctional melanocytic activity, alone or accompanied by scattering of malignant melanocytes within the epithelium, is diagnostic of primary esophageal melanoma. When present, it is observed at the periphery of the tumor and is the sole feature that allows differentiation from metastases involving the lamina propria and epithelium. Melanoma is composed of large, loosely cohesive, round to polygonal to spindle-shaped tumor cells arranged in nests, fascicles, and sheets. The malignant melanocytes typically possess abundant granular cytoplasm and eccentric, markedly pleomorphic nuclei often with huge nucleoli. Intranuclear cytoplasmic invaginations (pseudoinclusions) are also characteristic, as is multinucleation. The presence of intracytoplasmic pigment granules is extremely variable, but when discernible in histologic sections, it is highly suggestive of melanoma.

Experience with cytologic brushings of esophageal melanomas is rare [15]. Melanomas typically yield highly cellular cytologic specimens composed of large, obviously malignant cells occurring singly or in small, loosely cohesive aggregates. Neoplastic cells manifest a wide variation in size, shape, and pigmentation, but characteristically have distinct cellular borders and abundant cytoplasm that appears green and granular in Papanicolaou-stained preparations. Melanin may appear as distinct, dark brown granules or as dispersed, extremely fine flecks that impart a dusky hue to the cytoplasm. Eccentrically located, markedly pleomorphic nuclei with massive nucleoli are characteristic. Nuclei vary from vesicular to hyperchromatic, but coarsely clumped, marginated chromatin is frequently the predominant pattern. Intranuclear cytoplasmic inclusions are characteristic. Multinucleated tumor cells, as well as giant bizarre forms, are not uncommon.

## Leukemia

The initial presentation of leukemia in an esophageal cytologic specimen is quite rare. Fulp et al. [34] presented the clinical and morphologic features of three adults with acute myeloblastic leukemia who presented with dysphagia unrelated to reflux esophagitis, infectious esophagitis, or chemotherapy-associated mucocytis. The patients underwent both endoscopic brushings and biopsies. In all three patients, both the histologic and cytologic specimens were diagnostic of leukemic involvement. In all three, the biopsies demonstrated leukemic elements within the mucosa. The cytologic specimens from all three patients also contained numerous individually dispersed malignant leukocytes (Color Plate 44). Blasts were easily recognized by their round nuclei, distinct nucleoli, and extremely high N/C ratios. One to four small nucleoli were apparent within the evenly distributed, moderately stained chromatin. Within the smears, a distinct absence of intercellular cohesion and nuclear molding was apparent. In neither the histologic nor cytologic specimens was another cause of esophagitis identified.

## REFERENCES

1. Achkar E, Carey W. The cost of surveillance for adenocarcinoma complicating Barrett's esophagus. Am J Gastroenterol 1988;83:291
2. Adami B, Eckardt VF, Paulini K. Sampling error and observer variation in the interpretation of esophageal biopsies. Digestion 1979;19:404
3. Adeslstein DJ, Forman WB, Beavers B. Esophageal carcinoma: a six-year review of the Cleveland Veterans Administration Hospital experience. Cancer 1984;54:918
4. Akdamar K, et al. Clinical analysis of reflux esophagitis in symptomatic patients. Gastrointest Endosc 1973;19:172
5. American Society of Gastrointestinal Endoscopy. The role of endoscopy in the surveillance of premalignant conditions of the upper gastrointestinal tract. Guidelines for clinical application. Gastrointest Endosc 1988;34:185
6. Ashenburg C, Rothstein FC, Dahms BB. Herpes esophagitis in the immunocompetent child. J Pediatr 1986;108:584
7. Ballem CM, Fletcher HW, McKenna RD. The diagnosis of esophagitis. Am J Dig Dis 1960;5:88
8. Behar J, Sheahan DC. Histologic abnormalities in reflux esophagitis. Arch Pathol 1975;99:3987
9. Berry AV, Baskind AF, Hamilton DG. Cytologic screening for esophageal cancer. Acta Cytol 1981;25:135
10. Berthrong M, Fajardo LE. Radiation injury in surgical pathology: II. Alimentary tract. Am J Surg Pathol 1981;5:153
11. Biddlestone LR, Barham, Wilkinson, Barr H, Shepherd NA. The histopathology of treated Barrett's esophagus. Squamous reepithelialization after acid suppression and laser and photodynamic therapy. Am J Surg Pathol 1998;22:239
12. Black DD, et al. Esophagitis in infants. Morphometric histologic diagnosis and correlation with measures of gastroesophageal reflux. Gastroenterology 1990;98:1408
13. Bozymski EM, Herlihy KJ, Orlando RC. Barrett's esophagus. Ann Intern Med 1982;97:103
14. Briggs JC, Ibrahim NBN. Oat cell carcinoma of the esophagus: a clinicopathologic study of 23 cases. Histopathology 1983;7:261
15. Broderick PA, Allegra SR, Corvese N. Primary malignancy melanoma of the esophagus. A case report. Acta Cytol 1972;16:159
16. Brown LF, Goldman H, Antonioli DA. Intraepithelial eosinophils in endoscopic biopsies of adults with reflux esophagitis. Am J Surg Pathol 1984;8:899
17. Buss DH, Scharyj M. Herpes virus infection of the esophagus and other visceral organs in adults. Incidence and clinical significance. Am J Med 1979;66:457
18. Chadwick LM, Kurinczuk JJ, Hallam LA, Brennan BA, Forbes D. Clinical and endoscopic predictors of histological esophagitis in infants. J Paediatr Child Health 1997;33:388
19. Christensen W, Sternberg SS. Adenocarcinoma of the upper esophagus arising in ectopic gastric mucosa. Am J Surg Pathol 1987;11:397
20. Collins BJ, et al. Oesophageal histology in reflux esophagitis. J Clin Pathol 1985;38:1265
21. Collins JSA, et al. Assessment of esophagitis by histology and morphometry. Histopathology 1989;14:381
22. Cusso X, Mones-Xiol J, Vilardell F. Endoscopic cytology of cancer of the esophagus and cardia: a long-term evaluation. Gastrointest Endosc 1989;35:321
23. Dahms BB, Rothstein FC. Barrett's esophagus in children: a consequence of chronic gastroesophageal reflux. Gastroenterology 1984;86:318
24. Dawsey et al. Esophageal cytology and subsequent risk of cancer. A prospective follow-up study from Linxian, China. Acta Cytol 1994;38:183
25. DeNardi FG, Riddell RH. The normal esophagus. Am J Surg Pathol 1991;15:296
26. Deprew WT, et al. Herpes simplex ulcerative esophagitis in a healthy subject. Am J Gastroenterol 1977;68:381
27. Dowlatshahi K, et al. Evaluation of brush cytology as an independent technique for detection of esophageal carcinoma. J Thorac Cardiovasc Surg 1985;89:848
28. Eastwood GL. Histologic changes in gastroesophageal reflux. J Clin Gastroenterol 1986;8:45
29. Falk GW, et al. Surveillance of Barrett's esophagus for dysplasia and cancer with balloon cytology. Gastroenterology 1997;112:1787
30. Fennerty MB, et al. Screening for Barrett's esophagus by balloon cytology. Am J Gastroenterol 1995;90:1230
31. Fink SM, et al. Reassessment of esophageal histology in normal subjects: a comparison of suction and endoscopic techniques. J Clin Gastroenterol 1983;5:177
32. Frierson HF Jr. Histologic criteria for the diagnosis of reflux esophagitis. Pathol Annu 1992;27:87
33. Friesen CA, Zwick DL, Streed CJ, Zalles C, Roberts CC. Grasp biopsy, suction biopsy, and clinical history in the evaluation of esophagitis in infants 0–6 months of age. J Pediatr Gastrointerol Nutr 1995;20:300
34. Fulp SR, et al. Leukemic infiltration of the esophagus. Cancer 1993;71:112
35. Geboes K, et al. Lymphocytes and Langerhans cells in the human oesophageal epithelium. Virchows Arch A Pathol Anat Histopathol 1983;401:45
36. Geboes K, et al. Vascular changes in the esophageal mucosa. An early histologic sign of esophagitis. Gastrointest Endosc 1980;26:29
37. Gefter WB, et al. Candidiasis in the obstructed esophagus. Radiology 1981;138:25
38. Geisinger KR. Endoscopic biopsies and cytologic brushings of the esophagus are diagnostically complementary. Am J Clin Pathol 1995;103:295
39. Geisinger KR. Histopathology of human reflux esophagitis and experimental esophagitis in animals. In Castell DO, ed, The Esophagus, 2nd ed, Boston: Little, Brown, and Company, 1995;481–503
40. Geisinger KR. Alimentary tract (esophagus, stomach, small intestine, colon, rectum, anus, biliary tract). In Bibbo M, ed, Comprehensive Cytopathology, 2nd ed. Philadelphia: WB Saunders, 1997:413
41. Geisinger KR, Biscotti CV. The complementary role of exfoliative cytology in the management of patients with Barrett's esophagus. Pathol Case Rev 1997;2:98
42. Geisinger KR, Teot LA, Richter JE. A comparative cytopathologic and histologic study of atypia, dysplasia, and adenocarcinoma in Barrett's esophagus. Cancer 1992;69:8
43. Geisinger KR, Sheppard E, Teot LA, Raab SS. Histopathologic practices for esophageal biopsies: survey results and implications for surveillance in patients with Barrett's esophagus. Am J Clin Pathol 1998;110:219
44. Goldman H, Antonioli DA. Mucosal biopsy of the esophagus, stomach, and proximal duodenum. Hum Pathol 1982;13:423
45. Greco FA, et al. Adriamycin and enhanced radiation reaction in normal esophagus and skin. Ann Intern Med 1976;85:294
46. Greenbaum E, Schreiber K, Shu YJ, Koss LG. Use of the esophageal balloon in the diagnosis of carcinomas of the head, neck and upper gastrointestinal tract. Acta Cytol 1984;28:9
47. Greenson JK. Macrophage aggregates in cytomegalovirus esophagitis. Hum Pathol 1997;28:375
48. Haggitt RC. Adenocarcinoma in Barrett's esophagus: a new epidemic? Hum Pathol 1992;23:475
49. Haggitt RC. Barrett's esophagus, dysplasia, and adenocarcinoma. Hum Pathol 1994;25:982
50. Hameeteman W, et al. Barrett's esophagus: development of dysplasia and adenocarcinoma. Gastroenterology 1989;96:1249
51. Hamilton SR, Smith RRL. The relationship between columnar epithelial dysplasia and invasive adenocarcinoma arising in Barrett's esophagus. Am J Clin Pathol 1987;87:301
52. Hanson JT, Thoreson C, Morrissey JF. Brush cytology in the diagnosis of upper gastrointestinal malignancy. Gastrointest Endosc 1980;26:33
53. Hassall E, Weinstein WM, Ament MG. Barrett's esophagus in childhood. Gastroenterology 1985;89:1331
54. Hoda SA, Hajdu SI. Small cell carcinoma of the esophagus. Cytology and immunohistology in four cases. Acta Cytol 1992;36:113

55. Hopwood D, Milne G, Logan KR. Electron microscopic changes in human esophageal epithelium in esophagitis. J Pathol 1979;129:161

56. Horai T, et al. A cytologic study on small cell carcinoma of the esophagus. Cancer 1978;41:1890

57. Hughes JH, Cohen MB. Is the cytologic diagnosis of esophageal glandular dysplasia feasible? Diagnost Cytopathol 1998;18:312

58. Hyams JC, Ricci A Jr., Leichtner AM. Clinical and laboratory correlates of esophagitis in young children. J Pediatr Gastroenterol Nutr 1988;7:52

59. Ibrahim NBN, Briggs JC, Corbishley CM. Extrapulmonary oat cell carcinoma. Cancer 1984;54:1645

60. Isaac DW, Parham DM, Patrick CC. The role of esophagoscopy in diagnosis and management of esophagitis in children with cancer. Med Pediatr Oncol 1997;28:299

61. Ismail-Beigi F, Pope CE. Distribution of the histological changes of gastroesophageal reflux in the distal esophagus of man. Gastroenterology 1974;66:1109

62. Ismail-Beigi F, Horton PF, Pope CE II. Histological consequences of gastroesophageal reflux in man. Gastroenterology 1970;58:163

63. Jabbari M, et al. The inlet patch: heterotopic gastric mucosa in the upper esophagus. Gastroenterology 1985;89:352

64. Jacobs DH, et al. Esophageal cryptococcosis in a patient with hyperimmunoglobulin E-recurrent infection (Job's) syndrome. Gastroenterology 1984;87:201

65. Jarvis LR, Dent J, Whitehead R. Morphometric assessment of reflux esophagitis in fiberoptic biopsy specimen. J Clin Pathol 1985;38:44

66. Jawalekar K, Tretter P. Primary malignant melanoma of the esophagus. Report of two cases. J Surg Oncol 1979;12:19

67. Jennings FL, Arden A. Acute radiation effects in the esophagus. Arch Pathol 1960;69:407

68. Jenkins DW, Fisk DE, Byrd RB. Mediastinal histoplasmosis with esophageal abscess. Gastroenterology 1976;70:109

69. Jessurun J, et al. Intracytoplasmic plasma proteins in distended esophageal squamous cells (balloon cells). Mod Pathol 1988;1:175

70. Johnson LF, DeMeester TR, Haggitt RC. Esophageal epithelial response to gastroesophageal reflux. A quantitative study. Dig Dis 1978;23:498

71. Katada N, et al. Apoptosis is inhibited early in the dysplasia–carcinoma sequence of Barrett esophagus. Arch Surg 1997;132:728

72. Keighley MRB, et al. Comparison of brush cytology before or after biopsy for diagnosis of gastric carcinoma. Br J Surg 1992;66:246

73. Kelly VJ, Lazenby AJ, Rowe PC, Yardley JH, Perman JA, Sampson HA. Eosinophilic esophagitis attributed to gastroesophageal reflux: improvement with an amino acid-based formula. Gastroenterology 1995;109:1503

74. Klotz DA, Silverman L. Herpes virus esophagitis consistent with herpes simplex, visualized endoscopically. Gastrointest Endosc 1974;21:71

75. Knuff TG, et al. Histologic evaluation of chronic gastroesophageal reflux. An evaluation of biopsy methods and diagnostic criteria. Dig Dis Sci 1984;29:194

76. Kobayashi S, Kasugai T. Endoscopic and biopsy criteria for the diagnosis of esophagitis with a fiberoptic esophagoscope. Dig Dis 1974;19:345

77. Kodsi BE, et al. Candida esophagitis. A prospective study of 27 cases. Gastroenterology 1976;71:715

78. Komorowski RA, Leincke JA. Comparison of fiberoptic endoscope and Quinton tube esophageal biopsies in esophagitis. Gastrointest Endosc 1978;24:154

79. Lasser A. Herpes simplex virus esophagitis. Acta Cytol 1977;21:301

80. Lightdale CJ, et al. Herpetic esophagitis in patients with cancer. Ante mortem diagnosis by brush cytology. Cancer 1977;39:223

81. Lin BPC, Harmata PA. Gastric and esophageal brush cytology. Pathology 1983;15:393

82. Liu SF, et al. Esophageal balloon cytology and subsequent risk of esophageal and gastric-cardia cancer in a high-risk Chinese population. Int J Cancer 1994;57:775

83. Mangano MM, et al. Nature and significance of cells with irregular nuclear contours in esophageal mucosal biopsies. Mod Pathol 1992;5:191

84. McDonald GB, Brand DL, Thorning DR. Multiple adenomatous neoplasms arising in columnar lined (Barrett's) esophagus. Gastroenterology 1977;72:1317

85. McManus JPA, Webb JN. A yeast-like infection of the esophagus caused by *Lactobacillus acidophilus*. Gastroenterology 1975;68:583

86. Miller DP, Everett ED. Gastrointestinal histoplasmosis. J Clin Gastroenterol 1979;1:233

87. Mineur PH, et al. Bronchoesophageal fistula caused by pulmonary aspergillosis. Eur J Respir Dis 1985;66:360

88. Mitros FA. Inflammatory and neoplastic diseases of the esophagus. In Appelman HD, ed, Pathology of the Esophagus, Stomach and Duodenum. New York: Churchill-Livingstone, 1984

89. Moersch RN, Ellis FH Jr, McDonald JR. Pathologic changes occurring in severe reflux esophagitis. Surg Gynecol Obstet 1959;108:476

90. Nash G, Ross JS, Herpetic esophagitis. A common cause of esophageal ulcers. Hum Pathol 1974;5:339

91. Nelson RS, Lanza C. Malignant melanoma metastatic to the upper gastrointestinal tract. Gastrointest Endosc 1978;24:156

92. Novak JM, et al. Effects of radiation on the human gastrointestinal tract. J Clin Gastroenterol 1979;1:9

93. Ohno S, Mori M, Tsutsui S, et al. Growth patterns and prognosis of submucosal carcinoma of the esophagus. A pathologic study. Cancer 1991;68:335

94. O'Morchoe PJ, Lee DC, Korak CA. Esophageal cytology in patients receiving cytotoxic drug therapy. Acta Cytol 1983;27:630

95. Owensby LC, Stammer JL. Esophagitis associated with herpes simplex infection in an immunocompetent host. Gastroenterology 1978;74:1305

96. Palmer ED. Subacute erosive (peptic) esophagitis. Arch Pathol 1955;59:51

97. Paull A, et al. The histologic spectrum of Barrett's esophagus. N Engl J Med 1976;295:476

98. Phillips TL, Fu K. Quantification of combined radiation therapy and chemotherapy effects on critical normal tissues. Cancer 1976;37:1186

99. Provenzale D, Kemp JA, Arora S, Wong JB. A guide for surveillance of patients with Barrett's esophagus. Am J Gastroenterol 1994;89:670

100. Qazi FM, et al. Symptomatic congenital gastroenteric duplication cyst of the esophagus containing exocrine and endocrine pancreatic tissues. Am J Gastroenterol 1990;85:65

101. Reid BJ, et al. Endoscopic biopsy can detect high-grade dysplasia and early adenocarcinoma in Barrett's esophagus without recognizable neoplastic lesions. Gastroenterology 1988;94:81

102. Reid BJ, et al. Observer variation in the diagnosis of dysplasia in Barrett's esophagus. Hum Pathol 1988;19:166

103. Robertson CS, et al. Value of endoscopic surveillance in the detection of neoplastic change in Barrett's esophagus and associated carcinoma. Br J Surg 1988;75:760

104. Robey SS, Hamilton SR, Gupta PK, Erozan YS. Diagnostic value of cytopathology of Barrett esophagus and associated carcinoma. Am J Clin Pathol 1988;89:493

105. Rosen P, Hajdu SI. Visceral herpesvirus infection in patients with cancer. Am J Clin Pathol 1971;56:459

106. Sampliner RG, et al. Squamous mucosa overlying columnar epithelium in Barrett's esophagus in the absence of anti-reflux surgery. Am J Gastroenterol 1988;83:510

107. Schmidt HG, et al. Dysplasia in Barrett's esophagus. J Cancer Res Clin Oncol 1985;110:145

108. Schwartz DA, Wilcox CM. Atypical cytomegaloviral inclusions in gastrointestinal biopsy specimens from patients with the acquired immunodeficiency syndrome: diagnostic role of *in situ* nucleic acid hybridization. Hum Pathol 1992;23:1019

109. Seefeld U, et al. Esophageal histology in gastroesophageal reflux. Morphometric findings in suction biopsies. Dig Dis 1977;22:956

110. Singh SP, Odze RD. Multinucleated epithelial giant cell changes in esophagitis: a clinico-pathologic study of 14 cases. Am J Surg Pathol 1998;22:93

111. Shah SM, Schaefer RF, Araoz E. Cytologic diagnosis of herpetic esophagitis. A case report. Acta Cytol 1977;21:109

112. Shehata WM, Meyer RL. The enhancement effect of irradiation by methotrexate. Cancer 1980;46:1349

113. Shen Q, et al. Cytologic screening for esophageal cancer. Results from 12,877 subjects from a high-risk population in China. Int J Cancer 1993;54:185

114. Shu YJ, Cytology of the esophagus: an overview of esophageal cytopathology in China. Acta Cytol 1983;27:7

115. Shu YJ. The Cytopathology of Esophageal Carcinoma Precancerous Lesions and Early Cancer. New York: Masson, 1985

116. Shub MD, et al. Esophagitis: a frequent consequence of gastroesophageal reflux in infancy. J Pediatr 1985;107:881

117. Shurbaji MS, Erozan YS. The cytopathologic diagnosis of esophageal adenocarcinoma. Acta Cytol 1991;35:189

118. Spechler SJ. Endoscopic surveillance for patients with Barrett esophagus: does the cancer risk justify the practice? Ann Intern Med 1987; 106:902

119. Spechler SJ. Barrett's esophagus: what's new and what to do. Am J Gastroenterol 1989;84:220

120. Spechler SJ, Goyal RK. Barrett's esophagus. N Engl J Med 1986; 315:462

121. Spin FP. Adenomas of the esophagus. A case report and review of the literature. Gastrointest Endosc 1973;20:26

122. Springer DJ, DaCosta LR, Beck IT. A syndrome of acute self-limiting ulcerative esophagitis in young adults probably due to herpes simplex virus. Dig Dis Sci 1979;24:535

123. Takubo K, et al. Primary malignant melanoma of the esophagus. Hum Pathol 1983;14:727

124. Teot LA, Ducatman BS, Geisinger KR. Cytologic diagnosis of cytomegaloviral esophagitis. A report of three acquired immunodeficiency syndrome-related cases. Acta Cytol 1993;37:93

125. Thompson JJ, Zinsser KR, Enterline HT. Barrett's metaplasia and adenocarcinoma of the esophagus and gastroesophageal junction. Hum Pathol 1983;14:42

126. Tummala V, et al. The significance of intraepithelial eosinophils in the histologic diagnosis of gastroesophageal reflux. Am J Clin Pathol 1987;87:43

127. Van Asche C, et al. Columnar mucosa in the proximal esophagus. Gastrointest Endosc 1988;34:324

128. Walsh TJ, Belitsos NJ, Hamilton SR. Bacterial esophagitis in immunocompromised patients. Arch Intern Med 1986;146:1345

129. Wang HH, Ducatman BS, Thibault S. Cytologic features of premalignant glandular lesions in the upper gastrointestinal tract. Acta Cytol 1991;35:199

130. Wang HH, Johasson JG, Ducatman BS. Brushing cytology of the upper gastrointestinal tract. Obsolete or not? Acta Cytol 1991;35:195

131. Wang HH, et al. Barrett's esophagus. The cytology of dysplasia in comparison to benign and malignant lesions. Acta Cytol 1992;36:60

132. Wang HH, Sovie S, Zeroogian JM, Spechler SJ, Goyal RK, Antonioli DA. Value of cytology in detecting intestinal metaplasia and associated dysplasia at the gastroesophageal junction. Hum Pathol 1997;28: 465

133. Weiden PL, Schuffler MD. Herpes esophagitis complicating Hodgkin's disease. Cancer 1974;33:1100

134. Weinstein WM, Bogoch ER, Bowes KL. The normal human esophageal mucosa: a histological reappraisal. Gastroenterology 1975;68:40

135. Winter HS, et al. Intraepithelial eosinophils: a new diagnostic criterion for reflux esophagitis. Gastroenterology 1982;83:818

136. Yardley JH. Biopsy findings in low-grade reflux esophagitis. In Skinner DB, et al., eds, Gastroesophageal Reflux and Hiatal Hernia. Boston: Little, Brown 1972

137. Zargar SA, et al. Prospective comparison of the value of brushings before and after biopsy in the endoscopic diagnosis of gastroesophageal malignancy. Acta Cytol 1991;35:549

*The Esophagus*, Third Edition,
edited by D. O. Castell and J. E. Richter.
Lippincott Williams & Wilkins, Philadelphia © 1999.

CHAPTER 9

# Disorders Causing Oropharyngeal Dysphagia

Ian J. Cook

Oropharyngeal dysphagia, the commonest cause of which is stroke, carries a high morbidity, mortality, and cost. Oropharyngeal dysphagia occurs in one-third of all stroke patients [112, 244, 260]. It is common in the chronic care setting, with up to 60% of nursing home occupants having feeding difficulties [100, 212], of whom a substantial proportion have dysphagia. Other special populations, such as those with head injuries, Parkinson's disease or Alzheimer's disease, have a 20% to 40% prevalence of oropharyngeal dysphagia [6, 96, 110, 112, 162, 255]. In our aging population, oropharyngeal dysphagia is a large and growing problem, the consequences of which can be severe: malnutrition, aspiration, choking, pneumonia, and death. The cost implications are significant, and it is recognized that the resulting complications significantly increase the chance of institutionalization and hospital readmission following stroke [217, 218]. Responsiveness to currently available treatments is extremely variable and unpredictable, in many instances with response being dependent upon several factors including the underlying cause of the dysphagia, the severity and nature of the mechanical dysfunction, the degree of cognitive dysfunction, and the prognosis of the underlying disease [55].

Pharyngeal dysphagia differs from esophageal dysphagia in several important respects. Because airway protection is such an integral part of the oropharyngeal swallow, pharyngeal dysfunction carries a high risk of aspiration and its life-threatening sequelae. Hence, assessment of aspiration risk and its treatment becomes important parts of the management strategy in these patients. Gravity makes an important contribution to esophageal transport [127], while oral and pharyngeal transport relies solely on locally generated muscular forces [123]. Esophageal dysfunction arises almost invariably from primary disease of the esophagus. In contrast, pharyngeal dysphagia most commonly arises from neurogenic or myogenic diseases in which dysphagia is frequently

a part of a wider neurological syndrome, making it necessary for the clinician to consider a wide range of diagnostic possibilities and appropriate investigations. Finally, pharyngeal dysphagia, more so than esophageal dysphagia, is a problem that frequently demands a multidisciplinary management approach which may involve the radiologist, gastroenterologist, neurologist, speech–language pathologist, otolaryngologist, and dietician.

## PRESENTATION AND CLINICAL ASSESSMENT OF OROPHARYNGEAL DYSPHAGIA

It is a common mistake for the clinician, confronted with a patient reporting bolus holdup in the neck, to assume that the patient has pharyngeal dysphagia. If dysfunction does relate to the oral or pharyngeal region, the patient can localize accurately the site of such dysfunction which correlates well with radiological localization of the problem [156]. However, distal esophageal obstruction can give rise to a sensation of the bolus catching either in the retrosternal region or in the cervical region in 15% to 30% of cases [78, 194, 253]. Hence, a perception by the patient of apparent bolus holdup in the neck has low diagnostic specificity and cervical localization per se does not help the clinician to distinguish pharyngeal from esophageal causes of dysphagia. Nonetheless, a careful history can reliably distinguish esophageal from pharyngeal dysphagia in the majority of cases. The clinician may mistake the purely sensory symptom of globus for pharyngeal dysphagia. Globus is an extremely common, nonpainful sensation of a lump or fullness in the throat of unknown etiology in which deglutitive food bolus transport is unimpaired [50, 234]. Indeed, globus sensation is usually most apparent to the patient between meals, is not necessarily related to the act of swallowing, and is usually alleviated by eating. The minority of affected patients who do report associated dysphagia may have associated esophageal dysmotility [177]. A number of pharyngeal and esophageal radiological appearances have been described in association with globus, but none has been proven to have a causative relationship with the symptom [202].

I. J. Cook: University of New South Wales, Kensington, New South Wales 2052, and Department of Gastroenterology, St. George Hospital, Kogarah, New South Wales 2217, Australia.

The patient with pure globus sensation, without pain, dysphagia, or weight loss, generally only requires otolaryngological evaluation to exclude local inflammatory or infiltrative disorders, followed by explanation and reassurance.

Due to the complexity of functions served by the upper aerodigestive tract, oropharyngeal dysphagia should be considered to be one component of a multidimensional symptom complex. The patient with oropharyngeal dysphagia may have oral or pharyngeal dysfunction or both. Typical symptoms of oral dysfunction might include drooling from the mouth or spillage of food due to poor labial and facial muscle function, sialorrhea or xerostomia, difficulty with swallow initiation, piecemeal swallows, and dysarthria. Typical symptoms of pharyngeal dysfunction include an immediate sense of bolus holdup localized to the neck; postnasal regurgitation; the need to swallow repeatedly to clear food or fluid from the pharynx; coughing or choking during meals, suggesting aspiration; and dysphonia. Pain on swallowing or persistent sore throat may indicate malignancy. Immediate expectoration of an offending bolus is indicative of bolus retention in the hypopharyngeal or cricopharyngeal region. Delayed regurgitation of old food is typical of a large pharyngeal diverticulum. Dysphagia solely for solids is indicative of a structural lesion such as a stenosis, web, or tumor. However, distinction between dysphagia for liquids and solids is of little diagnostic value in distinguishing oropharyngeal dysphagia from esophageal dysphagia because it is the specific type of mechanical pharyngeal dysfunction, rather than the presence of pharyngeal dysfunction, which dictates which bolus type generates most symptoms.

The circumstances of symptom onset, duration, and progression of dysphagia provide useful diagnostic information. For example, malignant dysphagia usually presents with a relatively short history of progressive dysphagia and is frequently associated with weight loss. A sudden onset of dysphagia, often in association with other neurological symptoms or signs, usually indicates a cerebrovascular cause, such as stroke. A subacute or more insidious onset is more consistent with disorders such as inflammatory myopathy, myasthenia, or amyotrophic lateral sclerosis. Oropharyngeal dysphagia usually has a neurological basis. A prior history of stroke may be obtained. Symptoms of bulbar muscle dysfunction or other brainstem symptoms, such as vertigo, nausea, vomiting, hiccup, tinnitus, diplopia, and drop attacks, should be sought. More widespread neuromuscular symptoms, such as dysarthria, diplopia, limb weakness, and fatigability, are variably present in motor neuron disease, myasthenia, and myopathy. The patient may report tremor, ataxia, or unsteadiness, which might indicate an underlying movement disorder such as Parkinson's disease (Table 9–1).

Xerostomia is frequently accompanied by dysphagia and is a common symptom in the elderly, being present in 16% of men and 25% of women [188]. Dysphagia is attributed to loss of the lubricating qualities of saliva. Dry mouth may be accompanied by dry eyes, inflammatory arthropathy (e.g., rheumatoid arthritis, Sjögren's syndrome), a prior history

**TABLE 9–1.** *Etiology of oropharyngeal dysphagia*

Central nervous system
  Stroke
  Extrapyramidal syndromes (Parkinson's, Huntington's chorea, Wilson's disease)
  Head trauma
  Brainstem tumors
  Alzheimer's disease
  Multiple sclerosis
  Cerebral palsy
  Amyotrophic lateral sclerosis
  Drugs (phenothiazines, benzodiazepines)
Peripheral nervous system
  Spinal muscular atrophy
  Guillain-Barré syndrome
  Poliomyelitis
  Post-polio syndrome
  Diphtheria
  Drugs (botulinum toxin, procainamide, cytotoxics)
Myogenic
  Myasthenia gravis
  Botulism
  Dermatomyositis
  Polymyositis
  Mixed connective tissue disease
  Sarcoidosis
  Thyrotoxic myopathy
  Paraneoplastic syndromes
  Myotonic dystrophy
  Oculopharyngeal muscular dystrophy
  Drugs (amiodarone, alcohol, cholesterol-lowering drugs)
Structural disorders
  Posterior (Zenker's) pharyngeal diverticulum
  Lateral pharyngeal diverticulum
  Cricopharyngeal bar
  Cricopharyngeal stenosis
  Cervical web
  Oropharyngeal tumor
  Head and neck surgery
  Radiotherapy
  Cervical osteophyte

of head and neck radiotherapy, or concurrent medications displaying anticholinergic side effects. A detailed drug history is also important as a number of centrally acting drugs can impair oropharyngeal dysfunction and can cause tardive dyskinesia with masticatory and swallowing difficulties (Table 9–2).

The aims of the physical examination in the dysphagic patient are to (a) identify features of underlying systemic or metabolic disease when present; (b) localize where possible the neuroanatomical level and severity of a causative neurological lesion when present; and (c) detect adverse sequelae, such as pulmonary sepsis or nutritional deficiency, which are important indicators of the severity of dysphagia. In addition to the diagnostic assessment, an assessment by a speech–language pathologist will provide further information about language, cognitive and behavioral dysfunction, as well as the strength and range of movement of the muscles involved in speech and swallowing. This information will

**TABLE 9–2.** *Drugs associated with oropharyngeal dysphagia*

Centrally acting drugs
  Phenothiazines[a]
  Metoclopramide[a]
  Benzodiazepines[a] (nitrazepam, clorazepate, alprazolam)
  Antihistamines[a]

Drugs acting at neuromuscular junction
  Botulinum A toxin[a]
  Procainamide[a]
  Penicillamine
  Erythromycin
  Aminoglycosides

Drugs toxic to muscle
  Amiodarone[a]
  Alcohol[a]
  HMG-CoA reductase inhibitors[a]
  Cyclosporin
  Penicillamine
  Other (colchicine, L-tryptophan, emetine, chloroquine, steroids, cimetidine, ipecac)

Miscellaneous, mechanism presumed neuromyopathic
  Digoxin[a]
  Trichloroethylene[a]
  Vincristine[a]

Drugs influencing salivation
  Inhibit salivation[a] (anticholinergics, antidepressants, antipsychotics, antihistamines, antiparkinsonian drugs, antihypertensives, diuretics)
  Enhance salivation[a] (anticholinesterase, nitrazepam, clozapine)

[a] Indicates that specific reports of drug-related dysphagia exist.
HMG-CoA, hepatic hydroxymethylglutaryl coenzyme A.

directly influence decisions as to the patient's suitability for swallow therapy and the type of therapy adopted [156].

A careful neurological examination is mandatory unless a certain cause of dysphagia is apparent. However, examination, even when combined with magnetic resonance imaging, is frequently unremarkable despite videoradiographic demonstration of severe impairment of the pharyngeal swallow [29], and the absence of neurological signs does not preclude significant pharyngeal neuromuscular dysfunction. When present, physical findings in affected patients might include cranial nerve dysfunction, cerebellar dysfunction, or signs of movement disorder or muscle disease. The clinician should remember that the gag reflex is absent in 20% to 40% of healthy adults [67] and, in the patient, is predictive of neither pharyngeal swallow efficiency, severity of swallow dysfunction, nor adequacy of deglutitive airway protection [142, 143]. Nasal speech is indicative of soft palatal dysfunction, which commonly results in deglutitive postnasal regurgitation. Tremor and gait disturbances may reflect an extrapyramidal movement disorder the commonest causing dysphagia being Parkinson's disease [80, 146]. Muscle fasciculation, wasting, and weakness or fatigability should be sought to detect underlying motor neuron disease, myopathy, or myasthenia.

The examiner should palpate the neck for masses, lymph nodes, or a goiter. Sometimes a pharyngeal pouch can be felt, nearly always on the left, and may be compressed, causing regurgitation of a small amount of food residue into the pharynx with an audible ''gurgle.'' Signs of prior surgery, tracheostomy, and radiotherapy are usually obvious when present. The oral cavity, including natural dentition or dentures, tongue, and oropharynx, should be inspected.

Examination of the eyes and ocular movements is relevant. Bilateral ptosis might indicate a myopathy or myasthenia, and unilateral ptosis, if associated with Horner's syndrome (descending sympathetic tract), is typical of lateral medullary infarction causing dysphagia. Eye signs, sweating, tremor, and tachycardia of thyrotoxicosis may be present in patients with thyrotoxic myopathy causing pharyngeal dysfunction. The typical features of thyrotoxicosis, however, may not be present in the elderly or in individuals taking beta-adrenergic antagonists, and dysphagia may be the only presenting symptom of thyrotoxicosis [25]. With the index and middle fingers resting lightly on the hyoid and laryngeal cartilage, respectively, axial motion of the larynx and hyoid bone should be noted while the patient takes a sip of water. Inadequate laryngeal ascent is frequently seen in neurogenic dysphagia; it impairs airway protection during the swallow and can be associated with aspiration. Aspiration will often (but not invariably) cause coughing or choking during the swallow. Radiological studies have shown that aspiration is underestimated by roughly 50% on the basis of clinical assessment alone [159, 222]. A video barium swallow, therefore, is vital to confidently establish the risk of significant aspiration in most [157].

## EVALUATION OF THE OROPHARYNGEAL SWALLOW

### Videofluoroscopy

Static films of the oropharynx obtained during a standard barium swallow can readily identify structural causes of dysphagia, such as diverticula, webs, stenoses, or cancers (Figs. 9–1, 9–2). However, static films frequently detect various anomalies, such as osteophytes or a cricopharyngeal bar, which may or may not be linked causatively with the patient's dysphagia. These entities must be interpreted with caution as they are usually not the cause of the patient's dysphagia (see below). Static films may also provide important clues to oral or pharyngeal dysfunction, such as barium pooling in the valleculae or pyriform sinuses or aspiration of contrast; but because of the rapidity and complexity of the oropharyngeal swallow, static films are inadequate to define any disturbance of the mechanics of the swallow. The most commonly utilized radiographic method to achieve this is the videofluoroscopic swallow study, frequently referred to as a modified barium swallow [156, 158]. This test acquires dedicated lateral and anteroposterior views of the oral and pharyngeal phases of the swallow and permits standard

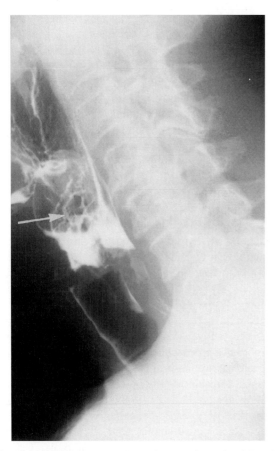

**FIG. 9–1.** Hypopharyngeal carcinoma *(arrow)* arising from the aryepiglottic fold and presenting with pharyngeal dysphagia and aspiration during meals.

and slow-motion replay of the swallow to define the mechanisms and severity of dysfunction and, if desired, the influence of modifications to bolus consistency, postures, and other swallow maneuvers on bolus flow and clearance. Videofluoroscopy is a sensitive means of confirming oropharyngeal dysfunction if its presence is uncertain on the basis of history. This technique will provide information on the presence and severity of the major categories of dysfunction, such as an absent or delayed pharyngeal swallow response, timing of aspiration if present, velopharyngeal competence, and impaired pharyngeal clearance of contrast (Table 9–3). One of the most important pieces of information provided by videofluoroscopy is the presence, timing, and severity of aspiration, which is frequently silent. Identification of these mechanisms will assist the therapist in deciding on specific swallow therapies. On the other hand, videofluoroscopy does not permit the quantification of pharyngeal contractile forces and intrabolus pressure nor the detection of incomplete upper esophageal sphincter (UES) relaxation, which can occur despite normal UES opening [2].

### Nasoendoscopy

Fiberoptic nasoendoscopy is the optimal method for identifying and biopsying mucosal abnormalities and is manda-

tory in all cases in which malignancy is suspected. In the workup of the patient with dysphagia, the gastroenterologist will frequently examine the laryngopharynx during routine fiberoptic esophagogastroduodenoscopy. However, the standard gastroscope passed orally is frequently very unreliable in the detection of glottic and pharyngeal cancers [91]. If there is any doubt about a possible malignancy, fiberoptic nasoendoscopy or even examination under anesthesia is recommended. Nasoendoscopy is less well suited to the assessment of swallow mechanics than videofluoroscopy but can detect the absence of or profound delay in initiating the pharyngeal swallow response and can provide indirect evidence of aspiration [140, 181].

### Manometry

Intraluminal manometry can quantify pharyngeal deglutitive forces and detect failure of UES relaxation and the relative coordination of pharyngeal contraction with UES relaxation [2, 38, 51, 186]. Pharyngeal manometry is technically

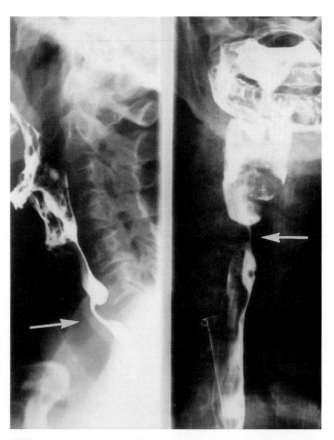

**FIG. 9–2.** Radiograph of a patient with longstanding dysphagia caused by cricopharyngeal stenosis. Note that the reduction in sphincter lumen is circumferential, indicating that this lesion is not a simple cricopharyngeal bar. The lateral view **(left)** also demonstrates the early formation of a pouch above the stenosed cricopharyngeus. The patient had significant benefit from cricopharyngeal myotomy, and histopathology of the resected muscle showed hypertrophy only without fibrosis. (From ref. 51, with permission.)

**TABLE 9–3.** *Mechanisms of oropharyngeal dysphagia*

| Dysfunction | Mechanism | Etiology |
| --- | --- | --- |
| **Oral phase** | | |
| Drooling | Poor lip closure | Facial muscle weakness |
| Poor oral clearance | Lingual dysfunction | Central lesion, myopathy |
| | Delayed swallow initiation | Afferent or central lesion |
| Premature bolus spill | Incompetent glossopalatal closure | Myopathy, palatal surgery |
| **Pharyngeal phase** | | |
| Postnasal regurgitation | Velopharyngeal incompetence | Central, Xth nerve, myopathy |
| Laryngeal penetration/aspiration | Reduced laryngeal elevation | Suprahyoid muscle dysfunction |
| | Incomplete epiglottal closure | Suprahyoid muscle dysfunction, tumor |
| | Impaired vocal cord closure | Medullary or Xth nerve lesion |
| | Impaired pharyngeal clearance | Central lesion, myopathy |
| Impaired pharyngeal propulsion | Absent or delayed pharyngeal response | Central lesion |
| | Impaired tongue base motion | Central lesion, myopathy |
| | Impaired constrictor muscle action | Central lesion, myopathy |
| Increased outflow resistance | Failed UES relaxation | Medullary lesion |
| | Loss of UES compliance | Cricopharyngeal fibrosis or hypertrophy |
| | Impaired hyoid traction | Suprahyoid muscle dysfunction |

UES, upper esophageal sphincter.

more demanding and more complex than esophageal manometry because of transducer requirements for high-fidelity recording, extreme longitudinal and radial asymmetry of intraluminal pressures recorded from within the pharynx while swallowing, and unpredictable structural movements during the pharyngeal swallow response, which have the effect of displacing the pressure sensor from its preswallow position [90, 116, 129, 207]. Manometry has been combined concurrently with videofluoroscopy by some investigators, which then permits correlation of motion of anatomical structures with the resulting intraluminal pressures [53, 130, 171, 186]. This technique permits identification of intrabolus pressure, which is an indirect measure of UES compliance [54, 65]. Impaired UES opening can also be distinguished from impaired sphincter relaxation, and weak propulsive pharyngeal forces can be distinguished from increased outflow resistance as manifest by high intrabolus pressure. Identification of some manometric abnormalities, particularly failed UES relaxation or elevated intrabolus pressure, may influence management decisions, particularly relating to the advisability of cricopharyngeal myotomy or dilatation [1, 2, 51, 186, 230]. However, it remains to be proven that such intervention in this context influences clinical outcome.

## THE NORMAL AND ABNORMAL SWALLOW

Voluntary initiation of the oropharyngeal swallow requires synthesis of sensory queues from the oropharynx into both the cerebral cortex and the medulla [173]. The interneuronal pool within the medulla, the so-called medullary swallow center, then orchestrates the entire sequence of motor responses, predominantly via the lower cranial nerves, that constitutes the oropharyngeal swallow. The pharyngeal swallow is a rapid sequence of responses involving propulsive forces appropriately coordinated with valving functions. These valving functions regulate antegrade and retrograde flow to and from the esophagus through the UES, control

bolus exit from the oral cavity (glossopalatal closure mechanism), and prevent laryngeal penetration and nasopharyngeal regurgitation (velopharyngeal closure mechanism). Sequential contact of the tongue against the palate propels the bolus into the pharynx. As the bolus passes the tonsillar arches, the pharyngeal swallow response is initiated and involves velopharyngeal closure, hyolaryngeal elevation with laryngeal closure, and relaxation and then opening of the UES [53, 130, 208]. Tongue pulsion combined with pharyngeal constrictor action then propels the bolus through the UES into the esophagus and the progressive pharyngeal contraction clears the pharynx of any residue [128, 131].

Oropharyngeal dysphagia results from disturbances in one or more of these functions and can manifest in several ways (Table 9–3). Swallow initiation may be delayed or absent. Aspiration may manifest as coughing or choking. Nasopharyngeal regurgitation may be reported. Excessive postswallow residue commonly necessitates repeated swallows to effect clearance or the patient may describe the bolus holding up in the neck. It is usual for several of these dysfunctions to manifest simultaneously in the dysphagic patient. Furthermore, none of these phenomena is specific for any particular disease process. Therefore, while it is convenient to categorize neurogenic oropharyngeal dysphagia according to the underlying disease, it is more useful in the evaluation and management of individual patients to conceptualize the disorder in functional terms. With several important exceptions (see below), management will be based more on these mechanisms of dysfunction than on the underlying disease causing the dysphagia (Table 9–3).

## STRUCTURAL CAUSES OF OROPHARYNGEAL DYSPHAGIA

### Tumors, Head and Neck Surgery, Radiotherapy

Intrinsic tumors of the tongue, palate, pharynx, tonsil, and glottis may present with dysphagia (Fig. 9–1). Radiology and nasoendoscopy are imperative for diagnosis [91]. Much less commonly, extrinsic tumors of the head and neck, particularly of the thyroid, can also cause dysphagia if they reach a substantial size [46, 238]. Surgical resection of head and neck cancer very commonly causes oropharyngeal dysphagia. The impact of head and neck cancer surgery on swallowing varies markedly among individuals and depends upon many factors, including extent of surgical resection; whether flap reconstruction is required; which muscular, bony, or cartilaginous structures are removed or deranged; whether surgery causes collateral damage to innervation; and whether surgery is accompanied by radiotherapy, which damages both muscles and nerves [245]. Because tongue base motion is important in the generation of pharyngeal propulsive forces, the extent of oral tongue and tongue base resection is the most important variable determining dysphagia severity in those undergoing surgery for oral cancer [160, 170]. Mandibular resection and oropharyngeal flap reconstructions, for example, seem to have a lesser impact on swallow function than does lingual resection. The degree of preservation of tongue base motion is also an important predictor of recovery of swallow function following laryngeal surgery [161].

Laryngectomy, with or without radiotherapy, can cause dysphagia due to a combination of anatomical derangements and pharyngeal muscular dysfunction [161, 172, 180]. Following laryngectomy, the middle and inferior constrictors are reconstituted anteriorly with their opposite number and with the tongue base in a "T" configuration. Partial breakdown of this repair gives rise to a pseudodiverticulum, or a pouch-like defect, anterior to the pharyngeal chamber at the tongue base, in which food boluses become trapped, thereby impairing pharyngeal clearance. Following removal of the cricoid cartilage, the free margins of the cricopharyngeus muscle are approximated anteriorly, converting the sphincter lumen from an oval to a smaller ring-like structure [251]. This alteration in its configuration and diameter significantly reduces the extent of UES opening and increases outflow resistance. Pharyngeal stenosis at the superior surgical closure site is also common [180]. Intrinsic pharyngeal muscle and nerve damage from the surgery, frequently exacerbated by radiotherapy, may impair pharyngeal propulsive forces. Head and neck surgery for benign disease is a less common cause of dysphagia, which is a reported complication following anterior cervical fusion [32, 224], carotid endarterectomy, and ventral rhizotomy for spasmodic torticollis [31, 83].

Radiotherapy is well recognized to cause structural and functional damage to oral and pharyngeal structures. Careful videofluoroscopic or manometric studies demonstrate a range of disturbances, including pharyngeal dysmotility, muscular weakness, and incoordination, to account for dysfunction in both oral and pharyngeal phases [87, 94, 141]. It is not uncommon for radiation-induced dysphagia to manifest clinically more than 10 years after administration of the radiotherapy [209]. Radiation-induced xerostomia is an important contributor to swallow dysfunction in the cancer patient as the salivary glands are extremely radiosensitive.

## Postcricoid Web, Stenosis, and the Cricopharyngeal Bar

A postcricoid web is a thin, shelf-like, usually eccentric but sometimes circumferential constriction which occurs in the proximal few centimeters of the esophagus and is comprised of a thin layer of mucosa and submucosa. Webs typically present with dysphagia for solids, but because of their very proximal location, deglutitive aspiration may occur. One consecutive series of 1,134 videofluoroscopic examinations reported a cervical esophageal web in 7.5% of patients investigated for dysphagia and that occurrence was twice as common in women as in men [85]. The web has been associated with iron deficiency anemia, in which case the terms Paterson–Brown-Kelly and Plummer-Vinson syndromes have been applied [243]. The incidence of this syndrome appears to have declined markedly in recent decades, and webs certainly occur in the absence of iron deficiency [43]. Squamous carcinoma is a recognized complication of this syndrome [44]. Webs are frequently more readily appreciated on barium swallow than they are endoscopically. Indeed, inadvertent disruption of the lesion at endoscopy and a somewhat retrospective appreciation of its existence are quite common. The lesion is often visible only transiently on standard barium swallow and is usually better visualized on video- or cinefluoroscopy.

A cricopharyngeal bar is an extremely common incidental radiological finding, the clinical significance of which is very controversial. There is no universally accepted term used to describe the cricopharyngeal bar. Frequently adopted but erroneous terminology applied to it include achalasia, spasm, and hypertrophy. The former two manometric terms have been inappropriately applied to radiological appearances. Indeed, careful manometric evaluation of a group of patients with cricopharyngeal bars confirmed normal resting UES pressure and complete deglutitive UES relaxation [65]. The term *hypertrophy* is applicable only if histopathological examination of the cricopharyngeus muscle confirms hypertrophy because the radiological appearance of fibrotic and hypertrophic stenoses can be indistinguishable (Fig. 9–2). A cricopharyngeal bar has been reported in 5% to 19% of patients undergoing pharyngeal cine- or videoradiography [45, 59, 86, 126, 205], and in patients undergoing videofluoroscopy, dysphagia is no more prevalent in those individuals found to have a cricopharyngeal bar (13%) than it is in those without one [59]. Inevitably, the cricopharyngeal bar will turn up in the investigation of many patients with dysphagia but causes dysphagia in the minority. In one series of 124 patients, a cricopharyngeal bar was identified in 24 (19%); esophageal pathology that could have accounted for dysphagia was found in all but one of these, and in at least eight (33%) the esophageal lesions almost certainly accounted for the dysphagia [126]. Pharyngeal motor dysfunction may co-

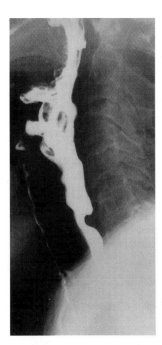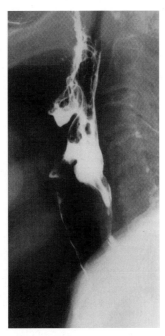

**FIG. 9–3.** Cricopharyngeal bar in a patient with dysphagia and deglutitive aspiration. Lateral radiographs taken during the swallow **(left)** and after the swallow **(right).** The predominant cause of the dysphagia in this case is coexistent pharyngeal motor dysfunction, clearly evident on videofluoroscopy. The indirect evidence for neurogenic pharyngeal dysfunction is the extremely poor pharyngeal clearance manifesting as postswallow hypopharyngeal and vallecular pooling **(right)** and tracheal aspiration of contrast.

exist with a cricopharyngeal bar, and in this context, the accompanying neurogenic pharyngeal dysfunction is the dominant mechanism of the dysphagia (Fig. 9–3). Notwithstanding, the argument that the cricopharyngeal bar might cause holdup of the swallowed bolus is plausible. Careful radiological and manometric measurements of the sphincter zone in these patients demonstrate normal manometric UES relaxation but restricted UES opening and increased resistance to bolus flow across the sphincter [65, 220]. In some cases, however, the postcricoid narrowing may only be apparent, being accounted for by widening of the gullet above and below the cricopharyngeus [82]. Histological examination of the cricopharyngeus muscle retrieved from patients undergoing myotomy for a cricopharyngeal bar has shown muscle fiber degeneration and interstitial fibrosis in some cases [10, 58, 247], similar to that found in the cricopharyngeus retrieved from Zenker's diverticulum patients at surgery [52]. Furthermore, cricopharyngeal myotomy in some patients with a cricopharyngeal bar can relieve dysphagia.

The clinical significance of the entity remains controversial, but it is the author's opinion that a cricopharyngeal bar can assume pathophysiological and functional significance under the following three circumstances. First, if the constriction is circumferential (i.e., visible on both anteroposterior and lateral radiographs) and if additional esophageal or pharyngeal abnormalities have been ruled out by appropriate

radiological, manometric, and endoscopic investigation, the descriptor *cricopharyngeal stenosis* is a reasonable one to apply to such a circumferential lesion because the term makes no unsubstantiated assumptions about the underlying pathogenesis and could be applicable to a fibrotic, hypertrophic, or other histopathological process (Fig. 9–2). Second, if a posterior hypopharyngeal diverticulum is present, the cricopharyngeal bar can assume significance. Third, if coexistent pharyngeal neuromuscular dysfunction is identified, the functional significance of the combined abnormalities is likely to be greater than that of the cricopharyngeal bar in isolation (Fig. 9–3).

These structural lesions, when considered the cause of symptoms, are treated by mechanical disruption, by either cricopharyngeal myotomy or dilatation. Cricopharyngeal myotomy reduces resting sphincter tone by approximately 50% [18, 211, 230]. The fact that myotomy does not abolish tone suggests that therapeutic benefit is derived from the increased capacity for sphincter opening and decreased resistance to transsphincteric flow [54, 211]. Myotomy is most efficacious when applied to patients with structural disorders which limit opening of the cricopharyngeus in association with preserved pharyngeal contractility, as seen in webs and stenoses [120, 153]. Data supporting efficacy of either dilatation or myotomy for cervical esophageal webs and postcricoid stenosis are also consistently favorable, albeit uncontrolled [152, 153, 249]. However, repeated dilatations over many years seem to be required in at least 40% of such patients, and in one study, 20% eventually required myotomy [152, 249].

## Lateral Pharyngeal Diverticula

Pharyngeal diverticula are most conveniently classified according to anatomical site. Broadly speaking, these anatomical structures can be lateral or posterior. Lateral pharyngeal diverticula, or pharyngoceles, are frequently bilateral, are more common in the elderly, and occur at the level of the vallecula in an area of relative weakness through the thyrohyoid membrane at a site that is relatively poorly supported by cartilage or muscle. Because this anomaly is a common incidental radiological finding, symptoms may be erroneously attributed to it and the clinician should carefully consider alternative causes of dysphagia and/or regurgitation in these patients. Lateral diverticula protrude from the lateral wall of the midpharynx and should not be confused with the typical posterior, hypopharyngeal (Zenker's) diverticulum which arises just above the proximal margin of the cricopharyngeus. Lateral diverticula may be congenital or, more commonly, acquired. Congenital lateral pouches are true branchial cleft cysts, representing an embryological remnant of the third pharyngeal pouch corresponding to the thyrohyoid membrane [4]. The area of relative weakness is bounded by the hyoid bone superiorly, at a site where there is incomplete overlap of the thyrohyoid muscle anteriorly and the inferior constrictor muscle inferiorly [154, 206]. At this site, the thyrohyoid membrane is also perforated by the superior laryngeal artery and the internal laryngeal branch of the superior laryngeal nerve. It is controversial whether these lateral diverticula cause symptoms as they are a common incidental finding. However, there are sporadic case reports of successful alleviation of dysphagia following surgical ligation or removal of the diverticulum [166, 189].

### Zenker's Diverticulum

The posterior hypopharyngeal pouch, Zenker's diverticulum, arises in the posterior hypopharyngeal wall through an area of relative muscular weakness (Killian's dehiscence) just proximal to the upper margin of the cricopharyngeus muscle. Patients are usually elderly, with the median age at presentation being in the eighth decade [54]. Presenting symptoms include dysphagia combined with varying degrees of regurgitation depending on the size of the pouch. Regurgitation of food particles ingested many hours earlier is often reported. Aspiration symptoms and recurrent chest infections are common features. Audible gurgling during the swallow may be present.

Since Zenker and von Ziemssen [261] first hypothesized in 1878 that herniation of the pouch was due to increased hypopharyngeal pressures, there has been much debate about its pathogenesis. Initially it was believed that UES incoordination, specifically premature sphincter closure, in some cases combined with early UES relaxation, was the cause of the proposed elevated hypopharyngeal pressure [3, 89, 148]. The validity of those early observations is questionable, however, because UES relaxation profiles were recorded

with a discrete sidehole positioned within the sphincter without appreciation of its deglutitive axial mobility [116]. Other theories proposed include UES spasm [113], failure of UES relaxation [115], and a second swallow against a closed sphincter [148, 254]. There has been no consistent demonstration of any of these phenomena, and a number of subsequent carefully conducted manometric studies reported normal or low basal sphincter tone and normal pharyngosphincteric coordination [54, 134].

A more likely explanation is based on evidence showing that UES opening is restricted by an intrinsic cricopharyngeal muscle disease [52]. Simultaneous videofluorography and manometry confirmed normal pharyngosphincteric coordination, normal UES tone, and complete UES relaxation but that UES opening is restricted during the swallow [54] (Fig. 9–4). That study showed that inadequate UES opening markedly increases hypopharyngeal intrabolus pressure during transsphincteric bolus flow. It is possible that such a rise in hypopharyngeal pressure just proximal to the sphincter might contribute to pouch herniation. The likely cause of inadequate sphincter opening is muscle fiber degeneration and fibroadipose tissue replacement confined to the cricopharyngeus muscle [52]. These combined observations suggest that Zenker's diverticulum is due to a poorly compliant but normally relaxing UES which cannot fully distend during the process of sphincter opening. Further evidence supporting this concept lies in the finding that cricopharyngeal myotomy, effectively a curative surgical procedure, normalizes both the extent of UES opening and the hypopharyngeal intrabolus pressure [211] (Fig. 9–5).

Treatment is cricopharyngeal myotomy, either alone or in

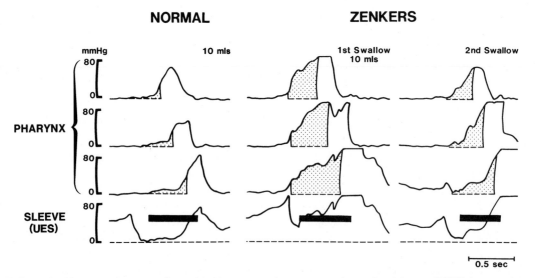

**FIG. 9–4.** Manometric traces from the pharynx and upper esophageal sphincter (UES) in a patient with a hypopharyngeal (Zenker's) diverticulum **(right)** compared with that of a healthy subject **(left)**. Recordings were synchronized with concurrent videofluoroscopy to permit identification of UES opening and bolus flow across the sphincter **(black horizontal bar)**. Resting UES tone, recorded by a perfused sleeve sensor, is normal and UES relaxation is complete in response to a "dry" swallow (second swallow on **right**). Note also the marked increase in hypopharyngeal intrabolus pressure *(stippled)* compared to that in the control subject. (From ref. 54, with permission.)

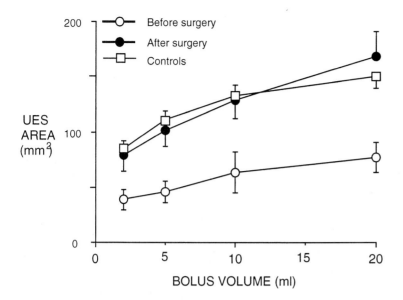

**FIG. 9–5.** Upper esophageal sphincter (UES) opening is restricted in patients with Zenker's diverticulum. Shown are maximal UES areas, calculated from radiologically determined sagittal and transverse diameters, for swallowed bolus volumes of from 2 to 20 mL. Note that for all bolus volumes swallowed, UES opening is restricted in Zenker's patients when compared to controls. Following surgery, including cricopharyngeal myotomy, the maximal UES opening capability returns to normal. (From ref. 211, with permission.)

combination with pouch resection or suspension [120]. The early observation that cricopharyngeal dilatation by bougienage gave temporary relief of dysphagia [118] prompted the introduction of cricopharyngeal myotomy [213]. Simple dilatation can afford symptomatic benefit of variable duration [118, 139, 183]. Cricopharyngeal myotomy is the key element for successful long-term relief of dysphagia, and it has been established that resection of the pouch alone is inadequate treatment and that myotomy is the essential element in treatment of this condition [12, 35, 103, 105, 136, 192, 216]. Indeed, excellent symptomatic results can be achieved from myotomy alone [120, 136]. Regression of the intact pouch can be observed following myotomy [84, 88], and radiological recurrence of the pouch is reduced after myotomy [89]. No controlled trials of the efficacy of surgical treatment for Zenker's diverticulum exist. However, the consistency of published response rates of 80% to 100% is in keeping with the strong clinical impression that surgery is nearly always curative in this disorder [8, 18, 76, 147, 153, 211, 256]. Myotomy via the endoscopic route is used less commonly but is an effective alternative treatment for Zenker's diverticulum. Endoscopic therapy can be performed with a rigid esophagoscope under general anesthesia [48, 70, 258] or under conscious sedation using a flexible endoscope [178]. Although the endoscopic technique has traditionally been reserved for the elderly patient with significant comorbidity, mediastinitis, hemorrhage, or restenosis complicate about 6% in the largest series [258].

### Cervical Osteophytes

Cervical osteophytes are a common incidental finding in the dysphagic patient, occurring in 6% to 30% of the elderly [19, 199]. On the other hand, only 0.7% of patients with cervical disc disease report dysphagia [228]. Hence, the finding of prominent osteophytes should prompt a careful search

for an alternative cause of dysphagia, which will be found in the majority. Nonetheless, if prominent, osteophytes can cause dysphagia, which is correctable by surgical removal of the bony spur [26, 135, 137]. The major mechanism of dysphagia is mechanical compression of the posterior pharyngeal wall, but associated periesophageal inflammation induced by pharyngoesophageal motion over the cervical exostoses (predominantly over the C3–6 vertebrae) might contribute as well [190, 219]. Development of osteophytes may be related to DISH (diffuse idiopathic skeletal hyperostosis), ankylosing spondylosis, infectious spondylosis, previous surgical fusion of the cervical vertebrae, or local trauma or it may be of idiopathic origin [104, 224]. Surgical treatment of cervical osteophytes remains controversial, and appropriate objective criteria have not been consistently used to assess results. Complications of surgical excision include vocal fold paresis, vertebral disc prolapse, fistula, hematoma, infection, aspiration, and Horner's syndrome [252]. In view of these limitations, most feel surgery should be performed only for those with severe dysphagia in whom conservative treatment has failed [104].

### NEUROGENIC CAUSES OF OROPHARYNGEAL DYSPHAGIA

#### Stroke

Stroke is the commonest cause of oropharyngeal dysphagia. Oropharyngeal dysphagia occurs in approximately one-third of all strokes [112, 244, 260]. Because of the bilateral innervation of the lower cranial nerves, it was previously believed that the swallow is not significantly affected by a lesion confined to a single hemisphere. Although much more common and more severe in bilateral or brainstem stroke, dysphagia affects 25% to 40% of patients in the acute phase of a single-hemisphere stroke [6, 96, 98, 111, 239].

Of stroke patients with dysphagia, 45% to 68% are dead

within 6 months, largely due to dysphagia-related nutritional and pulmonary complications [6, 203]. In addition to a higher mortality, dysphagia infers a higher risk of infection, poor nutrition, longer hospital stay, and institutionalization [96, 218, 260]. The most prevalent complication of stroke-related pharyngeal dysphagia is aspiration pneumonia, occurring in one-third of all patients and in 67% of those with brainstem stroke [112, 244, 260]. Hence, determining the risk of aspiration in this population is an important aim in management. Unfortunately, bedside evaluation underestimates the prevalence of deglutitive aspiration. Radiography detects aspiration not evident at the time of bedside assessment in 42% to 60% of patients [101, 112, 151, 222, 239]. In addition, an absent or depressed gag reflex does not have predictive value for aspiration as only 60% of aspirators have an impaired gag reflex [112]. Similarly, while dysphonia has a 91% sensitivity for aspiration, it has a positive predictive value of only 58%. Radiographic demonstration of an absent pharyngeal swallow response or a delayed response combined with a poor pharyngeal contraction carries the highest risk of aspiration [112, 239]. These facts underpin the importance of videofluoroscopy as being the only certain way of detecting aspiration, and if such gross features of pharyngeal dysfunction are demonstrated along with aspiration, immediate introduction of nonoral feeding is indicated. Typical videofluoroscopic findings are difficult in initiating the swallow, a delayed or absent pharyngeal swallow response, pharyngeal weakness with poor pharyngeal clearance and postswallow pooling in vallecula and pyriform sinuses, and aspiration. Brainstem stroke, particularly lesions in the rostral medulla, can result in a true failure of UES relaxation, detectable manometrically [56].

## Parkinson's Disease

Dysphagia in Parkinson's disease is common and associated with considerable morbidity from nutritional and pulmonary sequelae [15, 34, 37, 42, 77, 79, 80, 149, 248]. The true prevalence of dysphagia in Parkinson's is uncertain but may be as high as 52% [77, 80, 95, 106, 138, 149]. Drooling of saliva is even more common than dysphagia, being reported in up to 78% of patients [77, 80, 124]. Although symptoms are referable to the oropharynx in the majority, esophageal dysfunction is also common in Parkinson's [36, 41, 81, 92]. The majority of investigators who have examined the relationships among symptoms, severity of disease, and dysphagia have found that neither the duration of the disease, the severity of underlying disease, nor specific cardinal parkinsonian features correlate with severity or mechanism of dysphagia [2, 34, 81, 198].

Preparatory and oral phase dysfunction is common in Parkinson's. Impaired preparatory lingual movements and mastication, piecemeal swallows, increased oral residue, preswallow spill, and swallow hesitancy are common radiological observations [2, 145, 155, 227]. Lingual tremor appears to be specific for extrapyramidal movement disorders including Parkinson's disease [2, 34, 81]. All Parkinson's patients with dysphagia and many without dysphagia demonstrate one or more radiological indicators of pharyngeal dysfunction, such as postswallow contrast coating of the pharyngeal wall, vallecula and pyriform sinus pooling, abnormal pharyngeal wall motion, and impaired UES opening [2, 146]. Intra- and/or postswallow aspiration occurs in one-third of those with dysphagia, and silent aspiration has been reported in up to 15% of those reporting neither dysphagia nor symptoms of aspiration [2, 13, 34, 198].

Manometric studies may demonstrate diminished pharyngeal contraction pressures, pharyngosphincteric incoordination, or synchronous pressure waves; and failure of UES relaxation is common, occurring in up to 25% of cases [2, 115, 250]. Failed UES relaxation, while relatively common, is not the major determinant of dysphagia in Parkinson's as its presence does not correlate with the severity of either the associated motor disorder or the dysphagia [2]. Impaired pharyngeal bolus transport is the major determinant of dysphagia in Parkinson's disease.

Cricopharyngeal myotomy would seem to be a logical treatment in view of the high prevalence of failed UES relaxation. A favorable response to myotomy has been reported in a small series, many of whom had additional structural abnormalities, but more data are required before surgery can be recommended for the condition [20]. Similarly, there has been little systematic evaluation of the responsiveness of dysphagia to antiparkinsonian medication. The acute effect of central dopaminergic stimulation on pharyngeal mechanics is controversial. An early study assessed swallow function cineradiographically and reported no difference in swallow function following acute administration of oral levodopa (L-Dopa) compared to placebo [37]. A subsequent study using videofluoroscopy found that central dopaminergic stimulation by apomorphine improved pharyngeal bolus clearance acutely in roughly 50% of patients with mild disease [236]. Bushmann et al. [34] studied the acute effects of L-Dopa using videofluoroscopy and a clinical rating. While they found general improvement in parkinsonian motor features, such improvement was not an indicator of improved swallow function. In that study, 15% of those with abnormal videofluoroscopic studies demonstrated acute improvement following oral administration of L-Dopa. Hunter et al. [114] studied subjective dysphagia symptoms and videofluoroscopic parameters before and after acute administration of oral L-Dopa and apomorphine. Despite an unequivocal motor response to both drugs, there was no or minimal detectable change in oropharyngeal swallow function. These findings strongly suggest that parkinsonian dysphagia is not solely related to nigrostriatal dopamine deficiency.

The longer-term effects of therapy for Parkinson's on swallow function also remain unclear. It has been the experience of the author that the dysphagia is relatively unresponsive to antiparkinsonian drug therapy. Nevertheless, evidence for a good clinical response to drug therapy exists in isolated case reports [233]. Optimal pharmacotherapy generally improves the patients' ability to feed themselves by minimizing hand tremor and bradykinesia; treatment of mood disturbance, when present, may also improve feeding behavior and appetite. Appropriate timing of medication, 1 hour prior to meals, seems logical and was found to be beneficial in at lease one case report [93]. One study found that a combination of L-Dopa and swallow therapy improved swallow function, but it is uncertain to what extent improvement could be attributed to pharmacotherapy per se [34].

## Motor Neuron Disease

Oropharyngeal dysphagia commonly complicates motor neuron disease, affecting the majority of cases at some stage [169]. In the commonest variant of this disease, amyotrophic lateral sclerosis (ALS), there is degeneration of motor neurons in the cortex, brainstem, and spinal cord, leading to both upper and lower motor neuronal weakness. Bulbar involvement with dysarthria and dysphagia is a primary manifestation in 25% to 30% of cases of ALS [231]. The onset of the disease is insidious. Early symptoms include coughing or choking during liquid swallows, followed by progressive dysphagia and weight loss. The sequence of involvement of the bulbar musculature is relatively predictable in that the tongue is generally involved early and nearly always before the pharyngeal muscles. Aspiration pneumonia is a common complication and, when coupled with diminished respiratory muscle reserve, is the most common cause of death [24, 179].

Videofluoroscopic findings are variable and depend on the stage of disease [23]. By the time dysphagia is a significant problem, lingual dysfunction is almost invariably present and manifests as repetitive tongue movements, premature retrolingual bolus spill, and significant retention of barium in the oral sulci, requiring several swallows for clearance. The pharyngeal swallow response may be delayed and is eventually lost with markedly impaired bolus clearance from the pharynx and intra- and postswallow aspiration of contrast. There have been few systematic manometric studies of these patients. However, UES relaxation appears to be complete and sphincter spasm is not a feature [165] (I. J. Cook, *unpublished data*).

Although the disease is inexorably progressive, leading to death with a median survival of 3 years [179], the rate of disease progression is quite variable [226]. One study has shown a close temporal correlation among speech, swallowing, and lung vital capacity and noted a rapid deterioration in swallowing with the onset of compromised speech intelligibility [226]. These findings suggest that vital capacity and speech are useful prognostic indicators which guide the clinician as to the timing of intervention with swallow therapy and consideration of non-oral feeding.

## Poliomyelitis and Post-polio Syndrome

Although less common than the spinal involvement in this disease, bulbar poliomyelitis carries a much greater mortality, primarily from depression of respiratory muscles associated with an inability to clear pharyngeal secretions. Pharyngeal involvement with dysphagia probably occurs in around 60% of cases of bulbar poliomyelitis [164]. Dysphagia, when present, involves the neurons of the nucleus ambiguus in the medulla with variable involvement of the adjacent reticular formation. Furthermore, the rostrocaudal level of involvement in poliomyelitis determines the likelihood of dysphagia occurring in that involvement of the rostral nucleus ambiguus has a much stronger correlation with dysphagia than involvement of the mid- or distal medulla [5]. Cineradiographic swallow studies in affected patients commonly show velopharyngeal incompetence affecting speech and causing deglutitive, postnasal regurgitation. Abnormal pharyngeal wall motion reflecting constrictor muscle and suprahyoid muscle dysfunction is commonly seen and results in impaired pharyngeal bolus clearance [22].

Since the widespread introduction of vaccination, acute poliomyelitis is now rarely seen. However, a late onset and very slowly progressive muscular weakness, the post-polio syndrome, is now recognized in some patients who have partially or totally recovered from acute poliomyelitis many years before [60]. Typically, the post-polio syndrome manifests 25 to 35 years after the original attack of poliomyelitis. Patients report an insidious onset of new fatigability, muscle wasting, weakness, and sometimes muscle pain. Although these symptoms are generally most prominent in previously affected muscles, regions not previously involved with the original attack may be affected. Only 50% of those with post-polio dysphagia experienced dysphagia at the time of their acute poliomyelitis [27, 214]. One survey determined the prevalence of dysphagia in a polio survivors support group to be 18% [47]. The videofluoroscopic features are not specific for this syndrome and may include those described in poliomyelitis, such as velopharyngeal incompetence, pharyngeal weakness, and silent aspiration. Silent aspiration is reported in up to 50% of these patients [27]. Additionally, while pharyngeal dysfunction is the most common deficit, it is recognized that oromotor dysfunction is also common, affecting about half of these patients [47, 117, 125, 221]. It is now appreciated that in people affected by post-polio syndrome motor neurons continue to undergo damage and that slowly progressive deterioration of swallow function can occur once the syndrome is apparent [221].

## MYOGENIC CAUSES OF OROPHARYNGEAL DYSPHAGIA

### Myasthenia Gravis

Myasthenia usually has an insidious onset and protean manifestations. Muscles most frequently involved include the facial, laryngeal, pharyngeal, and respiratory groups, but limb muscles are usually affected also. Facial and pharyngeal weakness is present in 70%, and dysphagia affects 30% to 60% of cases [72, 187]. Dysphagia is present at diagnosis in around 20% of cases [187, 242] and may dominate the clinical picture, being the sole presenting symptom in 6% to 17% of affected individuals [99, 201]. The so-called fatigable flaccid dysarthria, manifest by hypernasal speech (velopharyngeal incompetence), imprecise articulation, and breathiness, reflects bulbar dysfunction and is usually prominent in those with dysphagia [72, 133]. Progressive difficulty chewing and swallowing during the course of a long meal may also be reported [72, 133]. The ocular features of palpebral ptosis and diplopia are usually but not invariably present. Atrophy of the tongue may be prominent also [215]. Diagnosis may be apparent from typical clinical signs, including fatigability, but should be considered in any dysphagic patient, even though typical ocular signs may be absent.

Diagnosis is confirmed by detecting acetylcholine receptor (AChR) antibodies, which are present in 85% overall [184]. The finding of AChR antibodies is highly specific and virtually diagnostic, but antibodies may be absent in up to 50% of patients without typical ocular signs. The Tensilon (edrophonium) stimulation test may be positive. The diagnosis may also be made electomyographically using repetitive nerve stimulation and single-fiber electromyography (EMG) recording, which is the most sensitive diagnostic test [72, 184, 185]. Pharyngeal pressure recordings during the Tensilon test may be useful to quantify the response, particularly if the response as judged by other muscle groups is equivocal (I. J. Cook, *unpublished data*). Videoradiographic examination reveals obvious features of virtually all of the muscle groups involved, including both oral and pharyngeal phases and the suprahyoid muscles responsible for hyolaryngeal ascent [133, 182]. Poor oral delivery with incomplete oral clearance, premature bolus spill, deglutitive velopharyngeal incompetence, abnormal pharyngeal wall motion with aspiration, and vallecula and pyriform sinus pooling are characteristic features. Subnormal hyolaryngeal ascent results in incomplete epiglottal inversion, further predisposing to aspiration.

The response of pharyngeal swallow dysfunction to medical therapy (acetylcholinesterase inhibitor and immunosuppressive drugs) is very variable and may occur at a different rate and less satisfactorily than that of other muscle groups. For example, in one report of eight elderly men whose primary symptoms of myasthenia gravis were dysarthria and dysphagia, in only three did dysphagia respond satisfactorily, the remaining five requiring long-term enteral feeding tubes [133]. Some have reported dramatic improvement in hypopharyngeal bolus clearance in response to edrophonium [242], but this is not a consistent observation. Even in those with a satisfactory clinical response, the videofluoroscopic improvement following therapy may be marginal, which casts doubt on the use of videofluoroscopy in assessing the progress of these patients [133]. Notwithstanding the frequently disappointing response to medical therapy, establishing the diagnosis does influence management as it always warrants drug therapy, a search for thymoma, and avoidance of risk factors for myasthenic crisis, to which the dysphagic patient is frequently exposed, including respiratory tract infections, anesthesia, and surgery.

## Inflammatory Myopathies

Dysphagia is a frequent and sometimes the presenting symptom, occurring in 30% to 60% of cases of inflammatory myopathy [61, 72, 119, 257]. The inflammatory myopathies comprise three major and distinct groups: polymyositis, dermatomyositis, and inclusion body myositis [61]. Pharyngeal dysphagia can occur in the mixed connective tissue disease overlap syndrome in up to 20% of cases [109, 237]. In this syndrome, patients may display the clinical features of polymyositis, along with those of lupus, Sjögren's syndrome, or scleroderma, and antibodies to extractable nuclear antigen are detectable. The clinical features of inflammatory myopathy generally include a subacute or chronic and progressive symmetrical, proximal, muscular weakness. The characteristic rash (Gottron's sign) over the extensor surfaces of the metacarpophalangeal and interphalangeal joints is typical of dermatomyositis. The classic violaceous (heliotrope) rash of dermatomyositis is typically seen in the periorbital area, often with prominent palpebral edema; the upper torso; over the knuckles; and around the nail beds.

Diagnosis is confirmed by abnormalities in one or more of muscle enzymes, EMG, or muscle biopsy. Serum creatine phosphokinase (CPK) is the most sensitive enzyme, but alanine aminotransferase (ALT), aspartate aminotransferase (AST), lactate dehydrogenase (LDH), and aldolase are also sensitive indicators of muscle injury. The CPK level generally parallels disease activity, but the CPK is frequently normal even in active disease [61]. At the time of presentation, CPK is raised in around 70% of cases [237] but is elevated in 95% at some time in the course of the disease [17]. Elevations in plasma C-reactive protein and erythrocyte sedimentation rate are common but nonspecific. Antinuclear antibody (ANA) is detectable only in around 25% but is much more likely to be present (85% to 90%) if the myositis occurs as part of an overlap syndrome [237]. Rheumatoid factor is rarely positive in pure myositis but is detectable in 50% of those cases which are associated with connective tissue disease [237]. Needle EMG is useful in excluding neurogenic disorders and will demonstrate features consistent with inflammatory myositis in 85% to 90% [237]. However, the EMG changes observed are not always specific for inflammatory myopathy and recordings may reveal a mixed neuropathic and myopathic picture [7]. Hence, muscle biopsy is required to definitively establish the presence of myositis and to distinguish among dermatomyositis, polymyositis, and inclusion body myositis. Notwithstanding, muscle biopsy is diagnostic in only 80%, emphasizing that diagnosis of myositis can be elusive and the need for complete clinical, biochemical, and laboratory evaluation in all suspected cases [237]. Selection of the site for muscle biopsy is important, and attempts should be made to sample those muscles that are not yet atrophic, but that are involved clinically or electromyographically. The inflammatory process may be quite patchy and is occasionally apparently confined to the pharyngeal musculature [210]. If cricopharyngeal myotomy is undertaken in suspected cases without prior confirmation of the diagnosis by the above techniques, fresh muscle samples should be obtained from the cricopharyngeus and other neck muscles (e.g., omohyoid, sternomastoid) for histological examination.

The videofluoroscopic features are variable. A number of observers have reported limitation of UES opening with or without a cricopharyngeal bar in patients with polymyositis [68, 115, 195]. The significance of this is uncertain and may reflect reporting bias of a common and obvious anatomical anomaly (see above), or the incomplete UES opening might simply represent diminished pharyngeal propulsive forces. However, histological examination of the cricopharyngeus muscle in affected patients has confirmed that the inflammatory myopathies can involve this particular muscle [195, 240] and that a rather focal inflammatory myopathy can affect the cricopharyngeus without the usual biochemical, EMG, or histological evidence of muscle involvement elsewhere [210]. Pharyngeal dysfunction is almost universal in radiological studies of patients with dysphagia due to inflammatory myopathy [102, 115, 122]. Aspiration and limited hyolaryngeal motion are also common. Oral phase dysfunction is less common but occurs in at least 60% in our experience (I. J. Cook, *unpublished data*).

Very few systematic manometric studies of pharyngeal function in polymyositis exist, and those reported were done when techniques of questionable fidelity were in use [57, 223]. Low resting UES pressure with normal relaxation and markedly reduced pharyngeal contraction pressures seem to be common, but not consistent, findings [108, 132, 204].

The mainstay of treatment for inflammatory myopathies is immunosuppressive therapy with steroids in the first instance, with azathioprine or methotrexate as second-line or steroid-sparing agents. Despite the lack of controlled efficacy trials, a significant number of patients respond favorably to these agents. Inclusion body myositis is generally resistant to standard therapies, although high-dose intravenous immunoglobulin may be helpful [64]. Reports of response of swallow function to drug therapy are anecdotal but generally favorable. Similarly, cricopharyngeal myotomy might have a role in treatment, but there has been no systematic evaluation of this [66, 68, 195].

## Toxic and Metabolic Myopathies

Hyperthyroidism is a well-recognized cause of myopathy which is believed to be due to mitochondrial dysfunction [246]. Muscle weakness affects 80% of thyrotoxic patients, and men are affected more commonly than women [246]. The myopathy of thyrotoxicosis can cause pharyngeal dysphagia, which is generally slowly progressive and may be the presenting feature of this endocrinopathy [25, 176]. Although uncommon, this condition should always be considered, particularly in the elderly where the more classical thyrotoxic features may be absent, because it is a reversible cause of dysphagia [25, 229]. Serum CPK is not increased, in contrast to the myopathy of myxedema in which CPK is usually increased but weakness is uncommon [197]. The response of limb muscle function to specific treatment of thyrotoxicosis is usually excellent. Although published data are limited, there are case reports of resolution of pharyngeal dysphagia with return to the euthyroid state [25], and this has also been the anecdotal experience of the author. A number of drugs capable of causing toxic or inflammatory myopathy should be considered in the assessment of the patient with dysphagia as removal of the drug generally reverses the dysphagia (Table 9–2).

## Oculopharyngeal Muscular Dystrophy

Taylor [232], who was the first to describe this rare syndrome in 1915, originally postulated that the disorder was a neuropathy. Oculopharyngeal muscular dystrophy has subsequently been shown to be a myopathy affecting nearly exclusively the bulbar muscles and the levator muscles of the eyes [241]. The disease usually presents between the ages of 40 and 70 years, most often initially with bilateral ptosis followed some years later by dysphagia. The ptosis usually develops before, or sometimes simultaneously with, the dysphagia, but it is unusual for the dysphagia to develop first. The disease is very slowly progressive. Variable but mild facial weakness may develop, as may a minor degree of ophthalmoplegia, and limb muscle weakness is occasionally present. However, the pharyngeal and levator palpebral involvement always dominates the clinical picture. The disorder is inherited in an autosomal dominant fashion. There is a high incidence in French Canadians. However, it has been well documented in many other racial groups, including the Italian, Spanish, English, Armenian, Australian, Norwegian, and Japanese populations [16, 69, 200].

Dystrophic changes in muscle biopsy have been demonstrated by light and electron microscopy on levator, pharyngeal, and vastus lateralis muscles [16, 69, 121, 191, 196, 200]. Although the findings are variable, a number of investigators report histological and ultrastructural features which suggest that this disorder is a heterogeneous syndrome and that it may be a manifestation of mitochondrial myopathy [69, 191, 196]. Histopathological findings in cricopharyngeus muscle specimens must be interpreted with caution, however, because the normal cricopharyngeus muscle demonstrates features which, if identified in limb muscle, would be consistent with a mitochondrial myopathy [52]. Nonetheless, the reported changes of cricopharyngeal muscle fiber degeneration and fibrosis are definitely pathological [69], and such changes in the cricopharyngeus would be expected to impair sphincter opening and compliance and might account for the reported favorable response to cricopharyngeal myotomy in this disease [73, 230]. Elevated levels of immunoglobulins G and A are frequently found in the serum of these patients [196]. The major differential diagnoses are myasthenia gravis and mitochondrial myopathies.

Videoradiographic findings include relative preservation of oral function, incomplete UES opening, pharyngeal weakness with impaired pharyngeal bolus clearance, variable aspiration, and postnasal regurgitation. Manometric recordings have generally shown a normally relaxing UES which is sometimes hypotensive and markedly reduced pharyngeal pressure wave amplitudes [39, 40, 75, 115, 230]. Although the syndrome is a disease of striated muscle, manometric abnormalities have also been described in the esophagus. A high prevalence of nonpropulsive, simultaneous pressure waves and failed peristalsis is reported [40, 69, 235], which is associated with delayed esophageal isotope clearance [230, 235].

Due to its late onset and slow progression, the prognosis of oculopharyngeal muscular dystrophy is generally good and the disease in many cases does not adversely influence life expectancy. This syndrome is one homogenous condition in which the results of cricopharyngeal myotomy appear to be fairly consistently favorable [74, 230]. Despite the lack of controlled trials of efficacy of myotomy, this procedure appears to be appropriate in cases with severe dysphagia.

## DRUGS CAUSING OROPHARYNGEAL DYSPHAGIA

It is important for the clinician to obtain a detailed drug history from the patient who has oropharyngeal dysphagia because a range of drugs can act either centrally or peripherally to impair neural function, neuromuscular transmission, muscle function, or salivary secretion and thereby cause dysphagia (Table 9–2). Drugs can impair swallow function indirectly by either inhibiting or enhancing salivary flow.

Centrally acting drugs with dopamine antagonist action, such as phenothiazines and metoclopramide, can cause extrapyramidal movement disorders such as dystonia and dyskinesia, resulting in dysphagia. Phenothiazines in particular can cause tardive dyskinesia, in which choreoathetoid movements of the tongue can severely impair swallowing [97, 107, 175]. This syndrome, which is frequently irreversible, is characterized by repetitive, involuntary tongue movements which render the masticatory process and oral delivery ineffective. These centrally acting drugs may also impair pharyngeal propulsive and clearance functions by causing a clinical picture similar to Parkinson's disease [9, 144]. Benzodiazepines such as nitrazepam, alprazolam, and clorazepate [30, 150, 259] have been documented to cause oropharyngeal dysphagia. Nitrazepam, a drug frequently used to treat myoclonic epilepsy, has been associated with fatalities in children, probably due to a combination of excessive salivation, poor pharyngeal clearance, and bronchospasm resulting in fatal respiratory distress [150, 259].

A number of drugs can produce a myasthenic syndrome. Botulinum A toxin (Botox), when injected into the neck muscles to treat spasmodic torticollis, may cause pharyngeal dysphagia, presumably due to regional spread of the toxin to adjacent muscles [21, 33, 49]. Other drugs capable of causing a myasthenic syndrome include penicillamine [167], large doses of aminoglycosides [72], and procainamide [174]. In some cases, anti-AChR antibodies are detectable [167]. The myasthenia and dysphagia, if present, are reversible on cessation of the offending drug. Erythromycin may aggravate neuromuscular function in existing myasthenia gravis and should be avoided in this condition [168].

Drugs are a relatively common cause of myopathy, which may be complicated by oropharyngeal dysphagia. A drug can cause either an inflammatory or a toxic myopathy (Table 9–2). Penicillamine [71] and zidovudine [63], for example, can cause an endomysial inflammation similar to that observed in polymyositis, although recent evidence shows that zidovudine is primarily toxic to muscle mitochondria [62]. A number of drugs capable of causing a reversible toxic myopathy should also be considered as some of these have been linked specifically with dysphagia. Amiodarone-induced thyroid myopathy may present as dysphagia [11]. The cholesterol-lowering hepatic hydroxymethylglutaryl coenzyme A reductase inhibitors (e.g., lovastatin, simvastatin) are a relatively common cause of toxic myopathy [62, 163] and may cause oropharyngeal dysphagia associated with elevated CPK levels (I. J. Cook, *unpublished observations*).

## MANAGEMENT OF OROPHARYNGEAL DYSPHAGIA

Because oropharyngeal dysphagia can be the presenting or accompanying manifestation of one of a large number of systemic diseases (Table 9–1), a multidisciplinary strategy is frequently necessary to achieve optimal management. Furthermore, the accompanying neurological impairment, by limiting the patient's cognitive and physical competence, can compromise the ability to understand and cooperate with the process of investigation and therapy. Broadly speaking, the aims of management are to identify and treat an underlying primary disease where possible and then try to compensate or circumvent the specific mechanical disturbances responsible for the dysphagia [55]. Hence, there is no single strategy appropriate for all cases nor, indeed, for dysphagia caused by a single disease process because the mechanical disturbances are generally neither homogeneous nor specific for a particular disease. However, there are logical, generic management principles which are widely applicable, while specific surgical or rehabilitative swallow therapies should be tailored to the individual case.

The first step is to confirm that oropharyngeal dysphagia is a problem and to identify the underlying cause. A careful history will generally distinguish oropharyngeal dysphagia from globus, xerostomia, and esophageal dysphagia. History and physical examination may provide clues of a treatable systemic, metabolic, or drug-related disorder. They will also identify the pulmonary and nutritional sequelae of dysphagia. Based on this information, the clinician can prioritize subsequent investigations, including laboratory tests and imaging techniques, to verify a systemic, metabolic, or neuromyogenic disease when present. Laboratory tests should attempt to detect treatable metabolic diseases (e.g., thyrotoxicosis, Cushing's disease, drugs), inflammatory myopathies, and myasthenia.

The second step is to identify the structural or neuromyogenic mechanisms of oropharyngeal dysfunction. Structural disorders are generally readily detected by radiographic or endoscopic evaluation. Identification of a neoplasm or a Zenker's diverticulum will dictate surgery. A cervical web or a cricopharyngeal stenosis will prompt dilatation or, in some cases, cricopharyngeal myotomy. Identification of a cricopharyngeal bar or cervical osteophytes should prompt a careful search for a coexistent or alternative explanation for dysphagia but may, in some circumstances, warrant dilatation or surgery, respectively (see above). The evidence supporting the efficacy of mechanical disruption (usually surgical) for structural disorders is consistently favorable [55]. Nasoendoscopic examination of the laryngopharynx is mandatory if neoplasm is suspected. Nasoendoscopy may also provide useful indirect information about some aspects of pharyngeal dysfunction and aspiration [140]. In some instances, particularly in the assessment of disorders with a high prevalence of failed UES relaxation such as Parkinson's disease and medullary lesions (Fig. 9–6), pharyngeal manometry with or without concurrent videofluoroscopy may allow further delineation of the underlying mechanism of dysfunction [2, 38, 56]. In some instances manometry is able to identify abnormalities which are not apparent on videofluoroscopy [2, 186], but whether such decisions based on manometric findings can influence outcome remains unproven [1].

The third management objective is to determine the risk of aspiration pneumonia, which is the primary factor in the decision as to whether and when gastrostomy feeding should be instituted. The risk of aspiration and its complication is determined by videofluoroscopic examination because clinical estimation of aspiration underestimates this risk by about 50% [222]. The decision on the advisability of gastrostomy feeding is also influenced by the likelihood that therapeutic maneuvers, which may be tested during videofluoroscopy, will reduce or eliminate aspiration, the natural history of the underlying disease, and the patient's cognitive ability [203, 217, 218].

Finally, after exclusion of structural lesions and underlying treatable diseases and having established the safety of oral feeding, specific "local" therapy should be considered. The therapeutic options open are dietary modification, swallow therapy, surgery, or a combination of all three. While the data supporting the efficacy of cricopharyngeal myotomy for structural cricopharyngeal disorders are strong, the outcome following myotomy for neuromyogenic dysphagia is far less certain. There are no controlled trials of cricopharyngeal myotomy in neurogenic dysphagia, but the available evidence suggests an overall response rate of around 60% with an operative mortality of 1% to 2% [193, 230]. A number of indicators have been proposed which might predict a favorable outcome from myotomy, such as intact swallow initiation, "adequate" lingual and pharyngeal propulsive

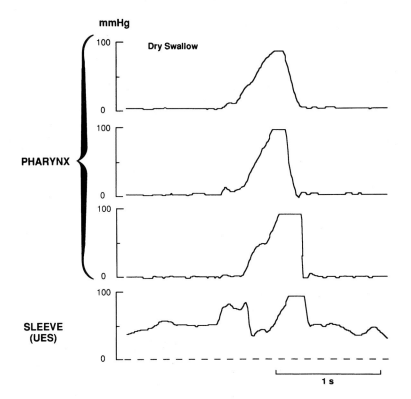

**FIG. 9–6.** Example of a manometric trace from a patient with syringobulbia and dysphagia. Note the incomplete upper esophageal sphincter relaxation in response to a dry swallow.

forces, radiographic and/or manometric evidence of increased outflow resistance at the UES, and a relatively good prognosis for the underlying neurological disease [1, 28, 225]. However, myotomy has not been proven conclusively to influence outcome in neurogenic dysphagia or to have any preoperative variables that predict response to myotomy. Hence, the decision to undertake myotomy remains largely empiric at present. In some instances, both because non-oral feeding does not necessarily eliminate the risk of aspiration pneumonia and because of the need to eliminate aspiration of oral secretions, surgical procedures aimed at minimizing aspiration (epiglottoplasty, partial or total cricoid excision, laryngeal suspension, vocal fold medialization, glottic closure, laryngotracheal diversion, or laryngectomy) may be necessary [14].

Current swallow therapy strategies include dietary modification and manipulation of swallowing posture or swallowing technique. Modifications of swallowing technique are intended to strengthen weak oropharyngeal muscle groups, thereby improving their speed and range of movement, and/or to selectively modify the mechanics of the swallow to facilitate bolus flow and minimize aspiration. In applying swallow therapies, the speech–language pathologist will use videofluoroscopy to define the relevant mechanism of dysfunction and to examine the acute effects of therapeutic strategies designed to eliminate or compensate for that dysfunction [158]. Simple dietary modification can reduce the risk of aspiration pneumonia and should be instituted if an aspiration risk is apparent [101]. There are reasonable data supporting the biological plausibility of the remaining swallow strategies, but the limited available controlled efficacy data are inconclusive [55]. On the other hand, swallow therapy has not been proven to be ineffective, and based on the demonstration of biological plausibility for specific therapeutic techniques, the consistency of the low-grade evidence suggesting efficacy, the relatively low cost, and the absence of either risk or any better alternative in many instances, it is appropriate to institute swallow therapy under the supervision of a speech–language pathologist. Clearly, large-scale controlled trials are necessary to clarify the appropriateness of all current treatment strategies on neurogenic oropharyngeal dysphagia.

## REFERENCES

1. Ali GN, Wallace KL, Laundl TM, Hunt DR, deCarle DJ, Cook IJ. Predictors of outcome following cricopharyngeal disruption for pharyngeal dysphagia. Dysphagia 1997;12:133
2. Ali GN, Wallace KL, Schwartz R, de Carle DJ, Zagami A, Cook IJ. Mechanisms of oral-pharyngeal dysphagia in patients with Parkinson's disease. Gastroenterology 1996;110:383
3. Ardran GM, Kemp FH, Lund WS. The aetiology of the posterior pharyngeal diverticulum: a cineradiographic study. J Laryngol Otol 1964;78:333
4. Bachman AL, Seaman WB, Macken KL. Lateral pharyngeal diverticula. Radiology 1968;91:774
5. Baker AB, Matzke HA, Brown JR. Poliomyelitis III. Bulbar poliomyelitis; a study of medullary function. Arch Neurol Psychiatry 1950;62:257
6. Barer DH. The natural history and functional consequence of dysphagia after hemisphere stroke. J Neurol Neurosurg Psychiatry 1989;52:236
7. Barkhaus PE, Nandedkar SD, Sanders DB. Quantitative EMG in inflammatory myopathy. Muscle Nerve 1990;13:247
8. Barthlen W, Feussner H, Hannig C, Holscher AH, Siewert JR. Surgical therapy of Zenker's diverticulum: low risk and high efficiency. Dysphagia 1990;5:13
9. Bashford G, Bradd P. Drug-induced Parkinsonism associated with dysphagia and aspiration: a brief report. J Geriatr Psychiatry Neurol 1996;9:133
10. Benedict EB, Sweet RH. Dysphagia due to hypertrophy of the cricopharyngeus muscle or hypopharyngeal bar. N Engl J Med 1955;253:1161
11. Berbegal J, Lluch V, Morera J, de Gracia MC. Dysphagia as the presentation of amiodarone-induced hyperthyroidism [Letter]. Med Clin (Barc) 1993;100:437
12. Bingham DC. Cricopharyngeal achalasia. Can Med Assoc J 1963;89:1071
13. Bird MR, Woodward MC, Gibson EM, Phyland DJ, Fonda D. Asymptomatic swallowing disorders in elderly patients with Parkinson's disease: a description of findings on clinical examination and videofluoroscopy in sixteen patients. Age Ageing 1994;23:251
14. Blitzer A, Krespi YP, Oppenheimer RW, Levine TM. Surgical management of aspiration. Otolaryngol Clin North Am 1988;21:743
15. Blonsky ER, Logemann JA, Boshes B, Fisher HB. Comparison of speech and swallowing function in patients with tremor disorders and in normal geriatric patients: a cinefluorographic study. J Gerontol 1975;30:299
16. Blumbergs PC, Chin D, Burrows D, Burns RJ, Rice JP. Oculopharyngeal dystrophy: clinicopathological study of an Australian family. Clin Exp Neurol 1982;19:102
17. Bohan A, Peter JB, Bowman RL, Pearson CM. A computer-assisted analysis of 153 patients with polymyositis and dermatomyositis. Medicine 1977;56:255
18. Bonavina L, Khan NA, DeMeester TR. Pharyngoesophageal dysfunctions. The role of cricopharyngeal myotomy. Arch Surg 1985;120:541
19. Bone RC, Nahum AM, Harris AS. Evaluation and correlation of dysphagia-producing cervical osteophytosis. Laryngoscope 1974;84:2045
20. Born LJ, Harned RH, Rikkers LF, Pfeiffer RF, Quigley EM. Cricopharyngeal dysfunction in Parkinson's disease: role in dysphagia and response to myotomy. Mov Disord 1996;11:53
21. Borodic GE, Joseph M, Fay L, Cozzolino D, Ferrante RJ. Botulinum A toxin for the treatment of spasmodic torticollis: dysphagia and regional toxin spread. Head Neck 1990;12:392
22. Bosma JF. Studies of the disabilities of the pharynx resultant from poliomyelitis. Ann Otol Rhinol Laryngol 1953;64:529
23. Bosma J, Brodie D. Disabilities of the pharynx in amyotrophic lateral sclerosis as demonstrated by cineradiography. Radiology 1969;92:97
24. Bowman K, Meurman T. Prognosis of amyotrophic lateral sclerosis. Acta Neurol Scand 1967;43:489
25. Branski D, Levy J, Globus M, Aviad I, Keren A, Chowers I. Dysphagia as a primary manifestation of hyperthyroidism. J Clin Gastroenterol 1984;6:437
26. Bridger AG, Stening WA, Bridger GP. Cervical osteophytes: an unusual cause of dysphagia. Aust N Z J Surg 1996;66:261
27. Buchholz D. Dysphagia in post-polio patients. Birth Defects 1987;23:55
28. Buchholz DW. Cricopharyngeal myotomy may be effective treatment for selected patients with neurogenic oropharyngeal dysphagia. Dysphagia 1995;10:255
29. Buchholz DW. Clinically probable brainstem stroke presenting primarily as dysphagia and nonvisualized by MRI. Dysphagia 1993;8:235
30. Buchholz D, et al. Two cases of benzodiazepine induced pharyngeal dysphagia. In Proceedings of the Dysphagia Res Society Conference, 1994
31. Buchholz DW. Oropharyngeal dysphagia due to iatrogenic neurological dysfunction. Dysphagia 1995;10:248
32. Buchholz DW, Jones B, Ravich WJ. Dysphagia following anterior cervical fusion. Dysphagia 1993;8:390

33. Buchholz DW, Neumann S. The swallowing side effects of botulinum toxin type A injection in spasmodic dysphonia. Dysphagia 1997;12:59

34. Bushmann M, Dobmeyer SM, Leeker L, Perlmutter JS. Swallowing abnormalities and their response to treatment in Parkinson's disease. Neurology 1989;39:1309

35. Butcher RB, Larabee WF. Surgical treatment of hypopharyngeal (Zenker's) diverticulum. Arch Otolaryngol 1989;105:254

36. Byrne KG, Pfeiffer R, Quigley EM. Gastrointestinal dysfunction in Parkinson's disease. A report of clinical experience at a single center. J Clin Gastroenterol 1994;19:11

37. Calne DB, Shaw DG, Spiers AS, Stern GM. Swallowing in Parkinsonism. Br J Radiol 1970;43:456

38. Castell J, Dalton C, Castell D. Pharyngeal and upper esophageal sphincter manometry in humans. Am J Physiol 1990;258:G173

39. Castell JA, Castell DO, Duranceau A. Pharyngeal and upper esophageal sphincter (UES) manometric characteristics of patients with oculopharyngeal muscular dystrophy (OPMD). Gastroenterology 1991;100:A39

40. Castell JA, Castell DO, Duranceau CA, Topart P. Manometric characteristics of the pharynx, upper esophageal sphincter, esophagus, and lower esophageal sphincter in patients with oculopharyngeal muscular dystrophy. Dysphagia 1995;10:22

41. Castell JA, Li Q, Gideon RM, Hurtig H, Stern M, Castell DO. Esophageal dysfunction in Parkinson's disease. Gastroenterology 1994;106:A60

42. Chen MYM, Peele VN, Donati D, Ott DJ, Donofrio PD, Gelfand DW. Clinical and videofluoroscopic evaluation of swallowing in 41 patients with neurologic disease. Gastrointest Radiol 1992;17:95

43. Chen TSN, Chen PSY. Rise and fall of the Plummer-Vinson syndrome. J Gastroenterol Hepatol 1994;9:654

44. Chisolm M. The association between webs, iron, and post-cricoid carcinoma. Postgrad Med 1974;50:215

45. Clements JL, Cox GW, Torres WE, Weens HS. Cervical esophageal webs: a roentgen anatomic correlation. Am J Roentgenol 1974;121:221

46. Close LG, Costin BS, Kim EE. Acute symptoms of the aerodigestive tract caused by rapidly enlarging thyroid neoplasms. Otolaryngol Head Neck Surg 1983;91:441

47. Coelho CA, Ferranti R. Incidence and nature of dysphagia in polio survivors. Arch Phys Med Rehabil 1991;72:1071

48. Collard JM. Zenker's diverticulum: stapling esophago-diverticulostomy by endoscopy. Dis Esophagus 1994;7:66

49. Comella CL, Tanner CM, DeFoor HL, Smith C. Dysphagia after botulinum toxin injections for spasmodic torticollis: clinical and radiologic findings. Neurology 1992;42:1307

50. Cook IJ. Globus—real or imagined? Gullet 1991;1:68

51. Cook IJ. Cricopharyngeal function and dysfunction. Dysphagia 1993;8:244

52. Cook IJ, Blumbergs P, Cash K, Jamieson GG, Shearman DJ. Structural abnormalities of the cricopharyngeus muscle in patients with pharyngeal (Zenker's) diverticulum. J Gastroenterol Hepatol 1992;7:556

53. Cook IJ, et al. Opening mechanisms of the human upper esophageal sphincter. Am J Physiol 1989;257:G748

54. Cook IJ, et al. Pharyngeal (Zenker's) diverticulum is a disorder of upper esophageal sphincter opening. Gastroenterology 1992;103:1229

55. Cook IJ, Kahrilas PJ. American Gastroenterological Association technical review on management of oropharyngeal dysphagia. Gastroenterology 1998;(in press)

56. Cook IJ, Wallace KL, Zagami AS, Enis JM. Mechanisms of pharyngeal dysphagia in lateral medullary syndrome (LMS). Gastroenterology 1996;110:A650

57. Creamer B, Andersen HA, Code CF. Esophageal motility in patients with scleroderma and related diseases. Gastroenterologia (Basel) 1956;86:763

58. Cruse JP, Edwards DAW, Smith JF, Wyllie JH. The pathology of cricopharyngeal dysphagia. Histopathology 1979;3:223

59. Curtis DJ, Cruess DF, Berg T. The cricopharyngeal muscle: a videorecording review. Am J Roentgenol 1984;142:497

60. Dalakas M, et al. A long term follow-up study of patients with postpoliomyelitis neuromuscular symptoms. N Engl J Med 1986;314:954

61. Dalakas MC. Polymyositis, dermatomyositis and inclusion body myositis. N Engl J Med 1991;325:1487

62. Dalakas MC. Inflammatory and toxic myopathies. Curr Opin Neurol Neurosurg 1992;5:645

63. Dalakas MC, Illa I, Pezeshkpour GH, Laukaitis JP, Cohen B, Griffin JL. Mitochondrial myopathy caused by long term zidovudine therapy. N Engl J Med 1990;322:1098

64. Dalakas MC, Sonies B, Dambrosia J, Sekul E, Cupler E, Sivakumar K. Treatment of inclusion-body myositis with IVIg: a double-blind, placebo-controlled study [see comments]. Neurology 1997;48:712

65. Dantas RO, Cook IJ, Dodds WJ, Kern MK, Lang IM, Brasseur JG. Biomechanics of cricopharyngeal bars. Gastroenterology 1990;99:1269

66. Darrow DH, Hoffman GT, Barnes GJ, Wiley CA. Management of dysphagia in inclusion body myositis. Arch Otolaryngol Head Neck Surg 1992;118:313

67. Davies AE, Kidd D, Stone SP, MacMahon J. Pharyngeal sensation and gag reflex in healthy subjects. Lancet 1995;345:487

68. Dietz F, Logeman JA, Sahgal V, Schmid FR. Cricopharyngeal muscle dysfunction in the differential diagnosis of dysphagia in polymyositis. Arthritis Rheum 1980;23:491

69. Dobrowski JM, Zajtchuk JT, LaPiana FG, Hensley SD. Oculopharyngeal muscular dystrophy: clinical and histopathologic correlations. Otolaryngol Head Neck Surg 1986;9:131

70. Dohlman G, Mattson O. The endoscopic operation for hyopharyngeal diverticula. Arch Otolaryngol 1960;71:744

71. Doyle DR, McCurley TL, Sergent JS. Fatal polymyositis in D-penicillamine treated rheumatoid arthritis. Ann Intern Med 1983;98:327

72. Dumitru D. Electrodiagnostic Medicine. Philadelphia: Hanley and Blefus, 1995

73. Duranceau A, Forand MD, Fateux JP. Surgery in oculopharyngeal muscular dystrophy. Am J Surg 1980;139:33

74. Duranceau A, Lafontaine ER, Taillefer R, Jamieson GG. Oropharyngeal dysphagia and operations on the upper esophageal sphincter. Surg Annu 1987;19:317

75. Duranceau CA, Letendre J, Clermont RJ, Levesque HP, Barbeau A. Oropharyngeal dysphagia in patients with oculopharyngeal muscular dystrophy. Can J Surg 1978;21:326

76. Duranceau A, Rheault MJ, Jamieson GG. Physiological response to cricopharyngeal myotomy and diverticulum suspension. Surgery 1983;94:655

77. Eadie MJ, Tyrere JH. Alimentary disorder in Parkinsonism. Aust Ann Med 1965;14:13

78. Edwards D. Discriminatory value of symptoms in the differential diagnosis of dysphagia. Clin Gastroenterol 1976;5:49

79. Edwards LL, Eamonn BS, Quigley MM, Pfeiffer RF. Gastrointestinal dysfunction in Parkinson's disease: frequency and pathophysiology. Neurology 1992;42:726

80. Edwards LL, Pfeiffer RF, Quigley EMM, Hofman R, Balluff M. Gastrointestinal symptoms in Parkinson's disease. Mov Disord 1991;6:151

81. Edwards LL, Quigley EM, Harned RK, Hofman R, Pfeiffer RF. Characterization of swallowing and defecation in Parkinson's disease. Am J Gastroenterol 1994;89:15

82. Ekberg O. Dimension of the pharyngo-esophageal segment in dysfunction of the cricopharyngeal muscle. Acta Radiol Diagn 1986;27:539

83. Ekberg O, Bergqvist D, Takolander R, Uddman R, Kitzing P. Pharyngeal function after carotid endarterectomy. Dysphagia 4:151

84. Ekberg O, Lindgren S. Effect of cricopharyngeal myotomy on pharyngoesophageal function: pre- and postoperative cineradiographic findings. Gastrointest Radiol 1987;12:1

85. Ekberg O, Malmquist J, Lindgren S. Pharyngo-oesophageal webs in dysphageal patients. A radiologic and clinical investigation in 1134 patients. Rofo Fortschr Geb Rontgenstr Nuklearmed 1986;145:75

86. Ekberg O, Nylander B. Dysfunction of the cricopharyngeal muscle. Radiology 1982;143:481

87. Ekberg O, Nylander G. Pharyngeal dysfunction after treatment for pharyngeal cancer with surgery and radiotherapy. Gastrointest Radiol 1983;8:97

88. Ellis FH, Crozier RE. Cervical esophageal dysphagia. Indications for and results of cricopharyngeal myotomy. Ann Surg 1981;194:279

89. Ellis FH, Schlegal JF, Lynch VP, Payne WS. Cricopharyngeal myotomy for pharyngoesophageal diverticulum. Ann Surg 1969;170:340

90. Ergun GA, Kahrilas PJ, Logemann JA. Interpretation of pharyngeal manometric recordings: limitations and variability. Dis Esophagus 1993;6:11

91. Fenton JE, Hone S, Gormley P, O'Dwyer TP, Timon CI. Hypopharyngeal tumours may be missed on flexible oesophagogastroscopy. BMJ 1995;311:623

92. Fisher RA, et al. Esophageal motility in neuromuscular disorders. Ann Intern Med 1965;63:229

93. Fonda D, Schwarz J, Clinnick S. Parkinsonian medication one hour before meals improves symptomatic swallowing: a case study. Dysphagia 1995;10:165

94. Gaze M, Wilson J, Gilmour H, MacDougall R, Maran A. The effect of laryngeal irradiation on pharyngoesophageal motility. Int J Radiat Oncol Biol Phys 1991;21:1315

95. Goetz CG, Lutge W, Tanner CM. Autonomic dysfunction in Parkinson's disease. Neurology 1986;36:73

96. Gordon C, Hewer RL, Wade DT. Dysphagia in acute stroke. BMJ 1987;295:411

97. Gregory RP, Smith PT, Rudge P. Tardive dyskinesia presenting as severe dysphagia. J Neurol Neurosurg Psychiatry 1992;55:1203

98. Gresham SL. Clinical assessment and management of swallowing difficulties after stroke. Med J Aust 1990;153:397

99. Grob D, Brunner NG, Namba T. The natural course of myasthenia gravis and effect of therapeutic measures. Ann NY Acad Sci 1981;377:652

100. Groher ME. The prevalence of swallowing disorders in two teaching hospitals. Dysphagia 1986;1:3

101. Groher ME. Bolus management and aspiration pneumonia in patients with pseudobulbar dysphagia. Dysphagia 1987;1:215

102. Grunebaum M, Salinger H. Radiologic findings in polymyositis-dermatomyositis involving the pharynx and upper oesophagus. Clin Radiol 1971;22:97

103. Gullane PJ, Willett JM, Heenaman H, Greenway RE, Ruby RE. Zenker's diverticulum. Arch Otolaryngol 1983;12:53

104. Halama AR. Surgical treatment of oropharyngeal swallowing disorders. Acta Otorhinolaryngol Belg 1994;48:217

105. Harrison MS. The aetiology, diagnosis and surgical treatment of pharyngeal diverticula. J Laryngol 1958;72:523

106. Hartelius L, Svensson P. Speech and swallowing symptoms associated with Parkinson's disease and multiple sclerosis: a survey. Folia Phoniatr Logop 1994;46:9

107. Hayashi T, Nishikawa T, Koga I, Uchida Y, Yamawaki S. Life-threatening dysphagia following prolonged neuroleptic therapy. Clin Neuropharmacol 1997;20:77

108. Hellemans J. Pelemans W, Vantrappen G. Pharyngoesophageal swallowing disorders and the pharyngoesophageal sphincter. Med Clin North Am 1981;65:1148

109. Hietaharju A, Jaaskelainen S, Kalimo H, Hietarinta M. Peripheral neuromuscular manifestations in systemic sclerosis (scleroderma). Muscle Nerve 1993;16:1204

110. Horner J, Alberts MJ, Dawson DV, Cook GM. Swallowing in Alzheimer's disease. Alzheimer Dis Assoc Disord 1994;8:177

111. Horner J, Massey E. Silent aspiration following stroke. Neurology 1988;38:317

112. Horner J, Massey EW, Riski JE, Lathrop DL, Chase KN. Aspiration following stroke: clinical correlates and outcome. Neurology 1988;38:1359

113. Hunt PS, Connell AM, Smiley TB. The cricopharyngeal sphincter in gastric reflux. Gut 1970;11:303

114. Hunter PC, Crameri J, Austin S, Woodward MC, Hughes AJ. Response of parkinsonian swallowing dysfunction to dopaminergic stimulation. J Neurol Neurosurg Psychiatry 1997;63:579

115. Hurwitz AL, Nelson JA, Haddad JK. Oropharyngeal dysphagia: manometric and cine-esophagographic findings. Am J Dig Dis 1975;20:313

116. Isberg A, Nilsson ME, Schiratzki H. Movement of the upper esophageal sphincter and a manometric device during deglutition, a cineradiographic investigation. Acta Radiol Diagn 1985;26:381

117. Ivanyi B, Phoa SS, de Visser M. Dysphagia in postpolio patients: a videofluorographic follow-up study. Dysphagia 1994;9:96

118. Jackson C, Shallow TA. Diverticula of esophagus, pulsion, traction, malignant and congenital. Ann Surg 1926;83:1

119. Jacob H, et al. The esophageal motility disorder of polymyositis. A prospective study. Arch Intern Med 1983;143:2262

120. Jamieson GG, Duranceau AC, Payne WS. Pharyngo-esophageal diverticulum. In Jamieson GG, ed, Surgery of the Oesophagus. Edinburgh: Churchill Livingstone, 1988:435

121. Johnson CC, Kuwabara T. Oculopharyngeal muscular dystrophy. Am J Ophthalmol 1974;77:872

122. Johnson ER, McKenzie SW. Kinematic pharyngeal transit times in myopathy: evaluation for dysphagia. Dysphagia 1993;8:35

123. Johnson F, Shaw D, Gabb M, Dent J, Cook I. Influence of gravity and body position on normal oropharyngeal swallowing. Am J Physiol 1995;269:G653

124. Johnston BT, Li Q, Castell JA, Castell DO. Swallowing and esophageal function in Parkinson's disease. Am J Gastroenterol 1995;90:174

125. Jones B, Buchholz DW, Ravich WJ, Donner MW. Swallowing dysfunction in the postpolio syndrome: a cinefluorographic study. Am J Roentgenol 1992;158:283

126. Jones B, Ravich WJ, Donner MW, Kramer SS. Pharyngoesophageal interrelationships: observations and working concepts. Gastrointest Radiol 1985;10:225

127. Kahrilas P, Dodds W, Hogan W. Effect of peristaltic dysfunction on esophageal volume clearance. Gastroenterology 1988;94:73

128. Kahrilas P, Logemann J, Shezhang L, Ergun G. Pharyngeal clearance during swallowing: a combined manometric and videofluoroscopic study. Gastroenterology 1992;103:128

129. Kahrilas PJ, Clouse RE, Hogan WJ. American Gastroenterological Association technical review on the clinical use of esophageal manometry. Gastroenterology 1994;107:1865

130. Kahrilas PJ, Dodds WJ, Dent J, Logemann JA, Shaker R. Upper esophageal sphincter function during deglutition. Gastroenterology 1988;95:52

131. Kahrilas PJ, Lin S, Logemann JA, Ergun GA, Facchini F. Deglutitive tongue action: volume accommodation and bolus propulsion. Gastroenterology 1993;104:152

132. Kilman WJ, Goyal RK. Disorders of pharyngeal and upper esophageal sphincter motor function. Arch Intern Med 1976;136:592

133. Kluin KJ, Bromberg MB, Feldman EL, Simmons Z. Dysphagia in elderly men with myasthenia gravis. J Neurol Sci 1996;138:49

134. Knuff TE, Benjamin SB, Castell DO. Pharyngoesophageal (Zenker's) diverticulum: a reappraisal. Gastroenterology 1982;82:734

135. Kodama M, Sawada H, Udaka F, Kameyama M, Koyama T. Dysphagia caused by an anterior cervical osteophyte: case report. Neuroradiology 1995;37:58

136. Konowitz PM, Biller HF. Diverticulopexy and cricopharyngeal myotomy: treatment for the high risk patient with a pharyngoesophageal (Zenker's) diverticulum. Otolaryngol Head Neck Surg 1989;100:146

137. Krause P, Castro WH. Cervical hyperostosis: a rare cause of dysphagia. Case description and bibliographical survey. Eur Spine J 1994;3:56

138. Kuhlemeier KV. Epidemiology and dysphagia. Dysphagia 1994;9:209

139. Lahey FH. Pharyngo-esophageal diverticulum: its management and complications. Ann Surg 1946;124:617

140. Langmore SE, Schatz K, Olsen N. Endoscopic and videofluoroscopic evaluations of swallowing and aspiration. Ann Otorhinolaryngol 1991;100:678

141. Lazarus CL, et al. Swallowing disorders in head and neck cancer patients treated with radiotherapy and adjuvant chemotherapy. Laryngoscope 1996;106:1157

142. Leder SB. Gag reflex and dysphagia. Head Neck 1996;18:138

143. Leder SB. Videofluoroscopic evaluation of aspiration with visual examination of the gag reflex and velar movement. Dysphagia 1997;12:21

144. Leopold NA. Dysphagia in drug-induced parkinsonism: a case report. Dysphagia 1996;11:151

145. Leopold NA, Kagel MC. Prepharyngeal dysphagia in Parkinson's disease. Dysphagia 1996;11:14

146. Leopold NA, Kagel MC. Pharyngo-esophageal dysphagia in Parkinson's disease. Dysphagia 1997;12:11

147. Lerut T, Van Raemdonck D, Guelinckx P. Pharyngo-oesophageal diverticulum (Zenker's). Clinical therapeutic and morphological aspects. Acta Gastroenterol Belg 1990;53:330

148. Lichter I. Motor disorder in pharyngoesophageal pouch. J Thorac Cardiovasc Surg 1978;76:272

149. Lieberman AN. Dysphagia in Parkinson's disease. Am J Gastroenterol 1980;74:157

150. Lim HC, Nigro MA, Beierwaltes P, Tolia V, Wishnow R. Nitrazepam-induced cricopharyngeal dysphagia, abnormal esophageal peristalsis

and associated bronchospasm: probable cause of nitrazepam-related sudden death. Brain Dev 1992;14:309

151. Linden P, Siebens A. Dysphagia: predicting laryngeal penetration. Arch Phys Med Rehabil 1983;64:281

152. Lindgren S. Endoscopic dilatation and surgical myectomy of symptomatic cervical esophageal webs. Dysphagia 1991;6:235

153. Lindgren S, Ekberg O. Cricopharyngeal myotomy in the treatment of dysphagia. Clin Otolaryngol 1990;15:221

154. Liston SL. Lateral pharyngeal diverticula. Otolaryngol Head Neck Surg 1985;93:582

155. Logemann J, Blonsky ER, Boshes B. Lingual control in Parkinson's disease. Trans Am Neurol Assoc 1973;98:276

156. Logemann JA. Evaluation and Treatment of Swallowing Disorders. San Diego: College Hill Press, 1983

157. Logemann JA. The role of the speech language pathologist in the management of dysphagia. Otolaryngol Clin North Am 1988;21:783

158. Logemann JA. Role of the modified barium swallow in management of patients with dysphagia. Otolaryngol Head Neck Surg 1997;116:335

159. Logemann JA, et al. Impact of the diagnostic procedure on outcome measures of swallowing rehabilitation in head and neck cancer patients. Dysphagia 1992;7:179

160. Logemann JA, et al. Speech and swallow function after tonsil/base of tongue resection with primary closure. J Speech Hear Res 1993;36:918

161. Logemann JA, et al. Mechanisms of recovery of swallow after supraglottic laryngectomy. J Speech Hear Res 1994;37:965

162. Logemann JA, Blonsky ER, Boshes B. Dysphagia in parkinsonism. JAMA 1975;231:69

163. London SF, Gross KF, Ringel SP. Cholesterol-lowering agent myopathy (CLAM). Neurology 1991;41:1159

164. Lueck W, Calligan J, Bosma JF. Persistent sequelae of bulbar poliomyelitis. J Pediatr 1952;41:549

165. MacDougall G, Wilson JA, Pryde A, Grant R. Analysis of the pharyngoesophageal pressure profile in amyotrophic lateral sclerosis. Otolaryngol Head Neck Surg 1995;112:258

166. Mantoni M, Ostri B. Acquired lateral pharyngeal diverticulum. J Laryngol Otol 1987;101:1092

167. Masters CL, Dawkins RL, Zilko PJ, Simpson JA, Leedman RJ, Lindstrom J. Penicillamine-associated myasthenia gravis, antiacetylcholine receptor and antistriational antibodies. Am J Med 1977;63:689

168. May EF, Calvert PC. Aggravation of myasthenia gravis by erythromycin. Ann Neurol 1990;28:577

169. Mayberry JF, Atkinson M. Swallowing problems in patients with motor neuron disease. J Clin Gastroenterol 1986;8:233

170. McConnel FM, et al. Surgical variables affecting postoperative swallowing efficiency in oral cancer patients: a pilot study. Laryngoscope 1994;104:87

171. McConnel FMS, Cerenko D, Hersh T, Weil LJ. Evaluation of pharyngeal dysphagia with manofluorography. Dysphagia 1988;2:187

172. McConnel FMS, Cerenko D, Mendelsolm MS. Dysphagia after total laryngectomy. Otolaryngol Clin North Am 1988;21:721

173. Miller AJ. Neurophysiological basis of swallowing. Dysphagia 1986;1:91

174. Miller CD, Oleshansky MA, Gibson KF, Cantilena LR. Procainamide-induced myasthenia-like weakness and dysphagia. Ther Drug Monit 1993;15:251

175. Miller LG, Janovic J. Metoclopramide-induced movement disorders. Arch Intern Med 1989;149:2486

176. Ming RH, Dreosti LM, Tim LO, Segal I. Thyrotoxicosis presenting as dysphagia. A case report. South Afr Med J 1982;61:554

177. Moser G, et al. High incidence of esophageal motor disorder in consecutive patients with globus sensation. Gastroenterology 1991;101:1512

178. Mulder CJJ, den Hartog G, Robijn RJ, Thies JE. Flexible endoscopic treatment of Zenker's diverticulum: a new approach. Endoscopy 1995;27:438

179. Mulder D. The Diagnosis and Treatment of Amyotrophic Lateral Sclerosis. Boston: Houghton Mifflin, 1980

180. Muller-Miny H, Eisele DW, Jones B. Dynamic radiographic imaging following total laryngectomy. Head Neck 1993;15:342

181. Murray J, Langmore SE, Ginsberg S, Dostie A. The significance of oropharyngeal secretions and swallowing frequency in predicting aspiration. Dysphagia 1996;11:99

182. Murray JP. Deglutition in myasthenia gravis. Br J Radiol 1962;35:43

183. Negus VE. The etiology of pharyngeal diverticula. Johns Hopkins Hosp Bull 1957;100:209

184. Newson-Davis J. Myasthenia gravis and related syndromes. In Walton J, Karpati G, Hilton-Jones D, eds, Disorders of Voluntary Muscle. Edinburgh: Churchill Livingstone, 1994:761

185. Oh SJ, Kim DE, Kuruoglu R, Bradley RJ, Dwyer D. Diagnostic sensitivity of the laboratory tests in myasthenia gravis. Muscle Nerve 1992;15:720

186. Olsson R, Castell JA, Castell DO, Ekberg O. Solid-state computerized manometry improves diagnostic yield in pharyngeal dysphagia: simultaneous videoradiography and manometry in dysphagia patients with normal barium swallows. Abdom Imaging 1995;20:230

187. Osserman KE, Genkins G. Studies in myasthenia gravis: review of a 20 year experience in over 1200 patients. Mt Sinai J Med 1971;38:497

188. Osterberg T, Landahl S, Hedergard M. Salivary flow, saliva, pH and buffering capacity in 70 year old men and women. J Oral Rehabil 1984;11:157

189. Pace-Balzan A, Habashi SMZ, Nassar WY. View from within: radiology in focus. Lateral pharyngeal diverticulum. J Laryngol Otol 1991;105:793

190. Papandoulos SM, Chen JC, Fledenzer JA, Bucci MN, McGillicuddy JE. Anterior cervical osteophytes as a cause of progressive dysphagia. Acta Neurochirurg 1989;101:63

191. Pauzner R, Blatt I, Mouallem M, Ben-David E, Farfel Z, Sadeh M. Mitochondrial abnormalities in oculopharyngeal muscular dystrophy [see comments]. Muscle Nerve 1991;14:947

192. Payne SW, King RM. Pharyngo-esophageal (Zenker's) diverticulum. Surg Clin North Am 1983;63:815

193. Poirier NC, Bonavina L, Taillefer R, Nosadini A, Peracchia A, Duranceau A. Cricopharyngeal myotomy for neurogenic oropharyngeal dysphagia. J Thorac Cardiovasc Surg 1997;113:233

194. Polland WS, Bloomfield AL. Experimental referred pain from the gastrointestinal tract. Part I. The esophagus. J Clin Invest 1931;10:435

195. Porubsky ES, Murray JP, Pratt LL. Cricopharyngeal achalasia in dermatomyositis. Arch Otolaryngol 1973;78:428

196. Pratt MF, Meyers PK. Oculopharyngeal muscular dystrophy: recent ultrastructural evidence for mitochondrial abnormalities. Laryngoscope 1986;96:368

197. Ramsay ID. Thyrotoxic muscle disease. Postgrad Med J 1968;44:385

198. Robbins J, Logemann J, Kirshner H. Swallowing and speech production in Parkinson's disease. Ann Neurol 1986;19:283

199. Saffouri MH, Ward PH. Surgical correction of dysphagia die to cervical osteophytes. Ann Otol 1974;83:65

200. Salvesen R, Brautaset NJ. Oculopharyngeal muscular dystrophy in Norway. Survey of a large Norwegian family. Acta Neurol Scand 1996;93:281

201. Sanders DB, Howard JF. Disorders of neuromuscular transmission. In Bradley WG, Daroff RB, Fenichel GM, Marsden CD, eds, Neurology in Clinical Practice, vol 2 Boston: Butterworth-Heinemann, 1991:1819

202. Schima W, et al. Globus sensation: value of static radiography combined with videofluoroscopy of the pharynx and oesophagus. Clin Radiol 1996;51:177

203. Schmidt J, Holas M, Halvorson K, Reding M. Videofluoroscopic evidence of aspiration predicts pneumonia and death but not dehydration following stroke. Dysphagia 1994;9:7

204. Scobey MW. Secondary motility disorders. In Castell DO, Richter JE, Dalton CB, eds, Esophageal Motility Testing. Amsterdam: Elsevier Science, 1987:163

205. Seaman WB. Cineroentgenographic observations of the cricopharyngeus. Am J Roentgenol 1966;96:922

206. Seaman WB. Roentgenology of pharyngeal disorders. In Margulis AR, Burhenne HJ, eds, Alimentary Tract Roentgenology. St Louis: Crosby, 1973:305

207. Sears VW, Castell JA, Castell DO. Radial and longitudinal asymmetry of human pharyngeal pressures during swallowing. Gastroenterology 1991;101:1559

208. Shaker R, Ren J, Kern M, Dodds WJ, Hogan WJ, Li Q. Mechanisms of airway protection and upper esophageal shincter opening during belching. Am J Physiol 1992;262:G621

209. Shapiro BE, Rordorf G, Schwamm L, Preston DC. Delayed radiation-induced bulbar palsy. Neurology 1996;46:1604

210. Shapiro J, Martin S, DeGirolami U, Goyal R. Inflammatory myopathy causing pharyngeal dysphagia: a new entity. Ann Otol Rhinol Laryngol 1996;105:331

211. Shaw DW, Cook IJ, Jamieson GG, Gabb M, Simula ME, Dent J. Influence of surgery on deglutitive upper esophageal sphincter mechanics in Zenker's diverticulum. Gut 1996;38:806

212. Siebens H, et al. Correlates and consequences of eating dependency in institutionalized elderly. J Am Geriatr Soc 1986;34:192

213. Sieffert A. Zur Behardlung beginnender hypopharynx-diverykel. J Laryngol Rhinol Otol 1932;23:256

214. Silbergleit AK, Waring WP, Sullivan MJ, Maynard FM. Evaluation, treatment, and follow-up results of post polio patients with dysphagia. Otolaryngol Head Neck Surg 1991;104:333

215. Simpson JA. Myasthenia gravis and myasthenic syndromes. In Walton JN, ed, Disorders of Voluntary Muscle (4th ed). London: Churchill Livingstone, 1981:585

216. Skinner DB, Altorki N, Ferguson M, Little G. Zenker's diverticulum: clinical features and surgical management. Dis Esophagus 1988;1:19

217. Smithard DG, et al. The natural history of dysphagia following a stroke. Dysphagia 1997;12:188

218. Smithard DG, et al. Complications and outcome after acute stroke: does dysphagia matter? Stroke 1996;27:1200

219. Sobol SM, Rigual NR. Anterolateral extrapharyngeal approach for cervical osteophyte induced dysphagia. Ann Otol Rhinol Laryngol 1984;93:498

220. Sokol EM, Heitmann P, Wolf BS, Cohen BR. Simultaneous cineradiographic and manometric study of the pharynx, hypopharynx, and cervical esophagus. Gastroenterology 1966;51:960

221. Sonies BC, Dalakas MC. Dysphagia in patients with the post polio syndrome. N Engl J Med 1991;324:1162

222. Splaingard ML, Hutchins B, Sulton LD, Chaudhuri G. Aspiration in rehabilitation patients: videofluoroscopy vs bedside clinical assessment. Arch Phys Med Rehabil 1988;69:637

223. Stevens MB, Hookman P, Siegel CI, Esterly JR, Shulman LE, Hendrix T. Aperistalsis of the oesophagus in patients with connective tissue disorders and Raynaud's phenomenon. N Engl J Med 1964;270:1218

224. Stewart M, Johnston RA, Stewart I, Wilson JA. Swallowing performance following anterior cervical spine surgery. Br J Neurosurg 1995;9:605

225. St Guily JL, Zhang K-X, Perie S, Copin H, Butler-Browne GS, Barbet JP. Improvement of dysphagia following cricopharyngeal myotomy in a group of elderly patients. Ann Otol Rhinol Laryngol 1995;104:603

226. Strand EA, Miller RM, Yorkston KM, Hillel AD. Management of oral-pharyngeal dysphagia symptoms in amyotrophic lateral sclerosis. Dysphagia 1996;11:129

227. Stroudley J, Walsh M. Radiological assessment of dysphagia in Parkinson's disease. Br J Radiol 1991;64:890

228. Stuart D. Dysphagia due to cervical osteophytes. Int Orthop 1989;13:95

229. Sweatman MC, Chambers L. Disordered oesophageal motility in thyrotoxic myopathy. Postgrad Med J 1985;61:619

230. Taileffer R, Duranceau AC. Manometric and radionuclide assessment of pharyngeal emptying before and after cricopharyngeal myotomy in patients with oculopharyngeal dystrophy. J Thorac Cardiovasc Surg 1988;95:868

231. Tandan R, Bradley WG. Amyotrophic lateral sclerosis. Part I: Clinical features, pathology, and ethical issues in management. Ann Neurol 1985;18:271

232. Taylor EW. Progressive vagus-glossopharyngeal paralysis with ptosis. J Nerv Ment Dis 1915;42:129

233. Thomas M, Haigh RA. Dysphagia, a reversible cause not to be forgotten. Postgrad Med J 1995;71:94

234. Thompson W, Heaton K. Heartburn and globus on apparently healthy people. CMAJ 1982;126:46

235. Tiomny E, et al. Esophageal smooth muscle dysfunction in oculopharyngeal muscular dystrophy. Dig Dis Sci 1996;41:1350

236. Tison F, et al. Effects of central dopaminergic stimulation by apomorphine on swallowing disorders in Parkinson's disease. Mov Disord 1996;11:729

237. Tymms KE, Webb J. Dermatopolymyositis and other connective tissue diseases: a review of 105 cases. J Rheumatol 1985;12:1140

238. Van Ruiswyk J, Cunningham C, Cerletty J. Obstructive manifestations of thyroid lymphoma. Arch Intern Med 1989;149:1575

239. Veis S, Logemann J. Swallowing disorders in persons with cerebrovascular accident. Arch Phys Med Rehabil 1985;66:372

240. Verma A, Bradley WG, Adesina AM, Sofferman R, Pendlebury WW. Inclusion body myositis with cricopharyngeus muscle involvement and severe dysphagia. Muscle Nerve 1991;14:470

241. Victor M, Hayes R, Adams RD. Oculopharyngeal muscular dystrophy: a familial disease of late life characterized by dysphagia and progressive ptosis of the eyelids. N Engl J Med 1962;267:1267

242. Viets HR. Diagnosis of myasthenia gravis in patients with dysphagia. JAMA 1947;134:987

243. Waldenstrom J, Kjellberg S. Roentgenologic diagnosis of sideropenic dysphagia (Plummer-Vinson syndrome). Acta Radiol 1939;20:618

244. Walker AE, Robins M, Weinfield FD. Clinical findings: in the National Survey of Stroke. Stroke 1981;12(Suppl. 1):417

245. Walther EK. Dysphagia after pharyngolaryngeal cancer surgery. Part 1: Pathophysiology of postsurgical deglutition. Dysphagia 1995;10:275

246. Walton J, Karpati G, Hilton-Jones D. Disorders of Voluntary Muscle (6th ed). Edinburgh: Churchill Livingstone, 1994

247. Watson WL, Bancroft FW. Hypertrophic cricopharyngeal stenosis. Surg Gynecol Obstet 1936;62:621

248. Waxman MJ, Durfee D, Moore M, Morantz RA, Koller W. Nutritional aspects and swallowing function of patients with Parkinson's disease. Nutr Clin Pract 1990;5:196

249. Webb WA, McDaniel L, Jones L. Endoscopic evaluation of dysphagia in two hundred and ninety-three patients with benign disease. Surg Gynecol Obstet 1984;158:152

250. Weber J, et al. Esophageal manometry in patients with unilateral hemispheric cerebrovascular accidents or idiopathic Parkinsonism. J Gastrointest Motil 1991;3:98

251. Welch RW, Luckmann K, Ricks PM, Drake ST, Gates GA. Manometry of the normal upper esophageal sphincter and its alterations in laryngectomy. J Clin Invest 1979;63:1036

252. Welsh LW, Welsh JJ, Chinnici JC. Dysphagia due to cervical spine injury. Ann Otol Rhinol Laryngol 1987;96:112

253. Wilcox CM, Alexander LN, Clark WS. Localization of an obstructing esophageal lesion. Is the patient accurate? Dig Dis Sci 1995;40:2192

254. Wilson CP. Pharyngeal diverticula, their cause and treatment. J Laryngol Otol 1962;76:151

255. Winstein CJ. Neurogenic dysphagia: frequency, progression, and outcome in adults following head injury. Phys Ther 1981;63:1992

256. Witterick IJ, Gullane PJ, Yeung E. Outcome analysis of Zenker's diverticulectomy and cricopharyngeal myotomy. Head Neck 1995;17:382

257. Wortman RL. Inflammatory disease of muscle and other myopathies. In Kelley WN, Harris ED, Ruddy S, Sledge CB, eds, Textbook of Rheumatology, vol 2. Philadelphia: WB Saunders, 1997:1177

258. Wouters B, van Overbeek JJ. Endoscopic treatment of the hypopharyngeal (Zenker's) diverticulum [see comments]. Hepatogastroenterology 1992;39:105

259. Wyllie E, Wyllie R, Cruse RP, Rothner AD, Erenberg G. The mechanism of nitrazepam-induced drooling and aspiration. N Engl J Med 1986;314:35

260. Young EC, Durant-Jones L. Developing a dysphagia program in an acute care hospital: a needs assessment. Dysphagia 1990;5:159

261. Zenker FA, von Ziemssen H. Dilatations of the esophagus. In Cyclopaedia of the Practice of Medicine, vol III. London: Low, Marston, Searle and Rivington, 1878:46

The Esophagus, Third Edition,
edited by D. O. Castell and J. E. Richter.
Published by Lippincott Williams & Wilkins, Philadelphia, 1999.

# CHAPTER 10

# Achalasia

## Roy K. H. Wong and Corinne L. Maydonovitch

Achalasia is a motor disorder of the esophagus characterized by loss of esophageal peristalsis and failure of the lower esophageal sphincter (LES) to completely relax upon deglutition. This chapter will discuss the pathologic findings and pathophysiology of achalasia, as well as appropriate medical and surgical treatment, and review new advances in the possible treatment and assessment of achalasia.

## HISTORICAL PERSPECTIVE

In 1674, Sir Thomas Willis [386] recounted the case of a patient with a dilated esophagus who was successfully treated by dilation with a whale bone. Tyson and co-workers [368] described a dilated esophagus without evidence of a stricture, and von Mikulicz [379] estimated that at least 100 cases of cardiospasm had been reported. Initially, the term *simple ectasia* was used to describe the entity; however, because no stricture was noted on endoscopy, von Mikulicz [379] felt that *cardiospasm* was the etiologic factor. Hurst [190] was the first person to use the term *achalasia* in describing the inability of the LES to relax normally.

Initial attempts to explain the etiology of achalasia were both innovative and amusing. Bassler [21] and Jackson [192] theorized that the narrowed esophageal segment represented the tight crura of the diaphragm, and Zenker and von Ziemssen [402] and others suggested a loss of esophageal peristalsis as the primary disorder. Other postulated mechanisms included pressure by the tips of the lungs on the distal esophageal segment, encroachment on the esophagus by the "liver tunnel," twisting and kinking of the long esophagus, and fibrosis of tissue surrounding the esophagus [259–261].

The opinions and assertions contained herein are the personal views of the authors and are not to be construed as reflecting the views of the U.S. Department of the Army or Department of Defense. This work was written by government employees using government resources.

R. K. H. Wong and C. L. Maydonovitch: Gastroenterology Service, Walter Reed Army Medical Center, Washington D.C. 20307-5001.

## GROSS AND MICROSCOPIC PATHOLOGY OF THE ESOPHAGUS

In early achalasia, minimal esophageal dilation may be noted; however, esophagi as large as 16 cm have been reported in longstanding disease [223]. Histologically, epithelial thickening with basal cell hyperplasia, papillary elongation, widening of the stratified zone, and pathologic cornification has been reported, and in longstanding achalasia, small ulcers may extend into the submucosa or muscularis [223]. Endoscopic ultrasound reveals wall thickening proximal to the gastroesophageal junction over a 4-cm length in achalasia patients with tortuous esophagi [371]. Electron microscopy of the esophageal muscle may reveal surface membrane detachment of myofilaments and cellular atrophy and hypertrophy at the transition zone between the dilated and undilated esophagus [51, 170]. Other nonspecific ultrastructural findings include filament disarray, mottling of the fiber density in myocytes, thick and long cytoplasmic dense bodies, long dense plaques, and few nexus junctions [136].

## NEUROPATHOLOGIC FINDINGS

Eight neuropathic lesions have been described: (a) early on in the disease process, when the esophagus is not dilated, inflammation of the myenteric plexus without a decrease in myenteric ganglion cells or neurofibrosis, especially in patients with vigorous achalasia [149]; (b) later in the disease process, loss of ganglion cells within the myenteric plexus of the distal esophagus [49, 77, 80, 223, 252, 373] and middle third of the stomach [80]; (c) a decrease in varicose nerve fibers of the myenteric plexus [380]; (d) degenerative changes of the vagus nerve [49]; (e) quantitative and qualitative changes in the dorsal motor nucleus of the vagus [49, 209]; (f) marked decreases in small intramuscular nerve fibers, as well as a decrease in vasointestinal peptide (VIP) and neuropeptide Y immunostaining of nerve fibers [136, 380]; (g) paucity of vesicles in small nerve fibers [136]; and

(h) occasional intracytoplasmic inclusions (Lewy bodies) in the dorsal motor nucleus of the vagus and myenteric plexus [302].

Lendrum [223] examined 13 cadaveric esophagi with idiopathic esophageal dilation and noted an average of 0.31 ganglion cells per plexus, whereas the controls averaged six. Lendrum emphasized the fact that multiple observations of tissue were essential for accurate assessment of ganglion cells. A study utilizing silver stains noted the complete absence of argyrophilic neurons, with replacement of the myenteric plexus by Schwann cells. In two cases, only argyrophilic neurons were noted, but no inflammatory infiltration of the myenteric plexus or vagal damage was seen.

Cassella and co-workers [49] noted significantly fewer myenteric ganglion cells throughout the esophagus in seven of nine achalasia specimens when compared to control specimens, whereas two had fewer ganglion cells only in the distal 2 cm of the undilated portion of the esophagus. Specimens of patients having symptoms for longer than 10 years had fewer ganglion cells than those with symptoms of less than 10 years' duration. Csendes et al. [80] studied the myenteric plexus of 34 achalasia patients and noted normal jejunums but absence of plexus in 91% of distal esophagi and 20% of the middle third of the stomachs studied. Peak acid output was significantly decreased, and no correlation could be made between the number of ganglion cells present in the stomach and acid secretion. Anatomic and physiologic vagal nerve abnormalities have been reported. Wallerian degeneration of vagus nerves was noted on electron microscopy by Cassella and colleagues [50]. These findings were characteristic of experimental nerve transection with degeneration of myelin sheaths, disintegration of the axoplasm, and changes in Schwann cells. Light microscopic studies often showed no vagal degeneration [124, 223]. Utilizing the Hollander test to determine vagal nerve function, Wollam and associates [389] found no acid stimulation in eight of 32 patients and a delayed response in two patients, suggesting complete or partial vagotomy. Betazole stimulated acid in all patients, indicating normal parietal cell function. Dooley and colleagues [98] noted impaired acid secretion and release of pancreatic polypeptides in seven of 13 achalasia patients following sham feeding, while Annese and associates [12] noted increased gastric emptying with a liquid meal. Eckardt and co-workers [110] recently noted that some achalasia patients had autonomic defects of both the gastrointestinal and cardiovascular systems. Other neurologically mediated reflexes, such as transient LES relaxations, are altered in achalasia. Holloway and colleagues [180, 182] noted significantly fewer transient LES relaxations in achalasia patients versus normals following gastric distention and postulated a defect in the same inhibitory nerves affecting swallowing. Likewise, distention of the midesophagus results in impaired LES relaxation [288, 325] but preservation of proximal phases of contraction, suggesting a defect in the intrinsic inhibiting innervation but preservation of extrinsic vagal reflexes [288]. An abnormal belch reflex of the upper esopha-

geal sphincter (UES) has been documented and associated with an increase, rather than a decrease, in UES pressure following esophageal air installation in an achalasia patient [23, 239]. Others showed a significant reduction in gallbladder ejection fraction and emptying [12, 110, 180].

In a meticulous study, Cassella and co-workers [49] described less than ten dorsal motor nuclei per section in achalasia patients as compared to 30 to 60 nuclei in controls. Kimura [209] also noted degenerative vagal nuclear changes in two achalasia patients.

In ultrastructural studies on achalasia specimens, Friesen and colleagues [136] noted a consistent decrease in small intramuscular nerve fibers with an associated paucity of granules. These findings coincide with immunohistochemical studies which show decreases in VIP and neuropeptide Y in nerve fibers located in the longitudinal and circular muscles, indicating damage to the inhibiting motor neurons. In the myenteric plexus, varicose nerve fibers are uncommon while nonvaricose fibers and neuropeptide Y are present, suggesting damage to the intrinsic neurons but intact extrinsic nerve fibers [380].

Although pathologic findings in achalasia have been well substantiated and described from the brain to the most peripheral aspects of the lower motor neuron, the initial site of injury is unknown. Whether the primary site of the disease begins in the brain or esophageal myenteric plexus is open to speculation [176, 177].

## PHARMACOLOGIC STUDIES TO DETERMINE THE SITE OF DENERVATION

Normally, the LES is in a relative state of constant contraction, and in animals this results from the release of intracellular $Ca^{2+}$, a process which is regulated by inositol triphosphate [29]. Stimuli such as swallowing or esophageal distention initiate primary or secondary peristalsis, resulting in LES relaxation [56, 147]. Electrical signals initiating primary peristalsis begin in the dorsal motor nuclei of the vagus and are transmitted via long preganglionic vagal neurons to shorter postganglionic inhibitory neurons located near the LES. From animal [30, 157, 160] and human [221, 331] studies, VIP and dopamine-containing nerve fibers or nonadrenergic, noncholinergic (NANC) inhibitory neurons release the neurotransmitter VIP and dopamine, which stimulate VIP and dopamine-2 receptors. VIP stimulation activates intramuscular adenylate cyclase, which results in an increase in intracellular adenosine 3'5'-cyclic adenosine monophosphate (cAMP) concentration and LES relaxation. Depending on the type of stimulus, increased concentrations of intracellular 3'5'-cyclic guanosine monophosphate (cGMP) are also associated with LES relaxation. In opossums, electrical and nitroprusside stimulations result in increased cGMP levels and LES relaxation, whereas VIP, isoproterenol, and dopamine increase cAMP levels with concomitant LES relaxation [265, 359]. The intermediate mechanism by which VIP induces LES relaxation is not completely understood. In isolated guinea pig gastric fundic muscle cells, VIP released presynaptically stimulates intracellular nitric oxide synthase (NOS) and the production of nitric oxide (NO), resulting in muscle relaxation. However, NO diffusion from the smooth muscle cells back to the presynaptic region enhances the presynaptic secretion of VIP [165]. In isolated rabbit gastric smooth muscle, VIP acts through a receptor-mediated G protein to activate NOS [266]. Immunohistochemical studies indicate that NOS may also be localized in the neurons of the myenteric plexus and may thus enhance VIP release or have direct effects on smooth muscle relaxation via NO production [72].

It is apparent that in achalasia the inhibitory mechanisms of the circular LES muscle are impaired. Studies from isolated LES muscle strips from achalasia patients suggest that the absence of ganglionic inhibitory stimulation results in unopposed LES contraction [252]. Likewise, during electrical field stimulation, circular muscle strips from achalasia patients contract rather than relax, while stimulation of longitudinal muscles of achalasia patients and controls results in relaxation [360]. This effect on the circular muscle resulted from muscarinic receptor activation. LES hypersensitivity to exogenous gastrin in achalasia patients suggested denervation of the LES [64], although intravenous gastrin decreases LES pressure in aganglionic Chagas' disease patients [277]. Morphine and secretin decrease LES pressure in achalasia patients [278], while intravenous cholecystokinin (CCK) paradoxically increases LES pressure [95]. The inhibitory effect of CCK is probably neurally mediated as it is abolished by tetrodotoxin. Intravenous VIP infusion results in decreased LES pressure and increased LES relaxation only in patients with achalasia but not in normal controls [167]. Ultimately, the neuropathic abnormalities of achalasia result in VIP and NO depletion of the myenteric plexus and nerve fiber connections of the LES and distal esophagus [5] as measured by immunohistochemistry for VIP and reduced nicotinamide adenine dinucleotide phosphate (NADPH) diaphorase, a marker of neuronal NOS [245, 380].

In the opossum, destruction of the esophageal myenteric plexus with benzalkonium compounds results in an achalasia-like esophagus manometrically, histologically, pharmacologically, and biochemically. The LES of these esophagi were unresponsive to infused arginine and showed a decrease in NADPH diaphorase activity but an increase in cholinergic nerve bundles, suggesting greater cholinergic input in the face of a markedly damaged NOS system, which would result in a hypertensive LES [141, 335].

## ETIOLOGY

Close review of case studies indicates that there may be several etiologies to "idiopathic achalasia." Present data implicate familial [208, 229, 232, 267], autoimmune [252], infectious [195, 310, 311], or environmental causes. Review of achalasia case studies shows an age distribution for the disease of between birth and the ninth decade of life, occur-

ring rarely during the first two decades of life. Mean ages for achalasia patients in case studies ranged between 30 and 60 years, with a peak in the 40s [186], an incidence of 0.4 to 1.1 per 100,000 [107, 139, 242, 243, 341], and a prevalence of 7.9 to 12.6 per 100,000 population [243].

Reports of familial achalasia represent less than 1% of all achalasia cases. In 1984, Zimmerman et al. [404] counted 66 reported cases of familial achalasia, and subsequently 20 more cases have been reported in the literature. Most reported familial cases are horizontally transmitted, occurring in the pediatric age group and between siblings and even monozygotic twins [38, 109, 345]. Many of the horizontally transmitted cases result from consanguineous unions with reports from northwest Mexico [174] and India [84] and from among French Canadian/North American [244] and Apache [384] native populations. With an early childhood onset, usually before age 5, associated anomalies can occur, such as adrenocorticotropic hormone insensitivity, alacrima, microcephaly, Sjögren's syndrome, short stature, nerve deafness, vitiligo, hyperlipoproteinemia, and autonomic and motor neuropathy [10, 57, 114, 115, 122, 142, 162, 163, 171, 174, 188, 203, 217, 249, 255, 270, 293, 295, 315, 333, 348, 365, 377, 381]. The likely mode of inheritance in these reports is autosomal recessive, with full penetrance in the homozygous form. In a recent startling linkage study, the gene for the triple A syndrome was localized to chromosome 12q13 near the type II keratin gene cluster [381].

Of the vertically transmitted cases, only five reports are noted in the literature [53, 208, 244, 403, 404]. Unlike horizontally transmitted achalasia, vertically transmitted achalasia is rarer, occurring in a significantly older population (range, 37 to 72 years; mean age, 56 years) and probably has a different etiology.

While familial achalasia represents less than 1% of the achalasia population, the majority of cases have no obvious etiology. Mayberry and Atkinson [241] studied 167 families of patients with achalasia to determine the familial occurrence of the disease. Of 447 siblings contacted, none had achalasia, although the Mendelian principle would predict 112 affected siblings if achalasia were an autosomal recessive disorder.

Misiewicz and colleagues [252] suggested an autoimmune etiology when they noted round cell infiltration of ganglion cells only in mildly dilated distal esophagi. Similarly, Goldblum and colleagues [149] noted myenteric inflammation with ganglion cells in three patients with vigorous achalasia but no ganglion cells in eight patients exhibiting classic achalasia with mild to moderate esophageal dilation. Monocytic infiltration of myenteric ganglion cells was also noted by Lendrum [223] and Cassella and co-workers [49]. In studies from our laboratory at Walter Reed Army Medical Center (WRAMC) [393], we found an association between achalasia and a class II histocompatibility antigen, Dqw1, which also suggested an autoimmune process. We theorized that an infectious or toxic inflammatory process stimulated interferon-γ release, thereby inducing class II antigen expression on neural tissue. Recognized as foreign antigens, T lymphocytes would ultimately destroy the neural tissue. An insidious process, the neuropathology could mimic a long-term degenerative neurologic disorder, initially associated with lymphocytic infiltration but eventually resulting in Schwann cell replacement. Further data to support an autoimmune process come from two studies which noted serum antibodies to neurons of the myenteric plexus in 39% to 64% of patients with achalasia. In one study [378], none of the normal and gastroesophageal reflux disease (GERD) patients had antibodies, while in the other study, 4/54 healthy controls, 2/22 peptic esophagitis and myasthenia gravis patients, and none of the Hirschspring's or esophageal cancer patients had antibodies [346]. Antibodies stained both the NADPH-positive (NOS) and -negative neurons [378].

Pursuing the possibility of an infectious etiology, Jones and associates [195] performed complement fixation tests to measles virus in achalasia patients and noted significantly higher antibody titers in achalasia patients as compared to controls. Likewise, Robertson and co-workers [310] found a significant correlation between varicella-zoster complement fixation titers in 58 achalasia patients versus 40 controls. A subsequent study utilizing DNA hybridization techniques to identify varicella-zoster in esophageal tissue was positive in three of nine achalasia specimens but negative in 20 matched controls [311]. Recent studies utilizing polymerase chain reaction techniques examined 13 achalasia myotomy specimens for herpes, measles, and human papillomavirus and found no evidence of viral particles [32].

An association between neurologic disorders and achalasia has also been described. Qualman and colleagues [302] noted Lewy bodies in degenerating ganglion cells of the myenteric plexus and vagal dorsal motor nucleus in patients with achalasia and Parkinson's disease. Also, two separate case reports [264] describe achalasia associated with hereditary cerebellar ataxia, and a large epidemiologic study noted an association between Parkinson's disease, depressive disorders, and other myoneural disorders [341]. From these studies, one can suggest that there are probably three general etiologic categories of achalasia: (a) idiopathic achalasia, which represents approximately 98% of cases reported; (b) familial achalasia, which is genetically transmitted; and (c) achalasia associated with degenerative neurologic diseases, such as Parkinson's disease and cerebellar ataxia. Other disease states associated with achalasia have been reported (Table 10–1), but their role as possible etiologies of achalasia are unlikely.

**TABLE 10–1.** *Diseases associated with achalasia or achalasia-like presentation*

| Disease | References |
| --- | --- |
| Unconjugated hyperbilirubinemia | 130 |
| Hirschsprung's disease | 18 |
| Congenital tracheoesophageal fistula | 272 |
| Adrenocorticotropic hormone insensitivity–alacrima | 115, 122, 142, 162, 163, 217, 255, 270, 295, 333, 348, 377 |
| Cerebellar ataxia, optic atrophy, microcephaly, mental retardation | 56, 267 |
| Hereditary nervous system degeneration | 230 |
| Double pylorus | 196 |
| Neurofibromatosis | 132 |
| Parkinson's disease | 302 |
| Hypertrophic osteoarthropathy | 67 |
| Barrett's esophagus | 219 |
| Tetanus | 92 |
| Focal nodular hyperplasia | 343 |
| Small cell carcinoma | 301 |
| Pregnancy | 125, 317 |
| Rumination | 231 |
| Beta mannosidosis | 155 |
| Sarcoidosis | 37 |
| Esophageal intramural pseudodiverticulosis | 99 |
| CREST syndrome | 140 |
| Post-polio dysphagia | 24 |
| Varicella | 52 |
| Multiple endocrine neoplasia type 2B | 145 |
| Ectodermal dysplasia syndrome | 326 |
| Autoimmune polyglandular syndrome type II | 138 |
| Sigmoid megacolon, epilepsy | 358 |

## CLINICAL PRESENTATION

The clinical presentation of achalasia varies depending on the duration of the disease process. However, there are common symptoms of achalasia patients regardless of the disease progression.

At WRAMC, 34 patients over a 4-year period were determined to have achalasia. Ages ranged from 12 to 76 years, with two-thirds being from 20 to 40 years and seven older than 50 years. Men outnumbered women by a 2:1 ratio, which is expected in a military population.

In our patients, the mean duration of symptoms at the time of evaluation was $2.6 \pm 2.5$ years, while others have noted means up to 4.4 years [16]. Forty-two percent had symptoms for less than 1 year and 32% for 2 to 3 years. Two patients had symptoms for as long as 12 years prior to presentation. Symptomatic complaints varied in type and in degree. As shown in Fig. 10–1, of 34 patients seen at WRAMC, all had solid food dysphagia. However, symptoms of regurgitation, chest pain, and heartburn were not uncommon and at times misleading to the primary physician, who misdiagnosed achalasia for gastroesophageal reflux [119, 186], esophageal spasm, or dyspepsia. On the other hand, Eckardt et al. [112] felt that the mean delay in the diagnosis of achalasia of $4.7 \pm 6.4$ years related to misinterpretation of typical findings and not to atypical symptoms.

Although solid food dysphagia was the most common and prominent symptom in all patients, many also described varying degrees of liquid dysphagia and one study noted that 97% of patients with achalasia had liquid dysphagia at presentation [186]. The onset of dysphagia was usually

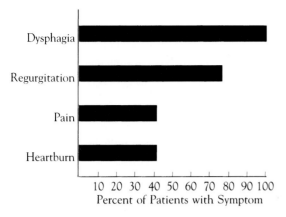

**FIG. 10–1.** Symptoms of 34 achalasia patients evaluated at Walter Reed Army Medical Center.

confined at first to solids but later included liquids. Dysphagia was described as a fullness in the chest during a meal, with a filling and even overflow sensation as the meal progressed. In many patients, the dysphagia seemed to increase in severity, reaching a plateau over time, whereas other patients noted increasing symptoms that led to significant weight loss. Two patients had such mild symptoms of dysphagia that they did not seek medical attention for 12 years.

Historically, it was difficult to quantitate the degree of dysphagia, although the length of time it takes to eat a similar quantity and consistency of food prior to the onset of symptoms is a good measure of dysphagia. Bodily maneuvers and techniques used by patients to improve their dysphagia include (a) head back position while maintaining an upright posture associated with a Valsalva maneuver; (b) drinking carbonated beverages, which increases intraesophageal pressure, although some patients refrain from this technique because of chest pain and regurgitation [398]; (c) belching; (d) drinking alcoholic beverages or warm liquids; and (e) smoking marijuana. Cigarette smoking had no effect, and leafy vegetables caused severe dysphagia in two patients.

The second most common symptom was regurgitation. Regurgitated food was described as undigested, nonbilious, and generally nonacidic. However, fermented intraesophageal contents may taste and become acidic over time [76, 339]. During sleep or early in the morning, many patients were awakened by coughing or choking spells resulting from regurgitation of a characteristic white, foamy material representing the accumulation of intraesophageal saliva. Surprisingly, no patients developed aspiration pneumonia despite nocturnal regurgitation, but this may be related to the relatively young population studied as others have noted more pulmonary complications [341]. Regurgitation sometimes occurred when patients tried "pumping" food down with liquids or when vomiting was voluntarily induced to relieve chest discomfort or to empty the esophagus prior to going to bed. Patients adapted to these problems by elevating the head of the bed at night and refraining from eating large meals prior to bedtime. Substernal chest pain was noted in

42% of patients, with studies indicating that chest pain is more frequently seen in younger patients [61] and less likely to be associated with dysphagia, regurgitation, and weight loss. The pain may be described as a squeezing, pressure-like sensation substernally that, at times, radiated to the neck, arms, jaws, and back, occurring nocturnally and postprandially. The xiphoid region was the most common location of pain.

Surprisingly, the symptom of classic pyrosis is a common complaint, noted in 42% of patients in our study and 36% in other studies [186]. Heartburn was not generally relieved by antacids, did not occur postprandially, and showed no evidence of gastroesophageal reflux in those patients undergoing 24-hour pH monitoring. In some patients, the heartburn did not migrate up and down retrosternally but seemed to be diffuse in one location. Interestingly, Smart and colleagues [340] suggested that achalasia may be associated with gastroesophageal reflux, and Ellis [116] reoperated on four cases of achalasia misdiagnosed as having gastroesophageal reflux. Spechler et al. [342] noted that achalasia patients who complained of heartburn had lower LES pressures than those without heartburn and that in some patients heartburn disappears with the onset of dysphagia, suggesting that GERD was present prior to the development of achalasia. On the other hand, achalasia patients may have an abnormal esophageal afferent sensory pathway as the usual arousal mechanisms during nocturnal acid exposure seem impaired [327].

**TABLE 10–2.** *Complications of achalasia*

| Complication | References |
|---|---|
| Esophagocardiac fistula | 41 |
| Esophageal squamous cell carcinoma | 58, 168, 197, 313, 332, 396 |
| Suppurative pericarditis | 135 |
| Postmyotomy Barrett's esophagus | 6, 127 |
| Distal esophageal diverticulum | 101 |
| Stridor with upper airway obstruction | 8, 9, 54, 68, 97, 148, 281, 353, 363, 367, 383 |
| Bezoar of the esophagus | 235 |
| Neck mass (bullfrog neck) | 164, 216 |
| Esophageal varices | 211 |
| Esophageal foreign body | 289 |
| Pulmonary *Mycobacterium fortuitum* | 17, 187, 202, 320 |
| Pneumopericardium | 41 |
| Esophagobronchial fistula | 133, 388 |
| Submucosal dissection esophagus | 184 |
| Esophageal perforation | 47 |
| Small cell carcinoma | 301 |
| Hiccups | 322 |
| Respiratory failure | 207 |
| Sudden death | 126 |
| Gastroesophageal intussusception | 390 |
| Esophageal bleed | 262 |

Weight loss was noted in 84% of patients with a marked variability and a mean of 13 lb. Weight loss best described the severity of achalasia, whereas weight gain correlated well with degree of improvement in esophageal emptying after treatment. Some patients maintained their weight, despite having a megaesophagus with large amounts of retained contents, while other obese patients who were successfully dilated lost weight from dieting.

While most presentations of achalasia are typical and confined to problems of dysphagia, important complications can occur in patients with large esophagi and longstanding disease. These complications are associated with three major physiologic processes: (a) displacement of mediastinal structures by the esophagus, (b) esophageal ulcerations and perforations through the esophageal wall, and (c) aspiration of esophageal contents (Table 10–2).

## PATHOPHYSIOLOGIC FEATURES

LES pressures vary in patients with achalasia. In our patients, the mean end-expiratory LES pressure was 24 + 2 mm Hg, ranging from 15 to 57 mm Hg (normal, 15 ± 5). One might expect patients with higher sphincter pressures to have more symptoms, greater weight loss, and decreased esophageal emptying; however, we and others [247] found a poor correlation between LES pressure and esophageal emptying. This suggests that other factors play a role in esophageal emptying, such as (a) the pressure generated in the distal esophagus by a fluid column, (b) changes in LES pressure over time, (c) the sensitivity and compliance of the esophagus, and (d) the intraesophageal pressure rise associated with a swallowed bolus.

Observations of radiologic studies in patients with achalasia show that the height of the barium column affects esophageal emptying [375]. As the barium column rises, the pressure generated in the distal esophagus increases until it exceeds the LES pressure and results in esophageal emptying. Esophageal emptying decreases and eventually stops as the pressure generated by height of the barium column is less than the LES pressure. This implies that the pressure generated by the height of the column should be reflected in the distal esophagus. Hence, an LES pressure of 10 and 20 mm Hg should sustain a water column with a height of 13.6 and 27 cm, respectively. If this calculation were completely correct, more patients should complain of regurgitation and food overflow as the average esophageal length is only 25 cm. Obviously, LES pressure is not the only factor affecting esophageal emptying.

In achalasia, LES response to endogenous hormones is paradoxical and relates to the loss of various inhibitory stimuli [95]. LES pressure results from the intrinsic contractile characteristics of LES smooth muscle [159, 226] in addition to the intrinsic (NANC), extrinsic (vagal), and hormonal stimuli which fluctuate throughout the day [156, 158, 304]. Patients typically note that emotionally stressful conditions promote dysphagia, and they will seek a quiet, relaxed atmo-

sphere when consuming meals. Foregoing meals for fear of esophageal pain or the embarrassment of regurgitating food in front of people is not unusual and may be an explanation for further weight loss. Recent biofeedback [324] and neuroanatomic [69] studies tend to corroborate these observations, suggesting that the central nervous system probably modulates esophageal function through extensive brain–gut neural pathways.

Esophageal sensitivity to distention may cause weight loss in some patients. Early in the disease process, when the esophagus is relatively undilated, pain and discomfort may be associated with eating. Because of regurgitation to relieve the pain, patients may develop a fear of eating and lose weight because of a decreased intake rather than impaired esophageal emptying. Adam's group [2] found that as the esophagus dilates, few symptoms of pain are noted.

Dilation probably results from the neuropathic changes in the esophagus and the pressure exerted on the esophageal wall from retained food contents. As the esophagus dilates, the esophageal wall loses its tone and the compliance increases. Also, because of the dilation, the height of the food column decreases for the same quantity of ingested material, resulting in less distal esophageal pressure, less esophageal emptying, and more stasis.

Contractions in the mid- and distal portions of the esophagus are frequently noted with and without swallows. These contractions may either promote esophageal emptying or encourage regurgitation, depending on whether intraesophageal pressures overcome the LES or cricopharyngeal sphincter. During swallowing, a fluid-filled esophagus can effectively transmit pharyngeal contraction pressures to the distal esophagus and improve emptying. In recent 24-hour esophageal ambulatory manometric study, peristaltic activity was noted in a surprising 27% of achalasia patients, but the study did not determine whether these peristaltic waves were effective at clearing the esophagus of food [44].

## RADIOLOGIC FINDINGS

In most instances, the diagnosis of achalasia is considered following a barium swallow. Early in the disease process, the esophagus may be undilated with evidence of spasm or tertiary contractions (Fig. 10–2). At this point in time, the barium swallow may be nonspecific or normal, and hence, some investigators have advocated mixing the barium with food, such as rice, to make the study more physiologic and sensitive to a physiologic obstruction [321]. Videofluoroscopy is also more sensitive at diagnosing motor disorders of the esophagus [284, 319], especially if the procedure is performed in the supine position, where gravity will not influence the flow of barium. As the disease progresses, a dilated, sometimes tortuous esophagus with a smooth, tapered "bird beak" becomes a characteristic finding. Barium typically empties into the stomach intermittently with movement of barium up and down the esophagus in vigorous achalasia. On chest x-ray or barium swallow, an air-fluid

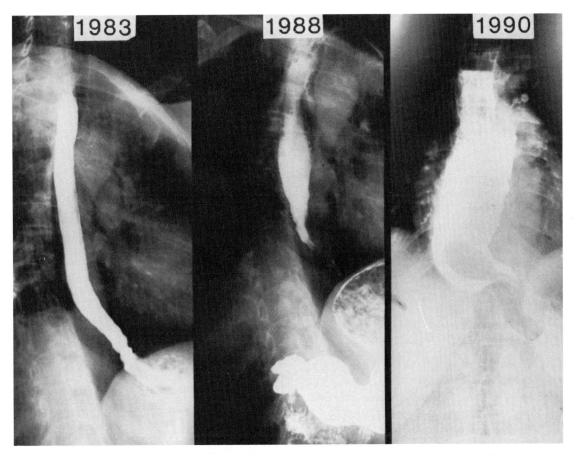

**FIG. 10–2.** Progressive dilation of the esophagus over 8 years in an achalasia patient.

level with retained food material may be seen. The distal esophageal mucosa is smooth without mucosal irregularities, nodularities, or an abrupt "shelf," suggesting carcinoma. If possible, distended views of a barium-filled gastric cardia should be obtained to rule out adenocarcinoma of the stomach. Hiatal hernia, which is relatively uncommon (6% to 14%) when compared to the normal population [31, 151, 218, 247], should be sought for because of the possible increased perforation risk during dilation, although this impression has been disputed [275]. On chest x-ray, absence of a gastric air bubble is noted in over 50% of patients, depending on esophageal size [273, 375], while mediastinal widening and/or an associated double density in an area to the right of the heart may be noted [374]. In patients with longstanding achalasia, chest x-ray may reveal pulmonary interstitial disease related to chronic aspiration.

Computerized tomography (CT) more graphically depicts these changes, with tracheal deviation to the right and anteriorly, flattening of the tracheal wall, and displacement of great vessels laterally in the area of the sternal notch. In the middle and lower esophagus, CT scans may be interpreted as a mass in the right or left hemithorax [356]. Endoscopic ultrasound studies revealed a thicker LES muscle in achalasia patients, measuring 31 mm as compared to 22 mm for normal subjects, utilizing a 20-mHz probe [251]. Addition-

ally, endoscopic ultrasound is more sensitive than CT at determining a submucosal etiology for achalasia [356], although a recent CT study suggested that an asymmetric wall diameter of greater than 10 mm at the gastroesophageal junction (GEJ) is very suggestive of pseudoachalasia [48], while a negative CT in the face of clinical suspicion for cancer should not deter further workup [361]. Classic thickening of the second and third hypoechoic layers (mucosa and submucosa) is very suggestive of an infiltrating lesion, whereas thickening of the fourth hyperechoic area represents the thicker muscularis propria (8 to 16 mm) noted in achalasia [91]. Utilizing a simple technique, Dodds and colleagues [96] determined that amyl nitrite radiographically opened the LES in achalasia but not in pseudoachalasia.

## ENDOSCOPY

Endoscopy should be performed in all achalasia patients, especially those (a) aged 50 years or older, (b) with a history of familial carcinoma, (c) with a strong history of smoking and alcohol intake, (d) with a history of gastroesophageal reflux, and (e) with a suspicious barium swallow. The endoscopic appearance of the esophageal mucosa varies depending on the degree of esophageal stasis and how well the esophagus had been lavaged prior to the procedure. In most cases, the mucosa will appear normal; however, mild erythema, whitish plaques, and punctate ulcers may be noted in a dilated esophagus that has acted as a reservoir for retained particulate matter. Endoscopy should not be employed to assess peristaltic contractions or mild esophageal dilation as esophageal manometry and barium swallow are more definitive.

Generally, resistance is noted at the GEJ, which yields to a gentle forward pressure as the endoscope "pops" into the stomach. Resistance requiring undue force to overcome is very suspect for carcinoma or peptic stricture, especially since smaller-diameter endoscopes are currently being employed [361]. Particular attention should be paid to determining the presence of a hiatal hernia, which can add to the risk of perforation during pneumatic dilation [374]. A retroflex view of the GEJ should be made to note any mucosal abnormalities, which should be biopsies for histologic examination.

## MANOMETRIC DESCRIPTION AND 24-HOUR pH

Esophageal manometry is definitive in differentiating achalasia from other esophageal motor disorders but cannot differentiate between primary achalasia and secondary achalasia due to cancer or other causes of secondary achalasia. Characteristic manometric findings of achalasia include (a) normal to elevated resting LES pressures; (b) abnormal relaxation upon deglutition; (c) lack of esophageal peristalsis upon deglutition replaced by simultaneous, low-amplitude (less than 50 mm Hg), single-peaked, widened contractions; and (d) a positive gastroesophageal gradient [44, 75]. A typical manometric tracing in achalasia is shown in Fig. 10–3. Katz and co-workers [206] have noted an apparent complete LES relaxation in 30% of achalasia patients studied. Manometrically, such relaxations were significantly shorter when compared to normal controls. Clinically, these patients did not have as severe dysphagia and may have represented an earlier phase of the disease process. While the term *vigorous achalasia* has been used loosely to identify patients with more chest pain and a very contractile esophagus, studies indicate that there is no objective clinical, manometric, or radiologic evidence for this distinction [150, 357]. Reports in the literature also indicate that nonspecific motor abnormalities, esophageal spasm, and segmental aperistalsis [248] may eventually progress to achalasia. UES abnormalities have also been noted with increased residual (UES) pressure upon swallowing [90], decreased duration of sphincter relaxation, and a more rapid pharyngeal contraction after UES relaxation [102].

Scleroderma may be manometrically confused with achalasia because of poor or absent distal esophageal aperistalsis [169, 282], although LES pressure should be abnormally low. Also, processes which obstruct the distal esophagus, such as antireflux procedures, Angelchik prosthesis, and obstructing tumors of the distal esophagus which do not invade

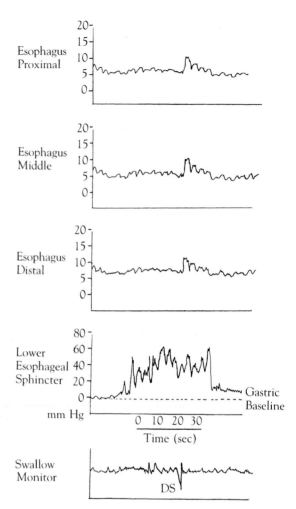

**FIG. 10–3.** Typical manometric tracing for achalasia. Four pressure recordings of the proximal, middle, and distal esophagus and the lower esophageal sphincter are shown. The **bottom tracing** is a pneumogram for swallowing. Low-amplitude, simultaneous contractions are displayed in the three esophageal leads. The lower esophageal sphincter recording displays a hypertensive pressure (40 mm Hg) that incompletely relaxes with a swallow and a positive gastroesophageal gradient (+7). *DS,* dry swallow.

the myenteric plexus, may rarely result in esophageal aperistalsis and could thus be misinterpreted as achalasia.

Twenty percent of 24-hour pH studies in achalasia have been noted to be abnormal [329], but the tracings may be difficult to interpret as retained contents in the esophagus undergo fermentation, resulting in a gradual decrement in pH, at times below pH 4 [76, 327, 329]. Hence, only sudden drops in intraesophageal pH apart from ingesting acidic foods should be considered gastroesophageal reflux. One study showed that 24-hour pH tracings in aperistaltic esophagi are reproducible [328].

## DIFFERENTIAL DIAGNOSIS

The two major differential diagnoses in achalasia are carcinoma and Chagas' disease. Chagas' disease, endemically found in Central and South America, is caused by the hemo-flagellate protozoan *Trypanosoma cruzi*. This disease should be suspected in patients who have traveled or lived in rural areas of South or Central America.

The most common malignancy mimicking achalasia is gastric carcinoma of the distal esophagus. Clinically, patients are older than 50 years, with recent dysphagia and weight loss of less than 1 year in duration [366]. Radiologically, the esophagus resembles early achalasia with mild dilation and, in some instances, a sudden acute distal taper with mucosal irregularities at the GEJ. Esophageal motility studies may be entirely characteristic for achalasia, especially in regard to failure of relaxation of LES as a result of mechanical obstruction by the tumor. Esophageal peristalsis is often absent and is attributed to invasion of the myenteric plexus by the tumor or distal esophageal obstruction. Unfortunately, one can never be certain that achalasia does not result from underlying malignancy [361]. Specific criteria have been suggested [366], although their predictive value is low [316]. Aggressive approaches to obtain tissue, amyl nitrite inhalation during barium swallow to determine the presence of LES relaxation [200], CT scanning, and endoscopic ultrasound [91] in suspected cases are reasonable.

As noted in Table 10–3, the causes of secondary achalasia are not always associated with LES tumor invasion. Even the diagnosis of gastroesophageal reflux [186] with subsequent fundoplication has been reported [119]. Anorexia nervosa [100, 300] and rumination [231] have also been misdiagnosed for achalasia. Nausea and vomiting attributed to pregnancy but caused by achalasia has also been reported [317, 389].

## TREATMENT

### Medical Therapy

Medical treatment for achalasia has focused on dilation of the obstructed, distal esophagus and recently intrasphincteric injection of botulism toxin. In the past and even more recently, transient relief was noted with fixed-diameter bougies, prompting the development of dilators which expanded once positioned in the LES.

### *Pneumatic Dilation with Polyethylene Dilator*

Because rubber dilators with expanding latex bags are no longer being manufactured, most physicians are using polyethylene balloon dilators with dilators sizes of 3.0, 3.5, and 4.0 cm.

According to the dilation technique utilized at WRAMC, after an overnight fast, the patient is taken to the radiologic suite, where the procedure is performed. Esophageal lavage with a wide-bore tube to clear retained contents may be required for patients with moderately to severely dilated esophagi. Enough intravenous medication is administered to highly sedate the patients so that the degree of pain experienced during the procedure will not influence future decisions for further dilations. Premedications include intravenous meperidine, 75 to 200 mg; midazolam, 2 to 6 mg; and in some instances, droperidol, 2.5 to 5.0 mg. Nasal $O_2$ is administered to maintain $O_2$ saturation above 90%. Upper endoscopy is performed, and retained contents are aspirated with gentle suction and lavage through the endoscope. All gastric contents should be aspirated and the endoscope should be positioned in the antrum, after a clear retroflexed view of the GEJ has been obtained to exclude cancer. Air insufflation should be kept to a minimum, and both the esophagus and stomach should be decompressed prior to passing the guide wire as intraabdominal gas may obscure visualization of the expanding air-filled balloon. A stiff guide wire (Amplatz or Savory wire) is then passed through the biopsy channel and positioned in the antrum, and the endoscope is withdrawn while advancing the guide wire to maintain its position. To allow greater mobility during the dilation, a 20-inch extension tube with a four-way stopcock is attached to the balloon insufflation orifice. Utilizing this technique, the bag, which contains between 40 and 100 cc of air, can be completely deflated with a 100 cc syringe prior to esophageal intubation and removal of the bag. The dilator is passed over the guide wire and advanced into the mouth so that the angle of the dilator as it enters the posterior pharynx is obtuse and not perpendicular to the spine. The patient may need to tilt the head backward to obtain this angle, which allows more of the force applied to the dilator to be

**TABLE 10–3.** *Causes of secondary achalasia*

| Cause | References |
|---|---|
| Adenocarcinoma of the stomach with and without involvement of the esophagus | 121, 134, 173, 316, 366 |
| Hodgkin's disease | 26, 45 |
| Hepatocellular carcinoma | 307 |
| Sarcoidosis | 104 |
| Congenital lower esophageal diaphragmatic web | 4 |
| Amyloidosis | 73, 222, 349 |
| Pancreatic pseudocysts | 395 |
| Adenocarcinoma of the lung | 152 |
| Prostate carcinoma | 108 |
| Squamous cell carcinoma of the esophagus | 313 |
| Anderson-Fabry disease | 308 |
| Postvagotomy achalasia | 294 |
| Mesothelioma | 153, 323 |
| Highly selective vagotomy | 105 |
| Chagas' disease | — |
| Esophageal lymphangioma | 352 |
| Reticulum cell sarcoma | 83 |
| Eosinophilic esophagitis | 55, 215 |
| Esophageal leiomyomatosis | 191, 237 |
| Breast carcinoma | 175 |
| Renal cell carcinoma | 236 |
| Brainstem metastasis | 1 |
| *Candida* esophagitis and transient achalasia | 34 |

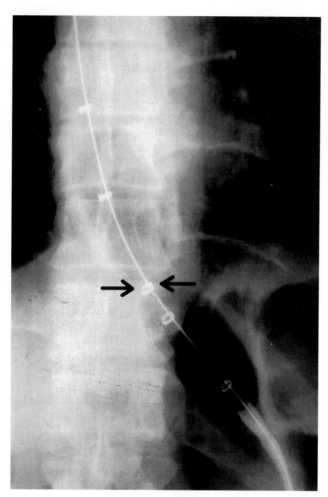

**FIG. 10–4.** Radiograph of a polyethylene dilator in the distal esophagus. Note that the radiographic indentation surrounding the pneumatic dilator *(arrows)* is positioned in the center of the dilator.

directed caudally toward the distal esophagus. With the use of stiffer guide wires, there is less difficulty in advancing the dilator through a tortuous GEJ because the stiff wire maintains a straighter pathway for the dilator to enter the GEJ. If the dilator cannot be advanced through the GEJ because the dilator tip is acutely angled, the guide wire should be slowly withdrawn while the dilator is advanced. This maneuver will straighten the bend at the GEJ and allow for easier passage. After 50% of the balloon is intubated beyond the convergence of the diaphragms, the bag is slowly inflated so that the indentation or waist created by the LES is positioned in the center of the bag. To obtain this radiographic image, several minutes of partially inflating and deflating the bag and repositioning the dilator may be required (Fig. 10–4). Once centered, the bag is rapidly inflated and held in place for 60 seconds. With large dilators, the bag will tend to migrate downward, requiring gentle upward traction on the dilator to keep the dilator centered. This aspect of the dilation is extremely important because if the dilator is not centered, the LES, which is at least 3 cm long, may not be

maximally ruptured or stretched by the dilator. Since we employ the technique of graduated dilations, the initial dilator size is always the smallest (3.0 cm diameter) and only enough air is inflated to fully expand the dilator and obliterate the waist deformity on the bag (≈7 psi). Each patient will require different dilation pressures to obliterate the waist deformity because of intrinsic differences in LES pressures, dilator size, and esophageal distendability. We do not feel that pressure is important in determining efficacy of dilation nor is it the cause of esophageal perforation but, rather, the outer diameter of a fully expanded bag. Immediately following the dilation, naloxone and flumazenil are administered to awaken the patient so that the patient can stand at 45 degrees and drink gastrograffin (30 cc) to determine the presence of an esophageal perforation. If no perforation is noted, 90 cc of barium is administered to generate a higher barium column and fully distend the distal esophagus. Small and large perforations may not otherwise be detected as the large, collapsed esophagus can easily accept and partially empty 30 cc of gastrograffin without generating enough pressure to detect a perforation site. Employing this radiologic technique, recognition of a perforation is noted within a few minutes of the dilation and can guide further intervention if necessary.

Other dilation techniques include the use of a pneumatic dilator, which surrounds the shaft of an endoscope (Witzel balloon) and is visually positioned across the LES while the endoscope is in the retroflexed position [387]. Others have used direct endoscopic visualization to position the Rigiflex achalasia balloon [213] without the use of fluoroscopy.

### Results of Pneumatic Dilation

The objective of forceful dilation is to stretch and rupture only enough circular LES muscle to allow the passage of solids and liquids without concomitant esophageal perforation or subsequent gastroesophageal reflux. Each LES muscle fiber has a unique length-tension characteristic, and the degree to which it can be stretched without complete rupture varies and is unknown. Whether a rapid, maximal, short-duration stretch is more efficacious than a rapid, submaximal, long-duration stretch is unknown because of nonstandardized approaches to pneumatic dilation (Table 10–4).

**TABLE 10–4.** *Factors that may affect the outcome of pneumatic dilation*

Premedication—effect on lower esophageal sphincter and dilation outcome
  Anticholinergics (atropine)
  Analgesics (meperidine, morphine)
  Muscle relaxants (diazepam)
Size of dilator bag
Graduated versus single-size dilation
Rate of inflation—effect on outcome and complications
Dilation pressure
Duration of dilation—length of time dilator remains inflated
Number of repeat dilations in a single session (how many repeats are considered safe in a single session?)

In viewing the literature, several comments concerning pneumatic dilation can be made (Tables 10–5, 10–6). Csendes and colleagues [78] utilized one of the largest dilators (5-cm diameter) and could only maintain complete expansion (620 to 780 mm Hg, 12 to 15 psi) for 3 to 5 seconds because of severe pain experienced by the patients. Patients refused subsequent dilations because of pain intensity, which is consistent with a previous study reporting increasing pain with larger dilators [391]. Blood was noted on the dilator, and although no frank perforations were reported, one patient developed gastroesophageal reflux. This report suggests that the LES and adjacent circular muscles and/or esophageal mucosa will not completely rupture during a short (3 to 5 seconds), rapid, large dilation. Cox and coworkers [74] dilated with a 3-cm dilator to 780 mm Hg (15 psi) for 1 minute but repeated the dilation three to five times during one session. They noted no perforations and reported good short-term results, suggesting that a submaximal stretch repeated several times may weaken esophageal circular muscle.

Others have utilized the technique of graduated pneumatic dilations. Vantrappen et al. [373] and Van Goidsenhoven et al. [372] increased the dilator size from 3.0 to 5.0 cm over a few days, while we [394], Kadakia and Wong [199], and Levine et al. [225] increased the dilator size from 2.7 to 4.0 cm over months to years depending on clinical response. Vantrappen et al. [373] noted three perforations in 133 patients, Van Goidsenhoven et al. [372] noted seven perforations in 57 patients, we [394] noted no perforations in 30 patients with 64 dilations, Kadakia and Wong [199] noted no perforations in 29 patients with 35 dilations, and Levine et al. [225] noted no perforations in 62 patients with 71 dilations. In all of these studies, greater than 80% efficacy was noted, suggesting that gradually increasing the dilator size is an effective form of therapy, but perforations may occur if large sizes are repeated too soon or prior to testing longer-term clinical efficacy.

Another important factor affecting dilation efficacy is the pressure employed during dilation. Investigators such as Kurlander et al. [212], Vantrappen et al. [375], Van Goidsenhoven et al. [372], Witzel [387], and Frimberger et al. [137] employed large Sippy, Mosher, and polyurethane dilators and insufflated with pressures of 200 to 400 mm Hg (3.8 to 7.7 psi). These pressures are insufficient to fully expand the latex balloon dilator in the patient as a similar Hurst-Tucker dilator requires at least 6 to 7 psi to fully distend at atmospheric pressure and 12 to 15 psi to fully dilate within the patient [78, 394]. These studies indicate that the maximal dilation diameters may not be attained during dilation, and therefore, comparison of dilation efficacy between these and other studies is difficult. However, polyethylene balloons are stiffer with lower compliance and are fully dilated in patients at 7 to 8 psi.

Most reports indicate significant improvement in dysphagia following pneumatic dilation, but length of follow-up and quantitative assessment methods are not always reported. At WRAMC [394], good to excellent long-term (mean, 18 months) improvement was noted in 40% of patients following a 2.7-cm-diameter dilation, with an additional 26%, 10%, and 11% of patients improving following dilation with 3.3-, 3.7-, 4.1-cm dilations, respectively. Thirteen percent of patients required surgery in this young population (mean age, 37 years). In large, long-term studies with 2 to 16 years' follow-up, 65% to 80% of patients have good to excellent results and 10% to 30% of patients have fair to poor results [266, 375]. In a recent study by Katz et al. [205], 85% of patients noted good to excellent results after a mean follow-up of 6.5 years, with 94% of patients undergoing a single pneumatic dilation. However, short-term studies note greater improvement following dilation, suggesting that dysphagia gradually worsens over time [74, 137, 143, 193, 224, 344, 387, 394]. Physiologically, LES pressures decrease following dilation but almost always increase over time and may be the reason for increased dysphagia [79].

The requirement for repeat pneumatic dilations seems to depend on several factors. Witzel [387] and Frimberger et al. [137] used a large dilator (4.0 cm) but only insufflated between 3.8 and 7.7 psi with a need to redilate in 50% to 70% of cases. Dellipiani and Hewetson [88] and Lishman and Dellipiani [227], using a modified Brown-McHardy dilator with diameters probably ranging between 3.5 and 4.0 cm, insufflated to 15 psi with a subsequent redilation requirement of less than 10%. Dellipiani and Hewetson [88], however, had perforation and gastroesophageal rates of 9% and 8%, respectively. Gelfond and Kozarek [143], using two polyurethane dilator sizes of 3.0 and 3.5 cm, noted a 30% versus 7% redilation requirement, respectively. Although only 5 to 12 psi (mean, 7.16) was employed, polyurethane dilators require less pressure to fully expand as strict radiographic observations to insure complete insufflation were reported. Our longer-term dilation studies indicate that fully expanded 2.7- and 3.3-cm dilators will have redilation rates of 60% and 33%, respectively, although our method of graduated dilation is extremely safe, with ultimate long-term success of 87% [394]. Employing the technique of graduated dilations, Kadakia and Wong [199] noted redilation rates of 38%, 21%, and 7% following dilation with polyethylene dilators of 3.0, 3.5, and 4.0 cm, respectively.

Interestingly, many investigators [111, 128, 283, 297, 309, 334, 375] agree that older patients respond favorably to pneumatic dilations when compared to younger patients, with one study reporting contrary results [146]. Vantrappen et al. [375] also reported better results in patients with a long history of dysphagia (mean duration, 8.2 years) compared to patients with a mean dysphagia history of 2.5 years, while Ponce et al. [296] noted no difference in dilation efficacy between patients with classic versus vigorous achalasia.

Immediately following dilation, LES pressure decreases but, over time, increases in varying degrees [65, 143]. A decrement in LES pressure postdilation of greater than 50% or an absolute end expiratory pressure of less than 10 mm Hg results in symptomatic improvement and in one study

**TABLE 10–5.** *Technique of forceful dilation of the cardia in treating achalasia*

| Study | Dilator | Premedication | Dilator diameter (cm) | Pressure[a] | Duration | No. of dilations during hospitalization |
|---|---|---|---|---|---|---|
| Kurlander et al. [212] | Sippy | — | 2.38–4.78[b] | 5.8 psi (300 mm Hg) | 3 min | Several |
| van Goidsenhoven et al. [372] | Sippy | — | 3–5[c] | First at 200 mm Hg/1 min | Second at 300 mm Hg/1 min | 2–4 |
| Bennett and Hendrix [27] | Hurst-Tucker | Atropine, opiate | 3.0 | 9–15 psi (465–533 mm Hg) | 30–60 sec | 1–2 total, not more than 2 per session |
| Sanderson [254] | Plummer | — | — | 9.5–10.3 psi (490–533 mm Hg) | Several seconds | — |
| Vantrappen et al. [375] | Sippy | — | See [372] | See [372] | — | 3.16–3.26 |
| Heimlich [171A] | Mosher | Scopolamine, meperidine | — | 1.38 kg/cm (1,013 mm Hg) | 5 min | — |
| Witzel [387] | Polyurethane attached to endoscope | Light sedation | 4.0 | 5.8 psi (300 mm Hg) | 2 min | Several prior to 2-min dilation |
| Frimberger et al. [137] | Rubber, nylon bag attached to endoscope | Meperidine, diazepam | 4.0 | 3.8–7.7 psi (200–400 mm Hg) | — | Probably several |
| Fellows et al. [128] | Rider-Moeller | General anesthesia | — | 5.4–5.8 psi (280–300 mm Hg) | 3 min | 1 |
| Csendes et al. [78] | Mosher | Atropine, 0.5 mg | 5.0 | 12–15 psi (620–780 mm Hg) | 3–5 sec | 2 |
| Jacobs et al. [193] | Modified Rider-Moeller | Diazepam | — | 12–15 psi (620–780 mm Hg) | — | 1 |
| Lishman and Dellipiani [227] | Modified Brown-McHardy | Omnopon, chlorpromazine, atropine | — | 15 psi (780 mm Hg) | 15 sec | 2 |
| Dellipiani and Hewetson [88] | Modified Brown-McHardy, hourglass balloon | Diazepam | 3.0 | 15 psi (780 mm Hg) | 15–20 sec | 1 |
| Cox et al. [74] | Polyurethane | Diazepam | 3.0 | 2–15 psi (105–108 mm Hg) | 60 sec | 1 |
| Levine et al. [225] | Polyurethane | — | 3.0 | 15 psi (780 mm Hg) | 60 sec | 3–5 |
| Wong and Maydonovitch [394] | Hurst-Tucker | Meperidine | 2.7, 3.1, 3.7, 4.1[d] | 9–15 psi (460–780 mm Hg) | 60 sec | 1 |
| Adams [2] | Rider-Moeller | Diazepam | — | 5.8 psi (300 mm Hg) | 3 min | 1 |
| Gelfond and Kozarek [143] | Polyurethane | None | 3.0 3.5 | 5–12 psi ($\bar{X}$ = 7.16 psi) (258–620 mm Hg) | 30 sec | 1 |
| Stark et al. [344] | Brown-McHardy | — | 3.5 | >9 psi (>465 mm Hg) | 60 sec | 1 |
| | Polyurethane | — | 3.5 | | | |
| Kadakia and Wong [199] | Polyethylene | Meperidine, diazepam | 3.0, 3.5, 4.0 | Mean, 8.8 psi | 60 sec | 1 |

$\bar{X}$ = mean of population.
[a] 1 psi = 51.7 mm Hg; 1 kg/cm = 14.2 psi.
[b] Diameter increased by 0.4 cm.
[c] Diameter increased by 3.5, 3.8, 4.0, 4.2, and 4.5 cm.
[d] If poor clinical response at 1 month or greater, the next dilator size was employed (3.3, 3.7, 4.1 cm). No more than one dilation per hospitalization.

**TABLE 10–6.** *Results of forceful dilation of the cardia in treating achalasia*

| Study | Year | No. of patients (% total) | Excellent | Fair | Poor | No. of perforations | Surgery for complications |
|---|---|---|---|---|---|---|---|
| Kurlander et al. [212] | 1963 | 62 | 32 | 56 | 8 | 10 | — |
| van Goidsenhoven et al. [372] | 1963 | 57 | 98 | — | 2 | 7 | — |
| Bennett and Hendrix [27] | 1970 | 48 | 70 | 11 | 19 | 3 | 1 |
| Sanderson [254] | 1970 | 408 | 81 | — | 19 | 14 | 10 |
| Vantrappen et al. [375] | 1971 | 133 | 77 | 17 | 6 | 3 | 1 |
| Heimlich [171A] | 1978 | 25 | 84 | — | 16 | — | — |
| Witzel [387] | 1981 | 39: 9 (23%),[b] 30 (77%)[c] | — 90 — | | 10 | 0 | 0 |
| Frimberger et al. [137] | 1981 | 11: 3 (27%),[a] 3 (27%),[b] 4 (36%),[c] 1 (9%)[d] | 88 | 18 | — | 0 | 0 |
| Csendes et al. [78] | 1981 | 18: 12 (66%),[a] 3 (17%),[b] 3 (17%),[f] 1 (7%)[g] | 66 | — | 40 | 0 | 0 |
| Lishman and Dellipiani [227] | 1982 | 18: 2 (11%)[g] | 55 | 33 | 11 | 0 | 0 |
| Fellows et al. [128] | 1983 | 63: 37 (59%),[a] 9 (14%),[b] 5 (7.9%),[c] 5 (7.9%),[d] 2 (3.1%),[e] 5 (7.9%)[f] | — 61 — | | 39 | — | 1 (1.6%) |
| Jacobs et al. [193] | 1983 | 30: 25 (83%),[a] 5 (17%),[b] 2 (7%)[f] | — 83 — | | 17 | 1 | 0 |
| Dellipiani and Hewetson [88] | 1986 | 45: 38 (84%),[a] 2 (4%),[b] 2 (4%),[c] 4 (8%)[g] | 53 | 31 | 16 | 4 | 1 |
| Cox et al. [74] | 1986 | 8: 7 (87.5%),[a] 1 (12.7%)[b] | — 88 — | | 13 | 0 | 0 |
| Levine et al. [225] | 1987 | 17 | — 100 — | | | 2(?) | |
| Wong and Maydonovitch [394] | 1989 | 30: 12 (40%),[a] 8 (27%),[b] 3 (10%),[c] 2 (7%),[d] 5 (17%)[f] | — 83 — | | 17 | 0 | 0 |
| Adams [2] | 1989 | 44: 32 (72%),[a] 10 (22%),[b] 2 (6%)[c] | | | | 7 tears, 2 complete ruptures | 0 |
| Gelfond and Kozarek [143] | 1989 | 10 (3.0 cm): 7 (70%),[a] 2 (20%)[b] | — 70 — | | 30 | 0 | 0 |
| | | 14 (3.5 cm): 13 (93%),[a] 1 (7%)[a,f] | — 93 — | | 7 | | |
| Stark et al. [344] | 1990 | 10 Brown-McHardy (3.5 cm) | 100 | — | | 0 | 0 |
| | | 10 polyurethane (3.5 cm) | 70 | — | 30 | 0 | |
| Kadakia and Wong [199] | 1993 | 29: 18 (62%),[a] 5 (17%),[b] 4 (14%),[c] 2 (7%)[f] | — 93 — | | 7 | 0 | 0 |

[a] One dilation.
[b] Two dilations.
[c] Three dilations.
[d] Four dilations.
[e] More than four dilations.
[f] Failed; underwent myotomy.
[g] Developed gastroesophageal reflux.

was the single most valuable factor predicting long-term clinical response [12]. Relaxation of the LES with swallowing does not return after dilation and neither does coordinated esophageal peristalsis [128, 375], although recent reports seem to suggest otherwise in small numbers of patients [78, 79, 81, 214, 298].

Gastroesophageal reflux is not a significant problem, as noted in numerous older dilation reports, although recent 24-hour pH studies shed new insight on acid reflux. Vantrappen and co-workers [375] found no evidence of reflux utilizing a modified reflux test. Bennett and Hendrix [27] noted that 17% of patients had symptoms and radiologic evidence for reflux but found no evidence of peptic stricture. Csendes and associates [79] reported a single case of gastroesophageal reflux in a dilation series of 18 patients, while Dellipiani et al. [88] noted gastroesophageal reflux in four of 45 dilated patients and one with a peptic stricture. Shoenut et al. [330] studied achalasia patients pre- and postdilation and myotomy with 24-hour pH monitoring. There were no significant differences between pre- and posttreatment gastroesophageal reflux in either form of therapy, although 12/32 patients had a percent total time of greater than 6% following treatment. Benini et al. [25] noted that 22% (5/22) of patients undergoing pneumatic dilation developed GERD on 24-hour pH monitoring, but postdilation LES pressures and gastric emptying were similar between the reflux and nonreflux groups. Only esophageal clearance of acid was delayed in the GERD group. Endoscopically, one patient had grade I esophagitis and another had an esophageal ulcer. Burke et al. [42] studied this problem in eight achalasia patients and found two patients with abnormal pH studies before and two following dilation. In one patient, the abnormal pH profile was related to acidic residue and a lactate concentration of greater than 2 mmol/L. There was no clinical correlation between chest pain, heartburn, and intraesophageal acid reflux. The mild GERD noted following dilation was of no clinical significance.

In longer prospective evaluation of 40 achalasia patients, Wehrmann et al. [382] showed a significant increase in the number and duration of reflux episodes postdilation, but only one patient reported having heartburn and one asymptomatic patient was noted to have esophagitis. While these data suggest that a certain degree of gastroesophageal reflux does occur pre- and postdilation, the clinical manifestations are minimal.

It is surprising that more esophageal perforations have not been reported as the physiologic basis of dilation success depends on the traumatic disruption of esophageal mucosa and muscle. Endoscopic ultrasound studies at the level of the diaphragm immediately following pneumatic dilation reveal mucosal and submucosal thickening which resolves in 24 hours [318]. Indeed, blood on the dilator and severe pain during dilation have been clinical hallmarks of dilation success and probably represent mucosal and muscular tears. Nair et al. [268] noted that repeat dilations, a psi of greater than 11, blood on the dilator, fever, and chest pain of greater

than 4 hours' duration were factors associated with esophageal perforation. Borotto and colleagues [36] identified two risk factors for esophageal perforation: minimal weight loss and high-amplitude esophageal contractions of greater than 50 mm Hg in the distal esophagus. The reported incidence of esophageal perforation varies from 0% to 15%, with most studies reporting rates between 0% and 4%. Of 70 reported perforations, 64% of patients did well with conservative treatment, while 26% underwent surgery, with a 4% mortality rate (Table 10–6). As noted in Table 10–6, the reported incidence of esophageal perforation has decreased over the last 10 years, which may relate in part to the use of fixed-sized polyethylene dilators or to the awareness of dilator size. However, because polyethylene dilators are stiffer (low compliance) as compared with the older, softer, latex dilators (higher compliance), concern that these dilators have caused more perforations has arisen. Eckardt et al. [113] noted that the overall morphologic and symptomatic complication rate was higher at 32%. Morphologic complications in 12/67 (18%) patients included one perforation, two intramural hematomas, and nine diverticula at the GEJ following dilation, while symptomatically ten patients (15%) had prolonged postdilation pain. While not significant, patients who had postdilation pain tended to do slightly better, while those with traumatic diverticula did worse over 10 years. However, many patients in this study did not receive conscious sedation and the diverticula were not associated with any symptoms or complications, so the actual complication rate may not be as high as reported. To ensure a safe dilation, a graduated size technique should be utilized beginning with the smallest diameter (3.0 cm), and caution should be exercised in patients with hiatal hernias.

A study comparing dilation efficacy between two different dilators of similar size (3.5 cm) and technique was performed [344]. Clinical and quantitative parameters assessing success were significantly better following dilation with a Brown-McHardy versus the newer polyurethane dilators. These differences may relate to the length of the bag (Brown-McHardy, 15 cm versus polyurethane, 10 cm) or the ability to position the LES radiographically in the center of the dilator. In another comparative study between a 4.0-cm-diameter, latex (high-compliance) balloon and a 3.5-cm-diameter rigid (low-compliance) balloon, there was no significant difference in overall outcome [263]. Although, the diameter of the latex balloon was larger, an inflation pressure of 6 psi was used, which may not result in complete distention of the balloon.

### Treatment of Esophageal Perforations

In a careful radiographic study, Adams and colleagues [3] noted four major postdilation findings: (a) linear mucosal tears; (b) contained perforations penetrating beyond the muscular wall; (c) diverticular mucosal outpouching just proximal to, within, or below the LES; and (d) free perforations into the mediastinum, pleural space, or peritoneal cavity. In most instances, linear tears are asymptomatic, requiring no therapy, but when symptomatic they can be treated conservatively with nothing by mouth and intravenous antibiotics [254]. One recent study used metallic clips to close a small, confined perforation [385]. Patients with contained perforations beyond the muscular wall should be treated with intravenous antibiotics, receive nothing by mouth, and nasogastric suction proximal to the perforation. In most studies, free perforations require immediate thoracic surgery and drainage; however, medical treatment with hyperalimentation and intravenous antibiotics has been successful [47, 250, 351]. Special emphasis should be placed on aspirating and removing debris from the esophagus prior to dilation as a prophylactic measure should a complete perforation occur. Pricolo et al. [299] suggest that postdilation esophageal perforations can probably be surgically managed by repair of the perforation alone without the addition of an esophagomyotomy. Most perforations occur in the distal left lateral aspect of the esophagus and are noted on an anterior radiographic projection. However, lateral projections are required to exclude posterior perforations. Cadaveric studies [43, 233] suggest that Mallory-Weiss-like mucosal tears tend to occur within the GEJ, whereas muscle tears occur in the less distensible distal esophageal body. Sites of esophageal perforation originate 5 to 10 mm proximal to or 5 mm distal to the squamocolumnar junction [223], extending from a few millimeters up to 10 cm or more. This information suggests that the LES muscle is relatively resistant to complete tears, with the proximal and distal musculature most prone to perforation. To have a free perforation, tearing of both mucosa and musculature must occur; otherwise, linear tears or mucosal diverticular or wall hematomas are radiographically noted.

Postdilation barium swallows have been utilized to determine dilation efficacy and to identify esophageal perforations. Ott and colleagues [276] noted a change in lumen size from 4.2 to 7.5 mm at the GEJ but no correlation between lumen size and clinical improvement. Intramuscular hematoma and perforations were noted in nine patients, with one hematoma progressing to a free perforation 5 hours later. In another study, postdilation esophageal emptying of 8 ounces of barium did not predict dilation efficacy [220]. Agha and Lee [7] and Csendes et al. [78] noted that a gastroesophageal lumen size of 8 to 10 mm following dilation or surgery resulted in a good clinical response. Others have reported the unusual occurrence of esophageal perforation several hours following a normal postdilation barium swallow, attributing this to ischemic necrosis [400]. Some have advocated abandoning postdilation radiographic studies and inpatient admissions, citing evidence that if radiographic studies were performed only on persistently symptomatic patients, perforations would not be missed and the surgical outcome would remain unchanged [19, 43, 59]. On the other hand, Nair and colleagues [268] noted that three of four perforations were immediately identified with postprocedure barium studies, resulting in immediate interventional treatment.

## Surgery

Since Heller's first bilateral longitudinal myotomy for achalasia in 1914 [172], the technical approach to the treatment of achalasia has changed dramatically, although a single anterior lateral myotomy or modified Heller myotomy is the usual therapy. Conceptually, surgery seems to be the ideal treatment for achalasia as an LES myotomy is performed under ''controlled'' conditions. However, incising enough muscle to relieve dysphagia but not cause gastroesophageal reflux is difficult to gauge. If the entire sphincter is completely disrupted, free gastroesophageal reflux will result, but an incomplete myotomy results in recurrent dysphagia. By adding an antireflux procedure, reflux can be prevented, but dysphagia may recur with a tight wrap, especially since there is no esophageal peristalsis.

With the advent of fiberoptic techniques to perform surgery, the morbidity of achalasia surgery has decreased significantly to the point where the majority of achalasia surgery is performed laparoscopically. In one study [11], the median hospital stay and interval to resume normal activity were significantly shorter with the laparoscopic approach, although the mean intraoperative time was shorter, with the open approach requiring 125 minutes versus 178 minutes for the laparoscopic approach. Initial studies in 1993–1994 were performed thoracoscopically [290]. However, this approach is technically more difficult as a double lumen endotracheal tube needs to be intubated to deflate the left lung. With the patient in the right lateral position, the fiberscope enters the thorax perpendicular to the esophagus, thus making dissection at the distal esophagus more difficult [183]. In the past 3 years, over 95% of articles concerning achalasia surgery have described the laparoscopic approach, which also allows for a more magnified view of the GEJ as compared with a thoracotomy or laparotomy [66].

The same technical questions concerning open thoracotomies and laparotomies still exist when performing laparoscopic surgery. How long should the length of the abdominal LES and thoracic myotomy be, and should an antireflux procedure be performed? Two surgical approaches representing the extremes of therapy still exist. A complete LES myotomy includes a 1- to 5-cm incision distal to the GEJ, in which case an antireflux procedure must be performed [106, 228, 399]. The other approach would be to perform a myotomy a few millimeters distal to the GEJ and not include an antireflux procedure [116, 118–120, 271]. In the literature, most myotomies are performed by extending the incision 1 to 2 cm distal to the GEJ, in addition to including an antireflux procedure. Of the recent laparoscopic antireflux procedures (Table 10–7), the Dor procedure is the most commonly performed, probably because it is easier to mobilize the stomach and fashion an anterior fundoplication [11, 15, 35, 66, 86, 123, 201, 240, 253, 257, 291, 303, 376, 397]. This procedure also results in a looser wrap and is therefore less prone to result in dysphagia. Other antireflux procedures with equally effective results include Toupet [71, 303, 350], Nissen [87, 189], and Rossetti [70] fundoplications.

**TABLE 10–7.** *Techniques and results of laparoscopic/thorascopic myotomy*

| Reference | n | Surgery | Antireflux | Complications | Operative time | Results | 24-hr pH manometry | Esophageal emptying | Hospital days | Follow-up |
|---|---|---|---|---|---|---|---|---|---|---|
| 350 | 12 | Laparo Heller | Toupet (9) Heller alone (3) | 2 perforations repaired | 115 min | Good-excellent, 3 | 2 of 3 Heller's alone; pH ⊕ Toupet's ⊖ LESp (33.4 → 19) mm Hg | | 1.6 | 16 months |
| 312 | 9 | Laparo Heller Just below EGJ | No antireflux | | 105 min | Excellent | pH; 4 performed, all ⊕ | | | x = 14 (12–21) |
| 11 | 17 17 | Laparo Heller vs. open Heller | Dor Dor | 1 dysphagia 1 GERD | Laparo 178 min Open 125 min | | | | Laparo: 4 days Open: 10 days | |
| 253 | 14 | Laparo Heller | Dor | 3 conversions to open postoperative bleeding | x̄ = 120 min (75–210) | Excellent, 12; good, 2 | 5, Normal pH 7, Normal manometry 7, Barium meal | 7 normal | 4 (3–18) | |
| 291 | 40 | Laparo Heller | Dor | 13% conversions 5% postop conversions 8% asympt. GERD | 120 min | | | | | |
| 85 | 1 | Laparo Heller: 6 cm proximal, 2 cm distal GEJ | Anterior (Dor) | | | | Preop, 52 mm Hg S/P, 18 mm Hg BAS, no reflux | | | Intraoperative manometry |
| 397 | 4 | Laparo Heller | Dor | 1 leak 5 days later | 99 | 1 yr: no reflux, doing well | 24 hr ⊕ 4/4 patient Preop, 56 mm Hg S/P, 5 mm Hg | | 2 | 1 year |
| 201 | 3 | Laparo Heller | Dor | | | | LESp, 12 mm Hg at end of surgery Pneumoperitoneum did not affect LESp during intraop manometry | | | |
| 66 | 8 a 12 b 7 c | a: Laparo Heller Dor, 8 b: Laparo, 12 having previous dilations c: Laparo, 7 | Dor | group a = 75%, no dysphagia group b = 83%, no dysphagia | | | 6 in group b had normal 24-hr pH | | | 1–113 Laparo allows for magnified view of esophagus |
| 86 | 12 | Laparo | Dor | 10, disappearance of dysphagia 2, partial relief | | | Preop LESp 26.3 S/P, 15.5 mm Hg | | 5 (4.7–6.7) | |

| | | | | | | | S/P change in LESp | | Back to work: Thoraco 42 days vs. Laparo 12 days |
|---|---|---|---|---|---|---|---|---|---|
| 303 | 39 | Thoraco-Dor, 4 Laparo-Dor, 6 Laparo Toupet, 29 | Dor 2–3 cm below GEJ | Mild dysphagia 44% Toupet 78% Dor ? More scar over myotomy with Dor | | | Dor = 16.4 Toupet = 14.8 mm Hg Symptom HB Dor = 67% Toupet = 22% | Thoraco 4 vs. Laparo 2 | Thoraco 42 days vs. Laparo 12 days |
| 40 | 27 | Laparo Heller | None | 1 mucosal tear, treated with conversion to open | | Good 81% Moderate 19% | Reduction LESp pH 1 case, reflux | 5.5 | 1–4 yr |
| 161 | 26 | Laparo Heller | Anterior fundoplication | 1 perforation | 3.5 hr | Satisfied 90% Somewhat 10% Mild dysphagia 33% | Improved clearance pH 6/7 normal | 5.0 | |
| 15 | 43 | Laparo Heller | Dor | | | Excellent 88.4% Good 4.6% Poor 4.6% Esophagus size decreased | LESp 26.6 → 8.8 mm Hg S/P pH 5.7% abnormal 2/35 = 5.7% 1 case esophagitis | | x = 12 mo; (3–43) |
| 183 | 10 | Thoroscopy, 3 Laparo, 7 | | 1 converted to open thoraco 2° to perforation 1 repeat myotomy 2° to dysphagia 2 perforations in previously dilated patients | 125 (79–160) | Excellent 80% Good 20% Fair 10% | | 2 (1.5–3) | Converted to laparo because simpler anesthetic and surgical management |
| 257 | 21 | Laparo | | | | | | | |
| 336 | 25 | Laparo | Short cardiomyotomy | 2 mucosal tears | | Excellent 76% Good 20% Fair 4% | | 2.75 (1–13) | 1–7 yr |
| 189 | 40 | Laparo: 7 no previous Rx, 21 previous PD, 1 Botox, 6 PD + BT, 2 previous transthoracic myotomies, 3 previous laparo fundoplications | Myotomy: 6 cm above, 1 cm below GEJ, 32 postfundoplications, 7 anterior fundoplications, 1 patient with no fundoplication | 6 mucosal lacerations, 2 postoperative pneumonias, 1 moderate hemorrhage from esophageal ulcer | 3.3 | Dysphagia gone 90% Regurgitation gone 95% | | | |

PD, pneumatic dilation; BT, botulinum toxin; Laparo, laparoscopic; GEJ, gastroesophageal junction; GERD, gastroesophageal reflux disease; asympt., asymptomatic; LESp, lower esophageal sphincter pressure; thoraco, thoracotomy.

Recently, there were at least 26 publications representing over 464 patients undergoing laparoscopically modified Heller myotomies [11, 15, 35, 40, 46, 66, 70, 85, 86, 123, 161, 183, 189, 201, 253, 257, 258, 291, 303, 312, 336–338, 350, 376, 397]. Most studies averaged between ten and 20 patients (range 1 to 43), with excellent results noted in over 70% of patients. Of these publications, there are no randomized controlled studies comparing different antireflux techniques or studies comparing techniques not utilizing an antireflux procedure. Several studies [66, 303] presented experience concerning a thoracoscopic versus laparoscopic approach. The most frequent complication reported during surgery was an esophageal perforation or mucosal tear, at 4.5% [35, 40, 70, 123, 161, 183, 189, 257, 258, 336, 350, 397]. This complication was easily managed and repaired if identified at the time of surgery, at which time, in some institutions, intraesophageal methylene blue was routinely infused into the distal esophagus prior to closure to identify a possible perforation. Conversion to open laparotomy was reported in 2.1%, although this figure may be low [40, 183, 253, 291]. Other less frequent complications include hemorrhage from an esophageal ulcer 2 weeks following surgery [189].

The operative times for performing a laparoscopic Heller myotomy ranged from 99 to 210 minutes, with most ranging between 120 and 160 minutes, and the operative times did not seem to vary with the type of antireflux procedure performed. The average hospital stay was 2 to 5 days (range 1 to 18 days), with patients being able to return to work much sooner as compared with open procedures [11]. Shorter hospital stays were noted in patients undergoing laparoscopic versus thoracoscopic procedures, and the time required for a patient to assume normal activities was significantly longer for those patients undergoing a thoracoscopic myotomy [303]. Pre- and post-operative LES pressures showed significant decrements, ranging between 8.5 and 19 mm Hg [15, 40, 85, 86, 303, 338, 350, 397].

Few laparoscopic surgical series included intraesophageal 24-hour pH monitoring, and if pH monitoring was performed, it included only a segment of the cases undergoing surgery [66, 240, 253, 312, 338, 350, 397]. In two studies in which only modified Heller myotomies were performed [312, 347], reflux as measured by 24-hour pH was noted in 26% of patients, with only two patients having symptoms. Anselmino et al. [15], who performed laparoscopic Heller-Dor operations, studied 35/43 patients with 24-hour pH and noted a 5.7% reflux rate, with one patient having grade II esophagitis and the other being symptomatic. Raiser et al. [303] compared a laparoscopically performed Dor and Toupet antireflux procedure and noted less dysphagia and GERD symptoms utilizing the 270-degree Toupet procedure. Both ends of the fundoplication were sutured to the edges of the myotomy, which allowed the myotomy to remain open and the esophageal mucosa to bulge through the myotomy. Boulez et al. [40] performed Heller myotomies in 27 patients without antireflux procedures and noted good

results in 81% of cases, with slight reflux in three and dysphagia in two. Some have argued that the posterior fundoplication is more efficacious than a Dor procedure at preventing dysphagia. These authors believe that by suturing both ends of a posterior fundoplication to the myotomy incision, the myotomy will remain open and not close secondary to fibrosis, as might occur with an anterior fundoplication like the Dor procedure [303]. Other antireflux procedures reported in the older literature include a Belsey Mark IV [228], Collis repair, and diaphragmatic flap [399]. Although extremely time-consuming, intraoperative esophageal manometry has been performed to guide the extent of LES myotomy [178] and tailor antireflux repair [210]. Patients with mean LES pressures of 6.2 mm Hg had significantly less dysphagia versus those with LES pressures of 15.1 mm Hg, although the incidence of GERD was higher in the low LES pressure group [60, 280].

There is little reason to believe that the degree of GERD and dysphagia will be significantly different between open and laparoscopically performed myotomy. In the older thoracotomy literature, a range of 3% to 52% for GERD was noted [269, 305, 355], as was a dysphagia rate of 0.9% to 25% related mostly to peptic strictures [33, 118, 119], rather than an incomplete myotomy, and these figures are similar to those in the laparoscopic literature. In a small number of patients with postmyotomy-associated GERD, Barrett's esophagus may also be noted [6, 127]. Previous pneumatic dilations or esophageal perforations do not seem to affect the outcome of surgery [129, 183], although severe inflammation and scarring of the GEJ may be associated with intrasphincteric botulinum toxin injection [185]. Questions concerning length of hospital stay and morbidity are no longer issues as laparoscopically performed procedures are clearly more cost-effective and less morbid. So the major question today is whether laparoscopically performed procedures are as durable as open procedures, but this answer can only be determined over time.

In a larger reoperative achalasia study [117], reasons for repeat surgery were as follows: (a) inadequate myotomy, 37%; (b) gastroesophageal reflux, 29%; (c) previous antireflux surgery, 12%; (d) carcinoma, 8%; (e) megaesophagus, 6%; (f) paraesophageal surgery, 2%; and (g) incorrect diagnosis, 8%. Two-thirds of previous antireflux procedures were Nissen fundoplications and one-third were Belsey Mark IV procedures. All four incorrectly diagnosed patients had a previous Nissen fundoplication for what was misdiagnosed to be gastroesophageal reflux. Midesophageal squamous cell carcinoma was noted in three of four patients and adenocarcinoma of the GEJ in one patient, occurring 17 to 27 years following initial surgery. Recalcitrant dysphagia with megaesophagus required esophagogastrectomy, with patients having significant improvement. Similarly, in a series concerning complex achalasia problems [274] esophagectomies were performed for incomplete myotomies, megaesophagus, and failed myotomies with antireflux procedures.

## Pharmacologic and Newer Forms of Therapy

Because of low morbidity and ease of administration, several pharmacologic agents have been used to treat achalasia. In 1930, Ritvo and McDonald [306] administered amyl nitrate to an achalasia patient undergoing a barium swallow and noted immediate relaxation of the cardia. Subsequently, isosorbide dinitrate [314] and nifedipine [20, 62, 63, 144, 362] have been shown to decrease LES pressure by 47% to 63%, improve esophageal emptying, and reduce symptoms associated with achalasia. Likewise, DiMarino and Cohen [93], Becker and Burakoff [22], Wong et al. [392], Triadafilopouslos et al. [364], and Marzio et al. [238] have shown that beta agonists, phosphodiesterase inhibitors, calcium antagonists, and anticholinergics can significantly lower LES pressure and, in some cases, improve esophageal emptying. However, despite the initial interest in pharmacologic agents as a means of treatment, long-term experience and studies indicate that pharmacotherapy be used as a temporizing measure prior to more definitive treatment. Chronic therapy in the elderly [354] or in the pediatric age group [234] is an area of potential usefulness.

Intriguing reports of symptomatic improvement associated with decrements in LES pressure and increases in serum VIP concentrations have been noted following transcutaneous nerve stimulation of the hand [198]. Shabsin et al. [324] reported relief of chest pain in a vigorous achalasia patient following behavioral pain management, suggesting that while specific anatomic abnormalities exist in achalasia, other physiologic mechanisms in the body may be recruited to improve esophageal emptying. An interesting method of therapy using intrasphincteric injection of ethanolamine has been reported [256]. Three to four sessions were given over a 2- to 3-month period, and symptomatic long-term improvement was noted, as was a marked decrement in LES pressure. Fibrotic strictures which were easily dilated were noted in approximately 20% of patients treated.

### Botulinum Toxin

Intrasphincteric injection of the LES with botulinum toxin (Botox) represents a new and exciting therapeutic modality for the treatment of achalasia. The toxin binds to the presynaptic, parasympathetic nerve endings in the smooth muscle, producing a chemical cholinergic denervation of the LES, essentially blocking the release of acetylcholine across the neuromuscular junction [94, 194]. Reversal of the effect of botulinum toxin relates to sprouting of new terminal axons which form synaptic junctions adjacent to muscles [279].

Botox (botulinum toxin type A, Purified Neurotoxin Complex, 100 units/vial; Allergen Inc., Irvine, CA/Mougins, France) is kept at $-5°C$ prior to reconstitution and is gently diluted with 4 to 5 mL of preservative-free, sterile saline, being careful not to form bubbles during the mixing process, which would decrease the potency of the toxin [39]. Once reconstituted, the toxin should be kept at 2° to 8°C and used within 4 hours. Caution should be exercised in patients receiving aminoglycosides as these medications may potentiate the effect of the toxin. The average total dose used per session ranges between 80 and 100 units, with a concentration of 20 to 25 units per mL. Twenty to 25 units are injected into each quadrant of the LES via a sclerotherapy needle placed through the endoscope. In one study of four patients [179], the intrasphincteric botulinum toxin was administered via direct ultrasound guidance. Antibodies to the toxin may form, especially when larger doses are administered in frequent successions over a 1-month period [39].

Recognizing the pharmacologic attributes of botulinum toxin, Pasrischa et al. [287] studied the effects of Botox injection into the LES, first in piglets and then in patients with achalasia [285, 286]. Subsequently, there have been several trials ranging from 16 to 60 patients [14, 82, 131, 154, 285, 286, 369] (Table 10–8). Most trials have included patients with previous pneumatic dilations [82, 131, 154, 285] and some with modified Heller myotomies [82, 154].

The overall results of intrasphincteric botulinum toxin injection for achalasia are excellent within the first month of treatment, followed by a gradual but persistent decrease in efficacy. Within the first month of treatment, the efficacy ranged from 70% to 100% [14, 131, 154, 285], dropping to 55% to 69% and 52% to 75% at 2 and 6 months, respectively. At 1 year or greater, the efficacy of a single injection ranged from 3.2% to 36% [14, 131, 285]. In larger studies [82, 131, 285], the efficacy at 6 months and 1 year could be improved to 50% to 60% with two or more repeat treatments.

All studies measuring LES pressure [14, 82, 285] showed a marked decrement, ranging between 30% and 50% within the first month of therapy. Likewise, esophageal emptying and symptom scores for dysphagia, regurgitation, and retrosternal pain were significantly better following treatment within the first month. Responders tended to be older (51 to 55 years) in comparison to nonresponders (41 to 49 years) [82, 131, 285], and in one study [285] older patients and patients with vigorous achalasia did significantly better following botulinum toxin treatment. Immediate symptomatic improvement following botulinum toxin injection within the first 24 hours ranged between 38% and 46% [82, 131] and between 72% and 90% within the first week of injection [131, 285]. Interestingly, symptomatic improvement continued up to 2 months following treatment in a small group of patients [131]. Even patients with previous Heller myotomies and a primary Nissen fundoplication secondary to a misdiagnosis improved [13, 154].

Mild chest pain was the most frequent, untoward effect, seen in 16% to 22% [82, 285] of patients, with many of these patients having previous histories of chest pain. Rarely, the chest pain can be extremely severe, resulting in admission to the cardiac care unit to rule out a myocardial infarction. Severe GERD was seen in one patient and marked paraesophageal inflammation and adhesions in two patients undergoing modified Heller myotomy within 2 weeks and

**TABLE 10–8.** *Results of botulinum toxin treatment of achalasia*

| Reference | n | Previous dilation (D) or Heller (H) | Total Botox dose (units) | Response time | Response rate, 0–2 wk (%) | Overall response rate to Botox Rx (%) | | | | Response rate to 2nd Botox Rx (%) | | Side effects |
|---|---|---|---|---|---|---|---|---|---|---|---|---|
| | | | | | | 1 mo | 2–3 mo | 6 mo | >1 yr | Initial failure | Initial success | |
| 285 | 31 | 55% D | 80[a] | 90% 1st wk | 90 | | 55 | 65[b] | 3.2, 29+ | 79 | 21 (3/14) | 5 Chest pain<br>1 HB |
| 131 | 60 | 50% (D + H) | 80–100[c] | 38% in 24 hr<br>34% in 1 wk<br>7.5% in 2 wk<br>3.7% in 3 wk<br>9.4% in 4 wk<br>7.5% in 2 mo | 70 | 70 | | | 36<br>54[b] | 20 (1/5) | 85.7 (6/7)<br>80 (4/5)[c] | 1 Skin rash<br>1 Skin rash |
| 82 | 55 | No H, previous D not stated | 80[b] | 46% in 24 hr | 75 | | 69 | 60[b]<br>52 | | 27 (2/11) | 57.1 (4/7) | 12 Chest pain |
| 154 | 16 | 1 D, 2 H, 1 D+H, 1 Nissen | 80[c] | | | 75 | | 56[b] | | 0 (0/2) | 100 (2/2) | Wall inflammation, adhesions (2)<br>GERD (1) |
| 14 | 8 BT<br>8 D | No D or H | 100[b] | | | 100 | | 75<br>100[b] | 12.5<br>100[b] | | 100 (7/7) | Chest pain:<br>1 placebo<br>1 BT<br>1 PD |
| 369 | 22 BT<br>20 D | No D or H | 100[b] | | | 63 | 50 | 36 | 32 | 67 (4/6) | 33 | |

[a] Some up to four injections.
[b] Some up to two injections.
[c] Some up to three injections.
D, previous pneumatic dilations; H, previous Heller myotomies; BT, previous botulism toxin injection; GERD, gastroesophageal reflux disease; HB, Heartburn.

3 months following injection [185]. Transient skin rashes were noted in two patients [131, 285].

These studies indicate that intrasphincteric botulinum toxin is very effective therapy for achalasia, which persists for 3 to 6 months. However, there is a significant decrement in efficacy beyond 6 months and further injections are required to maintain efficacy. In one long-term study, as many as four treatments were administered, yet the overall efficacy was 29% at 1 to 2 years [285]. In a few patients, the efficacy of botulinum toxin may persist for over 1 year. However, the majority of patients will require repeated injections between 3 and 9 months [82, 131, 154, 285]. Also, while repeat injections may be efficacious for patients who respond initially, the duration of efficacy of subsequent injection may decrease as antibodies develop [94] or because of intrinsic characteristics of the smooth muscle. Hence, the major advantages of botulinum toxin treatment are that it is relatively simple to administer, has excellent early results with minimal side effects, and may be the treatment of choice for older debilitated patients, in whom the complications of pneumatic dilation or the morbidity of surgery cannot be tolerated. The major disadvantages are that patients who do not respond initially are unlikely to respond to further treatments, exacerbations of dysphagia following injections are expected and occur between 3 and 9 months, and subsequent injections may be less efficacious and of shorter duration, although this point is debatable [369].

Pseudoachalasia has also been treated with botulinum toxin injection [103, 131, 370]. Improvement was noted in 42% cases reported. Of the cases that responded, there were two lung cancers, with one encasing the esophagus and adenopathy at the GEJ [131] and the other being stage III [13]. A case of gastric adenocarcinoma of the cardia, cirrhosis, and severe varices also responded initially to botulinum toxin injection. In two cases [103, 370], the response was brief, lasting 3 to 4 weeks, while one lasted 5 months [131].

## Esophageal Emptying Studies

Improvement in dysphagia and weight gain are good indicators of response to treatment; however, various attempts have been made to quantify esophageal emptying. Vantrappen and associates [375] administered barium (200 mL) to patients after dilation and measured the height of the esophageal barium column at 10 and 20 seconds. Likewise, a recent study by de Oliveira et al. [89], who performed area calculations of a barium column by multiplying the height by the width, noted an excellent correlation between observers. This measurement was used in patients undergoing therapy for pneumatic dilation, and the results correlated with patients who had good versus poor dilation results. Gross and colleagues [166] used scintigraphy to monitor clearance of a meal consisting of 250 mL of milk and cornflakes radiolabeled with technetium 99m diethylenetriamine pentaacetic acid. Differences in esophageal emptying could clearly be noted between treated and untreated patients (Fig. 10–5). Berger and McCallum [28] devised a similar study utilizing a radiolabeled egg salad sandwich meal to quantitate esophageal emptying following dilation, surgery, and nifedipine administration.

In many studies, esophageal emptying did not always correlate with symptomatic improvement or with LES pressure measurements after treatment [144, 181]. This inconsistency may result from the fact that in very large esophagi the meal fills the distal esophagus without generating a substantial food column. No significant change is noted between pretreatment and posttreatment because there is little change in the height of the food column or in the hydrostatic pressure which promotes emptying.

## Medical Versus Surgical Therapy

While botulinum toxin therapy is probably the simplest and safest form of treatment for achalasia, it has become

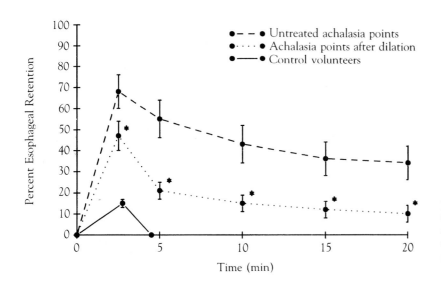

FIG. 10–5. Esophageal emptying curve for a radiolabeled test meal (technetium 99m diethylenetriamine pentaacetic acid) in ten achalasia patients before and after dilation and seven control volunteers. A significant decrease in esophageal retention is shown after pneumatic dilation at all time points. Asterisk indicates $p < 0.05$.

increasingly evident that chronic botulinum toxin therapy is required to maintain remission [14, 82, 131, 285, 369]. When the cost of Botox ($422.52 per 100-unit vial) and endoscopy is combined and multiplied by repeated therapy, the overall cost-effectiveness diminishes greatly. In the study by Pasricha et al. [285], a total of 50 injections resulted in a long-term efficacy of only 29% in 31 patients after 1 year or more of therapy. Likewise, in a randomized study comparing Botox versus pneumatic dilation, Vaezi et al. [369] noted an overall success rate of 32% after one or two injections ($n = 22$) and a 70% success rate for a single pneumatic dilation ($n = 20$) after 1 year of follow-up. No complications were noted, and improvement correlated with LES pressure and esophageal emptying only in the patients undergoing pneumatic dilation. Esophageal symptoms seem to have been blunted by the botulinum toxin as there was poor correlation between symptoms and physiologic studies in these patients. In a randomized study by Annese et al. [14], a 12% versus 100% remission rate in the Botox ($n = 8$) versus pneumatic dilation ($n = 8$) groups, respectively, was noted after one injection and several initial dilations. Following a second injection in seven patients, all patients responded so that the remission rate was 100% at around 12 months. On the other hand, Kadakia et al. [199] noted a 93% long-term response rate after 46 pneumatic dilations, utilizing graduated dilators in 29 patients. When combining three studies [199, 225, 394] which employed the technique of graduated pneumatic dilations, 121 achalasia patients had an overall long-term efficacy of over 80% with no esophageal perforations.

These data suggest that over time pneumatic dilation may be the most cost-effective form of medical therapy for achalasia and as safe as botulinum toxin therapy if a graduated dilation system is followed. On the other hand, if the first dilation starts with a balloon diameter of 3.5 to 4.0 cm, the esophageal perforation rate will range between 2% and 5% [382], and caution should be exercised in dilating patients with hiatal hernias. The therapeutic niche for botulinum toxin may be the debilitated patient who is a poor surgical candidate and is too sick to undergo pneumatic dilations.

Now that laparoscopic Heller myotomies can be performed with markedly less morbidity and cost, surgery becomes a more attractive alternative for the treatment of achalasia. The operative results should not be different from open thoracotomies or laparotomies and the major complications of GERD and dysphagia will persist. These procedures should be performed at major centers by a surgeon experienced in doing laparoscopic myotomies. There is an art to performing a myotomy, whether combined with an antireflux procedure or alone. Recurrent dysphagia associated with a tight wrap represents a net loss in outcome to the patient and physician as reoperations for achalasia are always more difficult. Erring on the side of a looser wrap, such as a Dor or Toupet, may not be unreasonable as histamine receptor antagonists and proton pump inhibitors are now readily available to treat mild GERD.

## ESOPHAGEAL CANCER

Older literature indicates that the prevalence of squamous cell carcinoma of the esophagus in patients with achalasia ranges from 1.7% to 20% [204]. Unfortunately, most studies have different population sizes and mean follow-up times, are retrospective, utilize different criteria for the diagnosis of cancer, are performed in geographically different locations, and do not consider risk factors such as smoking or alcohol ingestion. Three recent studies [16, 58, 292] with relatively large population sizes and a total of 497 patients noted one esophageal carcinoma for an overall prevalence of 0.2%. Mean follow-up times ranged between 3.6 and 6.0 years, and these studies suggest that surveillance is not feasible. On the other hand, Meijssen et al. [246] prospectively studied 195 achalasia patients with surveillance endoscopy at 3 months and 1, 2, 7, and 10 years postdilation. Carcinoma was discovered in the middle third of the esophagus in three patients at 5, 19, and 28 years following the onset of dysphagia, with the age of the patients being 89, 37, and 77 years (mean age, 68 years), respectively. The overall incidence of cancer was 3.4 per 1,000 patients per year, which was calculated to be a 33-fold increase when compared with controls. This is the most comprehensive surveillance study in the literature and suggests that there is a significant increase in squamous cell carcinoma in achalasia. However, even with achalasia as an underlying disease, the development of squamous cell carcinoma of the esophagus is multifactorial, and only when large, well-controlled studies are performed can cost-effective screening criteria be developed. Presently, if screening is to be performed, older patients and patients with long histories of dysphagia seem to be at greatest risk, although exceptions to these general guidelines exist in the literature [401].

## REFERENCES

1. Abello R, Yeakley JW, Goodman P. Secondary achalasia in a patient with brainstem metastases from lung carcinoma. J Clin Gastroenterol 1992;14:176
2. Adams CWM, et al. Achalasia of the cardia. Guys Hosp Rep 1961;110:191
3. Adams H, Roberts GM, Smith PM. Oesophageal tears during pneumatic balloon dilatation for the treatment of achalasia. Clin Radiol 1989;40:53
4. Adeyemo A, Oluwole SF, AdeKunle A. Lower esophageal diaphragm and achalasia in an adult. An unusual association. Scand J Thorac Cardiovasc Surg 1984;18:271
5. Aggestrup S, et al. Lack of vasoactive intestinal peptide nerves in esophageal achalasia. Gastroenterology 1983;84:924
6. Agha FP, Keren DF. Barrett's esophagus complicating achalasia after esophagomyotomy. J Clin Gastroenterol 1987;9:232
7. Agha FP, Lee HH. The esophagus after endoscopic pneumatic balloon dilatation for achalasia. Am J Roentgenol 1986;146:25
8. Akhter J, Newcomb RW. Tracheal obstruction secondary to esophageal achalasia. J Pediatr Gastroenterol Nutr 1988;7:769
9. Ali GN, Cook IJ, deCarle DJ, Jorgensen JO, Hunt DR. Esophageal achalasia and coexistent upper esophageal sphincter-relaxation disorder presenting with airway obstruction. Gastroenterology 1995;109:1328
10. Allgrove J, et al. Familial glucocorticoid deficiency with achalasia of the cardis and deficient tear production. Lancet 1978;1:1284
11. Ancona E, et al. Esophageal achalasia: laparoscopic versus conventional open Heller-Dor operation. Am J Surg 1995;170:265

12. Annese V, et al. Gallbladder function and gastric liquid emptying in achalasia. Dig Dis Sci 1991;36:1116
13. Annese V, et al. Perendoscopic injection of botulinum toxin is effective in achalasia after failure of myotomy or pneumatic dilation. Gastrointest Endosc 1996;44:461
14. Annese V, et al. Controlled trial of botulinum toxin injection versus placebo and pneumatic dilation in achalasia. Gastroenterology 1996;111:1418
15. Anselmino M, et al. One-year follow-up after laparoscopic Heller-Dor operation for esophageal achalasia. Surg Endosc 1997;11:3
16. Arber N, et al. Epidemiology of achalasia in central Israel. Rarity of esophageal cancer. Dig Dis Sci 1993;38:1920
17. Aronchick JM, Miller WT, Epstein DM, Gefter WB. Association of achalasia and pulmonary *Mycobacterium fortuitum* infection. Radiology 1986;160:85
18. Badrawy R, Akon-Bieh A. Congenital achalasia of the esophagus in children. J Laryngol Otol 1975;89:697
19. Barkin JS, Guerlrand M, Reiner DK, Goldberg RI, Philips RS. Forceful balloon dilation an outpatient procedure for achalasia. Gastrointest Endosc 1990;36:123
20. Bartolotti M, Labo G. Clinical and manometric effects of nifedipine in patients with esophageal achalasia. Gastroenterology 1981;80:39
21. Bassler A. Cardiospasms: what it is—what it seems to be. NY State J Med 1914;14:9
22. Becker BS, Burakoff R. The effect of verapamil on lower esophageal sphincter pressure effect in normal subjects and those with achalasia. Gastroenterology 1981;80:1107A
23. Becker DJ, Castell DO. Acute airway obstruction in achalasia. Possible role of defective belch reflex. Gastroenterology 1989;97:1323
24. Benini L, et al. Achalasia. A possible late cause of postpolio dysphagia. Dig Dis Sci 1996;41:516
25. Benini L, et al. Pathological esophageal acidification and pneumatic dilitation in achalasic patients. Too much or not enough? Dig Dis Sci 1996;41:365
26. Benjamin SB, Castell DO. Achalasia and Hodgkin's disease: a chance association? J Clin Gastroenterol 1981;3:175
27. Bennett JR, Hendrix TR. Treatment of achalasia with pneumatic dilatation. Mod Treat 1970;7:1217
28. Berger K, McCallum RW. Nifedipine in the treatment of achalasia. Ann Intern Med 1982;96:61
29. Biancani P, et al. Acute experimental esophagitis impairs signal transduction in cat lower esophageal sphincter circular muscle. Gastroenterology 1992;103:1199
30. Biancani P, Walsh JH, Behar J. Vasoactive intestinal polypeptide. A neurotransmitter for lower esophageal sphincter relaxation. J Clin Invest 1984;73:963
31. Binder HJ, et al. Rarity of hiatal hernia in achalasia. N Engl J Med 1965;272:680
32. Birgisson S, Richter JE, Rice TW, Goldblum JR, Galinski MS. Achalasia is not associated with measles or known herpes and human papilloma viruses. Dig Dis Sci 1997;42:300
33. Black J, Vorbach AN, Collis J. Results of Heller operation for achalasia of the esophagus: the importance of hiatal hernia. Br J Surg 1976;63:949
34. Bode CP, Wahn V, Lubke H, Koletzko S, Schroten H. Transient achalasia-like esophageal motility disorder after *Candida* esophagitis in a boy with chronic granulomatous disease. J Pediatr Gastroenterol Nutr 1996;23:320
35. Bonavina L, Peracchia A, Segalin A, Rosati R. Laparoscopic Heller-Dor operation for the treatment of oesophageal achalasia: technique and early results. Ann Chir Gynaecol 1995;84:165
36. Borotto E, et al. Risk factors of oesophageal perforation during pneumatic dilatation for achalasia. Gut 1996;39:9
37. Boruchowicz A, et al. Sarcoidosis and achalasia: a fortuitous association [Letter]? Am J Gastroenterol 1996;91:413
38. Bosher LP, Shaw A. Achalasia in siblings. Clinical and genetic aspects. Am J Dis Child 1981;135:709
39. BOTOX (botulinum toxin type A) purified neurotoxin complex. Allergan, Inc. September 1995 (package insert)
40. Boulez J, Espalieu P, Meeus P. Heller's esocardiomyotomy without anti-reflux procedure by the laparoscopic approach. Analysis of a series of 27 cases. Ann Chir 1997;51:232
41. Breatnach E, Han SY. Pneumopericardium occurring as a complication of achalasia. Chest 1986;90:292
42. Burke CA, Falk GW, Achkar E. Effect of pneumatic dilation on gastroesophageal reflux in achalasia. Dig Dis Sci 1997;42:998
43. Burt CAV. Pneumatic rupture of the intestinal canal with experimental data showing mechanism of perforation and pressure applied. Arch Surg 1931;22:875
44. Buttin JW, et al. A study of esophageal pressures in normal persons and patients with cardiospasm. Gastroenterology 1953;23:278
45. Buyukpamukcu M, Buyukpamukcu N, Cevik N. Achalasia of the oesophagus associated with Hodgkin's disease in children. Clin Oncol (R Coll Radiol) 1982;8:73
46. Cade RJ, Martin CJ. Thoracoscopic cardiomyotomy for achalasia. Aust N Z J Surg 1996;66:107
47. Cameron JL, et al. Selective nonoperative management of contained intrathoracic disruptions. Ann Thorac Surg 1978;27:404
48. Carter M, Traube M, Burrell MI, Smith RC, Deckmann RC. Differentiation of achalasia from pseudoachalasia by computed tomography. Am J Gastroenterol 1997;92:624
49. Cassella RR, et al. Achalasia of the esophagus: pathologic and etiologic considerations. Ann Surg 1964;160:474
50. Cassella RR, Ellis FH Jr, Brown AL. Fine structure changes in achalasia of the esophagus: I. Vagus nerves. Am J Pathol 1965;46:279
51. Cassella RR, Ellis FH, Brown AL. Fine-structure changes in achalasia of the esophagus: II. Esophageal smooth muscle. Am J Pathol 1965;46:467
52. Castex F, Cortot A, Paris JC, Colombel JF, Talbodec N, Guillemot F. Association of an attack of varicella and an achalasia [Letter]. Am J Gastroenterol 1995;90:1188
53. Chawla K, Chawla SK, Alexander LL. Familial achalasia of the esophagus in mother and son: a possible pathogenetic relationship. J Am Geriatr Soc 1979;27:519
54. Chijimatsu Y, et al. Airway obstruction in achalasia. Chest 1980;78:348
55. Chou CH, Lin XZ, Chow NH, Wu MH, Shin JS. Eosinophilic gastroenteritis with esophageal involvement. J Formos Med Assoc 1996;95:403
56. Christensen J. Motor functions of the pharynx and esophagus. In Johnson LR, ed, Physiology of the Gastrointestinal Tract. New York: Raven Press, 1987:595
57. Chu ML, Axelrod FB, Berlin D. Allgrove syndrome: documenting cholinergic dysfunction by autonomic tests. J Pediatr 1996;129:156
58. Chuong JJH, DuBovik S, McCallum RW. Achalasia as a risk factor for esophageal carcinoma. A reappraisal. Dig Dis Sci 1984;29:1105
59. Ciarolla DA, Traube M. Achalasia. Short-term clinical monitoring after pneumatic dilation. Dig Dis Sci 1993;38:1905
60. Clemente G, Picciocchi A, Nuzzo G, Granone P, D'Ugo D. Intraoperative esophageal manometry in surgical treatment of achalasia: a reappraisal. Hepatogastroenterology 1996;43:1532
61. Clouse RE, Abramson BK, Todorczuk JR. Achalasia in the elderly. Effects of aging on clinical presentation and outcome. Dig Dis Sci 1991;36(2):225
62. Coccia G, Bortolotti M, Michetti P, Dodero M. Prospective clinical and manometric study comparing pneumatic dilatation and sublingual nifedipine in the treatment of oesophageal achalasia. Gut 1991;32:604
63. Coccia G, Bortolotti M, Michetti P, Dodero M. Return of esophageal peristalsis after nifedipine therapy in patients with idiopathic esophageal achalasia. Am J Gastroenterol 1992;87:1705
64. Cohen S, Fisher R, Tuch A. The site of denervation in achalasia. Gut 1972;13:556
65. Cohen S, Lipshutz W, Hughes W. Role of gastrin supersensitivity in the pathogenesis of lower esophageal sphincter hypertension in achalasia. J Clin Invest 1971;50:1241
66. Collard JM, Kestens PJ, Salizzoni M, Lengele B, Romagnoli R. Heller-Dor procedure for achalasia: from conventional to video-endoscopic surgery. Acta Chir Belg 1996;96:62
67. Collier DH, Zulman JI. Hypertrophic osteoarthropathy associated with achalasia. Am J Med 1986;81:355
68. Collins MP, Rabie S. Sudden airway obstruction in achalasia. J Laryngol Otol 1984;98:207
69. Collman PI, Tremblay L, Damant NE. The central vagal efferent supply to the esophagus and lower esophageal sphincter of the cat. Gastroenterology 1993;104:1430
70. Corcione F, et al. Surgical laparoscopy with intraoperative manometry in the treatment of esophageal achalasia. Surg Laparosc Endosc 1997;7:232

71. Cosentini E, et al. Achalasia. Results of myotomy and antireflux operation after failed dilatations. Arch Surg 1997;132:143

72. Costa M, et al. Projections and chemical coding of neurons with immunoreactivity for nitric oxide synthase in the guinea-pig small intestine. Neurosci Lett 1992;14:121

73. Costigan DJ, Clouse RE. Achalasia-like esophagus from amyloidosis. Successful treatment with pneumatic bag dilatation. Dig Dis Sci 1983;28:763

74. Cox J, Buckton GK, Bennett JR. Balloon dilatation in achalasia: a new dilator. Gut 1986;27:986

75. Creamer B, Olsen AM, Code CF. The esophageal sphincters in achalasia of the cardia (cardiospasm). Gastroenterology 1957;33:293

76. Crookes PF, DeMeester TR, Corkill S. Gastroesophageal reflux in achalasia. When is reflux really reflux? Dig Dis Sci 1997;42:1354

77. Csendes A, Smok G, Braghetto I, Ramirez C, Velasco N, Henriquez A. Gastroesophageal sphincter pressure and histological changes in distal esophagus in patients with achalasia of the esophagus. Dig Dis Sci 1985;30:941

78. Csendes A, Velasco N, Braghetto I, Henriquez A. A prospective randomized study comparing forceful dilation and esophagomyotomy in patients with achalasia of the esophagus. Gastroenterology 1981;80:789

79. Csendes A, et al. Late results of a prospective randomized study comparing forceful dilation and oesophagomyotomy in patients with achalasia. Gut 1989;30:299

80. Csendes A, et al. Histological studies of Auerbach's plexuses of the oesophagus, stomach, jejunum, and colon in patients with achalasia of the oesophagus: correlation with gastric acid secretion, presence of parietal cells and gastric emptying of solids. Gut 1992;33:150

81. Cucchiara S, et al. Return of peristalsis in a child with esophageal achalasia treated by Heller's myotomy. J Pediatr Gastroenterol Nutr 1986;5:150

82. Cuilliere C, et al. Achalasia: outcome of patients treated with intrasphincteric injection of botulinum toxin. Gut 1997;41:87

83. Davis JA, Kantrowitz PA, Chandler HL, Schatzki SC. Reversible achalasia due to reticulum-cell sarcoma. N Engl J Med 1975;293:130

84. Dayalan M, Chettur L, Ramatnishman MS. Achalasia of the cardia in siblings. Arch Dis Child 1972;47:115

85. Decanini TC, Galicia JA, Varela GG. Laparoscopic esophagomyotomy and antireflux procedure with intraoperative manometry. Surg Laparosc Endosc 1996;6:398

86. Delgado F, et al. Laparoscopic treatment of esophageal achalasia. Surg Laparosc Endosc 1996;6:83

87. Del Genio A, Mugione P, Zampiello P, Izzo G, Maffettone V, Di Martino N. Failure of surgical treatment for achalasia: diagnosis and treatment. Ann Ital Chir 1995;66:587

88. Dellipiani AW, Hewetson KA. Pneumatic dilatation in the management of achalasia: experience of 45 cases. QJM 1986;58:253

89. de Oliveira JM, et al. Timed barium swallow: a simple technique for evaluating esophageal emptying in patients with achalasia. AJR Am J Roentgenol 1997;169:473

90. DeVault KR. Incomplete upper esophageal sphincter relaxation: association with achalasia but not other esophageal motility disorders. Dysphagia 1997;12:157

91. Deviere J, et al. Endoscopic ultrasonography in achalasia. Gastroenterology 1989;96:1210

92. Dhiman RK, et al. Transient achalasia of esophagus in tetanus. Indian J Gastroenterol 1992;11:139

93. DiMarino AJ, Cohen S. Effect of an oral beta$_2$-adrenergic agonist on lower esophageal sphincter pressure in normal subjects and in patients with achalasia. Dig Dis Sci 1982;27:1063

94. Di Simone MP, et al. Onset timing of delayed complications and criteria of follow-up after operation for esophageal achalasia [published erratum appears in Ann Thorac Surg 1996;62:632]. Ann Thorac Surg 1996;61:1106

95. Dodds WJ, Dent J, Hogan WJ, Patel GK, Toouli J, Arndorfer RC. Paradoxical lower esophageal sphincter contraction included by cholecystokinin-octapeptide in patients with achalasia. Gastroenterology 1981;80:327

96. Dodds WJ, Stewart ET, Kishk SM, Kahrilas PJ, Hogan WJ. Radiologic amyl nitrite test for distinguishing pseudo achalasia from idiopathic achalasia. Am J Roentgenol 1986;146:21

97. Dominguez F, et al. Acute upper-airway obstruction in achalasia of the esophagus. Am J Gastroenterol 1987;82:362

98. Dooley CP, Taylor IL, Valenzuela JE. Impaired acid secretion and pancreatic polypeptide release in some patients with achalasia. Gastroenterology 1983;84:809

99. Dua KS, Shaker R, Arndorfer R, Stewart E. Esophageal intramural pseudodiverticulosis associated with achalasia. Am J Gastroenterol 1996;91:1859

100. Duane PD, Magee TM, Alexander MS, Heatley RV, Losowsky MS. Oesophageal achalasia in adolescent women mistaken for anorexia nervosa. BMJ 1992;305:43

101. Duda M, et al. Etiopathogenesis and classification of esophageal diverticula. Int Surg 1985;70:291

102. Dudnick RS, Castell JA, Castell DO. Abnormal upper esophageal sphincter function in achalasia. Am J Gastroenterol 1992;87:1712

103. Dufour JF, Fawaz KA, Libby ED. Botulinum toxin injection for secondary achalasia with esophageal varices. Gastrointest Endosc 1997;45:191

104. Dufresne CR, Jeyasingham K, Baker RR. Achalasia of the cardia associated with pulmonary sarcoidosis. Surgery 1983;94:32

105. Duntemann TJ, Dresner DM. Achalasia-like syndrome presenting after highly selective vagotomy. Dig Dis Sci 1995;40:2081

106. Duranceau A, LaFonteine ER, Vallieres B. Effects of total fundoplication on function of the esophagus after myotomy for achalasia. Am J Surg 1982;143:28

107. Earlam RJ, Ellis FH, Nobrega FT. Achalasia of the esophagus in a small urban community. Mayo Clin Proc 1969;44:478

108. Eaves R, Lambert J, Rees J, King RW. Achalasia secondary to carcinoma of prostate. Dig Dis Sci 1983;28:278

109. Echrich JD, Winans CS. Discordance for achalasia in identical twins. Am J Dig Dis 1979;245:221

110. Eckardt VF, Bernhard G, Koop H, Roder R, Liewen H, Stenner F. Autonomic dysfunction in patients with achalasia. Neurogastroenterol Motil 1995;7:55

111. Eckardt VF, Krause J, Bolle D. Gastrointestinal transit and gastric acid secretion in patients with achalasia. Dig Dis Sci 1989;34:665

112. Eckardt VF, Westermeier T, Junginger T, Kohne U. Risk factors for diagnostic delay in achalasia. Dig Dis Sci 1997;42:580

113. Eckardt VF, Westermeier T, Kanzier G. Complications and their impact after pneumatic dilation for achalasia: prospective long-term follow-up study. Gastrointest Endosc 1997;45:349

114. Efrati Y, Mares AJ. Infantile achalasia associated with deficient tear production. J Clin Gastroenterol 1985;7:413

115. Ehrich E, Aranoff G, Johnson WG. Familial achalasia associated with adrenocortical insufficiency, alacrima, and neurological abnormalities. Am J Med Genet 1987;26:637

116. Ellis FH Jr. Oesophagomyotomy for achalasia: a 22-year experience. Br J Surg 1993;80:882

117. Ellis FH, Crozier RE, Gibb SP. Reoperative achalasia surgery. J Thorac Cardiovasc Surg 1986;92:859

118. Ellis FH, Crozier RE, Watkins E. Operation of esophageal achalasia. Result of esophagomyotomy without an antireflux operation. J Thorac Cardiovasc Surg 1984;88:344

119. Ellis FH, Gibb SP, Crozier RE. Esophagomyotomy for achalasia of the esophagus. Ann Surg 1980;192:157

120. Ellis FH Jr, Watkins E Jr, Gibb SP, Heatley GJ. Ten to 20-year clinical results after short esophagomyotomy without an antireflux procedure (modified Heller operation) for esophageal achalasia. Eur J Cardiothorac Surg 1992;6:86

121. el-Newihi HM, Achord JL, Mihas AA, Dellinger GW. Gastric cancer and pernicious anemia appearing as pseudoachalasia. South Med J 1996;89:906

122. el-Rayyes K, Hegab S, Besisso M. A syndrome of alacrima, achalasia, and neurologic anomalies without adrenocortical insufficiency. J Pediatr Ophthalmol Strabismus 1991;28:35

123. Esposito PS, Santelices AA, Sleeman D, Sosa JL. Laparoscopic management of achalasia. Am Surg 1997;63:221

124. Etzel E. Megaesophagus and its neuropathology. A clinical and anatomopathological research. Guys Hosp Rep 1937;87:158

125. Faloon T. Achalasia in pregnancy. A case of a rare coexistence. Can Fam Physician 1993;39:1182

126. Fassina G, Osculati A. Achalasia and sudden death: a case report. Forensic Sci Int 1995;75:133

127. Feczko PJ, Ma CK, Halpert RD, Batra SK. Barrett's metaplasia and dysplasia in postmyotomy achalasia patients. Am J Gastroenterol 1983;78:265

128. Fellows IW, Ogilvie AL, Atkinson M. Pneumatic dilation in achalasia. Gut 1983;24:1020

129. Ferguson MK, Olak J, Reeder LB. Results of myotomy and partial fundoplication after pneumatic dilation for achalasia. Ann Thorac Surg 1996;62:327

130. Fevery J, Heiwegh KP, DeGrote J. Unconjugated hyperbilirubinemia in achalasia. Gut 1974;15:121

131. Fishman VM, et al. Am J Gastroenterol 1996;91:1724

132. Foster PN, Stewart M, Lowe JS, Atkinson M. Achalasia-like disorder of the oesophagus in von Recklinghausen's neurofibromatosis. Gut 1987;28:1522

133. Frank MS, Brandt LJ, Haas K, Parker JG. Malignant esophago-pulmonary fistula complicating achalasia. Am J Gastroenterol 1979;71:206

134. Fredens K, et al. Severe destruction of esophageal nerves in a patient with achalasia secondary to gastric cancer: a possible role of eosinophil neurotropic protein. Dig Dis Sci 1989;34:292

135. French T, Kench P, Swanepoel A, Hewitson R, Gelb A. Achalasia with suppurative pericarditis. A case report. Am J Gastroenterol 1974; 62:536

136. Friesen DL, Henderson RD, Hanna W. Ultrastructure of the esophageal muscle in achalasia and diffuse esophageal spasm. Am J Clin Pathol 1983;79:319

137. Frimberger E, et al. Results of treatment with the endoscope dilator in 11 patients with achalasia of the esophagus. Endoscopy 1981;13:173

138. Fritzen R, Scherbaum WA, Bornstein SR. Megaoesophagus in a patient with autoimmune polyglandular syndrome type II. Clin Endocrinol (Oxf) 1996;45:493

139. Galen EA, Switz DM, Zfass AM. Achalasia. Incidence and treatment in Virginia. Va. Med 1982;109:183

140. Garrigues V, Berenguer J, Valverde J, Galvez C, Ponce J. Achalasia-like syndrome as the first manifestation in a patient with CREST syndrome. Eur J Gastroenterol Hepatol 1996;8:289

141. Gaumnitz EA, Singaram C, Sweet MA, Osinski MA, Bass P. Electrophysiological and pharmacological responses of chronically denervated lower esophageal sphincter of the oppossum. Gastroenterology 1995;109:789

142. Geffner ME, et al. Selective ACTH insensitivity, achalasia, and alacrima: a multisystem disorder presenting in childhood. Pediatr Res 1983;17:532

143. Gelfond MD, Kozarek RA. An experience with polyethylene balloons for pneumatic dilation in achalasia. Am J Gastroenterol 1988;84:924

144. Gelfond M, Rozen P, Gilat T. Isosorbide dinitrate and nifedipine treatment of achalasia: a clinical, manometric and radionuclide evaluation. Gastroenterology 1982;83:963

145. Ghosh P, Quigley EM, Gallagher TF, Linder J. Achalasia of the cardia and multiple endocrine neoplasia 2B. Am J Gastroenterol 1994;89:1880

146. Ghosh S, Palmer KR, Heading RC. Achalasia of the oesophagus in elderly patients responds poorly to conservative therapy. Age Ageing 1994;4:280

147. Gidda JS. Control of esophageal peristalsis. Viewpoint Dig Dis 1985; 17:13

148. Givan DC, Scott PH, Eigen H, Grosfeld JL, Clark JH. Achalasia and tracheal obstruction in a child. Eur J Respir Dis 1985;66:70

149. Goldblum Jr, Richter JE, Rice TW. Histopathologic features in esophagomyotomy specimens from patients with achalasia. Gastroenterology 1996;111:648

150. Goldenberg SP, Burrell M, Fette GG, Vos C, Traube M. Classic and vigorous achalasia: a comparison of manometric, radiographic, and clinical findings. Gastroenterology 1991;101:743

151. Goldenberg SP, Vos C, Burrell M, Traube M. Achalasia and hiatal hernia. Dig Dis Sci 1992;37:5628

152. Goldin NR, Butnd TW, Ferrante WA. Secondary achalasia: association with adenocarcinoma of the lung and reversal with radiation therapy. Am J Gastroenterol 1983;78:203

153. Goldschmiedt M, Peterson WL, Spielberger R, Lee EL, Kurtz SF, Feldman M. Esophageal achalasia secondary to mesothelioma. Dig Dis Sci 1989;34:1285

154. Gordon JM, Eaker EY. Prospective study of esophageal botulinum toxin injection in high-risk achalasia patients. Am J Gastroenterol 1997;92:1812

155. Gourrier E, et al. Beta mannosidosis: a new case. Arch Pediatr 1997; 4:147

156. Goyal RK, McGuigan JE. Is gastrin a major determinant of basal lower esophageal sphincter pressure? A double-blind controlled study using high titer gastrin antiserum. J Clin Invest 1976;57:291

157. Goyal RK, Rattan S. Mechanism of the lower esophageal sphincter relaxation. Action of prostaglandin E2 and the ophylline. J Clin Invest 1973;52:337

158. Goyal RK, Rattan S. Nature of the vagal inhibitory innervation to the lower esophageal sphincter. J Clin Invest 1975;55:1119

159. Goyal RK, Rattan S. Genesis of basal sphincter pressure: effect of tetrodotoxin on lower esophageal sphincter pressure in opossum *in vivo*. Gastroenterology 1976;71:62

160. Goyal RK, Rattan S. VIP as a possible neurotransmitter of non-cholinergic non-adrenergic inhibitory neurones. Nature 1980;288:379

161. Graham AJ, Storseth C, Clifton JC, Dong SR, Worsley DF, Finley RJ. Laparoscopic esophageal myotomy and anterior partial fundoplication for the treatment of achalasia. Ann Thorac Surg 1997;64:785

162. Grant DB, et al. Neurological and adrenal dysfunction in the adrenal insufficiency/alacrima/achalasia (3A) syndrome. Arch Dis Child 1993;68:779

163. Grant DB, Dunger DB, Smith I, Hyland K. Familial glucocorticoid deficiency with achalasia of the cardia associated with mixed neuropathy, long-tract degeneration and mild dementia. Eur J Pediatr 1992; 151:85

164. Green AT, Grainger SL, Thompson RPH. Bullfrog neck in achalasia. Br J Hosp Med 1990;43:70

165. Grider JR, Murthy KS, Jin JG, Makhlouf GM. Stimulation of nitric oxide from muscle cells by VIP: prejunctional enhancement of VIP release. Am J Physiol 1992;G774

166. Gross RR, Johnson LF, Kaminski RJ. Esophageal emptying in achalasia quantitated by a radioisotope technique. Dig Dis Sci 1979;24:945

167. Guelrud M, Rossiter A, Souney PF, Rossiter G, Fanikos J, Mujica V. The effect of vasoactive intestinal polypeptide on the lower esophageal sphincter in achalasia. Gastroenterology 1992;103:377

168. Hankins JR, McLaughlin JS. The association of carcinoma of the esophagus with achalasia. J Thorac Cardiovasc Surg 1975;69:355

169. Hanna SM. A case of scleroderma presenting as cardiospasm. Postgrad Med 1972;48:236

170. Harman JW, O'Hegarty MT, Byrnes CK. The ultrastructure of human smooth muscle: I. Studies of cell surface and connections in normal and achalasia esophageal smooth muscle. Exp Mol Pathol 1962;1:204

171. Havarkamp F, Zerres K, Rosskamp R. Three siblings with achalasia and alacrima: a separate entity different from triple-A syndrome. Am J Med Genet 1989;34:289

171A. Heimlich JJ, O'Connor TW, Flores DC. Case for pneumatic dilation in achalasia. Occurrence 23 years after esophagomyotomy. Dig Dis Sci 1984;29:1006

172. Heller E. Extramukose Kardioplastik beim chronischen Kardiospasmus mit Dilatation Oesophagus. Mitt Grenzgeb Med Chir 1914;27:141

173. Helm JF, et al. Carcinoma of the cardia masquerading as idiopathic achalasia. Gastroenterology 1982;82:1082A

174. Hernandez A, Reynoso MC, Soto F. Achalasia microcephaly syndrome in a patient with consanguineous parents. Clin Genet 1989;36: 456

175. Herrera JL. Esophageal metastasis from breast carcinoma presenting as achalasia. Am J Med Sci 1992;303:321

176. Higgs B, Ellis FH Jr. The effect of bisternal supranodosal vagotomy on canine esophageal function. Surgery 1965;58:828

177. Higgs B, Kerr FWL, Ellis FH Jr. The experimental production of esophageal achalasia by electrolytic lesions in the medulla. J Thorac Cardiovasc Surg 1965;50:613

178. Hill LD, Asplund CM, Roberts PN. Intraoperative manometry: adjunct to surgery for esophageal motility disorders. Am J Surg 1984; 147:171

179. Hoffman BJ, Knapple WL, Bhutani MS, Verne GN, Hawes RH. Treatment of achalasia by injection of botulinum toxin under endoscopic ultrasound guidance. Gastrointest Endosc 1997;45:77

180. Holloway RH, Dodds WJ, Helm JF, Hogan WJ, Dent J, Arndorfer RC. Integrity of cholinergic innervation to the lower esophageal sphincter in achalasia. Gastroenterology 1986;90:924

181. Holloway RH, Krosin G, Lange RC, Baue AE, McCallum RW. Radionuclide esophageal emptying of a solid meal to quantitate results of therapy in achalasia. Gastroenterology 1983;84:771

182. Holloway RH, Wayman JB, Dent J. Failure of transient lower esophageal sphincter relaxation in response to gastric distention in patients with achalasia: evidence for neural mediation of transient lower esophageal sphincter relaxation. Gut 1989;30:762

183. Holzman MD, Richards WO, Holcomb GW III, Eller RF, Ladipo JK, Sharp KW. Laparoscopic surgical treatment of achalasia. Am J Surg 1997;173:308

184. Hooper TL, Gholkar J, Smith SR, Manns JJ, Moussalli H. Recurrent

submucosal dissection of the oesophagus in association with achalasia. Postgrad Med J 1986;62:955

185. Horgan S, Hudda K, Eubanks T, McAllister J, Pellegrini CA. Does botulinum toxin injection make esophagomyotomy a more difficult operation? Surg Endosc 1998 (in press)

186. Howard PJ, Maher L, Pryde A, Cameron EW, Heading R. Five year prospective study of the incidence, clinical features, and diagnosis of achalasia in Edinburgh. Gut 1992;33:1011

187. Howard RS II, Woodring JH, Vandiviere HM, Dillon ML. *Mycobacterium fortuitum* pulmonary infection complicating achalasia. South Med J 1991;84:1391

188. Hubschmann K. Achalasia, alacrimia and cortisol deficiency—Allgrove syndrome. Klin Padiatr 1995;207:126

189. Hunter JG, Waring JP, Branum GD, Trus TL. Laparoscopic Heller myotomy and fundoplication for achalasia. Ann Surg 1997;225:655

190. Hurst AF. The treatment of achalasia of the cardia; so-called "cardiospasm." Lancet 1927;1:618

191. Idenburg FJ, Akkermans LM, Smout AJ, Kooijman CD, Obertop H. Leiomyoma of the distal oesophagus mimicking achalasia. Neth J Surg 1991;43:79

192. Jackson C. The diaphragmatic pinchcock in so-called cardiospasm. Laryngoscope 1922;32:139

193. Jacobs JB, Cohen NL, Mattel S. Pneumatic dilatation as the primary treatment for achalasia. Ann Otol Rhinol Laryngol 1983;92:353

194. Jankovic J, Brin MF. Therapeutic uses of botulinum toxin. N Engl J Med 1991;324:1186

195. Jones DB, Mayberry JF, Rhodes J, Munro J. Preliminary report of an association between measles virus and achalasia. J Clin Pathol 1983; 36:655

196. Jorge Ad, D'iaz M. Double pylorus and esophageal achalasia. Endoscopy 1976;8:208

197. Just-Viera JO, Haight C. Achalasia and carcinoma of the esophagus. Surg Gynecol Obstet 1969;128:1081

198. Kaada B. Successful treatment of esophageal dysmotility and Raynauds' phenomenon in systemic sclerosis and achalasia by transcutaneous nerve stimulation. Scand J Gastroenterol 1987;22:1137

199. Kadakia SC, Wong RKH. Graded pneumatic dilation using Rigiflex achalasia dilators in patients with primary esophageal achalasia. Am J Gastroenterol 1993;88:34

200. Kahrilas PJ, Kishk SM, Helm JF, Dodds WJ, Harig JM, Hogan WJ. Comparison of pseudoachalasia and achalasia. Am J Med 1987;82: 439

201. Kamiike W, et al. Intraoperative manometry during laparoscopic operation for esophageal achalasia: does pneumoperitoneum affect manometry? World J Surg 1996;20:973

202. Karsell PR. Achalasia, aspiration, and atypical mycobacteria. Mayo Clin Proc 1993;68:1025

203. Kasirga E, et al. Four siblings with achalasia, alacrimia and neurological abnormalities in a consanguineous family. Clin Genet 1996;49: 296

204. Katz P. Esophageal carcinoma and achalasia: another call for screening? Am J Gastroenterol 1993;88:783

205. Katz PO, Gilbert J, Castell DO. Pneumatic dilation is effective long-term treatment for achalasia. Dig Dis Sci 1998;43:1973–1977

206. Katz PO, Richter JE, Cowan R, Castell DO. Apparent complete lower esophageal sphincter relaxation in achalasia. Gastroenterology 1986; 90:978

207. Kendall AP, Lin E. Respiratory failure as presentation of achalasia of the oesophagus. Anaesthesia 1991;46:1039

208. Kilpatrick ZM, Miller SS. Achalasia in mother and daughter. Gastroenterology 1972;62:1042

209. Kimura K. The nature of idiopathic esophagus dilatation. Jpn J Gastroenterol 1929;1:199

210. Kotoh F. Follow-up study of patients with achalasia treated by long myotomy + partial fundopexy + posterior fixation based on intraoperative manometry. Nippon Kyobu Geka Gakkai Zasshi 1991;39:2117

211. Kraft AR, Frank HA, Glotzer DJ. Achalasia of the esophagus complicated by varices and massive hemorrhage. N Engl J Med 1973;288: 405

212. Kurlander DJ, et al. Therapeutic value of the pneumatic dilator in achalasia of the esophagus: long-term results in sixty-two living patients. Gastroenterology 1963;45:604

213. Lambroza A, Schuman RW. Pneumatic dilation for achalasia without fluoroscopic guidance: safety and efficacy. Am J Gastroenterol 1995; 90:1226

214. Lamet M, Fleshler B, Achkar E. Return of peristalsis in achalasia after pneumatic dilation. Am J Gastroenterol 1985;80:602

215. Landres RT, Kuster GGR, Strum WB. Eosinophilic esophagitis in a patient with vigorous achalasia. Gastroenterology 1978;74:1298

216. Lane TG, Wu WC, Ott DJ. Achalasia presenting as a neck mass. Ann Intern Med 1981;94:786

217. Lanes R, et al. Glucocorticoid and partial mineralocorticoid deficiency associated with achalasia. J Clin Endocrinol Metab 1980;50:268

218. Laub W, Achkar E. Hiatal hernia in patients with achalasia. Am J Gastroenterol 1987;82:1256

219. Lee FI, Bellary SV. Barrett's esophagus and achalasia. A case report. J Clin Gastroenterol 1991;13:559

220. Lee JD, Cecil BD, Brown PE, Wright RA. The Cohen test does not predict outcome in achalasia after pneumatic dilation. Gastrointest Endosc 1993;39:157

221. Lefebvre RA. Nitric oxide in the peripheral nervous system. Ann Med 1995;27:379

222. Lefkowitz JR, Brand DL, Schuffler MD, Brugge WR. Amyloidosis mimics achalasia effect on lower esophageal sphincter. Dig Dis Sci 1989;34:630

223. Lendrum FC. Anatomic features of the cardiac orifice of the stomach with special reference to cardiospasm. Arch Intern Med 1937;59:474

224. Levine ML, Dorf BS, Moskowitz G, Bank S. Pneumatic dilatation in achalasia under endoscopic guidance: correlation pre- and post-dilatation by radionuclide scintiscan. Am J Gastroenterol 1987;82: 311

225. Levine ML, Moskowitz GW, Dorf BS, Bank S. Pneumatic dilation in patients with achalasia with a modified Gruntzig dilator (Levine) under direct endoscopic control: results after 5 years. Am J Gastroenterol 1991;86:1581

226. Lipshutz W, Highes W, Cohen S. The genesis of lower esophageal sphincter pressure: its identification through the use of gastrin antiserum. J Clin Invest 1972;51:522

227. Lishman AH, Dellipiani AW. Management of achalasia of the cardia by forced pneumatic dilation. Gut 1982;23:541

228. LIttle AG, Sorian A, Ferguson MK, Winans CS, Skinner DB. Surgical treatment of achalasia: results with esophagomyotomy and Belsey repair. Ann Thorac Surg 1988;45:489

229. London FA, Raab DE, Fuller J. Achalasia in three siblings. Mayo Clin Proc 1977;52:97

230. Longstreth GF, Walker FD. Megaesophagus and hereditary nervous system degeneration. J Clin Gastroenterol 1994;19:125

231. MacKalski BA, Keate RF. Rumination in a patient with achalasia. Am J Gastroenterol 1993;88:1803

232. Mackler D, Schneider R. Achalasia in father and son. Dig Dis Sci 1978;23:1042

233. Mackler SA. Spontaneous rupture of the esophagus: an experimental and clinical trial. Surg Gynecol Obstet 1952;95:345

234. Maksimak M, Perlmutter DH, Winter HS. The use of nifedipine for the treatment of achalasia in children. J Pediatr Gastroenterol Nutr 1986;5:883

235. Mamel JJ. Bezoar of the esophagus occurring in achalasia. Gastrointest Endosc 1984;30:317

236. Manela FD, Quigley EM, Paustian FF, Taylor RJ. Achalasia of the esophagus in association with renal cell carcinoma. Am J Gastroenterol 1991;86:1812

237. Marshall JB, Diaz-Arias AA, Bochna GS, Vogele KA. Achalasia due to diffuse esophageal leiomyomatosis and inherited as an autosomal dominant disorder. Report of a family study. Gastroenterology 1990; 98:1358

238. Marzio L, Grossi L, DeLaurentiis MF, Cennamo L, Lapenna D, Cuccurullo F. Effect of Cimetropium bromide on esophageal motility and transit in patients affected by primary achalasia. Dig Dis Sci 1994; 39:1389

239. Massey BT, Hogan WJ, Dodds WJ, Dantas R. Alteration of the upper esophageal sphincter belch reflex in patients with achalasia. Gastroenterology 1992;103:1574

240. Mattioli FP, Tassone U, Bozzano PL, Spigno L, Pandolfo N. Heller's intervention for esophageal achalasia. Ann Ital Chir 1995;66:579

241. Mayberry JF, Atkinson M. A study of swallowing difficulties in first degree relatives of patients with achalasia. Thorax 1985;40:391

242. Mayberry JF, Atkinson M. Studies of incidence and prevalence of achalasia in the Nottingham area. QJM 1985;56:451

243. Mayberry JF, Rhodes J. Achalasia in the city of Cardiff from 1926 to 1977. Digestion 1980;20:248

244. McKusick VA. Mendelian Inheritance in Man. Baltimore: Johns Hopkins University Press, 1978

245. Mearin F, et al. Patients with achalasia lack nitric oxide synthase in the gastro-oesophageal junction. Eur J Clin Invest 1993;23:724

246. Meijssen MA, Tilanus HW, Van Blankenstein M. Achalasia complicated by oesophageal squamous cell carcinoma: a prospective study in 195 patients. Gut 1992;33:155

247. Meshkinpour H, Kaye L, Elias A, Glick ME. Manometric and radiologic correlations in achalasia. Am J Gastroenterol 1992;87:1567

248. Meshkinpour H, Mason RG. Achalasia evolving from segmental aperistalsis. Dysphagia 1992;7:166

249. Micetic-Turk D, Tomazic D. Achalasia with absent tear production. Acta Paediatr 1995;84:835

250. Michel L, Grillo HC, Malt RA. Operative and non-operative management of esophageal perforations. Ann Surg 1981;194:57

251. Miller LS, et al. High-resolution endoluminal sonography in achalasia. Gastrointest Endosc 1995;42:545

252. Misiewicz JJ, Waller SL, Anthony PP, Gummer JW. Achalasia of the cardia: pharmacology and histopathology of isolated cardiac sphincteric muscle from patients with and without achalasia. QJM 1969;38:17

253. Mitchell PC, et al. Laparoscopic cardiomyotomy with a Dor patch for achalasia. Can J Surg 1995;38:445

254. Molina EG, Barkin JS, Reiner DK, Grauer L. Conservative management of esophageal nontransmural tears after pneumatic dilation for achalasia. Am J Gastroenterol 1996;91:15

255. Moore PS, Couch RM, Perry YS, Shuckett EP, Winter JS. Allgrove syndrome: an autosomal recessive syndrome at ACTH insensitivity, achalasia and alacrima. Clin Endocrinol (Oxf) 1991;34:107

256. Moreto M, Ojembarrena E, Rodriguez ML. Endoscopic injection of ethanolamine as a treatment for achalasia: a first report. Endoscopy 1996;28:539

257. Morino M, Garrone C, Festa V, Rebecchi F. Laparoscopic Heller cardiomyotomy with intraoperative manometry in the management of oesophageal achalasia. Int Surg 1995;80:332

258. Morino M, Garrone C, Festa V, Rebecchi F. Preoperative pneumatic dilatation represents a risk factor for laparoscopic Heller myotomy. Surg Endosc 1997;11:359

259. Mosher HP. Liver tunnel and cardiospasm. Laryngoscope 1922;32:348

260. Mosher HP. Cardiospasm. Med J 1923;26:240

261. Mosher HP. Fibrosis of the terminal portion of the esophagus: cardiospasm. Proc Int Assembly Inter St Postgrad MA North Am 1931;6:95

262. Mosley RG, Singaram C, Sengupta A, Reichelderfer M. Innervation of an esophageal ectatic submucosal blood vessel in achalasia and a comparison with normals. Am J Gastroenterol 1994;89:1874

263. Muehldorfer SM, Ell C, Hahn EG. High and low compliance balloon dilators in patients with achalasia: a randomized prospective comparative trial. Gastrointest Endosc 1996;4:398

264. Murphy MS, Gardner-Medwin D, Eartham EJ. Achalasia of the cardia associated with hereditary cerebellar ataxia. Am J Gastroenterol 1989;84:1329

265. Murray JA, Du C, Ledlow A. Guanylate cyclase inhibitors: effect on tone, relaxation and cGMP content of the lower esophageal sphincter. Am J Physiol 1992;263:G97

266. Murthy KS, Makhlouf GM. Vasoactive intestinal peptide/pituitary adenylate cyclase-activating peptide-dependent activation of membrane-bound NO synthase in smooth muscle mediated by pertussis toxin-sensitive $G_{i1-2}$. J Biol Chem 1994;269:15977

267. Nagler RW, et al. Achalasia in fraternal twins. Ann Intern Med 1963;59:906

268. Nair LA, et al. Complications during pneumatic dilation for achalasia or diffuse esophageal spasm. Analysis of risk factors, early clinical characteristics, and outcome. Dig Dis Sci 1993;38:1893

269. Nemir P Jr, Fallahnejad M, Bose B, Jacobowitz D, Frobese AS, Hawthorne HR. A study of the cause of the esophagus in childhood. Surgical treatment in 35 cases, with special reference to familial cases and glucocorticoid deficiency association. Hepatogastroenterology 1991;38:510

270. Nihoul-Fékété C, Bawab F, Lortat-Jacob S, Arhan P. Achalasia of the esophagus in childhood. Surgical treatment in 35 cases, with special reference to familial cases and glucocorticoid deficiency association. Hepatogastroenterology 1991;38:510

271. Okike N, Payne WS, Neufeld DM, Bernatz PE, Pairolero PC, Sanderson DR. Esophagomyotomy versus forceful dilation for achalasia of the esophagus: results in 899 patients. Ann Thorac Surg 1979;28:199

272. Olivet RT, Payne WS. Congenital H-type tracheoesophageal fistula complicated by achalasia in an adult: report of a case. Mayo Clin Proc 1975;50:464

273. Orlando RC, Call DL, Bream CA. Achalasia and absent gastric air bubble. Ann Intern Med 1978;88:60

274. Orringer MB, Stirling MC. Esophageal resection for achalasia: indications and results. Ann Thorac Surg 1989;47:340

275. Ott DJ, Hodge RG, Chen MY, Wu WC, Gelfand DW. Achalasia associated with hiatal hernia: prevalence and potential implications. Abdom Imaging 1993;18:7

276. Ott DJ, Wu WC, Gelfand DW, Richter JE. Radiographic evaluation of the achalasic esophagus immediately following pneumatic dilation. Gastrointest Radiol 1984;9:185

277. Padovan W, Godoy RA, Dantas RO, Meneghelli UG, Oliveira RB, Troncon LE. Lower oesophageal sphincter response to pentagastrin in chagasic patients with megaoesophagus and megacolon. Gut 1980;21:85

278. Pagini R, et al. Lower oesophageal sphincter hypersensitivity to opioid receptor stimulation in patients with idiopathic achalasia. Gut 1993;34:16

279. Pamphlett R. Early terminal and nodal sprouting of motor axons after botulinum toxin. J Neurol Sci 1989;92:181

280. Pandolfo N, Mattioli FP, Bozzano PL, Spigno L, Bortolotti M. Manometric assessment of Heller-Dor operation for esophageal achalasia. Hepatogastroenterology 1996;43:160

281. Panzini L, Traube M. Stridor from tracheal obstruction in a patient with achalasia. Am J Gastroenterol 1993;88:1097

282. Park RH, McKillop JH, Belch JJ, Faichney A, MacKenzie JF. Achalasia-like syndrome in systemic sclerosis. Br J Surg 1990;77:46

283. Parkman HP, et al. Pneumatic dilatation or esophagomyotomy treatment for idiopathic achalasia: clinical outcomes and cost analysis. Dig Dis Sci 1993;38:75

284. Parkman HP, Fisher RS, Krevsky B, Miller DL, Caroline DF, Maurer AH. Optimal evaluation of patients with nonobstructive esophageal dysphagia. Manometry, scintigraphy, or videoesohagography? Dig Dis Sci 1996;41:1355

285. Pasricha PJ, Rai R, Ravich WJ, Hendrix TR, Kalloo AN. Botulinum toxin for achalasia: long-term outcome and predictors of response. Gastroenterology 1996;110:1410

286. Pasricha PJ, Ravich WJ, Hendrix TR, Sostre S, Jones B, Kalloo AN. Intrasphincteric botulinum toxin for the treatment of achalasia. N Engl J Med 1995;332:774

287. Pasricha PJ, Ravich WJ, Kalloo AN. Effects of intrasphincteric botulinum toxin on the lower esophageal sphincter in piglets. Gastroenterology 1993;105:1045

288. Paterson WG. Esophageal and lower esophageal sphincter response to balloon distention in patients with achalasia. Dig Dis Sci 1997;42:106

289. Patrick A, Campbell IW, Fraser MS, Smith DH, Walbaum PR. Achalasia presenting a foreign body obstruction. Arch Dis Child 1984;59:576

290. Pellegrini CA, Leichter R, Patti M, Somberg K, Ostroff JW, Way L. Thoracoscopic esophageal myotomy in the treatment of achalasia. Ann Thorac Surg 1993;56:680

291. Peracchia A, Chella B, Bonavina L, Fumagalli U, Bona S, Rosati R. Laparoscopic treatment of functional diseases of the esophagus. Int Surg 1995;80:336

292. Peracchia A, Segalin A, Bardini R, Ruol A, Bonavina L, Baessato M. Esophageal carcinoma and achalasia: prevalence, incidence and results of treatment. Hepatogastroenterology 1991;38:514

293. Phillip M, Schulman H, Hershkovitz E. Adrenal insufficiency after achalasia in the triple-A syndrome. Clin Pediatr (Phila) 1996;35:99

294. Pierandozzi JS, Ritter JH. Transient achalasia: a complication of vagotomy. Am J Surg 1966;111:356

295. Pombo M, et al. Glucocorticoid deficiency with achalasia of the cardia and lack of lacrimation. Clin Endocrinol (Oxf) 1985;23:237

296. Ponce GJ, Berenguer LJ, Galvez CC, Valverde dela OJ, Pertejo PV, Garrigues GV. Are there clinical differences between typical and vigorous achalasia and response to pneumatic dilatation? Gastroenterol Hepatol 1995;18:315

297. Ponce J, Berenguer J, Sala T, Pertejo V, Garrigues V. Individual prediction of response to pneumatic dilation in patients with achalasia. Dig Dis Sci 1996;41:2135

298. Ponce J, Miralbés M, Garrigues V, Berenguer J. Return of esophageal peristalsis after Heller's myotomy for idiopathic achalasia. Dig Dis Sci 1986;31:545

299. Pricolo VE, Park CS, Thompson WR. Surgical repair of esophageal perforation due to pneumatic dilatation for achalasia. Is myotomy really necessary? Arch Surg 1993;128:540

300. Prior AJ. Oesophageal achalasia mistaken for anorexia nervosa. BMJ 1992;305:833

301. Proctor DD, Fraser JL, Mangano MM, Calkins DR, Rosenberg SJ. Small cell carcinoma of the esophagus in a patient with longstanding primary achalasia. Am J Gastroenterol 1992;87:664

302. Qualman SJ, Haupt HM, Yang P, Hamilton SR. Esophageal Lewy bodies associated with ganglion cell loss in achalasia. Similarity to Parkinson's disease. Gastroenterology 1984;87:848

303. Raiser F, et al. Heller myotomy via minimal-access surgery. An evaluation of antireflux procedures. Arch Surg 1996;131:593

304. Rattan S, Goyal RK. Neural control of the lower esophageal sphincter. Influence of the vagus nerves. J Clin Invest 1974;54:899

305. Rees JR, Thorbjarnarson B, Barnes WH. Achalasia: results of operation in 84 patients. Ann Surg 1970;171:195

306. Ritvo M, McDonald EJ. Value of nitrites in cardiospasm (achalasia of esophagus): preliminary report. AJR 1930;43:500

307. Roark G, Shabot M, Patterson M. Achalasia secondary to hepatocellular carcinoma. J Clin Gastroenterol 1983;5:255

308. Roberts DH, Gilmore IT. Achalasia in Anderson-Fabry's disease. J R Soc Med 1984;77:430

309. Robertson CS, Fellows IW, Mayberry JF, Atkinson M. Choice of therapy for achalasia in relation to age. Digestion 1988;40:244

310. Robertson CS, Martin BAB, Atkinson M. Possible role of herpes viruses in the etiology of achalasia of the cardia. Gut 1990;30:A731

311. Robertson CS, Martin BA, Atkinson M. Varicella-zoster virus DNA in the oesophageal myenteric plexus in achalasia. Gut 1993;34:299

312. Robertson GS, Veitch PS, de Caestecker J, Wicks AC, Lloyd DM. Laparoscopic Heller's cardiomyotomy without an antireflux procedure. Br J Surg 1995;82:957

313. Rock LA, Latham PS, Hankins JR, Nasrallah SM. Achalasia associated with squamous cell carcinoma of the esophagus: a case report. Am J Gastroenterol 1985;80:526

314. Rozen P, Gelfond M, Salzman S, Baron J, Gilat T. Radionuclide confirmation of the therapeutic value of isosorbide dinitrate in relieving the dysphagia in achalasia. J Clin Gastroenterol 1982;4:17

315. Rozycki DL, Ruben RJ, Rapin I, Spiro AJ. Autosomal recessive deafness associated with short stature, vitiligo, muscle wasting and achalasia. Arch Otolaryngol 1971;93:194

316. Sandler RS, Bozymski EM, Orlando RC. Failure of clinical criteria to distinguish between primary achalasia and achalasia secondary to tumor. Dig Dis Sci 1982;27:209

317. Satin AJ, Twickler D, Gilstrap LC. Esophageal achalasia in late pregnancy. Obstet Gynecol 1992;79:812

318. Schiano TD, Miller LS, Dabezies M, Cohen S, Parkman HP, Fisher RS. Use of high-resolution endoscopic ultrasonography to assess esophageal wall damage after pneumatic dilation and botulinum toxin injection to treat achalasia. Gastrointest Endosc 1996;44:151

319. Schima W, et al. Globus sensation: value of static radiography combined with videofluoroscopy of the pharynx and oesophagus. Clin Radiol 1996;51:177

320. Schulz KT, Fischer P. Coincidence of lung diseases caused by *Mycobacterium fortuitum* and esophageal achalasia. Pneumologie 1992;46:576

321. Schwickert HC, et al. Motility disorders of the esophagus: diagnosis with barium-rice administration. Eur J Radiol 1995;21:131

322. Seeman H, Traube M. Hiccups and achalasia. Ann Intern Med 1991;115:711

323. Seki H, et al. Malignant pleural mesothelioma presenting as achalasia. Intern Med 1994;33:624

324. Shabsin HS, Katz PO, Schuster MM. Behavioral treatment of intractable chest pain in a patient with vigorous achalasia. Am J Gastroenterol 1988;83:970

325. Shafik A. Esophago-sphincter inhibitory reflex: role in the deglutition mechanism and esophageal achalasia. J Invest Surg 1996;9:37

326. Shimohashi N, Nawata H, Umeda F, Hashimoto T, Yamaguchi H, Furukawa M. Ectodermal dysplasia syndrome in siblings with true keloids stenosis of the esophagus after operations for congenital achalasia and renovascular hypertension due to stenosis of renal artery. Intern Med 1995;34:406

327. Shoenut JP, Kryger MH, Micflikier AB, Kerr P, Orr WC, Yamashiro Y. Effect of severe gastroesophageal reflux on sleep stage in patients with aperistaltic esophagus. Dig Dis Sci 1996;41:372

328. Shoenut JP, Micflikier AB, Aldor TA, Yaffee CS, Goldenberg DJ. Reproducibility of ambulatory esophageal pH monitoring in the aperistaltic esophagus. Dysphagia 1996;11:248

329. Shoenut JP, Micflikier AB, Yaffe CS, Den Boer B, Teskey JM. Reflux in untreated achalasia patients. J Clin Gastroenterol 1995;20:6

330. Shoenut JP, Yaffe CS, Duerksen D. A prospective assessment of gastroesophageal reflux before and after treatment of achalasia patients: pneumatic dilation versus transthoracic limited myotomy. Am J Gastroenterol 1997;92:1109

331. Sigala S, et al. Different neurotransmitter systems are involved in the development of esophageal achalasia. Life Sci 1995;10:1311

332. Sigurgeirsson B, Jóhannsson KB, Haroarson S, Onundarson PT, Thorgeirsson G. Acute thoracic inlet obstruction in achalasia with adenoid cystic and squamous cell carcinoma. Ann Thorac Surg 1985;40:516

333. Simila S, Kokkonen J, Kaski M. Achalasia sicca-juvenile Sjogren's syndrome with achalasia and gastric hyposecretion. Eur J Pediatr 1978;129:175

334. Simmons DB, Griffin JW Jr, Schuman BM. Achalasia in patients over 65. J Fla Med Assoc 1997;84:101

335. Singaram C, Snipes RL, Bass P, Gaumnitz EA, Sweet MA. Evaluation of early events in the creation of amyenteric oppossum model of achalasia. Neurogastroenterol Motil 1996;8:351

336. Sinha S, Chattopadhyay TK. Short segment oesophago-cardiomyotomy for achalasia cardia. Trop Gastroenterol 1997;18:34

337. Slim K, Chipponi J, Lechner C, Le Roux S, Pezet D. Heller's myotomy by laparoscopic approach for megaesophagus. Ann Chir 1995;49:287

338. Slim K, Mathieu S, Boulant J, Chipponi J, Peret D. Laparoscopic myotomy for primary esophageal achalasia: prospective evaluation. Hepatogastroenterology 1997;44:11

339. Smart HL, Foster PN, Evans DF, Slevin B, Atkinson M. Twenty four hour oesophageal acidity in achalasia before and after pneumatic dilation. Gut 1987;28:883

340. Smart HL, Mayberry JF, Atkinson M. Achalasia following gastro-oesophageal reflux. J R Soc Med 1986;79:71

341. Sonnenberg A, Massey BT, McCarty DJ, Jacobsen SJ. Epidemiology of hospitalization for achalasia in the United States. Dig Dis Sci 1993;38:233

342. Spechler SJ, Goyal RK, Ruben RA, Rosenberg SJ, Souza RF. Heartburn in patients with achalasia. Gut 1995;37:305

343. Spinelli C, et al. Focal nodular hyperplasia of the liver associated with cardial achalasia, situs viscerum inversus and gastric mucosal ectopia in the duodenum. Minerva Chir 1991;46:765

344. Stark GA, Castell DO, Richter JE, Wu WC. Prospective randomized comparison of Brown-McHardy and microinvasive balloon dilators in treatment of achalasia. Am J Gastroenterol 1990;85:1322

345. Stein DT, Knauer CM. Achalasia in monozygotic twins. Dig Dis Sci 1982;27:636

346. Storch WB, et al. Autoantibodies to Auerbach's plexus in achalasia. Cell Mol Biol (Noisy-le-grand) 1995;41:1033

347. Streitz JM Jr, Tilden RL, Aas JA, Glick ME, Williamson WA, Ellis FH Jr. Objective assessment of gastroesophageal reflux after short esophagomyotomy for achalasia with the use of manometry and pH monitoring. J Thorac Cardiovasc Surg 1996;111:107

348. Stuckey BG, Mastaglia FL, Reed WD, Pullan PT. Glucocorticoid insufficiency, achalasia, alacrima with autonomic and motor neuropathy. Ann Intern Med 1987;106:62

349. Suris X, Moyà F, Panés J, del Olmo JA, Solé M, Muñoz-Gómez J. Achalasia of the esophagus in secondary amyloidosis. Am J Gastroenterol 1993;88:1959

350. Swanstrom LL, Pennings J. Laparoscopic esophagomyotomy for achalasia. Surg Endosc 1995;9:290

351. Swedlund A, Traube M, Siskind BN, McCallum RW. Nonsurgical management of esophageal perforation from pneumatic dilation in achalasia. Dig Dis Sci 1989;34:379

352. Tamada R, Sugimachi K, Yaita A, Inokuchi K, Watanabe H. Lymphangioma of the esophagus presenting symptoms of achalasia—a case report. Jpn J Surg 1980;10:59

353. Tasker AD. Achalasia: an unusual cause of stridor. Clin Radiol 1995;50:496

354. Thomas E, Lebow RA, Gubler RJ, Bryant LR. Nifedipine for the poor-risk elderly patient with achalasia: objective response demonstrated by solid meal study. South Med J 1984;77:394

355. Thomson D, Shoenut JP, Trenholm BG, Teskey JM. Reflux patterns following myotomy without fundoplication for achalasia. Ann Thorac Surg 1987;43:550

356. Tishler JM, Shin MS, Stanley RJ, Koehler RE. CT of the thorax in patients with achalasia. Dig Dis Sci 1983;28:692

357. Todorczuk JR, Aliperti G, Staiano A, Clouse RE. Reevaluation of manometric criteria for vigorous achalasia. Is this a distinct clinical disorder? Dig Dis Sci 1991;36:274

358. Tokumine F, et al. A rare case of achalasia coexistent with sigmoid megacolon and associated with epilepsy. J Gastroenterol 1994;29:637

359. Torphy TJ, Fine CF, Burman M, Barnette MS, Ormsbee HS III. Lower esophageal sphincter relaxation is associated with increased cyclic nucleotide content. Am J Physiol 1986;251:G786

360. Tottrup A, et al. Effects of postganglionic nerve stimulation in oesophageal achalasia: an *in vitro* study. Gut 1990;31:17

361. Tracey JP, Traube M. Difficulties in the diagnosis of pseudoachalasia. Am J Gastroenterol 1994;89:2014

362. Traube M, Dubovik S, Lange RC, McCallum RW. The role of nifedipine therapy in achalasia: results of a randomized, double-blind, placebo controlled study. Am J Gastroenterol 1989;84:1259

363. Travis KW, Saini VK, O'Sullivan PT. Upper airway obstruction and achalasia of the esophagus. Anesthesiology 1981;54:87

364. Triadafilopoulos G, Aaronson M, Sackel S, Burakoff R. Medical treatment of esophageal achalasia. Double-blind crossover study with oral nifedipine, verapamil, and placebo. Dig Dis Sci 1991;36:260

365. Tuck JS, Bisset RA, Doig CM. Achalasia of the cardia in childhood and the syndrome of achalasia alacrima and ACTH insensitivity. Clin Radiol 1991;44:260

366. Tucker HJ, Snape WJ, Cohen S. Achalasia secondary to carcinoma: manometric and clinical features. Ann Intern Med 1978;39:315

367. Turkot S, Oren S, Lebovici O, Ben Valid E, Kogan J, Golzman B. Acute upper-airway obstruction in a patient with achalasia. Ann Emerg Med 1997;29:687

368. Tyson J, Martin E, Evans JS Jr. Diffuse dilation of the esophagus due to cardiospasm. N Y Med J 1904;80:731

369. Vaezi M, Richter J, Wilcox M, Schroeder P, Slaughter R. One year follow-up: pneumatic dilatation more effective than botulinum toxin. Gastroenterology 1997;112:A318

370. Vallera RA, Brazer SR. Botulinum toxin for suspected pseudoachalasia. Am J Gastroenterol 1995;90:1319

371. Van Dam J, Rice TW, Achkar E, Sivak MV Jr, Falk GW. Endosonographic evaluation of the patient with achalasia: appearance of the esophagus using the echoendoscope. Endoscopy 1995;27:185

372. Van Goidsenhoven GE, et al. Treatment of achalasia of the cardia with pneumatic dilations. Gastroenterology 1963;45:326

373. Vantrappen G, et al. Manometric studies in achalasia of the cardia, before and after pneumatic dilations. Gastroenterology 1963;45:317

374. Vantrappen G, Hellemans J. Diseases of the Esophagus. New York: Springer, 1974:341

375. Vantrappen G, Hellemans J, Deloof W, Valembois P, Vandenbroucke J. Treatment of achalasia with pneumatic dilations. Gut 1971;12:268

376. Vara-Thorbec C, Herrainz R. Esophageal achalasia: laparoscopic Heller cardiomyotomy. Int Surg 1995;80:376

377. Várkonyi A, Julesz J, Szüts P, Tóth I, Faredin I. Simultaneous occurrence of selective ACTH insensitivity, achalasia and alacrima accompanied by hyperlipoproteinaemia. Acta Paediatr Hung 1992;32:31

378. Verne GN, Eaker EY, Sallustio JE. Anti-myenteric neuronal antibodies in patients with achalasia. A prospective study. Dig Dis Sci 1997;42:307

379. von Mikulicz J. Ueber Gastroskopie und Oesophagoskopie. Miu Ver Aeszte Niede Oest Wien 1882;8:41

380. Wattchow DA, Costa M. Distribution of peptide-containing nerve fibers in achalasia of the oesophagus. J Gastroenterol Hepatol 1996; 11:478

381. Weber A, et al. Linkage of the gene for the triple A syndrome to chromosome 12q13 near the type II keratin gene cluster. Hum Mol Genet 1996;5:2061

382. Wehrmann T, Caspary WF, Lembcke B, Jung M, Jacobi V. Pneumatic dilation in achalasia with a low-compliance balloon: results of a 5-year prospective evaluation. Gastrointest Endosc 1995;42:31

383. Westbrook JL. Oesophageal achalasia causing respiratory obstruction. Anaesthesia 1992;7:38

384. Westly CR, et al. Infantile achalasia inherited as an autosomal recessive disorder. J Pediatr 1975;87:243

385. Wewalka FW, Haidinger D, Clodi PH. Endoscopic clipping of esophageal perforation after pneumatic dilation for achalasia. Endoscopy 1995;27:608

386. Willis T. Pharmaceutice Rationalis sive Diatriba do Medicamentorum Operationibus in Humano Corpore. London: Hagae Comitis, 1674

387. Witzel L. Treatment of achalasia with a pneumatic dilator attached to a gastroscope. Endoscopy 1981;13:176

388. Wolf EL, Frager D, Goldman MJ, Parker JG, Beneventano TC. Achalasia complicated by esophagobronchial fistula. Am J Gastroenterol 1985;80:584

389. Wollam GL, Maher FT, Ellis FH Jr. Vagal nerve function in achalasia of the esophagus. Surg Forum 1967;18:362

390. Wong MD, Lucas CE, Ledgerwood AM, Davidson SB. Retrograde gastroesophageal intussusception complicating chronic achalasia. Arch Surg 1995;130:1009

391. Wong RK, Maydonovitch CL. Utility of parameters measured during pneumatic dilation as predictors of successful dilation. Am J Gastroenterol 1996;91:1126

392. Wong RK, Maydonovitch C, Garcia JE, Johnson LF, Castell DO. The effects of terbutaline sulfate, nitroglycerin and aminophylline on lower esophageal sphincter pressure and esophageal emptying in patients with achalasia. J Clin Gastroenterol 1987;9:386

393. Wong RK, Maydonovitch CL, Metz SJ, Baker JR, Jr. Significant Dqwl association in achalasia. Dig Dis Sci 1989;34:349

394. Wong RKH, Maydonovitch CL. Efficacy of graduated pneumatic dilations in achalasia: a six year prospective study. Am J Gastroenterol 1989;84:1153

395. Woods CA, Foutch PG, Waring JP, Sanowski RA. Pancreatic pseudocyst as a cause of secondary achalasia. Gastroenterology 1989; 96:235

396. Wychalis AR, et al. Achalasia and carcinoma of the esophagus. JAMA 1971;215:1638

397. Xynos E, Vassilakis JS, Chrysos E, Petrakis I, Tzovaras G. Laparoscopic Heller's cardiomyotomy and Dor's fundoplication for esophageal achalasia. J Laparoendosc Surg 1996;6:253

398. Yang P, et al. The effect of carbonated beverages on esophageal clearance in achalasia. Gastroenterology 1982;82:1215A

399. Yong-Xian Y. Treatment of esophageal achalasia (cardiospasm) with diaphragmatic graft: report of 44 patients. Ann Thorac Surg 1983; 35:249

400. Zegel HG, Kressel HY, Levine GM, Rosato EF. Delayed esophageal perforation after pneumatic dilation for treatment of achalasia. Gastrointest Radiol 1979;4:219

401. Zeigler K, et al. Endoscopic appearance of the esophagus in achalasia. Endoscopy 1990;22:1

402. Zenker F, von Ziemssen H. Handbuch der speziallen Pathologie and Therapie. Leipzig: FWC Vogel, 1876

403. Zhou CW. Association of esophageal carcinoma with achalasia: report on 7 cases. Chung Hua Chung Liu Tsa Chih 1992;14:127

404. Zimmerman FH, Rosenweig NS. Achalasia in a father and son. Am J Gastroenterol 1984;79:506

The Esophagus, Third Edition,
edited by D. O. Castell and J. E. Richter.
Lippincott Williams & Wilkins, Philadelphia © 1999.

# CHAPTER 11

# Nonachalasia Motility Disorders

## Philip O. Katz and June A. Castell

The term *motility disorder* has been traditionally used to describe abnormal motility patterns demonstrated when esophageal manometry is performed, primarily in patients with unexplained (noncardiac) chest pain and nonobstructive dysphagia. Classification of these "disorders" has been a subject of some controversy. New research into the potential pathogenesis of unexplained chest pain and the increase in the number of esophageal manometric studies performed as part of the preoperative evaluation for minimally invasive surgery for gastroesophageal reflux have led to new debate over the classification and clinical relevance of these spastic motility disorders. While these contraction abnormalities can be separated manometrically from the pattern seen in normal subjects, their clinical importance is not always clear as many patients will demonstrate them in the manometry laboratory but lack correlation with the presenting symptoms. Treatment may reduce symptoms—particularly chest pain or reflux—without change in manometric abnormalities, suggesting that these may be markers of sensory abnormalities and not reflective of a true disease state.

Recent investigations, primarily from our laboratory, have led to a revised classification of esophageal motility abnormalities based on manometric abnormalities that differ significantly from accepted normal findings. These primary esophageal motility abnormalities can now be classified based on their predominant contraction patterns, as listed in Table 11–1. Achalasia, the only true primary motility disorder documented with certainty, is discussed in detail in Chapter 10. The other abnormalities include incoordinated motility [diffuse esophageal spasm (DES)], hypercontractile motility [hypertensive lower esophageal sphincter (HLES) and nutcracker esophagus (NE)], and hypocontractile motility, a category that includes hypotensive LES and ineffective

esophageal motility (IEM). The latter represents a reclassification of the large category formerly termed nonspecific esophageal motility disorders (NEMDs). This chapter will review these motility abnormalities in detail and put into perspective their clinical meaning.

## GENERAL OVERVIEW, PREVALENCE AND PRESENTATION

Although the precise prevalence of esophangeal motility abnormalities is unknown, one study of 1,161 adult patients referred for evaluation of chest pain or dysphagia found a motility abnormality in 33% [78]. They were found more commonly in patients with dysphagia (132 of 251 or 53%) than in those with chest pain (255 of 910 or 28%). The type of esophageal motility abnormality varied depending on the patient's presenting complaint (Fig. 11–1). Another study, of 83 children and young adults aged 1 to 20 years evaluated with motility studies for chest pain, found a motility abnormality in 25%. The distribution of abnormalities in this group was different from that of the study outlined in Fig. 11–1. Achalasia and DES were seen in 14 (66%), while NE and HLES were seen in only two patients each. The remaining four patients had a hypotensive LES [65].

An esophageal motility abnormality should be suspected in any patient who presents with dysphagia, chest pain, or odynophagia. Unfortunately, there are no specific signs or symptoms that allow the clinician to make a definitive diagnosis of a motility disorder based solely on the history. Dysphagia for both solids and liquids suggests a motility abnormality, but a structural lesion must be ruled out by a barium swallow or upper endoscopy. Chest pain of esophageal origin (see Chapter 36) is indistinguishable from chest pain of coronary artery disease; heart disease must be excluded before a diagnosis of esophageal pain can be entertained. Odynophagia (painful swallowing) should signal a search for infectious, pill-induced, or reflux esophagitis. Primary esophageal motility abnormalities rarely present with this

P. O. Katz: Department of Medicine, Chest Pain and Swallowing Center, Graduate Hospital, Philadelphia, Pennsylvania 19146.

J. A. Castell: Department of Medicine, Graduate Hospital, Philadelphia, Pennsylvania 19146.

**TABLE 11–1.** *Classification of primary esophageal motility abnormalities*

| Functional defect | Descriptive term | Manometric findings |
|---|---|---|
| Aperistalsis | Achalasia (a true disorder; see Chapter 10) | Absent distal peristalsis[a] <br> Elevated resting LES pressure (>45 mm Hg)[b] <br> Incomplete LES relaxation (residual pressure >8 mm Hg)[b] <br> Elevated baseline esophageal pressure[b] |
| Incoordinated motility | Diffuse esophageal spasm | Simultaneous contractions ≥20% wet swallows, with intermittent peristalsis[a] <br> Repetitive contractions (≥3 peaks)[b] <br> Prolonged-duration contractions (>6 sec)[b] <br> Retrograde contractions[b] <br> Isolated incomplete LES relaxations[b] |
| Hypercontractile | Nutcracker esophagus | Increased distal peristaltic amplitude (≥180 mm Hg)[a] <br> Increased distal peristaltic duration (>6 sec)[b] |
| | Hypertensive LES | Resting LES pressure >45 mm Hg[a] <br> Incomplete LES relaxation (residual pressure >8 mm Hg)[b] |
| Hypocontractile | Ineffective esophageal motility | Increased nontransmitted peristalsis (≥30%)[c] <br> Distal peristaltic amplitude,[c] <30 mm Hg in ≥30 swallows |
| | Hypotensive LES | Resting LES pressure <10 mm Hg[a] |

LES, lower esophageal sphincter.
[a] Required for diagnosis.
[b] May be seen, not required.
[c] Either or both may be seen.

symptom. The physical examination will help rule out other causes of dysphagia, odynophagia, and chest pain; but it will not help in diagnosing or classifying primary esophageal motility abnormalities. An esophageal motility abnormality may be suggested by findings on barium radiography; however, a manometric examination is required for a precise diagnosis.

### RADIOLOGY

An esophageal motility abnormality may be suggested by findings seen on a barium swallow. When carefully performed, with videofluoroscopy, the barium study can be sensitive and specific for the presence of a motility abnormality. A study using simultaneous videofluoroscopy and manometry in 11 subjects found high concordance between the fluoroscopic and manometric assessments of peristalsis [108]. The positive and negative predictive values of fluoroscopy for a motility abnormality were 93% and 98%, respectively, when individual barium swallows were compared with manometry. If two or more abnormal swallows were required for diagnosis, complete agreement that a motility abnormality was present was seen between fluoroscopy and manometry. Small bolus size (5- or 10-mL swallows), which greatly reduces radiation exposure, still resulted in 92% agreement between modalities.

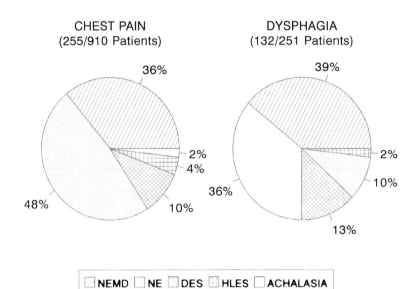

FIG. 11–1. Pie diagram describing the prevalence of esophageal motility disorders in patients with noncardiac chest pain **(left)** and those with dysphagia **(right)**. *NEMD,* nonspecific esophageal motility disorder; *HLES,* hypertensive lower esophageal sphincter; *DES,* diffuse esophageal spasm; *NE,* nutcracker esophagus.

This same study attempted to interpret the significance of tertiary activity [108], a fluoroscopic finding that is often difficult to interpret. It is seen frequently in association with esophageal motility abnormalities but often is seen radiographically when manometry is normal. The authors classified tertiary activity as segmental or nonsegmental based on complete or incomplete obliteration of the esophageal lumen. Nonsegmental tertiary activity did not differentiate between normal or abnormal primary peristalsis seen manometrically; segmental (or severe) tertiary activity, manifested by esophageal coiling (Fig. 11–2) or rosary-bead appearance, was almost always associated with abnormal peristalsis when manometry was performed. Milder forms of tertiary activity are therefore not indicative of motility abnormalities and should not be classified as esophageal spasm.

This study suggests that a well-performed videofluoroscopic study with five individual barium swallows is accurate for diagnosing an esophageal motility abnormality, particularly if two swallows are abnormal and severe segmental tertiary activity is seen. Although the radiograph appears highly sensitive for diagnosing an esophageal motility ab-

normality, the findings are nonspecific and do not distinguish between the manometrically defined disorders of peristalsis. Few radiologists will take the time and meticulous care required to perform the barium study with this accuracy, so manometry is required for final classification of the motility abnormality.

Endoscopy plays little role in the evaluation of patients with suspected motility abnormalities. It is used in conjunction with radiologic studies to evaluate patients with suspected structural dysphagia and to rule out esophagitis or Barrett's esophagus in patients with gastroesophageal reflux disease (GERD) but will not aid in diagnosis of an esophageal motility abnormality.

Accurate classification of primary esophageal motility abnormalities requires a well-performed manometric study, with assessment of LES pressure and relaxation as well as esophageal body contraction and duration with ten 5-mL water swallows. Using a standardized technique (see Chapter 5), a well-defined set of normal values has been obtained in 95 subjects [122]. Using this as a baseline, the primary esophageal motility abnormalities discussed subsequently can be accurately classified (Table 11–1).

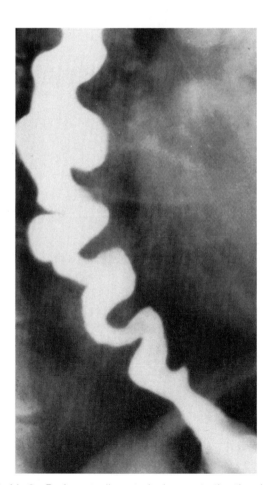

**FIG. 11–2.** Barium swallow study demonstrating the characteristic "corkscrew" appearance of diffuse esophageal spasm.

## INCOORDINATED MOTILITY (DIFFUSE ESOPHAGEAL SPASM)

The first description of esophageal spasm is attributed to Osgood [106], who in 1889 described six patients who had attacks of "sudden and often intense constriction in the epigastrium; if the pain occurred at the table, with an arrest of the food at the cardiac orifice, and perfect consciousness on the part of the patient of this arrest, the food, however, after an instance delay, passing on into the stomach." The use of the term *diffuse esophageal spasm* as a diagnosis for this clinical presentation likely stems from this description. Early radiographic descriptions come from Moersch and Camp [99], who first used the phrase *diffuse spasms of the distal esophagus*. The first manometric descriptions were by Creamer and colleagues [48] in 1958 and Roth and Fleshler in 1964 [125]. The commonly used clinical syndrome of DES was defined by Fleshler in 1967 [58] as a "clinical syndrome characterized by symptoms of substernal distress or dysphagia or both, the radiographic appearance of localized, nonprogressive waves (tertiary contractions), *and* an increased incidence of non-peristaltic contractions recorded by intraluminal manometry." This complete description continues to be accurate today.

DES is a disorder seen in patients with unexplained chest pain or dysphagia associated with disordered peristalsis and severe tertiary activity on barium swallow. Manometrically it is characterized by incoordinated motility, that is, simultaneous distal esophageal contractions intermixed with normal peristalsis [117]. DES has inappropriately been used as a catchall diagnosis for all esophageal disorders associated with unexplained chest pain or tertiary activity in patients with dysphagia who are examined by barium swallow. Early studies suggested that DES accounted for 15% to 18% of esophageal motility disorders seen in patients with chest pain [45, 111, 117]. When accurately classified manometrically, DES is actually uncommon. One study of 1,161 patients with noncardiac chest pain or dysphagia found that DES comprised only 10% of the motility abnormalities when defined manometrically [78] (Figs. 11–1, 11–3) A more recent, large study by Dalton et al. [50] found a prevalence of only 3%. Our own data suggest that this latter figure is closer to the real prevalence. DES is seen at any age, most commonly in patients older than 50, without gender predominance [92, 96, 98].

## Etiology and Pathophysiology

The etiology of DES is not known. Familial clustering [62, 82, 83] has been reported, suggesting a genetic link for this disorder in some individuals.

Evidence suggesting neural dysfunction has been found in some patients with DES [34]. Administration of methacholine, a cholinergic agonist (2 to 6 mg), was followed by reproduction of typical chest pain in four of 14 patients with DES and ''replacement of normal peristaltic pressure by repetitive and simultaneous contractions typical of DES'' in one study [86]. Normal control subjects had no pain or significant motility abnormalities when receiving twice the dose used in DES (10 mg). Another study found a significant increase in amplitude and duration of esophageal contractions in DES patients compared with healthy control subjects when intravenous edrophonium (100 $\mu$g per kg) and subcutaneous bethanechol (40 $\mu$g per kg) were given to DES patients [93]. Chest pain was reproduced in six of eight patients with edrophonium and in three of six patients with bethanechol. Ergonovine (0.5 to 1.0 mg) produced ''esophageal spasm'' in 22 of 44 patients with DES compared with four of ten control subjects in one study [7]. Chest pain was experienced by 22 of 47 patients and two of ten control subjects. Unfortunately, ergonovine also can cause coronary artery spasm, which precludes use of this drug in routine clinical practice [31]. Pentagastrin, at a dose of 6 $\mu$g/kg subcutaneously, was shown to produce a significant increase in mean LES pressures, amplitude of contractions, and repetitive wave activity in nine patients with DES [104]. These changes were not seen in 25 healthy control subjects. In addition, four of nine patients with DES also had reproduction of their chest pain, compared with none of the control subjects. Gastrin used in physiologic concentrations did not demonstrate these effects [88].

One study [17] found a shorter latency of simultaneous and spontaneous contractions in patients with DES compared to controls. It was suggested that the shorter latency of simultaneous contractions may result from a defective deglutitive inhibitory reflex. Preliminary observations indi-

cate that nitric oxide may play a role in the inhibition of ethanol-induced esophageal smooth muscle contractility [57]. Konturek and coauthors [85] studied five patients with DES and compared the effects of intravenous glyceryl trinitrate (GTN), L-arginine, and saline on esophageal contractions and symptoms. They demonstrated a dose-dependent increase in the latency period after swallowing. No change was seen in amplitude of esophageal contractions; however, duration of contractions decreased from 11.2 $\pm$ 4.85 to 5.4 $\pm$ 0.85 with GTN. This was accompanied by a decrease in swallow-induced symptoms. No change was seen with saline or arginine. The authors suggested that patients with DES may have an impaired process of nitric oxide synthesis or degradation.

Studies using recombinant human hemoglobin (rHb1.1) given intravenously have shown that this agent, which inactivates nitric oxide, can alter the timing of esophageal peristalsis in the opposum such that contractions became nearly simultaneous along the length of the smooth muscle [47a]. In a study from the same laboratory, rHb1.1 (0.11 to 0.15 g per kg) was administered intravenously to nine human volunteers. Manometry was performed 30 and 60 minutes after infusion. Amplitude and duration of esophageal contraction increased in all subjects. Simultaneous contractions developed in eight of nine subjects. These observations support the hypothesis that nitric oxide is an important mediator of esophageal peristalsis [99a].

In summary, these investigations suggest that the esophagus of patients with DES shows a hypersensitivity response to cholinergic and hormonal stimulation. This enhanced esophageal sensitivity may be mediated by a defect in neural inhibition possibly related to decreased available nitric oxide. Whether these effects are seen with other motility abnormalities is not known.

## Clinical Presentation

Recurrent chest pain and dysphagia are the most common presenting symptoms. Chest pain is variable in frequency, intensity, and location. Often, a pattern indistinguishable from cardiac angina, including relief with nitroglycerin, is seen. The pain may be associated with meals and is rarely exertional [35, 92, 102]. Dysphagia is intermittent, nonprogressive, and associated with liquids and solids and may be precipitated by stress, hot or cold liquids, or rapid eating [95]. Aspiration or regurgitation is usually not seen with DES. A rare patient has been reported with swallow syncope [26, 125]. Food impaction [48] and fear of eating [64] have been reported in patients with spastic disorders. These symptoms should raise suspicion of the abnormality; the diagnosis requires confirmation by radiology and manometry.

## Radiographic Findings

Radiographic findings are variable. Many examinations are normal. Disruption of primary peristalsis distal to the

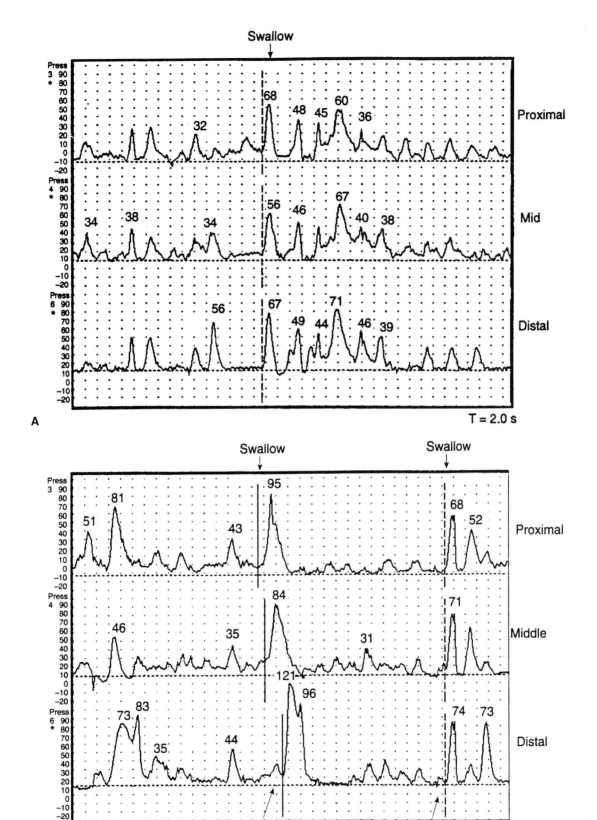

**FIG. 11–3.** Diffuse esophageal spasm. **A:** This tracing shows an esophageal motility pattern typical of the patient with esophageal spasm. The *cursor* marks the beginning of the contraction wave initiated by the swallow. This wave is followed by multiple spontaneous, simultaneous contractions. The amplitudes of these contractions, however, are not particularly high. There is also a great deal of contractile activity between swallows. **B:** This tracing shows another pattern common to patients with spasm. Their motility study will show a variety of wave types. Here, the *solid cursor* marks a peristaltic wave while the *dotted cursor* marks a simultaneous wave. (From ref. 38a, with permission.)

219

aortic arch and in esophageal smooth muscle and severe tertiary activity are the most common abnormalities. Proximal propagation of a bolus is usually normal. Tertiary activity produces the rosary-bead appearance or esophageal coiling seen in Fig. 11–2. The LES region is usually normal radiographically.

A study of 17 patients undergoing a barium swallow within 1 week of a manometric diagnosis of DES revealed several interesting and important findings [40]. Four of 17 patients had normal peristalsis radiographically despite a mean frequency of only 53% normal peristalsis at manometry. Radiographic diagnosis of DES was made in only six patients. In ten patients, the disorder was labeled nonspecific motility disorder, and in one a diagnosis of achalasia was made. Tertiary activity was seen in 12 of 17 patients, four of whom were classified as mild, four moderate, and four severe. Esophageal wall thickness was normal. The authors emphasized several important points; DES is a dynamic disease, a normal radiographic study does not rule out the diagnosis, and tertiary activity may not be seen or be mild. A barium swallow cannot make a diagnosis of a specific esophageal motility abnormality.

**Manometric Findings**

The manometric study is the only way to accurately diagnose DES. Incoordinated motility is the primary finding. Our current criteria require the presence of simultaneous contractions in 20% or greater of wet swallows intermixed with some normal peristalsis. If all contractions are simultaneous, the diagnosis is achalasia. This definition is based on a review by Richter and Castell [117], in which increased simultaneous contractions were the only consistent finding described in published studies of patients with DES (Fig. 11–3). These criteria are reinforced by the observation that simultaneous contractions are rarely seen in normal subjects (four of 95 studied) and none had simultaneous contractions in more than 10% of wet swallows [122]. Simultaneous contractions may be seen with other disorders. Diabetes [69], scleroderma [47], amyloidosis [126], idiopathic pseudo-obstruction [128], alcoholic neuropathies [147], and gastroesophageal reflux [5, 135] are all associated with simultaneous contractions. These disorders are manometrically indistinguishable from symptomatic DES.

Two recent studies suggest that there may be two distinct populations of patients with DES based on symptom presentation and amplitude of simultaneous contractions. Allen and DiMarino [10] recently reviewed 60 patients who met the manometric criteria for DES and evaluated contraction amplitude in both peristaltic and simultaneous contractions. These authors found a bimodal distribution based on each individual patient's highest amplitude of simultaneous contractions. A clear separation was demonstrated: 29/60 had highest simultaneous contraction of 74 mm Hg or less, while 31 had simultaneous amplitudes of 100 mm Hg or greater. Group 1 patients had lower mean LES pressure, mean peri-staltic esophageal amplitude, and mean simultaneous amplitude than patients in group 2. Patients with higher-amplitude simultaneous contractions (group 2) had a greater incidence of chest pain.

We recently reviewed our experience in 35 patients with DES presenting between 1989 and 1996 [131]. Manometric tracings were analyzed for distal esophageal amplitudes of peristaltic and simultaneous contractions, number of simultaneous contractions, and LES pressure and relaxation. Fifteen patients presented with dysphagia, 20 with chest pain. Those with chest pain had higher mean and maximal peristaltic amplitude as well as higher mean amplitude of simultaneous contractions than patients with dysphagia. There was a trend toward higher maximum amplitude of simultaneous contractions in those with chest pain (Table 11–2). LES parameters were not different in the two patient groups. The clear separation in amplitude of simultaneous contractions reported by Allen and DiMarino [10] was not seen. The results of these two reports suggest that patients with a manometric pattern of DES comprise two groups based on amplitude of distal esophageal contraction: those with chest pain have higher pressures and those with dysphagia lower pressures. The pathogenesis of this difference requires further study.

Other manometric findings observed in patients with DES are outlined in Table 11–1. Repetitive waves (three peaks) are seen in only 0.1% of wet swallows in healthy subjects [122]. Dalton and associates [50] found repetitive contractions (three peaks or more in 12 of 56 21%) patients with DES. Early studies of DES reported high-amplitude contractions or waves of prolonged duration [23, 48, 81]. A recent retrospective study in which manometric findings in patients with DES were reviewed found high-amplitude (at least 180 mm Hg) contractions in only two (4%) of 56 patients [50], and increased wave duration was rare. Spontaneous contractions, once thought to be a common motility finding in DES, occurred in 50% of healthy subjects [122]. LES function and pressure are normal in most patients with DES [115]. However, several studies have reported abnormal LES pressure and/or relaxation in 12% to 45% of patients [7, 32, 50, 51, 93, 135].

**Ambulatory 24-Hour Manometry**

Stein [133] compared the diagnostic value of 24-hour ambulatory manometry to that of stationary manometry in patients with esophageal dysmotility and noncardiac chest pain. In this study, 108 patients and 25 healthy control subjects were evaluated. Overall, the diagnostic agreement between the two types of manometry was only 51%. If this number is augmented by the 13 patients in whom DES and NE were interchanged and the 11 in whom normal and NE were interchanged, the agreement between these two technologies is 75%. These findings underscore the hypothesis that these motility abnormalities are interrelated phenomena.

**TABLE 11–2.** *Motility findings in patients with diffuse esophageal spasm based on presenting symptoms*

|  | Chest pain ($n = 15$) | Dysphagia ($n = 20$) | |
|---|---|---|---|
| Mean peristaltic amplitude (mm Hg) | 145 ± 22 | 93 ± 22 | $p = 0.02$ |
| Maximal peristaltic amplitude (mm Hg) | 207 ± 26 | 132 ± 13 | $p = 0.02$ |
| Mean simultaneous amplitude (mm Hg) | 136 ± 23 | 73 ± 8 | $p = 0.02$ |
| Mean simultaneous amplitude (mm Hg) | 182 ± 28 | 177 ± 16 | $p = 0.06$ |

From ref. 131, with permission.

A recent study of 390 consecutive patients evaluated with both ambulatory and stationary manometry underscores the difficulties in interpretation of ambulatory manometry [14]. The authors compared the frequency of DES during the ambulatory study with a stationary study. Using the criteria in Table 11–1, 55 patients (14%) had two or more simultaneous contractions, meeting criteria for DES. For the ambulatory study, the authors defined DES by the presence of high-amplitude, prolonged-duration, multiple-peaked contractions that were associated with chest pain. By this definition, only 16 patients (4%) were diagnosed as having DES. Only 2 (12%) had a manometric diagnosis of spasm as defined in Table 11–1. Only two of the 55 patients with DES during the stationary study had evidence of DES in the ambulatory study. Of the others, 20 had NEMD, 19 GERD, and 14 normal ambulatory manometry.

### Long-term Course

In general, the prognosis is excellent. The few studies that have evaluated DES over time suggest a dynamic disorder. The same manometric diagnosis was found in only 33% of patients in two studies [4, 114] that repeated manometry in DES patients. Patients were followed for a mean of 3.5 and 3.7 years in these studies. Transition to achalasia has been documented and is believed to occur in 3% to 5% of patients [87, 143]. This should not be distressing as treatment of achalasia is usually very successful. Symptoms generally remain stable and may spontaneously improve. No association has been seen between malignancy and DES.

### HYPERCONTRACTILE MOTILITY

#### Nutcracker Esophagus

This manometric abnormality, seen predominantly in patients with noncardiac chest pain, was first described 1977 [28]. In this study, high-amplitude peristaltic contractions (HAPCs) were demonstrated in 41% of patients with noncardiac chest pain. The term *nutcracker esophagus* was first proposed by Benjamin and Castell in 1980 [19] following a study in which they reported patients with noncardiac chest pain and esophageal contractions exceeding 400 mm Hg [21]. Others have used terms such as *supersqueezer* and *hypertensive peristalsis,* but *nutcracker esophagus* has evolved as the most common term used to describe this entity.

The manometric abnormality is defined as average (usu-

ally of ten swallows) distal esophageal peristaltic pressures greater than two standard deviations above normal (i.e., greater than 180 mm Hg) in a symptomatic patient [122]. Prolonged-duration contractions have also been described in NE patients, particularly in one large series [67]. We classify cases of prolonged-duration contractions and normal amplitudes as a hypercontractile motility abnormality and believe this is part of the spectrum of NE. Using this definition, NE has been described in 27% to 48% of patients evaluated by manometry for noncardiac chest pain [28, 67, 78, 100, 105, 137] (Table 11–3). In the largest series (910 patients), NE was clearly the most common disorder (Fig. 11–1), seen in 48% of chest pain patients who had a motility abnormality.

### Etiology

The etiology is unknown. The occasional transition to other motility abnormalities or achalasia raises speculation that this abnormality lies at the beginning of a spectrum of disease that ends in achalasia [13, 19, 110]. Of particular interest is the association of psychologic profiles and symptom overlap with patients with irritable bowel syndrome (IBS) [119]. In this study, the Millon behavior inventory—a psychologic instrument shown to be useful in patients with organic disease—was given to patients with NE, IBS, or structural esophageal disease and to normal controls. Psychologic profiles were similar in patients with NE and IBS, showing high scores on scales measuring somatization, anxiety, and depression. Clouse and Lustman [42] found psychiatric abnormalities by *Diagnostic and Statistical Manual* (DSM II) criteria in more than 30% of their patients with esophageal motility abnormalities surveyed with a diagnostic interview. NE patients with chest pain have been found to have lower pain thresholds during esophageal balloon distention [116]. This is similar to the finding in patients with IBS undergoing rectal balloon distention studies [11]. Both groups of patients seem to be generally sensitive to a variety of esophageal stimuli, some of which normally do not cause chest pain in healthy subjects. The high prevalence of abdominal pain, constipation, flatus, and other lower gastrointestinal symptoms in this patient population suggests a generalized functional disorder, the irritable gut syndrome. Perhaps some patients express their symptoms predominantly in the chest, whereas some do so in the abdomen.

### Presentation

Ninety percent of patients present with chest pain. Dysphagia is a less prominent symptom [78]. Symptom inten-

**TABLE 11–3.** *Manometric abnormalities in patients with chest pain (percentage of total motility abnormalities)*

| Reference | NE (%) | DES (%) | Achalasia (%) | NEMD (%) | HLES (%) |
|---|---|---|---|---|---|
| Katz et al. [78] | 48 | 10 | 2 | 36 | 4 |
| Herrington et al. [67] | 38 | 12 | 5 | 33 | 12 |
| Brand et al. [28] | 41 | 14 | 10 | 35 | — |
| Traube et al. [137] | 27 | 23 | 27 | — | 23 |
| Orr and Robinson. [105] | 28 | 7 | 10 | 55 | — |

NE, nutcracker esophagus; DES, diffuse esophageal spasm; NEMD, nonspecific esophageal motility abnormality; HLES, hypertensive lower esophageal sphincter.

sity, frequency, and location vary. Most patients seek attention for a chest pain syndrome, are evaluated by an internist or cardiologist, and are referred to a gastroenterologist after cardiac disease is ruled out. Associated symptoms include depression, anxiety, and somatization; but these are not readily apparent on routine evaluation. Separation from other esophageal motility abnormalities or cardiac chest pain is not possible by history alone. NE has been reported in association with a meat impaction [29] and diffuse intramural diverticulosis [144]. The physical examination is invariably normal, unless diseases unrelated to the esophagus are present.

### Radiology

By definition, all patients have normal peristalsis, so barium studies should be normal; tertiary waves and hiatal hernia are occasionally seen [41, 107]. Radionuclide esophageal emptying studies should also be normal; however, conflicting results [49, 70, 124] have been published. One study [124], using simultaneous manometry and radionuclide esophageal emptying studies, found that radionuclide transit was normal. Two studies have shown prolonged transit time, particularly in the distal esophagus [22, 53]. Perhaps these patients have other contraction abnormalities not seen at the time of initial manometry.

### Manometry

The diagnosis of NE requires manometry. As stated earlier, contraction amplitude must be greater than two standard deviations above normal, with all contractions peristaltic (Fig. 11–4). Prolonged-duration contractions and increased LES pressure are occasionally seen [38, 56, 67] but are not required features.

The location of the manometric abnormality in the distal esophagus also has been a subject of controversy. In general, NE is regarded as a diffuse process with increased amplitude seen throughout the smooth muscle portion of the esophagus [38]. However, one study described NE as affecting only isolated regions of the distal esophageal smooth muscle [60]. An additional study [28] found HAPCs at multiple levels (every 2 cm) of the esophagus. Benjamin et al. [21] used a stationary location at 2 and 7 cm from the LES in their original descriptive paper. Most experts use the combined mean pressure of the two distal recording sites [38], usually 3 and 8 cm above the LES.

A recent study compared the prevalence and clinical features of patients with either segmental HAPCs (localized to one transducer) or the traditional diffuse contraction abnormalities of NE (found at both distal esophageal transducers) (Fig. 11–4) [2]. The prevalence and the clinical features of patients with HAPC, whether localized to one distal transducer (segmental) or diffuse (both transducers), were the same. In addition, the authors [2] observed HAPC in areas of the esophagus (at 13 cm above the LES) not previously described.

### Manometric Course

Patients with NE have a tendency to show different manometric findings during long-term follow-up studies. Dalton and co-workers [49] studied manometric tracings of 24 patients with NE who had an average of 4.6 studies during a mean period of 32 months. The consistency of the diagnosis of NE varied considerably. Only 54% of these patients had initial diagnosis confirmed during all follow-up studies. Another manometric follow-up study of 25 patients with NE [3] documented change from the initial finding of NE into another manometric pattern, including DES, NEMD, and normal tracings. Evolution of NE into DES [100, 136] and achalasia [13, 110] has been reported in single case studies.

### Clinical Importance of Nutcracker Esophagus

NE has undergone repeated evaluation and redefinition over its existence as a discrete diagnostic entity. It has been suggested that it may not be a true disorder but merely a manometric curiosity [76]. This suggestion is based on several criteria. First, chest pain is seldom seen during a manometric examination when the high pressure is generated. Second, reduction in pressures—either by pharmacologic agents or with time—does not correlate with improvement in chest pain. Finally, no abnormality in contraction sequence can be consistently demonstrated by radiographic or radionuclide emptying studies, suggesting little alteration in physiology.

What evidence do we have that NE is real, and how does

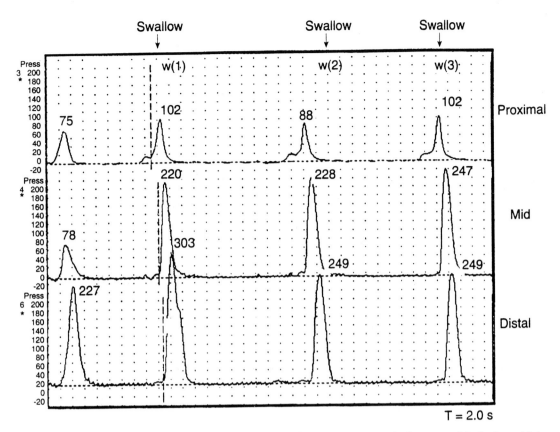

FIG. 11–4. Nutcracker esophagus. This tracing illustrates the most typical manometric feature, high-amplitude distal peristalsis. The *cursors* mark the beginning of the wave and show clear peristalsis; however, the amplitudes are well in excess of the normal range, not to exceed 180 mm Hg. (From ref. 38a, with permission.)

it fit in the clinical spectrum of esophageal abnormalities? NE is the most common manometric abnormality seen when patients with noncardiac chest pain are studied and is seen rarely in patients with dysphagia [78]. These patients have reproduction of their chest pain with edrophonium, acid, or balloon provocation more frequently than patients with other esophageal motility abnormalities [78]. NE appears to be a marker for noncardiac chest pain, even if it is not the cause. Evolution into manometric patterns consistent with ineffective esophageal motility (see below) or DES has been reported in several patients in one study that examined NE patients on up to three occasions over a 1-year period [49]. Other reports have shown transition of NE to DES or achalasia [2, 13, 49, 100], suggesting that this abnormality is part of a spectrum of esophageal motility abnormalities. In addition to being a potential marker for chest pain, the variability in pressures over multiple studies [49] and long-term follow-up studies may give some insight into the interaction of esophageal motility abnormalities, stress, and noncardiac chest pain. Though no difference in chest pain scores could be demonstrated with nifedipine versus placebo (see below), the observation that most patients improved with time is important. Decrease in physician visits by 77%, elimination of medication in 45%, and decrease in pain frequency [49]

(seemingly related to good physician–patient interaction) suggest a stress-related or psychologic component to chest pain syndromes, a situation common in IBS. Psychologic profiles, based on measurement scales used to assess patients with organic illness, demonstrate that patients with NE tend to be hypochondriacal, to react to stress-related events with increased symptoms, and to seek medical care earlier than controls [119]. Depression, anxiety, and somatization are seen with increased frequency in this group [119], which can be correlated with esophageal response to laboratory stressors. Cold pressor, noise, and stressful interviews have been shown to increase esophageal contraction amplitude [12, 149] and trigger simultaneous contractions in normal subjects. This has been confirmed in patients with NE who have shown increased contraction amplitude following similar stressors [3].

The place of NE in the spectrum of esophageal motility abnormalities remains to be clarified but cannot be dismissed as unimportant [37] (Table 11–4). Currently, we can say with certainty that it is a well-defined manometric entity, commonly found in patients examined for noncardiac chest pain, particularly at their first visit [49]. The cause is unknown and, as in IBS, may be closely related to stress. The long-term outlook is good. Improvement can usually be

**TABLE 11–4.** *Nutcracker esophagus: the evidence*

| For | Against |
|---|---|
| HAPCs are the most common manometric abnormality in chest pain patients | No correlation between HAPC and chest pain |
| Increase in response to provocative agents (edrophonium, balloon) greater compared to other EMAs | Reduction in HAPC correlates poorly with improvement in symptoms |
| Transition to DES, achalasia seen | No demonstrable transit abnormality |

HAPC, high-amplitude peristaltic contraction; EMA, esophageal motility abnormality; DES, diffuse esophageal spasm.

achieved with frequent physician–patient interaction, i.e., good old-fashioned rapport. It might be best to consider NE pressures as a marker for chest pain syndrome for which the esophagus is the offending organ, analogous to the increase in rectal motility (three to six cycles per minute) in patients with IBS [43].

## HYPERTENSIVE LOWER ESOPHAGEAL SPHINCTER

HLES is an uncommon manometric abnormality of unknown etiology defined as increased resting LES pressure (two standard deviations above normal, usually greater than 45 mm Hg) with normal residual pressure associated with normal peristaltic sequence. HAPCs or prolonged-duration peristaltic contractions have also been described, indicating some overlap with NE. An example of HLES is shown in Fig. 11–5.

Described as early as 1960 [46], this abnormality is typically seen in patients being evaluated for unexplained chest pain. Dysphagia can be the presenting symptom [78]. The frequency of HLES ranges from 0.5% to 2.8% [15, 66, 78, 79] in reported series. It may be seen in patients with gastroesophageal reflux. A recent study reviewed manometric and pH recordings from 349 consecutive patients studied over a 3-year period to determine the frequency of HLES in patients with gastroesophageal reflux. Eighteen patients were identified, representing 5.2% of all patients with reflux seen in the study period [79]. A recent preliminary study found HLES in close to 10% of patients with abnormal gastroesophageal reflux by pH monitoring [59]. The finding of HLES in patients with reflux disease does not appear to influence therapy. Psychologic abnormalities have been described in these patients, suggesting a stress-related component and further

overlap with NE [146]. Perhaps HLES is another manometric marker for esophageal chest pain.

### Manometry

Functional abnormalities of the LES, including impaired relaxation and increases in residual pressure (Fig. 11–5B), have been described in some studies [61, 79, 147]. In addition, about 50% of the patients also had HAPC in the distal esophagus. This finding raises the possibility that NE and HLES may be part of the same spectrum of hypercontractile dysmotility of the distal esophagus. Two older studies, using open-tipped catheters, demonstrated that the LES in patients with this abnormality contracted with excess force following a swallow [46, 63]. No studies examining the long-term manometric course of patients with HLES are presently available.

### Radiology

Barium swallow is usually normal, though up to 50% may demonstrate a hiatal hernia. Radionuclide emptying studies are also usually normal [134, 138], confirming functionally normal esophageal transit. The mechanism of dysphagia or chest pain is therefore unknown.

## NONSPECIFIC ESOPHAGEAL MOTILITY DISORDERS

This category of motility abnormality has been used to describe manometric patterns that are clearly abnormal but do not fit one of the abnormalities outlined in this chapter. They have been grouped into this broad category and typically include low-amplitude peristalsis (less than 30 mm Hg), nontransmitted contractions (more than 20% of wet swallows), spontaneous contractions, prolonged-duration contractions (longer than 6 seconds), isolated incomplete LES relaxation, retrograde contractions, or triple-peaked contractions [20, 36, 45, 68, 80]. Abnormalities in this broad diagnostic category are seen with high frequency in patients with chest pain, dysphagia, and gastroesophageal reflux. In most reports, this manometric diagnosis is the first or second most common in patients with unexplained chest pain [28, 67, 78, 105].

In an attempt to further clarify these NEMDs, Leite et al. [90] reviewed the manometric records of 600 consecutive patients referred to one laboratory over a 2.5-year period to identify all patients classified as NEMD. Sixty-one pa-

**FIG. 11–5. A:** Hypertensive lower esophageal sphincter (LES): baseline pressure. This tracing shows a station pull-through of a patient with a hypertensive LES. The resting pressure of the LES, calculated as the mean pressure between the cursors, is 54 mm Hg. **B:** Hypertensive LES: relaxation. The hypertensive LES most commonly does not relax to gastric baseline following a swallow, as shown in this tracing. These four swallows show a residual pressure of about 7 mm Hg. Peristaltic activity above the LES is normal. (From ref. 38a, with permission.)

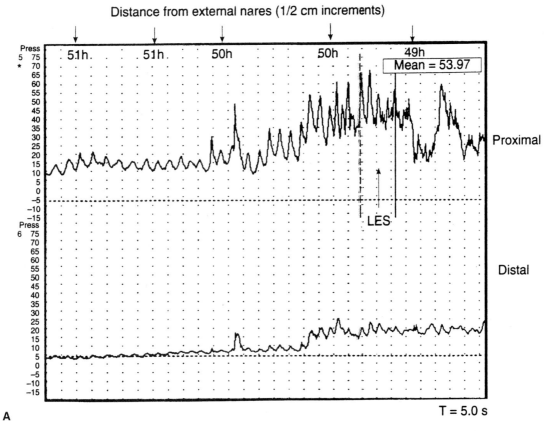

A

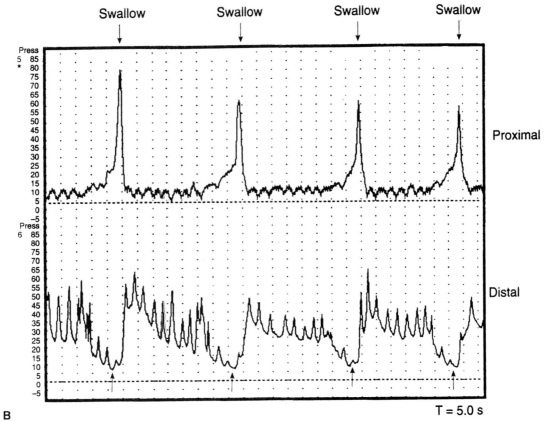

B

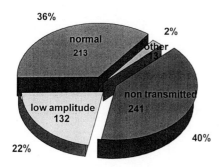

**FIG. 11–6.** Distribution of 599 wet swallows in 61 patients with nonspecific esophageal disorder. Other contractions are either triple or retrograde.

tients—30 men, 31 women, mean age 49 years (range 23 to 78)—were classified as NEMD in this time period. Five hundred ninety-nine wet swallows from these 61 tracings were reviewed. Two hundred thirteen (36%) were normal. One hundred thirty-two (22%) were low-amplitude (<30 mm Hg), 241 (40%) nontransmitted, and only 13 (2%) triple-peaked on retrograde (Fig. 11–6). Sixty of 61 patients (98%) had contraction amplitudes of less than 30 mm Hg, either low-amplitude or nontransmitted, in 30% or more of their wet swallows. Because amplitudes below 30 mm Hg result in ineffective propagation of a bolus [77], these patients were considered to be abnormal based on the ineffective contractions. The median number of ineffective swallows in these 60 patients was six (range three to ten). Though 10/61 (16%) also had incomplete LES relaxation, nine of these ten also

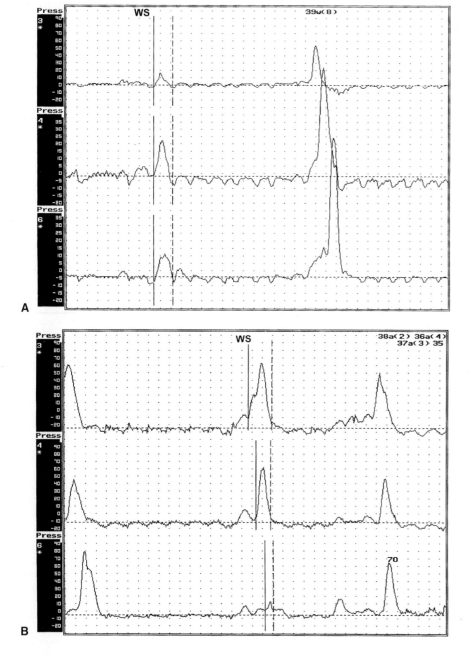

**FIG. 11–7.** Examples of ineffective esophageal motility tracings.

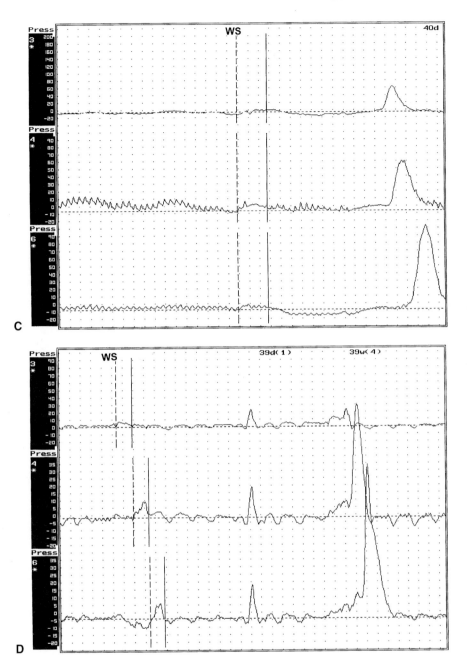

FIG. 11–7. *(continued)*

had ineffective motility. Leite et al. [90] thus suggested that the diagnosis of NEMD be replaced by the more accurate description of IEM, a distinct manometric abnormality defined by 30% or more wet swallows with amplitudes of less than 30 mm Hg (Fig. 11–7). This newly described abnormality is discussed subsequently.

## INEFFECTIVE ESOPHAGEAL MOTILITY

After the seminal observation by Leite et al. [90], several studies have been performed to further characterize IEM. The reproducibility of this entity was assessed by reviewing manometric tracings of 16 patients with motility studies diagnosed as IEM who had follow-up studies. The median

time between motility studies was 14 months (range 2 to 32 months). The tracings were blinded and reread. Twelve of 16 (75%) were again interpreted as IEM, 3/16 (18.8%) were normal (2, 2, and 0 contractions of less than 30 mm Hg), and 1/16 had DES on the repeat study [112].

The amplitude of effective contractions in 24 patients with IEM (41 studies) was compared to contraction amplitudes in 35 patients with normal motility [112]. All studies were coded and the reader blinded to the diagnosis. The mean distal esophageal amplitude of effective contractions in IEM patients was $75 \pm 44$ mm Hg (x $\pm$ SD) compared to $104 \pm 46$ mm Hg in normal tracings ($p < 0.0001$). The mean distal amplitude of the effective contraction fell as the number of ineffective swallows increased ($r = 0.92$) (Fig. 11–8).

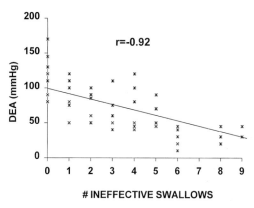

FIG. 11–8. Comparison of distal esophageal amplitude (DEA), effective contraction 3 and 8 cm above lower esophageal sphincter, with number of ineffective (amplitude less than 30 mm Hg) swallows.

## Ineffective Esophageal Motility and Gastroesophageal Reflux Disease

IEM is commonly associated with GERD, particularly GERD associated with respiratory symptoms. In addition, these patients have markedly delayed esophageal clearance compared to patients with other motility abnormalities. Leite et al. [90] found that 35/60 IEM patients in their study had GERD symptoms (19 men, 16 women; median age 45.5 years) and compared them to 153 patients (46 men, 69 women; median age 56 years) with other manometric findings: normal = 30, DES = 14, NE = 37, HLES = 29, systemic sclerosis = 43. All patients had ambulatory pH monitoring. The pH studies were read blindly and the median time pH less than 4 and median acid clearance time in minutes per episode were compared, both upright and recumbent. The recumbent time pH less than 4 and recumbent acid clearance were greater for IEM than all groups except scleroderma ($p < 0.01$) (Figs. 11–9, 11–10). The frequency

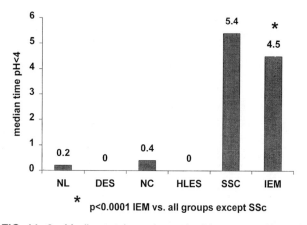

FIG. 11–9. Median total esophageal acid exposure (time pH less than 4) in patients with primary motility abnormalities and scleroderma. NL, normal ($n = 42$); DES, diffuse esophageal spasm ($n = 14$); NE, nutcracker esophagus ($n = 37$); HLES, hypertensive lower esophageal sphincter ($n = 35$); SSC, systemic sclerosis ($n = 43$).

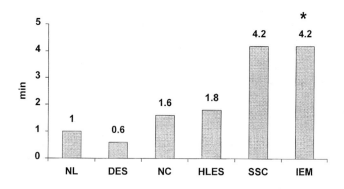

* p<0.01 IEM vs. all group except SSc

FIG. 11–10. Median esophageal acid clearance in minutes per episode in patients with normal motility (NL), diffuse esophageal spasm (DES), nutcracker esophagus (NE), hypertensive lower esophageal sphincter (HLES), ineffective esophageal motility (IEM), and systemic sclerosis (SSC).

of IEM in GERD patients with various symptom presentations was assessed in a recent preliminary study [59]. Ninety-eight consecutive patients with respiratory symptoms and abnormal reflux on prolonged pH monitoring were reviewed: 43 with chronic cough, 13 asthma, and 42 laryngitis. Sixty-six patients with abnormal prolonged pH monitoring studies and no respiratory manifestations were used as a control group. As previously found, IEM was the most common motility abnormality in all GERD patients and the frequency of IEM was significantly higher in the cough and asthma patients ($p \leq 0.01$) than reflux controls (Table 11–5). Total esophageal clearance time (upright and supine) was significantly longer in patients with GERD-associated respiratory symptoms than in the reflux control group (1.51 minutes per episode versus 0.72 minutes per episode, $p = 0.01$).

## Summary

IEM is a distinct manometric entity characterized by a hypocontractile esophagus. It is defined as distal esophageal contraction amplitude of less than 30% mm Hg (low-amplitude or non-transmitted contractions) in 30% or more of wet swallows and replaces NEMD in the classification of esophageal motility abnormalities (Table 11–1). IEM is a reproducible manometric finding of generalized low amplitude in which overall contraction amplitudes are lower than in patients with normal manometry. It is highly associated with GERD, especially in GERD patients with respiratory symptoms.

## TREATMENT OPTIONS

Treatment of patients with esophageal motility abnormalities must be individualized. The frequency and intensity of symptoms and emotional and physical limitations all must

**TABLE 11–5.** *Ineffective motility and gastroesophageal reflux disease*

| Symptom | Pts | IEM (%) | DES (%) | NE (%) | LLESP (%) | HLESP (%) |
|---|---|---|---|---|---|---|
| Cough | 43 | 48.8[a] | 4.7 | 4.7 | 9.3 | 7 |
| Asthma | 13 | 53.3[a] | 0 | 7.6 | 15.4 | 0 |
| Laryngitis | 42 | 31 | 2.4 | 2.4 | 9.5 | 9.5 |
| Reflux control | 66 | 19.6 | 1.5 | 1.5 | 12.5 | 15.2 |

[a] $p < 0.01$ compared to reflux control patients.

Pts, patients; IEM, ineffective esophageal motility; DES, diffuse esophageal spasm; NE, nutcracker esophagus; LLESP, low lower esophageal sphincter pressure; HLESP, high lower esophageal sphincter pressure.

be assessed in developing a treatment plan. Clinical trials have not been numerous, contain small numbers of patients, and are not, but for a few, well controlled; so treatment must often be based on experience rather than hard data. Symptom relief and improving quality of life should be the primary goals. Multiple therapies may be useful (Table 11–6), as discussed subsequently.

### Nonpharmacologic Therapy

Reassurance plays a key role. The patient with a motility abnormality and unexplained chest pain in whom heart disease has been ruled out should be told that the heart is normal or, if dysphagia is a primary symptom, that no malignancy or other structural lesion is present. Ward and colleagues [146] have shown that if a patient is aware that a definite diagnosis of esophageal chest pain has been made, anxiety about the pain and the number of physician visits will decrease. A strong trend toward improvement in chest pain

was also demonstrated, according to patients' self-report questionnaires. Richter and colleagues [123] found that awareness of esophageal etiology coupled with supportive follow-up from a health professional was as effective as nifedipine in relief of chest pain in patients with NE. Clinical experience supports these trials.

Psychologic intervention, with counseling or biofeedback, has been shown to reduce symptoms in a case report of a patient with DES and one with achalasia [89, 129]. The frequency of psychologic abnormalities seen in chest pain patients, especially those with NE, suggests a role for psychotherapy in these disorders, though the precise role has not been studied.

### Nitrates

Nitrates cause smooth muscle relaxation [6] but have no effect on peristalsis in normal subjects [84, 135]. They were first used in DES in the late 1940s. This early study found

**TABLE 11–6.** *Potential therapies for esophageal motility abnormalities*

| Treatment modality | Dose | Mode of administration |
|---|---|---|
| Reassurance | | |
| Nitrates | | |
|   Nitroglycerin | 0.4 mg sublingually | Usually before meals and as needed to prevent attacks |
|   Isosorbide | 10–30 mg orally | 30 min before meals |
| Visceral analgesic | | |
|   Imipramine | 50 mg orally | Bedtime |
| Sedatives, antidepressants | | |
|   Alprazolan | 2–5 mg orally | q.i.d. |
|   Trazodone | 50 mg orally | t.i.d. or q.i.d. |
| Calcium channel blockers[a] | | |
|   Nifedipine | 10–30 mg | q.i.d. |
|   Diltiazem | 60–90 mg | q.i.d. |
| Smooth muscle relaxant[a] | | |
|   Hydralazine | 25–50 mg orally | t.i.d. |
|   Botulinum toxin[d] | 80 U | Injection into LES via endoscopy |
| Static dilatation | 56–60 French bougie | Repeat as needed |
| Pneumatic dilatation[b] | | |
| Esophagomyotomy[c] | | |

q.i.d., Four times daily; t.i.d., three times daily; LES, lower esophageal sphincter.
[a] Orthostatic hypotension is a common complication of this class of drugs.
[b] May be indicated if dysphagia is a prominent symptom.
[c] Rarely indicated (intractability).
[d] Single uncontrolled study.

that amyl nitrate caused a decrease in radiographic abnormalities and reduced chest pain associated with DES [127]. This effect disappeared when the drug was stopped. An acute decrease in chest pain or dysphagia was demonstrated within minutes of administration of sublingual nitroglycerin in a single case report [103]. High-amplitude, repetitive contractions were reduced within minutes, and this effect persisted for almost 30 minutes. No effect on simultaneous waves could be demonstrated. This was the first demonstration of a manometric response to nitrates. Several other small trials have demonstrated a decrease in esophageal amplitude and relief of symptoms of DES with nitrates [96, 109, 130, 135]. All were uncontrolled but report improvement in symptoms for up to 4 years. Konturek et al. [85] have recently reported improvement in swallow-induced dysphagia and a decrease in duration of contractions with intravenous GTN in five subjects with DES. No effect was seen with L-arginine or placebo. In clinical practice, short-acting nitrates are often used when there is a predictable pattern of symptoms, primarily for rapid treatment.

## Anticholinergic Agents

Agents such as atropine [52, 113], hyoscyamine [9, 75], propantheline [23, 71], and cimetropium bromide [16] cause a decrease in peristalsis. The latter agent has been tested in patients with NE and caused a significant decrease in distal esophageal and LES pressures in eight patients [16]. Symptoms were not assessed. Trazodone hydrochloride, an antidepressant with anticholinergic properties, has been shown to reduce symptoms compared to placebo in patients with chest pain and esophageal motility abnormalities in an 8-week trial. No change was seen in motility abnormalities, suggesting that this effect was by a mechanism other than abnormalities [44]. The use of these or other anticholinergic agents that do not affect esophageal peristalsis [24] in the treatment of esophageal motility abnormalities is largely unstudied.

## Calcium Channel Blockers/Vasodilators

The most popular agents used in the treatment of esophageal motility abnormalities are calcium channel blockers. These drugs have been shown to decrease the amplitude of contractions in the esophageal body and reduce LES pressure in studies in healthy control subjects [25, 72, 121, 139]. This effect is probably caused by preventing calcium influx into smooth muscle in both the resting and stimulated states. Though many of the available studies have been done in patients with NE, several studies have involved DES patients.

Blackwell and co-workers [25] were able to demonstrate that sublingual nifedipine could abort acute chest pain attacks and decrease the frequency and severity of chest pain when taken in a 20-mg dose three times daily. In this study, decreased amplitude and decreased frequency of simultaneous contractions could be demonstrated. Another study showed decreased frequency of chest pain attacks but no overall decrease in the frequency or severity of chest pain in a 12-week clinical trial with nifedipine [8]. A case report demonstrated a return to normal peristalsis as well as reductions in chest pain frequency and amplitude and in duration of contraction in a patient treated with nifedipine 10 mg three times daily [101]. Twenty patients with NE were treated in a 14-week crossover study with 10 to 30 mg nifedipine three times daily or placebo [123]. Nifedipine decreased esophageal amplitude, duration of contractions, and LES pressure compared to placebo; however, no difference in symptom relief was seen in either group.

Diltiazem decreases amplitude and duration of esophageal contractions in patients with NE. Symptom improvement in chest pain has been demonstrated in an open label trial in patients with NE [120]. A placebo-controlled study of diltiazem in patients with NE compared 60 to 90 mg four times daily with placebo in a randomized, double-blind crossover trial in 14 patients [39]. Decrease in esophageal contraction amplitude and duration and improvement in chest pain scores were seen with diltiazem compared to placebo. Another report [54] described conflicting results, with diltiazem 60 mg three times daily in eight patients in a 10-week crossover trial versus placebo. No change in chest pain was seen compared to placebo.

Hydralazine, an arterial smooth muscle relaxant [1], improved symptoms in three patients with DES [94] at oral doses of 75 to 200 mg per day. No other trials are available.

## Sedatives/Tranquilizers

Patients with chest pain and abnormal esophageal motility have a high incidence of psychiatric disturbances, such as depression and panic disorders [42, 43, 91]. Experimentally induced stress produces significant changes in esophageal peristalsis [132, 142, 151], suggesting that psychoactive medications might be useful in the management of patients with chest pain and/or dysphagia and esophageal dysmotility. In a 6-week double-blind, controlled trial with trazodone (an antidepressant) to treat chest pain in patients with a variety of motility abnormalities (mostly nonspecific), patients receiving low-dose trazodone (100 to 150 mg per day) obtained significant symptomatic improvement compared with those on placebo [44]. No change was seen in motility patterns, despite improvement in pain. Side effects such as priapism may limit the use of this drug.

Alprazolam (a benzodiazepine analog) also has been used successfully in a limited number of patients with noncardiac chest pain, though motility abnormalities were not documented in the study [18]. A recent placebo-controlled study of patients with chest pain and normal coronary arteries showed that the tricyclic antidepressant imipramine significantly decreased the frequency of pain episodes [33]. Although 17 (43%) of the 40 study patients had NE or NEMD, the symptom response was not related to the presence of esophageal motility. Whether therapy should be aimed at symptoms only (chest pain/dysphagia) or should also take into consideration the specific type of spastic motility pattern remains to be determined. We often use these medications in symptomatic patients regardless of the specific motility abnormality.

## Esophageal Bougienage

The effects of mercury bougienage in a group of nine patients with NE were evaluated in a prospective, double-blind, crossover clinical trial comparing a "placebo" dilator (24 French) to a "therapeutic" dilator (54 French) [148]. Only temporary (less than 4 weeks) subjective improvement was noted with both treatments. Esophageal motility abnormalities were not changed after either dilator intervention.

## Botulinum Toxin

Success of this agent in patients with achalasia prompted an uncontrolled study [97] with 15 patients with DES, NE, HLES, or NEMD unresponsive to treatments with anticholinergics, nitrates, or calcium channel blockers and antireflux therapy. All patients were treated with intrasphincteric botulinum toxin and followed for 270 days. Overall, ten had LES dysfunction (incomplete relaxation). Good to excellent response to chest pain and/or dysphagia was seen in 11/15 patients at 1 month after treatment. At 120 days, there was no significant difference between pre- and posttreatment scores. Five patients had sustained response for 9 months without retreatment. Long-term response without need for repeat injection cannot be inferred from this uncontrolled trial. Botulinum toxin should be used with caution in these patients until more data are available.

## Pneumatic Dilatation

Nine patients with DES and LES dysfunction who had dysphagia and chest pain unresponsive to medical therapy with nitrates and anticholinergic agents as well as bougienage were treated with pneumatic dilatations using a Brown-McHardy dilator at pressures of 8 to 12 psi for 15 seconds in one study [55]. Symptomatic improvement occurred in eight of nine patients but only for dysphagia. Mean follow-up was about 3 years. One case report described effective use of pneumatic dilatation in a patient with HLES [138].

Beneficial effects of pneumatic dilatation were described in 53 patients with dysphagia and "suspected esophageal motor disorders" [27]. Only two patients in this group had documented DES. Fifteen patients had achalasia, and the remaining subjects did not undergo esophageal motility testing. Another study [74] evaluated a Rigiflex balloon dilator (Microvasive) to treat 20 patients with DES and symptoms of chest pain and dysphagia in whom conventional medical therapy had failed. Balloon dilatations were performed by radiologists under fluoroscopic guidance, using either 30- or 35-mm-diameter, 8-cm-length balloons. The esophagus was dilated with undetermined hand pressure "from the LES to above the level of the aortic arch, no attempt being made to dilate the LES itself." If symptoms recurred, a second balloon dilatation was performed. Complete relief of symptoms was obtained in eight patients, with improvement reported in six additional subjects. Two patients had a second dilatation. Five patients were treatment failures. One patient had an esophageal perforation requiring surgery. Four of five patients who failed dilatation had been diagnosed with reflux during 24-hour ambulatory pH testing. Only one of ten patients who were successfully treated and had pH monitoring had evidence of reflux. The mean follow-up was 3.4 years. This technique of dilatation is not recommended.

## Surgery

Use of esophagomyotomy for treatment of NE is considerably limited, although it has been described as effective in case reports [30, 73, 140, 141]. Limited experience with DES is available as well. Surgery should be reserved for patients with severe symptoms causing major compromise in lifestyle who cannot be improved with the measures described previously [118]. Surgical approaches to motility abnormalities are covered in Chapter 18.

## Suggested Approach to Therapy

Given the available data, we suggest the following approach. Time frames are arbitrary. Reassurance is an important part of all treatment programs. The generally nonprogressive and benign nature of the disease should be emphasized. The presence of GERD should prompt an aggressive trial of antireflux therapy (see Chapter 19). If this is unsuccessful and the patient has mild intermittent symptoms with a demonstrable precipitating event (e.g., meals, stress, or exercise), treatment can be on an as-needed basis to abort attacks. Sublingual nitrates or nifedipine may be useful in this situation. Patients with unexplained chest pain with depressive or anxiety components can be treated with trazodone, 50 to 100 mg three times daily, or imipramine, 50 mg at bedtime. Early psychologic intervention (testing, counseling) should be considered.

Patients refractory to these measures or those with persistent, frequent dysphagia or pain can be treated with diltiazem, 60 to 90 mg three times daily; nifedipine, 10 to 20 mg three times daily; or sustained-release preparations. Postural hypotension and gastrointestinal side effects may occur. Only severely refractory patients and those with LES dysfunction should be considered for botulinum toxin, pneumatic dilatation, or myotomy. Choosing between these options is difficult because of the paucity of studies. Botulinum toxin should be considered for the elderly patient and/or those patients with multiple medical problems, who would be poor surgical candidates. It would otherwise make sense to attempt dilatation first, as in achalasia, particularly in patients with elevated LES pressure and incomplete relaxation, proceeding to myotomy if dilatation fails. Agents available and useful in the treatment of esophageal motility disorders are outlined in Table 11–6.

## REFERENCES

1. Achem SR, Kolts BE. Current medical therapy for esophageal motility disorders. Am J Med 1992;92(suppl 5A):98S
2. Achern SR, Kolts BE, Burton L. Segmental versus diffuse nutcracker esophagus: an intermittent motility pattern. Am J Gastroenterol 1993; 88:847
3. Achem SR, et al. Segmental aperistalsis: association with chest pain and dysphagia. Presented to the Third International Poly-disciplinary Congress on Primary Esophageal Motility Disorders, Paris, France, June 1990
4. Achem SR, et al. Esophageal motor disorders: patterns and understanding in a state of flux. Gastroenterology 1991;100:A24
5. Achem SR, et al. Chest pain associated with nutcracker esophagus: a preliminary study of the role of gastroesophageal reflux. Am J Gastroenterol 1993;88:187
6. Ahlner J, Axelsson KL. Nitrates. Mode of action at a cellular level. Drugs 1987;33(suppl 4):32
7. Alban-Davies H, et al. Diagnosis of oesophageal spasm by ergometrine provocation. Gut 1982;23:89
8. Alban-Davies H, et al. Nifedipine for relief of esophageal chest pain? N Engl J Med 1982;307:1274
9. Allen M, et al. Comparison of calcium channel blocking agents and an anticholinergic agent on esophageal function. Aliment Pharmacol Ther 1987;1:153
10. Allen M, Dimarino AJ. Manometric diagnosis of diffuse esophageal spasm Dig Dis Sci 1996;41:1346
11. Almy TP, et al. Alteration in colonic function in man under stress. 111. Experimental production of sigmoid spasm in patients with spastic constipation. Gastroenterology 1949;12:437
12. Anderson KO, et al. Stress induced alteration of esophageal pressures in healthy volunteers and noncardiac chest pain patients. Dig Dis Sci 1989;34:83
13. Anggiansah A, et al. Transition from nutcracker esophagus to achalasia. Dig Dis Sci 1990;35:1162
14. Barham C, et al. Diffuse esophageal spasm: diagnosis by ambulatory 24 hour manometry. Gut 1997;41:151
15. Bassotti G, et al. Isolated hypertensive lower esophageal sphincter. Clinical and manometric aspects of an uncommon esophageal motor abnormality. J Clin Gastroenterol 1992;14:285
16. Bassotti O, et al. Manometric evaluation of cimetropium bromide activity in patients with the nutcracker oesophagus. Scand J Gastroenterol 1988;23:1079
17. Behar J, Biancani P. Pathogenesis of simultaneous esophageal contractions in patients with motility disorders. Gastroenterology 1993; 105:111
18. Beitman BD, et al. Alprazolam in the treatment of cardiology patients with atypical chest pain and panic disorder. J Clin Psychopharmacol 1988;8:127
19. Benjamin SB, Castell DO. The "nutcracker esophagus" and the spectrum of esophageal motor disorders. Curr Concepts Gastroenterol 1980;5:3
20. Benjamin SB, Castell DO. Esophageal causes of chest pain. In Castell DO, Johnson LF, eds, Esophageal Function in Health and Disease. New York: Elsevier Science, 1983:85
21. Benjamin SB, Gerhardt DC, Castell DO. High amplitude, peristaltic esophageal contractions associated with chest pain and/or dysphagia. Gastroenterology 1979;77:478
22. Benjamin SB, et al. Prolonged radionuclide transit in "nutcracker esophagus." Dig Dis Sci 1983;28:775
23. Bennett JR, Hendrix TR. Diffuse esophageal spasm: a disorder with more than one cause. Gastroenterology 1970;59:273
24. Blackwell JN, Dalton CB, Castell DO. Oral pirenzepine does not affect esophageal pressures in man. Dig Dis Sci 1986;31:230
25. Blackwell JN, et al. Effect of nifedipine on esophageal motility and gastric emptying. Digestion 1981;21:50
26. Bortolotti M, Cirignotta F, Labo G. Atrioventricular block induced by swallowing in a patient with diffuse esophageal spasm. JAMA 1982;248:2297
27. Bourgeois N, et al. Management of dysphagia in suspected esophageal motor disorders. Dig Dis Sci 1991;36:268
28. Brand DL, Martin D, Pope CE. Esophageal manometrics in patients with anginal type chest pain. Am J Dig Dis 1977;23:300
29. Breumelhof R, et al. Food impaction in nutcracker esophagus. Dig Dis Sci 1990;35:1167
30. Brown M, Stacier MS, May ES. Esophageal myotomy and treatment of "nutcracker esophagus." Am J Gastroenterol 1987;82:1331
31. Buxton A, et al. Refractory ergonovine induced coronary vasopasm: importance of intracoronary nitroglycerin. Am J Cardiol 1980;46:329
32. Campo S, Traube M. Lower esophageal sphincter dysfunction in diffuse esophageal spasm. Am J Gastroenterol 1989;84:928
33. Cannon RO, et al. Imipramine in patients with chest pain despite normal coronary angiograms. N Engl J Med 1994;330:1411
34. Casella RR, Ellis H, Brown AL. Diffuse spasm of the esophagus: fine structure of esophageal smooth muscle and nerve. JAMA 1965;191: 379
35. Castell DO. Achalasia and diffuse esophageal spasm. Arch Intern Med 1976;136:571
36. Castell DO. Shortened relaxation of the LES. Primary motility of the esophagus. 450 questions. 450 answers. In Giuli R, McCallum R, Skinner D, eds, Primary Motility Disorders of the Esophagus. London: John Libbey, 1991:850
37. Castell DO. The nutcracker and the ostrich. Am J Gastroenterol 1993; 88:1287
38. Castell DO. The nutcracker esophagus. The hypertensive lower esophageal sphincter, and nonspecific esophageal motility disorders. In Castell DO, Castell JA, eds, Esophageal Motility Testing (2nd ed). Norwalk, CT: Appleton & Lange, 1994:135
38a.Castell JA, Gideon RM, Castell DO. Esophagus. In MM Schuster, ed, Atlas of GI Motility in Health and Disease (1st ed). Baltimore: Williams & Wilkins, 1993
39. Cattau EL Jr, et al. Diltiazem therapy for symptoms associated with nutcracker esophagus. Am J Gastroenterol 1991;86:272
40. Chen YM, et al. Diffuse esophageal spasm: radiographic and manometric correlation. Radiology 1989;170:807
41. Chobanian SJ, et al. Radiology of the nutcracker esophagus. J Clin Gastroenterol 1986;8:230
42. Clouse RE, Lustman PJ. Psychiatric illnesses and contraction abnormalities of the esophagus. N Engl J Med 1986;31:131
43. Clouse RE, Lustman PJ, Reidel WL. Correlation of esophageal motility abnormalities with neuropsychiatric status in diabetics. Gastroenterology 1986;90:1146
44. Clouse RE, et al. Low-dose trazodone for symptomatic patients with esophageal contraction abnormalities. Gastroenterology 1987;92: 1027
45. Clouse RE, Staiano A. Contraction abnormalities of the esophageal body in patients referred for manometry. Dig Dis Sci 1983;28:784
46. Code CF, et al. Hypertensive gastroesophageal sphincter. Staff Meet Mayo Clin 1960;35:391
47. Cohen S. The gastrointestinal manifestations of scleroderma; pathogenesis and management. Gastroenterology 1980;79:155
47a.Conklin JL, et al. Effect of recombinant human hemoglobin on opossum esophageal muscle. Am J Physiol 1991;261:G1012
48. Creamer B, Donoghue FE, Code CF. Pattern of esophageal motility in diffuse spasm. Gastroenterology 1958;34:782
49. Dalton CB, Castell DO, Richter JE. The changing faces of the nutcracker esophagus. Am J Gastroenterol 1988;83:623
50. Dalton CB, et al. Diffuse esophageal spasm (DES): a rare motility disorder not characterized by high amplitude contractions. Dig Dis Sci 1991;36:1025
51. DiMarino AJ, Cohen S. Characteristics of lower esophageal sphincter function in symptomatic diffuse esophageal spasm. Gastroenterology 1974;66:1
52. Dodds WJ, et al. Effect of atropine on esophageal motor function in humans. Am J Physiol 1981;240:G290
53. Drane WE, et al. "Nutcracker" esophagus: diagnosis with radionuclide esophageal scintigraphy versus manometry. Radiology 1987; 163:33
54. Drenth JPH, Bos LP, Engels LGJB. Efficacy of diltiazem in the treatment of diffuse esophageal spasm. Aliment Pharmacol Ther 1990;4: 411
55. Ebert EC, et al. Pneumatic dilation in patients with symptomatic diffuse esophageal spasm and lower esophageal sphincter dysfunction. Dig Dis Sci 1983;28:481

56. Ferguson MK, Little AG. Angina-like chest pain associated with high-amplitude peristaltic contractions of the esophagus. Surgery 1988; 104:713

57. Fiedier JT, Brand TR, Fields JZ. Does nitric oxide mediate ethanol (E) induced inhibition of contractivity in the esophagus. Gastroenterology 1993;104:A507

58. Fleshler B. Diffuse esophageal spasm. Gastroenterology 1967;52:559

59. Fouad YM, Khoury R, Hattlebakk JG, Katz PO, Castell DO. Ineffective esophageal motility (IEM) is more prevalent in reflux patients with respiratory symptoms [Abstract]. Gastroenterology 1968;114

60. Freidin N, et al. Segmental high amplitude peristaltic contractions in the distal esophagus. Am J Gastroenterol 1989;84:619

61. Freidin N, et al. The hypertensive lower esophageal sphincter: manometric and clinical aspects. Dig Dis Sci 1989;34:1063

62. Frieling T, et al. Family occurrence of achalasia and diffuse spasm of the oesophagus. Gut 1988;29:1595

63. Garrett JM, Godwin DH. Gastroesophageal hypercontracting sphincter. Manometric and clinical characteristics. JAMA 1969;208:992

64. Gillies M, Nicks R, Skyring A. Clinical, manometric, and pathologic studies in diffuse esophageal spasm. BMJ 1967;2:527

65. Glassman MS, et al. Spectrum of esophageal disorders in children with chest pain. Dig Dis Sci 1992;37:663

66. Graham DY. Hypertensive lower esophageal sphincter: a reappraisal. South Med J 1978;71(suppl 1):31

67. Herrington JP, Bums TW, Balart LA. Chest pain and dysphagia in patients with prolonged peristaltic contractile duration of the esophagus. Dig Dis Sci 1984;29:134

68. Hogan WF, Caflisch CR, Winship DH. Unclassified esophageal motor disorders simulating achalasia. Gut 1969;10:234

69. Hollis JB, Castell DO, Braddon RL. Esophageal function in diabetes mellitus and its relationship to peripheral neuropathy. Gastroenterology 1977;73:1098

70. Holloway RH, et al. Detection of esophageal motor disorders by radionuclide transit studies. Dig Dis Sci 1989;34:905

71. Hongo M, Traube M, McCallum RW. Comparison of effects of nifedipine, propantheline bromide, and the combination on esophageal motor function in normal volunteers. Dig Dis Sci 1984;29:300

72. Hongo M, et al. Effects of nifedipine on esophageal motor function in humans: correlation with plasma nifedipine concentration. Gastroenterology 1984;86:8

73. Horton ML, Goff JS. Surgical treatment of nutcracker esophagus. Dig Dis Sci 1986;31:878

74. Irving D, et al. Management of diffuse esophageal spasm with balloon dilatation. Gastrointest Radiol 1992;17:189

75. Jaup BH, et al. Effect of pirenzepine compared with atropine and L-hyoscyamine on esophageal peristaltic activity in humans. Scand J Gastroenterol 1982;17:233

76. Kahrilas PJ. Nutcracker esophagus: an idea whose time has gone? Am J Gastroenterol 1993;88:167

77. Kahrilas PJ, Dodds WJ, Hogan WJ, Kern M, Arndorfer RC, Reece A. Esophageal peristaltic dysfunction in peptic esophagitis. Gastroenterology 1986;92:897

78. Katz PO, et al. Esophageal testing of patients with noncardiac chest pain and/or dysphagia. Results of a three year experience with 1161 patients. Ann Intern Med 1987;106:593

79. Katzka D, Sidhu M, Castell DO. Hypertensive lower esophageal sphincter pressures and gastroesophageal reflux: apparent paradox that is not unusual. Gastroenterology 1995;90:280

80. Kaye MD. Dysfunction of the lower esophageal sphincter in disorders other than achalasia. Am J Dig Dis 1973;18:734

81. Kaye MD. Anomalies of peristalsis in idiopathic diffuse oesophageal spasm. Gut 1981;22:217

82. Kaye MD, Derneules JE. Achalasia and diffuse oesophageal spasm in siblings. Gut 1979;20:811

83. Kaye MD, Johnson WF. Sororal occurrence of diffuse esophageal spasm. Am J Dig Dis 1976;21:901

84. Kikendall JW, Mellow MH. Effect of sublingual nitroglycerin and long-acting nitrate preparations on esophageal motility. Gastroenterology 1980;79:703

85. Konturek JW, et al. Diffuse esophageal spasm: a malfunction that involves nitric oxide? Scand J Gastroenterol 1995;30:1041

86. Kramer P, et al. Oesophageat sensitivity to mecholyt in symptomatic diffuse spasm. Gut 1967;8:120

87. Kramer P, Harris LD, Donaldson RM Jr. Transition from symptomatic diffuse spasm to cardiospasm. Gut 1967;8:115

88. Lane WH, Ippoliti AF, McCallum RW. Effect of gastrin heptadeca-peptide (017) on oesophageal contractions in patients with diffuse oesophageal spasm. Gut 1979;20:756

89. Latimer PR. Biofeedback and self-regulation in the treatment of diffuse esophageal spasm: a single-case study. Biofeedback Self Regul 1981;6:181

90. Leite L, et al. Ineffective esophageal motility (IEM): the primary finding in patients with nonspecific esophageal motility disorder. Dig Dis Sci 1997;42:1859

91. Lustman PJ, Griffith LS, Clouse RE. Psychiatric illness in diabetes mellitus: relationship to symptoms and glucose control. J Nerv Ment Dis 1986;174:736

92. McCord G, Staiano A, Clouse R. Achalasial diffuse spasm and nonspecific motor disorders. Baillieres Clin Gastroenterol 1991;5:307

93. Mellow M. Symptomatic diffuse esophageal spasm: manometric follow-up and response to cholinergic stimulation and cholinesterase inhibition. Gastroenterology 1977;73:237

94. Mellow MH. Effect of isosorbide and hydralazine in painful primary esophageal motility disorders. Gastroenterology 1982;83:364

95. Melzer E, et al. Assessment of the esophageal wall by endoscopic ultrasonography in patients with nutcracker esophagus. Gastrointest Endosc 1997;46:223

96. Millaire A, et al. Nitroglycerin and angina with angiographically normal coronary vessels: clinical effects and effects on esophageal motility. Arch Mal Coeur Vaiss 1989;82:63

97. Miller LS, et al. Treatment of symptomatic nonachalasia esophageal motor disorders with botulinum toxin at the lower esophageal sphincter. Dig Dis Sci 1996;41:2025

98. Milov DE, Cynarmon H, Andres J. Chest pain and dysphagia in adolescents caused by diffuse esophageat spasm. J Pediatr Gastroenterol Nutr 1989;9:450

99. Moersch HJ, Camp JD. Diffuse spasm of the lower part of the esophagus. Ann Otol Rhinol Laryngol 1934;43:1165

99a. Murray JA, et al. The effects of recombinant human hemoglobin on esophageal motor function in humans. Gastroenterology 1995;109:1241

100. Narducci F, et al. Transition from nutcracker esophagus to diffuse esophageal spasm. Am J Gastroenterol 1985;80:242

101. Nasrallah SM. Nifedipine in the treatment of diffuse esophageal spasm. Lancet 1982;2:1285

102. Nelson JB, Castell DO. Esophageal motility disorders. Dis Mon 1988; 34:297

103. Orlando RC, Bozymski EM. Clinical and manometric effects of nitroglycerin in diffuse esophageal spasm. N Engl J Med 1973;289:23

104. Orlando RC, Bozymski EM. The effects of pentagastrin in achalasia and diffuse esophageal spasm. Gastroenterology 1979;77:472

105. Orr WC, Robinson MG. Hypertensive peristalsis in the pathogenesis of chest pain: further exploration of the ''nutcracker esophagus.'' Am J Gastroenterol 1982;77:604

106. Osgood H. A peculiar form of esophagismus. Boston Med Surg J 1889;120:401

107. Ott DJ, et al. Radiologic and manometric correlation in ''nutcracker'' esophagus. AJR Am J Roentgenol 1986;147:692

108. Ott DJ, et al. Esophageal motility: assessment with synchronous video fluoroscopy and manometry. Radiology 1989;173:419

109. Parker WA, MacKinnon GL. Nitrates in the treatment of diffuse esophageal spasm. Drug Intell Clin Pharm 1981;15:806

110. Paterson WG, Beck IT, Da Costa LR. Transition from nutcracker esophagus to achalasia: a case report. J Clin Gastroenterol 1991;13:554

111. Patterson DR. Diffuse esophageal spasm in patients with undiagnosed chest pain. J Clin Gastroenterol 1982;4:415

112. Peghini P, Katz PO, Ko A, Gideon M, Castell J, Castell D. Ineffective esophageal motility (IEM) is a reproducible manometric entity, and affects all swallows. Gastroenterology 1997;112:A255

113. Phaosawasdi K, et al. Cholinergic effects on esophageal transit and clearance. Gastroenterology 1981;81:915

114. Rhoton AJ, et al. The natural history of diffuse esophageal spasm (DES): a long term follow-up study. Am J Gastroenterol 1992;87:A1256

115. Richter JE. Diffuse esophageal spasm. In Castell DO, Casteli JA, eds, Esophageal Motility Testing (2nd ed). Norwalk, CT: Appleton & Lange, 1994:122

116. Richter JE, Barish CF, Castell DO. Abnormal sensory perception in patients with esophageal chest pain. Gastroenterology 1986;91:485

117. Richter JE, Castell DO. Diffuse esophageat spasm: a reappraisal. Ann Intern Med 1984;100:242
118. Richter JE, Castell DO. Surgical myotomy for nutcracker esophagus: to be or not to be? Dig Dis Sci 1987;32:95
119. Richter JE, et al. Psychological comparison of patients with nutcracker esophagus and irritable bowel syndrome. Dig Dis Sci 1986;31:131
120. Richter JE, et al. Effects of oral calcium blocker, diltiazem, on esophageal contractions. Dig Dis Sci 1984;29:64915
121. Richter JE, et al. Nifedipine: a potent inhibitor of contractions in the body of the human esophagus. Gastroenterology 1985;89:549
122. Richter JE, et al. Esophageal manometry in 95 healthy adult volunteers. Dig Dis Sci 1987;32:583
123. Richter JE, et al. Oral nifedipine in the treatment of noncardiac chest pain with the nutcracker esophagus. Gastroenterology 1987;93:21
124. Richter JE, et al. Relationship of radionuclide liquid bolus transport and esophageal manometry. J Lab Clin Med 1987;109:217
125. Roth HP, Fleshler B. Diffuse esophageal spasm. Ann Intern Med 1964;61:914
126. Rubinow A, et al. Esophageal manometry in systemic amyloidosis. A study of 30 patients. Am J Med 1983;75:951
127. Scheinmel A, Priviteri CA, Poppel MH. A study of the effect of certain drugs on curling of the esophagus. AJR Am J Roentgenol 1949;62:807
128. Schuffler MD, Pope CE II. Esophageal motor dysfunction in idiopathic intestinal pseudoobstruction. Gastroenterology 1976;70:677
129. Shabsin HS, Katz PO, Schuster MM. Behavioral treatment of intractable chest pain in a patient with vigorous achalasia. Am J Gastroenterol 1988;83:970
130. Shafran I, et al. Segmental esophageal spasm: a variant of diffuse esophageal spasm. Gastroenterology 1979;76:1243(A)
131. Srinivasan R, et al. Diffuse esophageal spasm (DES) includes two distinct subgroups of patients. Am J Gastroenterol 1997;92:1604
132. Stacher G, Schmierer C, Landgraf M. Tertiary esophageal contractions evoked by acoustic stimuli. Gastroenterology 1979;44:49
133. Stein HI. Clinical use of ambulatory 24-hour esophageal motility monitoring in patients with primary esophageal motor disorders. Dysphagia 1993;8:105
134. Sullivan SN. The supersensitive hypertensive lower esophageal sphincter. Precipitation of pain by small doses of intravenous pentagastrin. J Clin Gastroenterol 1986;8:619
135. Swamy N. Esophageal spasm: clinical and manometric response to nitroglycerin and long acting nitrates. Gastroenterology 1977;72:23
136. Traube M, Aaronson RM, McCallum RW. Transition from peristaltic esophageal contractions to diffuse esophageal spasm. Arch Intern Med 1986;146:1844
137. Traube M, Abibi R, McCallum RW. High amplitude peristaltic esophageal contractions associated with chest pain. JAMA 1983;250:2655
138. Traube M, Lagarde S, McCallum RW. Isolated hypertensive lower esophageal sphincter: treatment of a resistant case by pneumatic dilatation. J Clin Gastroenterol 1984;6:139
139. Traube M, et al. Effects of nifedipine in achalasia and patients with high-amplitude esophageal contractions. JAMA 1984;252:1733
140. Traube M, et al. Surgical myotomy in patients with high-amplitude peristaltic esophageal contractions—manometric and clinical effects. Dig Dis Sci 1987;32:16
141. Tummala V, Baue AE, McCallum RW. Surgical myotomy in patients with high-amplitude peristaltic contractions: manometric and clinical effects. Dig Dis Sci 1987;32:16
142. Valori RM. Nutcracker, neurosis, or sampling bias. Gut 1990;31:736
143. Vantrappen G, et al. Achalasia, diffuse esophageal spasm, and related motility disorders. Gastroenterology 1979;76:450
144. Walker S, Hippeli R, Goes R. Diffuse esophageal intramural pseudodiverticulosis and nutcracker esophagus in a 54 year old man. Klin Wochenschr 1990;68:187
145. Ward BW, et al. Long-term follow-up of symptomatic status of patients with noncardiac chest pain; is diagnosis of esophageal etiology helpful? Am J Gastroenterol 1987;82:215
146. Waterman DC, et al. Hypertensive lower esophageal sphincter: what does it mean? J Clin Gastroenterol 1989;11:139
147. Winship DH, et al. Deterioration of esophageal peristalsis in patients with alcoholic neuropathy. Gastroenterology 1968;55:173
148. Winters C, et al. Esophageal bougienage in symptomatic patients with the nutcracker esophagus—a primary esophageal motility disorder. JAMA 1984;252:363
149. Young LD, et al. The effects of psychological and environmental stressors on peristaltic esophageal contractions in healthy volunteers. Psychophysiology 1987;24:132

*The Esophagus*, Third Edition,
edited by D. O. Castell and J. E. Richter.
Lippincott Williams & Wilkins, Philadelphia © 1999.

CHAPTER 12

# Neoplasms of the Esophagus

## David E. Fleischer and Nadim G. Haddad

Some facts about esophageal neoplasms have not changed over the past several decades: (a) Most tumors are malignant; (b) dysphagia is the usual presenting symptom; (c) Most patients who present with symptoms are incurable; and (d) surgery offers the best chance for cure. However, there are some important new matters to consider. Esophageal cancer (EC) is no longer synonymous with squamous cell carcinoma. Adenocarcinoma of the esophagus and esophagogastric junction—the fastest growing cancer—is now more frequent in the United States. Esophageal cancer exhibits significant racial variation. Squamous cell carcinoma is more common in blacks and adenocarcinoma is more common in whites [33]. The most important prognostic factor for EC is the stage of the disease at the time of diagnosis. That means that the best hope for improving survival is linked to earlier diagnosis—not better surgical, radiologic, or endoscopic techniques. As the genetic changes are better understood, the options for newer treatment modalities will expand. The aim of this chapter is to review information about all esophageal neoplasms, although the emphasis will be on squamous cell and adenocarcinoma.

## ESOPHAGEAL MALIGNANCIES

Esophageal malignancy is a difficult problem for both the patient and the physician. As with most cancers, there is the adjustment a patient must make to the realization that he or she has a terminal disease. Perhaps more difficult, however, is dealing with the way this disease affects the quality of the patient's remaining life. The progressive inability to swallow and intermittent regurgitation deprive the patient of certain social graces that quickly render him or her an outcast, particularly at mealtime. Because the disease is almost always advanced by the time symptoms occur, curative therapy is the exception, and the physician's efforts are predominantly palliative and supportive.

D. Fleischer: Division of Gastroenterology, Georgetown University Medical Center, Washington, D.C. 20007.

N. G. Haddad: Trad Hospital, Klemenceau, Beruit, Lebanon.

### Squamous Cell Carcinoma

#### Demographics

In the United States, the overall annual incidence of squamous cell carcinoma is 2.6 per 100,000 population [211]. The age-specific rates are extremely low in persons younger than 40 years and continue to rise with each decade of life. The incidence of esophageal cancer varies among different racial groups; squamous cell cancer is four to five times higher in blacks than whites and has become the second most common malignancy among black men younger than 55 [20]. Age-adjusted mortality for squamous cell carcinoma has remained relatively steady among whites, whereas for blacks the rate has approximately doubled over the same 30-year period [20]. In whites and blacks, men are more commonly affected than women, with male-female ratios of 3 to 4:1 [34, 211]. Approximately 10,000 new cases of esophageal cancer are diagnosed yearly in the United States. The overall 5-year survival rate for this disease, which has remained relatively steady at approximately 5%, may be improving slightly among whites [171].

#### Epidemiology and Etiology

From an epidemiologic viewpoint, esophageal cancer is one of the most interesting malignancies. The wide geographic and cultural variation in incidence of squamous cell cancer of the esophagus suggests that environmental exposure is causally important [154]. Regions with a high incidence are generally located in poor parts of the world (Table 12–1). Worldwide, there are remarkable geographic variations in incidence [48, 63, 82]. In China, where approximately 60% of the world's cases occur annually, the incidence is clustered into sharply demarcated geographic areas. One can be in an endemic area where the incidence of esophageal cancer is unparalleled by any other fatal tumor anywhere in the world, yet travel a mere few hundred miles to an area where the incidence is low. In Central Asia, there is an esophageal cancer belt extending from northern Sinkiang

**TABLE 12–1.** *Worldwide incidence of esophageal cancer*

| Region | Locality | Incidence per 100,000 | |
|---|---|---|---|
| | | Men | Women |
| Asia | | | |
| China | Linxian | 132 | 120 |
| | Yangcheng | 130 | 84 |
| | Tianjin | 16 | 8 |
| India | Kashmir | 42 | 28 |
| | Bombay | 11 | 9 |
| | Bangalore | 6 | 5 |
| Europe | | | |
| Northern Europe | | 4 | 2 |
| Eastern Europe | | 4 | 2 |
| France | Calvados | 26 | — |
| United Kingdom | England/Wales | 6 | 3 |
| South America | | | |
| Uruguay | | 40 | — |
| Brazil | Porto Alegre | 26 | 8 |
| North America | | | |
| United States | Los Angeles | 16 | 4 |
| | Washington, D.C.: blacks | 17 | 5 |
| | Washington, D.C.: whites | 4 | 1 |
| Africa | | | |
| Transkei | | 37 | 21 |

through the former Soviet Union's republics of Kazakhstan, Uzbekistan, and Turkmenistan, and including northern Afghanistan and the northeastern area (Caspian littoral) of Iran [48]. Areas of high and low incidence are intermingled in eastern and southern Africa, and the disease is rare in the remaining parts of the continent. The incidence is particularly high in the Transkei of South Africa. High rates are also noted in the Indian subcontinent, and intermediate to high rates exist in the Caribbean and part of Latin America [201]. In the United States, where the disease is relatively uncommon, urban black men seem particularly affected, especially in Washington, D.C., and along coastal South Carolina [28, 63, 148]. Marked regional clustering has also been reported among Alaskan natives [109].

The geographic variations in the incidence and mortality of esophageal cancer suggest that various environmental factors are important in the etiology of this disease. The relationship between esophageal cancer in humans and gullet cancer in chickens best illustrates this hypothesis. In the Chinese counties of Linxian, Fanxian, and Hunyuanxian, the incidence of esophageal cancer in humans is 131.8, 23.7, and 1.3 per 100,000, respectively [209, 210]. In Zhongxiang county, though no cases of gullet cancer in chickens were found among poultry belonging to the native people of Hubei province, several cases of esophageal cancer were detected among Henan immigrants, who have an incidence of esophageal cancer four times that of the native population [209]. Since the prevalence and pathologic findings of esophageal cancer were similar between humans and chickens, and since the chickens usually shared the same food sources and envi-

ronment as their owners, dietary and environmental factors appear to be important in pathogenesis. A variety of potential factors have been identified.

Another thesis focuses on polycyclic aromatic hydrocarbons which are given off when soft coal is burned—particularly from cooking. Since many cooking areas are unventilated and the incidence of EC is equal in women (who usually do not smoke cigarettes) and men (who often do), this thesis has epidemiologic appeal [160].

*Nutrition*

Worldwide, nutritional deficiencies have been implicated in the pathogenesis of esophageal cancer. Low levels of retinol, riboflavin, ascorbic acid, and alpha-tocopherol are prevalent in the population of Linxian, China, where esophageal cancer is endemic [211]. In Japan, poor food variety has been identified as a risk-enhancing factor, and combinations of fruits, vegetables, and fresh meat appear to be risk-reducing factors [132]. Low intake of fruits, particularly citrus fruits, and, accordingly, vitamin C intake, has been repeatedly associated with an increased risk of esophageal cancer [28, 69, 148]. Deficiencies in various mineral elements such as selenium [96], zinc [209], and molybdenum [23, 29, 209] also have been cited as possible etiologic factors. Generally poor nutrition was also a predictor of risk for esophageal cancer among black men in Washington, D.C., although no specific micronutrient deficiency was identified [148, 219]. These deficiencies are believed to make one more susceptible to the carcinogenic effects of exogenous factors.

*Environmental Carcinogens*

Because nitrates and nitrites can be converted within the body to carcinogenic N-nitrosamines, they are suspected etiologic factors in the development of esophageal cancer. Higher nitrate and nitrite content in plants may be caused by low molybdenum levels in the soil, because molybdenum functions as a cofactor for the plant enzyme nitrate reductase [29, 209]. The apparent risk reduction brought about by citrus fruits may be due to the inhibition of endogenous nitrosation by vitamin C [119]. The high prevalence of esophageal cancer in Gassim region, Saudi Arabia, has been linked to contamination of water by impurities such as petroleum oils [7].

*Alcohol and Tobacco*

In Western countries where the overall risk for esophageal cancer is comparatively low, numerous epidemiologic studies have linked alcohol and tobacco use with the development of esophageal cancer [28, 111, 137, 201, 215, 218]. Ethanol was estimated to be causally associated with approximately 80% of the neoplasms among esophageal cancer subjects, and the relative risk increases with the amount of alcohol consumed [148, 218]. Of the three types of alcoholic beverages, the association with esophageal cancer is strongest with liquor, intermediate with wine, and weakest with beer. Since there is an inverse relationship between the caloric intake of alcohol and a wholesome diet, alcohol may increase the risk of esophageal cancer by reducing nutrient intake. The risks associated with tobacco use appear to increase with the number of cigarettes smoked per day, duration of smoking, and tar content [111, 215]. Ex-smokers have a reduced risk compared to current smokers and after 10 years their risk is similar to the risk for those who have never smoked [28, 111, 215]. A synergistic effect for the combined habit of alcohol drinking and tobacco smoking or chewing has been reported [137, 192]. Among well-nourished, nondrinking, nonsmoking men in Europe and North America, esophageal cancer virtually does not occur [48]. Opium smoking, perhaps via the carcinogenic potential of substances formed by pyrolysis, has been implicated in the etiology of esophageal cancer in northern Iran [66].

## Achalasia

On the basis of numerous case reports in the literature, esophageal carcinoma is believed to be associated with achalasia. The prevalence of esophageal cancer in patients with achalasia is approximately 3% to 6%. The average duration between symptoms and detection of esophageal malignancy is 17 years, and esophageal cancer appears to occur at an earlier age in achalasic patients than in the general population [32]. Intervention may alter the natural history of this association; in patients treated with dilation or esophagomyotomy, esophageal cancer developed at a rate only slightly higher than that for the general population [207]. Current guidelines for clinical application of endoscopy suggest endoscopic surveillance is indicated in the untreated patient, but if effective dilation or myotomy has been performed early in the course of disease, surveillance is unnecessary [8]. Although the association of achalasia with risk of subsequent esophageal cancer has gained wide acceptance, this has recently been questioned. A retrospective evaluation of patients with esophageal cancer and a prospective study of patients with achalasia failed to substantiate the purported association [40].

## Chronic Esophagitis

Chronic injury to the esophagus appears to increase the risk of esophageal cancer. Endoscopic surveys in Iran and China showed that chronic esophagitis (a different entity from the chronic reflux esophagitis seen in Western countries) is much more prevalent (65% to 80% of subjects) in areas where esophageal cancer is endemic [43, 44, 216]. In addition, atrophy of the epithelium was noted in 10% and dysplasia in 4% of subjects. Conversely, low-risk populations had a low prevalence of chronic esophagitis (28%), rare atrophy of the epithelium, and no dysplasia [44]. These findings suggest that in high-risk areas, there is a propensity

for chronic severe esophagitis to develop and then to progress through the histologic phases of atrophy, dysplasia, and finally, cancer. These precursor lesions are seen in young individuals and have been associated with the consumption of burning hot beverages, a family history of esophageal cancer, and infrequent consumption of fresh fruit [36, 203]. The consumption of mate, a tea made from the herb *Llex paraguensis,* which is drunk at very hot temperatures, has been associated in a dose–response relationship with the risk of esophageal cancer in Uruguay [51, 201].

## Caustic Injury

It has been estimated that the incidence of esophageal cancer among patients with a history of caustic ingestion is 1,000-fold greater than that of the general population [92, 104]. Squamous cell carcinoma is the rule and usually occurs in the midesophagus at the level of the tracheal bifurcation [94]. Most cases of corrosion carcinoma present some four to five decades after the initial injury and 10 to 20 years earlier than in the general population [9]. Increasing dysphagia and a change in the ability to dilate a chronic corrosion stricture that was easily dilated in the past should alert the physician to the possibility of carcinoma [110]. Theoretically, the natural history of esophageal cancer is favorably altered by the scarred esophagus. Since the esophageal lumen is less distensible, dysphagia is more likely to present earlier in the course of the disease. Because of the damage to submucosal lymphatics and the presence of dense scar tissue within the esophageal wall, lymphatic spread of the disease and direct extension are less likely to occur before the appearance of symptoms [110]. Diagnosis and therapy should be aggressively pursued in these patients.

## Human Papillomavirus

The link between human papillomavirus (HPV) and esophageal cancer continues to be explored. Although no definitive etiologic role has been established, the link is intriguing [127, 131, 181]. Morphologic evidence of HPV and evidence of viral antigen have been found in a high percentage of esophageal cancer specimens [73, 84, 85, 105, 183]. Using DNA probes, HPV DNA was detected in 72% of patients in a high-risk area of northern China who had cytologic evidence of precancerous lesions [35]. A hypothesis has been put forth to explain these findings. In normal human esophageal mucosa, Langerhans' cells and intraepithelial lymphocytes are believed to coexist in a symbiotic relationship with keratinocytes. The immunocompetent cells function to defend the integrity of the esophageal mucosa through the detection and eradication of foreign antigenic material. The cytopathic effect of HPV overwhelms this mucosal defense symptom, and colonization of the mucosa occurs. The vast majority of these lesions are flat (noncondylomatous) and form an acanthotic form of cellular proliferation. Glycogenic acanthosis, heretofore believed to be a benign lesion of no clinical significance, may represent a morphologic variant of HPV infection. In the setting of persistent infection, nutritional deficiencies, or various exogenous cofactors, HPV-induced cytopathic changes may progress to dysplasia, which then sets the stage for the development of *in situ* carcinoma [131]. The accepted association of HPV and squamous cell cancer of the cervix makes this an intriguing hypothesis.

### Genetic Factors

The biology of esophageal cancer is complex and molecular changes are being elucidated with increased frequency. Much research has centered around p53, a tumor suppressor gene located on the p arm of chromosome [17, 64]. Mutation and allelic losses are common abnormalities in many human neoplasms. p53 has been implicated in the control of cell cycle, DNA repair and synthesis, cell differentiation, genomic stability, and apoptosis. p53 overexpression also correlates with increased intratumoral vessel density, a measure of neoangiogenesis. A study in China and Hong Kong evaluating p53 tumor suppressor genes with analyses by single-strand conformation polymorphism and DNA sequencing showed that 42% contained mutations in exons 5 to 8 of the p53 gene [122]. Chinese esophageal carcinomas are often associated with genetic alterations which may be attributed to specific dietary or environmental carcinogens that affect Chinese, but not non-Chinese. Another study from Hong Kong evaluated squamous cell esophageal carcinoma specimens to determine a link between HPV and p53 mutation [108]. In those Hong Kong patients no link was found. Wang and colleagues found p53 mutations in the early stages of human esophageal carcinogenesis and postulated that independent somatic mutations in different regions of the esophagus might be key molecular events in multifocal esophageal carcinogenesis [205]. p53 protein was overexpressed in the nonmalignant mucosa of patients after gastrectomy (68%) and in patients with advanced achalasia (44%). Both types of patients are considered to be at increased risk for squamous cell cancer of the esophagus. Increased p53 levels were seen in all patients with dysplasia [162].

Chaves et al. [37] and Uchino et al. [193] looked at how p53 overexpression correlates with both tumor behavior and overall prognoses. Chaves et al. found specific staining for p53 in 57% of esophageal cancer patients. p53 was noted in areas of adjacent epithelium with both low-grade and high-grade dysplasia. Uchino et al. showed that p53 correlates with poorer patient survival.

Hori et al. studied genetic polymorphisms of tobacco- and alcohol-related metabolizing enzymes in patients with esophageal cancer and found that the ADH2/ADH2 and ALDH2/ALDH2 genotypes were significantly higher in esophageal cancer patients than controls [87].

Tylosis, an autosomal dominant disorder characterized by hyperkeratosis of the palms and soles, appears to be the only well-documented genetic association with esophageal cancer [164, 169, 170]. It is estimated that affected family members have a 95% chance of developing cancer at some point in their lives, provided they do not die from some other cause [89].

### Miscellaneous

Esophageal cancer also has been associated with a number of other risk groups. Patients who have a history of ionizing radiation [168], head and neck cancer [13, 67], Plummer-Vinson syndrome [208], celiac disease [165], and thyroid disease [12] have been reported to be at increased risk for developing esophageal cancer. The postulated association between esophageal carcinoma and prior gastrectomy appears to be incidental [107]. The risk for esophageal cancer appears to be increased among women who receive radiation for breast cancer [1].

## Natural History

### Presentation

The symptoms of esophageal cancer are nonspecific and similar regardless of the histologic subtype. Dysphagia is the most common presentation [149]. Typically, difficulty swallowing is noted with solid foods first and then, over a period of weeks to months, progresses to include semisolids and eventually liquids. Patients seem to tolerate or ignore this symptom for some time before seeking medical attention. Odynophagia (retrosternal pain associated with swallowing) is the next-most-common symptom. It may be caused by an ulcerated area in the tumor or invasion of the surrounding mediastinal structures. If it is the latter, the implications are more ominous. Constant pain in the midback or midchest also portends mediastinal invasion. Regurgitation of food immediately after swallowing may occur as the growing neoplasm narrows the esophageal lumen. The constitutional symptoms of anorexia and weight loss are often present by the time the patient seeks medical attention. Hoarseness may occur with proximal tumors. Hematemesis is uncommon.

Physical examination may reveal entirely normal findings, and in general is not very useful in this disease. The rarity of tylosis makes the search for thickened and fissured palms and soles or onycholysis unrewarding. Temporal wasting, dehydration, and inanition are commonly seen. It is not clear whether this is simply malnutrition resulting from an obstructed esophageal lumen or whether the tumor secretes a factor that promotes cachexia. The ability of patients to gain weight after successful palliation of dysphagia suggests the former. It is important to look for physical signs that may alter one's therapeutic approach, such as supraclavicular or cervical adenopathy, a discrete abdominal mass, or fullness that may indicate involvement of the celiac nodes or metastatic disease to the liver. Clubbing of the fingers may be seen, but is not specific for esophageal cancer [143, 195].

Anemia may result from chronic occult blood loss. A chest x-ray may reveal mediastinal widening or pulmonary nodules or evidence of aspiration pneumonia.

The midesophagus is the most common site for esophageal squamous cell carcinoma. The distal esophagus is a close second, and the upper esophagus is a distant third.

### Complications

Obstruction of the esophageal lumen promotes aspiration pneumonitis. This is a common problem and may lead to the patient's death. Because the thoracic esophagus has no serosa and lies in close proximity to other vital mediastinal structures, local tumor growth may be associated with a number of complications. Contiguous involvement of the tumor with the tracheobronchial tree may lead to the formation of an esophago-airway fistula. Esophagomediastinal and esophagopleural fistulas also are seen. Rarely, exsanguination may occur if the tumor erodes into a major vessel such as the descending thoracic aorta. Vocal cord paralysis may be seen with involvement of the recurrent laryngeal nerve.

### Metastatic Spread

Early lymphatic spread of esophageal cancer is characteristic. In general, lesions of the cervical and upper esophagus involve the cervical, supraclavicular, or mediastinal nodes; middle and lower esophageal lesions involve the mediastinal, paratracheal, and abdominal lymph nodes; and lesions of the cardia metastasize to the upper gastric, paraceliac, and paraaortic nodes (Fig. 12–1) [2, 128]. Because of the extensive submucosal lymphatic network within the esophagus, however, longitudinal spread frequently results in lymphatic metastases outside of these "expected" anatomic drainage patterns. Spread to superior gastric lymph nodes has been reported in 31.8% of patients with upper esophageal tumors, and superior mediastinal nodes have been involved in 33% of patients with lower esophageal tumors [3, 93]. Hematogenous spread usually goes to the liver (32%) and lungs (21%), but a variety of other sites may be involved, including (but not limited to) bone (8%), kidney (7%), omentum or peritoneum (5%), adrenal glands (4%), stomach (4%), and heart (4%) (Fig. 12–2) [123, 128].

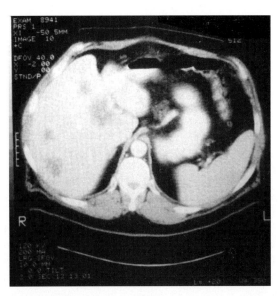

FIG. 12–2. Computed tomography scan of the abdomen. Multiple filling defects in the liver represent metastatic disease from squamous cell carcinoma of the esophagus.

### Clinical Prognostic Factors

Survival of women exceeds that of men [179], and experimental evidence supports a hormonal basis for this difference, with estrogens inhibiting and androgens enhancing tumor growth [197]. The disease seems to be more aggressive in younger patients. Malignancy-associated hypercalcemia, which may occur in up to 28% of patients with squamous cell cancer of the esophagus [213], also has been linked to an unfavorable clinical outcome [106]. Histologic grade does not appear to be a major factor associated with the outcome of squamous cell carcinoma [173]. Evidence of host immunity, such as infiltration of the tumor with Langerhans' cells, may indicate a more favorable outcome [125].

All of these clinical factors are of interest, but it is important to emphasize that the extent of disease spread at the time of diagnosis is the single most important prognostic factor. This emphasizes the importance of staging and the potential for screening to enhance the likelihood of earlier diagnoses.

### Diagnosis

Because the prognosis is dismal when a clinical diagnosis (based on signs and symptoms) of esophageal cancer can be

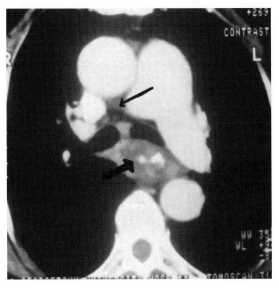

FIG. 12–1. Computed tomography scan of the thorax. The esophageal wall is thickened (*wide arrow*) and paraaortic lymph nodes are present (*thin arrow*).

made, and since diagnosis and treatment of early (subclinical) esophageal cancer has resulted in a 5-year survival rate of 90% [209], there has been considerable interest in the screening of asymptomatic patients.

### Mass Screening

In high-risk areas such as China, population screening has enabled subclinical detection of early esophageal cancer [209]. A nylon mesh-covered balloon, inserted transorally into the stomach, is inflated and pulled back through the esophagus. Epithelial cells that become debrided and trapped within the nylon mesh are then subjected to cytologic evaluation. Of the cancers detected by this method, three-fourths are at an early stage. A study in Linxian by Roth et al. compared the traditional mesh-covered Chinese balloon to an American-made sponge sampler [159]. The specificity of both devices was 99%, but the Chinese balloon, which is larger and more abrasive, was better. In 1998, Barrios carried out a study with a Brazilian balloon which is intermediate in size between the Chinese balloon and the American sponge and the results are encouraging (personal communication). In patients in whom the cytology is positive, endoscopic evaluation can be performed. The value of endoscopy is increased by the use of mucosal staining with Lugol's iodine. Normal squamous mucosa, which contains glycogen, is stained green-brown by Lugol's, but dysplastic or neoplastic tissue, which is deplete of glycogen, does not stain, and these unstained areas can be biopsied. Dawsey et al. found that 23% of patients with severe dysplasia and 55% with moderate dysplasia were identified only after staining [47]. Ban et al. studied asymptomatic Japanese patients with a history of cigarette smoking and alcohol intake and found an increased incidence of abnormalities with staining [15].

Balloon cytology has been evaluated in a group of high-risk U. S. veterans (older than 40 years, alcohol abuse, cigarette smokers). It was found to be of limited value because of the difficulty of distinguishing dysplasia from inflammation [77]. A more recent study by Strader et al., also in a U.S. veterans hospital, examined direct endoscopic screening with iodine staining [178]. The yield was higher in older patients.

### Selective Screening

In the United States, the age-adjusted incidence of esophageal cancer (3.2 per 100,000 population) is too small to justify mass screening. Selective screening via endoscopy with biopsy and cytology every 1 to 3 years has been recommended for specific risk groups [8, 117]. The groups most likely to be encountered in the United States include patients with achalasia and lye strictures (Barrett's esophagus and adenocarcinoma are discussed elsewhere). Annual surveillance is also recommended for the rare patient with tylosis or Plummer-Vinson syndrome. Although screening of head and neck cancer patients for simultaneous esophageal cancer

was found to be low yield and did not convey any survival advantage, all but one of the esophageal cancers in this retrospective study were symptomatic at the time of diagnosis, and patients were not screened for metachronous lesions subsequent to the initial evaluation. Head and neck cancer patients should be included among the high-risk patients selected for screening. Horiuchi et al. screened 676 patients with head and neck cancer for esophageal cancer. Primary esophageal cancer was found in 5.5% of patients. Patients with cancer of the oral cavity or pharynx had significantly more esophageal cancer (11%) than those with laryngeal or sinusoid cancer (2%) [88].

### Esophagoscopy

Endoscopic evaluation is necessary in the evaluation of all patients whose signs, symptoms, or radiologic appearance are suggestive of esophageal malignancy. The majority of symptomatic lesions will exhibit moderate to severe luminal encroachment, often with ulcerated centers and heaped-up edges (Fig. 12–3). Esophageal dilation may be necessary to view the distal extent of the lesion. Early lesions may be very subtle or almost normal in their appearance. Focal areas of elevation, depression, or color change may be the only indication of malignancy [129]. In fact, the early changes of esophageal cancer are often so subtle that many skilled endoscopists who rarely see early cancer may not recognize them (Color Plate 45). Lugol's solution can be used to delineate abnormal areas likely to be malignant. Unstained areas therefore represent abnormal mucosa and have a higher likelihood of malignancy (Color Plate 46). Vital staining has also been attempted with toluidine blue, although the experience is much more limited than with Lugol's and the benefit not as clear. The results of one study were disappointing, with a positive predictive value of only 33% and a negative predictive value of 89% [95]. In addition to enabling visual observation, endoscopy allows cytologic and histologic eval-

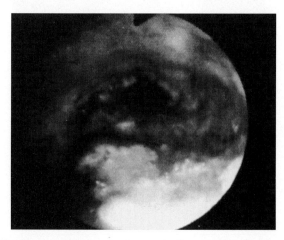

**FIG. 12–3.** Endoscopy demonstrating typical features of esophageal cancer. The lumen is narrowed and irregular. (See also Plate 47.)

uation of the lesion through brushings and biopsy. The most accurate diagnosis is achieved using a combination of biopsy and cytology [45].

### Upper Gastrointestinal Series

Radiographic evaluation of the esophagus and the proximal part of the stomach using a barium swallow remains a useful test in the evaluation and management of esophageal malignancy. Double-contrast esophagography is required to demonstrate small esophageal tumors. Because of the test's relatively low sensitivity, a normal-appearing barium esophagogram should not be used to exonerate the esophagus in symptomatic patients. Radiographic evaluation using a barium-impregnated food bolus, such as bread or marshmallow, may help define the location where normal peristalsis is disrupted. Although this modality may demonstrate the location, severity, and extent of luminal narrowing, only disruption of the esophageal axis appears helpful in deciding on resectability (Fig. 12–4) [130].

### Staging

#### Computed Tomography/Magnetic Resonance Imaging

Although computed tomography (CT) is commonly employed in the pretreatment staging of esophageal cancer, enthusiasm is waning because the sensitivity is not high. Per-

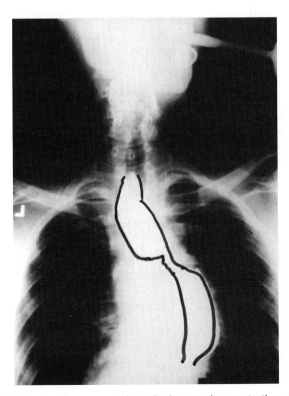

**FIG. 12–4.** Upper gastrointestinal x-ray demonstrating disruption of the esophageal axis. This finding argues against resectability.

haps the most important and reliable function of CT is the detection of distant, extranodal metastases or recurrent tumor. Metastatic disease to the liver may be apparent as low-attenuating lesions. In decreasing order of frequency, lung, adrenal, and kidney masses also may be seen. Histologic confirmation of these findings via needle biopsy is often necessary.

A determination of the extent of local or regional tumor and invasion of adjacent mediastinal structures is made by evaluating the mediastinal fat planes. Depending on the degree of esophageal distention, normal esophageal wall thickness is approximately 3 to 5 mm, and carcinomas may exhibit focal or circumferential wall thickening [74]. Transmural invasion into the mediastinum may be evident as a soft-tissue density. Invasion of the tracheobronchial tree may appear as displacement, compression, or disruption of the airway by tumor. One may be able to predict aortic invasion if the fat plane between the esophagus and aorta has been replaced by tumor; the likelihood increases with the degree of contact between these structures [144]. However, detection of transmural tumor extension is made more difficult in the cachectic patient, in whom mediastinal fat planes are diminished, and CT has been shown to have limited usefulness in the preoperative assessment of resectability based on these parameters [124, 150, 202].

Assessment of lymph node involvement by CT is also often inaccurate [124, 150]. Determination of nodal involvement is made on the basis of size. Since lymph nodes may have microscopic invasion, and since benign inflammatory changes may enlarge lymph nodes, there is an unacceptably high degree of inaccuracy in diagnosing nodal involvement by tumor [112, 124]. This is especially true in some areas where esophageal cancer metastasizes frequently, such as periesophageal and subdiaphragmatic nodes. CT often leads to "understaging" the cancer, and more extensive disease is found at the time of attempted curative resection. The utility of magnetic resonance imaging for the assessment of the extent of spread of esophageal carcinoma has been limited due to image degradation by esophageal motion and flow artifact from adjacent cardiovascular structures, but this may change with improvements in technology, such as gating techniques and shortening of scan times [150].

### Endoscopic Ultrasonography

Endoscopic ultrasonography (EUS) is a hybrid technology that houses an ultrasonic transducer at the tip of an endoscope and provides detailed ultrasonic images of the wall of the gastrointestinal tract and surrounding structures. Therefore, it is ideally suited for staging of esophageal cancer. The depth of penetration of tumors into the wall can be assessed, as can lymph nodes in proximity to the gastrointestinal wall (Fig. 12–5). Preliminary reports on its use in the pretreatment staging of esophageal cancer are encouraging. This modality was evaluated in patients with esophageal cancer and was found to have an accuracy of 74% to 92% with

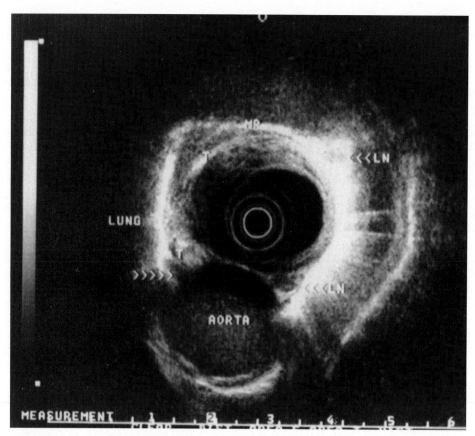

**FIG. 12–5.** Endoscopic ultrasound view of an esophageal cancer. *T,* Tumor; *MP,* muscularis propria; *LN,* lymph node.

regard to depth of tumor invasion [180, 188] (Table 12–2). The reported accuracy of EUS in determining the N stage of esophageal cancer is 74% to 88% (Table 12–3). Although alterations in echogenicity may aid in discrimination, differentiation of enlarged benign lymph nodes for micrometastases remained problematic, with a specificity of only 56% [188]. Because of the limited depth of penetration by ultrasound, detection of distant metastases is poor. The reported accuracy of M stage by EUS is 68% to 70% [24, 117, 187]. The staging accuracy was found to be 86% when CT was used to assess the M stage and EUS was used for T- and N-stage determination. Inability to traverse the malignant stenosis may hinder a thorough evaluation in 12% to 63% of patients (Table 12–4) [46]. This does limit the ability of

**TABLE 12–3.** *Esophageal cancer: accuracy of endoscopic ultrasonography N-stage determination*

| | No. | N-stage accuracy (%) |
|---|---|---|
| Rice, 1991 [155] | 80 | 74 |
| Tio et al., 1989 [187] | 74 | 80 |
| Botet et al., 1991 [24] | 50 | 88 |
| Dittler, 1993 [52] | 167 | 73 |
| Grimm, 1993 [68] | 63 | 86 |

**TABLE 12–2.** *Esophageal cancer: accuracy of endoscopic ultrasonography T-stage determination*

| | No. | T-stage accuracy (%) |
|---|---|---|
| Rice, 1991 [155] | 80 | 74 |
| Takemoto et al., 1986 [185] | 12 | 75 |
| Tio et al., 1989 [187] | 74 | 89 |
| Botet et al., 1991 [24] | 50 | 92 |
| Hordjik et al., 1993 [86] | 41 | 76 |
| Kalantzis et al., 1992 [97] | 28 | 82 |

**TABLE 12–4.** *Esophageal cancer: strictures not permitting passage of endoscope*

| | No. | Percent stricture |
|---|---|---|
| Rice et al., 1991 [155] | 52 | 12 |
| Takemoto et al., 1986 [185] | 16 | 12.5 |
| Vilgrain et al., 1990 [202] | 46 | 50 |
| Tio et al., 1989 [187] | 74 | 26 |
| Dancygier and Classen, 1989 [46] | 24 | 62.5 |
| Heyder and Lux, 1986 [82] | 42 | 36 |
| Grimm et al., 1992 [68] | 67 | 21 |
| Dittler, 1993 [52] | 253 | 30 |
| Van Dam et al., 1993 [199] | 79 | 27 |

EUS to accurately determine tumor stage. Rice and colleagues [156] reported an unacceptably high rate of perforation when dilation was performed to permit passage of the echoendoscope. In our experience at Georgetown University Hospital, 13 patients with advanced esophageal cancer (T3, T4) underwent EUS/dilation simultaneously and there were no observed perforations [99].

Two important advances in endoscopic ultrasonography have enhanced the evaluation of esophageal cancer: through-the-scope catheter probes and fine-needle aspiration. The development of 12-MHz and 20-MHz catheter probes (Fig. 12–6) which can be passed through the biopsy channel allows strictures which previously prevented advance of the EUS endoscope to be evaluated [189]. Another advance relates to fine-needle aspiration. One of the criticisms, or perhaps unfulfilled hopes, for EUS has been that it does not provide histologic diagnosis. Using a linear scanning echoendoscope (Pentax FG-32UA, FG-36 UX), one can sample periesophageal or celiac lymph nodes with a 23-gauge aspiration needle (Fig. 12–7). Harada and colleagues sampled 112 lymph nodes in 77 patients and improved sensitivity, specificity, and accuracy for lymph node staging [76].

Another new technique, three-dimensional EUS, was first reported by Kallimanis and coauthors [98]. This has the potential to enhance diagnostic accuracy by using specially developed software to reconstruct a three-dimensional image from a two-dimensional EUS (Fig. 12–8). As software becomes more sophisticated, even more potential will be realized.

*Bronchoscopy*

A large percentage of patients with esophageal malignancy have involvement of the tracheobronchial tree that can be documented by bronchoscopy. It should be considered for

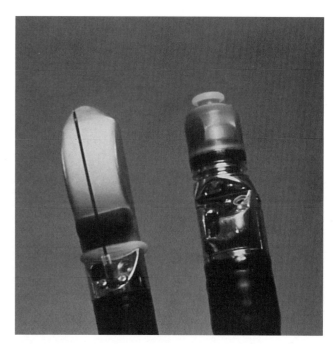

**FIG. 12–7. Left:** linear scanning echoendoscope used for ultrasound evaluation and fine-needle aspiration (Pentax Corp.). **Right:** Radial scanning echoendoscope (Olympus Corp.).

tumors of the cervical esophagus and midesophagus. One study found evidence of impingement or invasion in approximately 34% of preoperative evaluations [39]. The incidence of respiratory tree involvement was directly related to tumor length, and positive bronchoscopic findings were present in 47% of tumors longer than 10 cm. Esophageal cancers in the cervical and upper thoracic region tend to involve the trachea, whereas those in the midthoracic region tend to involve the left main stem bronchus. Vocal cord paralysis is suggestive of entrapment of the recurrent laryngeal nerve by tumor.

*Laparoscopy*

In detecting the presence of intraabdominal metastases in patients with esophageal cancer, laparoscopy was determined to have a sensitivity of 88%, a specificity of 100%, and an overall accuracy of 96% [206]. With regard to liver metastases, this modality proved to be significantly more sensitive and more accurate than either ultrasonography or CT and had the advantage of providing histologic confirmation of findings. Laparoscopy was also better than ultrasonography at detecting intraabdominal nodal metastases. Despite this sensitivity and specificity, laparoscopy is generally not employed in the evaluation of most patients with esophageal cancer.

***Traditional Therapies***

*General Principles*

The therapeutic approach to esophageal cancer is not standardized. The bulk of the literature on the subject is retro-

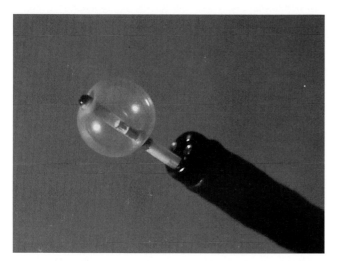

**FIG. 12–6.** Endoscopic ultrasound catheter probe (Olympus Corp.). This 20-MHz probe is shown passing through the endoscopic channel and can be placed directly over the area to be studied.

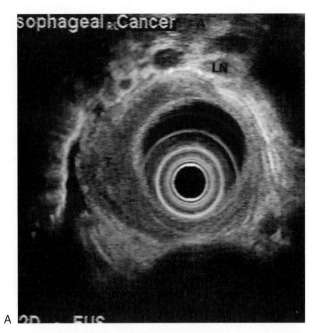
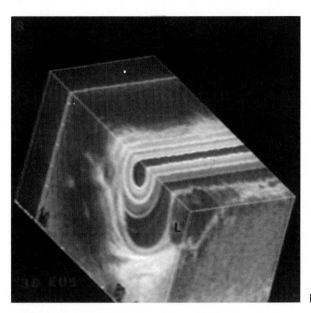

**FIG. 12–8. A:** A two-dimensional view of an esophageal cancer by conventional endoscopic ultrasound (EUS). **B:** A three-dimensional view of the same lesion. *T,* Tumor; *PF,* pleural fluid; *I,* invasion.

spective, uncontrolled, or anecdotal, and often is written from a single perspective, depending on whether the author's experience is surgical, radiologic, oncologic, or endoscopic. Results of recent prospective studies have improved the outlook for selected groups of patients; however, the morbidity and mortality associated with these therapeutic approaches are significant, and by comparison the handful of 5-year survivors seems a Pyrrhic victory. Since most patients who are discovered to have esophageal cancers are diagnosed after symptoms occur, the real hope for altering the prognosis will be realized by screening asymptomatic individuals. Given the limitations of available knowledge, most recommendations on the therapy of esophageal cancer are more philosophic than scientific. In an area such as this where no axioms exist, it is reasonable to base the choice of therapy on two determinations: (a) the stage of the patient's cancer, and (b) the patient's general medical condition.

There is a strong association between the anatomic extent of tumor spread and prognosis. Regardless of the therapeutic approach, patients with stage I of II tumors live considerably longer than those with stage III or IV disease (Table 12–5) [16]. Tumor, node, and metastasis (TNM) classification proved to be among the strongest independent predictor of long-term survival among 657 patients operated on during the period 1960 through 1984 [121]; the more advanced the anatomic extent of disease, the poorer was the prognosis. Similar studies in Japan and China showed that the depth of tumor invasion into the esophageal wall was associated with survival; the greater the depth of invasion, the worse was the prognosis [91, 213, 214]. This observation, along with improvements in imaging techniques, has been the impetus for making depth of invasion the principal criterion

for clinical classification, replacing size, circumferential involvement, and obstruction in the old TNM classification [175]. Patients whose tumors invade neighboring structures have even lower survival rates [91]. With regard to lymph node status, patients with evidence of involvement have one-half to one-third the chance of surviving 5 years as do patients without lymph node metastases [3, 167, 213, 215]. The presence of organ metastases is frequently associated with death within 6 months.

Clinical parameters are also important in selecting a therapeutic approach to esophageal cancer. Advanced age, coexisting pulmonary disease, tachycardia, clinical dehydration, and hepatomegaly were found to be independent variables that adversely affect outcome following surgical treatment [121]. Hepatomegaly was associated with congestive heart failure rather than metastatic disease.

As mentioned previously, the therapeutic approach to esophageal cancer is not standardized. Radiotherapy, chemotherapy, surgery, or endoscopic therapy may be used alone, but it is more common for a multimodality approach to be used, and for the treatment to be coordinated by the different subspecialists. For the purpose of clarity, the treatment options will be discussed separately, then by combination. Endoscopic management is discussed separately in Chapter 4.

*Radiotherapy*

The greatest experience in treating esophageal cancer with ionizing radiation has been with external-beam radiotherapy. The biologic effect of radiation on the tumor is directly proportional to the dose administered, and the amount that can

**TABLE 12–5.** *American Joint Committee on Cancer staging of esophageal cancer*[a]

Primary tumor (T)
  TX, primary tumor cannot be assessed
  T0, no evidence of primary tumor
  Tis, carcinoma *in situ*
  T1, tumor invades lamina propria or submucosa
  T2, tumor invades muscularis propria
  T3, tumor invades adventitia
  T4, tumor invades adjacent structures
Regional lymph nodes (N)
  NX, regional lymph nodes cannot be assessed
  N0, no regional lymph node metastasis
  N1, regional lymph node metastasis
Distant metastasis (M)
  MX, presence of distant metastasis cannot be assessed
  M0, no distant metastasis
  M1, distant metastasis

Stage grouping

| Stage | T | N | M |
|---|---|---|---|
| Stage 0 | Tis | N0 | M0 |
| Stage 1 | T1 | N0 | M0 |
| Stage IIA | T2 | N0 | M0 |
|  | T3 | N0 | M0 |
| Stage IIB | T1 | N1 | M0 |
|  | T2 | N1 | M0 |
| Stage III | T3 | N1 | M0 |
|  | T4 | Any N | M0 |
| Stage IV | Any T | Any N | M1 |

[a] From Bears et al. [16].

be delivered is limited by the tolerance of adjacent normal tissue. The minimum dose required for radical therapy is 50 Gy, and 60 Gy is regarded as the maximum dose [53].

Historically, radiotherapy has been regarded as palliative; therefore, the patient population tends to be biased toward more advanced disease. Nevertheless, overall 5-year survival rates of 6% to 9% [53, 54, 135] rival those of many surgical series, and local control of disease and effective palliation of dysphagia can be achieved in the majority (60% to 80%) of patients. Like surgical results, treatment efficacy appears directly related to the anatomic extent of the disease [57]. Complete resolution of dysphagia has been achieved in more than three-fourths of patients with lesions smaller than 5 cm, but in only 29% of patients with lesions larger than 9 cm [57]. Efficacy does not appear to be related to the degree of tumor differentiation [141]. While no prospective randomized controlled studies compared the two approaches, patients regarded as operative candidates who received radiotherapy had a 5-year survival rate of 14% [54].

Analysis of patterns of failure indicate that most patients (83%) die of persistent disease at the primary site [59]. Even in patients with stage I disease, local recurrence occurred in 25%, recurrence outside of the radiation port (but within the esophagus) was noted in 25%, and distant metastatic disease was seen in another 25% [57]. Sixty-four percent of patients with stage II or III disease exhibited local recurrence [57]. In contrast to results in the thoracic esophagus, the cervical esophagus and postcricoid region seem particularly amena-

ble to megavoltage irradiation, with 5-year survival rates approaching 19% [135].

Radiotherapy is associated with a number of potential complications. In contrast to surgery, treatment-related fatality is exceedingly rare. The principal morbidity is fibrous stricture formation in the esophagus, which may occur in up to 44% of patients [135]. Skin burns, leukopenia, pulmonary fibrosis, cardiomyopathy, and rarely, transverse myelitis leading to paraplegia also may occur [53, 57, 135]. If pretreatment staging suggests that the tumor has infiltrated the tracheobronchial tree or thoracic aorta, radiotherapy may promote fistulous tracts between the structures [53] and should not be employed as part of the patient's treatment.

Intracavitary radiation (brachiotherapy), alone or in combination with external-beam radiotherapy is being evaluated with renewed interest in esophageal cancer because of technical advances in the available isotopes and methods of administration [59, 65]. Theoretical advantages include a higher radiation dose to the local tumor bed and lower exposure to other vital mediastinal structures. Ninety percent of patients experience improvement in swallowing lasting 3 months or longer, and improvements in odynophagia and weight gain are also significant. Radiation esophagitis is common and may be severe and persistent in some patients. Preliminary results show survival statistics of 33% at 1 year, 26% at 2 years, and 19% at 3 years [59]. All patients with evidence of distant metastases died within 8 months of treatment.

*Chemotherapy*

Systemic chemotherapy would appear to be a logical approach to the treatment of esophageal cancer, because surgical and autopsy data indicate the disease is almost always widespread at the time of diagnosis. Unfortunately, the response of esophageal squamous cell cancer to chemotherapy is poor. Single-agent chemotherapy has been associated with response rates of approximately 15% to 20% that are short-lived [100]. Combination chemotherapy using cisplatin, vindesine, and bleomycin has achieved response rates in one-third of patients with extensive disease; however, the median duration of response remains low (7 months), and the toxicities of this regimen include renal dysfunction, nausea, vomiting, alopecia, peripheral neuropathy, pulmonary fibrosis, and neutropenia with susceptibility to infection [102]. Similar to treatment efficacy seen with other modalities, response rates, median survival times, and ability to tolerate chemotherapy are better in patients with local or regional disease. Substitution of mitoguazone for bleomycin reduced the pulmonary toxicity, but median duration of remission in patients with extensive disease dropped to 3 months and myelosuppression remained the major dose-limiting toxicity [103]. No study has shown an improved patient survival. Given the short life span of patients with esophageal cancer and the low response rates, high toxicity, and ineffectiveness of chemotherapy to change survival in advanced disease, administration of chemotherapy alone to these patients currently seems irrational.

## Multimodality Therapy

The disappointing results achieved with surgery, radiotherapy, and chemotherapy alone have led to recent attempts to combine various modalities in the hopes of achieving superior results.

### Preoperative Chemotherapy

The 5-year survival rate for 34 patients with local or regional disease treated with cisplatin, vindesine, and bleomycin followed by esophagectomy was 17.6% [101]. Partial responses were noted in 63%, resectability rate was 83%, and preoperative chemotherapy was not associated with an increase in operative complications or mortality [102]. A subsequent prospective study that compared preoperative and postoperative chemotherapy (consisting of cisplatin, vindesine, and bleomycin) to operation alone showed no overall improvement in survival [158]. Nevertheless, the preoperative response rate was 47%, and these patients had a significantly prolonged survival time (median, longer than 20 months) when compared with either nonresponders (median, 6.2 months) or patients receiving only operation (median, 8.6 months). It is noteworthy that patients who responded to chemotherapy had a prerandomization weight loss of less than 10% and that chemotherapy did not improve the resectability rate or increase the postoperative complication rate. Survival benefit appears confined to patients who respond to preoperative chemotherapy.

### Preoperative Radiotherapy

Radiotherapy is used in a preoperative fashion in the hope that reduction of the tumor size may permit a more complete resection. Retrospective analyses support that contention by demonstrating resectability and 5-year survival rates that are nearly twice those of historical controls without adversely affecting operative mortality [167, 213]. Kelsen [100] randomized 96 patients with local or regional squamous cell carcinoma to receive either preoperative radiotherapy or preoperative chemotherapy. When surgery was performed on day 56, a response rate of 64% was seen with radiotherapy versus 55% with chemotherapy (not statistically significant), and no difference was noted in the operability or resectability rates. The results of four additional trials which show no benefit with preoperative radiation are summarized in a recent publication [27].

### Preoperative Chemotherapy and Selective Postoperative Therapy

Thirty-five patients with potentially resectable lesions were treated with 5-fluorouracil (5-FU) and cisplatin. Complete responses were seen in 37% and partial responses in another 20%, and 27 patients underwent surgical resection. Selective postoperative chemotherapy or radiotherapy was given to 69%. The 3-year survival rate for patients who had resection was 54%, nearly double the historical control rate. Factors associated with increased survival were the complete clinical response to chemotherapy, absence of esophageal wall penetration, and either the absence of tumor or only microscopic disease in the surgical specimen. Although there was a trend favoring survival in patients who received postoperative chemotherapy and radiotherapy, this did not reach statistical significance [83].

### Postoperative Radiotherapy

Postoperative radiotherapy has been compared with the combination of preoperative and postoperative radiotherapy in a prospective, randomized multicenter trial [90]. Patients treated with surgery followed by radiotherapy survived longer than did those treated with radiation preoperatively and postoperatively, although this did not reach statistical significance. In three other trials, postoperative radiation therapy was compared to surgery alone [60, 186, 220]. Doses between 30 and 48 Gy were used. In no instance was the postoperative treatment of benefit.

### Preoperative Concurrent Chemotherapy and Radiotherapy

Since some chemotherapeutic agents exhibit both cytotoxic and radiosensitizing properties, chemotherapy and radiotherapy have been used concurrently in the hope of improving results [80], Parker and co-workers [141] added mitomycin C and 5-FU to preoperative radiotherapy. Only 33 of 129 patients were able to complete the preoperative concurrent therapies and undergo resection. Although one-third of these patients had no evidence of tumor present in the surgical resection, there was no significant increase in 5-year survival rates (15%, 1984) compared to historical control patients treated with preoperative radiotherapy alone (10%, 1975). Investigators at Wayne State University switched their chemotherapy regimen from 5-FU and mitomycin C to 5-FU and cisplatin in the hope of combating distant disease in addition to enhancing the effects of radiation [113]. Although the studies were performed sequentially and subjects were not randomized, substitution of cisplatin for mitomycin C in conjunction with preoperative radiotherapy increased the median survival time from 12 to 24 months [79, 113]. With either regimen, however, the only correlation with improved survival was the ability of preoperative therapy to eradicate all evidence of cancer at the time of esophagectomy. This therapy alters the natural history of the disease; in 80% of patients in whom recurrent disease develops, it does so in distant sites outside of the radiation port.

Because of these encouraging results, the Southwest Oncology Group evaluated the efficacy of radiotherapy (30 Gy) and chemotherapy (5-FU and cisplatin) administered prior to surgery [146]. Toxicity included a variety of gastrointestinal symptoms, mucositis, and myelosuppression; most cases were of moderate severity, but some were severe or life-threatening. Overall, the results were discouraging, with an operability rate of 63%, resectability rate of 49%, and surgical mortality of 11%. The combined modality approach may have benefited 17% of patients who exhibited a complete response (median postsurgical survival time of 32 months); however, the overall median survival time was only 14%, and only 16% of eligible patients survived 3 years [146].

Forastiere and associates [61] utilized preoperative cisplatin, vinblastine, and 5-FU in conjunction with radiotherapy followed by transhiatal esophagectomy. Of the 43 selected patients with local or regional esophageal cancer entered into the study, myelosuppression with severe leukopenia developed in 93% of patients, and there were 2 septic deaths. A variety of nonhematologic toxicities were encountered and included esophagitis and secondary dysphagia (86%), weight loss (19%), diarrhea (60%), and nausea, vomiting, and anorexia. The operability rate was 95%, 84% of tumors were completely resected, and a complete response was noted in 24% of patients. There was a 59% survival rate at 2 years, with results for adenocarcinoma more favorable than for squamous cell carcinoma.

In a study by Nusheim and coauthors [138], 47 patients with esophageal cancer were treated preoperatively with simultaneous radiotherapy and chemotherapy (5-FU, cisplatin). Ninety-four percent of patients completed a full course of therapy, 88% had lesions that were resectable, and actuarial survival was significantly better than that of the 1980 to 1985 historical control patients [138].

In a small study by LePrise et al., 86 patients with squamous cell cancer were randomized [114]. There were no differences between the survival in the two groups. Bosset et al. gave preoperative radiation and cisplatin to 282 patients with squamous cell cancer [23]. There was no difference in survival. Although there was improved local control, it came at a cost of significantly raised operative modality. The Wayne State group studied 100 patients with esophageal cancer, 25 of whom had squamous cell cancer [196]. The overall 3-year survival was higher in the combined treatment group (32% vs. 15%), but the results are not statistically significant.

## Chemoradiotherapy without Surgery

Several studies have compared combined radiation and chemotherapy (CMT) to radiation alone. These are summarized in Table 12–6. Three of the five studies showed no statistically significant benefit [6, 10, 55, 161, 172]. A study by Sischy et al. shows a 15% 5-year survival in the CMT group and a 9% survival in the group receiving only radiation ($p < 0.05$) [172]. A multicenter study by the Radiation Therapy Oncology Group (RTOG) compared radiation alone to a lower dose of radiation combined with cisplatin and 5-FU [80]. The intention of giving a lower dose of radiation in the CMT arm was to reduce acute toxicity. Despite this, however, only 50% of patients randomized to the CMT arm completed all four cycles. At 3 years there were no survivors in the radiation arm, but 31% in the combined arm. This study has been recently updated and confirms a 5-year survival of 30% in the CMT arm [6]. From this study, it appears that concurrent CMT is superior to radiation alone. It should be emphasized that three studies showed no benefit and the RTOG study was associated with significant toxicity.

In a nonrandomized trial, Coia et al. [41] treated 50 patients, 30 of whom had stage I or II disease and 20 of whom had more advanced disease. The former group was treated for potential cure. The median time to relapse was 10 months, and a 32% 5-year survival was reported. In the latter group the overall median survival was 8 months.

### Hyperthermochemoradiotherapy

Matsuda [126] in Japan recently reported on ten patients with early-stage esophageal carcinoma who were treated with hyperthermochemoradiotherapy without surgery because of concurrent medical illnesses. Five patients experienced no local recurrence for 12 to 70 months, three died of other medical conditions without evidence of esophageal cancer, and two died of recurrent disease 20 to 27 months after diagnosis. All ten patients tolerated the treatment well without systemic side effects. Therefore, hyperthermochemoradiotherapy deserves serious consideration for patients with small malignant lesions of the esophagus who, for various reasons, are unable to undergo surgery [126].

### Endoscopic Palliation

Despite the encouraging results obtained with multimodality therapy, the majority of patients with esophageal can-

**TABLE 12–6.** *Randomized trials of radiation and radiation with concurrent chemotherapy[a]*

| Study | Number of patients | | 5-year survival | | Significance |
|---|---|---|---|---|---|
| | RT | CMT | RT | CMT | |
| Russel, 1988 [161] | 69 | 75 | 6 | 12 | NS |
| Araujo et al., 1997 [10] | 31 | 28 | 6 | 16 | NS |
| Sischy et al., 1990 [172] | 62 | 65 | 9 | 15 | $p < 0.05$ |
| Earle et al., 1980 [55] | 37 | 40 | 12 | 11 | NS |
| Al-Sarraf et al., 1997 [6] | 60 | 69 | — | — | $p < 0.0001$ |

[a] RT, Radiation therapy; CMT, combined radiation and chemotherapy.

cer continue to require some form of palliation. In many patients, either the anatomic extent of tumor or coexisting medical problems will preclude surgical intervention. In others, refractory or recurrent disease will culminate in malignant dysphagia and its associated complications. Consequently, a variety of nonsurgical endoscopic methods have been developed to improve the quality of the patient's remaining life [200]. These are discussed in Chapter 4.

## Adenocarcinoma

### Demographics

Two decades ago adenocarcinoma of the esophagus was uncommon, with an age-adjusted incidence in the United States of 0.4 per 100,000. The incidence of adenocarcinoma has been rising steadily and it now accounts for at least half of all esophageal cancers in the United States [5, 21]. This seems to most closely follow the trend for the rising incidence of Barrett's esophagus found in 12% of patients who undergo endoscopy for gastroesophageal reflux disease. Two decades ago the mean age at diagnosis was 64 years, but is now most commonly seen in the sixth decade [22]. The disease exhibits a strong race and sex bias. Ninety percent of cases occur in men [22, 115, 211], and it is more common in whites.

There is a clear site preference for adenocarcinoma; 90% of cases affect the distal third of the esophagus, the disease is very uncommon in the upper two-thirds of the esophagus, and it is rare in the cervical esophagus [22, 33, 58, 81, 120]. Differentiation of primary esophageal adenocarcinoma in the distal esophagus from upward extension of gastric adeno-

carcinoma arising in the cardia may be difficult [174]. The gross characteristics of the tumor are similar to those of squamous cell carcinoma [128].

### Epidemiology and Etiology

It has been conjectured that primary esophageal adenocarcinoma arises from a number of sources: (a) from islands of heterotopic gastric mucosa or cardiac glands, (b) within esophageal glands scattered in the submucosa, or (c) within mucosa that undergoes glandular metaplasia following injury [11, 174]. A number of observations implicate Barrett's epithelium as the major precursor of adenocarcinoma of the esophagus (Fig. 12–9). Columnar-lined esophagus has been observed in 69% to 86% of patients with adenocarcinoma [72]. The areas adjacent to and remote from the invasive adenocarcinoma often exhibit a spectrum of abnormalities ranging from mild dysplasia to carcinoma-in-situ. Conversely, the overall prevalence of adenocarcinoma at the time of diagnosis of Barrett's esophagus is approximately 10% [31, 176]. Prospective evaluation has suggested that the incidence of adenocarcinoma in patients with Barrett's esophagus is 40 to 125 times that expected in the general population [31, 75]. Barrett's esophagus is discussed in Chapter 26.

In addition to classic Barrett's esophagus, there is a concern that patients with short-segment Barrett's may also be at risk. In combined data from the Cleveland Clinic and the University of Arizona it was suggested that the risk for adenocarcinoma was the same [139]. It has also been suggested that intestinal metaplasia occurring in the cardia is a

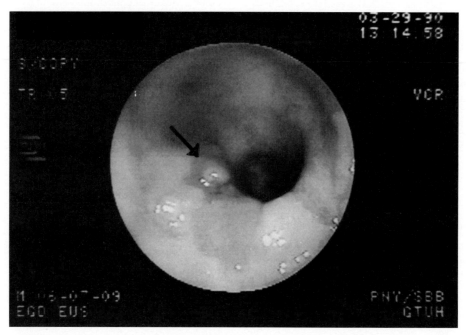

**FIG. 12–9.** Endoscopic view of a Barrett's epithelium. The nodule (*arrow*) represents carcinoma that has developed at the columnosquamous junction.

precursor to adenocarcinoma, just as intestinal metaplasia is a required precursor in the distal esophagus.

In pathologic specimens, areas of Barrett's adenocarcinoma are usually contiguous to areas of dysplasia, suggesting a linear progression from normal squamous mucosa to specialized intestinal metaplasia to dysplasia to carcinoma. Disturbances in gene expression probably mediate the individual transitions; as with squamous carcinoma, p53 overexpression, as well as $4N$ populations, increased aneuploidy, decreased apoptosis, and ultimately altered gene expression [164]. Whatever potential molecular markers may have for future diagnosis and treatment, they fall short today. For example, in the study by Schneider et al. only 46% of patients with Barrett's cancer had p53 mutations, so p53 alone cannot be used for screening [163].

### Natural History

The presentation of adenocarcinoma of the esophagus is similar to that of squamous cell carcinoma. Patients generally present with dysphagia, regurgitation, substernal chest pain, and weight loss, in decreasing order of frequency. It has been suggested that patients are less malnourished at the time of diagnosis in comparison to patients with squamous cell carcinoma. Medical history often suggests long-standing symptoms of gastroesophageal reflux [78]. Because the lesions occur most commonly in the distal esophagus, invasion into the tracheobronchial tree and the formation of esophago-airway fistulas are less frequently encountered. This is not to imply a better outcome, for adenocarcinoma appears to have a natural history and prognosis similar to those for squamous cell carcinoma [152, 191].

Early lymphatic spread is the rule. The prevalence of lymph node metastases in patients with adenocarcinoma of the distal esophagus and cardia was found to be 75% in parahiatal nodes, 66% in left gastric artery nodes, and 54% in splenic artery nodes [50]. As with squamous cell carcinoma, longitudinal spread is common and wide resection margins are important (e.g., paraesophageal nodes are involved in 20% of cases). Historically, overall 5-year survival rates are lower than 5% [33, 191], and patients with advanced disease who are deemed unresectable and treated with supportive care survive an average of 3 to 5 months [58, 191].

### Therapy

Most series on the treatment of esophageal cancer do not stratify patients based on histologic subtype. Consequently, it is difficult to know whether adenocarcinoma should be treated any differently from squamous cell carcinoma. Surgical resection is believed to offer the best chance of long-term survival. In one study of 69 patients, surgery was attempted in 24 patients (35%); of those, resection was possible in 11 (16% of all the patients, or 46% of those in whom surgery was attempted). The 5-year survival rate for those 11 patients was 18% [33]. Survival statistics for adeno-

carcinoma of the cardia or arising in Barrett's esophagus are similar to those for squamous cell carcinoma. Because of the patterns of local extension, surgical success appears dependent on near-total resection of the involved organ (whether esophagus or stomach) and with extensive resection of the adjacent normal structures [50].

Radiotherapy of adenocarcinoma appears to palliate symptoms effectively, but does not appear to prolong survival [33, 55, 58]. The median survival time for patients treated with palliative or radical radiotherapy was 6 to 12 months [33, 191]. More recent studies employing combined radiotherapy and chemotherapy (5-FU and mitomycin C) in more favorably staged patients showed a 2-year actuarial survival rate of 50%, not significantly different from that of squamous cell carcinoma [41].

Information regarding the effectiveness of chemotherapy in esophageal adenocarcinoma is sparse. No single chemotherapeutic agent appears to be best; however, resistance to chemotherapy may be related to expression of a multidrug resistance gene that acts as a drug efflux pump for a variety of antineoplastic agents [157]. Multimodality combination therapy appears to offer the best chance of improving survival. Among 21 patients with local or regional adenocarcinoma of the esophagus, gastroesophageal junction, or cardia who were treated with concurrent cisplatin, vinblastine, 5-FU, and radiotherapy prior to transhiatal esophagectomy, 56% were alive at 36 months after resection [60]. A study by Urba et al. was quoted in a previous section on preoperative concurrent chemotherapy and radiotherapy for squamous cell carcinoma [196]. The 3-year survival was 32% in the combined treatment group and 15% in the surgery-alone group. Seventy-five percent of those patients had adenocarcinoma. In a randomized control study of preoperative concurrent CMT in adenocarcinoma of the esophagus only reported by Walsh et al. the preoperative regime consisted of two courses of 5-FU and cisplatin and 40 Gy of radiotherapy followed by surgery [204]. The median survival in the combined arm was 16 months compared with 11 months for surgery along ($p = 0.001$). Twenty-five percent of patients assigned to the combined arm had a pathologic complete remission.

Palliative endoscopic approaches are similar to those described for squamous cell carcinoma. However, since they are always distal in the esophagus there are a few distinctions. These tumors generally damage the vagus nerve so that patients tend to have delayed gastric emptying in addition to swallowing problems. This means the potential for esophageal reflux is greater, particularly after a stent is placed. Since the placement of a prosthesis will generally cross the esophagogastric junction, there are some technical considerations and migration is more frequent.

## OTHER MALIGNANT TUMORS

### Adenoid Cystic Carcinoma

The prevalence of this tumor is approximately 1 in 10,000 esophageal tumors. It occurs most commonly in elderly men and its presentation and site preference are similar to those of squamous cell carcinoma [128]. It is usually located in the middle one-third of the esophagus. Although it shares histologic features with adenoid cystic carcinomas of the salivary gland, distant metastases dominate the clinical course, and the prognosis is poor [142].

**Sarcomas**

Sarcomas of the esophagus account for approximately 0.8% of all esophageal tumors [49]. Epidermoid carcinoma with spindle cell features is the more common variety and includes carcinosarcoma and pseudosarcoma. Clinical diagnosis is suggested by evidence of a large polypoid lesion within the esophagus. Differentiation between these two is impossible on clinical grounds. Histologically, the sarcomatous and carcinomatous areas intermingle in carcinosarcoma, whereas these areas are separate from, but adjacent to, one another in pseudosarcoma. Both the carcinomatous and sarcomatous elements of carcinosarcomas may metastasize, whereas usually only the carcinomatous elements of pseudosarcomas metastasize [58, 153]. Although the depth of invasion of carcinosarcomas remains limited despite their large size, 5-year survival rates are not convincingly better than with squamous cell carcinoma, probably because of the high rate of lymph node and hematogenous metastases [94].

Another type of esophageal sarcoma is true sarcoma arising from mesenchymal tissue. This group includes leiomyosarcomas, rhabdomyosarcomas, and fibrosarcomas. Leiomyosarcoma is the most common primary esophageal sarcoma [38, 62], reported at 0.5% of all esophageal malignancies. This lesion may be polypoid or infiltrating. Patients usually present with dysphagia of several years' duration,

which may be related to the slow growth of the tumor. The overlying mucosa is usually normal, but focal ulcerations may be found occasionally. Diagnosis is suspected by radiography, endoscopy, and EUS, but histologic examination is required to differentiate this from leiomyoma (Fig. 12–10). Although it has no preference for either sex, women appear to have a better prognosis. Surgical resection is the preferred therapy.

Kaposi's sarcoma of the esophagus was a rare disease until the emergence of the acquired immunodeficiency syndrome (AIDS) epidemic. Most commonly patients have numerous skin lesions and other foci in the digestive tract. The lesions are usually found incidentally, but rarely may present with bleeding or dysphagia. They have the typical red-purple raised endoscopic appearance. Endoscopic treatment with coagulation or injection or chemotherapy has been used.

**Lymphoma**

Despite its rarity, accurate diagnosis of primary esophageal lymphoma is important because it is potentially curable. In most patients, esophageal involvement by lymphoma is secondary. Malignant mediastinal lymph nodes may cause narrowing of the esophageal lumen by external compression or the esophageal wall may be invaded directly by tumor. About ten cases of isolated primary esophageal lymphoma have been published [184]. Retrosternal pain with consumption of alcohol (so-called Hoster's phenomenon) may occur in the presence of primary Hodgkin's disease of the esophagus; however, the nonspecificity of this symptom and the rarity of this lesion probably negate its clinical usefulness [177]. Primary histiocytic lymphoma of the esophagus also has been reported [17]. In otherwise healthy patients, long-

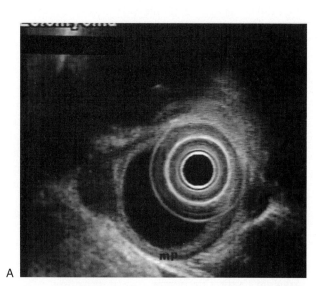
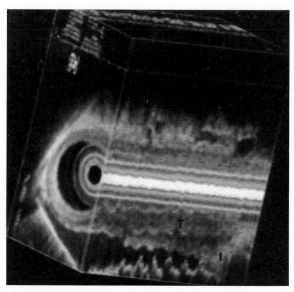

**FIG. 12–10. A:** Leiomyoma (*L*) seen by two-dimensional endoscopic ultrasound (EUS). **B:** Leiomyoma seen by a three-dimensional EUS cut into three Cartesian axes with intersection inside the tumor. *MP,* Muscularis propria.

term survival can be achieved with radiation and chemotherapy. The advent of AIDS has brought about an increase in the frequency of primary esophageal lymphoma [18]. The lesions may be seen as a mass or as an ulcer which can be indistinguishable from an infectious ulcer.

## Endocrine Cell Tumors (Apudomas)

Apudomas are rare in the esophagus (0.8% to 2.4% of malignant esophageal neoplasm). Primary small-cell (oat cell) carcinoma is the more common variety, and like oat cell carcinoma in the lung, rapid and widespread dissemination of malignancy is the rule; hence surgery is ineffective [136]. Despite responses to multidrug combination chemotherapy and radiotherapy, death results from distant metastases after a median survival time of 7.5 months [19, 30]. Malignant carcinoid is an even rarer apudoma variant. The tumor may be submucosal and exhibit metastases to regional lymph nodes. Argentaffin staining may be negative [128, 170].

## Primary Malignant Melanoma

Primary malignant melanoma, an extremely rare tumor, occurs primarily in older persons of either sex [128], accounting for only 0.1% of primary esophageal cancer [25, 30]. Neighboring melanosis or melanocytic dysplasia is generally required to distinguish it from metastatic disease. The lesions are usually polypoid, large, focally ulcerated, and mostly covered by intact squamous mucosa and occur in the lower esophagus. Tumor behavior is similar to melanomas elsewhere in the body; most patients die from distant metastases, and the 5-year survival rate is approximately 4% [71]. The most common presentation is with dysphagia, although occasionally hematemesis may occur. At the time of presentation, 40% of patients have already metastasized, primarily to regional lymph nodes, liver, lung, or bones.

## Adenosquamous Carcinoma

Adenosquamous carcinoma is a rare tumor that exhibits infiltrating elements of both adenocarcinoma and squamous carcinoma; however, these elements are not intimately mixed [58]. When mature squamous epithelium is present, it is termed an adenocanthoma [58, 152].

## Mucoepidermoid Carcinoma

Mucoepidermoid carcinoma is believed to be a rare variant of adenocarcinoma that may arise from the esophageal mucous glands. Mucus-secreting cells are seen within squamous cell carcinoma [58].

## Primary Esophageal Carcinoid Tumor

This is an extremely rare lesion with a variety of clinical features that mimic more common lesions [30, 170]. Histopathologic studies are required for confirmation, and this diagnosis is usually a surprise to the clinician.

## Metastatic Esophageal Tumors

Malignant tumors originating outside the gastrointestinal tract may metastasize to the digestive system. They usually present with signs of obstruction, and endoscopically a bulging mass is seen. Unless they break through the submucosa, bleeding is not a common problem. If the tumor is submucosal, the diagnosis will be missed if only overlying mucosa is biopsied.

Breast carcinoma metastasizes to the esophagus and usually is seen as a submucosal mass. The average interval between the primary diagnosis of breast cancer and metastasis is 8 years. Therapy should focus on radiation therapy or chemotherapy for the primary neoplasm. Endoscopic treatment for dysphagia may involve stent placement if the disease is circumferential. Dilation is usually not effective.

Lung cancer also may involve the esophagus by either metastasis or contiguous spread. Squamous cell carcinoma is the most common, followed by oat cell and large-cell carcinoma. Esophageal involvement may be discovered when the patient is asymptomatic or it may cause obstruction. It may also present as a tracheoesophageal fistula. If dysphagia is present, tumor ablation can be used, but it is more difficult than treating primary esophageal cancer. Because the involvement is often asymmetric, stenting is often not effective. Specialized stents with cuffs have been used, but they also tend to migrate. Often radiation or chemotherapy is employed. The risk of creating a fistula is higher than with primary esophageal cancer.

Malignant melanomas may also metastasize to the upper digestive tract. The stomach is the most common site, but they also spread to the esophagus. If the lesion is pigmented, it appears black endoscopically. Amelanotic melanomas may be indistinguishable from carcinoma or lymphoma. Biopsies are diagnostic. Bleeding or obstruction may be the presenting symptom. Prognosis is poor because the finding of this metastatic tumor implies dissemination. Survival beyond 1 year is uncommon. Treatment is seldom of benefit. There is a limited role of resection.

## Benign Tumors of the Esophagus

With some exceptions, benign tumors of the esophagus have similar natural histories. Usually, the neoplasms are asymptomatic and slow growing, with most cases discovered incidentally. In time, large or strategically located tumors may become symptomatic. Dysphagia is the most frequent presentation. Less common presenting symptoms include odynophagia, retrosternal pain, immediate postdeglutition regurgitation, anorexia, and weight loss. On rare occasions, respiratory complaints contribute to the presentation and include cough, dyspnea, sore throat, hiccups, or even recurrent pneumonia. Since these nonspecific symptoms are more commonly associated with esophageal malignancies, the diagnosis of a benign, treatable lesion is usually a delightful surprise [77, 147].

Benign esophageal lesions are often classified as either intramural-extramucosal or mucosal-intraluminal. This is a clinical classification based on the roentgenographic appearance of a barium-filled esophagus. An intramural-extramucosal tumor appears as a smooth, extrinsic mass projecting into the lumen from the esophageal wall, with relatively sharp angles. Mucosal-intraluminal lesions are less common and appear as smooth-filling defects within the esophageal lumen, commonly on a stalk.

## Intramural-Extramucosal Tumors

### Leiomyomas

Leiomyomas are the most common benign esophageal tumors, accounting for two-thirds of benign esophageal tumors and being reported in up to 5% of autopsy specimens [147, 166]. They usually affect the distal two-thirds of the esophagus [147], probably because the muscularis propria is comprised predominantly of smooth muscle in its distal third, skeletal muscle in its upper third, and a variable composition in the middle thrid. The tumor is most often single; however, multiple leiomyomas have been reported. As with leiomyomas elsewhere in the body, they may be oval to round and of variable size (3 to 8 cm in largest dimension). Mediastinal calcification may be present in a minority of patients [70]. By virtue of their intramural location, these tumors are usually covered by intact normal squamous mucosa. Unlike leiomyomas in the stomach, they rarely ulcerate, and bleeding is seldom encountered. Most leiomyomas are discovered incidentally on a barium esophagogram or endoscopy. However, patients with leiomyomas that do become symptomatic usually present with insidiously progressive dysphagia or retrosternal pain. Incidental asymptomatic lesions can be followed clinically, as the risk of malignant transformation is minimal. Surgical enucleation should be considered for symptomatic lesions, and esophageal resection with its higher morbidity and mortality is avoided whenever possible.

About 10% of reported leiomyomas require surgical removal. Enucleation is associated with a 1.8% mortality [147]. Snare and electrocautery techniques were not considered safe as nonsurgical therapy for submucosal tumors of the esophagus. A report by Eda and colleagues [56] indicated that submucosography (radiopaque contrast injected intramurally around the lesion) and EUS can determine the extent of the tumor in relation to the esophageal wall thickness. This precise determination may prevent complications of nonsurgical treatment (electrocautery alone or electrocautery and absolute alcohol injection). By EUS, leiomyoma appears as a hypoechoic mass arising from the fourth hypoechoic layer (muscularis propria) (see Fig. 12–12). An attempt has been made to differentiate leiomyosarcoma from leiomyoma

on the basis of size, shape, and sonographic appearance. However, EUS disclosed no unique feature that would permit an exact diagnosis, especially when the lesion is larger than 3 cm in diameter [212]. An EUS scoring system has been devised to help with that distinction. Five parameters are included: size over 30 mm, nodular shape, presence of an anechoic area, heterogeneous internal echo, and presence of an ulceration 0.5 mm deep. A score of three or more out of five suggests malignancy. The sensitivity is 100%. The specificity is 73%. Fibromas and hemangiomas are very rare and are also usually located within the musculature of the esophageal wall. Surgery is the therapy for leiomyoma whenever it is symptomatic or if there is a question of malignancy. Endoscopic resection is generally contraindicated, but may be attempted in the rare pedunculated leiomyoma.

### Esophageal Cysts

Esophageal cysts are congenital abnormalities, probably resulting from the sequestration of cell nests during the ingrowth of mesoderm that ordinarily separates the foregut from the lower respiratory tract during embryogenesis [134]. The sequestered cell nests develop into intramural cysts, are commonly lined by ciliated epithelium, and become filled with a thick, mucoid material. The majority of patients are asymptomatic or have nonspecific complaints. Symptoms may occur with increasing cyst size; however, a sudden onset of symptoms is usually secondary to acute inflammation or infection. Respiratory symptoms are more common in infants and children [147]. Endoscopic evaluation may enable one to make the diagnosis by demonstrating a blue, smooth, round shape beneath intact mucosa. Symptomatic cysts should be managed with surgical enucleation or excision when the patient's medical condition permits.

## Mucosal-Intraluminal Tumors

### Fibrovascular Polyps

Fibrovascular polyps are slow-growing benign tumors composed of various admixtures of fibrovascular tissue, adipose tissue, and myxoid or collagenous fibrous stoma and are covered by normal squamous epithelium. They almost always originate in the upper esophagus, are commonly asymptomatic for long periods of time, and may attain "giant" proportions (10 to 20 cm in length). Three-fourths of cases are described in elderly men. Since these tumors are usually on a stalk, they may be regurgitated into the hypophyarynx, where they can cause laryngeal obstruction and result in sudden death by asphyxiation. Therefore, definitive surgical excision should be considered in all patients [14]. Endoscopic neodymium–yttrium aluminum garnet laser ablation has been reported, but is potentially dangerous since the stalk may have a large vessel within it [133].

## Granular Cell Tumors

The histogenesis of granular cell tumors is unclear. Current opinion favors a neural origin, with Schwann cells being the most likely candidate. Nearly two-thirds of such tumors are located in the distal third of the esophagus. They may also be found in the tongue, skin, and breast. They are typically submucosal in location and are almost always benign, with exceptional cases exhibiting low-grade malignant potential. Endoscopically they appear as broad-based yellow or yellow-white tumors with intact overlying mucosa. Because they lie directly under a thin layer of squamous epithelium, endoscopic biopsies are usually diagnostic. Histologically they are characterized by large polygonal or fusiform cells, with eosinophilic cytoplasm arranged in compact nests. Immunohistochemically they stain positive with s-100, supporting the neural origin. Dysphagia is the most common symptom, chest pain is rare, and the majority of cases are asymptomatic. Since these lesions are slow growing and the malignant potential is very low, conservative management is indicated for asymptomatic lesions. Surgical excision is recommended for symptomatic lesions or when malignancy is suspected. Fewer than 30 malignant granular cell tumors have been reported. They are distinguishable by size (greater than 4 cm) and histologically by increased nuclear pleomorphism and mitotic activity.

## Inflammatory Pseudotumors

Inflammatory pseudotumors are composed of inflamed fibrous and granulation tissue and appear as localized, polypoid masses. Although nonneoplastic, the lesion is discussed here for the purpose of differential diagnosis. The histogenesis of these pseudotumors appears to be an overly exuberant reparative response to mucosal injury. The lesions appear histologically as proliferating fibrous tissue and reactive blood vessels accompanied by an inflammatory infiltrate. They are typically found in the middle and distal esophagus and have been associated with mucosal ulcers [118].

## Lymphangiomas

Lymphangioma are benign tumors that very rarely involve the esophagus. The tumor may be distinguished endoscopically from other benign lesions by its intraluminal location, cystic translucent appearance, and ease of compressibility with closed biopsy forceps. Histologic confirmation should be possible with endoscopic biopsy. Since malignant degeneration is not a feature of lymphangiomas in general, a conservative approach is usually warranted unless symptoms are problematic [26].

## Squamous Cell Papillomas

Squamous cell papillomas of the esophagus are rare benign tumors that have a pale, gray-white polypoid endoscopic appearance [190]. They may be single or multiple and vary in size. Endoscopic removal by snare polypectomy is usually adequate therapy [217]. The pathogenesis of esophageal squamous papilloma (ESP) is not known, but chronic mucosal irritation and infection with HPV are two proposed etiologies. Using DNA *in situ* hybridization techniques, Politoske [145] was able to identify the HPV in a patient with ESP. In one study, HPV type 16 was detected in 50% of the papillomas tested using the polymerase chain reaction technique. Patients with ESPs commonly had an associated chronic and often severe form or esophageal mucosal irritation such as esophagitis or Barrett's esophagus [140]. Although ESP is usually considered a benign lesion [151], malignant degeneration in large ESPs has been reported [198]. Recently, several other studies showed the presence of HPV in squamous carcinoma of the esophagus [35]. However, further studies of the relationship between HPV and malignant degenerated squamous papillomas and between HPV and esophageal cancer are needed.

## Lipomas

Lipomas may occur anywhere in the gastrointestinal tract, but they are rare in the esophagus. They usually originate in the submucosa and protrude into the lumen with increasing growth, often becoming pedunculated. They usually occur in the cervical esophagus and may become symptomatic when they are regurgitated into the hypopharynx, where asphyxiation may occur with laryngeal obstruction [4].

## REFERENCES

1. Ahsan H, Neugut A. Radiation therapy for breast cancer and increased risk for esophageal carcinoma. Ann Int Med 1988;128:114
2. Aikou T, Shimzu H. Difference in main lymphatic pathways from the lower esophagus and gastric cardia. Jpn J Surg 1989;19:290
3. Akiyama H, et al. Principles of surgical treatment for carcinoma of the esophagus. Analysis of lymph node involvement. Ann Surg 1981;194:438
4. Allen MS, Talbot WH. Sudden death due to regurgitation of a pedunculated esophageal lipoma. J Thorac Cardiovasc Surg 1967;65:756
5. Alpern HD, Buell C, Olson J. Increasing percentage of adenocarcinoma in primary carcinoma of the esophagus (letter) Am J Gastroenterol 1989;84:574
6. Al-Sarraf M, et al. Progress report of combined chemotherapy vs. radiotherapy in patients with esophageal cancer. J Clin Oncol 1997;15:277
7. Amer MH, et al. Water contamination and esophageal cancer at Gassim region, Saudi Arabia. Gastroenterology 1990;98:1141
8. American Society for Gastrointestinal Endoscopy. The role of endoscopy in the surveillance of premalignant conditions of the upper gastrointestinal tract (ASGE publication no. 1002). Gastrointest Endosc 1998;34:18S
9. Appelqvist P, Salmo M. Lye corrosion carcinoma of the esophagus: a review of 63 cases. Cancer 1980;45:2655
10. Araujo C, et al. A randomized trial comparing radiation therapy vs. radiation therapy plus chemotherapy in carcinoma of the esophagus. Cancer 1997;67:2258
11. Armstrong RA, Blalock JB, Carrera GM. Adenocarcinoma of the middle third of the esophagus arising from ectopic gastric mucosa. J Thorac Surg 1959;37:398
12. Arnott SJ, et al. The association of squamous esophageal cancer and thyroid disease. Br J Cancer 1971;25:33

13. Atabek U, et al. Impact of esophageal screening in patients with head and neck cancer. Am Surg 1990;56:289

14. Avezzano EA, et al. Giant fibrovascular polyps of the esophagus. Am J Gastroenterol 1990;85:299

15. Ban M, et al. Early detection of esophageal cancer in alcoholics. Endoscopy 1998 (in press)

16. Beahrs OH, et al, eds, Manual for Staging of Cancer (3rd ed). Philadelphia: Lippincott, 1988

17. Berman MD, et al. Primary histiocytic lymphoma of the esophagus. Dig Dis Sci 1979;24:883

18. Bernal A, delJunco GW. Endoscopic and pathologic features of esophageal lymphomas. Gastrointest Endosc 1986;32:96

19. Beyer KL, et al. Primary small-cell carcinoma of the esophagus. Report of 11 cases and review of the literature. J Clin Gastroenterol 1991;13:135

20. Blot WJ, Fraumeni JF Jr. Trends in esophageal cancer. Mortality among U.S. blacks and whites. Am J Public Health 1987;77:296

21. Blot W, Deversa S, Fraumeni J. Continuing climbing rates of esophageal adenocarcinoma. JAMA 1993;270:1320

22. Bosch A, Frias Z, Caldwell L. Adenocarcinoma of the esophagus. Cancer 1979;43:1557

23. Bosset J, Gignoux M, Triboulet J. Chemotheradiotherapy followed by surgery alone vs. surgery alone for squamous cell cancer of the esophagus. N Engl J Med 1997;337:161

24. Botet JF, et al. Preoperative staging of esophageal cancer: comparison of endoscopic US and dynamic CT. Radiology 1991;181:419

25. Boulafendis D, et al. Primary malignant melanoma of the esophagus in a young adult. Am J Gastroenterol 1985;80:417

26. Brady PG, Milligan FD. Lymphangioma of the esophagus—diagnosis by endoscopic biopsy. Dig Dis 1973;18:423

27. Brierly J and Oza A. Radiation and chemotherapy in the management of malignant esophageal structures. Gastrointest Endosc Clin N Am 1998;8:451

28. Brown LM, et al. Environmental factors and high risk of esophageal cancer among men in coastal South Carolina. J Natl Cancer Inst 1988;80:1620

29. Burrell RJW, Roach WA, Shadwell A. Oesophageal cancer in the Bantu of the Transkei associated with mineral deficiency in garden plants. J Natl Cancer Inst 1966;36:201

30. Caldwell CF, Bains MS, Burt M. Unusual malignant neoplasms of the esophagus. J Thorac Cardiovasc Surg 1991;101:100

31. Cameron AJ, Ott BJ, Payne WS. The incidence of adenocarcinoma in columnar-lined (Barrett's) esophagus. N Engl J Med 1985;313:857

32. Carter R, Brewer LA. Achalasia and esophageal carcinoma. Am J Med 1985;313:857

33. Cederqvist C, et al. Adenocarcinoma of the oesophagus. Acta Chir Scand 1980;146:411

34. Chalasani N, Wo J, Waring P. Racial differences in histology, location and risk factors of esophageal cancer. J Clin Gastroenterol 1998;26:11

35. Chang F, et al. Detection of human papillomavirus DNA in cytologic specimens derived from esophageal precancer lesions and cancer. Scand J Gastroenterol 1990;25:383

36. Chang-Claude JC, et al. An epidemiological study of precursor lesions of esophageal cancer among young persons in high-risk population in Huixian, China. Cancer Res 1990;50:2268

37. Chaves P, et al. p53 protein expression in esophageal squamous cell cancer. J Surg Oncol 1997;65:3

38. Choh JH, Khazei AH, Ihm HJ. Leiomyosarcoma of the esophagus: report of a case and review of the literature. J Surg Oncol 1986;32:223

39. Choi TK, et al. Bronchoscopy and carcinoma of the esophagus 1. Am J Surg 1984;147:757

40. Chuong JJH, DuBovik S, McCallum RW. Achalasia as a risk factor for esophageal carcinoma. Dig Dis Sci 1984;29:1105

41. Coia LR, Engstrom PF, Paul A. Nonsurgical management of esophageal cancer: report of a study of combined radiotherapy and chemotherapy. J Clin Oncol 1987;5:1783

42. Coutinho DS, et al. Granular cell tumors of the esophagus: a report of two cases and review of the literature. Am J Gastroenterol 1985;80:758

43. Crepsi M, et al. Oesophageal lesions in northern Iran: a premalignant condition? Lancet 1979;2:217

44. Crepsi M, et al. Precursor lesions of oesophageal cancer in a low-risk population in China: comparison with high-risk populations. Int J Cancer 1984;34:599

45. Cusso X, Mones-Xiol J, Vilardell F. Endoscopic cytology of cancer of the esophagus and cardia: a long-term evaluation. Gastrointest Endosc 1989;35:321

46. Dancygier H, Classen M. Endoscopic ultrasonography in esophageal diseases. Gastrointest Endosc 1989;35:220

47. Dawsey S, et al. Mucosal iodine staining improves endoscopic visualization of squamous dysplasia and squamous cell carcinoma of the esophagus in Linxian, China. Cancer 1998 (in press)

48. Day NE. The geographic pathology of cancer of the oesophagus. Br Med J 1984;40:329

49. DeMeester TR, Skinner DB. Polypoid sarcomas of the esophagus. Ann Thorac Surg 1975;20:405

50. DeMeester TR, Zaninotto G, Johansson K. Selective therapeutic approach to cancer of the lower esophagus and cardia. J Thorac Cardiovasc Surg 1988;95:42

51. DeStefani E, et al. Mate drinking, alcohol, tobacco, diet, and esophageal cancer in Uruguay. Cancer Res 1990;50:426

52. Dittler H, et al. Role of endoscopic ultrasonography in esophageal carcinoma. Endoscopy 1993;25:156

53. Earlam R, Cunha-Melo JR. Oesophageal squamous cell carcinoma: II. A critical review of radiotherapy. Br J Surg 1980;67:457

54. Earlam RJ, Johnson L. Oesophageal cancers: a surgeon uses radiotherapy. Ann R Coll Surg Engl 1990;72:32

55. Earle JD. A controlled evaluation of combined radiation and bleomycin therapy for squamous cell carcinoma of the esophagus. Int J Radiat Oncol Biol Phys 1980;6:821

56. Eda Y, et al. Endoscopic treatment for submucosal tumors of the esophagus: studies in 23 patients. Gastroenterol Jpn 1990;25:411

57. Elkon D, Lee M, Hendrickson FR. Carcinoma of the esophagus: sites of recurrence and palliative benefits after definitive radiotherapy. Int J Radiat Oncol Biol Phys 1978;4:615

58. Faintuch J, Shepard KV, Levin B. Adenocarcinoma and other unusual variants of esophageal cancer. Semin Oncol 1984;11:196

59. Flores AD, et al. Impact of new radiotherapy modalities on the surgical management of cancer of the esophagus and cardia. Int J Radiat Oncol Biol Phys 1989;17:937

60. Fok M, et al. Postoperative radiation therapy for carcinoma of the esophagus. Surgery 1991;113:138

61. Forastiere AA, et al. Concurrent chemotherapy and radiation therapy followed by transhiatal esophagectomy for local-regional cancer of the esophagus. J Clin Oncol 1990;8:119

62. Franklin GO, et al. Esophageal leiomyosarcoma. NY State J Med 1982;87:1100

63. Fraumeni JF Jr, Blot WJ. Geographic variation in esophageal cancer mortality in the United States. J Chronic Dis 1977;30:759

64. Galipeau P, et al. 17p (p53) allelic losses, 4N populations, and progression to aneuploidy in Varrett's esophagus. Proc Natl Acad Sci USA 1996;93:7081

65. George FW III. Radiation management in esophageal cancer. Am J Surg 1980;139:795

66. Ghadirin P, et al. Oesophageal cancer studies in the Caspian littoral of Iran: some residual results, including opium use as a risk factor. Int J Cancer 1985;35:593

67. Goldstein HM, Zonoza J. Association of squamous cell carcinoma of the head and neck with cancer of the esophagus. Am J Roentgenol 1978;131:791

68. Grimm H, et al. Endosonography to preoperative locoregional staging of esophageal and gastric cancer. Endoscopy 1993;25:224

69. Guo W, et al. Correlations of dietary intake and blood nutrient levels with esophageal cancer mortality in China. Nutr Cancer 1990;13:131

70. Gutman E. Posterior mediastinal calcification due to esophageal leiomyoma. Gastroenterology 1972;63:665

71. Guzman RP, et al. Primary malignant melanoma of the esophagus with diffuse melanocytic atypia and melanoma in situ. Am J Clin Pathol 1989;92:802

72. Haggitt RC, et al. Adenocarcinoma complicating columnar epithelium-lined (Barrett's) esophagus. Am J Clin Pathol 1978;70:1

73. Hale MJ, Liptz TR, Paterson AC. Association between human papillomavirus and carcinoma of the oesophagus in South African blacks. S Afr Med J 1989;76:329

74. Halvorsen RA, Thompson WM. Computed tomographic evaluation of esophageal carcinoma. Semin Oncol 1984;11:113

75. Hameeteman W, et al. Barrett's esophagus: development of dysplasia and adenocarcinoma. Gastroenterology 1989;96:1249

76. Harada W, Wiersema M, Wiersema L. Endosonography guided fine needle aspiration biopsy in the evaluation of lymphadenopathy. Gastrointest Endosc 1997;45:31

77. Harrington SW, Moersch HJ. Surgical treatment and clinical manifestations of benign tumors of the esophagus with report of seven cases. J Thorac Surg 1944;13:394

78. Hawe A, et al. Adenocarcinoma in the columnar epithelial lined lower (Barrett) oesophagus. Thorax 1973;28:511

79. Herskovic A, et al. Chemo-radiation with and without surgery in the thoracic esophagus: the Wayne State experience. Int J Radiat Oncol Biol Phys 1988;15:655

80. Herskovic A, Marty K, Al-Sarraf M. Combined chemotherapy and radiotherapy vs. radiotherapy alone in patient with cancer of the esophagus. N Engl J Med 1992;326:1593

81. Hesketh PJ, et al. The increasing frequency of adenocarcinoma of the esophagus. Cancer 1989;64:526

82. Heyder N, Lux G. Malignant lesions of the upper gastrointestinal tract. Scand J Gastroenterol Suppl 1986;123:47

83. Hilgenberg AD, et al. Preoperative chemotherapy, surgical resection, and selective postoperative therapy for squamous cell carcinoma of the esophagus. Ann Thorac Surg 1988;45:357

84. Hille JJ, et al. Human papillomavirus infection related to oesophageal carcinoma in black South Africans. S Afr Med J 1986;69:417

85. Hille, JJ, et al. Human papillomavirus and carcinoma of the esophagus (letter). N Engl J Med 1985;312:1707

86. Hordjik M, et al. Influence of tumor stenosis on T staging for esophageal cancer. Endoscopy 1993;25:171

87. Hori H, Kawano T, Endo M, Yuasa Y. Genetic polymorphisms of tobacco and alcohol related metabolizing enzymes and human esophageal squamous cell carcinoma susceptibility. T Clin Gastroenterol 1997;25:568

88. Horiuchi M, Makuuchi H, Machimura T. Survival benefit for screening for early esophageal carcinoma in head and neck patients. Digest Endosc 1998;10:110

89. Howel-Evans W, et al. Carcinoma of the oesophagus with keratosis palmaris et plantaris (tylosis). Q J Med 1958;27:413

90. Iizuka T, et al. Preoperative radioactive therapy for esophageal carcinoma. Chest 1988;93:1054

91. Iizuka T, et al. Parameters linked to ten-year survival in Japan of resected esophageal carcinoma. Chest 1989;96:1005

92. Isolauri J, Markkula H. Lye ingestion and carcinoma of the esophagus. Acta Chir Scand 1989;155:269

93. Isono K, et al. The treatment of lymph node metastasis from esophageal cancer by extensive lymphadenectomy. Jpn J Surg 1990;20:151

94. Iyomasa S, et al. Carcinosarcoma of the esophagus: a twenty-case study. Jpn J Clin Oncol 1990;20:99

95. Jacob P, et al. Natural history and significance of esophageal squamous cell dysplasia. Cancer 1990;65:2731

96. Jaskiewicz K, et al. Selenium and other mineral elements in populations at risk for esophageal cancer. Cancer 1988;62:2635

97. Kalantzis N, et al. EUS and CT in preoperative classification of esophageal cancer. Endoscopy 1992;24:653A

98. Kallimanis G, et al. Three dimensional ultrasound: a new technique for better diagnostic accuracy of endoscopic ultrasonography. Gastrointest Endosc 1993;39:252(A)

99. Kallimanis G, et al. Endoscopic ultrasound (EUS) for staging esophageal cancer with or without esophageal dilation—is clinically important—and safe. Gastroenterology 1994;104:A414

100. Kelsen D. Chemotherapy of esophageal cancer. Semin Oncol 1984;11:159

101. Kelsen D. Neoadjuvant therapy of esophageal cancer. Cancer Surg 1989;32:410

102. Kelsen D, et al. Cisplatin, vindesine, and bleomycin chemotherapy of local-regional and advanced esophageal carcinoma. Am J Med 1983;75:645

103. Kelsen DP, et al. Cisplatin, vindesine, and mitoguazone in the treatment of esophageal cancer. Cancer Treat Rep 1986;70:255

104. Kirvanta UK. Corrosion carcinoma of the esophagus: 381 cases of corrosion and nine cases of corrosion carcinoma. Acta Otolaryngol (Stockh) 1952;42:89

105. Kulski J, et al. Human papilloma virus DNA in oesophageal carcinoma (letter). Lancet 1986;2:683

106. Kuwano H, et al. Hypercalcemia related to the poor prognosis of patients with squamous cell carcinoma of the esophagus. J Surg Oncol 1989;42:229

107. Kuwano H, et al. Occurrence of esophageal carcinoma after gastrectomy. J Surg Oncol 1989;41:77

108. Lam K, et al. Presence of human papillomavirus in squamous cell cancer and its relation to p53 mutation. Hum Pathol 1997;28:657

109. Lanier AP, Kilkenny SJ, Wilson JF. Oesophageal cancer among Alaskan natives 1955–1981. Int J Epidemiol 1985;14:75

110. Lansing PB, Ferrante WA, Ochsner JL. Carcinoma of the esophagus at the site of lye stricture. Am J Surg 1989;118:108

111. La Vecchia C, et al. Tar yields of cigarettes and the risk of oesophageal cancer. Int J Cancer 1986;38:381

112. Lea JW, Prager RL, Bender HW. The questionable role of computed tomography in preoperative staging of esophageal cancer. Ann Thorac Surg 1984;38:479

113. Leichman L, et al. Combined preoperative chemotherapy and radiation therapy for cancer of the esophagus: the Wayne State University, Southwest Oncology Group and Radiation Therapy Oncology Group experience. Semin Oncol 1984;11:178

114. LePrise E, et al. A randomized study of radiation, chemotherapy, and surgery for localized squamous cell carcinoma. Cancer 1993;73:1779

115. Levi F, et al. The consumption of tobacco, alcohol and the risk of adenocarcinoma in Barrett's oesophagus. Int J Cancer 1990;45:852

116. Lightdale CJ, Winawer SJ. Screening diagnosis and staging of esophageal cancer. Semin Oncol 1984;11:101

117. Lightdale CJ, et al. Diagnosis of recurrent upper gastrointestinal cancer at the surgical anastomosis by endoscopic ultrasound. Gastrointest Endosc 1989;35:407

118. LiVolsi VA, Perzin KH. Inflammatory pseudotumors (inflammatory fibrous polyps) of the esophagus: a clinicopathologic study. Dig Dis 1975;20:475

119. Lu S, et al. Urinary excretion of N-nitrosamino acids and nitrate by inhabitants of high- and low-risk areas for esophageal cancer in northern China: endogenous formation of nitrosoproline and its inhibition by vitamin C. Cancer Res 1986;46:1485

120. Lund O, et al. Time-related changes in characteristics of prognostic significance in carcinomas of the oesophagus and cardia. Br J Surg 1989;76:1301

121. Lund O, et al. Risk stratification and long-term results after surgical treatment of carcinomas of the thoracic esophagus and cardia. J Thorac Cardiovasc Surg 1990;99:200

122. Lung M, et al. p53 mutational spectrum of esophageal carcinomas from 5 different locales in China. Cancer Epidemiol Biomarkers Prevention 1996;5:277

123. Mann NS, Sachdev AJ. Carcinoma of the esophagus and hypercalcemia. Am J Gastroenterol 1977;67:135

124. Markland CG, et al. The role of oesophageal carcinoma. Eur J Cardiothorac Surg 1989;3:33

125. Matsuda H, et al. Immunohistochemical evaluation of squamous cell carcinoma antigen and S-100 protein-positive cells in human malignant esophageal tissues. Cancer 1990;65:2261

126. Matsuda H, et al. Hyperthermo-chemo-radiotherapy as a definitive treatment for patients with early esophageal carcinoma. Am J Clin Oncol 1992;15:509

127. Miller B, et al. Human papillomavirus type 16 DNA in esophageal carcinomas from Alaskan natives. Int J Cancer 1997;71:218

128. Ming S. Tumors of the esophagus and stomach. In Atlas of Tumor Pathology. Washington, DC: Armed Forces Institute of Pathology, 1973:23

129. Misumi A, et al. Role of Lugol dye endoscopy in the diagnosis of early esophageal cancer. Endoscopy 1990;22:12

130. Mori S, et al. Preoperative assessment of resectability for carcinoma of the thoracic esophagus. Ann Surg 1979;190:100

131. Morris H, Price S. Langerhans' cells, papillomaviruses, and oesophageal carcinoma. S Afr Med J 1986;69:413

132. Nakachi K, et al. The joint effects of two factors in the aetiology of oesophageal cancer in Japan. J Epidemiol Community Health 1988;42:355

133. Naveau S, et al. Successful ablation of a large fibrovascular polyp of the esophagus by endoscopic Nd:YAG laser therapy. Gastrointest Endosc 1989;35:254

134. Nehme AE, Rbiah F. Ciliated epithelial esophageal cyst: case report and review of the literature. Am Surg 1977;43:114

135. Newaishy GA, et al. Results of radical radiotherapy of squamous cell carcinoma of the oesophagus. Clin Radiol 1982;33:347

136. Nichols GL, Kelsen DP. Small cell carcinoma of the esophagus. Cancer 1989;64:1531

137. Notani PN. Role of alcohol in cancers of the upper alimentary tract: use of models in risk assessment. J Epidemiol Community Health 1988;42:187

138. Nusheim KS, et al. Preoperative chemotherapy and radiotherapy for esophageal carcinoma. J Thorac Cardiovasc Surg 1982;103:887

139. O'Connor B, Falk G, Richter J. Risk of adenocarcinoma in long-segment and short-segment Barrett's esophagus. Gastroenterology 1998;114:A245

140. Ode R, et al. Esophageal squamous papillomas: a clinicopathologic study of 38 lesions and analysis for human papillomavirus by the polymerase chain reaction. Am J Surg Pathol 1993;17:803

141. Parker EF, et al. Chemotherapy, radiation therapy, and resection for carcinoma of the esophagus. J Thorac Cardiovasc Surg 1989;98:1037

142. Petursson SR. Adenoid cystic carcinoma of the esophagus. Cancer 1986;57:1464

143. Peyman MA. Achalasia of cardia, carcinoma of oesophagus and hypertrophic pulmonary osteoarthropathy. Br Med J 1959;1:23

144. Picus D, et al. Computed tomography in the staging of esophageal carcinoma. Radiology 1983;146:433

145. Politoske E. Squamous papilloma of the esophagus associated with the human papillomavirus. Gastroenterology 1992;102:668

146. Poplin E, et al. Combined therapies for squamous cell carcinoma of the esophagus, a Southwest Oncology Group study (SWOG-8037). J Clin Oncol 1987;5:622

147. Postlethwait RW. Benign tumors and cysts of the esophagus. Surg Clin North Am 1983;63:925

148. Pottern LM, et al. Esophageal cancer among black men in Washington, DC. I. Alcohol, tobacco, and other risk factors. J Natl Cancer Inst 1981;67:777

149. Puhakka HJ, Aitsalo K. Oesophageal carcinoma: endoscopic and clinical findings in 258 patients. J Laryngol Otol 1988;102:1137

150. Quint LE, Francis IR, Glazer M. Computed tomography and magnetic resonance imaging. In Margulis AR, Burhenne HJ, eds, Alimentary Tract Radiology (4th ed). St. Louis: Mosby, 1989:501

151. Quitadamo M, Benson J. Squamous papilloma of the esophagus: a case report and review of the literature. Am J Gastroenterol 1988;83:194

152. Raphael HA, Ellis FH Jr, Dockerty MB. Primary adenocarcinoma of the esophagus: 18-year review and review of literature. Ann Surg 1966;164:785

153. Razzuk MA, et al. Pseudosarcoma of the esophagus. J Thorac Cardiovasc Surg 1971;61:650

154. Ribeiro U, Pusner M, Safatle A, and Reynolds J. Risk factors for squamous cell carcinoma of the esophagus. Brit J Surg 1996;83:1174

155. Rice TW. Esophageal ultrasound in the preoperative staging of esophageal carcinoma. Cleveland Clinic Experience. Presented at Endoscopic Ultrasonography: A Tutorial, Cleveland, OH, March 21–22, 1991

156. Rice TW, Boyce GA, Sivak MV. Esophageal ultrasound and the preoperative staging of carcinoma of the esophagus. J Thorac Cardiovasc Surg 1991;101:536

157. Robey-Cafferty SS, Rutledge ML, Bruner JM. Expression of a multidrug resistance gene in esophageal adenocarcinoma. Am J Clin Pathol 1990;93:1

158. Roth JA, et al. Randomized clinical trial of preoperative and postoperative adjuvant chemotherapy with cisplatin, vindesine, and bleomycin for carcinoma of the esophagus. J Thorac Cardiovasc Surg 1988;96:242

159. Roth M, et al. Cytologic detection of esophageal squamous cell carcinoma using balloon cytology and sponge samplers in asymptomatic adults in Linxian, China. Cancer 1997;80:2047

160. Roth M, Strickland K, Wang G, Rothman M, Greenberg A, and Dawsey J. High levels of carcinogenic polycyclic aromatic hydrocarbons within food from Linxian, China. Eur J Cancer 1998;1:2449

161. Russel A, et al. Controlled clinical trial for the treatment of patients with inoperable esophageal cancer. Recent Results Cancer Res 1988;110:21

162. Safattle-Ribeiro A, Ribeiro V, Sakai P, et al. Integrated p53 histopathologic/genetic examination of premalignant lesions of the esophagus and stomach. Gastroenterology 1997;112:4016A

163. Schneider P, et al. Mutations of p53 in Barrett's esophagus and Barrett's cancer. J Thorac Cardiovasc Surg 1996;111:323

164. Schwindt WD, Bernhardt LC, Johnson SAM. Tylosis and intrathoracic neoplasms. Chest 1970;57:590

165. Selby WS, Gallagher ND. Malignancy in a 19-year experience of adult celiac disease. Dig Dis Sci 1979;24:684

166. Seremetis MG, et al. Leiomyomata of the esophagus. An analysis of 838 cases. Cancer 1976;38:2166

167. Shao L, et al. Results of surgical treatment in 6,123 cases of carcinoma of the esophagus and gastric cardia. J Surg Oncol 1989;42:170

168. Shiizu T, et al. Radiation-induced esophageal cancer: a case report and a review of the literature. Jpn J Surg 1990;20:97

169. Shine I, Allison PR. Carcinoma of the oesophagus with tylosis (keratosis palmaris et plantaris). Lancet 1966;1:951

170. Siegal A, Swarts A. Malignant carcinoid of oesophagus. Histopathology 1986;10:761

171. Silverberg E, Boring CC, Squires TS. Cancer statistics 1990. CA Cancer J Clinicians 1990;40:9

172. Sischy B, et al. Interim report of EST phase III protocol for evaluation of combined modalities for esophageal cancer. Prog Am Soc Clin Oncol 1990;105

173. Skinner DB, Dowlatshahi KD, DeMeester TR. Potentially curable cancer of the esophagus. Cancer 1982;50:2571

174. Smithers DW. Adenocarcinoma of the oesophagus. Thorax 1958;11:257

175. Sobin LH, Hermanek P, Hutter RV. TNM classification of malignant tumors. Cancer 1988;61:2310

176. Spechler SJ, et al. Adenocarcinoma and Barrett's esophagus—an overrated risk? Gastroenterology 1984;87:927

177. Stein HA, Murray D, Warner HA. Primary Hodgkin's disease of the esophagus. Dig Dis Sci 1981;26:457

178. Strader D, et al. Early detection of esophageal cancer/dysplasia in a high risk population via chromoscopy. Gastrointest Endosc 1997;45:A239

179. Sugimachi K, et al. Survival rates of women with carcinoma of the esophagus exceed those of men. Surg Gynecol Obstet 1987;164:541

180. Sugimachi K, et al. Endoscopic ultrasonographic detection of carcinomatous invasion and of lymph nodes in the thoracic esophagus. Surgery 1990;107:366

181. Suzuk L, Noffsinger A, Hui Y, Fenoglio C. Detection of human papillomavirus in esophageal squamous cell carcinoma. Cancer 1996;78:704

182. Syldesley WR. Oral leukoplakia associated with tylosis and esophageal carcinoma. J Oral Pathol 1974;3:62

183. Syrjanen KJ. Histological changes identical to those of condylomatous lesions found in esophageal squamous cell carcinomas. Arch Geschwulstforsch 1982;52:283

184. Taal BG, Van Heerde P, Somers R. Isolated primary esophageal involvement in lymphoma. Gut 1993;34:994

185. Takemoto T, et al. Endoscopic ultrasonography in the diagnosis of esophageal carcinoma with particular regard to staging it for operability. Endoscopy 1986;18(suppl 3):22

186. Teniere P, Hay J, Fingerhut A, Fagniez P. Postoperative radiation therapy does not increase survival after curative resection for squamous cell carcinoma of the esophagus. Surg Gynecol Obstet 1991;173

187. Tio TL, et al. Endosonography and computed tomography of esophageal carcinoma. Gastroenterology 1989;96:1478

188. Tio TL, et al. Esophagogastric carcinoma: preoperative TNM classification with endosonography. Radiology 1989;173:411

189. Tio TL, et al. High frequency balloon catheter ultrasound following chromoendoscopy in assessing esophageal dysplasia and cancer. Gastrointest Endosc 1997;45:635

190. Toet AE, et al. Squamous cell papilloma of the esophagus: report of four cases. Gastrointest Endosc 1985;31:77

191. Turnbull ADM, Goodner JT. Primary adenocarcinoma of the esophagus. Cancer 1968;22:915

192. Tuyns AJ, Pequinot G, Abbatucci JS. Le cancer de l'oseophage en Ille-et-Vilaine en fonction des niveaux de consommation d'alcool et de tabac. Des risques qui se multiplient. Bull Cancer 1977;65:45

193. Uchino S, et al. Prognostic significance of p53 mutation histopathologic/genetic examination of premalignant lesions of the esophagus and stomach. Gastroenterology 1997;112:4016A

194. Ueo H, Sugimachi K. Preoperative hyperthermo-chemoradiotherapy for patients with esophageal carcinoma or rectal carcinoma. Semin Surg Oncol 1990;6:8

195. Ullal SR. Hypertrophic osteoarthropathy and leiomyoma of the esophagus. Am J Surg 1972;123:356
196. Urba S, et al. A randomized trial comparing transhiatal esophagectomy to preoperative concurrent chemoradiation followed by esophagectomy in loco regional esophageal cancer. Proc Am Soc Clin Oncol 1995;14:194
197. Utsumi Y, et al. Role of estrogen receptors in the growth of human esophageal carcinoma. Cancer 1989;64:1189
198. Van Cutsem E, et al. Squamous papillomatosis of the oesophagus with malignant degeneration and demonstration of the human papilloma virus. Eur J Gastroenterol Hepatol 1991;3:561
199. Van Dam J, et al. High grade malignant stricture is predictive of esophageal tumor stage. Cancer 1993;71:2190
200. van Den Brandt-Gradel V, den Hartog Jager FCA, Tytgat GNJ. Palliative intubation of malignant esophagogastric obstruction. J Clin Gastroenterol 1987;9:290
201. Vassallo A, et al. Esophageal cancer in Uruguay: a case–control study. J Natl Cancer Inst 1985;75:1005
202. Vilgrain V, et al. Staging of esophageal carcinoma: comparison of results with endoscopic sonography and CT. Am J Roentgenol 1990;155:277
203. Wahrendorf J, et al. Precursor lesions of oesophageal cancer in young people in a high-risk population in China. Lancet 1989;2:1239
204. Walsh T, et al. A comparison of multimodality therapy and surgery for esophageal adenocarcinoma. N Engl J Med 1996;335:462
205. Wang L, Zhou Q, Hong J, Qui S, Yang C. p53 protein accumulation and gene mutations in a high incidence area of esophageal carcinoma in Henan, China. Cancer 1996;77:1244
206. Watt I, et al. Laparoscopy, ultrasound and computed tomography in cancer of the oesophagus and gastric cardia: a prospective comparison for detecting intraabdominal metastases. Br J Surg 1989;76:1036
207. Wychulis AR, et al. Achalasia and carcinoma of the esophagus JAMA 1971;215:1638
208. Wynder EL, et al. Environmental factors in cancer of the upper alimentary tract. Cancer 1957;10:470
209. Yang CS. Research on esophageal cancer in China: a review. Cancer Res 1980;40:2633
210. Yang CS, et al. Vitamin A and other deficiencies in Linxian a high esophageal cancer incidence area in northern China. J Natl Cancer Inst 1984;73:1449
211. Yang PC, Davis S. Incidence of cancer of the esophagus in the U.S. by histologic type. Cancer 1988;61:612
212. Yasuda K, Nakajima M, Kawai K. Endoscopic ultrasonographic imaging of submucosal lesions of the upper gastrointestinal tract. Gastrointest Endosc Clin North Am 1992;2:318
213. Ying-k'ai W, Kuo-chun H. Chinese experience in the surgical treatment of carcinoma of the esophagus. Ann Surg 1979;190:361
214. Ying-k'ai W, et al. Surgical treatment of esophageal carcinoma. Am J Surg 1980;130\9:805
215. Yu MC, et al. Tobacco, alcohol, diet, occupation, and carcinoma of the esophagus. Cancer Res 1988;48:3843
216. Zaridze DG, et al. Survey of a population with a high incidence of oral and oesophageal cancer. Int J Cancer 1985;36:153
217. Zeabart LE, Fabian J, Nord HJ. Squamous papilloma of the esophagus—a report of three cases. Gastrointest Endosc 1979;25:18
218. Ziegler RG. Alcohol–nutrient interactions in cancer etiology. Cancer 1986;58:1942
219. Ziegler RG, et al. Esophageal cancer among black men in Washington, DC: II Role of nutrition. J Natl Cancer Inst 1981;67:1199
220. Zieren H, Muller J, Jacobi C. Adjuvant postoperative radiation therapy after curative resection for squamous cell carcinoma of the esophagus. World J Surg 1995;19:444

The Esophagus, Third Edition,
edited by D. O. Castell and J. E. Richter.
Lippincott Williams & Wilkins, Philadelphia © 1999.

CHAPTER 13

# Surgical Therapy for Cancer of the Esophagus and Cardia

Jeffrey H. Peters and Tom R. DeMeester

The diagnosis of esophageal cancer is a devastating event for an individual. The American Cancer Society estimates that 12,300 new cases of esophageal cancer and 11,900 deaths from the disease will occur in 1998 [64]. Clearly, cure is a challenge. The clinician has two options: the first is to assume that most, if not all, esophageal tumors extending beyond the mucosa are systemic at the time of diagnosis, and thus palliation is the mainstay of therapy; the second is to select treatment with curative intent, recognizing that long-term survival will occur in the minority of patients. Increasing evidence suggests that cure is possible.

## EPIDEMIOLOGY OF ESOPHAGEAL CARCINOMA

In most Western countries, esophageal cancer was historically a disease of black men with long-standing tobacco and alcohol abuse. Histologically, nearly all were squamous cell carcinomas. Worldwide squamous cell carcinoma still accounts for the majority of esophageal carcinomas. Its incidence is highly variable, ranging from approximately 20 per 100,000 in the United States and Britain to 160 per 100,000 in certain parts of South Africa and the Honan province of China, and even 540 per 100,000 in the Guriev district of Kazakhstan. The environmental factors responsible for these localized high-incidence areas of squamous cell esophageal cancer have not been conclusively identified, though additives to local foodstuffs (nitroso compounds in pickled vegetables and smoked meats) and deficiencies (zinc and molybdenum) have been suggested.

Over the past several decades, a dramatic epidemiologic shift has occurred such that adenocarcinoma of the esophagus, once an unusual malignancy, now accounts for the majority of esophageal cancer in most Western countries (Fig. 13–1) [17, 92]. In contrast to squamous cell carcinoma, esophageal adenocarcinoma is a disease of white men in the sixth and seventh decades of life with gastroesophageal reflux disease. Men outnumber women 7 to 1 [8, 134], and whites outnumber blacks 20 to 1 [19, 103, 128]. Although smoking has been strongly implicated in the development of esophageal squamous cell cancer [77, 133], it is only weakly associated with the development of esophageal adenocarcinoma [135]. Alcohol appears not to be a significant factor [43].

The most significant risk factor is the presence of Barrett's esophagus [22, 105]. Barrett's esophagus represents metaplastic transformation of the squamous mucosa of the lower esophagus to intestinal-type columnar epithelium. It is an acquired condition secondary to the effects of chronic gastroesophageal reflux. Ten percent of patients with Barrett's esophagus will present with an esophageal adenocarcinoma [105]. Prospective studies suggest that in a cohort of patients with Barrett's esophagus approximately 1% per year will develop adenocarcinoma [52, 68, 107, 132].

A clear metaplasia–dysplasia–carcinoma sequence has been shown. Dysplasia is commonly found adjunct to areas of nondysplastic Barrett's, and high-grade dysplasia can be found adjacent to most adenocarcinomas of the esophagus [21, 73]. Prospective studies have documented the progression from nondysplastic Barrett's to low- and high-grade dysplasia and ultimately carcinoma in individual patients [52, 68]. In one of the few analyses of the direct clonal relationship between metaplasia, dysplasia, and carcinoma, Zhuang et al. studied APC gene alteration in patients with Barrett's esophagus [136]. Twelve specimens containing areas of normal epithelium, Barrett's metaplasia, dysplasia, and invasive adenocarcinoma were selected and deletion of the APC gene identified. The APC locus was deleted in five

---

J. H. Peters: Department of Surgery, University of Southern California School of Medicine, Section of General Surgery, University of Southern California University Hospital, and University of Southern California Healthcare Consultation Center, Los Angeles, California 90033.

T. R. DeMeester: Department of Surgery, University of Southern California Medical Center, Los Angeles, California 90033.

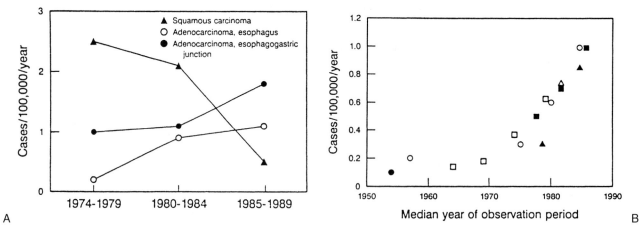

**FIG. 13–1. A:** Incidence of different types of esophageal cancer in Olmsted County, MN from 1974 to 1989. **B:** The incidence of adenocarcinoma of the esophagus in population-based studies: (●) Olmsted County, (○) Connecticut Cancer Registry, (■) National Cancer Institute Surveillance Epidemiology, and End Results Program, approximately 10% of the U.S. population, (□) Birmingham England, (▲) Canton Vaud, Switzerland. (From ref. 92, with permission.)

patients, two of which were female. In all five patients with loss of heterozygosity at the APC gene locus, the same allele was inactivated in the invasive carcinoma and dysplasia specimens. Further, LOH of the APC gene was present in Barrett's metaplasia adjacent to the dysplasia in two of the five patients. X-chromosome inactivation and clonal analysis from these two women showed that the inactivation was from the same clone of cells as the metaplastic, dysplastic, and carcinoma sections and all contained inactivation of the same allele.

## CLINICAL MANIFESTATIONS

Dysphagia and weight loss are by far the most common symptoms at the time of diagnosis. The complaint of dysphagia in patients older than 45 years should be investigated thoroughly since carcinoma is the most common cause of dysphagia in this age group. In a few patients, dysphagia does not occur and symptoms arise from invasion of the primary tumor into adjacent structures or from its metastasis. Extension of the primary tumor into the tracheobronchial tree can cause stridor, and if a tracheoesophageal fistula develops, coughing, choking, and aspiration pneumonia result. Severe bleeding from erosion into the aorta or pulmonary vessels occurs on rare occasions. Vocal cord paralysis may result from the invasion of either recurrent laryngeal nerve. Metastases are usually manifested by jaundice or bone pain.

Unfortunately, dysphagia usually presents late in the natural history of the disease because the lack of a serosal layer to the esophagus allows the smooth muscle to dilate with ease. As a result, the dysphagia becomes severe enough to motivate the patient to seek medical advice only when more than 60% of the esophageal circumference is infiltrated with cancer and the lumen is reduced to less than 12 mm in diameter. Due to this insidious onset, the disease is usually ad-

vanced at the time of diagnosis. Tracheoesophageal fistulas occur in up to 10% of patients on their first visit to the hospital, and greater than 40% will have evidence of distant metastases or recurrent nerve paralysis. With tumors of the cardia, anorexia and weight loss usually precede the onset of dysphagia.

## HISTORY OF SURGICAL TREATMENT OF ESOPHAGEAL CANCER

Carcinoma of the thoracic esophagus was well described by the early 19th century, but the thought of a transthoracic operation for its removal was stifled for several reasons. First, battle injuries had repeatedly demonstrated the lethal effects that ensued when a gaping hole in the chest resulted in collapse of the lung. As a consequence, surgeons feared to enter the pleural cavity. It was not until the early part of the 20th century that this fear was dispelled by an understanding of how lung expansion could be maintained with an open chest [74]. Second, surgeons observed that tugging or pinching the vagus nerve in the neck was promptly followed by slowing of the pulse and, in some situations, cardiac arrest. This was known as ''vagal collapse'' and gave rise to the fear that division of both vagi above the heart would cause instantaneous death [124]. The third observation was that patients who had escaped death from either injury to the vagi or the consequences of an open chest died from disruption of the esophageal anastomosis and subsequent infection of the pleural cavity. This gave rise to the concern that an intrathoracic anastomosis to any part of the esophagus was a potential source of great danger.

The first successful resection of a carcinoma of the thoracic esophagus was performed by Franz Torek [124]. General anesthesia was administered by a new technique: the tracheal insufflation of ether. The existing technique of a differential pressure chamber could not be used because the rubber cuff placed around the patient's neck used to create a subatmospheric pressure about the body precluded the planned construction of a cervical esophagostomy. Torek avoided injury to the vagi and the possibility of sudden death by carefully dissecting them off the esophagus. Pleural infection from an esophageal leak was circumvented by carefully closing the cardia and performing a cervical esophagostomy, thereby avoiding an intrathoracic anastomosis.

Torek's patient recovered and survived for another 13 years with continuity between the cervical esophagostomy and gastrostomy established via an external "rubber tube." This allowed the patient to swallow all varieties of food provided it was chewed into an almost liquid state. The successful establishment of normal alimentation via an esophagogastrostomy after an esophagectomy remained an unattainable goal until the report of Ohsawa in 1933 on successful resection with esophagogastrostomy in eight patients with carcinoma of the lower esophagus and cardia [82]. Marshall reported a similar procedure in one patient in 1938 [72]. No follow-up is available on Ohsawa's patients. Marshall's patient was reported to be plagued by persistent esophageal obstruction and esophagitis, which required repetitive dilation.

Adams and Phemister, from the University of Chicago, also realized the difficulty in constructing a dependable intrathoracic esophagogastric anastomosis and took the project to the laboratory. Only after a high degree of success was attained in dogs was a similar procedure applied to a patient with carcinoma of the thoracic esophagus. Their report, presented on April 5, 1938, before the Twenty-First Annual Meeting of the American Association for Thoracic Surgery in Atlanta, popularized the one-stage resection of thoracic esophageal cancer and intrathoracic esophagogastrostomy [1]. Despite the great strides made by these early pioneers, many of the problems they faced continue to plague today's esophageal surgeon. True, the fear of the "dreaded vagus collapse" has been overcome and the mortality associated with leakage and infection has been dramatically reduced. However, subsequent experience has shown that an intrathoracic anastomosis, as with Marshall's patient, is plagued with reflux, persistent esophagitis, and stricture.

The technique of standard esophagectomy was influenced by the publications of Sweet [116], Lewis [69], and Belsey [15]. Sweet advocated the left posterolateral thoracotomy approach for tumors of the lower esophagus, but this approach was not satisfactory when the malignancy extended cephalad and required division of the esophagus above the aortic arch. In such situations, the esophagus must be dissected out from behind the aortic arch and subclavian artery, and an esophagogastric anastomosis performed in the apex of the left chest. The anastomosis is technically demanding. Lewis performed the operation through separate upper midline abdominal and right thoracotomy incisions. This provided excellent visibility for both the abdominal and thoracic

portion, of the operation and the best exposure for performing a high intrathoracic anastomosis. He advocated two separate operations at the same sitting, with the closure of the abdominal incision and repositioning of the patient prior to performing the thoracic portion. Fisher et al. [37] modified Lewis's approach so that the abdominal and thoracic portions of the operation can be performed at the same time. The thoracic approach is through a right anterolateral incision in the third intercostal space, instead of the standard posterolateral incision. This approach allowed for both a laparotomy and a thoracotomy to be performed without repositioning or excessive twisting of the patient. It gave good exposure for performing an anastomosis high within the chest, but makes dissection of the lower third of the esophagus somewhat difficult. Belsey and Hiebert [15] reported on a technique by which the stomach is brought up through the esophageal hiatus from the right chest without using an abdominal incision. The gastric vessels are ligated sequentially as the stomach is pulled up through the hiatus. The drawback of this approach is that it did not allow for an adequate dissection of the abdominal lymph nodes.

Transhiatal esophagectomy was introduced by Turner [126], a British surgeon, in 1927. Its use was short-lived after general endotracheal anesthesia became popular and a transthoracic esophagectomy was feasible [118]. Transhiatal esophagectomy was repopularized in 1984 by Orringer [83, 84] for the resection of esophageal neoplasms. Based on his experience, there are few indications for opening the thorax in patients requiring an esophageal resection for malignant disease. In 1963 Logan [71] reported his experience with en bloc resection for carcinoma of the cardia and lower third of the esophagus. He thought that neglecting the principles of an en bloc resection meant being resigned to doing the same operation under direct vision. Employing the en bloc technique, Logan reported a 16% 5-year survival, which was better than other results reported at that time. Logan's operation was not widely adopted, partly because of the associated 21% operative mortality. Since that time, improvements have been made in the perioperative management of patients following major operations, so that more reasonable operative mortality rates can be anticipated. Akiyama et al. [5] in 1981 and Skinner [111] in 1983 revitalized interest in the en bloc resection for neoplasms of the esophagus and cardia. They were able to reduce the operative mortality to 1.4% and 11%, respectively, and Skinner reported a 33% 3-year survival for carcinoma of the lower esophagus and cardia. Logan, Akiyama, and Skinner all used the stomach to reestablish gastrointestinal continuity. For carcinomas of the lower esophagus and cardia, this represented the closest margin to the tumor and a potential weakness of the en bloc resection. After gaining experience with the techniques of Logan, Akiyama, and Skinner, DeMeester et al. further modified the en bloc approach to comply more faithfully with the principles of an en bloc resection [31]. This included (a) an operative approach to the patient to maximize operative exposure while at the same time allowing intraoperative staging of the tumor, so that the benefits of the curative resection were only applied to those who had favorable pathology, and (b) using the colon to reestablish gastrointestinal continuity in order to allow for a larger gastric resection.

## STAGING

Classification of tumors in the thoracic esophagus usually is not clinically possible and currently is based on imaging techniques. In our experience, computed tomographic (CT) scans are of little value in the staging of small tumors of the thoracic esophagus or cardia, and usually confirm clinical findings when extensive disease is present. Their usefulness in the evaluation of tumors of the cervical esophagus is no more than that of a clinical examination [33, 96, 97]. The technology of nuclear magnetic resonance imaging (MRI) so far has not been shown to be superior to CT scans for the classification of esophageal carcinomas [98].

In an analysis of 58 patients with early disease who underwent a potentially curative en bloc resection, only lymph node metastasis and tumor penetration of the esophageal wall had a significant and independent influence on prognosis [112]. Other factors such as tumor size, cell type, degree of cellular differentiation, and location of the tumor within the esophagus had no effect on survival of patients with resectable tumors. This indicated that resectable esophageal tumors which met the criteria of no wall penetration and/or no lymph node metastases could be defined as potentially curable regardless of their size, histologic grade, cell type, and location. The problem is how to determine accurately the extent of the disease before surgery.

### Current Staging Classifications

The current TNM (tumor, node, distant metastasis) staging classification of esophageal carcinoma has been challenged as inadequate. Most surgeons agreed that the 1983 TMN system left much to be desired. The third edition of

the manual for staging of cancer of the American Joint Committee on Cancer, published in 1988, attempted to provide a finer discrimination between stages than did the previous edition of 1983. Table 13–1 shows the definitions for the primary tumor, regional lymph nodes, and distant metastases as listed in the 1988 manual. Recently, Ellis et al., in a study comparing different staging criteria, showed that the new staging criteria of the American Joint Committee provided no better discrimination of the stages according to survival than did the earlier version [35]. The 5-year survival of stage IIA patients was similar to that of stage IIB patients, and the survival of stage IIB patients was similar to that of stage III patients. Similarly, they showed that there was no difference between the 5-year survival rates of patients with T1 and T2 disease; nor was there a difference between those with T3 and T4 disease. They did confirm the observation that the depth of wall penetration and extent of lymph node involvement were reliable independent predictors of survival.

Based upon survival analysis indicating tumor penetration and lymph node metastases as the major prognostic factors, the WNM (wall penetration, node, and distant metastasis) system for staging was developed by Skinner et al. [112]. The WNM system differs somewhat from the previous efforts to develop satisfactory staging criteria for carcinoma of the esophagus. Ellis et al. proposed the adoption of Skinner's WNM staging system with some modifications (Table 13–2). In the latter proposal, tumors limited to above the muscularis mucosa would be equivalent to Skinner's W0 designation, T1 and T2 tumors would equate to the W1 classification, and T3 and T4 tumors to the W2 classification. These classifications are illustrated in Fig. 13–2. Ellis et al. further reported a clear distinction between the 5-year survival of patients with negative nodes and those with fewer than five nodes involved, and a highly significant difference between the latter group and those with five or more nodes involved. Table 13–2 shows the definitions for the primary tumor,

**TABLE 13–1.** *Staging of cancer of the esophagus and cardia: American Joint Committee on Cancer 1988[a]*

| Stage | Classification[b] T | N | M | Number of patients | Five-year survival (%) | p value |
|---|---|---|---|---|---|---|
| 0 | Tis | $N_0$ | $M_0$ | 16 | 100 | } NS |
| I | $T_1$ | $N_0$ | $M_0$ | 22 | 78.9 | |
| IIA | $T_2$ | $N_0$ | $M_0$ | 80 | 37.9 | } 0.0021 |
| | $T_3$ | $N_0$ | $M_0$ | | | |
| IIB | $T_1$ | $N_1$ | $M_0$ | 39 | 27.3 | } NS |
| | $T_2$ | $N_1$ | $M_0$ | | | |
| III | $T_3$ | $N_1$ | $M_0$ | 218 | 13.7 | } 0.0001 |
| | $T_4$ | Any N | $M_0$ | | | |
| IV | Any T | Any N | $M_1$ | 33 | 0 | |
| Total | | | | 408 | | |

[a] From ref. 36, with permission.
[b] T, Tumor; N, node; M, metastasis.

**TABLE 13–2.** *Staging of cancer of the esophagus and cardia: modified WNM criteria[a]*

| Stage | Classification[b] | | | Number of patients | Five-year survival (%) | p value |
|---|---|---|---|---|---|---|
| | W | N | M | | | |
| 0 | $W_0$ | $N_0$ | $M_0$ | 38 | 88.2 | } 0.0002 |
| I | $W_0$ | $N_1$ | $M_0$ | 59 | 50.3 | |
| | $W_1$ | $N_0$ | $M_0$ | | | } 0.0005 |
| II | $W_1$ | $N_1$ | $M_0$ | 95 | 22.5 | |
| | $W_2$ | $N_0$ | $M_0$ | | | } 0.02 |
| III | $W_2$ | $N_1$ | $M_0$ | 183 | 10.7 | |
| | $W_1$ | $N_2$ | $M_0$ | | | |
| | $W_0$ | $N_2$ | $M_0$ | | | } 0.0001 |
| IV | Any W | Any N | $M_1$ | 33 | 0 | |
| Total | | | | 408 | | |

[a] From ref. 36, with permission.
[b] W, Wall penetration; N, node; M, metastasis.

regional lymph nodes, and distant metastasis for the Skinner et al. WNM staging system as modified by Ellis et al.

In a second publication, using an expanded base of 408 resected patients, Ellis et al. compared the 1988 staging criteria with their modified Skinner WNM system and showed evidence that a modified WNM staging system was more useful from a prognostic standpoint (Tables 13–1 and 13–2) [36]. Not only is the number of patients more evenly divided among the four stages in the modified Skinner system, but the comparison of the 5-year survival rates between stages is highly significant, with almost a 50% reduction in survival rates for each increasing stage. The major difference in the staging criteria of the proposed modification to the Skinner WNM system is the recognition that the number of nodes involved has a profound effect on prognosis. It is important to realize that Ellis has been a proponent of a limited resec-

tion and lymph node dissection. Thus, the data used to validate the modified staging system represent what the outcome would be for simple tumor removal. Consequently, they serve as an excellent basis for comparison with the results of the more extensive en bloc resection or a preoperative chemotherapy program.

**Endoscopic Ultrasound, Laparoscopic, and Thoracoscopic Staging**

Endoscopic ultrasound imaging of esophageal lesions has recently become available, and in experienced hands provides accurate information about the size and wall penetration of the tumor and the presence of lymph node metastasis [101, 123]. Staging via endoscopic ultrasound results in correct classification of the majority of patients into either early-, intermediate-, or late-stage groups, allowing appropriate treatment selection. Tumor penetration through the esophageal wall and the presence of metastatic nodal involvement can be accurately predicted in over 80% of patients. Differentiation of intramucosal from intramural tumors can be difficult [94]. The resolution of present-day endoscopic ultrasound systems is not sufficient to differentiate predictably the fine detail of tumor infiltration when limited to the esophageal wall. Detection of esophageal wall penetration is easier and is usually evident. Accurate prediction of nodal involvement can also be difficult. Although in general nodal involvement is correctly assessed in over 80% of patients, there is a tendency to overstage the status of the lymph nodes. Overstaging occurs because of the inability of endoscopic ultrasound to differentiate inflammatory from metastatic disease. Despite these limitations, most patients can be classified into an appropriate stage grouping. Unless one accepts the premise that the extent of the procedure has no influence on the overall survival of the patient, a tenet that remains far from proven, selection of patients for curative or palliative procedures is important. At present, endoscopic ultrasound provides the most accurate means of achieving this goal.

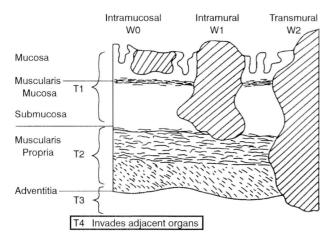

**FIG. 13–2.** Staging of the primary tumor according to the depth of invasion, using histologic landmarks: *intramucosal carcinoma* if it penetrates the glandular basement membrane, but is limited by the muscularis mucosae, *intramural carcinoma* if it penetrates through the muscularis mucosa, but not the muscularis propria, and *transmural carcinoma* if it penetrates through the muscularis propria.

Recently, thoracoscopic and laparoscopic staging of esophageal cancer has been recommended. Stein et al. have prospectively assessed the value of minimally invasive surgical staging in 127 consecutive patients with cancer of the esophagus and cardia [113]. Diagnostic laparoscopy and laparoscopic ultrasound revealed previously unknown findings in 22% in to 25% of patients with adenocarcinoma of the distal esophagus. Little was gained in patients with squamous cell carcinoma. They concluded that diagnostic laparoscopy with laparoscopic ultrasound and peritoneal lavage was safe and frequently provides therapeutically relevant new information in patients with locally advanced adenocarcinoma of the esophagus and cardia. A similar study was reported by the University of Maryland group [62]. These authors suggested that minimally invasive surgery be used to improve pretreatment staging prior to neoadjuvant therapy. Thoracoscopic staging was applied in 45 patients with biopsy-proven carcinoma of the esophagus, and laparoscopic staging was applied in the final 19 patients. Thoracoscopic staging was accurate in detecting the status of thoracic nodal involvement in 93% of patients. Laparoscopic staging was accurate in detecting lymph node metastases in 16 of 17 patients (94%). The authors concluded that thoracoscopic and laparoscopic staging are more accurate than existing staging methods (computed tomography and endoscopic ultrasound) and that in 6 of 19 patients in whom laparoscopic staging was used, unsuspected celiac lymph node metastases were detected. They suggested that the role of thoracoscopic and laparoscopic staging of esophageal cancer should be further evaluated in a multiinstitutional trial. If these results are confirmed and their cost is not prohibitive, then thoracoscopic and laparoscopic staging could become valuable tools to determine the extent of disease prior to therapy.

At the present time, despite the modern techniques of computed tomography, magnetic resonance imaging, endoscopic ultrasound, and laparoscopic and thoracoscopic technology, pretreatment staging still remains imprecise. This underscores the need for an intraoperative assessment of the potential for cure in each individual patient.

**Intraoperative Staging**

Intraoperative staging is designed for further selection of patients who before surgery were considered candidates for a curative resection. It is based on the observation that a patient with a tumor that penetrates through the esophageal wall or has multiple or distant lymph node metastases has a poor chance of survival. It requires an operative approach

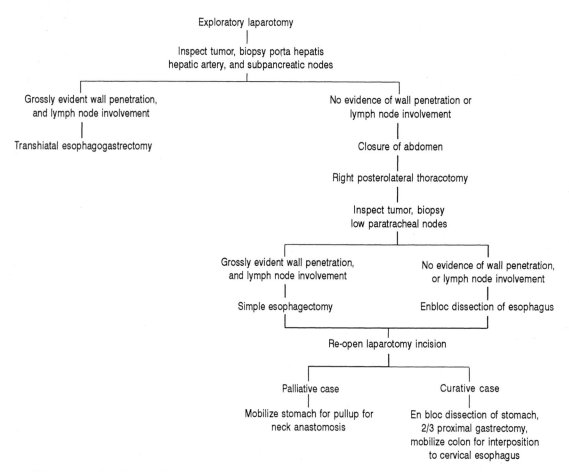

**FIG. 13–3.** Algorithm outlining the surgical procedure and intraoperative decisions. (From ref. 51.)

that allows switching from a curative to a palliative resection so that if, during the course of an operation, an incurable situation is identified, the surgeon can change to a palliative procedure. Figure 13–3 shows an algorithm of intraoperative decision making. A curative en bloc dissection is abandoned if it is discovered during the operation that the primary tumor is unresectable, cavitary spread of the tumor has occurred, distant organ metastases are present, the tumor extends through the mediastinal pleura, multiple gross lymph node metastases are present, or there is microscopic evidence of lymph node involvement at the margins of an en bloc resection, i.e., low paratracheal, portal triad, or subpancreatic peri-aortic lymph nodes. This algorithm is applied clinically to all patients with cancer of the lower esophagus and cardia. Our experience has shown that patients at a favorable stage of disease can be identified by a combination of preoperative and intraoperative staging with an accuracy of 86%. Preoperatively, patients are excluded from a curative resection on the basis of unequivocal findings of advanced disease observed on CT scan or endoscopy. If the findings are questionable, the patient is given the benefit of the doubt. The benefit of this selective approach is to provide an optimal chance for cure when appropriate, effective palliation when necessary, and the ability to switch from one to the other depending on the extent of disease encountered during the operation.

## TREATMENT OF ESOPHAGEAL CARCINOMA

Surgical resection is the mainstay of treatment of esophageal cancer. Although curative combination chemoradiotherapy without surgery has been reported [57], several factors limit its use. These include the inability to identify accurately patients curable without surgical resection, the prevalence of recurrence requiring subsequent surgical resection, a high treatment-related morbidity and mortality, whether cure is even possible with such treatment, and perhaps most importantly, the fact that long-term survival is the rule following curative resection in early-stage disease. For these reasons most authors presently consider such treatment investigational.

Historically there has been an aura of pessimism regarding the potential for cure of esophageal carcinoma. This has given rise to the attitude that palliation of dysphagia is the only reasonable therapeutic goal [114]. Consequently, surgical procedures of touted low operative mortality have been advocated as means of providing palliation by removal of the primary tumor without regard for the principles of cancer surgery. This not only runs counter to the strongly held principles of surgical oncology, but is contrary to the observation that cure is possible when the tumor extends transmurally or has spread to peritumoral nodes. In addition, the changing epidemiology of esophageal cancer and the declining morbidity and mortality of esophageal resection strongly support an attempt at cure whenever possible. With the increasing prevalence of adenocarcinoma associated with Barrett's

esophagus, patients are presenting at a younger age and with earlier stage tumors, both strong inducements for curative resection.

Making the selection for cure or palliation prior to resection has several benefits. It identifies the mission of the operation and emphasizes adequate surgery for cure and sufficient surgery for palliation. Furthermore, it does not conceal the benefits of surgery by reporting the survival of patients in which the procedure was done only for palliation. It also emphasizes the need for a more durable reconstruction of the gastrointestinal tract in patients operated on for cure and, finally, identifies candidates for multimodal therapy if surgical cure is not possible.

### Perioperative Management

Supportive measures are performed to improve the ability of the patient to tolerate the operation and to sustain him or her in the postoperative period. Advanced age, common in patients with esophageal cancer, is associated with decreased overall performance, regardless of the presence or absence of disease. In a study of marathon runners, who likely have a high cardiopulmonary reserve, Stones and Kozma found a rapidly decreasing performance after the age of 70 [114]. This decreased physical performance is manifested in increased operative mortality. Figure 13–4 is adopted from a study performed by Sikes and Detmer on 15,930 surgical cases, including both elective and emergency operations [108]. The graph demonstrates the effect of age on procedure-adjusted mortality. There is a steady increase in surgical mortality with advancing age and a precipitous rise in mortality over the age of 75 years.

Prior to proceeding with curative surgical therapy for carcinoma of the esophagus, it is important to confirm that the patient has sufficient cardiopulmonary reserve to tolerate the operation. The physiologic status of the patient will affect the extent of the surgery. It is futile to select an operation

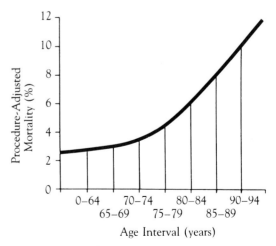

FIG. 13–4. The relationship between age and procedure-adjusted motility rate. (From ref. 108, with permission.)

that is aimed at increasing the long-term survival for a patient whose physiologic life expectancy is short. Respiratory function is best assessed by the forced expiratory volume $FEV_1$, which ideally should be 2 L or more. Any patient with an $FEV_1$ of less than 1.25 L is a poor surgical candidate because there is a 40% risk of dying from respiratory insufficiency within 4 years [32]. In such a patient the chance of long-term survival, even if the disease is cured, does not justify an extensive esophageal resection. Cardiac reserve can be assessed by gated radionucleotide-pool scan. This noninvasive study provides accurate information on wall motion and ejection fraction. If the latter is below 40% or decreases on exercise, a coronary arteriogram and ventriculogram may be indicated. A resting ejection fraction of less than 40% is an ominous sign. We would not advocate an extensive resection in such a patient, regardless of how favorable the pathology appears. Patients with mild congestive failure can be improved to some extent with vigorous medical management. Likewise, cessation of smoking, aggressive bronchopulmonary toilet, and bronchodilators may improve a marginal $FEV_1$. Patients with chronic lung disease do better if their operations are scheduled for the afternoon, thus allowing them to ambulate and cough up secretions that have accumulated in the lung overnight.

Patients undergoing esophageal resection are prone to developing postoperative respiratory failure mainly from interstitial pulmonary edema. Following surgical removal of the mediastinal lymphatics and nodes, lymph clearance of both lungs is compromised [119]. The lungs are supplied with a rich network of lymphatics that drain centrally toward the hilum. The direction of the flow is maintained by a series of strategically placed valves [125]. The disruption of these lymphatic channels, as occurs when the visceral mediastinal nodes are resected, leads to accumulation of interstitial lung water, which reduces alveolar volume and increases airway resistance. This phenomenon is manifested clinically by tachypnea, increased work of breathing, and eventually, respiratory failure. Rales may or may not be present, because the edema is mostly interstitial. Poor nutritional status may potentiate the problem. Guyton and Lindsey [50] demonstrated experimentally that if the serum proteins are normal, the left atrial pressure has to exceed 24 mm Hg before transudation into the alveoli develops. The critical left atrial pressure drops to 11 mm Hg when the serum proteins are low. As a consequence, a delicate balance must be maintained between minimizing the potential for pulmonary fluid accumulation and maximizing perfusion of the graft used for esophageal replacement.

Since the predominant symptom of esophageal carcinoma is dysphagia, the nutritional status of the patient is of paramount importance in determining the outcome [79]. Low serum proteins have a deleterious effect on the cardiovascular system, and a poor nutritional status affects the host resistance to infection and the rate of anastomotic and wound healing [54]. The simplest way to assess the nutritional status of the patient is to measure the serum albumin prior to any

hydration. A value below 3.4 g/dl indicates poor caloric intake and an increased risk of surgical complications, including anastomotic breakdowns [95].

Nutritional support can be provided in several ways. Oral intake is usually inadequate in patients with advanced esophageal cancer, and passage of a nasogastric tube can be difficult. The use of the gut for alimentation has several advantages over the intravenous route. These include better utilization of nutrients requiring a lower caloric intake [7], decreased incidence of metabolic, septic, and thrombotic complications, a tenfold decrease of cost per patient [70], and ease of performance in outpatients. In our experience, a feeding jejunostomy tube provides the most reliable and safest method for nutritional support in patients with esophageal carcinoma who cannot consume an oral diet and who have a functionally normal small bowel. A gastrostomy is inadvisable for these patients because it may interfere with the use of the stomach for reconstruction. The jejunostomy permits nutritional support early in the postoperative period and minimizes the danger of regurgitation into the pharynx and possible aspiration.

In severely malnourished patients, the catheter is placed as a separate procedure to allow for preoperative nutritional support. Catheter feedings are continued while the patient is investigated, thus saving valuable time. In the other patients, the jejunostomy is placed at the time of the esophageal resection and feeding is begun on the third postoperative day. It is started with 5% dextrose in water, and gradually advance, using a continuous drip infusion technique, to full-strength formula at a rate of 2,400 to 3,000 calories per day. As the patient resumes oral intake after surgery, the amount of nutritional support is tapered off. Patients who require nutritional support after discharge from the hospital are issued a portable pump that can be carried on a shoulder strap while they patient go about their daily activities. None of our patients have had any difficulty with the use of the pump at home over prolonged periods of time.

If the colon is chosen as esophageal substitute in patients undergoing en block resection or patients with previous gastric resection, the status of the colon is assessed preoperatively by colonoscopy. This is essential to exclude concomitant carcinoma of the colon, colonic polyps, and diverticulitis or colitis. Polyps, if found, are endoscopically removed and assessed histopathologically. Angiography of the superior and inferior mesenteric arteries provides precise information regarding the vascular supply of the colon and helps select the segment of colon to be used [30]. Mechanical cleansing is performed on the day prior to the operation with 1 to 2 gallons of osmotic diarrheal agents containing polyethyleneglycol. Oral nonabsorbable antibiotics are given in addition. Broad-spectrum parenteral antibiotic prophylaxis is started the day before surgery and is continued until 3 days after the operation. To prevent deep vein thrombosis and pulmonary emboli in the perioperative period, all patients are started on subcutaneous heparin at 5,000 units intramuscularly twice daily the day prior to esophageal resection.

A preoperative CEA level has been shown to be useful in determining recurrence during the postoperative follow-up.

## Surgical Resection

The extent of surgical resection for tumors of the thoracic esophagus is controversial. Many believe that the role of surgery should be limited to removing the primary tumor, with the hope that adjuvant therapy will increase cure rates by destroying systemic disease. This approach emphasizes the concept of biological predeterminism; that is, the outcome of treatment in esophageal cancer is determined at the time of diagnosis, and surgical therapy aimed at removing more than the primary tumor is not helpful. Lymph node metastases are considered simply markers of systemic disease, and the systematic removal of involved nodes is not beneficial.

Others believe that cure is possible and that, when possible, treatment should be selected with curative intent, recognizing that long-term survival will occur in the minority of patients. Akiyama, having dedicated a lifetime to the study and treatment of esophageal cancer states, ''Although it is commonly thought that lymphatic spread implies systemic disease, in practice malignancy can often be cured by removal of the involved lymph nodes'' (Fig. 13–5) [2]. This approach requires that the goal of surgery, cure or palliation, be identified prior to the operation, and emphasizes the prolongation of life as the endpoint of resection for cure and quality of the remaining life as the endpoint of resection for palliation [28]. An increasing number of centers around the world have now reported data suggesting a survival advantage with en bloc esophagectomy. This includes reports from Los Angeles [51], Tokyo [6], New York [11], Munich [58], and Leuven [67]. These studies have shown that, particularly for cancers of the lower esophagus and cardia, en bloc esophagogastrectomy results in significantly better survival than transhiatal or simple transthoracic esophagogastrectomy. It is unlikely that this can be explained by a bias in the stage of disease resected, a difference in operative mortality, or death from nontumor causes. Rather, it appears to be due to the type of operation performed. Options for esophageal resection include (a) transhiatal, (b) combined right thoracic and abdominal (Ivor Lewis), (c) left thoracoabdominal, and (d) en bloc, either two field or three field. The first three of these options include a simple esophagectomy without lymphadenectomy with reconstruction generally occurring via gastric interposition to the neck. The fourth involves a radical esophagectomy including mediastinal, upper abdominal (two field), and/or cervical (three field) lymphadenectomy.

### Simple Esophagectomy

In a simple esophagectomy whether by the transhiatal or transthoracic route, there is no specific attempt to remove lymph node-bearing tissue in the posterior mediastinum. The resection margin is generally limited by the esophageal wall. Stomach is used to reconstruct the gastrointestinal tract and no systematic upper abdominal lymphadenectomy is included.

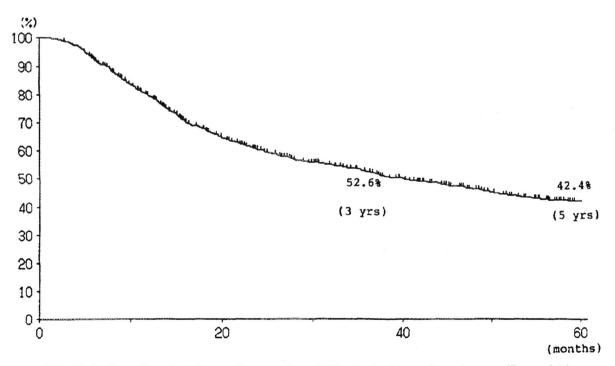

**FIG. 13–5.** Overall survival after curative resection of 913 patients with esophageal cancer. (From ref. 6.)

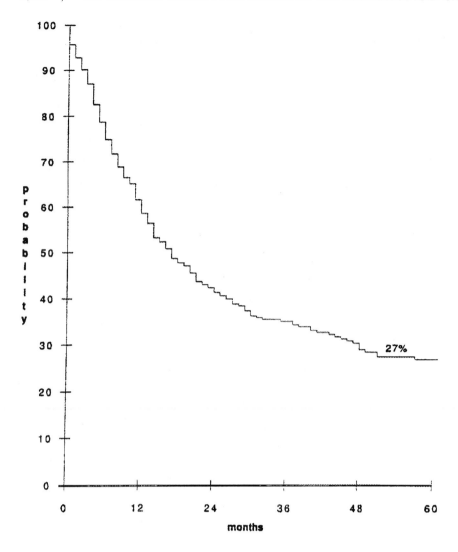

**FIG. 13–6.** Actuarial survival curve of 417 patients undergoing transhiatal esophagectomy for cancer of the intrathoracic esophagus and cardia. (From ref. 87.)

Transhiatal and transthoracic simple esophagectomy are nowadays essentially equivalent treatments. Cure is uncommon and occurs by chance. Actuarial survival over 5 years for patients undergoing transhiatal esophagectomy is shown in Fig. 13–6. Improvements in perioperative care including epidural analgesia and limited transfusion have resulted in no demonstrable morbidity advantage to the transhiatal approach. Numerous comparative series have shown equiva-lent survival (Table 13–3) and a similar prevalence of complications (Table 13–4) [18, 38, 47, 48, 53, 60, 76, 89].

### En Bloc Esophagectomy

A curative en bloc resection of the esophagus and cardia consists of the removal of a tissue block completely surrounded on all sides by normal tissue. Whatever extensions

**TABLE 13–3.** *Survival following transhiatal and transthoracic esophagectomy: collected series*

| Author | Year | N | Three-year survival (%) | | p value |
| | | | Transhiatal | Transthoracic | |
| --- | --- | --- | --- | --- | --- |
| Goldfaden et al. [47] | 1986 | 72 | 22 | 20 | NS |
| Hankins et al. [53] | 1989 | 78 | 24 | 11 | NS |
| Fok et al. [38] | 1989 | 210 | 15 | 27 | 0.04 |
| Moon et al. [76] | 1992 | 88 | 24 | 16 | NS |
| Jauch et al. [60] | 1992 | 86 | 25 | 22 | NS |
| Goldminc et al. [48] | 1993 | 67 | 32 | 17 | NS |
| Pac et al. [89] | 1993 | 238 | 30 | 26 | NS |
| Bolton et al. [18] | 1994 | 55 | 40 | 22 | NS |
| Total | | 894 | 26.5 | 20.1 | |

**TABLE 13–4.** *Prospective randomized trial of transhiatal versus transthoracic esophagectomy: mortality and morbidity*

| Complication | Transhiatal N = 18 | Transthoracic N = 16 |
|---|---|---|
| Mortality | 2 (6%) | 3 (10%) |
| Morbidity | 18 (56%) | 16 (46%) |
| Pulmonary infection | 6 (19%) | 7 (20%) |
| Pleural effusion | 11 (34%) | 4 (11%) |
| Anastomotic leak | 2 (6%) | 3 (9%) |
| Recurrent nerve palsy | 1 (3%) | 1 (3%) |
| Thoracic bleeding | 0 (0%) | 1 (3%) |
| Cervical abscess | 2 (6%) | 0 (0%) |
| Gastroplasty necrosis | 1 (3%) | 0 (0%) |
| Other | 3 (9%) | 5 (14%) |

[a] Data from Goldminc et al. [48].

of the primary tumor are present should be contained within the resected block. The esophagus is resected including a wide margin of periesophageal tissues and lymph node-bearing tissue. Two or three fields of lymphatic resection are included depending upon the location of the tumor; upper abdominal celiac and splenic nodes (field one), infracarinal posterior mediastinal (field two), and upper mediastinal and cervical (field three).

Rigorous data comparing simple and en bloc transthoracic esophagectomy are lacking. Comparison is difficult because the indication for surgery in the transhiatal group is only palliation, and cure, if achieved, is a chance phenomenon. Consequently, patients are not identified as having a curative operation, i.e., no evidence of gross tumor remaining in the chest or abdomen following the resection. Survival comparisons that have been reported show a significantly better survival in patients undergoing an en bloc resection (Figs. 13–7 and 13–8). It is unlikely that a randomized prospective study will be or could be done to answer the question.

*Lymph Node Metastasis*

Relevant to the decision of extent of resection is information regarding the incidence and patterns of nodal metastases for lower esophageal adenocarcinoma. Critical analysis of the patterns of lymph node metastases in the surgical specimens after transhiatal resection is inappropriate since a limited node dissection is performed, while detailed analysis of patients undergoing en bloc resection has only been reported for esophageal squamous cell carcinoma by Japanese investigators [2]. In a recent analysis of 43 patients undergoing curative en bloc resection for adenocarcinoma of the distal esophagus, lymph node metastases were present in 76% of patients [23]. Tumor depth was a good indicator of nodal involvement (Fig. 13–9). Eighty-nine percent of transmural tumors, 60% of intramural tumors, and 33% of intramucosal lesions had lymph node metastases at the time of resection. This is in agreement with the findings of Japanese investigators, who reported nodal involvement in 30% of 40 patients with intramucosal squamous cell carcinoma. This finding has implications in the management of patients with high-grade dysplasia, where the prevalence of unexpected adenocarcinoma is up to 50%.

Adenocarcinomas of the lower esophagus and cardia spread widely to regional nodes, most commonly to nodes along the lesser curvature, celiac axis, and parahiatal regions (Table 13–5). However, 10% had subcarinal nodes and 18% had involved nodes of the splenic hilum, along the splenic artery or along the greater curvature of the stomach. It is likely that the subcarinal and splenic nodes would remain following transhiatal resection. Further, the involved nodes along the greater curve of the stomach would, by necessity, be transposed into the chest if the stomach was used to reestablish gastrointestinal continuity. In addition, over 20% of patients had positive celiac axis nodes, an area not dissected by most surgeons during transhiatal esophagectomy.

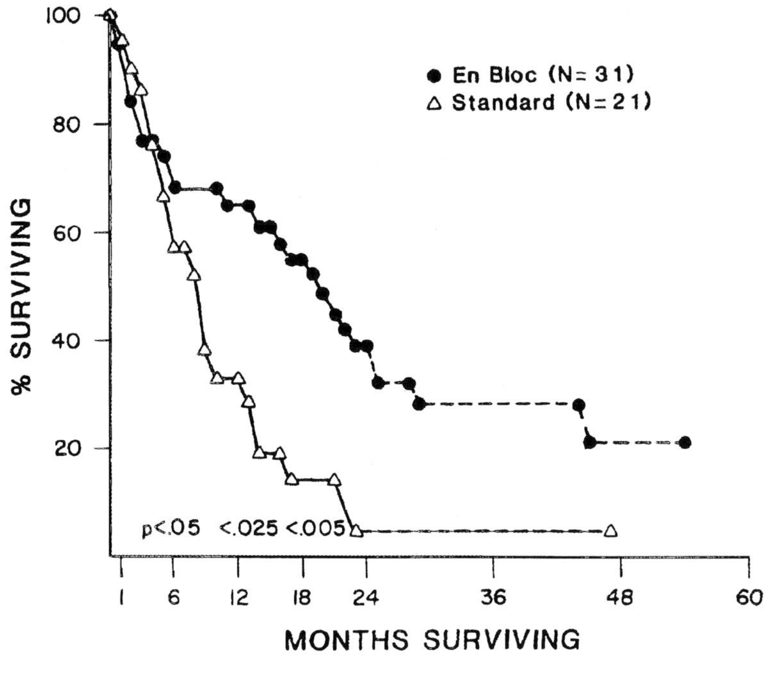

**FIG. 13–7.** Comparison of survival after en bloc and standard esophagectomy. The survival curves differ significantly at 6, 12, and 18 months. (From Skinner DB, Furgeson MK, Soriano A, Little AG Straszak VM. Selection of operation for esophageal cancer based on staging. Ann Surg 1986;204:391.)

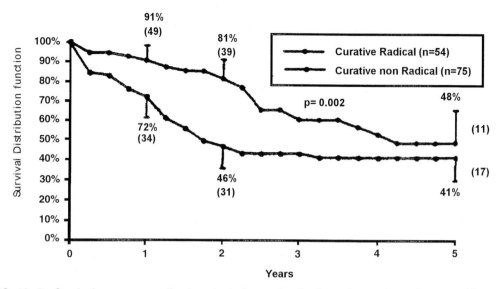

**FIG. 13–8.** Survival curves according to extent of resection for thoracic esophageal cancer. (From ref. 67.)

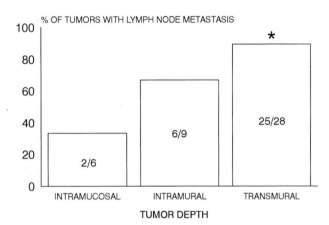

**FIG. 13–9.** Prevalence of lymph node metastases according to the depth of esophageal wall penetration by the tumor, *p < 0.01, $\chi^2$ = 9.3, 2 df. (From ref. 23.)

### Extent of Resection to Cure Disease Confined to the Mucosa

The development of surveillance programs for the detection of squamous cell carcinoma in endemic areas and for adenocarcinoma in patients with Barrett's esophagus has resulted in increasing numbers of patients with high-grade dysplasia and intramucosal esophageal cancer (Fig. 13–10). Several studies have shown that intraepithelial carcinoma, i.e., carcinoma *in situ* or high-grade dysplasia, and intramucosal tumors, i.e., invasive cancer limited by the muscular mucosa, are quite different in their biological behavior from submucosal tumors irrespective of their histology, whether squamous cell carcinoma or adenocarcinoma arising in Barrett's mucosa. Vessel invasion and lymph node metastasis do not occur in severe dysplasia, is uncommon in the intramucosal tumors, but is the rule in submucosal tumors. As a consequence, the 5-year survival for intramucosal tumors

**TABLE 13–5.** *Pattern of lymph node spread in resected tumors of the lower esophagus and cardia*

| Node location | Number of positive patients (n = 43) | Percent of positive patients | Number of positive nodes | Total number of nodes resected | Percent of nodes positive |
|---|---|---|---|---|---|
| Tracheobronchial | 1 | 2.3 | 1 | 42 | 2.4 |
| Subcarinal | 4 | 9.3 | 9 | 390 | 2.3 |
| Paraesophageal | 12 | 27.9 | 37 | 316 | 11.7 |
| Parahiatal | 15 | 34.8 | 35 | 247 | 14.2 |
| Splenic hilum | 1 | 2.3 | 3 | 39 | 7.7 |
| Splenic artery | 2 | 4.7 | 2 | 71 | 2.8 |
| Greater curve | 4 | 9.3 | 10 | 89 | 11.2 |
| Lesser curve | 18 | 41.8 | 64 | 261 | 24.5 |
| Left Gastric | 3 | 7 | 8 | 94 | 8.5 |
| Celiac | 9 | 20.9 | 25 | 60 | 41.6 |
| Hepatic | 1 | 2.3 | 6 | 21 | 28.5 |
| Portal | 1 | 2.3 | 2 | 84 | 2.4 |
| Right gastric | 1 | 2.3 | 4 | 47 | 8.5 |
| Retropancreatic | 0 | 0 | 0 | 23 | 0 |

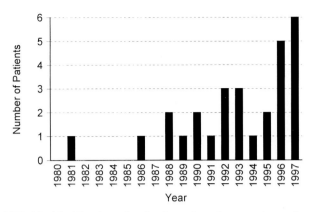

**FIG. 13–10.** Number of patients undergoing esophageal resection for intramucosal carcinoma each year at the University of Southern California Department of Surgery.

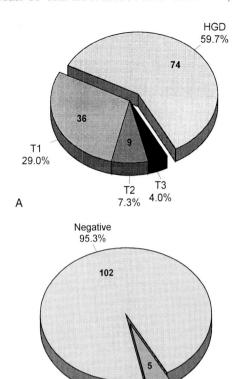

**FIG. 13–11.** Distribution of prognostic factors for patients undergoing esophagectomy for high-grade dysplasia. The data represent collected series of 125 patients. **A:** Wall penetration. **B:** Nodal status.

is significantly better than for submucosal tumors. These findings indicate that both severe dysplasia, i.e., carcinoma *in situ,* and intramucosal cancers, i.e., invasive cancer limited by the muscular mucosa, represent early malignant lesions of the esophagus. This has given rise to controversy over how to manage these early lesions.

High-grade dysplasia in Barrett's esophagus is a marker for the presence of invasive carcinoma in nearly half of the patients. This has been confirmed in our own studies from the University of Southern California as well as those from the Mayo Clinic, Johns Hopkins, and many other centers around the world (Table 13–6) [10, 34, 55, 91, 93, 102]. Most of these tumors are limited to the wall of the esophagus and few spread to regional lymph nodes (Fig. 13–11). Because it is not possible with present technology, including endoscopic ultrasound, to differentiate the patients who do or do not harbor a cancer, esophagectomy is the treatment of choice. Esophageal adenocarcinoma associated with high-grade dysplasia identified with surveillance endoscopy is highly curable. We and others have documented 5-year survival rates of 90% in this setting [93, 115]. Nonsurgical treatments of high-grade dysplasia, including endoscopic ablative therapy, have been proposed [88]. Most consider them to be investigational at the present stage of development and not standard care. Although these treatments should be investigated, few centers in the United States are capable of ablating Barrett's, the efficacy has not been established, and

clinical follow-up is not yet available to test firmly its efficacy.

A critical issue to be resolved is whether the depth of the lesion (intramucosal vs. submucosal) and the presence of regional nodal metastases can be correctly predicted prior to surgery. Accuracy of determining the depth of tumors confined to the esophageal wall using endoscopic ultrasound is questionable. In most hands, the resolution of the present-day endoscopic ultrasonographic system is not sufficient to predictably differentiate the fine detail of tumor infiltration when it is limited to the esophageal wall. Recent data from the author's experience suggests that in the absence of an

**TABLE 13–6.** *Prevalence of invasive carcinoma in resected specimens of patients with high-grade dysplasia: collected series*

| Author | Institution | Year published | Number of patients | Number with invasive cancer (%) |
|---|---|---|---|---|
| Altorki et al. [10] | Cornell | 1991 | 9 | 4 (45%) |
| Pera et al. [91] | Mayo Clinic | 1992 | 18 | 9 (50%) |
| Rice et al. [102] | Cleveland Clinic | 1993 | 16 | 6 (37%) |
| Peters et al. [93] | University of South California | 1994 | 9 | 5 (45%) |
| Edwards et al. [34] | Vanderbilt | 1996 | 11 | 8 (73%) |
| Heitmiller et al. [55] | Johns Hopkins | 1996 | 30 | 13 (43%) |

**TABLE 13–7.** *Histologic findings in the surgical specimen of patients with early esophageal adencocarcinoma with and without a visible mass on endoscopy*

| | Preoperative endoscopic biopsy[a] | | Postoperative surgical specimen histology | |
|---|---|---|---|---|
| Endoscopic finding | HGD | Intramucosal CA | Number of patients with penetration into muscularis propria | Number of patients with positive lymph nodes[b] |
| No visible lesion | 9 | 16 | 0 | 0 |
| Visible lesion | 2 | 4 | 2 | 4 |

[a] HGD, High-grade dysplasia; CA, carcinoma.
[b] Histologic and/or Immunohistochemical positive.

endoscopically visible lesion the tumors are predominantly intramucosal and nodal metastases are rare (Table 13–7). Whether this fact will suffice to select the extent of surgical resection awaits further study.

Patients with high-grade dysplasia and intramucosal carcinoma are best treated by a total esophagectomy removing all Barrett's tissue and any potential associated adenocarcinoma. Options include transhiatal esophagectomy or, more recently, vagal sparing esophagectomy. The vagal sparing approach is suitable only given confidence of the absence of regional nodal disease. Reconstruction is accomplished with either the stomach (transhiatal) or colon (vagal sparing) with the anastomosis in the neck. The mortality associated with this procedure should be less than 5%, and is minimal in centers experienced in esophageal surgery. Functional recovery is excellent, particularly in the vagal sparing group.

In the presence of an endoscopically visible lesion, the possibility of a submucosal tumor is high. Because tumors which invade through the muscularis mucosa into the submucosa have a 60% or more incidence of lymph node metastasis, it seems prudent to perform an en bloc esophagectomy for the treatment of visible lesions, regardless of the histologic findings on biopsy (i.e., high-grade dysplasia or intramucosal carcinoma). Recent studies indicate, however, that in early adenocarcinoma in Barrett's esophagus, metastases do not appear to involve the splenic artery nodes and the spleen. Splenic artery dissection consequently is not part of the en bloc resection in this condition [24], nor is extended gastric resection. Gastrointestinal continuity is reestablished by pulling the stomach up into the neck and performing an esophagogastrostomy. This approach, however, is not universally accepted.

In Japan, endoscopic mucosal resection has been utilized to resect squamous cell carcinomas after endoscopic ultrasound has been used to determined that the depth of the tumor is limited to the mucosa. High-frequency ultrasound (20 MHz) is used to accurately predict the depth of invasion. Surprisingly, large areas of squamous mucosa can be resected without perforation or bleeding, leaving the smooth surface of the muscularis mucosa intact. Reepithelization of the large, artificially induced ulcer is usually complete in 3 weeks. In order not to miss a squamous cancer that has invaded deeper than expected, it is important to examine carefully the deep margins of the resected specimen and perform

periodic endoscopic follow-up examinations with vital staining techniques. Multiple and widespread or circumferential squamous lesions are not applicable to this technique for fear of developing a stricture on healing. In this situation, those acquainted with endoscopic resection would advocate an esophagectomy.

## Surgical Approach Based upon Location of the Primary Tumor

### Cervical Esophageal Cancer

It has been estimated that 7% to 10% of primary malignant tumors of the esophagus occur in the cervical portion [110]. Czerny reported the first successful resection of a carcinoma of the cervical esophagus in 1877 [99]. Initially, it was hoped that the prognosis for patients with this disease might be better than for those with carcinoma of the thoracic esophagus. Unfortunately, this has not been proven true. Tumors in the cervical part of the esophagus, particularly those in the postcricoid area, are a well-defined pathologic entity in that the efferent lymphatics from the cervical esophagus drain directly into the paratracheal and deep cervical or internal jugular lymph nodes, with minimal flow in a longitudinal direction [26]. For all practical purposes, tumors of the cervical esophagus are managed as though they were head and neck tumors. Lesions that are not fixed to the spine, do not invade the vessels, and do not have fixed cervical lymph nodes metastases should be resected. If lymph node metastases are present, the resection should be considered palliative since cure at this stage of disease is rare. Low cervical lesions that reach the level of the thoracic inlet are usually unresectable owing to early invasion of the great vessels or the involvement of extensive length of the trachea. The length of the esophagus below the cricopharyngeal area is insufficient to allow palliative intubation or construction of a proximal anastomosis for a bypass procedure. Palliation of this tumor is very difficult, and patients with disease at this location have a very poor prognosis [61]. The larynx is often invaded with microscopic tumor and, in 94% of such cases, a total laryngectomy in combination with esophagectomy is necessary [63]. Experience has taught that the trachea should be removed even if gross tumor cannot be visualized. A simultaneous en bloc bilateral neck lymph node dissection is performed, sparing the jugular veins on both sides and reimplanting the parathyroid glands. The thoracic esophagus is removed by blunt dissection through a cervical and upper abdominal incision, and the continuity of the gastrointestinal tract is reestablished by pulling the stomach up through the esophageal bed. A permanent tracheostomy stoma is constructed in the lower flap of the cervical incision. Removal of the manubrium sterni for exposure to low cervical lesions facilitates the operation.

Early experience with resection of the cervical esophagus resulted in a high mortality rate, and reconstruction of the esophagus using neck flaps often required multiple operations [130]. Because of these complexities and the generally disappointing results, radiotherapy frequently was chosen. Immediate mortality decreased, but control of the tumor was not satisfactory [14]. The difference between the two forms of therapy is in the manner in which the disease recurs. Tumors treated initially with radiation therapy tend to recur locally as well as systematically, and the local disease becomes unmanageable, with erosion into neck vessels and trachea, resulting in hemorrhage and dyspnea. Patients who undergo surgical therapy have few local recurrences, provided total excision of the tumor was possible, but they succumb to metastatic disease. Colin and Spiro [25] reported a local failure rate of 80% after definitive radiation therapy and 20% of these patients required palliative surgery in order to control the local disease. Recent improvements in the techniques of immediate esophageal reconstruction have reduced the complications of the surgical treatment and have encouraged a more aggressive surgical approach [13]. The data reported by Colin and Spiro [25] suggest that an initial aggressive surgical resection yields longer survival than does radiation therapy (Fig. 13–12). However, tumor at the surgical margins, extensive involvement of the trachea, and vocal cord paralysis correlate with a significantly shorter survival following surgery. Their data also indicate that palliation

was achieved better with esophagectomy and immediate gastric pullup than with primary radiation therapy or chemotherapy (Fig. 13–13).

Cervical lesions that are totally unresectable are treated with radiation. If the patient has severe dysphagia, a colon bypass can be attempted with a proximal anastomosis made to the uninvolved piriform sinus. When there is extensive disease in the neck, or when there has been previous radiation therapy, the passage of the transplant through the thoracic inlet is usually impossible and the subcutaneous route must be used.

**Operative Technique**

The published works of Silver [109] and Akiyama et al. [4] are excellent guides on the surgical approach to carcinoma of the cervical esophagus, and our personal experience is based heavily on their observations. The patient is placed on the operating table in a manner that allows for simultaneous cervical, thoracic, and abdominal incisions (Fig. 13–14). The right hand is placed under the right buttock, and the right arm and forearm are cradled in a sheet along the side of the operating table. The right chest is elevated about 20 degrees by placing a folded sheet under the right scapula. This position allows for a right anterior thoracotomy to be made should it be necessary. The left arm is positioned alongside the body, and a padded shoulder brace is placed against the left arm to prevent the patient from slipping sideways when the table is rotated to the left to perform a thoracotomy. The table is initially rotated 20 degrees to the right, placing the patient in a horizontal position. In this position, simultaneous cervical and abdominal incisions can be made for resection of the cervical esophageal carcinoma and blunt dissection of the thoracic esophagus. The cervical esophagus is exposed through a transverse neck incision, and the neck is explored to determine whether the tumor is resectable.

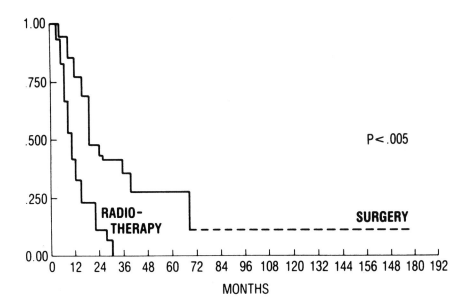

FIG. 13–12. Survival curves of patients with carcinoma of the cervical esophagus treated by surgery or radiotherapy at 5,000 rads or more. (From ref. 25, with permission.)

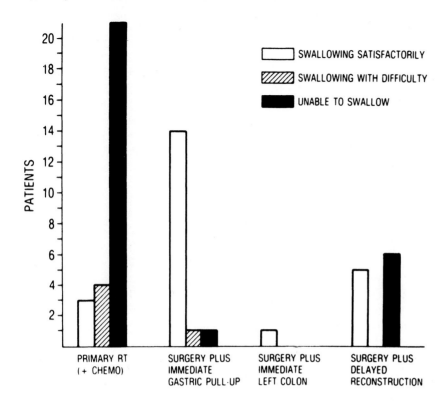

FIG. 13–13. Swallowing ability of patients following various therapies for carcinoma of the cervical esophagus. (From ref. 25, with permission.)

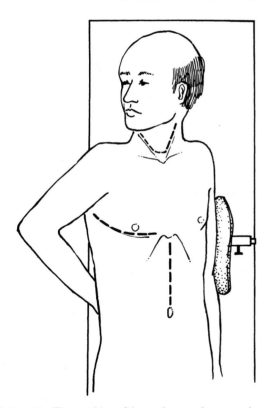

FIG. 13–14. The position of the patient on the operating table for resection of a cervical esophageal lesion. The position allows for an abdominal, anterolateral, thoracic, and cervical incision to be made without repositioning and redraping the patient. (From DeMeester TR, Barlow AP. Surgery and current management for cancer of the esophagus and cardia: Part II. Curr Probl Surg 1988;25:535, with permission.)

The tumor is removed if it or the cervical nodes are not fixed to the prevertebral fascia or adjacent vascular structures, and if the trachea can be divided at a level that will give a tumor-free margin and still allow enough length for a permanent cervical tracheostomy. If this is not possible, a mediastinal tracheostomy should be considered [42]. The opening of the larynx into the pharynx is closed and as much of the retrolaryngeal esophagus as possible is allowed to be retained. This will reduce the height at which the pharyngoesophageal anastomosis is performed.

In preparation for the gastric pullup, the gastrohepatic and the gastrocolic omental mesentery are divided in a manner that preserves the right gastric artery on the lesser curve and the right gastric epiploic vascular arcade along the greater curvature of the stomach. The short gastric vessels are divided, if possible, near the splenic hilum leaving the branches so as to provide collateral circulation along the proximal border of the greater curvature. The left gastric artery and its veins are divided near the celiac axis. The duodenum is mobilized by a Kocher maneuver (Fig. 13–15). The esophageal hiatus is enlarged by an anterior midline incision up underneath the pericardium to allow the surgeon to place her or his hand into the posterior mediastinum. The dissection of the thoracic esophagus is done digitally from both the abdominal and cervical incision in the manner described in the section on transhiatal esophagectomy.

In order to obtain adequate length of the stomach and prevent ischemia of the fundus, the cardia is encircled with a purse-string suture, ligated, and divided. The transected cardia is inverted into the stomach in a manner similar to inverting the stump of the appendix when performing an

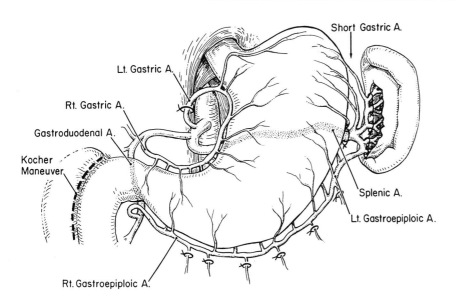

**FIG. 13–15.** Preparation of the stomach for pullup into the chest or neck showing ligation points of the left gastric, splenic, branches of splenic, and branches of right gastroepiploic arteries, and the incision for the Kocher maneuver. (From DeMeester TR, Barlow AP. Surgery and current management for cancer of the esophagus and cardia: Part II. Curr Probl Surg 1988;25:535, with permission.)

appendectomy. This maneuver preserves intragastric vascular anastomoses and maintains good vascularity to the very tip of the fundus.

The prepared stomach can easily be brought into the neck by suturing the fundus into the funnel of an inverted Mousseau-Barbin tube. A bowel bag, which has been divided approximately 3 to 4 inches from one end and cut so that one side and its bottom are open, is tied around the funnel so that the stomach is encased in the cellophane. The bag is lubricated with water, which greatly facilitates the movement of the stomach into the neck without it becoming ensnared in mediastinal structures. Prior to moving the stomach, it is helpful to stretch the organ wall by placing it under some tension. Care must be taken not to stretch the gastric vessels themselves. When this is done, the stomach usually reaches to the angle of mandible while lying on the anterior chest wall. After passing the stomach through the posterior mediastinum into the neck, a gastropharyngeal anastomosis is performed using a single layer of interrupted 4-0 polypropylene sutures.

If the stomach for some reason should not reach the pharynx, a helpful maneuver is to make a ''smile'' anterior gastric incision that when opened and reflected upward forms a flap to bridge the gap. The flap essentially extends the posterior wall of the stomach, and allows the central portion of the flap to be anastomosed with ease to the posterior pharyngeal tissue. The anterior portion of the anastomosis is completed by sewing the anterior walls of the stomach together along with the lateral portions of the flap, resulting in tubing of the fundus. For higher resections, the procedure can be reversed, giving more length on the anterior wall of the stomach and tacking the posterior wall to the prevertebral fascia. This leaves a raw area in the posterior pharynx that can be covered by pedicle flaps constructed in the mouth and slid down into the stomach, or the use of local skin flaps. The main advantage of a transhiatal esophagectomy performed at the time of resecting a cervical esophageal

tumor is that the entire esophagus is resected. This eliminates the possibility of tumor remaining in the distal esophageal stump, and removes any synchronous lesions in the thoracic esophagus. The completed procedure with a pharyngogastric anastomosis and permanent tracheostomy is shown in Fig. 13–16.

### Results

We have reported 15 of these procedures, with one operative death [29]. Although this procedure involves extensive surgery, it is tolerated better than a thoracic esophagectomy, particularly when associated with laryngectomy. This is probably due to the elimination of pulmonary complications that occur secondary to occult aspiration. Nonlethal complications which occurred early in our experience included one avascular necrosis of the stomach, necessitating its removal, one anastomotic disruption, two tracheal tears, and one mediastinal hemorrhage secondary to injury to the azygos vein. The latter required a thoracotomy to control bleeding.

Out of a combined group of patients reported by four authors, the operative mortality of 85 patients treated with transhiatal esophagectomy and gastric interposition for tumors of the cervical esophagus and hypopharynx was 7% [13, 29, 61, 63]. The most in-depth analysis of the procedure has been published by Kakegawa et al. [61]. They reported that total laryngectomy, combined with esophagectomy, is necessary in 94% of the patients and that 18% of the patients have intramural skip metastases, emphasizing the importance of total esophagectomy. They found that a transhiatal esophagectomy provided no particular advantage over a transthoracic one, except that the former could be done with the expectation of a lower operative mortality. Their 5-year survival of 23 patients resected with a concomitant transhiatal dissection was 22%, compared to 17% of 29 patients treated with a concomitant transthoracic esophagectomy.

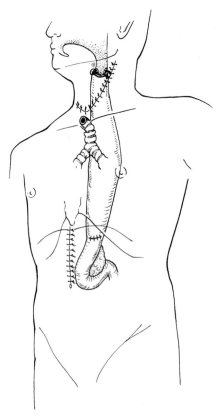

**FIG. 13–16.** Completed esophagolaryngectomy for cervical esophageal carcinoma showing pyloromyotomy, pharyngo-gastrostomy, and permanent tracheostomy. (From DeMeester TR, Barlow AP. Surgery and current management for cancer of the esophagus and cardia: Part II. Curr Probl Surg 1988;25:535, with permission.)

## Tumors of the Thoracic Esophagus above the Carina

Curative en bloc resection of tumors that arise within the upper or middle third of the thoracic esophagus is complicated by the close association of vital thoracic structures such as the trachea, aorta, arch vessels, and recurrent laryngeal nerves. Although an upper mediastinal lymphadenectomy is achievable, morbidity is high, particularly recurrent laryngeal nerve palsy and its associated respiratory complications. Nerve palsy and tracheostomy have been reported to be as high as 50% to 75% [80]. Consequently, in this location only tumors that have not penetrated the esophageal wall without obvious regional nodal metastasis are selected for curative resection.

Whether for cure or palliation, tumors above the carina are generally approached via a standard transthoracic esophagectomy. This allows careful dissection of the tumor off the trachea and minimizes the risk of tracheal injury. The thoracic portion is performed through a right posterolateral or anterolateral thoracotomy, depending on the location of the tumor. For cure, the thoracic lymphadenectomy is performed as completely as possible from the thoracic incision with the remaining high thoracic and left recurrent nodes

further dissected via the left neck incision, often with removal of a portion of the manubrium and left upper sternum. The thoracic incision is closed and the procedure completed via left neck and upper midline abdominal incisions. Proximal gastrectomy and splenectomy are not required, although a celiac lymphadenectomy is performed. Gastrointestinal continuity is reestablished by pulling up the stomach through the hiatus and anastomosing it to the esophagus in the neck.

### Results

The data on survival of transthoracic esophagogastrectomy for carcinoma of the esophagus are difficult to interpret because most reports do not identify whether the operation was done for cure or palliation, do not stratify their survival data as to the esophageal level involved with tumor, and mix adenocarcinoma of the cardia and squamous cell carcinoma of the body in their survival data. Tables 13–3 and 13–4 show results from reports with sufficient patient detail from senior authors with extensive experience in the management of this disease.

### Tumors of the Esophagus below the Carina

Most esophageal tumors occur in the esophagus below the carina. When expertise exists, a curative resection should be attempted whenever preoperative staging suggests favorable tumor characteristics. Clinical factors indicating an advanced stage of carcinoma that excludes cure by surgery are recurrent nerve paralysis, Horner's syndrome, persistent spinal pain, paralysis of the diaphragm, fistula formation, and malignant pleural effusion. Factors that make surgical cure unlikely are a tumor greater than 9 cm in length, abnormal axis of the esophagus on barium roentgenography (Fig. 13–17) [3], enlarged lymph nodes on CT, a weight loss greater than 20%, and loss of appetite. The endoscopic size of the tumor can be used as an approximation of the extent

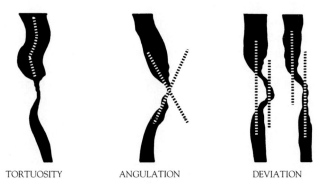

TORTUOSITY     ANGULATION     DEVIATION

**FIG. 13–17.** Three types of esophageal axis abnormalities originally described by Akiyama. The deviation is due to a carcinoma that has extended through the wall and caused contraction of periesophageal tissues. (From DeMeester TR, Barlow AP. Surgery and current management for cancer of the esophagus and cardia: Part I. Curr Probl Surg 1988;25: 477, with permission.)

Two-thirds gastrectomy and thoracic esophagectomy should be performed to incorporate the submucosal lymphatic spread of both organs in the specimen. Injection of the submucosal lymphatics of the esophagus with contrast medium shows that the length of longitudinal lymph flow is about six times the length of the transverse flow [26]. In the upper two-thirds of the esophagus, the lymph flow tends to move in a cephalad direction, and in the lower third, in

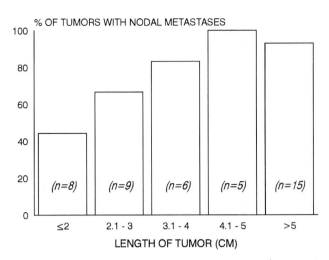

% OF TUMORS WITH NODAL METASTASES

**FIG. 13–18.** Prevalence of lymph node metastases according to the length of tumor in the pathology specimen. (From ref. 23.)

of disease, i.e., the presence of wall penetration and lymph node metastasis. Figure 13–18 shows the relationship of endoscopically measured tumor size to the presence of favorable staging for a curative resection, i.e., the absence of one or both of the limiting factors. In our experience, there is a high incidence of favorable parameters for tumors less than 4 cm in length, a lower incidence for tumors between 4 and 8 cm, and no favorable criteria for tumors greater than 8 cm in length [23]. Consequently, a tumor more than 8 cm long generally excludes curative resection; the finding of a small tumor should encourage an aggressive approach.

Resection margins for curative en bloc esophagectomy for tumors of the distal esophagus are limited anteriorly by the pericardium, laterally by the right and left mediastinal pleura, and posteriorly by the intercostal arteries, aorta, and anterior vertebral ligaments. The proximal margin is the carina and the inferior margin is a collar of diaphragmatic muscle around the esophageal hiatus, the celiac axis, and common hepatic artery. The specimen should consist of the distal esophagus, proximal stomach, spleen, and splenic artery together with the following nodal groups: subcarinal, inferior paraesophageal, parahiatal, left gastric, celiac, hepatic, and splenic artery nodes. Borders of such a resection are outlined in Fig. 13–19. Gastrointestinal continuity is reestablished with a colon interposition.

Arguments to support the more extensive resection are outlined in Table 13–8. Support for an extensive lymph node dissection as a necessary part of the curative resection includes the fact that survival of patients with other tumors that drain to the mediastinal lymphatics, i.e., squamous cell and adenocarcinoma of the lung, is dependent on the degree of lymph node metastasis. The removal of hilar lymph node metastasis in such patients is curative. In addition, studies indicate that patients with esophageal cancer and peritumoral nodes can be cured by resection that includes lymphadenectomy.

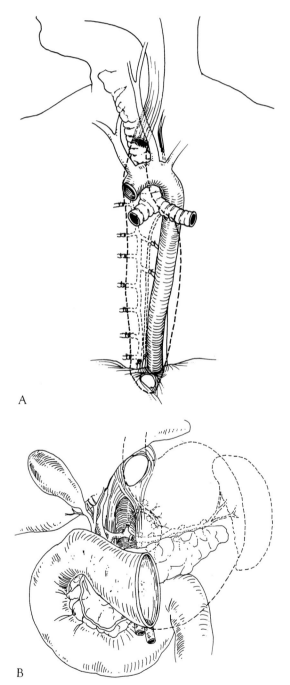

**FIG. 13–19. A:** Outline of the boundaries for the thoracic portion of an en bloc esophagogastrectomy. **B:** Outline of the boundaries for the abdominal portion of an en bloc esophagogastrectomy. (From ref. 31, with permission.)

**TABLE 13–8.** *Arguments to support extensive esophagectomy, gastrectomy, and lymph node dissection*

A. Arguments to support a more extensive esophagectomy
   1. Injection of submucosal contrast medium shows that the length of longitudinal lymph flow is six times the transverse flow
   2. At least 10 cm of grossly normal esophagus proximal to the tumor must be resected to prevent local recurrence
   3. Spatial relation indicates that for an adequate proximal margin a cervical anastomosis is almost always needed

B. Arguments to support a more extensive gastrectomy for tumors of the lower third of the esophagus or cardia
   1. No barrier exists to submucosal lymphatics between esophagus and stomach at the cardia
   2. Tumor cells in submucosal lymphatics can result in intragastric recurrence if too little of the stomach is resected
   3. Spatial relationships of the stomach do not allow for both adequate distal tumor margins and sufficient residual stomach to perform a cervical anastomosis

C. Arguments for lymph node dissection
   1. Survival of lung cancer patients with metastases to the hilar lymph nodes, i.e., a cancer that also metastasizes to mediastinal lymph nodes, is dependent on removal of involved nodes
   2. Patients with esophageal carcinoma and lymph node metastases are cured by resection, whereas, it is extremely rare for patients with lymph node metastases to be cured without their surgical removal
   3. Patients with esophageal and cardia cancer, like those with head and neck cancer, can die from lymph node metastasis alone
   4. Surgeons in China or Japan, who are incessant data keepers, accept unconditionally the benefit of lymph node dissection on survival in patients with carcinoma of the esophagus or stomach
   5. Forty-three percent of patients with esophageal carcinoma who have histologically node-negative disease have histochemical node-positive disease; further, after a median observation time of 12 months, patients with histochemical node-positive disease had a significantly shorter disease-free survival; on the basis of this finding, it is believed that when nodes are reported to be histologically free of tumor, more disease than what is currently appreciated is removed or left behind, depending on the extent of resection

a caudal direction. In the stomach, submucosal lymphatic channels contain valves that direct the lymph on the right side to the lesser curve nodes. The lymph on the left side is directed to the greater curvature nodes. Obstruction of the submucosal lymphatics along the lesser curve can cause reversal of lymph flow toward the greater curvature through extensive nonvalvular submucosal lymphatic channels. Consequently, cancers located in the lower esophagus or cardia can extend to a considerable length within the submucosal plexus superiorly in the esophagus, or inferiorly in several directions in the stomach. On the basis of this knowledge, the only means of assuring complete removal of all submucosal tumor spread is to resect a substantial portion of the stomach and the esophagus.

There is considerable support for this position in the literature. In patients with squamous cell carcinoma of the lower esophagus, a high esophageal anastomosis, and therefore a more extensive esophagectomy, tripled survival [45]. Similarly, Tam and associates [117] reported a high incidence of anastomotic recurrence when the proximal esophageal resected margin was less than 10 cm. Wong has shown that proximal anastomotic recurrence decreases as the length of the proximal margin increases. No recurrences were noted when the proximal margin was greater than 10 cm [131]. A similar emphasis on extensive esophageal resection can be made for adenocarcinoma of the cardia. Giuli and Sancho-Garnier [46], from the International Organization for Statistical Studies of the Esophageal Disease Data, reported a 19% 5-year survival rate for 360 patients with adenocarcinoma of the cardia. In 75% of the patients who had a late recurrence of tumor, it occurred, as with squamous cell tumors, in the residual portion of the esophagus. These findings would

encourage an extensive esophagectomy for cancers of the lower esophagus and cardia.

The need for an extensive gastric resection is similarly well documented. Squamous cell cancers of the lower esophagus infiltrate the stomach [90] and adenocarcinomas of the cardia infiltrate the esophagus. This is because the gastric cardia offers no barrier to the spread of carcinoma due to the anatomical continuity in the submucosa and muscle layers between the esophagus and stomach. This is in contrast to the gastroduodenal junction, where the submucosal continuity is greatly diminished by the pyloric glands and sphincter and provides considerable resistance to the spread of gastric cancer into the duodenum. Furthermore, the 15% incidence of positive splenic nodes for cancer of the lower esophagus would indicate that a considerable portion of spread is occurring transgastrically through the short gastric lymphatic channels and down along the splenic artery. The downward spread of esophageal cancer in the submucosal tissue of the stomach is not always obvious at operation. Clinically recurrent squamous cell carcinoma in the unresected portion of the stomach is considered unusual and is the basis for resecting less stomach in patients with this cancer type. We have, however, seen recurrent squamous cell carcinoma in the submucosa of the stomach used for esophageal replacement in patients who had total thoracic esophagectomy. Furthermore, we have seen carcinoma recur along the gastric suture line used to divide the stomach from the cardia. Wong has pointed out that because the esophagus is anastomosed to the fundus of the stomach, the stomach does not contribute to anastomotic recurrence. This is more due to inadequate esophageal resections. Instead, residual tumor at the gastric margin occurs along the lesser curve in the intrathoracic stomach and gives rise to back pain due to infiltration of the spine. In his experience, resection for cure failed to control local disease in 16% of his patients; half of the recurrences were at the esophagogastric anastomosis due to inadequate esophageal resection and half were in the intrathoracic stomach due to inadequate gastric resection [131]. To avoid intragastric recurrence, the resection should be at least 12 cm distal to visible tumor [75, 78]. This makes near total gastrectomy mandatory since the lesser curve of the stomach may be as short as 12 cm and the width of the fundus 10 cm [49, 121].

### Results

Recent data show that en bloc esophagogastrectomy results in significantly better 5-year survival despite the fact that postoperative pathologic staging showed that patients who underwent transhiatal esophagogastrectomy tended toward earlier disease (Fig. 13–20). Figs. 13–21 to 13–23 compare the actuarial survival following en bloc esophagogastrectomy and transhiatal esophagogastrectomy based on pathologic classification and stage of disease [51]. A clear survival advantage is observed in patients with early lesions following en bloc esophagogastrectomy, where the 5-year survival was 75%. This was less so for intermediate and late

lesions. Of interest, the results following transhiatal esophagogastrectomy were similar for early and intermediate disease, 19.8% and 21.0% at 2 years, respectively, and not much better than the 8.6% for late disease. Others have reported similar benefits of en bloc esophagectomy [6, 11, 41, 56, 58, 59, 67]. Table 13–9 shows operative mortality and survival data after en bloc resections performed by other authors.

Recent data show that in experienced hands, the morbidity and mortality of en bloc esophagectomy are equivalent to those for simple esophagectomy. Leru et al. compared the cause of death (Table 13–10) and complications in patients having curative nonradical, curative radical, and palliative esophagectomy [67]. There was no difference among the three groups of patients. Others have also shown that en bloc esophagectomy does not increase the prevalence of complications (Table 13–11) [11].

### Three-Field En Bloc Esophagectomy

Performing a more extended mediastinal dissection combined with a radical neck dissection has been advocated by some authors for the curative treatment of esophageal carcinoma [9, 80, 86] (Fig. 13–24). We have shown that the site of nodal recurrence following two-field en bloc resection

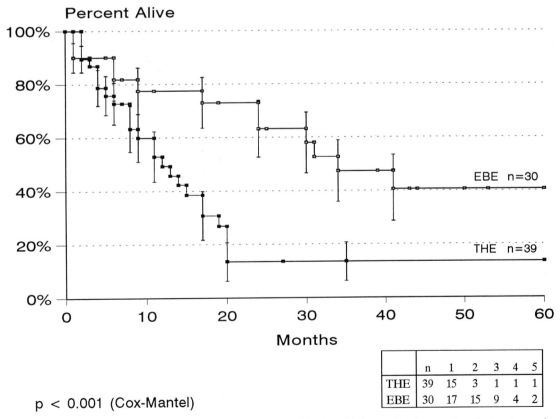

p < 0.001 (Cox-Mantel)

|      | n  | 1  | 2  | 3 | 4 | 5 |
|------|----|----|----|---|---|---|
| THE  | 39 | 15 | 3  | 1 | 1 | 1 |
| EBE  | 30 | 17 | 15 | 9 | 4 | 2 |

**FIG. 13–20.** Survival probabilities calculated by the Kaplan–Meier method according to the type of procedure performed. *EBE,* En bloc esophagogastrectomy; *THE,* transhiatal esophagogastrectomy. (From ref. 51.)

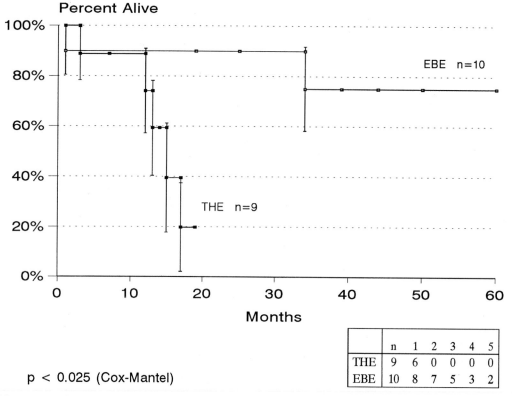

| | n | 1 | 2 | 3 | 4 | 5 |
|---|---|---|---|---|---|---|
| THE | 9 | 6 | 0 | 0 | 0 | 0 |
| EBE | 10 | 8 | 7 | 5 | 3 | 2 |

p < 0.025 (Cox-Mantel)

**FIG. 13–21.** Survival probabilities calculated by the Kaplan–Meier method according to the type of procedure performed in patients with early disease at the time of pathologic classification of removed specimen. *EBE,* En bloc esophagogastrectomy; *THE,* transhiatal esophagogastrectomy (From ref. 51.)

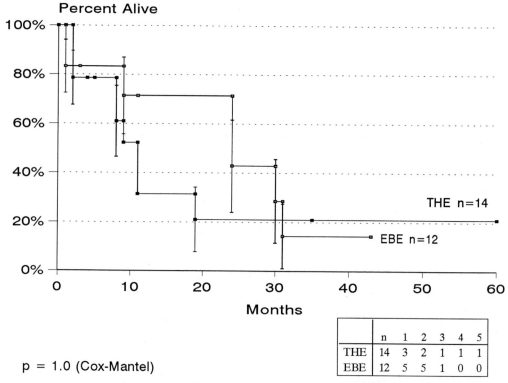

| | n | 1 | 2 | 3 | 4 | 5 |
|---|---|---|---|---|---|---|
| THE | 14 | 3 | 2 | 1 | 1 | 1 |
| EBE | 12 | 5 | 5 | 1 | 0 | 0 |

p = 1.0 (Cox-Mantel)

**FIG. 13–22.** Survival probabilities calculated by the Kaplan–Meier method according to the type of procedure performed in patients with intermediate disease at the time of pathologic classification of removed specimens. *EBE,* En bloc esophagogastrectomy; *THE,* transhiatal esophagogastrectomy. (From ref. 51.)

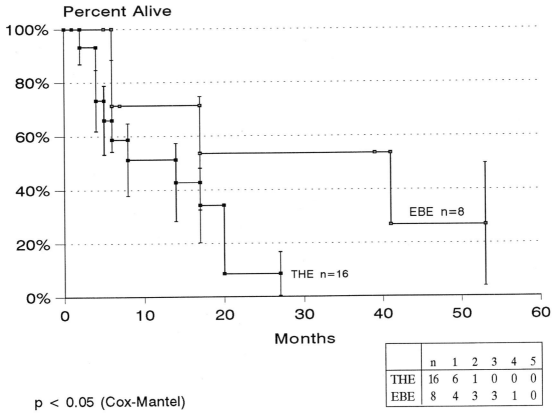

|      | n  | 1 | 2 | 3 | 4 | 5 |
|------|----|---|---|---|---|---|
| THE  | 16 | 6 | 1 | 0 | 0 | 0 |
| EBE  | 8  | 4 | 3 | 3 | 1 | 0 |

p < 0.05 (Cox-Mantel)

**FIG. 13–23.** Survival probabilities calculated by the Kaplan–Meier method according to the type of procedure performed in patients with late disease at the time of pathologic classification of removed specimen. *EBE*, En bloc esophagogastrectomy; *THE*, transhiatal esophagogastrectomy. (From ref. 51.)

**TABLE 13–9.** *Results of curative en bloc esophagectomy for tumors of the lower esophagus and cardia*

| Author | Year | N | Operative mortality (%) | Five-year actuarial survival (%) |
|--------|------|---|-------------------------|----------------------------------|
| Logan [71] | 1963 | 251 | 21 | 16 |
| Skinner [111] | 1983 | 31 | 9.7 | 22 |
| DeMeester et al. [31] | 1988 | 14 | 7 | 53 |
| Lerut et al. [67] | 1992 | 54 | 7.4 | 48 |
| Hagen et al. [51] | 1993 | 30 | 10 | 41 |
| Akiyama et al. [6] | 1994 | | | |
| Two field | | 84 | 5.2[a] | 39.3 |
| Three field | | 74 | | 48.0 |

[a] Data not limited to lower esophageal tumors.

**TABLE 13–10.** *Comparison of mortality and morbidity for en bloc versus standard esophagectomy*

| Morbidity | Curative nonradical (N = 75) | Curative en bloc (N = 54) | Palliative (N = 69) |
|-----------|------------------------------|---------------------------|---------------------|
| Death | 8 (10.6%) | 4 (7.4%) | 7 (10.1%) |
| Complications | 12 (16%) | 15 (27.6%) | 17 (24.6%) |

[a] Modified from Lerut et al. [67].

**TABLE 13–11.** *Comparison of mortality and morbidity for en bloc versus standard esophagectomy*

| Morbidity/mortality | Standard resection (N = 50) | En bloc resection (N = 78) |
|---------------------|-----------------------------|----------------------------|
| In-hospital death | 3 (6%) | 4 (5.1%) |
| Complications | | |
| Respiratory | 13 (26%) | 19 (24%) |
| Cardiac | 4 (8%) | 3 (3.8%) |
| Leaks | 8 (16%) | 10 (12.8%) |
| Recurrent nerve injury | 1 (2%) | 3 (3.8%) |
| Other | 8 (16%) | 11 (13%) |

[a] From Altorki et al. [11].

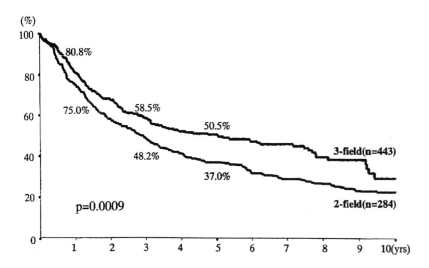

**FIG. 13–24.** Comparison of survival between two-field and three-field en bloc esophagectomy. (From Akiyama H, Tsurumaru M, Udagawa H, Kajiyama Y. Esophageal cancer. Curr Prob Surg 1997;34:765.)

was outside the limits of the resection in 80% of patients with recurrent disease [23]. All patients with thoracic nodal recurrence had the disease in their upper mediastinum or aortopulmonary window, suggesting that these recurrences arose from nodes lying along the recurrent laryngeal nerve chains and are not routinely removed by the en bloc dissection. Nishihara et al. recently reported a prospective randomized trial of two versus three field en bloc resections [80]. Two- and 5-year survival were significantly improved by the three-field resection (Table 13–12). Morbidity was significant, however, with over half of the patients in the three-field group suffering recurrent nerve palsy resulting in an astronomical 53% incidence of the need for tracheostomy (Table 13–13). The increased morbidity and the possibility of permanent hoarseness associated with this approach have discouraged its widespread application.

In summary, as the understanding of the pathology of esophageal cancer improves and experience with its resection increases, evidence is accumulating that for patients with an intramural tumor in the distal esophagus or cardia the best chance for cure is an en bloc esophagectomy and proximal gastrectomy with gastrointestinal continuity reestablished with a colon interposition. For patients with a tumor in the upper or cervical esophagus, the best chance for cure is an en bloc esophagectomy and a cervical lymph node dissection with gastrointestinal continuity reestablished with a gastric pullup. Table 13–14 presents a sum-

mary of the extent of resection for tumors extending various depths into the esophageal wall [27].

### Technique of En Bloc Resection for Cancer of the Lower Esophagus and Cardia

We perform the en bloc resection for carcinoma of the distal esophagus and cardia through three incisions and in the following order: right posterolateral thoracotomy, en bloc dissection of the esophagus below the aortic arch and mobilization of the esophagus above the aortic arch, closure of the thoracotomy, repositioning of the patient in the recumbent position, upper midline abdominal incision, en bloc dissection of the stomach and associated lymph nodes, left neck incision, proximal division of the esophagus, transhiatal removal of the previous en bloc dissected distal esophagus and mobilized proximal esophagus, distal division of the stomach, and reestablishment of gastrointestinal continuity with a left colon interposition.

The thoracic portion of the resection constitutes an en bloc removal of the distal thoracic esophagus below the aortic arch with its surrounding areolar tissue containing the low paratracheal, tracheobronchial, subcarinal, paraesophageal, and parahiatal lymph nodes; the thoracic duct; the azygos vein down to where it passes into the abdomen on the lateral surface of the vertebra; and a collar of diaphragmatic muscle around the esophageal hiatus. The block of tissue removed

**TABLE 13–12.** *Prospective randomized trial of extended cervical and mediastinal lymphadenectomy*

|  | Three field (N = 32) | Two field (N = 30) |
|---|---|---|
| Mean operating room time (min) | 487 ± 47 | 396 ± 43 |
| Mean blood loss (cc) | 850 ± 429 | 576 ± 261 |
| Rate of hospital deaths (%) | 3 | 7 |
| Two-year survival (%) | 83.3* | 64.8 |
| Five-year survival (%) | 66.2* | 48 |

*a* From Nishihara et al. [80].
* *p* < 0.192.

**TABLE 13–13.** *Prospective randomized trial of extended cervical and mediastinal lymphadenectomy: morbidity*

| Morbidity | Three field (N = 32) | Two field (N = 30) |
|---|---|---|
| Pulmonary complications | 6 (19%) | 5 (17%) |
| Recurrent nerve palsy | 18 (56%) | 9 (30%) |
| Phrenic nerve palsy | 4 (13%)* | 0 (0%) |
| Tracheostomy | 17 (53%)* | 3 (10%) |
| Anastomotic leak | 2 (6%) | 6 (20%) |

*a* From Nishihara et al. [80].
* *p* < 0.001.

**TABLE 13–14.** *Recommended surgical therapy for esophageal carcinoma*

| Lesion | Resection |
| --- | --- |
| Confined areas of high-grade dysplasia (intraepidermal cancer) | Endoscopic mucosal resection (at present only applicable to squamous carcinoma); vagal sparing esophagectomy |
| Widespread or circumferential area of high-grade dysplasia (intraepidermal cancer) | En bloc esophagectomy with appropriate lymph node dissection (see below) and preservation of the spleen; reconstruction with a gastric pullup |
| Tumor invading through the basement membrane, but not through the muscularis mucosa (intramucosal tumors) | |
| Tumor deeper than muscularis mucosa, but not through the esophageal wall (intramural tumors) | En bloc esophagectomy with appropriate systematic lymphadenectomy of the cervical, upper mediastinal (above tracheal bifurcation), lower mediastinal (below tracheal bifurcation), and abdominal nodes (for upper- and middle-third cancers, mediastinal dissection must include the node along the left recurrent nerve; for lower-third esophageal and cardia cancers, omit cervical and upper mediastinal node dissection, but include proximal stomach in the resection; for upper-third esophageal cancers, omit abdominal lymph node dissection); reconstruction with gastric pullup for middle- and upper-third tumors, and with colon interposition for lower-third and cardia tumors |
| Tumor extending through the muscularis propria (transmural tumors) | Same as for intramural tumors unless five or more lymph nodes are assumed to be involved, in which case a palliative transhiatal esophagectomy is done |

is limited anteriorly by the pericardium, laterally by the right and left mediastinal pleura, and posteriorly by the intercostal arteries, aorta, and anterior vertebral ligaments.

The abdominal portion of the resection constitutes an en bloc removal of all the posterior peritoneal periaortic areolar tissue down to the celiac axis and the superior border of the common hepatic and splenic artery, the greater omentum, and the proximal two-thirds of the stomach. In lesions that involve the cardia the spleen and splenic artery are included in the resection. The block of tissue includes lymph nodes along the left gastric artery, around the celiac axis, superior to and underneath the common hepatic artery, medial to the portal triad, in the greater omentum, and along the splenic artery down to the celiac axis. This extensive resection is done to incorporate in the surgical specimen all the potentially involved regional lymph nodes and submucosal lymphatics of the stomach and distal esophagus. The pancreas is not removed.

The first part of the procedure is to perform a right posterolateral thoracotomy through the seventh intercostal space along the upper border of the eighth rib. The intercostal branches of the azygos vein are divided from its arch down to where it passes into the abdomen on the lateral surface of the vertebra (Fig. 13–25). The segments of the posterior pleura between the ligated intercostal veins are divided with an incision parallel to the long axis of the spine. The posterior dissection is extended in the direction of the left chest along the intercostal arteries to the aorta and over the anterior surface of the aorta, through the left mediastinal pleura, and into the left pleural cavity (Fig. 13–26). To do so, the intact azygos vein and its surrounding tissues are retracted anteriorly, which allows the hemiazygos vein(s) to be seen as it crosses over the spine underneath the aorta to join the azygos vein. The hemiazygos vein must be identified, ligated, and divided. The aorta becomes visible when this vein is divided and serves as a guide for the extension of the posterior incision into the left side of the chest. Early division of the azygos vein at its junction with the superior vena cava is

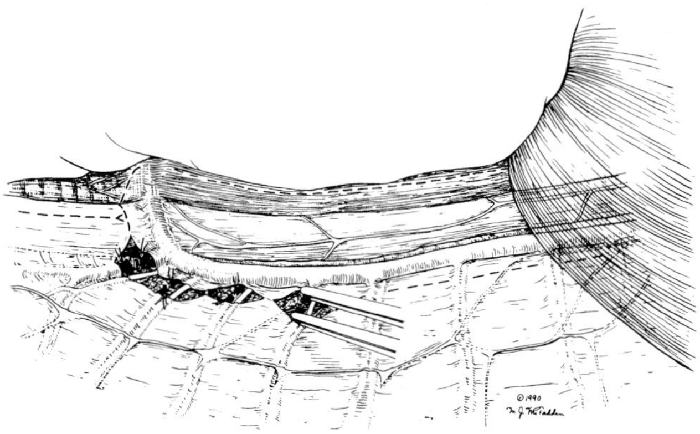

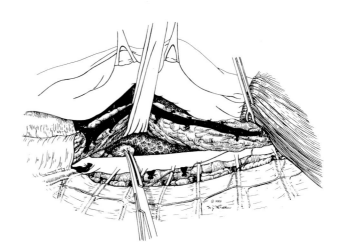

**FIG. 13–25.** En bloc esophagectomy: division of the intercostal veins over the course of the azygos vein.

**FIG. 13–26.** En bloc esophagectomy: dissection along the intercostal arteries.

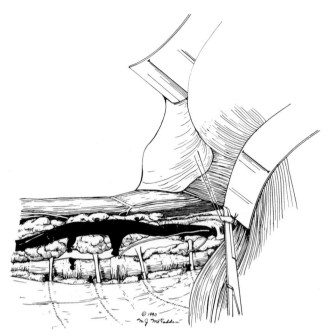

**FIG. 13–27.** En bloc esophagectomy: ligation of the thoracic duct.

avoided because it contributes to venous hypertension in the azygos system and excessive bleeding during the posterior mediastinal dissection. At the caudal end of the posterior pleural incision, where the azygos vein was ligated distally, the thoracic duct is identified, divided, and ligated (Fig. 13–27).

Anteriorly, the mediastinum is entered through a longitudinal pleural incision made parallel to the posterior margin of the trachea, hilum, and pericardium down to the diaphragm. The anterior dissection is extended across in the direction of the left chest along the posterior surface of the right main stem bronchus, trachea, left main stem bronchus, and the pericardium anterior to the subcarinal nodes (Fig. 13–28). To do so requires division of the azygos vein at its entry into the superior vena cava. When both the anterior

and posterior dissections of the posterior mediastinum are complete, the esophagus, encased in its periareolar tissues containing the paratracheal, subcarinal, paraesophageal, and parahiatal nodes, is pulled into the right thorax and freed by sharp division of a strip of left mediastinal pleura. Care must be taken to avoid damage to the left recurrent nerve near the aortic arch. The nerve can be identified as it comes underneath the aortic arch just above the left main stem bronchus. Its common course is to pass directly to the trachea without redundancy and to lie on the left posterolateral cartilaginous wall as it passes up into the neck. Identifying it underneath the aortic arch for mobilization of the proximal esophagus without damage to the nerve. Occasionally it follows the left lateral wall of the esophagus up into the neck. Inferiorly, a collar of diaphragmatic muscle is excised around the esophageal hiatus. Superiorly, the esophagus is bluntly dissected into the neck, but is not divided (Fig. 13–29). No attempt is made to do an en bloc dissection above the level of the aortic arch. Suspicious nodes above the aortic arch are biopsied and, if positive, the en bloc dissection is abandoned for a palliative procedure. When the dissection is complete, hemostasis is assured and the specimen left in the chest. The thoracotomy incision is closed.

Next, the patient is moved to the recumbent position. The previously inserted double-lumen endotracheal tube, used for selected deflation of the right lung, is removed and a single-lumen tube is inserted. The anterior neck, chest, and abdomen are prepared and draped, and an upper midline abdominal incision is made. Exposure for the abdominal dissection is facilitated by a Weinberg retractor that has been welded to a Balfour handle and attached to an overarm bar. The abdominal dissection begins with the removal of the greater omentum from the transverse mesocolon. The spleen along with the tail of the pancreas is mobilized to the midline in those patients in which it is to be removed. In those in which the spleen is not be to be removed the short gastrics are divided near the splenic hilum. The abdominal dissection continues along the left crus, where the thoracic dissection

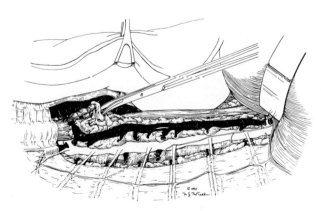

**FIG. 13–28.** En bloc esophagectomy: dissection of subcarinal lymph nodes.

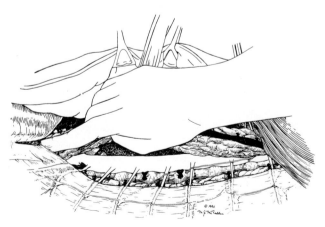

**FIG. 13–29.** En bloc esophagectomy: finger dissection of the proximal esophagus.

was discontinued. The excision of a collar of diaphragmatic muscle is continued down the margin of the left crus to the celiac axis. The pancreas is identified, and the splenic artery, along with its vein and associated lymph nodes, is dissected off the superior border of the tail of the gland. The splenic vein is ligated approximately midway down the pancreas, where it turns inferiorly and leaves the artery. Removal of the splenic artery, along with its associated lymph nodes, is continued down to the celiac axis, using the palpation of the pulse as a guide to the dissection. At its origin from the celiac axis, the splenic artery is divided, which allows for the identification of left gastric artery (Fig. 13–30). In patients in which the spleen is not removed the splenic artery is sceletonized and all retroperitoneal periaortic areolar tissue superior to it is removed with the specimen. In this situation the pancreas is left undisturbed.

On the right side, the gastrohepatic ligament is divided along the liver margin up to the esophageal hiatus (Fig. 13–31). Care must be taken not to interrupt a large aberrant hepatic artery that might be lying in this mesentery. If present, it is to be sceletonized back to its junction with the left gastric artery. The posterior peritoneal tissue underneath and along the superior border of the common hepatic artery, and the areolar tissue containing lymph nodes along the medial border of the portal triad, are swept toward the celiac axis. Dissection of a collar of diaphragmatic muscle around the esophageal hiatus, which was begun during the thoracic portion of the operation, is continued down the right crus. The dissection of the hiatus is completed with the division of the left gastric artery at its origin from the celiac artery or just proximal to a large aberrant hepatic branch.

The esophagus is exposed and divided in the neck through

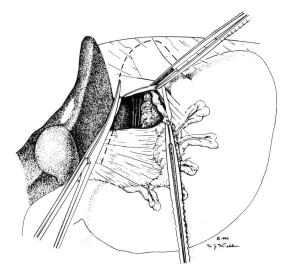

**FIG. 13–31.** En bloc esophagectomy: division of the gastrohepatic ligament and dissection of a collar of diaphragmatic muscle around the hiatus.

an incision made along the anterior border of the left sternocleidomastoid muscle. Care is taken to identify and protect the left recurrent laryngeal nerve. The dissection is carried out as described for the transhiatal resection. The cervical esophagus is divided leaving a length of 3 to 4 cm, and the specimen is removed from the posterior mediastinum transabdominally. The stomach is divided by a GIA stapler at the level of antrum (Fig. 13–32). Gastrointestinal continuity is reestablished between the proximal esophagus in the neck and the remaining gastric antrum in the abdomen with an isoperistaltic left colon transplant based on the left colic

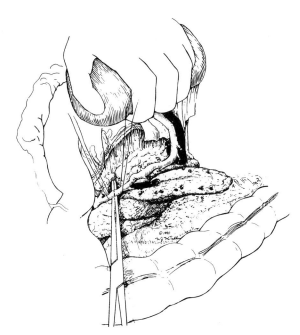

**FIG. 13–30.** En bloc esophagectomy: mobilization and division of splenic artery and splenic vein.

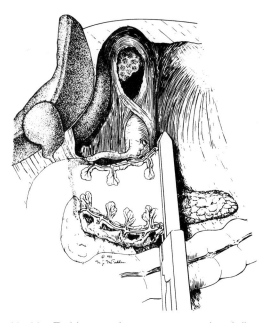

**FIG. 13–32.** En bloc esophagectomy: completed dissection of the abdominal portion of the en bloc resection. The stomach is divided by a stapler at the level of the antrum.

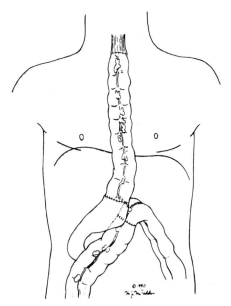

**FIG. 13–33.** En bloc esophagectomy: reconstruction of the gastrointestinal tract with left colon interposition after en bloc resection. Distal anastomosis is made to the antral portion of the stomach and proximal anastomosis to the esophagus in the neck. (From ref. 31, with permission.)

artery and the inferior mesenteric vein (Fig. 13–33) [30]. The retention of the antrum and the pyloric valve improves postoperative gastrointestinal function sufficiently to merit salvage. The colon transplant is pulled up through the posterior mediastinum with the aid of an upside-down Mousseau-Barbin tube encased in a trimmed cellophane bowel bag.

Of importance is that if the operation has lasted too long, if the patient is unstable, or if the arterial supply or venous drainage of the colon is not satisfactory, then the colon is not divided, an intramural jejunostomy tube is inserted, and a cervical esophagostomy is constructed. The divided proximal marginal and middle colic artery and vein will increase the collateral flow to the colon transplant and avoid the necessity of dissecting the base of the middle colic artery and vein at a later date. The transverse mesocolon should be opened wide and the entire small bowel brought through the opening so that the transverse colon lies under the small bowel low in the abdomen. The transverse colon is sutured to the low anterior abdominal wall to prevent its migration into the upper quadrant and adherence of the transverse mesocolon to the denuded splenic bed. The patient is discharged on jejunostomy tube feedings, and returns in 90 days for reestablishment of gastrointestinal continuity with the previously delayed isoperistaltic left colon graft through the substernal route. The one-stage operation is preferred because postoperative adhesions and scarring of the transverse mesocolon can limit the length of the colon transplant, but the reconstruction phase should not be done unless everything is satisfactory.

## PALLIATION OF ESOPHAGEAL CANCER

If a patient's lesion is considered incurable on preoperative or intraoperative evaluation, palliative therapy is provided only if the patient has symptoms that can be palliated. Since palliative surgery is usually followed by terminal illness, the objective of therapy is to provide adequate symptomatic relief with the lowest mortality and shortest hospital stay possible. It is well documented that if the patient is physiologically fit, a simple esophageal resection and reconstruction with an esophagogastrostomy offers the best palliation. It allows the patient to eat without dysphagia and prevents the local complications of perforation, hemorrhage, fistulization, and incapacitating pain from tumor infiltration. Occasionally, a patient will be cured by a palliative resection, but this should not be used as justification for the operative procedure in the absence of symptoms. A surgical resection for cure should be abandoned if cure is not possible and the patient has no symptoms to be palliated, provided the dissection is at a point where it is safe to do so. The decision for palliative esophageal resection and timing of the procedure should be made carefully, since at least 2 months of physical disability usually follows esophageal resection. Transhiatal esophagectomy is the most common procedure in the palliative setting.

If an obstructing tumor cannot be resected (a) owing to invasion of the trachea, aorta, or heart, (b) when distant organ metastases are present, or (c) when a patient's general condition precludes an extensive surgical procedure, relief of dysphagia by reestablishing the esophageal lumen is indicated. A variety of techniques are available, including bougienage, intubation, irradiation, laser ablation, and electrical coagulation, which can be used alone or in combination [100]. These techniques are discussed elsewhere in this volume. Surgical bypass is rarely indicated given modern alternate options.

### Technique of Transhiatal Esophagogastrectomy for Cancer of the Thoracic Esophagus

Patients with upper or midthoracic esophageal tumors and bronchoscopic evidence of a tracheobronchial invasion are not candidates for a transhiatal esophagectomy. Similarly, if, on exploration, the tumor is fixed to the aorta, pericardium, or the tracheobronchial tree, it is unwise to proceed with a transhiatal esophagectomy. In performing the transhiatal esophagectomy, the surgeon must be prepared to open the thorax and to resect the esophagus if the transhiatal approach becomes too dangerous and is aborted, or if complications occur during the transhiatal dissection.

The published work of Orringer [83, 87] is an excellent guide on the transhiatal resection, and our personal experience is heavily based on his work. The patient is placed on the operating table in the manner described for resection of a cervical esophageal cancer, i.e., the right chest is elevated 20 degrees and the right hand placed under the right buttock in order to have access to the right chest through an anterolateral thoracotomy, should that be necessary. A double-lumen endotracheal tube is used so that, should the chest need to be entered, one lung can be collapsed to facilitate the exposure.

The abdomen is entered through the upper midline incision. The surgeon's hand is inserted into the mediastinum through the diaphragmatic hiatus and grasps the tumor-containing portion of the esophagus to determine if it is fixed to the paravertebral fascia, pericardium, aorta, or tracheobronchial tree. Such fixation excludes resection by this route. Once it has been determined that the esophagus is mobile enough to be resected through the hiatus, the stomach is prepared as a substitute for the esophagus in the manner described for the resection of cervical esophageal tumors. If the tumor is at the gastroesophageal junction, the surgeon should proceed with the resection only if he or she is satisfied that there is sufficient stomach available to allow an adequate margin distal to the tumor with enough greater curvature to reach the neck.

After the stomach has been completely mobilized, the esophagogastric junction is encircled with a rubber drain. Downward traction on this drain by one hand tenses the esophagus as the other hand is inserted through the diaphragmatic hiatus and blunt gentle mobilization of the lower 10 cm of the esophagus from the mediastinum is carried out. When the esophageal tumor does not involve the distal esophagus, and after manual assessment of the tumor-containing esophagus through the diaphragmatic hiatus reveals

a resectable lesion, the esophagus, just above the esophagogastric junction, is divided with a GIA stapler and the lower end of the esophagus is grasped with a serrated bronchial clamp. The clamp, rather than the stomach, is then used for subsequent traction on the esophagus to minimize trauma to the stomach that will subsequently be used to replace the esophagus. A GIA stapler is used to divide the cardia near the gastroesophageal junction and the staple line is oversewn. Alternatively, a purse-string suture may be placed closely around the base of the cardia, and the gastroesophageal junction suture-ligated and inverted into the stomach. After 10 cm of distal esophagus has been mobilized, attention is turned to the neck.

A 7-cm incision is made along the anterior border of the left sternocleidomastoid muscle, starting at the suprasternal notch (Fig. 13–34). The sternohyoid and sternothyroid muscles are identified and divided at their sternoclavicular origin. This gives excellent exposure into the base of the neck. The carotid sheath and its contents are retracted laterally, and the thyroid, larynx, and trachea are retracted medially (Fig. 13–35). The recurrent laryngeal nerve is identified and protected. Care should be taken not to place a retractor directly on the nerve. The middle thyroid vein and inferior thyroid artery must also be divided.

A small indentation can be seen between the trachea and the esophagus just below the left recurrent laryngeal nerve. The dissection is begun in this area, with the scissors directed

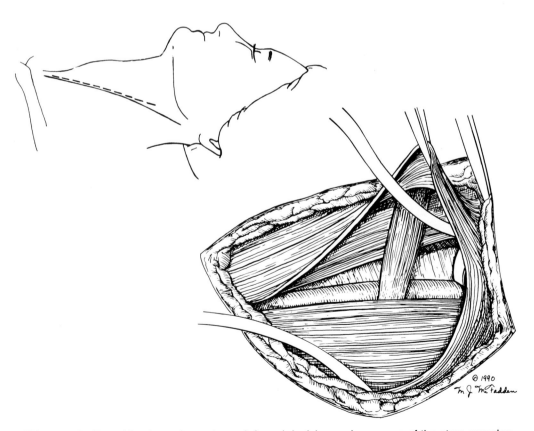

FIG. 13–34. Transhiatal esophagectomy: left neck incision and exposure of the strap muscles.

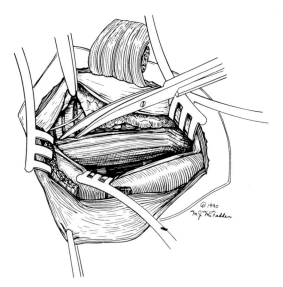

**FIG. 13–35.** Transhiatal esophagectomy: retraction of the carotid sheath laterally and the thyroid, larynx, and trachea medially. Demonstration of the left recurrent laryngeal nerve.

between the esophagus and trachea in a caudal direction. This is done so that the tip of the scissors reaches a point approximately 3 to 4 cm lower on the right side than on the left side of the esophagus. This is to avoid injury to the right recurrent nerve, which lies lateral to the esophagus at this point. The cervical esophagus is mobilized in this plane circumferentially and encircled with a rubber drain (Fig. 13–36). Upward traction is exerted on the drain, and blunt dissection of the upper esophagus from the posterior surface of the trachea is carried out.

The transhiatal dissection is then performed both from the neck and abdomen. The abdominal dissection is facilitated by enlarging the hiatus with a 2-cm incision made in the

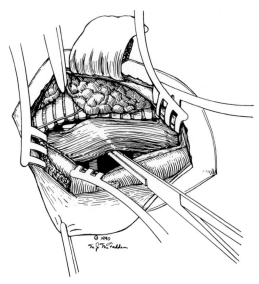

**FIG. 13–36.** Transhiatal esophagectomy: dissection of the cervical esophagus.

diaphragm anteriorly under the pericardium. Downward traction on the caudal esophagus is maintained by grasping the bronchial clamp with one hand as the opposite hand is inserted behind the esophagus and progressively advanced into the chest, sweeping away the loose areolar and periesophageal tissues and developing the prevertebral space to the level of the carina. The dissection is continued in the neck by upward traction on the rubber drain. The surgeon introduces her or his index and middle fingers through the neck incision along the paravertebral fascia and develops a paravertebral space. A clamp grasping a Kitner sponge dissector inserted into the superior mediastinum through the cervical incision facilitates the dissection. The esophagus is swept away from the paravertebral fascia from above until the Kitner sponge makes contact with the surgeon's hand inserted from below through the diaphragmatic hiatus. This completes the mobilization of the posterior esophagus from the prevertebral fascia. Blood pressure should be monitored during this maneuver because intermittent hypotension can occur from cardiac compression by the surgeon's abdominal hand.

The anterior dissection is performed as a mirror image of the posterior mobilization. The caudal end of the esophagus is retracted downward, and the opposite hand is inserted palm down through the diaphragmatic hiatus. The esophagus is swept away from the mediastinal structures by applying posterior pressure. To avoid injury to the posterior membranous trachea, the fingers and then a Kitner sponge dissector are inserted through the cervical incision anterior to the esophagus and behind the trachea until contact is made with a hand inserted from below. Anterior mobilization of the esophagus is then completed, leaving only the lateral esophageal attachments undivided.

Lateral mobilization of the upper 5 to 8 cm and the lower 8 to 10 cm of the intrathoracic esophagus can be achieved under direct vision through the cervical and abdominal incisions. To mobilize the remaining portion of the esophagus, the right hand is inserted through the diaphragmatic hiatus anterior to the esophagus and up into the superior mediastinum behind the trachea until the index and middle fingers can feel the circumferentially mobilized upper esophagus. The esophagus is trapped between the index and middle fingers, which are pressed posteriorly against the prevertebral fascia as a downward raking motion of the hand evulses any small remaining periesophageal attachments.

At times, dense attachments, usually branches of the vagal nerves, in and around the carina can prevent complete mobilization of the esophagus. These bands can be hooked by the fingers of the left hand or with a nerve hook and retracted toward the hiatus. Usually this will isolate the residual bands holding the midportion of the esophagus to allow them to be cut with large scissors inserted through the hiatus and guided to the bands by the left hand and fingers. This maneuver, however, generally is not necessary. After complete mobilization, the intrathoracic esophagus is delivered out of the cervical incision, or the abdominal incision after the cervical esophagus has been divided.

If the stomach is to be used for the reconstruction, the tip of the fundus that reaches most cephalad is identified and sutured to the side of an inverted funnel of a Mousseau-Barbin tube. The stomach is then wrapped in a bowel bag that has been cut to size and lubricated with saline. The tube is passed through the posterior mediastinum and up into the neck, pulling the stomach behind it. Very little traction is required when using these aids. Traction is placed on the cellophane bowel bag rather than the stomach itself. Once in the neck, the gastric fundus is suspended to the prevertebral fascia with 3-0 polypropylene sutures and the cervical esophagus is anastomosed to the anterior wall of the stomach in the manner described for the transthoracic esophagectomy. Prior to pulling the stomach up into the neck, the limbs of two Jackson-Pratt catheters are drawn into the posterior mediastinum via the cervical incision and out the esophageal hiatus. With the stomach in place, the catheters are positioned so that a portion of the drains extends through the esophageal hiatus into the abdomen. They are brought out through a stab incision in the anterior abdominal wall and are used to drain the posterior mediastinum, subphrenic area, and chest cavity, should that be necessary. A nasogastric tube is used to decompress the intrathoracic stomach and is passed across the anastomosis at the time of its construction.

Complications of transhiatal esophagectomy include pneumothorax, tracheal tear, hemorrhage, hoarseness from recurrent nerve injury, anastomotic disruption, chylothorax, and sympathetic pleural effusion. The most common intraoperative complication is entry into one or both pleural cavities during the mediastinal dissection. A tear of the posterior membranous trachea during the dissection can be disastrous, and management of this situation is greatly facilitated with the use of a double-lumen tube. It is advisable to do an anterolateral right thoracotomy and repair the tear directly. Exposure of the tear through this incision is excellent if ventilation to the right lung can be interrupted. Major intraoperative bleeding is an exception rather than the rule; if excessive, it is usually due to damage to the azygos vein and requires a thoracotomy to control.

## ADJUVANT THERAPY

### Adjuvant Radiation Therapy Alone

Adjuvant radiation therapy alone has been well studied and does not prolong survival [39, 40, 44]. Several prospective randomized studies have been performed without demonstrable benefit. Currently, the use of radiotherapy is restricted to patients who are not candidates for surgery. Palliation of dysphagia is short term, generally lasting only 2 to 3 months.

### Adjuvant Chemotherapy Alone

The use of chemotherapy in addition to surgical resection for esophageal cancer has been studied for decades [16, 65, 120]. Theoretically, effective systemic therapy would treat undetected systemic micrometastasis present at the time of diagnosis and improve survival. Recently this hypothesis has been supported by the observation of epithelial tumor cells in the bone marrow in 37% of patients with esophageal cancer who were resected for cure [122]. These patients had a greater prevalence of relapse at 9 months after surgery compared to those patients without such cells. Such studies emphasize that hematogenous dissemination of viable malignant cells occurs early in the disease and that systemic chemotherapy may be helpful if the cells are sensitive to the agent. Unfortunately, there has been no consistent demonstration of benefit with adjuvant chemotherapy alone, either given before or after surgery.

Three randomized prospective studies of neoadjuvant chemotherapy in squamous cell carcinoma have been completed. Each shows no survival benefit over surgery alone (Table 13–15) [81, 104, 106]. Similar studies for adenocarcinoma have not been done. For squamous cell tumors a complete response to chemotherapy occurred only in 6% of patients.

With the exception of the potential to improve resectability of tumors located above the carina, the benefits of preoperative chemotherapy are questionable. It is agreed that preoperative chemotherapy alone can potentially downstage the tumor, particularly squamous cell carcinoma. It also can potentially eliminate or delay the appearance of metastasis. However, there is no evidence that it can prolong survival of patients with resectable carcinoma of the esophagus. Most failures are due to distant metastatic disease, underscoring the need for improved systemic therapy. Further, postoperative septic and respiratory complications are more common in patients receiving chemotherapy.

### Combination Chemoradiotherapy

Preoperative chemoradiotherapy using cisplatin and 5-fluorouracil in combination with radiotherapy has been re-

TABLE 13–15. *Esophageal carcinoma: randomized preoperative chemotherapy versus surgery alone*[a]

| Authors | Year | $n$ = C/S | Cell type | Regimen[b] | CR (%) | Survival C vs. S |
|---|---|---|---|---|---|---|
| Roth et al. [104] | 1988 | 19/20 | Squamous | P, V, B | 6 | NS |
| Nygaard et al. [81] | 1992 | 50/41 | Squamous | P, B | — | NS |
| Schlag [106] | 1992 | 21/24 | Squamous | P, 5-FU | 5 | NS |

[a] C, Preoperative chemotherapy; S, surgery only; CR, complete response to chemotherapy.
[b] P, Cisplatin; V, vindesine; B, bleomycin; 5-FU, 5-fluorouracil.

**TABLE 13–16.** *Esophageal carcinoma: randomized preoperative chemoradiotherapy versus surgery alone*[a]

| Authors | Year | N = C/S | Cell type[b] | Regimen[c] | Survival C vs. S |
|---|---|---|---|---|---|
| Nygaard et al. [81] | 1992 | 47/41 | Squamous | P, B, 35 Gy | NS |
| LePrise et al. [66] | 1994 | 41/45 | Squamous | P, 5-FU, 20 Gy | NS |
| Apinop et al. [12] | 1994 | 35/34 | Squamous | P, 5-FU, 40 Gy | NS |
| Walsh et al. [129] | 1996 | 48/54 | AC | P, 5-FU, 40 Gy | $p = 0.01$ |
| Bosset et al. [20] | 1997 | 143/139 | Squamous | P, 18.5 Gy | NS |
| Urba et al. [127] | 1997 | 50/50 | Squamous + AC | P, 5-FU, V, 45 Gy | NS |

[a] Preoperative chemotherapy; S, surgery only.
[b] AC, Adenocarcinoma.
[c] P, Cisplatin; B, bleomycin; 5-FU, 5-fluorouracil; V, vinblastine.

ported by several investigators to be beneficial in both adenocarcinoma and squamous cell carcinoma of the esophagus [12, 20, 66, 127, 129]. There have been six randomized prospective studies, four with squamous cell, one with both squamous cell and adenocarcinoma, and one with only adenocarcinoma (Table 13–16). A survival benefit has been shown in two of the six studies. Complete response rates for adenocarcinoma range from 17% to 24%. Most studies have shown a survival benefit in the subset of patients with no residual tumor at the time of resection (i.e., complete response). Thus, up to 25% of patients may benefit, while 75% will not. The question is whether this justifies treatment of all patients, particularly in light of the substantial morbidity and mortality that has been associated with multimodal therapy.

Although the studies of Walsh et al. [129] and Urba et al. [129] are encouraging, the collective data do not support the recommendation of routine neoadjuvant combination therapy. Several concerns remain. First, it must be kept in mind that the majority of studies have not shown any benefit. The reports of both Walsh et al. and Urba et al. are interim analyses at 3 and 4 years, respectively. The data may change with further follow-up. In the study by Walsh et al., if one more death occurs in the multimodal group, the $p$ value will go from 0.01 to 0.03, and with two deaths, to greater than 0.05. In addition, some studies have shown that the rates of infection, anastomotic breakdown, incidence of adult respiratory distress syndrome, and long-term use of a respirator were greater in patients receiving adjuvant therapy as compared with surgery alone.

At present, the strongest predictors of outcome of patients with esophageal cancer are the anatomic extent of the tumor at diagnosis and the completeness of tumor removal by surgical resection. All other predictors or therapies pale by comparison. After incomplete resection of an esophageal cancer the 5-year survival rate is 0% to 5%. In contrast, after complete resection, independent of stage of disease, 5-year survival ranges from 15% to 40% according to selection criteria and stage distribution. Consequently the importance of early recognition and adequate surgical resection cannot be overemphasized.

## REFERENCES

1. Adams W, Phemister DB. Carcinoma of the lower thoracic esophagus. Report of a successful resection and esophagogastrostomy. J Thorac Surg 1938;7:621
2. Akiyama H. Esophageal cancer. Curr Probl Surg 1997;34:801
3. Akiyama H, Kogwe T, Itai Y. The esophageal axis and its relationship to the resectability of carcinoma of the esophagus. Ann Surg 1971; 176:30
4. Akiyama H, Hiyama M, Miyazono H. Total esophageal reconstruction after extraction of the esophagus. Ann Surg 1975;182:547
5. Akiyama H, et al. Principles of surgical treatment for carcinoma of the esophagus: analysis of lymph node involvement. Ann Surg 1981; 194:438
6. Akiyma H, Tsurumaru M, Udagawa H, Kajiyama Y. Radical lymph node dissection for cancer of the thoracic esophagus. Ann Surg 1994; 220:364
7. Allardyce D, Groves A. A comparison of nutritional responses from intravenous and enteral feedings. Surg Gynecol Obstet 1974;139:179
8. Alpern DA, Buell C, Olson J. Increasing percentage of adenocarcinoma in primary carcinoma of the esophagus (letter). Am J Gastroenterol 1989;84:574
9. Altorki NK, Skinner DB. Occult cervical nodal metastasis in esophageal cancer: preliminary results of three-field lymphadenectomy. J Thorac Cardiovasc Surg 1997;113:540
10. Altorki NK, Sunagawa M, Little AG, Skinner DB. High grade dysplasia in the columnar lined esophagus. Am J Surg 1991;161:97
11. Altorki NK, Girardi L, Skinner DB. En bloc esophagectomy improves survival for state III esophageal cancer. J Thorac Cardiovasc Surg 1997;114:948
12. Apinop C, Puttisak P, Preecha N. A prospective study of combined therapy in esophageal cancer. Hepato-Gastroenterol 1994;41:391
13. Baker JW Jr, Schechter GL. Management of paraesophageal cancer by blunt resection without thoracotomy and reconstruction with stomach. Ann Surg 1986;203:491
14. Beatty JD, DeBoer G, Rider WD. Carcinoma of the esophagus: pretreatment assessment, correlation of radiation treatment parameters with survival, and identification and management of radiation treatment failure. Cancer 1979;43:2254
15. Belsey RHR, Hiebert CA. An exclusive right thoracic approach for cancer of the middle third of the oesophagus. Ann Thorac Surg 1974; 18:1
16. Bhansali MS, Vaidya JS, Bhatt RG, Patil PK, Badwe RA, Desai PB. Chemotherapy for carcinoma of the esophagus; a comparison of evidence from meta-analyses of randomized trials and of historical control studies. Ann Oncol 1996;7:355
17. Blot WJ, Devesa SS, Kneller RW, Fraumeni JF Jr, Rising incidence of adenocarcinoma of the esophagus and gastric cardia, JAMA 1991; 265:1287
18. Bolton JS, Ochsner JL, Abdoh AA. Surgical management of esophageal cancer. A decade of change. Ann Surg 1994;219:475
19. Bosch A, Frias Z, Caldwell WL. Adenocarcinoma of the esophagus. Cancer 1979;43:1557
20. Bossett JF, et al. Chemoradiotherapy followed by surgery compared

with surgery alone in squamous cell cancer of the esophagus. N Engl J Med 1997;337:161

21. Cameron AJ, Carpenter HA. Barrett's esophagus, high-grade dysplasia, and early adenocarcinoma: a pathological study. Am J Gastroenterol 1997;92:586

22. Cameron AJ, Ott BJ, Payne WS. The incidence of adenocarcinoma in columnar-lined (Barrett's) esophagus. N Engl J Med 1985;313:857

23. Clark GWB, et al. Nodal metastases and recurrence patterns after en-bloc esophagectomy for adenocarcinoma. Ann Thorac Surg 1994;58:646

24. Clark GWB, et al. Is Barrett's metaplasia the source of adenocarcinomas of the cardia? Arch Surg 1994;129:609

25. Colin CF, Spiro RH. Carcinoma of the cervical esophagus. Changing therapeutic trends. Am J Surg 1984;148:460

26. DeMeester TR. Surgical anatomy of the esophagus. In Shields TW, ed, General Thoracic Surgery (2nd ed.). Philadelphia: Lea & Febiger, 1983

27. DeMeester TR. Esophageal carcinoma; current controversies. Semin Surg Oncol 1997;13:217

28. DeMeester TR, Barlow AP. Surgery and current management for cancer of the esophagus and cardia. Curr Probl Cancer 1988;12:241

29. DeMeester TR, Lafontaine ER. Surgical therapy. In DeMeester TR, Levin B, eds, Cancer of the Esophagus. Orlando, FL: Grune & Stratton, 1985

30. DeMeester TR, et al. Indications, surgical technique, and long-term functional results of colon interposition or bypass. Ann Surg 1988;208:460

31. DeMeester TR, Zaninotto G, Johansson KE. Selective therapeutic approach to cancer of the lower esophagus and cardia. J Thorac Cardiovasc Surg 1988;95:42

32. Diener CF, Burrows, B. Further observations on the course and prognosis of chronic obstructive lung disease. Am Rev Respir Dis 1975;111:719

33. Duignan JP, et al. The role of CT in the management of carcinoma of the oesophagus and cardia. Ann R Coll Surg Engl 1987;69:286

34. Edwards MJ, Gable DR, Lentsch AB, Richardson JD. The rationale for esophagectomy as the optimal therapy for Barrett's esophagus with high grade dysplasia. Ann Surg 1996;223:585

35. Ellis FH Jr, Watkins E Jr, Krasna MJ, Heatley GJ, Balogh K. Staging of carcinoma of the esophagus and cardia: a comparison of different staging criteria. J Surg Oncol 1993;52:231

36. Ellis FH, Heatley GJ, Krosna MJ, Williamson WA, Balogh K. Esophagogastrectomy for carcinoma of the esophagus and cardia: a comparison of findings and results after standard resection in three consecutive 8 year time intervals, using improved staging criteria. J Thorac Cardiovasc Surg 1997;113:836

37. Fisher DR, Brawley RK, Kiefer RF. Esophagogastrostomy in the treatment of carcinoma of the distal two-thirds of the esophagus. Ann Thorac Surg 1972;14:658

38. Fok M, Siu KF, Wong J. A comparison of transhiatal and transthoracic resection for carcinoma of the thoracic esophagus. Am J Surg 1989;158:414

39. Fok M, Sham JST, Choy D, Cheng SWK, Wong J. Postoperative radiotherapy for carcinoma of the esophagus; a prospective randomized controlled study. Surgery 1993;113:138

40. French University Association for Surgical Research, Tiniere P, Hay JM, Fingerhut A, Fagniez PL. Postoperative radiation therapy does not increase survival after curative resection for squamous cell carcinoma of the middle and lower esophagus as shown by a multicenter controlled trial. Surg Gynecol Obstet 1991;173:123

41. Fujita H, et al. Mortality and morbidity rates, postoperative course, quality of life, and prognosis after extended radical lymphadenectomy for esophageal cancer. Ann Surg 1995;222:654

42. Games MN, et al. Mediastinal tracheostomy. Ann Thorac Surg 1987;43:539

43. Gammon MD, et al. Tobacco, alcohol and socioeconomic status and adenocarcinomas of the esophagus and gastric cardia. J Natl Cancer Inst 1997;89:1277

44. Gignoux M, et al. The value of preoperative radiotherapy in esophageal cancer; results of a study of the EORTC. World J Surg 1987;11:426

45. Giuli, R. Surgical complications and reasons for failure. In DeMeester

TR, Levin B, eds, Cancer of the Esophagus. Orlando, FL: Grune & Stratton, 1985

46. Giuli R, Sancho-Garnier H. Diagnostic, therapeutic and prognostic features of cancers of the esophagus: results of the international prospective study conducted by the OESO group. Surgery 1986;99:614

47. Goldfadden D, Orringer MB, Appelman HD, Kalish R. Adenocarcinoma of the distal esophagus and gastric cardia; comparison of results of transhiatal esophagectomy and thoracoabdominal esophagogastrectomy. J Thorac Cardiovasc Surg 1986;91:242

48. Goldminc M, Maddern G, Le Prise EL, Meunier B, Campion JP, Launois B. Oesophagectomy transhiatal approach or thoracotomy—a prospective randomized trial. Br J Surg 1993;80:367

49. Goldsmith HS, Akiyama H. A comparative study of Japanese and American gastric dimensions. Ann Surg 1979;190:690

50. Guyton AC, Lindsey AW. Effect of elevated left atrial pressure and decreased plasma protein concentration on the development of pulmonary edema. Circ Res 1959;7:649

51. Hagen JA, Peters JH, DeMeester TR. Superiority of extended en bloc esophagogastrectomy for carcinoma of the lower esophagus and cardia. J Thorac Cardiovasc Surg 1993;106:850

52. Hameeteman W, Tytgat GNJ, Houthoff HJ, Van Den Tweel JG. Barrett's esophagus: development of dysplasia and adenocarcinoma. Gastroenterology 1989;96:1249

53. Hankins JR, et al. Carcinoma of the esophagus; a comparison of the results of transhiatal versus transthoracic resection. Ann Thorac Surg 1989;47:700

54. Heatly RV, Lewis MH, Williams RHP. Preoperative intravenous feeding: a controlled trial. Postgrad Med J 1979;55:541

55. Heitmiller RF, Redmond M, Hamilton SR. Barrett's esophagus with high grade dysplasia; an indication for prophylactic esophagectomy. Ann Surg 1996;224:66

56. Hennessy TPJ. Lymph node dissection. World J Surg 1994;18:367

57. Herskovic A, et al. Combined chemotherapy and radiotherapy compared with radiotherapy alone in patients with cancer of the esophagus. N Engl J Med 1992;326:1593

58. Holscher AH, Bollschwheiler E, Bumm R, Bartels H, Hofler H, Seiwert JR. Prognostic factors of resected adenocarcinoma of the esophagus. Surgery 1995;118:845

59. Hsu CP, et al. Clinical experience in radical lymphadenectomy for adenocarcinoma of the gastric cardia. J Thorac Cardiovasc Surg 1997;114:544

60. Jauch KW, Bacha EA, Denecke H, Anthuber M, Schildberg FW. Esophageal carcinoma; prognostic features and comparison between blunt transhiatal dissection and transthoracic resection. Eur J Surg Oncol 1992;18:553

61. Kakegawa T, Yamana H, Ando N. Analysis of surgical treatment for carcinoma situated in the cervical esophagus. Surgery 1985;97:150

62. Krasna MJ, Flowers JL, Attar S, McLaughlin J. Combined thoracoscopic laparoscopic staging of esophageal cancer. J Thorac Cardiovasc Surg 1996;111:880

63. Kron IL, et al. Blunt esophagectomy and gastric interposition for tumors of the cervical esophagus and hypopharynx. Am Surg 1986;52:140

64. Landis SH, Murray T, Bolden S, Wingo PA. Cancer statistics 1998. CA Cancer J Clinicians 1998;48:6

65. Law S, Fok M, Chow S, Chu KM, Wong J. Preoperative chemotherapy versus surgical therapy alone for squamous cell carcinoma of the esophagus; a prospective randomized trial. J Thorac Cardiovasc Surg 1997;114:210

66. Le Prise E, et al. A randomized study of chemotherapy radiation therapy and surgery versus surgery for localized squamous cell carcinoma of the esophagus. Cancer 1994;73:1779

67. Lerut T, et al. Surgical strategies in esophageal carcinoma with emphasis on radical lymphadenectomy. Ann Surg 1992;216:583

68. Levine DS, et al. An endoscopic biopsy protocol can differentiate high-grade dysplasia from early adenocarcinoma in Barrett's esophagus. Gastroenterol 1993;105:40

69. Lewis I. The surgical treatment of carcinoma of the oesophagus with special reference to a new operation for the growths of the middle third. Br J Surg 1946;34:18

70. Lim STK, et al. Total parenteral nutrition versus gastrostomy in preoperative preparation of patients with cancer of the esophagus. Br J Surg 1981;68:69

71. Logan A. The surgical treatment of carcinoma of the esophagus and cardia. J Thorac Cardiovasc Surg 1963;46:150

72. Marshall SF. Carcinoma of the esophagus: successful resection of lower end of esophagus with reestablishment of esophageal gastric continuity. Surg Clin North Am 1938;18:643

73. McArdle JE, Lewin KJ, Randall G, Weinstein W. Distribution of dysplasias and early invasive carcinoma in Barrett's esophagus. Hum Pathol 1992;23:479

74. Meade RH. Carcinoma of the esophagus. In A History of Thoracic Surgery. Springfield, IL: Thomas, 1961

75. Miller C. Carcinoma of the thoracic oesophagus and cardia. A review of 405 cases. Br J Surg 1962;49:507

76. Moon MR, Schulte WJ, Haasler GB, Condon RE. Transhiatal and transthoracic esophagectomy for adenocarcinoma of the esophagus. Arch Surg 1992;127:951

77. Morris-Brown L, et al. Environmental factors and high risk of EC among men in coastal South Carolina. J Natl Cancer Inst 1988;80:1620

78. Nicks R, Green D, McClatchie G. A clinicopathological study of some factors influencing survival in cancer of the oesophagus. A survey of 10 years experience. Aust NZ J Surg 1973;43:3

79. Nishi M, et al. Risk factors in relation to postoperative complications in patients undergoing esophagectomy or gastrectomy for cancer. Ann Surg 1988;207:148

80. Nishihira T, Hirayama K, Mori S. A prospective randomized trial of extended cervical and superior mediastinal lymphadenectomy for carcinoma of the thoracic esophagus. Am J Surg 1998;175:47

81. Nygaard K, et al. Pre-operative radiotherapy prolongs survival in operable esophageal carcinoma: a randomized multicenter study of pre-operative radiotherapy and chemotherapy. World J Surg 1992;16:1104

82. Ohsawa T. The surgery of the oesophagus. Arch Jpn Chir 1933;10:605

83. Orringer MB. Transhiatal esophagectomy without thoracotomy for carcinoma of the thoracic esophagus. Ann Surg 1984;200:282

84. Orringer MB. Transhiatal esophagectomy without thoracotomy for carcinoma of the esophagus. Adv Surg 1986;19:1

85. Orringer MB. Transthoracic vs transhiatal esophagectomy: what difference does it make? Ann Thorac Surg 1987;44:116

86. Orringer MB. Occult cervical nodal metastases in esophageal cancer: preliminary results of three-field lymphadenectomy (editorial). J Thorac Cardiovasc Surg 1997;113:538

87. Orringer MB, Marshall B, Stirling MC. Transhiatal esophagectomy for benign and malignant disease. J Thorac Cardiovasc Surg 1993;105:265

88. Overholt BF, Panjehpour M. Photodynamic therapy for Barrett's esophagus; clinical update. Am J Gastroenterol 1996;91:1719

89. Pac M, et al. Transhiatal versus transthoracic esophagectomy for esophageal cancer. J Thorac Cardiovasc Surg 1993;106:205

90. Papachristou DN, Fortner JG. Adenocarcinoma of the gastric cardia: the choice of gastrectomy. Ann Surg 1980;192:58

91. Pera M, Trastek VF, Carpente HA, Alen MS, Deschamps C, Pairolero PC. Barrett's esophagus with high grade dysplasia; an indication for esophagectomy? Ann Thorac Surg 1992;54:199

92. Pera M, Cameron AJ, Trastek VF, Herschel A, Carpenter HA, Zinsmeister AR. Increasing incidence of adenocarcinoma of the esophagus and esophagogastric junction. Gastroenterology 1993;104:510

93. Peters JH, Clark GWB, Ireland AP, Chandrasoma P, Smyrk T, De-Meester TR. Outcome of adenocarcinoma arising in Barrett's esophagus in endoscopically surveyed and non-surveyed patients. J Thorac Cardiovasc Surg 1994;108:813

94. Peters JH, et al. Selection of patients for curative or palliative resection of esophageal cancer based on preoperative endoscopic ultrasound. Arch Surg 1994;129:534

95. Piccone VA, et al. Esophagogastrectomy for carcinoma of the esophagus. Ann Thorac Surg 1979;28:369

96. Picus D, et al. Computed tomography in the staging of esophageal carcinoma. Radiology 1983;146:433

97. Quint LE, et al. Esophageal carcinoma: CT findings. Radiology 1985;155:171

98. Quint LE, Glazer GM, Orringer MB. Esophageal imaging by MR and CT: study of normal anatomy and neoplasms. Radiology 1985;156:727

99. Ravitch M. A Century of Surgery. Philadelphia: JB Lippincott Co, 1981

100. Reed CE. Comparison of different treatments for unresectable esophageal cancer. World J Surg 1995;19:828

101. Rice TW, Boyce GA, Sivak MV. Esophageal ultrasound and the preoperative staging of carcinoma of the esophagus. J Thorac Cardiovasc Surg 1991;101:536

102. Rice TW, Falk GW, Achkar E, Petras RE. Surgical management of high grade dysplasia in barrett's esophagus. Am J Gastroenterol 1993;88:1832

103. Rogers EL, Goldkin SF, Iseri OA, Bustin M, Goldkin L, Hamilton SR, Smith RRL. Adenocarcinoma of the lower esophagus. A disease primarily of white men with Barrett's esophagus. J Clin Gastroenterol 1986;8:613

104. Roth JA, et al. Randomized clinical trial of preoperative and postoperative adjuvant chemotherapy with cisplatin, vindesine, and bleomycin for carcinoma of the esophagus. J Thorac Cardiovasc Surg 1988;96:242

105. Sarr MG, Hamilton SR, Marrone GC, Cameron JL. Barrett's esophagus: its prevalence and association with adenocarcinoma in patients with symptoms of gastroesophageal reflux. Am J Surg 1985;149:187

106. Schlag PM, for the Chirurgische Arbeitsgemeinschaft fuer Onkologie der Deutschen Gesellschaft fuer Chirurgie Study Group. Randomized trial of preoperative chemotherapy for squamous cell cancer of the esophagus. Arch Surg 1992;127:1446

107. Sharma P, et al. Dysplasia in short-segment Barrett's esophagus: a prospective 3-year follow-up. Am J Gastroenterol 1997;92:2012

108. Sikes ED Jr, Detmer DE. Aging and surgical risk in older citizens of Wisconsin. Wisconsin Med J 1979;78:27

109. Silver CE. Surgical management of neoplasms of the larynx, hypopharynx and cervical esophagus. Curr Probl Surg 1977;14:2

110. Silverberg E. Cancer statistics 1983. CA Cancer J Clinicians 1983;16:33

111. Skinner DB. En bloc resection for neoplasms of the esophagus and cardia. J Thorac Cardiovasc Surg 1983;85:59

112. Skinner DB, Dowlatashy KD, DeMeester TR. Potentially curable cancer of the esophagus. Cancer 1982;50:2571

113. Stein HJ, Kraemer SJM, Feussner H, Fink U, Siewert JR. Clinical value of diagnostic laparoscopy with laparoscopic ultrasound in patients with cancer of the esophagus or cardia. J Gastrointest Surg 1997;1:167

114. Stones MJ, Kozma A. Adult age trends in record running performances. Exp Aging Res 1980;6:407

115. Streitz JM, Andrews CW, Ellis FH. Endoscopic surveillance of Barrett's esophagus; does it help? J Thorac Cardiovasc Surg 1993;105:383

116. Sweet RH. Late results of surgical treatment of carcinoma of the esophagus. JAMA 1954;155:422

117. Tam PC, et al. Local recurrences after subtotal esophagectomy for squamous cell carcinoma. Ann Surg 1987;205:189

118. Tanner NC. The present position of carcinoma of the oesophagus. cPostgrad Med J 1947;23:109

119. Thomas PA. Physiologic sufficiency of regenerated lung lymphatics. Ann Surg 1980;192:162

120. Thomas CR. Biology of esophageal cancer and the role of combined modality therapy. Surg Clin North Am 1997;77:1139

121. Thompson JC. The stomach and duodenum. In Sabiston DC Jr, ed, Davis-Christopher Textbook of Surgery (11th ed). London: Saunders, 1977

122. Thorban S, Rodeu JO, Nekarda H, Funk A, Pantel K, Siewert R. Disseminated epithelial tumor cells in bone marrow of patients with esophageal cancer: detection and prognostic significance. World J Surg 1996;20:567

123. Tio TL, Coene PLO, den Hartog Jager FCA, Tytgat GNJ. Preoperative TNM classification of esophageal carcinoma by endosonography. Hepatogastroenterol 1990;37:376

124. Torek F. The first successful case of resection of the thoracic portion of the esophagus for carcinoma. Surg Gynecol Obstet 1913;16:614

125. Trapnell DH. The peripheral lymphatics of the lungs. Br J Radiol 1963;36:660

126. Turner GG. Carcinoma of the oesophagus. The question of its treatment by surgery. Lancet 1936;130:67

127. Urba S, Orringer M, Turrisi A, Whyte R, Iannettoni M, Forastiere A. A randomized trial comparing surgery to preoperative concomitant chemoradiation plus surgery in patients with resectable esophageal cancer. Proc Am Soc Clin Oncol 1997;16:277a

128. Wang HH, Antonioli DA, Goldman H. Comparative features of esoph-

ageal and gastric adenocarcinomas: recent changes in type and frequency. Hum Pathol 1986;17:482

129. Walsh TN, et al. A comparison of multimodal therapy and surgery for esophageal adenocarcinoma. N Engl J Med 1996;335:462

130. Watson WL, Pool L. Cancer of the cervical esophagus. Surgery 1948; 23:893

131. Wong J. Esophageal resection for cancer: the rationale of current practice. Am J Surg 1987;153:18

132. Wright TA. High-grade dysplasia in Barrett's oesophagus. Br J Surg 1997;84:760

133. Wynder EL, Bross IJ. A study of etiological factors in cancer of the esophagus. Cancer 1961;14:389

134. Yang PC, Davis S. Incidence of cancer of the esophagus in the U.S. by histological type. Cancer 1988;61:612

135. Zhang ZF, Kurtz RC, Marshall JR. Cigarette smoking and esophageal and gastric cardia adenocarcinoma. J Natl Cancer Inst 1997;89: 1247

136. Zhuang Z, et al. Barrett's esophagus: metaplastic cells with loss of heterozygosity at the APC gene locus are clonal precursors to invasive adenocarcinoma. Cancer Res 1996;56:1961

*The Esophagus*, Third Edition,
edited by D. O. Castell and J. E. Richter.
Lippincott Williams & Wilkins, Philadelphia © 1999.

CHAPTER 14

# Esophageal Rings and Webs

Richard W. Tobin

Rings and webs are among the most common anatomic abnormalities of the esophagus. Although the majority of esophageal rings and webs do not cause symptoms, these structural lesions can cause some patients to have significant difficulties with dysphagia, regurgitation, and aspiration. The terms *esophageal ring* and *web* have often been used interchangeably in the literature, leading to some confusion. An "esophageal web" may best be defined as a thin, eccentric membrane of tissue which can occur anywhere in the esophagus but most commonly occurs in the anterior postcricoid area of the proximal esophagus. In contrast, "rings" are concentric and most commonly occur in the distal esophagus. The lower esophageal ring, often called a Schatzki's, or "B," ring, commonly occurs at the squamocolumnar junction defining the proximal border of a hiatal hernia. A different lower esophageal ring, the lower esophageal muscular, or "A," ring, may also be detected, particularly on radiographic contrast examination. This lower esophageal muscular ring is located about 2 cm proximal to the squamocolumnar junction and is rarely symptomatic. The "C" ring seen on radiographic studies refers to the indentation caused by the diaphragmatic crura and is never symptomatic. Radiographic and endoscopic illustrations of these lesions are available in Chapters 3 and 4. This chapter discusses the epidemiology, pathogenesis, diagnosis, and treatment of esophageal webs and rings.

## ESOPHAGEAL WEBS

### Epidemiology and Pathogenesis

The true prevalence of esophageal webs is unknown as most are felt to be asymptomatic and some require specialized tests for identification. In large retrospective studies using barium contrast examinations, esophageal webs can be found in 5% to 15% of selected patients presenting with

dysphagia [18, 73]. However, some of these webs may have been incidental findings unrelated to the symptom of dysphagia. Symptomatic esophageal webs do occur more commonly in women. An association between esophageal webs and iron deficiency anemia was first noted by the laryngologists Paterson [54] and Kelly [38] as well as the gastroenterologists Plummer and Vinson [69]. Thus, when esophageal webs are associated with iron deficiency anemia, glossitis, koilonychia, and, inconsistently, increased risk of pharyngeal and cervical esophageal cancer, the terms *Plummer-Vinson* and *Paterson-Kelly syndrome* are often applied [13, 32, 36, 47]. Pathologically, webs consist of mucosa and submucosa and are formed from connective tissue covered by normal squamous epithelium with occasional chronic inflammatory cells in the subepithelial tissues [20, 48].

Although the etiology of most esophageal webs is unknown, they are most commonly thought to be the remnants of incomplete vacuolation of the esophageal columnar epithelium during the early embryonic stage. The association with iron deficiency has long been described; however, at least one careful epidemiologic study did not show any correlation between iron deficiency and cervical esophageal web [19], and webs do not seem to consistently improve with iron therapy [8, 47, 54]. The development of esophageal webs has also been associated with thyroid disease [54], an esophageal duplication cyst [64], Zenker's diverticula [41], and several inflammatory states. Patients who develop chronic graft-versus-host disease after allogenic bone marrow transplantation may develop esophageal webs (Fig. 14–1), possibly due to the accretion of desquamated esophageal epithelium [43, 44]. Caution is advised when undertaking endoscopic procedures or esophageal dilation in patients with chronic graft-versus-host disease as perforation appears to be unusually common [44]. Patients with blistering skin diseases, such as cicatricial pemphigoid (mucous membrane pemphigoid) [3, 5, 49] and epidermolysis bullosa [1, 31, 50, 63], can develop esophageal webs. It has been suggested that psoriasis [28], idiopathic eosinophilic esophagitis [70], and Stevens-Johnson syndrome [55] may also be associated

R. W. Tobin: Department of Medicine, Division of Gastroenterology, University of Washington School of Medicine, Seattle, Washington 98195.

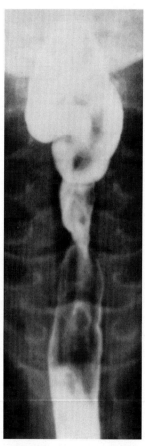

FIG. 14–1. Barium esophagram revealing the presence of an esophageal web and stricture in a patient with chronic graft-versus-host disease. (Courtesy of C. A. Rohrmann, Jr.)

esophageal webs. Barium swallow may detect the web, especially if careful attention is paid to the postcricoid area. However, videoradiography with lateral and anteroposterior views may be necessary to successfully identify a web. A web is usually best seen as a thin projection off the anterior surface of the postcricoid esophagus on the lateral view (see Chapter 3, Fig. 3–9). Endoscopic visualization is also possible but can be difficult due to the proximal location of most webs. Often, initial passage of the endoscope will pierce the web before its presence can be appreciated. In order to appreciate the web endoscopically, careful technique must be used to advance the scope slowly under direct visualization through the upper esophageal sphincter. The web appears as a thin, eccentric, membranous lesion which is covered by normal-appearing mucosa. The remainder of the esophagus is usually normal, although careful examination for the presence of heterotopic gastric mucosa should be performed. Differential diagnosis of the endoscopic diagnosis of an esophageal web includes inflammatory stenosis, postcricoid carcinoma, and postcricoid impression due to ventral venous plexus.

## Treatment

Most esophageal webs are asymptomatic and do not require therapy. Mild symptoms can often be alleviated by having the patient change dietary habits, cut and chew all food carefully, and eat more slowly. If simple dietary and eating manipulations are not totally successful at relieving symptoms related to an esophageal web, mechanical dilation is usually effective. Esophageal webs can be disrupted by passage of an endoscope or bougie [40, 73] or by inflation of an esophageal balloon [34, 40]. Successful treatment of a proximal esophageal web with neodymium:yttrium-aluminum-garnet (Nd:YAG) laser therapy has also been reported [39]. Surgical therapy has been performed in symptomatic patients with webs which are refractory to dilation [40] or associated with Zenker's diverticulum [41]. Patients with esophageal webs associated with iron deficiency, inflammatory conditions, or chronic-graft-versus host disease should be treated for these underlying conditions. Of note, contrast radiography of the esophagus after dilation may reveal persistent evidence of an esophageal web despite complete symptomatic relief [40].

## ESOPHAGEAL RINGS

### Epidemiology and Pathogenesis

Although esophageal rings can occur throughout the esophagus, the most common location is the distal esophagus. Lower esophageal rings were first described by Templeton in 1944 [66], and the first reports of symptomatic lower esophageal rings were by Ingelfinger and Kramer [35] and Schatzki and Gary [61] in 1953. As with esophageal webs, limited data are available on the epidemiology of

with esophageal web formation. First described in 1970 [72], recent studies have confirmed that heterotropic gastric mucosa in the proximal esophagus can be associated with web formation [10, 37, 71].

## Diagnosis

Most esophageal webs are asymptomatic and incidentally found on radiographic or endoscopic examination being performed for unrelated reasons. The most common presentation for a patient with a symptomatic esophageal web is longstanding dysphagia with dietary restriction. Less commonly, patients will present with nasopharyngeal reflux and/or aspiration. Spontaneous perforation of the esophagus associated with the presence of cervical webs has also been reported [4]. Patients with an esophageal web and iron deficiency may be diagnosed with Plummer-Vinson syndrome. Unless a patient has Plummer-Vinson syndrome or an inflammatory condition associated with web formation (such as a blistering skin disease or chronic graft-versus-host disease), physical examination is generally not helpful in establishing the diagnosis.

Radiography is the most sensitive method to diagnose

esophageal rings. The information available likely underestimates the true prevalence of these conditions because they are often asymptomatic and may require specialized tests for identification. Lower esophageal rings are found in about 6% to 14% of routine barium radiographs, but asymptomatic lower esophageal rings occur in approximately 0.5% of these examinations [60]. Although most esophageal rings are asymptomatic, lower esophageal rings are considered to be one of the most common causes of intermittent solid food dysphagia in adults. There appears to be no significant gender difference in the prevalence of lower esophageal rings. Most symptomatic rings occur after age 40.

Pathologically, esophageal rings have been defined as containing mucosa, submucosa, and muscle [56]. The classic lower esophageal ring, however, consists primarily of mucosa and submucosa [23]. Autopsy examination has revealed that the squamocolumnar junction lies at the free margin of the ring or marks its undersurface [23]. However, the exact anatomic relationship of the lower esophageal ring, the squamocolumnar junction, and the lower esophageal sphincter remains in debate [17, 26, 29, 30], primarily due to difficulties in accurately locating these structures during swallowing. Histopathologic examination of esophageal rings has revealed normal tissue, eosinophilic infiltration, basal cell hyperplasia, and hyperkeratosis with varying degrees of proliferative connective tissue [23, 57]. Occasional lymphocytes and plasma cells typical of chronic inflammation may extend for short distances above and below the ring.

The etiology of lower esophageal rings also remains controversial. Lower esophageal rings have been postulated to occur when a pleat of mucosa is formed by infolding of redundant esophageal mucosa due to shortening of the esophagus [65]. Lower esophageal rings have also been hypothesized to be congenital lesions [23]. However, the fact that patients with symptomatic esophageal rings do not present until later in life suggests that other factors may be important. Pill-induced esophageal inflammation may be a factor in the development and progression of esophageal rings [6], but it remains unclear if impacted medication causes ring formation or if a preexisting ring causes pill dysphagia and subsequent esophagitis. First suggested in 1978 [62], recent interest has again focused on the role of gastroesophageal reflux disease in the pathogenesis of lower esophageal rings. Although lower esophageal rings present without obvious surrounding reflux esophagitis and are thinner than peptic strictures, the spectrum of peptic esophageal strictures (see Chapter 27) and that of lower esophageal rings appear to overlap, thus making an association between lower esophageal rings and gastroesophageal reflux confusing. In a small retrospective study using endoscopy and barium radiography, the authors concluded that progression from normal esophagus to lower esophageal ring to an esophageal stricture associated with reflux esophagitis may occur [12]. In a prospective study of 20 consecutive patients with symptomatic lower esophageal rings, evidence for gastroesophageal reflux was documented by endoscopy or ambulatory esopha-

geal pH monitoring in 13 (65%) [42]. However, using esophageal manometry, Chen and colleagues [11] were unable to find a clear relationship between the presence of prolonged lower esophageal sphincter hypotension or esophageal dysmotility and lower esophageal rings, and a more recent study using ambulatory esophageal pH monitoring failed to show an increased prevalence of abnormal distal esophageal acid exposure in patients with hiatal hernia and lower esophageal rings compared to patients with hiatal hernia alone [53]. Unfortunately, although trials are available which support the use of acid suppression therapy to decrease the recurrence rate of peptic strictures (see Chapter 27), no such trials are currently available to document the effect of acid suppression on esophageal rings.

### Diagnosis

In 1963, Schatzki [59] reported that a patient's symptoms are somewhat predictable based on the luminal diameter of an esophageal ring. If the luminal diameter is less than 13 mm, patients almost always have dysphagia; if between 13 and 20 mm, patients may or may not have dysphagia; and if greater than 20 mm, patients rarely have symptoms from the esophageal ring. Patients with symptomatic esophageal rings commonly present with one of two clinical scenarios. The first scenario is that of long standing, intermittent dysphagia to solids. A meat or bread bolus obstructs the esophagus, causes discomfort, and makes the patient either regurgitate the bolus or swallow large amounts of fluid in an attempt to force the bolus into the stomach. After resolution of the obstruction, the patient can continue the meal without further difficulty. Patients with this presentation may have a gradual increase in the frequency of intermittent symptoms over a number of years and learn to carefully cut and chew food to avoid their symptoms. The second common presentation is the "steakhouse syndrome," in which the patient has sudden, unexpected obstruction of the esophagus with dysphagia and sometimes chest pain after swallowing a large bolus. Patients with this presentation are often seen in the emergency room because of an inability to swallow saliva or chest discomfort. Although barium radiography will confirm a food impaction in the esophagus in patients presenting with steakhouse syndrome, the barium will obscure views of the esophagus on the subsequent endoscopy which is often necessary to relieve the obstruction. In a patient with a known, symptomatic lower esophageal ring, spontaneous perforation of the esophagus has also been reported [46].

Generally, barium radiography is the best initial way to make the diagnosis of an esophageal ring (see Chapter 3, Figs. 3-19, 3-20). To optimally demonstrate esophageal rings radiographically, a large volume of low-viscosity barium suspension should be ingested by the patient. Low-volume and air-contrast examinations are suboptimal for the identification of most esophageal rings [51]. The best method involves placing the patient in the prone right anterior oblique position and use of the Valsalva maneuver to distend the lower esophageal segment as the patient swallows the barium. A solid bolus, such as a marshmallow [52] or barium tablet, can be helpful to identify the ring, estimate its lumen, and assess its physiologic significance. Although generally less sensitive than radiography, endoscopy can also be used to identify esophageal rings. Endoscopic detection of esophageal rings requires patience and persistent air insufflation on the part of the endoscopist. However, endoscopy does provide a more sensitive examination for associated mucosal changes, biopsy capability, and therapeutic options.

### Treatment

Patients with asymptomatic esophageal rings do not need treatment. As with esophageal webs, advising patients to change dietary habits, to cut and chew all food carefully, and to eat more slowly will often alleviate mild symptoms. If these measures are not adequate, mechanical bougienage is generally successful. Most commonly, passage of one large bougie (50 to 60 French) is used to disrupt the esophageal ring. Although convincing evidence is lacking, passage of a single large bougie is thought to be more effective than serial progressive dilation of esophageal rings because disruption rather than stretching of the ring is the desired outcome. Dilation with fluoroscopic visualization is recommended if the lumen distal to the ring cannot be visualized or if the ring is unyielding. Similar to esophageal webs, post-dilation barium study may still reveal the presence of the ring despite symptomatic relief. Long-term cure of symptomatic Schatzki's rings by passage of a single dilator appears to be uncommon, but repeat dilation is safe and effective [16, 24]. In a prospective study of 33 consecutive patients with symptomatic Schatzki's rings, all patients had relief of their dysphagia at 4-week follow-up after passage of a single Maloney bougie (46 to 58 French). However, the proportion of patients remaining symptom-free was only 68% at 1 year, 35% at 2 years, and 11% at 3 years of follow-up. Patients with symptomatic recurrences were successfully redilated, and no significant complications occurred with this strategy [16]. For recalcitrant esophageal rings, pneumatic dilation with an achalasia balloon may be necessary [56].

Other methods have been employed for esophageal rings that do not respond to mechanical dilation. In a study of seven patients with lower esophageal rings unresponsive to conventional esophageal dilation, electrocautery incision of the lower esophageal ring using a papillotome was successful at relieving dysphagia in all patients during a 36-month follow-up [9]. In this study, one patient did develop chest pain after treatment, and another had recurrent symptoms which required repeat incision at 6 months. In a different study of 17 patients with symptomatic lower esophageal rings, radial incisions in the ring using a sphincterotome were successful at relieving symptoms for a mean follow-up of 46 months in 14 patients. The remaining three patients responded to a second incision, and the only complication

reported was bleeding in one patient [25]. Using the Nd:YAG laser to incise symptomatic esophageal rings, good results were obtained in a study of 14 patients [33]. Surgical therapy for esophageal rings is rarely indicated. However, fracture of the ring digitally through a gastrostomy opening or actual segmental removal of parts of the ring has been advocated [14, 15].

## MISCELLANEOUS

### Feline Esophagus

Fine transverse folds occasionally seen by double-contrast barium study of the human esophagus have been termed *feline esophagus* due to their resemblance to folds seen regularly in the feline esophagus (Fig. 14-2) [22]. A pattern identical to the fine transverse folds seen in feline esophagus can be seen in surgical specimens as undulating folds of squamous mucosa created during esophageal shortening [21]. Feline esophagus is most commonly observed in asymptomatic patients as a normal radiologic variant or in patients with evidence of gastroesophageal reflux disease.

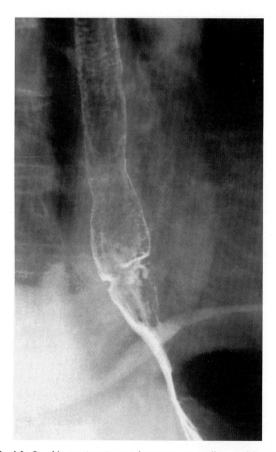

**FIG. 14–2.** Air-contrast esophagram revealing evidence of "feline esophagus" in the esophageal body. These fine transverse folds have been associated with gastroesophageal reflux disease, and a distal esophageal peptic stricture is present in this patient. (Courtesy of C. A. Rohrmann, Jr.)

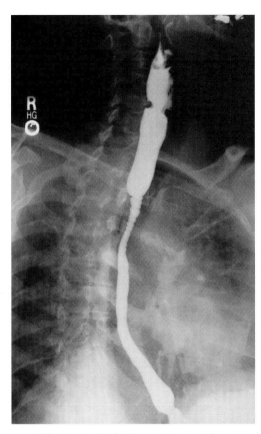

**FIG. 14–3.** Multiple esophageal rings.

## Multiple Esophageal Rings ("Ringed Esophagus")

In the absence of an obvious underlying inflammatory condition, multiple esophageal rings (Fig. 14-3) are a rare cause of dysphagia in adults [1, 45] and children [58]. In the small number of reported cases, there appears to be a male predominance and an association with gastroesophageal reflux and asthma [45]. The etiology of "ringed esophagus" remains unclear, but both gastroesophageal reflux [7, 45, 58] and congenital anomaly [27] have been implicated. Treatment with gentle bougienage is generally effective.

## Vascular Rings

Abnormal development of the branchial arch system can produce a ring which encircles the trachea and esophagus. Patients with vascular rings most commonly present with stridor or recurrent respiratory infections, but dysphagia may be the primary symptom in some patients [67]. Magnetic resonance imaging may be the current test of choice to delineate vascular rings [68]. Symptomatic patients often obtain excellent long-term results with surgical therapy [67].

## REFERENCES

1. Agarwal VP, Marcel BR. Multiple esophageal rings. Gastrointest Endosc 1990;36:147
2. Agha FP, Francis IR, Ellis CN. Esophageal involvement in epidermoly-sis bullosa dystrophica: clinical and roentgenographic manifestations. Gastrointest Radiol 1983;8:111
3. Al-Kutoubi MA, Eliot A. Oesophageal involvement in benign mucosa membrane pemphigoid. Clin Radiol 1984;35:131
4. Beggs D, Morgan WE. Spontaneous perforation of cervical oesophagus associated with oesophageal web. J Laryngol Otology 1989;103:537
5. Benedict EB, Lever WF. Stenosis of the esophagus in benign mucosa membrane pemphigus. Ann Otol Rhinol Laryngol 1952;61:1130
6. Bonavina L, DeMeester TR, McChesney L, Schwizer W, Albertucci M, Bailey RT. Drug-induced esophageal strictures. Ann Surg 1987; 206:178
7. Bousvaros A, Antonioli DA, Winter HS. Ringed esophagus: an association with esophagitis. Am J Gastroenterol 1992;87:1187
8. Brendenkamp JK, Castro DJ, Mickel RA. Importance of iron repletion in the management of Plummer-Vinson syndrome. Ann Otol Rhinol Laryngol 1990;99:51
9. Burdick JS, Venu RP, Hogan WJ. Cutting the defiant lower esophageal ring. Gastrointest Endosc 1993;39:616
10. Buse PE, Zuckerman GR, Balfe DM. Cervical esophageal web associated with a patch of heterotopic gastric mucosa. Abdom Imaging 1993; 18:227
11. Chen MYM, Ott DJ, Donati DL, Wu WC, Gelfand DW. Correlation of lower esophageal mucosal ring and lower esophageal sphincter pressure. Dig Dis Sci 1994;39:766
12. Chen YM, Gelfand DW, Ott DJ, Munitz A. Natural progression of the lower esophageal mucosal ring. Gastrointest Radiol 1987;12:93
13. Chisholm M. The association between webs, iron, and post-cricoid carcinoma. Postgrad Med J 1974;50:215
14. Eastridge CE, Pate J, Mann JA. Lower esophageal ring: experiences in treatment of 88 patients. Ann Thorac Surg 1984;103
15. Eastridge CE, Salazar J, Pate JW, Farrell G. Symptomatic lower esophageal ring: treatment of 24 patients. South Med J 1979;72:919
16. Eckardt VF, Kanzler G, Willems D. Single dilation of symptomatic Schatzki rings: prospective evaluation of its effectiveness. Dig Dis Sci 1992;37:577
17. Eckhardt VF, Adami B, Hucker H, Leeder H. The esophagogastric juction in patients with asymptomatic lower esophageal mucosal rings. Gastroenterology 1980;79:426
18. Ekkberg O, Nylander G. Webs and web-like formations in the pharynx and cervical esophagus. Diagn Imaging 1983;52:10
19. Elwood PC, Jacobs A, Pitman RG, Entwistle CC. Epidemiology of the Paterson-Kelly syndrome. Lancet 1964;2:716
20. Entwistle CC, Jacobs A. Histological findings in the Paterson-Kelly syndrome. J Clin Pathol 1965;18:408
21. Furth EE, Rubesin SE, Rose D. Feline esophagus. AJR Am J Roentgenol 1995;164:900
22. Gohel VK, Edell SL, Laufer I, Rhodes WH. Transverse folds in the human esophagus. Radiology 1978;128:303
23. Goyal RK, Glancy JJ, Spiro HM. Lower esophageal ring (first of two parts). N Engl J Med 1970;282:1298
24. Groskreutz JL, Kim CH. Schatzki's ring: long-term results following dilation. Gastrointest Endosc 1990;36:479
25. Guelrud M, Villasmil L, Mendez R. Late results in patients with Schatzki ring treated by endoscopic electrosurgical incision of the ring. Gastrointest Endosc 1987;33:96
26. Harris LD, Kelly E, Kramer P. Relation of the lower esophageal ring to the esophagogastric junction. N Engl J Med 1960;263:1232
27. Harrison CA, Katon RM. Familial multiple congenital esophageal rings: report of affected father and son. Am J Gastroenterol 1992;87:1813
28. Harty RF, Boharski MG, Harned RK. Psoriasis, dysphagia and esophageal webs or rings. Dysphagia 1988;2:136
29. Heitmann P, Wolf BS, Sokol EM, Cohen BR. Simultaneous cineradiographic-manometric study of the distal esophagus: small hernia and rings. Gastroenterology 1966;50:737
30. Hendrix TR. Schatzki's ring, epithelial junction, and hiatal hernia: an unresolved controversy. Gastroenterology 1980;79:584
31. Hillemeier C, Touloukian R, McCallum R, Gryboski J. Esophageal web: a previously unrecognized complication of epidermolysis bullosa. Pediatrics 1981;67:678
32. Hoffman RM, Jaffe PE. Plummer-Vinson syndrome: a case report and literature review. Arch Intern Med 1995;155:2008
33. Hubert G, Patrice T, Foultier MT, Le Bodic L. Dysphagie et anneau de Schatzki: traitement par le laser Nd-YAG chez 14 patients. Gastroenterol Clin Biol 1990;14:186

34. Huynh PT, de Lange EE, Shagger HA. Symptomatic webs of the upper esophagus: treatment with fluoroscopically guided balloon dilation. Radiology 1995;196:789

35. Ingelfinger FJ, Kramer P. Dysphagia produced by contractile ring in lower esophagus. Gastroenterology 1953;23:419

36. Jacobs A, Kilpatrick GS. The Paterson-Kelly syndrome. BMJ 1964;2:79

37. Jerome-Zapadka KM, Clarke MR, Sekas G. Recurrent upper esophageal webs in association with heterotopic gastric mucosa: case report and literature review. Am J Gastroenterol 1994;89:421

38. Kelly AB. Spasms at the entrance to the esophagus. J Laryngol Rhinol Otol 1919;34:285

39. Krevsky B, Pusateri JP. Laser lysis of an esophageal web. Gastrointest Endosc 1989;35:451

40. Lindgren S. Endoscopic dilatation and surgical myectomy of symptomatic cervical esophageal webs. Dysphagia 1991;6:235

41. Low DE, Hill LD. Cervical esophageal web associated with Zenker's diverticulum. Am J Surg 1988;156:34

42. Marshall JB, Kretschmar JM, Diaz-Arias AA. Gastroesophageal reflux as a pathogenic factor in the development of symptomatic lower esophageal rings. Arch Intern Med 1990;150:1669

43. McDonald GB, Sullivan KM, Plumley TF. Radiographic features of esophageal involvement in chronic graft-vs.-host disease. AJR Am J Roentgenol 1984;142:501

44. McDonald GB, Sullivan KM, Schuffler MD, Shulman HM, Thomas ED. Esophageal abnormalities in chronic graft-versus-host disease in humans. Gastroenterology 1981;80:914

45. McKinley MJ, Eisner TD, Fisher ML, Bronzo RL, Weissman GS. Multiple rings of the esophagus associated with gastroesophageal reflux. Am J Gastroenterol 1996;91:574

46. Miller S, Hines C, Ochsner JL. Spontaneous perforation of the esophagus associated with a lower esophageal ring. Am J Gastroenterol 1988;83:1405

47. Mohandas KM, Swaroop VS, Desai DC, Chir V, Nagral A, Iyer G. Upper esophageal webs, iron deficiency, anemia, and esophageal cancer [Letter]. Am J Gastroenterol 1991;86:117

48. Nakamura R, Watanabe M, Terashima M, Saito K, Iwasaki T. Dysphagia resulting from an upper esophageal web—a case report. Jpn J Surg 1991;21:676

49. Naylor MF, MacCarty RL, Rogers RS. Barium studies in esophageal cicatricial pemphigoid. Abdom Imaging 1995;20:97

50. Orlando RC, Bozymski EM, Briggaman RA, Bream CA. Epidermolysis bullosa: gastrointestinal manifestations. Ann Intern Med 1974;81:203

51. Ott DJ, Chen YM, Wu WC, Gelfand DW, Munitz HA. Radiographic and endoscopic sensitivity in detecting lower esophageal mucosal ring. AJR Am J Roentgenol 1986;147:261

52. Ott DJ, Kelley TF, Chen MYM, Gelfand DW, Wu WC. Use of a marshmallow bolus for evaluating lower esophageal mucosal rings. Am J Gastroenterol 1991;86:817

53. Ott DJ, Ledbetter MS, Chen MY, Koufman JA, Gelfand DW. Correlation of lower esophageal mucosal ring and 24-h pH monitoring of the esophagus. Am J Gastroenterol 1996;91:61

54. Paterson DR. A clinical type of dysphagia. J Laryngol Rhinol Otol 1919;34:289

55. Peters ME, Gourley G, Mann FA. Esophageal stricture and web secondary to Stevens-Johnson syndrome. Pediatr Radiol 1983;13:290

56. Pope CE. Rings, webs, and diverticula. In Yamada T, ed, Gastrointestinal Disease. Philadelphia: WB Saunders, 1993;419

57. Postlethwait RW, Musser AW. Pathology of the lower esophageal web. Surg Gynecol Obstet 1965;120:571

58. Rencken IO, Heyman MB, Perr HA, Gooding CA. Ringed esophagus (feline esophagus) in childhood. Pediatr Radiol 1997;27:773

59. Schatzki R. The lower esophageal ring. Long term follow-up of symptomatic and asymptomatic rings. Am J Roentgenol Radiat Ther Nucl Med 1963;90:805

60. Schatzki R, Gary JE. The lower esophageal ring. AJR Am J Roentgenol 1956;75:246

61. Schatzki R, Gary JE. Dysphagia due to diaphragm-like narrowing in lower esophagus ("lower esophageal ring"). Am J Roentgenol Radiat Ther Nucl Med 1953;70:911

62. Schmarschmidt BF, Watts HD. The lower esophageal ring and esophageal reflux. Am J Gastroenterol 1978;69:544

63. Sehgal VN, Jain VK, Bhattacharya SN, Broor SL, Mukherjee AK. Esophageal web in generalized epidermolysis bullosa. Int J Dermatol 1991;30:51

64. Snyder CL, Bickler SW, Gittes GK, Ramachandran V, Ashcroft KW. Esophageal duplication cyst with esophageal web and tracheoesophageal fistula. J Pediatr Surg 1996;31:968

65. Steinnon OA. The anatomic basis for the lower esophageal contraction ring: plication theory and its application. Am J Roentgenol Radiat Ther Nucl Med 1963;90:811

66. Templeton FE. X-ray examination of the stomach. In: A Description of the Roentgenologic Anatomy, Physiology and Pathology of the Esophagus, Stomach, and Duodenum. Chicago: University of Chicago Press, 1944;106

67. Van Son JAM, et al. Surgical treatment of vascular rings: the Mayo Clinic experience. Mayo Clin Proc 1993;68:1056

68. Van Son JAM, et al. Imaging strategies for vascular rings. Ann Thorac Surg 1994;57:604

69. Vinson PP. Hysterical dysphagia. Minn Med 1922;5:107

70. Vitellas KM, Bennett WF, Bova JG, Johnston JC, Caldwell JH, Mayle JE. Idiopathic eosinophilic esophagitis. Radiology 1993;186:789

71. Waring JP, Wo JM. Cervical esophageal web caused by inlet patch of gastric mucosa. South Med J 1997;90:554

72. Weaver GA. Upper esophageal web due to a ring formed by a squamocolumnar junction with ectopic gastric mucosa (another explanation on the Paterson-Kelly, Plummer-Vinson syndrome). Dig Dis Sci 1979;24:959

73. Webb WA, McDaniel L, Jones L. Endoscopic evaluation of dysphagia in two hundred and ninety-three patients with benign disease. Surg Gynecol Obstet 1984;158:152

*The Esophagus*, Third Edition, edited by D. O. Castell and J. E. Richter. Lippincott Williams & Wilkins, Philadelphia © 1999.

CHAPTER 15

# Esophageal Diverticula

Edgar Achkar

An esophageal diverticulum is a sac that protrudes from the esophageal wall. As in the rest of the gastrointestinal tract, a true diverticulum is one that contains all layers of the wall. A false diverticulum consists of mucosa, submucosa, and a few muscle fibers. Esophageal diverticula can be classified in many ways. They can be divided into congenital and acquired based on origin, into pulsion and traction based on etiology, or into false or true based on histology; but the simplest and most practical way is to classify them according to anatomy, into four categories: Zenker's diverticula; hypopharyngeal, midesophageal diverticula; epiphrenic diverticula; and intramural pseudodiverticulosis.

Esophageal diverticula have been described in all age groups, but they are most commonly seen in adults. Esophageal diverticula are rare, occurring in less than 1% of upper gastrointestinal roentgenograms and accounting for less than 5% of dysphagia cases [30].

Motor abnormalities of the esophagus are often associated with esophageal diverticula, but the belief that all diverticula are due to a motor disorder of the esophagus is not founded on solid evidence.

## ZENKER'S DIVERTICULUM

Zenker's diverticulum, also called pharyngoesophageal diverticulum, is described as an esophageal pouch. In fact, this type of diverticulum occurs in a location proximal to the esophagus, above the upper esophageal sphincter (UES), and should be considered as a hypopharyngeal diverticulum. The pharyngeal constrictor muscles form a funnel, and the mouth of the esophagus is like a transverse slit at the bottom of this funnel. At endoscopy, the larynx with its moving vocal cords is in the center, the pyriform sinuses are lateral, and the esophageal opening appears as a posterior slit. The fibers of the cricopharyngeus muscle run transversely and form the UES at the esophageal inlet. Above the cricopha-

ryngeus muscle, the walls of the hypopharynx contain oblique fibers of the inferior constrictor muscles. Between the transverse fibers of the cricopharyngeus muscle below and the oblique fibers of the inferior constrictors above, a triangular area containing fewer muscle fibers constitutes a region of relative weakness and is referred to as the triangle of Killian or Killian's dehiscence (Fig. 15–1). The mucosa of the hypopharynx is allowed to bulge posteriorly at Killian's triangle, and with time, a pouch may develop, forming a Zenker's diverticulum.

### Etiology and Pathogenesis

Several mechanisms have been invoked to explain the pathogenesis of Zenker's diverticulum, but none of them has been definitely proven. Age may play a role in the development of Zenker's diverticulum. A decrease in tissue elasticity leading to an increased weakness of the triangle of Killian may explain why Zenker's diverticulum is rarely seen in individuals younger than 40 years. Additionally, the prevalence of Zenker's diverticulum increases in the elderly, reaching 50% in the seventh and eight decades of life, particularly in women [97].

The most widely accepted mechanism for Zenker's diverticulum is a functional disturbance of the hypopharynx, such as increased resting pressure of the sphincter, lack of complete sphincter relaxation or incoordination between the sphincter and the hypopharynx. The UES is formed mainly by the cricopharyngeus muscle, with participation from fibers from the inferior portion of the inferior pharyngeal constrictors and some fibers of the cervical esophagus. The sphincter is shaped like a slit, not a circle, leading to marked radial asymmetry during tonic contractions. Normally, the UES is closed during tonic contraction and, immediately after a swallow, excitation of the muscle stops transiently and the UES relaxes, allowing passage of the bolus into the upper esophagus. UES function is under the influence of bolus volume as well as the nature of the upper esophageal contents [42, 58].

E. Achkar: Department of Gastroenterology, The Cleveland Clinic Foundation, Cleveland, Ohio, 44195.

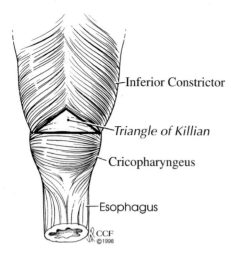

- Inferior Constrictor
- Triangle of Killian
- Cricopharyngeus
- Esophagus

CCF
©1998

**FIG. 15–1.** Triangle of Killian, an area of weakness that allows Zenker's diverticulum to develop.

Traditionally, the most frequently accepted hypothesis for the formation of a hypopharyngeal diverticulum is premature closure of the UES during swallowing, as shown by Ellis et al. [32]. The concept of "cricopharyngeal achalasia," i.e., failure of the sphincter to relax on time, was accepted for a long time as the reason for the development of Zenker's diverticula. Achalasia was demonstrated with the help of pharyngographs by Asherson in 1950 [3], and other authors, such as Sutherland [91], perpetuated this theory. Nilsson et al. [76] studied ten patients with symptomatic hypopharyngeal diverticulum using simultaneous radiography and manometry. Pressures were measured using triple microtransducers, allowing the authors to measure pressures at three levels of the UES, including the level immediately below the neck of the diverticulum. Cineradiography used simultaneously provided a correlation between the pressures generated and the passage of contrast material. Results showed that below the entrance of the diverticulum the sphincter pressure exceeded UES resting pressure as the bolus entered the pharynx. The authors concluded that this phenomenon represented incoordination. They also found within the UES, during swallowing, double pressure peaks, which they called a "split UES." These results were not found in all patients, and no asymptomatic controls were used. Nevertheless, Nilsson et al. [76] explained the pathogenesis of Zenker's diverticulum by pressures on the pharyngeal wall from the bolus forced against a contracted UES. Knuff et al. [60] compared nine patients with Zenker's diverticulum, with a mean age of 60 years, to a control group of 15 patients matched for age. Manometric measurements were obtained using a water-perfused system, which produces less reliable measurements than microtransducers. The tracings were analyzed into four time intervals, and the relationship of pharyngeal contractions to UES relaxation was studied. Using these four parameters, no difference between the two groups was found. However, there was a marked difference in mean UES resting pressure between patients with Zenker's diverticulum and those without. The authors had no explanation for the low resting pressure, but because of the absence of abnormal cricopharyngeal coordination, they questioned the concept that the diverticulum is the result of incomplete relaxation of the UES.

The notion of pharyngoesophageal incoordination or achalasia was contradicted further by Cook et al. [21], who studied 14 patients with diverticula and nine healthy, age-matched controls using simultaneous videoradiography and manometry. Manometric studies were obtained with a sleeve catheter equipped with metallic markers, allowing exact localization of the recording sites during radiography. There was no difference between patients and controls in timing of pharyngeal contractions and sphincter relaxation. However, the authors found a significantly reduced sphincter opening associated with greater intrabolus pressure, suggesting an impairment of UES opening. The authors concluded that Zenker's diverticulum is a disorder of longstanding diminished UES opening with increased hypopharyngeal pressures, eventually causing formation of the diverticulum. They dispelled the notion that UES opening is impaired by pharyngoesophageal incoordination or lack of sphincter relaxation. A histologic study carried out by the same group [20] seems to support the concept of diminished UES opening. Muscle strips were obtained from 14 patients with Zenker's diverticulum during surgical myotomy. Tissue was also obtained from ten control patients without history of dysphagia, nine from autopsy and one from a patient with laryngeal cancer. Of the 14 patients with Zenker's diverticulum, ten showed greater than 50% replacement of cricopharyngeal muscle fibers by fibrous adipose tissue. None of the controls showed similar findings. The authors thought that degenerative changes may account for the abnormality observed in patients with Zenker's diverticulum. Muscle degeneration would prevent the sphincter from opening completely because of decreased elasticity, while normally the UES should relax during normal swallowing as a result of external traction and propulsive forces within the sphincter. Lerut et al. [62] obtained biopsy specimens from 62 patients with Zenker's diverticulum and compared them to tissue obtained from 15 controls. Histologic and immunochemical studies were carried out on most specimens and contractility bath studies on all specimens of cricopharyngeus muscles. Reduced amplitude and lower contractions were found in eight patients with Zenker's diverticulum and not in the controls. Neurogenic and myogenic abnormalities were also found on histologic examination.

A study of another condition thought to be due to cricopharyngeal spasm or achalasia may shed some light on the pathogenesis of Zenker's diverticulum. A cricopharyngeal bar, which is detected as a marked indentation on esophagram, was also thought to be due to incoordination. Figure 15–2 illustrates a cricopharyngeal bar.

Dantas et al. [23] studied patients with cricopharyngeal bars who had a prominent indentation during radiography but in whom no diverticulum could be elicited. Six patients

# Color Plates

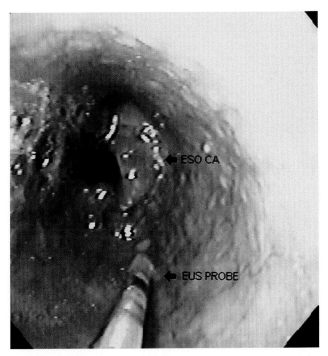

**COLOR PLATE 1.** Endoscopic ultrasound miniprobe in position in the esophagus for staging of a malignant stricture.

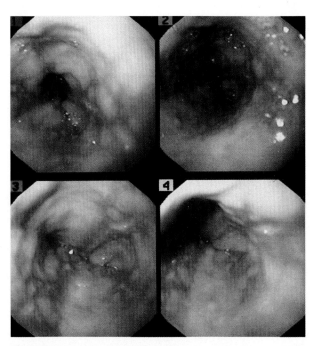

**COLOR PLATE 2.** Grade II esophagitis by the Savary-Miller New Endoscopic Grading System.

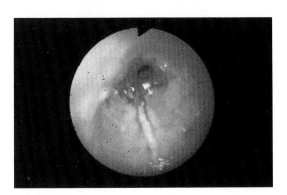

**COLOR PLATE 3.** Grade IV esophagitis by the Savary-Miller New Endoscopic Grading System. There is a long, linear ulceration proximal to a circumferential stricture. (Courtesy Drs. Marcon, Haber, Kortan, and Kandel.)

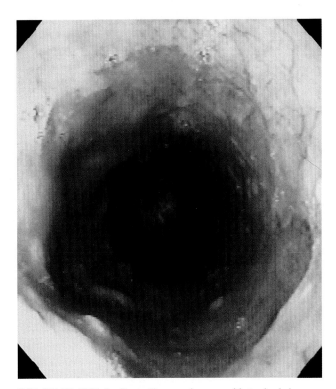

**COLOR PLATE 4.** Barrett's esophagus with typical demarcation between the white squamous mucosa and the salmon pink ectopic gastric mucosa.

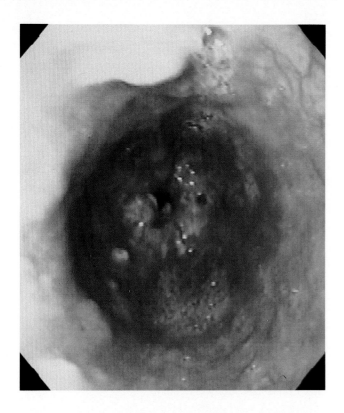

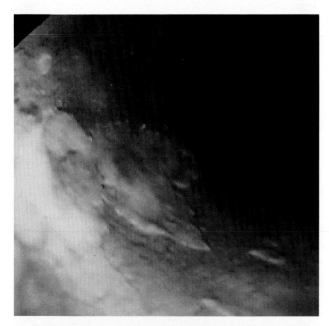

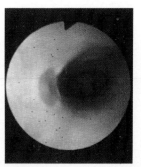

**COLOR PLATE 5.** Adenocarcinoma in the distal segment of a Barrett's esophagus. There is a 7-cm circumferential segment of ectopic gastric musosa leading to an area of adenocarcinoma with stricture at the gastroesophageal junction.

**COLOR PLATE 6.** Squamous islands in a segment of Barrett's esophagus. The squamous islands can be seen as focal areas of white squamous mucosa in a circumferential area of Barrett's.

**COLOR PLATE 7.** An inlet patch. This patch of reddish, velvety columnar mucosa is well circumscribed and has distinct borders. (Courtesy Drs. Marcon, Haber, Kortan, and Kandel.)

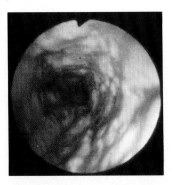

**COLOR PLATE 8.** Confluent candidiasis involving the entire esophagus. (Courtesy Drs. Marcon, Haber, Kortan, and Kandel.)

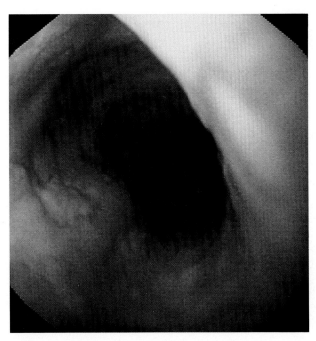

**COLOR PLATE 9.** Herpes simplex esophagitis with multiple upper esophageal ulcerations with raised edges.

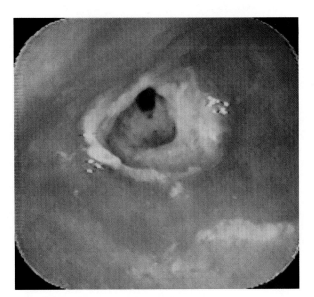

**COLOR PLATE 10.** Pill-induced ulceration with stricture. Circumferential ulceration with stricture formation in a patient taking alendronate sodium (Fosamax) tablets.

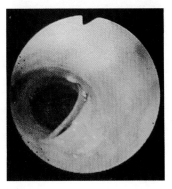

**COLOR PLATE 11.** Typical appearance of an esophageal web, which appears as a soft, mucosa-lined diaphragm oriented perpendicular to the esophageal wall. It is semilunar in shape and covered with a thin, semitransparent mucosa. (Courtesy Dr. Stanley Benjamin.)

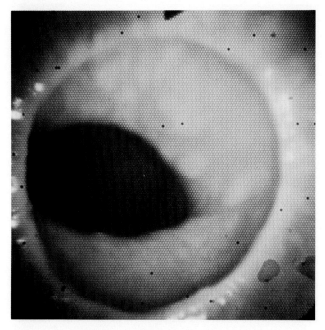

**COLOR PLATE 12.** Typical endoscopic appearance of Schatzki's ring.

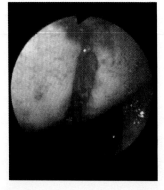

**COLOR PLATE 13.** Appearance of a deep Mallory-Weiss tear. This longitudinal laceration was located just below the Z line. (Courtesy Dr. Stanley Benjamin.)

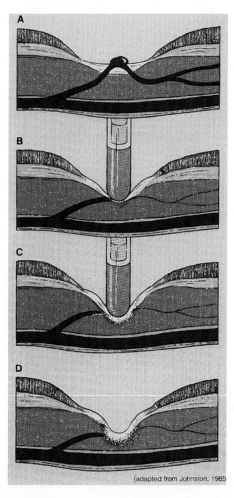

**COLOR PLATE 14.** Coaptive coagulation of a visible vessel. **A:** Anatomy of the visible vessel with feeding arteriole. **B:** Compression of a bleeding site or visible vessel tamponades and stops blood flow. **C:** Activation of heater probe or BECAP probe delivers thermal energy that creates coaptive coagulation and seals the site. **D:** Site remains sealed following probe removal. (From ref. XX with permission.)

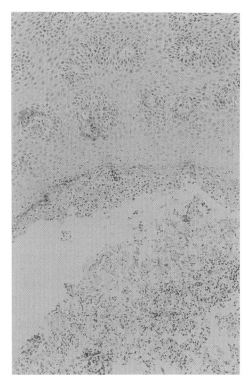

**COLOR PLATE 15.** *Candida* esophagitis. The hyperemic mucosa is coated by a pseudomembrane composed of fungal organisms, neutrophils, fibrin, and dead epithelial elements.

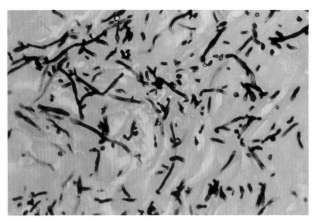

**COLOR PLATE 16.** *Candida* esophagitis. With the methenamine silver stain, both the pseudohyphae and the yeast cells are well demonstrated within this biopsy of the esophageal mucosa. The psuedohyphae appear as linear structures with indentations along their lengths creating a "sausage-link" appearance. Budding yeast cells are also readily delineated.

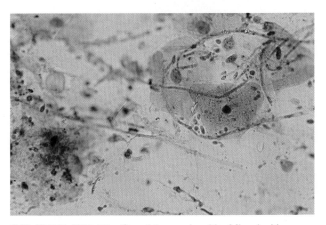

**COLOR PLATE 17.** *Candida* esophagitis. Mixed with superficial and intermediate squamous cells are yeast cells and pseudohyphae of *Candida.* With the Papanicolaou stain, the yeast cells and pseudohyphae are eosinophilic. The latter are delicate and show the irregular points of constriction along their lengths. A small number of neutrophils is also present.

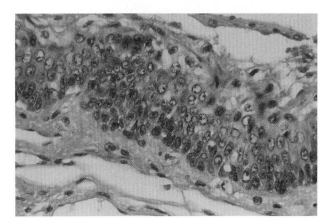

**COLOR PLATE 18.** Reparative atypia. This esophageal biopsy was from the edge of a peptic ulcer. The nuclei of most of the squamous cells are much larger than normal. Furthermore, they have distinct, but delicate membranes, vesicular chromatin, and obvious nucleoli. Cell borders are indistinct. Note, however, that there is a suggestion of maturation, as manifested by increased volumes of cytoplasm and lower nuclear-to-cytoplasmic ratios in the most superficial cells.

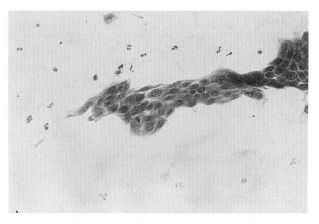

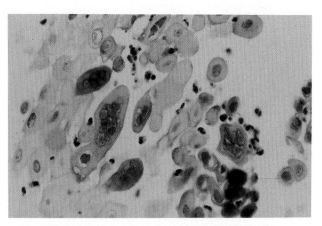

**COLOR PLATE 19.** Reparative atypia. This brushing displays a cohesive aggregate of altered squamous epithelium. This benign atypia is characterized by enlarged nuclei, distinct, but delicate membranes, pale, fine chromatin, and distinct nuclei. Within the aggregate is the classic "streaming" effect. Note the presence of a mitotic figure and neutrophils.

**COLOR PLATE 20.** Herpes esophagitis. This biopsy from the edge of an esophageal ulcer manifests the classic cytopathic alterations of herpes infection. Many of the infected squamous cells are markedly enlarged and contain multiple nuclei. Some of the nuclei are characterized by thickened nuclear membrane, a large eosinophilic inclusion body, and a surrounding halo. Other nuclei manifest the classic "ground glass" appearance. In both types of multinucleated squamous cells, the nuclei are characteristically compressed or molded against one another.

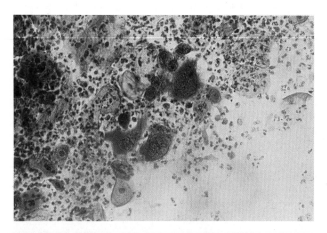

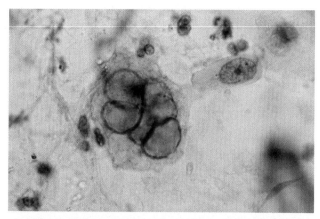

**COLOR PLATE 21.** Herpes esophagitis. Within an intense purulent inflammatory infiltrate are numerous isolated squamous cells. Several of them are herpes virocytes. They are larger than normal, contain multiple nuclei, and have dense green cytoplasm. Their nuclear membranes are thickened and "ground glass" chromatin is apparent in some nuclei, whereas inclusion bodies are present in others.

**COLOR PLATE 22.** Herpes esophagitis. This markedly enlarged multinucleated squamous cell shows the characteristic "ground glass" chromatin. It is characterized by a homogeneous, structureless pattern, and is associated with markedly thickened membranes. Note the prominent nuclear molding.

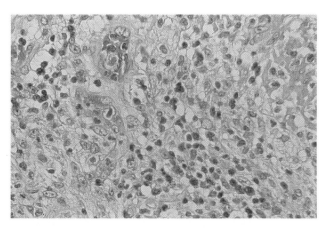

**COLOR PLATE 23.** Cytomegaloviral esophagitis. This is a biopsy from the base of an esophageal ulcer which manifests several different types of inflammatory cells. In addition, two endothelial cells show the classic changes of CMV infection. These include huge basophilic nuclear inclusions, thick, irregular membranes, and a broad, clear halo.

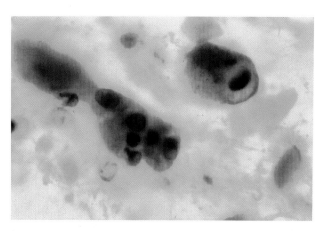

**COLOR PLATE 24.** Cytomegaloviral esophagitis. Compared to the adjacent epithelial cells, this isolated cytomegalovirus virocyte shows both nucleomegaly and cytomegaly. The normal landmarks in the enlarged nucleus are obliterated by the huge basophilic inclusion body and the surrounding halo. The thickened nuclear membrane results from chromatin condensation on the inner surface of the membrane.

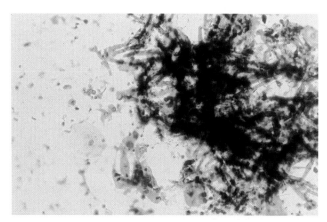

**COLOR PLATE 25.** *Aspergillus* esophagitis. This is a brushing from a leukemic individual who was severely leukopenic. These smears contained relatively few squamous epithelial cells and only a sparse number of inflammatory elements. This picture is dominated by a huge, deeply green-stained aggregate of the hyphae of *Aspergillus*. Compared to the pseudohyphae of *Candida,* they are thicker, cyanophilic, and show true septation.

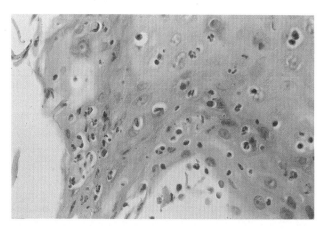

**COLOR PLATE 26.** Reflux esophagitis. Neutrophils are scattered within the squamous epithelium in large numbers. Many adjacent squamous cells manifest degenerative changes (e.g., pyknosis and cytoplasmic swelling).

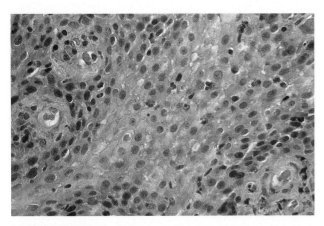

**COLOR PLATE 27.** Reflux esophagitis. Numerous intraepithelial eosinophils are present as an important diagnostic criterion of esophagitis.

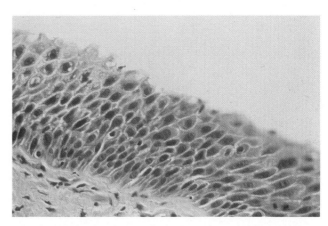

**COLOR PLATE 28.** Reflux esophagitis. In this area of hyperplasia, the basal cell zone occupies almost the full thickness of the epithelium. Mitotic figures are present, but inflammatory cells are not apparent. Overall, the thickness of the epithelium is reduced compared to normal.

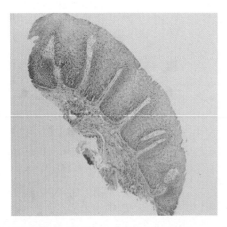

**COLOR PLATE 29.** Reflux esophagitis. The scanning magnification demonstrates prominent papillomatosis characterized by marked elongation of the connective tissue papillae of the lamina propria extending to within a few epithelial cell layers of the thickened squamous mucosa. Segmented leukocytes are absent from the epithelium.

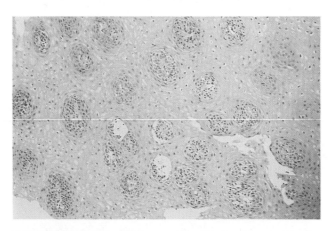

**COLOR PLATE 30.** Reflux esophagitis. Papillomatosis, and thus reflux esophagitis, may be diagnosed when a prominent increase in the number of papillary profiles is apparent in the proper clinical situation. Note the distinct absence of inflammatory elements within the squamous epithelium.

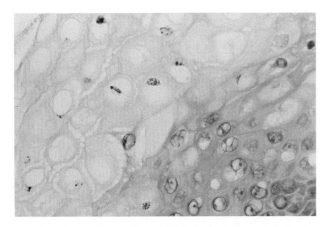

**COLOR PLATE 31.** Reflux esophagitis. A large array of balloon cells is present within the squamous epithelium. These cells have voluminous, pale-stained cytoplasm, and many of their nuclei show degenerative changes. Compare them with the adjacent squamous cells and their nuclei.

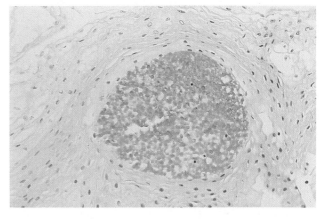

**COLOR PLATE 32.** Reflux esophagitis. The endothelial cell lining of this dilated blood vessel is not evident; instead, the erythrocytes appear to be opposed against degenerative squamous epithelial cells.

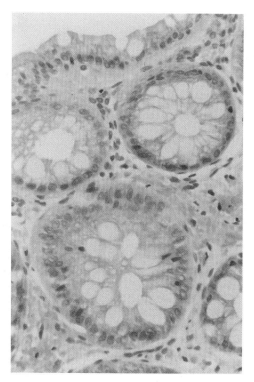

**COLOR PLATE 33.** Barrett's esophagus. Most of the cells lining the glands and many of those on the surface are goblet cells. They are characterized by bulbous distended cytoplasm ("cup-shaped"), mucus vacuoles, small basal nuclei, and low nuclear-to-cytoplasmic ratios.

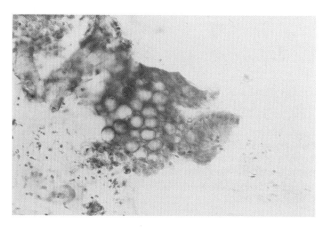

**COLOR PLATE 34.** Barrett's esophagus. This Papanicolaou-stained esophageal brushing shows the intestinal metaplasia of Barrett's esophagus. This is manifested by the presence of numerous goblet cells within the flat aggregate of glandular cells. The aggregate has sharply defined, smooth edges, in keeping with the preservation of intercellular cohesion. The goblet cells present as round, clear areas due to the abundant cytoplasmic mucus.

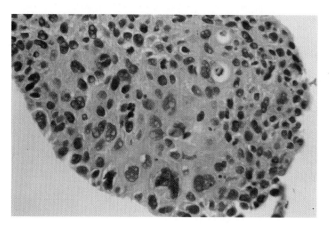

**COLOR PLATE 35.** Well-differentiated squamous cell carcinoma. The malignant cells in this biopsy specimen show a marked range in nuclear sizes and appearances. However, the nuclear chromatin is uniformly very darkly stained. The volume of dense eosinophilic cytoplasm varies remarkably from cell to cell.

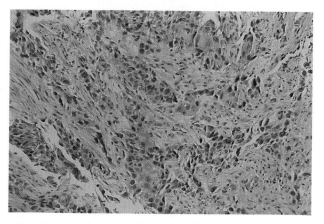

**COLOR PLATE 36.** Moderately differentiated squamous cell carcinoma. Irregularly shaped nests and cords of malignant cells infiltrate the wall of the esophagus. The tumor cells have hyperchromatic nuclei, dense cytoplasm, and relatively homogeneously high nuclear-to-cytoplasmic ratios. The host response is evident in the form of a desmoplastic response.

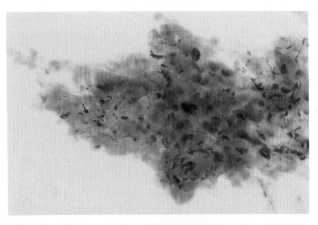

**COLOR PLATE 37.** Well-differentiated squamous cell carcinoma. This is an esophageal brushing from a tumor which histologically was well-differentiated squamous cell carcinoma. Intercellular cohesion is well preserved as demonstrated by the presence of a huge cellular aggregate and an absence of individually dispersed tumor cells. The cells are characterized by moderate to voluminous amounts of dense orangeophilic cytoplasm. In addition, nuclear hyperchromasia is readily apparent.

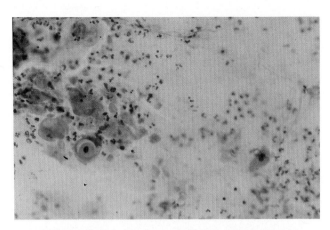

**COLOR PLATE 38.** Well-to-moderately differentiated squamous cell carcinoma. This is an esophageal brushing from a neoplasm which showed variable degrees of differentiation histologically. Intercellular cohesion is reduced compared to what is seen in Fig. 8-23. This manifests by the presence of individual malignant cells and small, loose clusters of such elements. The nuclei again are enlarged and hyperchromatic. In fact, some are extremely dense and pyknotic-like. A small pearl is evident.

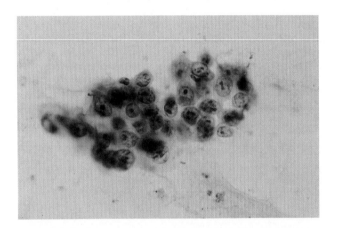

**COLOR PLATE 39.** Poorly differentiated squamous cell carcinoma. This loose cluster of malignant cells is characterized by huge solitary nuclei with large and multiple nucleoli. The cytoplasm is dense and cyanophilic. The nuclear-to-cytoplasmic ratios are uniformly high.

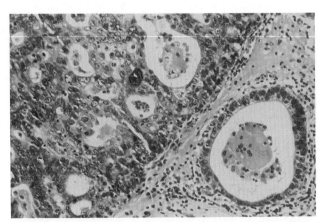

**COLOR PLATE 40.** Adenocarcinoma. Most of the field is occupied by a large, sheetlike arrangement on the malignant glandular cells. Within this sheet are a number of "back-to-back" glands in which adjacent gland lumens share the same carcinoma cells in their walls. This results in the classic cribriform pattern. Striking nuclear pleomorphism is obvious.

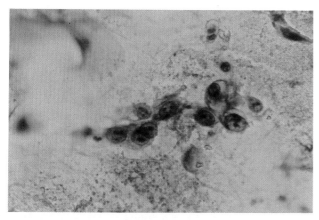

**COLOR PLATE 41.** Adenocarcinoma. This brushing shows a small, loose cluster of malignant glandular cells. These cells have high nuclear-to-cytoplasmic ratios, large nuclei, and prominent nucleoli. The cytoplasm in several of the tumor cells contains distinct cytoplasmic mucin vacuoles. In others, the cytoplasm has a delicate granular green appearance.

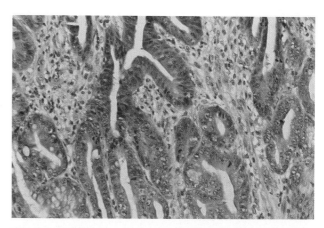

**COLOR PLATE 42.** Glandular dysplasia. High-grade dysplasia is apparent in this biopsy specimen. It is characterized by crowded and irregularly shaped branched glands. The latter are lined by cells with large hyperchromatic nuclei, little in the way of cytoplasmic mucin production, and high nuclear-to-cytoplasmic ratios. There is no evidence of stromal invasion.

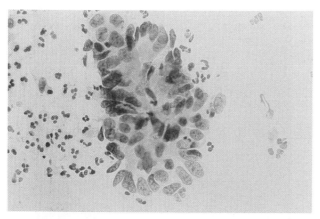

**COLOR PLATE 43.** Glandular dysplasia. This large, cohesive aggregate of abnormal glandular cells is present in a relatively clean background which contains a small number of neutrophils. The dysplastic glandular cells are characterized by large, often elongated nuclei. The latter have coarsely granular and evenly distributed chromatin and small, but distinct nucleoli. Cytoplasmic mucin production is not apparent. Note the absence of individually dispersed abnormal glandular cells.

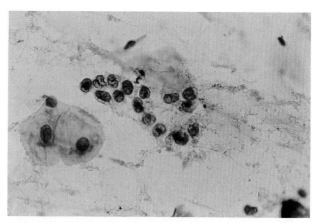

**COLOR PLATE 44.** Esophageal leukemia. This is a brushing from a patient with acute myeloblastic leukemia. A number of leukemic elements are present and are characterized by irregularly shaped, hyperchromatic nuclei, distinct nucleoli, and high nuclear-to-cytoplasmic ratios. Compared to the adjacent benign squamous epithelial cells, the nuclei are approximately the same size. Although the leukemic blasts are closely aggregated, true intercellular cohesion is absent.

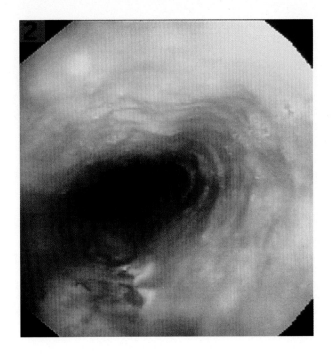

**COLOR PLATE 45.** Endoscopic view of early esophageal cancer. Only minimal change, a small erosion, is seen.

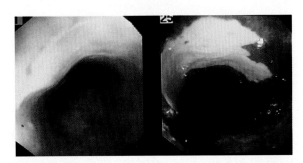

**COLOR PLATE 46.** Endoscopic view (**right**) of esophagus after stain with Lugol's iodine. Neoplastic area, deplete of glycogen, remains unstained. Endoscopic view on left before staining.

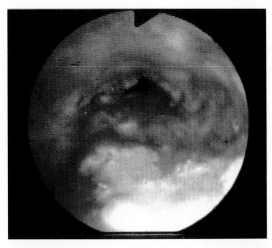

**COLOR PLATE 47.** Endoscopy demonstrating typical endoscopic features of esophageal cancer. The lumen is narrowed and irregular.

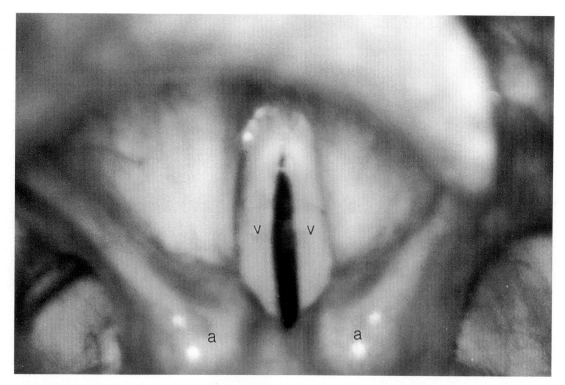

**COLOR PLATE 48.** Normal laryngoscopic examination showing the vocal fold (*v*) and arytenoids (*a*).

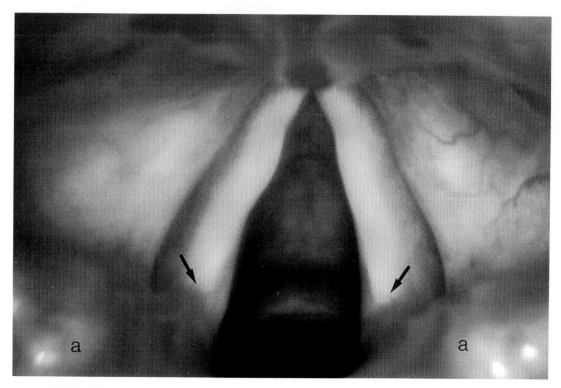

**COLOR PLATE 49.** Typical findings in a patient with gastroesophageal reflux laryngitis. Note the marked arytenoid erythema (a), which extends as hyperemia of the posterior portions of the vocal folds (arrows).

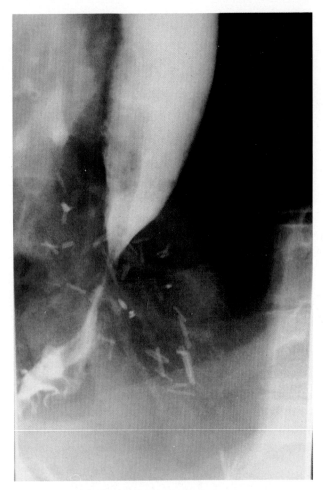

**COLOR PLATE 50.** Radiographic appearance of a fundoplication which is too tight.

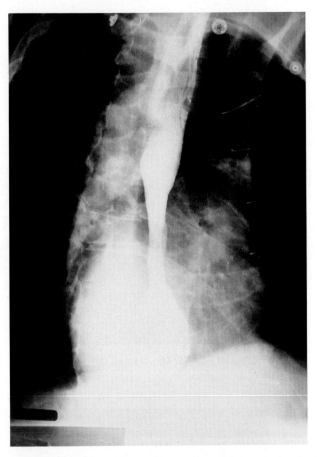

**COLOR PLATE 51.** The radiographic appearance of a short esophagus, which results from a combination of reflux esophagitis, poor acid clearance, dysmotility, stricturing, and fibrosis and is often associated with a large hiatial hernia.

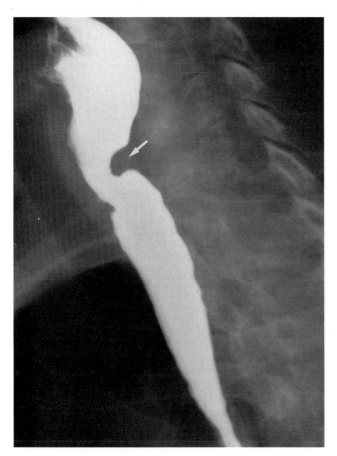

**FIG. 15–2.** Cricopharyngeal bar.

with bars underwent concurrent fluoroscopic and manometric examination of the pharynx and UES, as did eight volunteers. Patients with bars were found to have smaller openings of the UES during swallowing and increased intrabolus pressure when compared to controls. These findings indicate a reduced muscle compliance, preventing total relaxation of the cricopharyngeus. No evidence of spasm could be found and sphincter relaxation was complete during manometry. Studies such as this one and others performed on patients with Zenker's diverticulum indicate that it is best to abstain from using the term *cricopharyngeal achalasia* to describe these disorders. Although no single pathogenetic mechanism for the development of Zenker's diverticulum has been established, it appears that reduced UES compliance rather than cricopharyngeal incoordination accounts for the genesis of the pouch. The consistent finding in recent studies is increased intrabolus pressure in patients with Zenker's diverticulum [68].

Gastroesophageal reflux has been implicated in the genesis of Zenker's diverticulum. It was suggested that acid reflux leads to cricopharyngeal spasm and that eventually a pharyngoesophageal diverticulum will develop [54]. The UES is responsive to infusion of solutions in the esophagus and has been shown to react to the presence of acid. Gerhardt et al. [42] studied nine normal subjects, infusing different solutions in the esophagus. When 0.1 normal HCl was infused in the upper esophagus, high UES pressures were produced when compared to infusion of normal saline. Additionally, an increase in the rate of infusion resulted in further increases in pressure. These findings suggest that the UES acts as a barrier to acid reflux, possibly preventing aspiration. However, Vakil et al. [93] found that esophageal acid exposure did not affect UES pressure in normal volunteers or in patients with esophagitis. Although gastroesophageal reflux can result in throat symptoms such as cough, hoarseness, and globus as well as the lesion of posterior laryngitis, it is not known if anatomic abnormalities such as Zenker's diverticulum can result from chronic gastroesophageal reflux. Hunt et al. [54] found a greater resting UES pressure in patients with reflux esophagitis than in controls. In five patients with Zenker's diverticulum, the UES pressure was also elevated but there was no evidence of reflux esophagitis. Others have tried to use as evidence the presence of a hiatal hernia to establish a link between reflux and Zenker's diverticulum. Gage-White [41] showed a 39% occurrence of hiatal hernia in patients with Zenker's diverticulum compared to 16% in controls, suggesting that the two disorders may be due to a common pathophysiologic phenomenon. Resouly et al. [84] reported an increased occurrence of reflux symptoms in patients with pharyngeal pouches but did not show any objective results. At this point, there is no solid evidence that a direct relationship exists between Zenker's diverticulum and gastroesophageal reflux disease [39, 97]. Should patients with Zenker's diverticulum exhibit symptoms of heartburn or chest pain, they should be studied for the presence of acid reflux. However, we cannot support aggressive medical or surgical treatment of reflux disease as a way to avoid the development of Zenker's diverticulum.

## Clinical Features

Many pharyngoesophageal diverticula are asymptomatic and discovered by chance during radiologic evaluation. In general, symptoms of Zenker's diverticulum depend upon the stage of the disease. In the early phase, patients may complain only of a sensation of sticking in the throat or a sensation of vague irritation. They may also report intermittent cough, excessive salivation, and intermittent dysphagia, usually to solid foods. Some patients may present with such minor symptoms that they are dismissed as having "globus." Because of the vagueness of their symptoms, these patients are often labeled as *globus hystericus,* a very unfortunate term since some patients with globus turn out to have a significant pathology such as reflux, diverticula, or other disorders of the voluntary phase of swallowing.

When the sac becomes large, more severe symptoms develop. Dysphagia becomes more frequent. Regurgitation of food ingested several hours earlier is reported, and gurgling sounds occur upon swallowing. Patients learn to use special maneuvers to empty the pouch by pressing on the neck or coughing and clearing the throat. In rare cases, the pouch is so large that it obstructs the esophagus, but more frequently a bulging in the left side of the neck takes place. Pulmonary aspiration leading to pneumonia or lung abscess may occur but is rather infrequent [98].

Rare complications of Zenker's diverticulum have been described. Hendren et al. [48] reported massive bleeding in a diverticulum. Obstruction and tracheodiverticular fistula are rare. Isolated cases of squamous cell carcinoma associated with Zenker's diverticulum have been reported [8, 57]. In large series, the occurrence of carcinoma appears to be low; at the Mayo Clinic over a 53-year period, cancer was found only in 0.4% of 1,249 patients [52]. The diagnosis of cancer is rarely made clinically and is suspected usually because of a defect on x-ray [57]. Most patients with carcinoma report additional symptoms, such as weight loss and increasingly worsening dysphagia. Cancer appears to be more frequent in men and in longstanding cases. Because of the long period of time between the discovery of a diverticulum and the occurrence of a carcinoma, it is speculated that cancer results from chronic irritation and inflammation of the diverticulum due to stasis. The frequency of carcinoma arising in Zenker's diverticulum has been less frequent in recent years, perhaps because of more prompt treatment. Bowdler and Stell [8] reviewed the issue in 1987, finding only 38 cases in the English literature. Most of the cancers in these reports were squamous cell carcinoma, with an occasional basal cell or spindle cell carcinoma. Overall, the frequency of carcinoma arising in Zenker's diverticulum is not high enough to constitute by itself justification for surgery. From a practical standpoint, the decision to treat is based on the severity of symptoms.

## Diagnosis

A barium esophagram with special attention to the oropharyngeal phase of swallowing is the best diagnostic procedure for Zenker's diverticulum. Small diverticula may be missed, but careful evaluation with lateral and oblique views will detect even small pouches. The diverticulum protrudes posteriorly, and barium tends to fall into the pouch before progressing into the esophagus (Fig. 15–3). In the case of a very small diverticulum, the sac may be visible only during the phase of UES contraction and not during relaxation. Some authors have tried to classify Zenker's diverticula in stages or categories based on the size and shape of the diverticulum as well as the presence during contraction or relaxation of the UES. Ponette and Coolen [83] reviewed 143 patients with diverticula and attempted to relate the morphology of the pouch to upper sphincter function. These efforts to grade Zenker's diverticula based on shape and size result from the fact that barium studies will sometimes reveal a temporary posterior bulge at the level of or just above the UES. The bulge is not large enough and consistent enough through the study to be referred to as a diverticulum, and terms such as *transient diverticulum* and *early diverticulum* have been used [97]. Whether such changes represent a di-

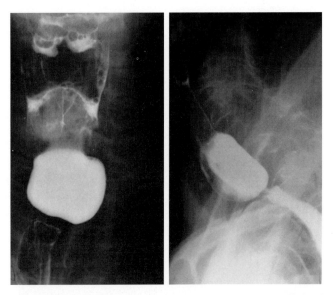

**FIG. 15–3.** Zenker's diverticulum, anteroposterior and lateral views.

verticulum or a manifestation of a cricopharyngeal bar which can be seen in association with a diverticulum (Fig. 15–4) or simply a trivial phenomenon can be argued. At any rate, such observations are of limited clinical importance and one must be guided by the patient's complaints. It is doubtful that a transient posterior bulge would cause significant throat

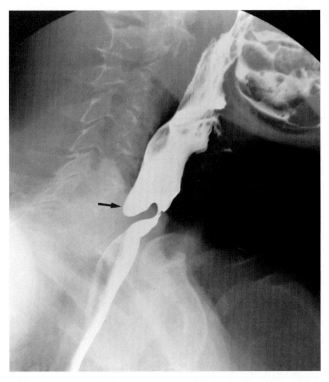

**FIG. 15–4.** Marked cricopharyngeal indentation with a posterial bulge *(arrow),* most likely representing a Zenker's diverticulum.

symptoms, and if dysphagia is truly present, a more careful evaluation of the voluntary phase of swallowing must be undertaken.

There is an area of weakness, distinct from Killian's triangle, located just below the cricopharyngeal muscle and called the Killian-Jamieson space [85]. Protrusions through this area of weakness are rare, but when they occur, they may be confused with a Zenker's diverticulum. However, a Killian-Jamieson diverticulum arises from the lateral wall, below the UES, and tends to be small (Fig. 15–5). Patients with Killian-Jamieson pouches are usually asymptomatic.

Endoscopy adds very little to the evaluation of pharyngoesophageal pouches. If it has to be performed for other reasons, caution should be exercised to not enter the diverticulum and risk a perforation [29].

Manometric testing of UES function has been recently refined, and accurate measurements with analysis of various phases of deglutition are possible [15]. However, the technique is of little value in the management of patients. Furthermore, manometry may be difficult to perform as the manometric catheter tends to coil in the diverticulum. There have been reports of low resting pressure of the sphincter [60, 71] as well as normal basal pressures [21] in patients with Zenker's diverticulum. The finding of cricopharyngeal incoordination is inconsistent, as discussed in the section on pathogenesis. Manometric testing of the cricopharyngeal area should be reserved for clinical research and is not necessary in evaluating patients with pharyngeal pouches [40].

## Treatment

Small Zenker's diverticula discovered by chance do not require any intervention and may be followed by periodic esophagrams. When needed, the only effective treatment of Zenker's diverticulum is surgical. Surgical techniques include, separately or in combination, diverticulopexy, diverticulectomy, and cricopharyngeal myotomy. Endoscopic treatment is emerging as an alternative to open surgery.

In the early 1900s, diverticulopexy became popular because attempts to excise the diverticulum in the 1800s were not encouraging. In diverticulopexy, the fundus of the diverticulum is attached high up in the neck to the prevertebral fascia after being dissected from surrounding tissues. By attaching the fundus of the diverticulum high in the neck, drainage is allowed to occur. A two-stage operation was also developed in which the diverticulum was ligated and an ostomy performed to allow drainage. In a second stage, the diverticulum was then resected. Various modifications to this operation were made to avoid infection and other complications. Today, diverticulopexy alone is rarely performed, while it is used sometimes in association with a myotomy. Diverticulectomy and myotomy, separately or together, constitute the most traditional approach to surgical treatment of Zenker's diverticulum [45]. At the Mayo Clinic, a one-stage pharyngoesophageal diverticulectomy with or without myotomy produced excellent results with only a 3.6% recurrence rate [80]. In an updated report in 1992, Payne [79] described his experience with over 900 patients treated for Zenker's diverticulum. Mortality was low at 1.2%, morbidity was 8%, and the rate of recurrence was still 3.6%. In the interval between the two reports, however, the surgical technique had varied from simple diverticulectomy to diverticulectomy associated with myotomy and, in some cases, myotomy alone without resection. Additionally, a mechanical stapling device was used in some cases. Therefore, it is difficult to conclude, based on this report, what is the single best technique to treat Zenker's diverticulum. When the diverticulum recurs, reoperation presents major technical difficulties, complications are more frequent, and mortality rises to 3.2% [51].

The open surgical technique involves usually a left cervical incision. The diverticulum once identified is retracted, dissected, and eventually resected and the point of insertion either sutured or stapled. When a myotomy is performed, it is done either before [10] or after [35] the diverticulectomy. Myotomy is extramucosal, dissecting the fibers of the cricopharyngeal muscles away from the mucosa. The incision is

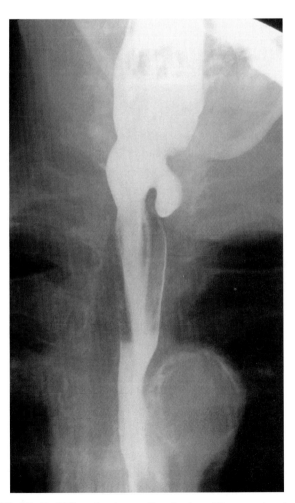

**FIG. 15–5.** Killian-Jamieson diverticulum. The pouch arises from the lateral esophageal wall below the upper esophageal sphincter.

extended 3 to 4 cm above the esophagus. Fegiz et al. [35] reported 15 patients with Zenker's diverticulum. Twelve were treated by resection only and three by resection and myotomy. The result was good in all three patients treated with a combined procedure. In the 12 treated by resection alone, results were good in eight and fair in three, with recurrence in one. Ellis and Crozier [31] treated ten patients, three of whom had undergone a diverticulotomy earlier. Cricopharyngeal myotomy was performed in all patients, but diverticulectomy was performed in only two and diverticulopexy in one. There were no complications and follow-up showed good results in all patients. Lerut et al. [62] justified the need to perform a cricopharyngeal myotomy by the pathophysiologic changes present in patients with Zenker's diverticulum. They asked two questions: Is a myotomy of the cricopharyngeus useful? How long should it be? The finding of abnormal contractility and abnormal histology led them to advocate the use of myotomy, emphasizing that the incision should be no less than 4 to 5 cm long. These authors reported 100 consecutive patients treated by myotomy and in the majority of cases, diverticulopexy. The mean follow-up was 4 years and morbidity was minimal. Schmit and Zuckerbraun [88] performed cricopharyngeal myotomy alone under local anesthesia. Good results occurred in 70% of patients and fair results in 17%. Because of these favorable results, they concluded that the operation under local anesthesia without resecting the diverticulum was safe and effective even though the size of the diverticulum had a mean of 3.3 cm with a range of 1 to 8 cm. It should be noted that patient follow-up was conducted by telephone and direct contact was possible in only 63%. Diverticulectomy with cricopharyngeal myotomy achieves good results, but the physiologic consequences of this anatomic disruption have not been rigorously analyzed. A videofluoroscopic study of 15 patients treated surgically showed that the process of swallowing becomes abnormal following surgery [100]. Among the changes observed are pooling of contrast material, aspiration, and premature closure of the cricopharyngeus muscle. In this study, seven patients reported absence of symptoms after surgery, while six had mild residual dysphagia, one reported no difference, and one felt that the symptoms were worse than preoperatively. There was no significant difference in the number of abnormalities recorded postoperatively between asymptomatic and symptomatic patients. Shaw et al. [90] studied eight patients pre- and postoperatively and showed that cricopharyngeal myotomy normalized UES opening by reducing hypopharyngeal intrabolus pressure.

Open surgical treatment of Zenker's diverticulum may result in complications such as fistulas, infection, vocal cord paralysis, and aspiration [51, 79, 88]. A technique of inversion of the diverticulum resulting in invagination rather than excision has been advocated to avoid complications [73]. This technique is reserved for small diverticula and can be carried out in a short period of time. However, some authors disagree with its usefulness [5]. Other technical variations

have also been suggested, such as the use of myotomy, diverticulectomy, and cervical esophagostomy with a feeding tube for the ostomy and removal of the feeding tube with closure of the esophagostomy in a second stage. This operation is advocated for severely debilitated patients [64].

Zenker's diverticulum may be treated endoscopically. Multiple reports have originated from non-U.S. centers [95]. Endoscopic treatment of pharyngeal pouches was tried without success in the early 1900s. In 1960, a technique using a rigid esophagoscope with a double lip was established. The endoscope is positioned so it rides over the bridge between the diverticulum and the esophageal lumen. This wall as well as the cricopharyngeus muscle are then transected at the same time, creating a communication between the diverticulum and the esophagus. In other words, rather than resecting or draining the diverticulum, a common cavity is created and the diverticulum now drains openly into the esophagus. Van Overbeek and Hoeksema [96], from The Netherlands, reported 211 cases in whom a satisfactory rate of 91.5% was found with few complications. The technique may be modified by using laser treatment for transection of the ridge rather than electrocoagulation [67]. Benjamin and Innocenti [7] treated 15 patients with a microsurgical laser procedure. A minor leak occurred in two patients only, and they responded to conservative treatment. Long-term results in this series appeared favorable, although no details were given on follow-up. Wouters and van Overbeek [99] compared their earlier experience with endoscopic electrocoagulation in 323 cases to the microendoscopic $CO_2$ laser treatment of 184 cases. They found the results to be comparable but thought that the laser technique produced less pain and allowed the patients to eat earlier. Another modification to the endoscopic treatment of Zenker's diverticulum involves the use of staples [18].

It is extremely difficult to conclude from reviewing the literature which operation constitutes the best treatment for Zenker's diverticulum. The inclusion of patients with Zenker's diverticulum as well as cricopharyngeal achalasia, neurologic disorders, and other abnormalities; the variations in technique; the use of historic controls; and the lack of consistent and objectively structured follow-up are some of the reasons for the confusion. At this point, it appears that endoscopic treatment with or without laser or stapling is not popular in the United States and that, in spite of the debate over the need for myotomy, most surgeons continue to perform it while excising the diverticulum unless it is very small. No causal relationship has been established between gastroesophageal reflux and Zenker's diverticulum. Antireflux surgery is therefore only appropriate when reflux is symptomatic [28, 39].

## MIDESOPHAGEAL DIVERTICULA

Midesophageal diverticula are given this name to distinguish them from epiphrenic diverticula, which occur in the most distal part of the esophagus, and because most diverticula are found in the midportion of the esophagus.

## Etiology and Pathogenesis

It is not known whether midesophageal diverticula are congenital. Most appear to develop in young and older adults. The development of esophageal diverticula in general has traditionally been explained by one of two mechanisms: traction or pulsion. This distinction was made in 1840 by Rokitansky [47]. A traction diverticulum is characteristically situated in the middle third of the esophagus and is thought to develop as a result of pulling of the esophageal wall by neighboring inflammatory or scar tissue. Therefore, a traction diverticulum is a true one as all layers of the esophagus are pulled out. A pulsion diverticulum, on the other hand, is thought to occur because of abnormal forces applied to a portion of the esophageal wall, resulting in an outpouching of mucosa through the muscle layer of the esophagus [13]. Zenker's diverticulum would be an example of pulsion diverticulum and so would the epiphrenic diverticulum, which will be discussed later. Midesophageal diverticula, based on this classification, could be of the traction or pulsion type.

Cross et al. [22] showed that most esophageal diverticula occur because of an area of spasm or because of lack of sphincter relaxation; they found motor abnormalities even in cases of isolated midthoracic diverticulum. Esophageal diverticula, which tend to be multiple, have been described in patients with achalasia, diffuse esophageal spasm, or other motor abnormalities [14]. Schima et al. [87] studied 30 patients with midesophageal diverticula, some they considered of the pulsion type and some of the traction type. Dysphagia was present in 22 patients. Esophageal manometry was performed in only 15 patients, but by associating cinefluoroscopy and manometry, the authors found a motor abnormality in 24 of 30 patients. Evander et al. [33] reported ten patients with motor abnormalities. Eight of these had epiphrenic diverticula. The two patients with midesophageal diverticula had no abnormality in lower esophageal sphincter (LES) function but showed occasional simultaneous or repetitive contractions in the thoracic esophagus. An important study was carried out by Dodds et al. [26] in 1975, who attempted to determine the importance of motor abnormalities in the genesis of midesophageal diverticula. The authors purposely chose six patients who had no evidence of esophageal motor disorder by radiology and manometry. Pressures were measured by four recording ports positioned radially around the lumen. In five of six patients, the orifice facing the mouth of the diverticulum recorded a lower pressure than the other three ports. In two patients, bizarre wave forms were seen with abrupt onset or offset of the contraction, and in two others, high peristaltic pressure amplitude greater than 250 mm Hg was found in the distal half of the esophagus. The radial asymmetry at the level of the diverticulum was attributed to the presence of the diverticulum, the bizarre forms were attributed to longitudinal motion of the diverticulum

during recording, and the high peristaltic pressure was thought to represent perhaps the reason leading to the diverticulum by forces pushing out the esophageal wall. This study does not prove that weakness at one point of the esophageal wall is the reason for the occurrence of diverticula as the pressure could be the result rather than the cause of the outpouching.

## Clinical Features

Most midesophageal diverticula are asymptomatic (Fig. 15–6). Indeed, the diverticulum tends to be small and points upward, making food accumulation rare. In some patients, chest pain and dysphagia are reported, but these are usually present in patients who have an esophageal motor disorder. Figure 15–7 illustrates a midesophageal diverticulum in a patient with diffuse esophageal spasm.

Gastroesophageal reflux is also noted in some patients with midesophageal diverticula [87]. Of the 30 patients Schima et al. [87] studied, five had gastroesophageal reflux. True diverticula were reported in a 5-year-old boy with hiatal hernia and a short esophagus [26].

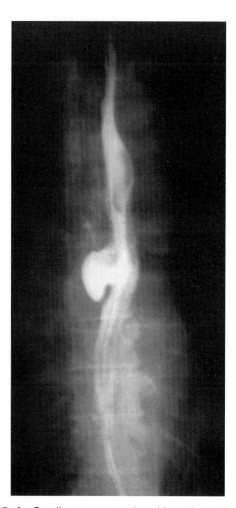

**FIG. 15–6.** Small, asymptomatic midesophageal diverticulum.

and other collagen vascular diseases. Wide-mouthed saccular pouches were seen at various levels of the esophagus.

## Diagnosis

Most midesophageal diverticula are discovered by chance during barium esophagram carried out for other reasons. Diverticula may be of various sizes and could be single or multiple [26, 56]. Figure 15–8 illustrates a case of multiple diverticula. In case of complication, radiology will determine the presence of a fistula. An intraluminal diverticulum may be missed by x-ray.

Endoscopy with today's flexible instruments is not contraindicated, but the procedure is not necessary for the diagnosis of diverticula.

## Treatment

Since most midesophageal diverticula are uncomplicated and cause no symptoms, treatment is not required. If treatment becomes necessary, the procedure of choice is diverticulectomy. It is imperative, however, to rule out an associ-

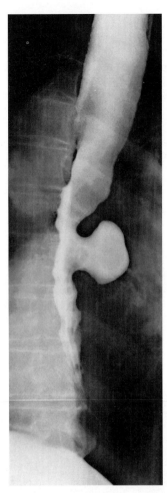

**FIG. 15–7.** Midesophageal diverticulum in a patient with diffuse esophageal spasm.

Complications are unusual. Spontaneous rupture, exsanguination [86], aspiration [2, 33], fistula formation [4], and carcinoma [36] have been reported. These complications are usually seen in patients with motor disorders or when, in the distant past, traction diverticula were associated with pulmonary tuberculosis [13]. Inflammatory lymph nodes around the esophagus account for the outpouching of the tissue.

Atypical diverticula of the esophagus have been reported. Herman and McAlister [49] found diverticula in two children who had developed strictures due to unsuspected foreign body ingestion. Diverticula were present above the foreign body. Saccular dilatation was reported in a patient following excision of an asymptomatic congenital cyst [65] and may also be seen postoperatively after repair of an esophageal perforation or laceration. Intraluminal diverticula which result in the appearance of a double esophageal lumen are difficult to diagnose, may result in dysphagia or esophagitis, and are of unknown origin [89]. Finally, in progressive systemic sclerosis, pseudodiverticula of the esophagus may develop. Clements et al. [17] reported five cases of unusual diverticula associated with progressive systemic sclerosis

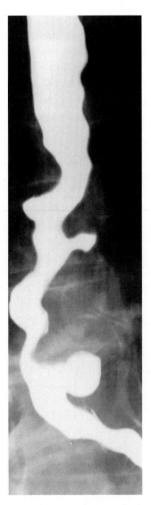

**FIG. 15–8.** Multiple mid- and lower esophageal diverticula.

ated esophageal motility disorder before contemplating surgery. If a motor disorder is present, diverticulectomy may be followed by a recurrence of the diverticulum and symptoms would not be relieved [37]. Altorki et al. [2] studied 20 patients with thoracic esophageal diverticula over a 20-year period and found that 45% had dysphagia, 55% regurgitation, and 25% pulmonary symptoms. Seventeen patients agreed to the operation, with successful results. However, 18 of the 20 patients had an associated motor disorder, such as achalasia, diffuse esophageal spasm, Zenker's diverticulum, and other nonspecific disorders.

Surgery is rarely necessary for midesophageal diverticula and, when indicated, is dictated by the presence of a motor abnormality or a complication [36]. Diverticulectomy with or without myotomy is the treatment of choice [37, 47]. Some surgeons add a fundoplication [33, 36].

## EPIPHRENIC DIVERTICULA

As the name indicates, epiphrenic diverticula arise near the diaphragm (Fig. 15–9). However, the epiphrenic segment of the esophagus has been defined by some as the distal 4 cm, by others 10 cm, and even by others as the distal one-third of the esophagus [11]. Most authors reserve the term *epiphrenic diverticulum* for those occurring in the distal 3 to 4 cm of the esophagus.

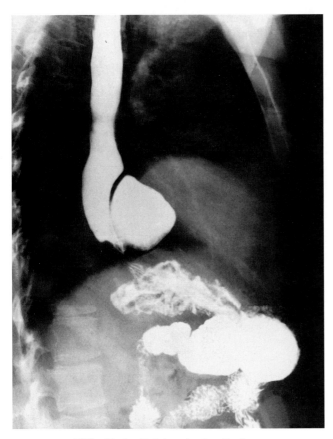

**FIG. 15–9.** Epiphrenic diverticulum.

### Etiology and Pathogenesis

The issue of traction and pulsion diverticulum was discussed earlier. For a long time, epiphrenic diverticula were thought to be of the pulsion type and were therefore labeled as pseudodiverticula. Such considerations have little clinical relevance. The important characteristic is that epiphrenic diverticula are almost always the result of an esophageal motor abnormality, such as incoordination between the distal esophagus and the LES, or a more diffuse abnormality, such as achalasia or diffuse esophageal spasm.

The strong association between epiphrenic diverticula and motor abnormalities of the esophagus was noted even in early reports. Bruggeman and Seaman [11] reported a motor abnormality in 48% of cases. It is probable that the proportion would have been higher had a method other than x-ray been used. In the same series, all patients with a diverticulum larger than 5 cm were found to have a significant abnormal motility disorder. Debas et al. [25] noted an abnormal motility disorder in 50 of 65 patients. This conclusion was reached based on manometry and roentgenology. However, only 36 patients had complete motility studies. In the 15 patients who did not appear to have an abnormal motility disorder, 13 had a hiatal hernia, five of whom had severe strictures.

### Clinical Features

Epiphrenic diverticula occur at all ages. The series of Bruggeman and Seaman [11] included 80 patients whose age ranged from 18 to 88 years, with 75% being between 41 and 70 years old.

Although the exact incidence of epiphrenic diverticula is not known, the condition does not appear to be too frequent. In 20 years, 160 patients were reported from the Mayo Clinic [1], and 80 patients were seen over a period of 18 years at the Columbia Presbyterian Medical Center [11]. The frequency is estimated to be 20% that of Zenker's diverticulum [6].

Patients with epiphrenic diverticula may be totally asymptomatic. Small diverticula may be discovered during an incidental roentgenographic examination. There appears to be no correlation between symptoms and size of the diverticulum. The presence and the severity of symptoms depend on the associated motor abnormality. It is imperative in patients with epiphrenic diverticula to obtain manometric studies in order to rule out a motility disorder. The most frequent abnormalities are achalasia and diffuse spasm [11, 25, 34], but other nonspecific abnormalities have been described as well [55]. Chest pain and regurgitation may also be presenting symptoms, particularly in giant diverticula [19]. Acute esophageal obstruction from food accumulating in the epiphrenic diverticulum has been reported [77]. Other complications are similar to those seen in midesophageal diverticula, such as perforation, fistula formation, and a rare case of carcinoma.

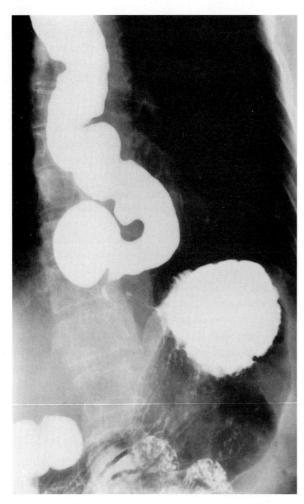

**FIG. 15–10.** Epiphrenic diverticulum in a patient with achalasia. The esophagus is dilated and tortuous, and other sacculations are seen.

### Diagnosis

An epiphrenic diverticulum is easily diagnosed on a barium roentgenogram. Multiple views should be taken in different positions to evaluate the size of the diverticulum and the site of its mouth. A video esophagram is helpful in subtle cases for identifying a motor abnormality. In patients with achalasia, the esophagus is tortuous and more than one diverticulum may be seen (Fig. 15–10). On computed tomography, a diverticulum will appear as a thin-walled or air-fluid-filled structure if an obstruction or motor disorder exists. The images may be confused with those of an abscess, a tumor, or a hiatal hernia [59].

Endoscopy, although not necessary, is helpful in diagnosing complications and esophageal inflammation. The procedure should be performed cautiously so that the endoscope does not inadvertently enter the cavity of the diverticulum.

Manometric studies are important to establish the presence of an associated motor abnormality. Usually, the area of the diverticulum will reveal low, poorly transmitted, or simultaneous contractions. Whether these changes are the result or the cause of the diverticulum is not known. Attention therefore should be given to the pressures and relaxation of the LES and abnormalities in peristalsis throughout the entire esophagus.

### Treatment

Small, asymptomatic epiphrenic diverticula probably do not require any treatment. However, the search for an associated motor abnormality should be carried out with the same intensity as in a symptomatic patient with a large diverticulum.

The goal of therapy should be to treat the motor disorder with the hope of avoiding further enlargement of the diverticulum (Fig. 15–11). The traditional treatment of an epiphrenic diverticulum consists of diverticulectomy alone or with myotomy [1, 6, 34, 53]. Surgical results are reported by most authors to be excellent, but little information is available about long-term follow-up. Hudspeth et al. [53] treated nine patients surgically and reported a follow-up of 94%, ranging from 3 months to 12 years, with good to excellent results in all patients as measured by symptom relief, weight gain, and absence of clinical recurrence. No details are given about radiographic appearance. On the other hand, Benacci et al. [6] operated on 33 patients, half of whom at least had had an associated motor disorder and had a follow-up in 29 patients ranging from 4 months to 15 years. The long-term results were good, but there were three operative deaths (9%) and an esophageal leak in 18%. All patients who showed an esophageal leak had had a diverticulectomy. In a related editorial, Orringer [78] pointed out the risks associated with surgical treatment of epiphrenic diverticula

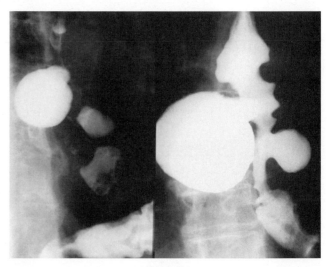

**FIG. 15–11.** Multiple epiphrenic diverticula are shown in two barium esophagograms taken 3 years apart in a 76-year-old man with solid-food dysphagia. The patient refused surgery at the time of the earlier study **(left)**. Note the progressive enlargement of the diverticula, which correlated with the patient's worsening symptoms.

and discussed the need to perform antireflux surgery in many patients. Diverticulectomy with myotomy in all patients is advocated by Mulder et al. [74].

It is quite difficult to assess the proper surgical technique for epiphrenic diverticula. Surgical series include a large proportion of patients with esophageal motor abnormalities. Some patients have been studied with manometry and many have not. It is not clear whether a diverticulectomy is necessary. Most authors agree that a diverticulectomy alone would result in a recurrence and advocate a long esophagomyotomy. The choice of operation should be based on the underlying disorder. For instance, in the case of a large, tortuous esophagus with esophageal sacculations due to achalasia, the addition of a diverticulectomy to myotomy would make no difference. If myotomy is not successful, esophagectomy should be considered.

## ESOPHAGEAL INTRAMURAL PSEUDODIVERTICULOSIS

Esophageal intramural pseudodiverticulosis is characterized by numerous minute, flask-like outpouchings along the esophageal wall.

### Etiology and Pathogenesis

Mendl et al. [70] described the condition as intramural diverticulosis due to herniation of the mucosa through gaps in the muscularis as a result of increased pressure. They likened the condition to the gallbladder sinuses of Rokitansky-Aschoff. Later studies using biopsy material and autopsy specimens revealed cystic dilatation of the esophageal gland ducts. The condition was thought to represent multiple mucous cysts of the submucosa, but since these pouches communicate with the lumen, the term *cyst* is not appropriate and the name *intramural pseudodiverticulosis* would be more accurate [9]. Hammon et al. [46] thought that the submucosal glands get impacted with inflammatory material secondary to stasis and suggested the term *esophageal adenitis*. Others thought that the pseudocystic dilatations were an exaggeration of normal anatomy, i.e., dilated glandular ducts [44]. Umlas and Sakhuja [92], studying carefully an esophagus obtained at autopsy, found thickening of the esophageal wall due to submucosal fibrosis at the level of a stricture, and the diverticular structures represented main excretory ducts of the submucosal glands rather than the glands themselves. Mederios et al. [69], who described two similar cases, proceeded to study 100 esophageal specimens collected during past autopsies as well as 20 cases obtained prospectively, in which sections were collected from various locations. The results of this study showed that in the random specimens obtained retrospectively dilated excretory ducts were found in 14% of cases and cysts in 7%. Comparatively, in the prospective study, 55% of specimens revealed dilated ducts and 15% cysts. In both groups, chronic inflammation was found in 65% to 67%. Additionally, cysts were found only

in patients over the age of 40. From these findings, Mederios et al. [69] concluded that the pathogenesis of intramural pseudodiverticulosis is extensive chronic inflammation leading to dilated ducts which in time develop small cysts and, when the cysts become large enough possibly decreased inflammation. They also pointed out that early changes of intramural pseudodiverticulosis were more common than described.

The frequent association of strictures in patients with pseudodiverticulosis and the frequent occurrence of pseudodiverticula above the stricture have been used as an argument to attribute the cause of the disorder to motor abnormalities. Various motor abnormalities have been described in these patients. Hammon et al. [46] found nonperistaltic contractions in two of three patients, and others have described nonspecific motility abnormalities [16]. One patient was reported with changes consistent with nutcracker esophagus [75], but esophageal motility may be normal in some cases [44, 46].

### Clinical Features

Intramural pseudodiverticulosis is a relatively rare condition. The exact prevalence is not known. In two large radiologic studies, it was present respectively in 0.09% [82] and 0.15% [63] of patients undergoing evaluation for a variety of conditions. Overall, less than 200 cases have been reported in the English literature [50].

The condition is found in both sexes. Most cases are discovered in the sixth and seventh decades, but a few cases have been reported in children and infants [24].

Patients with intramural pseudodiverticulosis present almost always with with dysphagia [9, 46, 66]. Dysphagia usually occurs with solid foods and may be abrupt [72].

When a stricture is associated with pseudodiverticulosis, it is most often proximal. In that case, pseudodiverticula occur above the stricture.

Other conditions have been described in association with intramural pseudodiverticulosis. Candidiasis is frequent and present in about 50% of cases. The presence of monilia may be attributed to stasis, which is quite frequent in cases of pseudodiverticulosis and does not seem to be the cause of the disease, even though chronic candidiasis may cause chronic esophageal inflammation [16, 46, 75].

Kochhar et al. [61] studied 59 patients with sequelae of corrosive acid injury and found 14 patients with esophageal intramural pseudodiverticulosis. The association with motor abnormalities has already been discussed. Pseudodiverticulosis was described in a case of achalasia [27]. Plavsic et al. [82] reviewed the esophagrams of 245 patients with carcinoma of the esophagus and compared them to 6,400 roentgenograms obtained for other reasons. They found intramural pseudodiverticulosis in 4.5% of patients with cancer compared to 0.09% in the control group. They concluded that there may be an increased risk of carcinoma in pseudodiverticulosis and stated that periodic surveillance for carcinoma may be worthwhile in patients with intramural pseudodiverticulosis. The coexistence of carcinoma and pseudodiverticulosis does not indicate a cause-and-effect relationship. Indeed, it is possible that pseudodiverticulosis is simply the result of stasis caused by obstruction from the carcinoma just as it is observed in benign strictures. There is no evidence that intramural pseudodiverticulosis constitutes a risk for cancer, and surveillance should not be recommended.

### Diagnosis

The diagnosis of esophageal intramural pseudodiverticulosis is usually made on a barium esophagram. The pouches are small, varying in length from 1 to 6 mm and usually less than 4 mm wide [61]. The neck of each diverticulum rarely measures more than 1 mm. The pouches are best seen when a double air contrast technique is performed [82]. Pseudodiverticulosis may be diffuse or segmental [38, 72, 92] (Figs. 15–12, 15–13).

Pseudodiverticulosis is not always recognized during en-

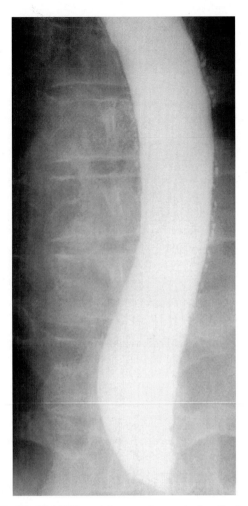

**FIG. 15–13.** Diffuse intramural pseudodiverticulosis.

doscopy, but visualization of pinpoint openings in the esophageal wall is easier since the advent of fiberoptic endoscopy [43, 66, 94].

Pearlberg et al. [81] described the computed tomographic (CT) features of esophageal intramural pseudodiverticulosis in one patient. They found marked thickening of the esophageal wall and loss of normal soft tissue planes with small intramural gas collections. The loss of soft tissue planes raised the question of malignancy, leading to a repeat endoscopy and biopsies which never confirmed the presence of a malignancy.

CT scanning does not seem to contribute to the diagnosis of pseudodiverticulosis and may create confusion in some cases. CT scans have been reported as normal [43] or showing thickening of the esophageal wall [94].

Esophageal manometry is indicated only in cases where a stricture is not present and when the radiographs suggest other abnormalities in the esophagus.

### Treatment

Intramural pseudodiverticulosis responds to esophageal dilatation with relief of symptoms for a few years [50, 66]. Some patients may require periodic dilatations [66].

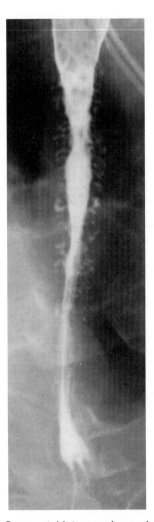

**FIG. 15–12.** Segmental intramural pseudodiverticulosis.

Medical treatment of candidiasis when present is appropriate and results in improvement [12] but is not always necessary [16]. In pseudodiverticulosis, treatment aims at relieving obstructive symptoms.

# REFERENCES

1. Allen TH, Clagett OT. Changing concepts in the surgical treatment of pulsion diverticula of the lower esophagus. J Thorac Cardiovasc Surg 1965;50:455

2. Altorki NK, Sunagawa M, Skinner DB. Thoracic esophageal diverticula. Why is operation necessary? J Thorac Cardiovasc Surg 1993;105:260

3. Asherson N. Achalasia of the cricopharyngeal sphincter: a record of cases, with profile pharyngograms. J Laryngol Otol 1950;64:747

4. Balthazar EJ. Esophagobronchial fistula secondary to ruptured traction diverticulum. Gastrointest Radiol 1977;2:119

5. Banerjee AJ, Westmore GA. Inversion of Zenker's diverticulum [Letter]. Head Neck 1994;16:291

6. Benacci JC, Deschamps C, Trastek VF, Allen MS, Daley RC, Pairolero PC. Epiphrenic diverticulum: results of surgical treatment. Ann Thorac Surg 1993;55:1109

7. Benjamin B, Innocenti M. Laser treatment of pharyngeal pouch. Aust N Z J Surg 1991;61:909

8. Bowdler DA, Stell PM. Carcinoma arising in posterior pharyngeal pulsion diverticulum (Zenker's diverticulum). Br J Surg 1987;74:561

9. Boyd RM, Bogoch A, Greig JH, Trites AEW. Esophageal intramural pseudodiverticulosis. Radiology 1974;113:267

10. Brouillette D, Martel E, Chen LQ, Duranceau A. Pitfalls and complications of cricopharyngeal myotomy. Chest Surg Clin N Am 1997;7:457

11. Bruggeman LL, Seaman WB. Epiphrenic diverticula. An analysis of 80 cases. AJR Am J Roentgenol 1973;119:266

12. Cantor DS, Riley TL. Intramural pseudodiverticulosis of the esophagus. Am J Gastroenterol 1982;77:454

13. Case records of the Massachusetts General Hospital. Weekly clinicopathological exercises. Case 7-1977. N Engl J Med 1977;296:384

14. Case records of the Massachusetts General Hospital. Weekly clinicopathological exercises. Case 32-1982. N Engl J Med 1982;307:426

15. Castell JA, Dalton BC, Castell DO. Pharyngeal and upper esophageal sphincter manometry in humans. Am J Physiol 1990;258:G173

16. Castillo S, Aburashed A, Kimmelman J, Alexander LC. Diffuse intramural esophageal pseudodiverticulosis. New cases and review. Gastroenterology 1977;72:541

17. Clements JL, Abernathy J, Weens HS. Atypical esophageal diverticula associated with progressive systemic sclerosis. Gastrointest Radiol 1978;3:383

18. Collard JM, Otte JB, Kestens PJ. Endoscopic stapling technique of esophagodiverticulostomy for Zenker's diverticulum. Ann Thorac Surg 1993;56:573

19. Conrad C, Nissen F. Giant epiphrenic diverticula. Eur J Radiol 1982;2:48

20. Cook IJ, Blumbergs P, Cash K, Jamieson GG, Shearman DJ. Structural abnormalities of the cricopharyngeus muscle in patients with pharyngeal (Zenker's) diverticulum. J Gastroenterol Hepatol 1992;7:556

21. Cook IJ, et al. Pharyngeal (Zenker's) diverticulum is a disorder of upper esophageal sphincter opening. Gastroenterology 1992;103:1229

22. Cross FS, Johnson GF, Gerein AN. Esophageal diverticula. Associated neuromuscular changes in the esophagus. Arch Surg 1961;83:525

23. Dantas RO, Cook IJ, Dodds WJ, Kern MK, Lang IM, Brasseur JG. Biomechanics of cricopharyngeal bars. Gastroenterology 1990;99:1269

24. Daud AS, O'Connor F. Oesophageal intramural pseudodiverticulosis: a cause of dysphagia in a 10-year-old boy. Eur J Pediatr 1997;156:530

25. Debas HT, Payne WS, Cameron AJ, Carlson HC. Physiopathology of lower esophageal diverticulum and its implications for treatment. Surg Gynecol Obstet 1980;151:593

26. Dodds WJ, Stef JJ, Hogan WJ, Hoke SE, Stewart ED, Arndorfer RC. Radial distribution of esophageal peristaltic pressure in normal subjects and patients with esophageal diverticulum. Gastroenterology 1975;69:584

27. Dua KS, Stewart E, Arndorfer R, Shaker R. Esophageal intramural pseudodiverticulosis associated with achalasia. Am J Gastroenterol 1996;91:1859

28. Duda M, Sery Z, Vojacek K, Rocek V, Rehulka M. Etiopathogenesis and classification of esophageal diverticula. Int Surg 1985;70:291

29. Duranceau A. Oropharyngeal dysphagia and disorders of the upper esopharyngeal sphincter. Ann Chir Gynaecol 1995;84:225

30. Ekberg O, Mylander G. Cineradiography of the pharyngeal phase of deglutition in 250 patients with dysphagia. Br J Radiol 1982;55:258

31. Ellis FH, Crozier RE. Cervical esophageal dysphagia. Indications for and results of cricopharyngeal myotomy. Ann Surg 1981;194:279

32. Ellis FH, Schlegel JF, Lynch VP, Payne WS. Cricopharyngeal myotomy for pharyngoesophageal diverticulitis. Ann Surg 1969;170:340

33. Evander A, Little AG, Ferguson MK, Skinner DB. Diverticula of the mid- and lower esophagus: pathogenesis and surgical management. World J Surg 1986;10:820

34. Falk G. Regurgitation in a patient with an esophageal diverticulum. Cleve Cleve Clin J Med 1994;61:409

35. Fegiz G, Paolini A, DeMarchi C, Tosato F. Surgical management of esophageal diverticula. World J Surg 1984;8:757

36. Fekete F, Vonns C. Surgical management of esophageal thoracic diverticula. Hepatogastroenterology 1992;39:97

37. Ferraro P, Duranceau A. Esophageal diverticula. Chest Surg Clin N Am 1994;4:741

38. Flora KD, Gordon MD, Lieberman D, Schmidt W. Esophageal intramural pseudodiverticulosis. Dig Dis 1997;15:113

39. Fuessner H, Siewert JR. Zenker's diverticulum and reflux. Hepatogastroenterology 1992;39:100

40. Fulp SR, Castell DO. Manometric aspects of Zenker's diverticulum. Hepatogastroenterology 1992;39:123

41. Gage-White L. Incidence of Zenker's diverticulum with hiatus hernia. Laryngoscope 1988;98:527

42. Gerhardt DC, Shuck TJ, Bordeaux RA, Winship DH. Human upper esophageal sphincter. Gastroenterology 1978;75:268

43. Gillessen A, Konturek J, Roos N, Domschke W. Esophageal intramural pseudodiverticulosis: a characteristically unusual path to diagnosis. Endoscopy 1996;28:640

44. Graham DY, Goyal RK, Sparkman J, Cagan ME, Pogonowska MJ. Diffuse intramural esophageal diverticulosis. Gastroenterology 1975;68:781

45. Grégoire J, Duranceau A. Surgical management of Zenker's diverticulum. Hepatogastroenterology 1991;39:132

46. Hammon JW Jr, Rice RP, Postlethwait RW, Young WG Jr. Esophageal intramural diverticulosis. Ann Thorac Surg 1974;17:260

47. Harrington SW. The surgical treatment of pulsion diverticula of the thoracic esophagus. Ann Surg 1949;129:606

48. Hendren WG, Anderson T, Miller JI. Massive bleeding in a Zenker's diverticulum. South Med J 1990;83:362

49. Herman TE, McAlister WH. Esophageal diverticula in childhood associated with strictures from unsuspected foreign bodies of the esophagus. Pediatr Radiol 1991;21:410

50. Herter B, Dittler HJ, Wuttge-Hannig A, Siewert JR. Intramural pseudodiverticulosis of the esophagus: a case series. Endoscopy 1997;29:109

51. Huang B, Payne WS, Cameron AJ. Surgical management for recurrent pharyngoesophageal (Zenker's) diverticulum. Ann Thorac Surg 1984;37:189

52. Huang B, Unni KK, Payne WS. Long-term survival following diverticulectomy for cancer in pharyngoesophageal (Zenker's) diverticulum. Ann Thorac Surg 1984;38:207

53. Hudspeth DA, Thorne MT, Conroy R, Pennell TC. Management of epiphrenic esophageal diverticula. A fifteen-year experience. Am Surg 1993;59:40

54. Hunt PS, Connell AM, Smiley TB. The cricopharyngeal sphincter in gastric reflux. Gut 1970;11:303

55. Hurwitz AL, Way LW, Haddad JK. Epiphrenic diverticulum in association with an unusual motility disturbance: report of surgical correction. Gastroenterology 1975;68:795

56. Jancu J, Marvan H. Multiple diverticula of the esophagus. Am J Gastroenterol 1973;60:408

57. Johnson JT, Curtin HD. Carcinoma associated with Zenker's diverticulum. Ann Otol Rhinol Laryngol 1985;94:324

58. Kahrilas PJ, Dodds WJ, Dent J, Logemann JA, Shaker R. Upper

esophageal sphincter function during deglutition. Gastroenterology 1988;95:52

59. Kim KW, Berkmen YM, Auh YH, Kazam E. Diagnosis of epiphrenic esophageal diverticulum by computed tomography. J Comput Assist Tomogr 1988;12:25

60. Knuff TE, Benjamin SB, Castell DO. Pharyngoesophageal (Zenker's) diverticulum: a reappraisal. Gastroenterology 1982;82:734

61. Kochhar R, Mehta SK, Nagi B, Goenka MK. Corrosive acid-induced esophageal intramural pseudodiverticulosis. Gastroenterology 1991; 13:371

62. Lerut T, van Raemdonck D, Guelinckx P, Dom R, Geboes K. Zenker's diverticulum: is a myotomy of the cricopharyngeus useful? How long should it be? Hepatogastroenterology 1992;39:127

63. Levine MS, Moolten DN, Herlinger H, Laufer I. Esophageal intramural pseudodiverticulosis: a reevaluation. AJR Am J Roentgenol 1986;147:1165

64. Louie HW, Zuckerbraun L. Staged Zenker's diverticulectomy with cervical esophagostomy and secondary esophagostomy closure for treatment of massive diverticulum in severely debilitated patients. Am Surg 1993;12:842

65. Mahajan RJ, Marshall JB. Severe dysphagia, dysmotility, and unusual saccular dilation (diverticulum) of the esophagus following excision of an asymptomatic congenital cyst. Am J Gastroenterol 1996;91: 1254

66. Mahajan SK, Warshauer DM, Bozymski EM. Esophageal intramural pseudodiverticulosis: endoscopic and radiologic correlation. Gastrointest Endosc 1993;39:565

67. Mahieu HF, deBree R, Dagli SA, Snel AM. The pharyngoesophageal segment: endoscopic treatment of Zenker's diverticulum. Dis Esophagus 1996;9:12

68. McConnel FMS, Hood D, Jackson K, O'Connor A. Analysis of intrabolus forces in patients with Zenker's diverticulum. Laryngoscope 1994;104:1571

69. Medeiros LJ, Doos WG, Balogh K. Esophageal intramural pseudodiverticulosis: a report of two cases with analysis of similar, less extensive changes in ''normal'' autopsy esophagi. Hum Pathol 1988;19: 928

70. Mendl K, McKay JM, Tanner CH. Intramural diverticulosis of the esophagus and Rokitansky-Aschoff sinuses in the gallbladder. Br J Radiol 1960;33:496

71. Migliore M, Payne H, Jeyasingham K. Pathophysiologic basis for operation on Zenker's diverticulum. Ann Thorac Surg 1994;57:1616

72. Montgomery RD, Mendl K, Stephenson SF. Intramural diverticulosis of the oesophagus. Thorax 1975;30:278

73. Morton RP, Bartley JRF. Inversion of Zenker's diverticulum: the preferred option. Head Neck 1993;15:253

74. Mulder DG, Rosenkranz E, DenBesten L. Management of huge epiphrenic esophageal diverticula. Am J Surg 1989;157:303

75. Murney RG, Linne JH, Curtis J. High-amplitude peristaltic contractions in a patient with esophageal intramural pseudodiverticulosis. Dig Dis Sci 1983;28:843

76. Nilsson ME, Isberg A, Schiratzki H. The hypopharyngeal diverticulum. Acta Otolaryngol (Stockh) 1988;106:314

77. Niv Y, Fraser G, Krugliak P. Gastroesophageal obstruction from food in an epiphrenic esophageal diverticulum. J Clin Gastroenterol 1993; 16:314

78. Orringer MB. Epiphrenic diverticula: fact and fable. Ann Thorac Surg 1993;55:1067

79. Payne WS. The treatment of pharyngoesophageal diverticulum: the simple and complex. Hepatogastroenterology 1992;39:109

80. Payne WS, Reynolds RR. Surgical treatment of pharyngoesophageal diverticulum (Zenker's diverticulum). Surg Rounds 1982;5:18

81. Pearlberg JL, Sandler MA, Madrazo BL. Computed tomographic features of esophageal intramural pseudodiverticulosis. Radiology 1983; 147:189

82. Plavsic BM, et al. Intramural pseudodiverticulosis of the esophagus detected on barium esophagograms: increased prevalence in patients with esophageal carcinoma. AJR Am J Roentgenol 1995;165:1381

83. Ponette E, Coolen J. Radiological aspects of Zenker's diverticulum. Hepatogastroenterology 1992;39:115

84. Resouly A, Braat J, Jackson A, Evans H. Pharyngeal pouch: link with reflux and oesophageal dysmotility. Clin Otolaryngol 1994;19:241

85. Rubesin SE, Yousem DM. Structural abnormalities. In Gore RM, Levine MS, Laufer I, eds, Textbook of Gastrointestinal Radiology. Philadelphia: WB Saunders, 1994:244

86. Schick A, Yesner R. Traction diverticulum of esophagus with exsanguination: report of a case. Ann Intern Med 1953;39:345

87. Schima W, et al. Association of midoesophageal diverticula with oesophageal motor disorders. Acta Radiol 1997;38:108

88. Schmit PJ, Zuckerbraun L. Treatment of Zenker's diverticula by cricopharyngeus myotomy under local anesthesia. Am Surg 1992;58:710

89. Schreiber MH, Davis M. Intraluminal diverticulum of the esophagus. AJR Am J Roentgenol 1977;129:595

90. Shaw DW, et al. Influence of surgery on deglutitive upper oesophageal sphincter mechanics in Zenker's diverticulum. Gut 1996;38:806

91. Sutherland HD. Cricopharyngeal achalasia. J Thorac Cardiovasc Surg 1962;43:114

92. Umlas J, Sakhuja R. The pathology of esophageal intramural pseudodiverticulosis. Am J Clin Pathol 1976;65:314

93. Vakil NB, Kahrilas PJ, Dodds WJ, Vanagunas A. Absence of an upper esophageal sphincter response to acid reflux. Am J Gastroenterol 1989;84:606

94. van der Putten ABMM, Loffeld RJLF. Esophageal intramural pseudodiverticulosis. Dis Esophagus 1997;10:61

95. van Overbeek JJM. Meditation on the pathogenesis of hypopharyngeal (Zenker's) diverticulum and a report of endoscopic treatment in 545 patients. Ann Otol Rhinol Laryngol 1994;103:178

96. Van Overbeek JJM, Hoeksema PE. Endoscopic treatment of the hypopharyngeal diverticulum: 211 cases. Laryngoscope 1982;92:88

97. Watemberg S, Landau O, Avrahami R. Zenker's diverticulum: reappraisal. Am J Gastroenterol 1996;91:1494

98. Welsh GF, Payne WS. The present status of one-stage pharyngoesophageal diverticulectomy. Surg Clin North Am 1973;53:953

99. Wouters B, van Overbeek JJM. Endoscopic treatment of the hypopharyngeal (Zenker's) diverticulum. Hepatogastroenterology 1992;39: 105

100. Zeitoun H, Widdowson D, Hammad Z, Osborne J. A video-fluoroscopic study of patients treated by diverticulectomy and cricopharyngeal myotomy. Clin Otolaryngol 1994;19:301

*The Esophagus*, Third Edition,
edited by D. O. Castell and J. E. Richter.
Lippincott Williams & Wilkins, Philadelphia © 1999.

CHAPTER 16

# Esophageal Manifestations in Systemic Diseases

Joseph Carl Yarze

Esophageal abnormalities can occur with a variety of systemic diseases. Heterogeneity of clinical manifestations occurs both within and between the various systemic diseases. In this chapter, a variety of systemic diseases that can affect the esophagus are reviewed, with an emphasis on systemic sclerosis (SSc).

## CONNECTIVE TISSUE DISEASES

### Systemic Sclerosis

SSc is a generalized connective tissue disorder which is characterized by obliterative small vessel vasculitis and proliferation of connective tissue with fibrosis of multiple organs, including the skin, heart, lungs, kidneys, and gastrointestinal tract. Although its etiology and pathogenesis are unknown, a recent hypothesis suggests that genetic susceptibility may interact with environmental stimuli to cause cellular immune activation and immune mediator release, with consequent endothelial injury, fibroblast proliferation, and ultimate end-organ damage [72]. In a historical account of the disease, Rodnan and Benedek [178] reviewed Curzio's monograph, which described the first convincing case of SSc in a 17-year-old woman. In this case, it is mentioned that ''her digestion was good and she found no inconvenience after eating.'' Involvement of the gastrointestinal tract was originally reported by Ehrmann [65] in 1903, when he described a patient with SSc who complained of dysphagia. Ehrmann postulated that changes similar to those affecting the skin were also present in the esophagus and other viscera.

Gastrointestinal tract involvement occurs in up to 90% of SSc patients and is the third most common clinical manifestation of the disease, following only skin changes and Raynaud's phenomenon (RP) [193]. In approximately 10% of patients, gastrointestinal symptoms may occur prior to the appearance of cutaneous manifestations [108]. Although

sclerodermatous gastrointestinal involvement may be asymptomatic [152, 179], approximately half of the patients experience serious, symptomatic gastrointestinal disease [42]. The esophagus is the most frequently affected gastrointestinal tract segment in SSc, followed in decreasing order of frequency by the anorectal region, small bowel, stomach, and colon.

### Pathologic Features

In 1924, Matsui [140] described sclerodermatous esophageal pathologic changes. Over the subsequent years, pathologic esophageal findings have been well described and include smooth muscle atrophy, sclerosis of arterioles, and collagen deposition in the lamina propria, submucosa, and serosa [45, 172, 205]. Normal striated muscle has been typically seen amid atrophic smooth muscle components in the proximal esophagus [11, 205]. Although occasional round cell inflammatory infiltrates involving Auerbach's myenteric plexus have been noted [57, 78, 205], consistent anatomic neuropathic lesions in the SSc esophagus have not been described [18, 172, 205]. A study performed by Cohen and colleagues [41] in 1972 has indirectly supported the presence of neural dysfunction in the pathogenesis of the functional esophageal abnormalities in SSc. In this investigation, the lower esophageal sphincter (LES) response to methacholine, edrophonium, and gastrin I was studied in patients with SSc. The study suggested that patients with less advanced SSc, as manifested by reduced peristaltic amplitude and LES pressure, have an abnormality in cholinergic neural function and a diminished LES response to cholinesterase inhibitor (edrophonium) with a somewhat preserved response to direct cholinergic receptor stimulation (with methacholine). Later in the disease, smooth muscle atrophy leads to aperistalsis and an absent response to even direct cholinergic stimulation. All patients showed diminished response to gastrin I (which acts by release of endogenous acetylcholine and requires an intact cholinergic nervous system), suggesting an abnormality in intrinsic cholinergic neural function. These findings appear to support the hypothesis that a neural

J. C. Yarze: Division of Gastroenterology, Department of Medicine, Glens Falls Hospital and Gastroenterology Associates of Northern New York, Glens Falls, New York 12801.

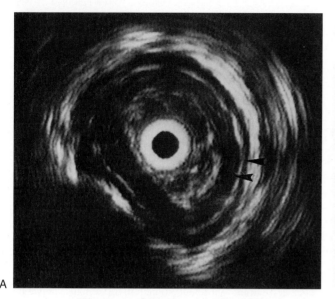
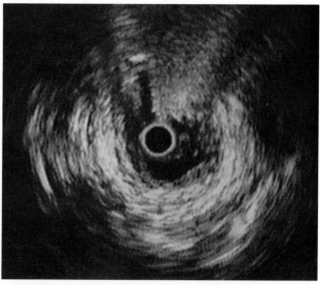

A                                                                          B

**FIG. 16–1. A:** Endoscopic ultrasound view of a normal distal esophagus, showing distinct hypoechoic outer longitudinal and inner circular layers of the muscularis propria (*arrowheads*). **B:** Endoscopic ultrasound view of the distal esophagus in a patient with scleroderma and distal aperistalsis. The muscularis propria has been widely replaced by connective tissue, indicated by the diffuse hyperechoic abnormality.

lesion may occur early in the disease course before the development of smooth muscle atrophy, which is characteristic of more advanced disease. Studies investigating other segments of the alimentary tract in SSc have also documented abnormal motor responses to mechanical stimulation, suggesting the presence of an early latent neural defect [14, 33, 59, 81, 83].

A recent study by Miller and colleagues [145] revealed a hyperechoic abnormality in the muscularis propria of the distal esophagus in SSc patients, utilizing high-resolution endoluminal sonography (Fig. 16–1). This hyperechoic abnormality (in the usually hypoechoic muscularis propria) correlated histologically with the presence of fibrosis. The degree of this hyperechoic abnormality also correlated with functional esophageal abnormalities, as determined by manometric and pH-monitoring studies. This study provided evidence that fibrosis in the muscularis propria may be prominent and of pathogenic importance, as regards the functional esophageal abnormalities in SSc.

### Clinical Features

Patients with sclerodermatous esophageal involvement may complain of pyrosis, regurgitation, and dysphagia. Although some authors have suggested that dysphagia may be more common [75, 93, 182, 192], most studies have documented heartburn as being the more prevalent symptom [2, 111, 128, 158, 210, 223]. The severe pyrosis experienced by these patients is due to reflux of acid across a relatively hypotonic LES, in conjunction with prolonged esophageal acid exposure time related to impaired esophageal peristalsis. Dysphagia may occur for a variety of reasons and may

reflect esophageal dysmotility, ulcerative esophagitis, a superimposed benign peptic stricture, a Barrett-related esophageal malignancy, or esophageal candidiasis. Esophageal dysmotility usually causes nonprogressive dysphagia to both liquids and solids. Benign peptic strictures are characteristically associated with gradually progressive dysphagia to solids and subsequently liquids. Esophageal malignancies typically cause rapidly progressive dysphagia in association with prominent weight loss. Severe acid-induced ulcerative esophagitis and infectious esophagitis are usually accompanied by prominent odynophagia.

Patients with SSc are known to be afflicted with severe, complicated gastroesophageal reflux (GER) disease (GERD). Although prior emphasis has been placed on LES hypotension, recent investigations have focused on the pathophysiologic importance of impaired esophageal peristalsis in determining the severity of SSc-related GERD [12, 151, 220, 223]. Zamost et al. [223] and Basilisco et al. [12] studied a total of 69 SSc patients and found esophagitis only in those with abnormal peristalsis. Colleagues and I [220] prospectively studied 36 SSc patients, utilizing a combination of computerized solid-state manometry and dual-channel ambulatory esophageal pH monitoring. The study population included 16 patients with diffuse and 20 with the limited variant of SSc, as classified by previously published criteria [120]. Patients were separated for analysis into two subgroups based on the absence or presence of distal esophageal peristalsis. In accord with previous studies [2, 73], we found a similar frequency of esophageal dysmotility in those with the diffuse and limited SSc variants. While LES pressures were similar in the patients with absent and retained peristalsis, those with aperistalsis had significantly greater distal esophageal acid exposure (Fig. 16–2A). Excessive proximal esophageal acid exposure was documented only in patients with absent distal esophageal peristalsis (Fig. 16–2B). Linear regression analysis revealed a poor correlation between resting LES pressure and esophageal acid exposure. While esophageal acid clearance times were significantly longer for patients with aperistalsis, those with retained peristalsis had a mean acid clearance time that was not significantly longer than that found in normal subjects. These observations suggest that the severity and extent of GER in SSc are most closely related to the integrity of distal esophageal peristalsis, with LES hypotension being a less critical factor.

Benign peptic strictures of the esophagus occur commonly in SSc as a consequence of severe GERD. The incidence of peptic strictures in published series has varied from 3% to 42% [36, 151, 160, 170, 223], and this wide variation likely reflects differences in patient selection.

Barrett's metaplasia of the esophagus (BE) is known to occur in 10% of patients with persistent, severe symptoms of GER. Given the high frequency of severe GER in SSc, a favorable milieu for the development of BE would be expected. A large retrospective study in which SSc patients with esophageal symptoms underwent endoscopy revealed a 37% prevalence of BE [105]. Another study that included 13 SSc patients, regardless of symptomatology, found BE in four (30%) [99]. Other studies did not find BE to be present in relatively large samples of SSc patients [220, 223]. A recent Danish study [87] investigated the use of omeprazole in the treatment of SSc patients whose GER was refractory to H2-receptor antagonist therapy. These investigators confirmed intestinal metaplasia of the esophagus in 36% of the 25 patients studied. These divergent results suggest that

different inclusion criteria in the various studies have likely introduced a prominent element of selection bias.

Considering that SSc is frequently accompanied by severe GER and a propensity for BE, one would expect a predisposition to esophageal adenocarcinoma. While the prevalence of esophageal adenocarcinoma in SSc has not been determined in a prospective manner, several reports have described an association between these diseases [100, 141, 156, 204]. A retrospective analysis of 680 patients with SSc found only one case of adenocarcinoma of the esophagus, which was considered to fall within the expected range for a control population [189]. The authors of this analysis [189] concluded that the incidence of esophageal adenocarcinoma was not increased in SSc, and surveillance procedures were not indicated [142, 189]. In the retrospective study by Katzka and co-workers [105], of 75 SSc patients, 24 underwent esophagoscopy and nine (37%) were found to have BE. Two patients in the group with BE had esophageal adenocarcinoma. The available data from retrospective studies suggest that the prevalence of esophageal adenocarcinoma in SSc is comparable to that in patients with idiopathic GER and BE, in which prevalence rates of 7% to 46.5% have been reported [26, 153, 171, 194–196, 216].

The association between RP and esophageal aperistalsis has raised the possibility that both may reflect an underlying autonomic nervous or vasomotor defect [24, 199]. Contrary to this hypothesis, Garrett and colleagues [75] found that the presence of RP was not useful in determining the prognosis or progression of esophageal involvement in SSc. Tsianos and colleagues [209] investigated the effects of peripheral cold exposure on esophageal motility in patients with rheumatologic conditions with and without associated RP. There was no difference in the manometric reaction to peripheral

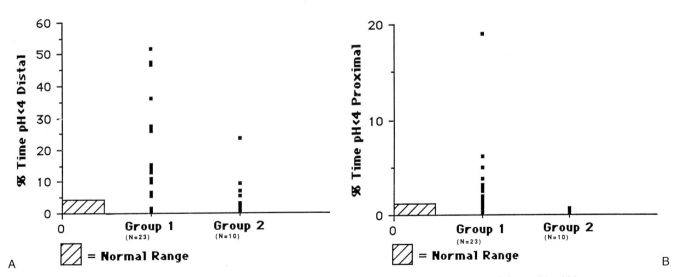

**FIG. 16–2. A:** Distal 24-hour esophageal acid exposure (expressed as percent of time with pH less than 4) as recorded for patients with scleroderma having absent (*group 1*) or retained (*group 2*) distal esophageal peristalsis. The normal range is included. **B:** Proximal 24-hour esophageal acid exposure (expressed as percent of time with pH less than 4) as recorded for scleroderma patients with absent (*group 1*) or retained (*group 2*) distal esophageal peristalsis. The normal range is included.

cold pressor testing between the two study groups. A recent study showed that episodes of RP did not worsen esophageal function [111]. In this investigation, Klein and co-workers [111] induced RP in nine patients with SSc and found no significant changes in esophageal function by manometric and scintigraphic testing. Although Belch and colleagues [17] showed that induction of RP decreased esophageal blood flow (by temperature studies), the observations of Klein et al. [111] suggest that such changes in esophageal perfusion have no clinically measurable effects on esophageal motility. A recent manometric investigation which included 150 patients with various rheumatic diseases [117] investigated the relation between esophageal dysmotility and RP. While approximately two-thirds of patients with RP demonstrated esophageal dysmotility, only half of those with manometric abnormalities had RP. The above findings suggest that in patients with rheumatologic diseases RP and esophageal dysmotility are not pathogenetically related and should be viewed as independent clinical phenomena.

Although involvement of the esophagus is not related to the overall prognosis in patients with SSc [5], esophageal dysmotility and consequent GER may be contributing pathogenetic factors to the pulmonary disease in these patients. Denis and colleagues [55] observed a significant decrease in lung compliance in SSc patients with impaired peristalsis and LES function when compared to patients with either normal esophageal motility or only impaired peristalsis. Although esophageal pH monitoring was not performed in this study, the results suggested that impaired esophageal motility in SSc may be related to the pulmonary fibrosis in this disease. Johnson and co-workers [99] performed a study that included esophageal pH monitoring, pulmonary function testing, and scintigraphic lung aspiration scanning. In this investigation, there was evidence for proximal GER and aspiration in the majority of patients. Furthermore, the degree of GER and severity of pulmonary disease were distinctly correlated. A recent retrospective analysis of 47 SSc patients who underwent extensive esophageal and pulmonary testing demonstrated no significant functional relationship between esophageal acid exposure and the severity of pulmonary disease (Fig. 16–3) [206]. This most recent evidence argues against acid microaspiration as being an important pathogenetic factor in the development of pulmonary disease in SSc.

A recent longitudinal study performed by Dantas and colleagues [50] has suggested that esophageal involvement in SSc is not necessarily a progressive phenomenon. In this investigation, 16 of 17 SSc patients had no difference in LES pressure or esophageal body peristaltic amplitude, velocity, or duration of contraction when studied manometrically at an interval of 9 to 111 months (median, 40 months). These results suggest that the inclusion of an appropriate control population is critical when studying the effects of drug intervention on esophageal motility in SSc.

### Diagnosis

The diagnosis of SSc is based on clinical criteria proposed by the American Rheumatism Association [137]. The major criterion for diagnosis of SSc is proximal scleroderma, which is defined as bilateral symmetric sclerodermatous changes in the skin proximal to the metacarpophalangeal or metatarsophalangeal joints. The minor criteria include sclerodactyly, digital pitting scars, and bibasilar pulmonary fibrosis. Systemic sclerosis is diagnosed if either the major criterion or at least two minor criteria are present. Scleroderma recently has been subclassified into diffuse and limited variants, based on the extent of cutaneous involvement [120].

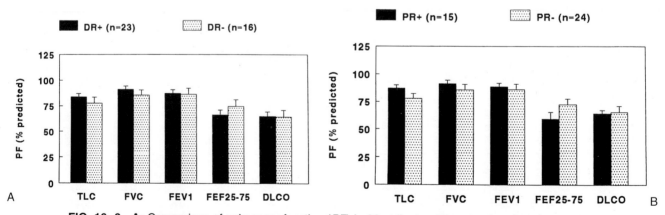

**FIG. 16–3. A:** Comparison of pulmonary function (*PF*) in 39 patients with systemic sclerosis: 23 with abnormal distal reflux (*DR+*) and 16 with normal distal reflux (*DR−*). No significant differences in any of the function test results were found between these two patient groups. **B:** Comparison of pulmonary function (*PF*) in 39 patients with systemic sclerosis: 15 with abnormal proximal reflux (*PR+*) and 24 with normal proximal reflux (*PR−*). No significant differences in any of the function test results were found between these two patient groups. *TLC*, total lung capacity; *FVC*, forced vital capacity; *FEV1*, forced expiratory volume in 1 second; *FEF25-75*, forced expiratory flow after 25% to 75% of vital capacity has been expelled; *DLCO*, carbon monoxide-diffusing capacity of the lungs.

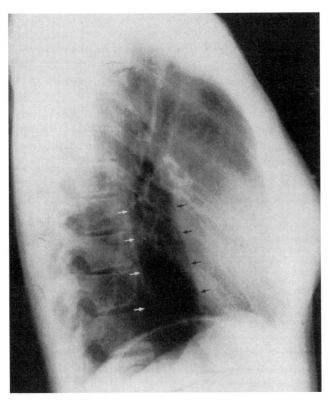

FIG. 16–4. A lateral chest radiograph of a patient with systemic sclerosis. The air-filled esophagus is outlined by *arrows* and results from incompetence of the lower esophageal sphincter in conjunction with a dilated, atonic esophagus. (From ref. 38, with permission.)

### Radiographic Findings

As the empty esophagus is normally a collapsed structure, it is usually not seen on plain chest roentgenograms. In SSc, a dilated and atonic esophagus may be visualized as a prominent air-filled structure [60, 94, 115, 135, 158], as illustrated in Fig. 16–4. The frequency with which an air esophagram is reported in SSc has varied considerably among studies. This variation is in large measure likely reflective of the definition employed (i.e., continuous versus ''skip'' air column). Studies which stringently define an air esophagram as being a reproducible, continuous air column note this radiographic finding to be present in ~15% of SSc patients [94, 158]. One study has suggested that although esophageal symptoms are inevitably present in SSc patients in whom an air esophagram is noted, this radiologic finding appears to be most closely related to the presence of regurgitation [158]. Air esophagrams are not specific to SSc and may also be seen in idiopathic achalasia, patients who practice esophageal speech (after total laryngectomy), and following chest surgery or chronic inflammatory disease involving the mediastinum [94]. Although more commonly noted in SSc, accompanying air in the gastric fundus may also be seen infrequently in achalasia [94]. Similarly, although more frequent in achalasia, a temporary air-fluid level may also be noted less commonly in SSc [94]. The presence of an esopha-

geal air-fluid level in known SSc should, however, heighten the clinician's awareness as to the possibility of a superimposed benign or malignant esophageal stricture.

Barium esophagrams are abnormal in the majority of SSc patients. Several studies which have compared barium radiography to esophageal manometry in SSc patients have corroborated that the former is a less sensitive method for detecting motility abnormalities [36, 69, 155, 215]. Barium radiography may suffer from its being necessarily subjective, but it clearly offers the advantage of yielding specific anatomic information. Barium radiographs often reveal esophageal dilation and a patulous gastroesophageal junction, with free reflux of contrast material into the proximal esophagus (Fig. 16–5). Diminished or absent primary peristaltic contractions in the smooth muscle-containing distal esophagus are often noted, and although contractions may move distally, they are often visualized as nonlumen-obliterating, with a portion of the barium bolus escaping proximally. Changes suggestive of erosive esophagitis and benign or malignant strictures may be identified in some patients.

Radionuclide scintigraphy has been reported to be useful for the quantitative assessment of esophageal function in patients with motility disorders [20, 69, 181]. Advantages of radionuclide scintigraphy include its noninvasive nature, low radiation exposure, objectivity, and excellent patient acceptance. The major drawbacks include its nonspecificity and its inability to provide anatomic information. Several studies have evaluated radionuclide scintigraphy in SSc and documented its usefulness in detecting esophageal dysfunction [3, 28, 52, 63, 111, 117, 214]. In SSc, radionuclide scintigraphy detects impaired esophageal function with a

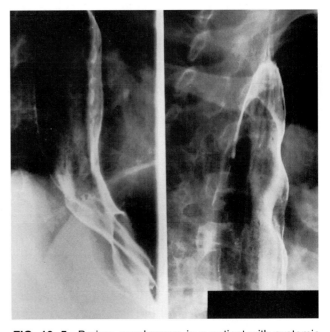

FIG. 16–5. Barium esophagram in a patient with systemic sclerosis. The esophagram reveals a dilated esophagus **(right)** and patulous gastroesophageal junction **(left)**.

sensitivity comparable to that of cineradiography and manometry. Given the above-mentioned considerations, radionuclide scintigraphy would appear to be most useful to quantitatively assess changes in esophageal function, as during therapeutic interventions.

### Manometric Findings

Esophageal manometric abnormalities are often noted prior to the evolution of symptoms in SSc. Up to 90% of SSc patients have demonstrable manometric abnormalities showing decreased frequency or amplitude of peristaltic contractions in the distal, smooth muscle-containing esophagus that may progress to aperitalsis but with retained contractions in the proximal, striated muscle portion (Fig. 16–6). A reduced LES pressure is often noted [36, 44, 62, 75, 106, 114, 215]. Recent studies suggest that, rather than being absent, LES pressures in these patients are usually in the lower range of normal [220, 223]. Incomplete LES relaxation has been noted [44, 106, 163] but appears to be uncommon [220]. Normal contraction pressures and peristalsis are usually present in the proximal (predominantly striated muscle) esophagus. Although the manometric pattern of distal

esophageal aperistalsis and LES hypotension is typical of sclerodermatous esophageal involvement, it is not specific for this entity and may be seen less commonly in a variety of rheumatologic and miscellaneous disorders [82, 134, 175, 184, 199, 207]. A recent single-center investigation [117] which studied 150 patients with a variety of rheumatogic disorders confirmed the prior impression that similar manometric abnormalities of the esophageal body and LES regions may be seen in other non-SSc rheumatologic diseases. Interestingly, although such esophageal manometric changes are noted less commonly in the other diseases, there is a broad overlap in frequency and, when found, the abnormalities may be of similar magnitude. This lack of specificity makes it imperative that the clinician consider a wide array of possible underlying disease states when confronted with a patient exhibiting such esophageal manometric abnormalities. Investigation of the pharyngeal and upper esophageal sphincter (UES) regions (composed of striated muscle) by standard water-perfused manometric techniques has been hampered by limitations that include the relatively low pressure-response times inherent to these systems. This may explain the divergent results that were noted previously when the UES in SSc was studied [44, 106, 198]. Colleagues and

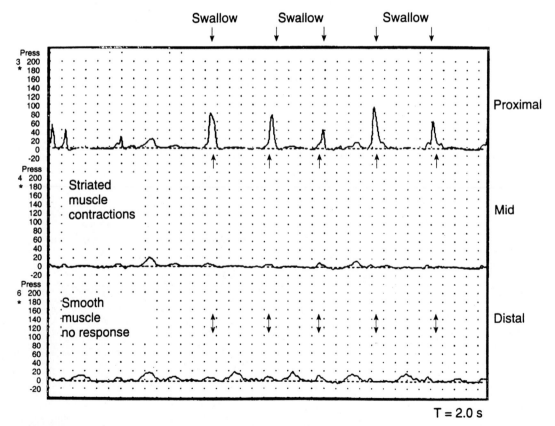

**FIG. 16–6.** Manometric tracing in a patient with scleroderma esophagus. In this tracing, the proximal transducer is located in the proximal striated muscle portion of the esophagus. The other two transducers are located in the mid- and distal smooth muscle portions. In response to a wet swallow, the striated muscle contracts but there is no peristaltic continuation of the contraction through the smooth muscle of the distal esophagus.

I [220] studied 36 SSc patients utilizing a solid-state computerized manometric system including a circumferential "sphincter transducer" with the capacity to detect pressure changes in excess of 2,000 mm Hg per second, which was previously shown to be necessary for the optimal evaluation of these regions [29]. Pharyngeal pressures, pharyngeal peristalsis, pharyngeal/UES coordination, and UES residual pressures were normal [220]. When analyzed with respect to the integrity of distal esophageal peristalsis, patients with aperistalsis had a significantly lower mean UES resting pressure and a shorter mean duration of UES relaxation. Cineradiographic, scintigraphic, and sonographic studies have recently documented oropharyngeal deglutition and cervical esophageal motility abnormalities in SSc [147, 203]. These subtle oropharyngeal and UES abnormalities may be related to the existence of a skeletal myopathy, which has been observed in patients with SSc [35, 116, 143].

Adamek and colleagues [1] have recently published the seminal study utilizing long-term, ambulatory esophageal manometry in SSc. This investigation revealed that 75% of 20 SSc patients demonstrated esophageal dysmotility when compared to a control group of 20 healthy volunteers (by descriptive and percentile analysis). The SSc patients did not undergo conventional stationary manometry, and the advantage of using prolonged ambulatory monitoring in this patient population remains unproven.

### Management

The treatment of SSc remains unsatisfactory. As the pathogenesis of SSc remains unknown, therapeutic trials have frequently focused upon suppressing the immune response in an attempt to counteract organ damage secondary to ischemia and fibrosis. Established approaches for the treatment of SSc have been reviewed in detail elsewhere [150] and include the use of disease-modifying agents, and therapy of specific end-organ involvement, and long-term psychotherapy.

D-Penicillamine is the drug which has been most extensively studied as a disease-modifying agent. It appears to provide at least partial benefit by improving cutaneous thickening, lung function, and cardiac output [53, 183]. In an uncontrolled trial [85] utilizing manometric assessment, the drug was unable to completely arrest the progression of esophageal involvement. Although there is no evidence to suggest that corticosteroids are beneficial in altering the outcome of SSc, other immunomodulatory agents have been studied, including chlorambucil, 5-fluorouracil, and methotrexate [150]. These drugs have predominantly been studied in the context of short-term, uncontrolled trials, and none has been directly compared to D-penicillamine. Several studies have investigated the use of cyclosporin A in SSc [37, 77, 224]. None of these studies show cyclosporin A to have a convincing beneficial effect on esophageal dysmotility, and all are limited by enrollment of small numbers of patients and lack of appropriate control populations. At present, the use of cyclosporin A cannot be recommended for the prevention or treatment of sclerodermatous esophageal involvement. Combined plasmapheresis and immunosuppressive drug therapy has been studied in a 2-year prospective, uncontrolled investigation which included 15 SSc patients [4]. The degree and extent of skin involvement significantly improved during the study. Although the authors conclude that their data support a beneficial effect on esophageal dysmotility, careful scrutiny of the esophageal cineradiographic and scintigraphic results suggests that a prominent placebo effect may have been responsible for the improvement in dysphagia noted in the majority of patients. Other disease-modifying agents which are experimental and under study include interferon, clotting factor XIII, pentoxifylline, and ketotifen, which ia an inhibitor of mast cell degranulation [150].

Several therapies are available for the treatment of sclerodermatous end-organ involvement [150]. The vasodilatory properties of calcium-channel blockers have been utilized to treat associated RP [102], and captopril has been used to manage the renal crisis in SSc [32, 125]. SSc-induced pulmonary hypertension is the long-term complication with the highest mortality. Although no standard therapy exists, treatment often includes a combination of cyclophosphamide and corticosteroids [197]. Physiotherapy remains an important component of the treatment regimen and should begin at an early stage of the disease. The goals of physiotherapeutic intervention depend on the disease stage, and results in large part depend on compliance.

Given that no disease-modifying agent has yet shown clear benefit in altering sclerodermatous esophageal involvement, management of the esophageal dysfunction associated with SSc has been directed toward treatment of GERD and its complications. Given that the SSc esophagus is characterized by diminished esophageal peristalsis in conjunction with a relatively hypotensive LES, there has been interest in the use of promotility agents that stimulate esophageal contractility and augment LES pressure. Ramirez-Mata and co-workers [173] performed a placebo-controlled study that assessed the effect of intravenous metoclopramide in 14 patients with esophageal involvement due to SSc. In this study, metoclopramide increased LES pressure in seven patients and peristalsis appeared in five of 11 patients who previously had had aperistalsis. The augmentation of LES pressure was, however, modest (approximate average, 5 mm Hg) and of questionable clinical significance. An increase in the amplitude of pressure waves was noted in the three patients who had esophageal hypomotility at baseline. Johnson and colleagues [98] studied 12 SSc patients and utilized esophageal manometric, scintigraphic, and pH-monitoring studies to assess the effect of intravenous metoclopramide infusion. Although LES pressure was noted to increase, the mean LES pressure after metoclopramide infusion was only slightly above the lower limit of normal, at 11 mm Hg. In this study, augmentation of peristaltic amplitudes was not seen and peristalsis was not induced in any patient who had aperistalsis prior to drug intervention. Although metoclopramide was associated with an increase in mean esophageal clearance (by scintigraphy) from 31% to 41%, the clearance value became normal in only one patient. The total number of reflux events and the 24-hour reflux scores were noted to decrease after metoclopramide treatment. Four SSc patients in this study had prolonged gastric emptying, and all responded to metoclopramide with normalization of the $t_{1/2}$ value. The above-cited results suggest that a subset of SSc patients may have a beneficial response to metoclopramide. The factors underlying this beneficial response appear to include an improvement in gastric emptying and a modest augmentation in LES pressure. Other investigators have also suggested that impaired gastric emptying in SSc may be an important factor in the development of upper gastrointestinal symptoms [128, 214].

Cisapride is a newer promotility agent, which stimulates gastrointestinal motility by facilitating acetylcholine release at the myenteric plexus [188]. Horowitz and co-workers [93] studied the effect of cisapride in eight SSc patients who had delayed gastric emptying. Although treatment with cisapride did not increase esophageal emptying, both gastric emptying and upper gastrointestinal symptoms were significantly improved. Limburg and colleagues [122] found that cisapride had no effect on LES pressure or distal esophageal motility in a small group of patients with either SSc or mixed connective tissue disease. Kahan and colleagues [103] performed a placebo-controlled crossover study that showed a significant increase in LES pressure (approximately 6 mm Hg) after intravenous cisapride injection.

A recent short-term study by Fiorucci and colleagues [68] investigated the acute effects of intravenous erythromycin administration on gastric emptying, as measured by gastric sonography, in both patients with SSc and normal controls. Prior to drug intervention, the SSc population had a prolonged $t_{1/2}$ gastric emptying. After administration of a single intravenous dose (2 mg per kg) of erythromycin lactobionate, the $t_{1/2}$ gastric emptying in SSc patients significantly improved and was similar to the value noted in normal controls prior to drug intervention.

Overall, it appears that metoclopramide and cisapride have little or no clinically significant effect in SSc with regard to improvement in esophageal peristalsis, esophageal emptying, and LES pressure. Promotility agents may, however, be useful in improving upper gastrointestinal symptoms in these patients by accelerating gastric emptying.

Given that promotility agents offer limited benefit in the treatment of SSc-related GER, therapy has focused on the use of phase 1 strategies or lifestyle modifications in conjunction with the use of medications that raise intragastric pH. Phase 1 and 2 therapies for GER are outlined in Chapters 24 and 25, respectively. The use of proton pump inhibitors appears to offer a significant benefit in the treatment of severe GER in SSc. Hendel and colleagues [87] treated 25 SSc patients who had severe GER with varying dosages of omeprazole for up to 5 years. Statistically significant relief

of symptoms and healing of esophagitis occurred. Since half of the patients in this study did not have endoscopic healing of esophagitis and other investigations demonstrated a poor correlation between symptom assessment and pH monitoring for GER in this patient population [12, 192], determining who requires treatment and the optimal mode of assessing the adequacy of therapy remain problematic. In this regard, routine ambulatory pH monitoring has been advocated [192] and may play a role in the diagnosis and treatment of GER in this patient population.

The development of worsening dysphagia may be related to the evolution of a peptic stricture which is amenable to dilation in a standard manner, as detailed in Chapter 27. The occurrence of worsening dysphagia in an SSc patient may also raise the specter of a Barrett-related malignancy, and esophagoscopic examination is necessary to definitively exclude this possibility. Lastly, superimposed esophageal candidiasis (EC) may similarly present with an exacerbation of dysphagia or the evolution of odynophagia. Hendel and colleagues [86, 87] have studied the occurrence of EC in SSc patients in detail. These investigators fastidiously screened for the presence of EC in a study which included patients with SSc, "idiopathic" GER (who were receiving long-term, potent acid-antisecretory therapy), and a dyspeptic control group referred for upper gastrointestinal endoscopic examination. The group of patients with SSc was subdivided into those who had received potent acid-antisecretory therapy for 2 months prior to study and those who had not yet been subjected to such treatment. The study showed that EC was infrequent in patients without SSc, whereas those with the disease were commonly afflicted. Eighty-nine percent of SSc patients receiving potent acid-antisecretory therapy had EC compared with 44% of SSc patients who had not yet received such treatment. These results suggest that that potent acid-antisecretory therapy increases the frequency of EC in patients with SSc, who are ordinarily predisposed to this disorder as a consequence of underlying esophageal dysmotility. The conclusions drawn from this investigation must be tempered by the understanding that patients in this study were carefully screened for the presence of EC. Due to the rapid, universal recurrence of EC after antimycotic therapy (fluconazole) is withdrawn, the authors ultimately decided not to consider the presence of asymptomatic mucosal candidiasis an indication for routine treatment. The occurrence of symptomatic EC would, however, appear to warrant an attempt at eradication utilizing an antimycotic agent.

With the advent of proton pump inhibitor therapy, failure of a medical antireflux regimen will likely become uncommon but may necessitate a surgical antireflux repair. Performing antireflux surgery to improve GER without exacerbating dysphagia may be difficult since these patients often have aperistalsis and compromised esophageal clearing capacity. Orringer and co-workers [159–161] performed Collis-Belsey and subsequently Collis-Nissen repairs in patients with SSc. A change to the latter procedure occurred due to an unacceptably high recurrence rate of reflux symptoms after Collis-Belsey operations. Mansour and Malone [132] reported recrudescence of reflux symptoms in all of their patients 4 years postoperatively and advocate esophageal replacement as initial surgical therapy. Unfortunately, the ability to perform a colon interposition procedure may be compromised if the sclerodermatous process has involved the large intestine. Poirier and colleagues [169] have published the most recent series on patients who underwent antireflux surgery in the setting of SSc. This study included 14 patients who underwent a variety of antireflux procedures (ten had a ''short'' Nissen repair) with exhaustive pre- and postoperative assessment, which included barium radiography, esophageal scintigraphy, manometry, pH monitoring, and endoscopic evaluation. Patient follow-up ranged from 8 to 181 months (mean, 65 months), and the authors noted a statistically significant postoperative improvement in reflux symptoms and 24-hour distal esophageal acid exposure time. There was no increase in the frequency of dysphagia, and there were no significant changes in manometric or scintigraphic parameters in the postoperative period. Although these results seem encouraging, in the postoperative period the mean distal esophageal acid exposure time remained abnormal (total = 7.5%) and eight of 14 patients (~60%) remained on acid-antisecretory therapy. The above results suggest that, especially given the availability of potent acid-suppressive therapy, caution remains in order when considering antireflux surgery in ''uncomplicated'' SSc-related GERD.

## Mixed Connective Tissue Disease

Mixed connective tissue disease (MCTD) is a syndrome characterized by overlapping clinical features of SSc, systematic lupus erythematosus, and polymyositis in association with high titers of antibodies directed against the ribonucleoprotein component of extractable nuclear antigen [191]. Although any region of the gastrointestinal tract may be affected in MCTD, the esophagus is the most commonly involved segment [134].

Heartburn, regurgitation, and dysphagia are the most common esophageal symptoms in MCTD [61, 134], and the majority of patients are symptomatic. Diminished esophageal peristalsis is noted radiographically in more than half of patients [117, 134]. Manometry is more sensitive than either symptom assessment or cineradiography in detecting esophageal abnormalities in this patient population [117]. Manometric abnormalities that have been observed with MCTD include a reduction in the amplitude of peristaltic waves throughout the esophageal body and a reduction in LES pressure [61, 70, 82, 117, 134, 184, 207]. Aperistalsis of the esophageal body may be seen in 17% to 29% of patients with MCTD [61, 117, 134]. Lapadula and colleagues [117] demonstrated incoordination of the pharyngeal and UES musculature in nearly one-third of 17 patients studied. UES resting pressures have been variously reported to be normal

[61] or low [82, 134]. Measurements of UES pressures in MCTD utilizing computerized circumferential sphincter transducers has not yet been reported and would likely clarify this issue, given the asymmetry of the UES. Jack and colleagues [96] recently studied a patient with MCTD and recurrent aspiration after a failed hiatal hernia repair, utilizing simultaneous esophageal and tracheal pH monitoring. Prolonged tracheal pH monitoring was shown to be safe and simple in this study, which included ten healthy control volunteers. Whether this technology is preferable to proximal esophageal pH monitoring remains to be proven. Although systematic investigation has not been performed, one would expect severe GERD in this patient population and aggressive treatment is warranted. There is some evidence to suggest that esophageal dysfunction in MCTD may improve with corticosteroid therapy [134, 166]. The question of whether corticosteroid therapy is useful only in patients with less advanced disease (and a presumably reversible inflammatory reaction in the esophageal musculature) has not yet been answered. In a short-term, placebo-controlled trial which included two patients with MCTD, intravenous cisapride was not shown to be of significant benefit in enhancing either LES pressure or motility of the esophageal body [122].

## Idiopathic Inflammatory Myopathies

The idiopathic inflammatory myopathies, which include polymyositis (PM), dermatomyositis (DM), and inclusion-body myositis (IBM), are a heterogeneous group of diseases of unknown pathogenesis that are characterized by mononuclear cell muscle inflammation. These inflammatory myopathies are pathogenetically, histologically, and clinically distinct and have recently been reviewed elsewhere in detail [6, 10, 46, 138]. In the past, it has been stressed that PM and DM affect striated muscle with consequent dysfunction of the cricopharyngeus and other muscles of the pharynx and proximal esophagus. Clinically, patients may experience oropharyngeal dysphagia and occasional nasopharyngeal regurgitation and aspiration [88, 101, 107]. The manometric correlates have been abnormalities referable to the proximal esophagus (where muscle is predominantly striated), which include decreased cricopharyngeal sphincter pressure and diminished pharyngeal and proximal esophageal peristaltic pressures [44, 210]. Masseter muscle weakness may occur, and consequent incomplete mastication may exacerbate swallowing difficulties. Although such oropharyngeal dysfunction may be demonstrable in nearly half of those tested [117, 168], esophageal and gastric smooth muscle dysfunction occurs with similar frequency and includes decreased frequency and amplitude of distal esophageal peristalsis, which is manifested as impaired esophageal and gastric emptying [54, 91, 97, 117, 210]. Esophageal aperistalsis has been reported [44] but is uncommon in PM and DM. The etiology of impaired smooth muscle activity is unclear, but the absence of abnormalities on histologic examination refutes atrophy, fibrosis, and lymphocytic infiltration as causes [54].

The presence of dysphagia has previously been shown to be associated with a poor prognosis in patients with PM/DM [21]. Improvement of dysphagia may be noted with treatment of myositis and reflux symptoms. Given the rarity of PM/DM, controlled trials assessing the effect of treatment on dysphagia have not been performed. On occassion, dysphagia may be caused by cricopharyngeal myositis and fibrosis. Symptoms related to cricopharyngeal myopathy may occur in the absence of clinically active peripheral myositis and may be amenable to surgical management (myotomy) [58, 101].

In contrast to PM and DM, IBM affects men more commonly and is clinically characterized by the insidious onset of muscle weakness, which is often asymmetrical [6]. The disease tends to affect elderly persons, typically presenting with the gradual evolution of weakness and atrophy, which most prominently affects the wrist and finger flexor and the knee extensor muscles. Dysphagia occurs in approximately 40% of patients with IBM [40, 126, 177, 218] and may precede the onset of symptomatic muscle weakness [126, 176, 218]. There continues to be lack of agreement regarding the mechanism of dysphagia in IBM. Darrow and colleagues [51] have enumerated multiple possible underlying factors which may contribute to dysphagia in these patients. These include impaired pharyngeal and cricopharyngeal muscular function, as well as impairment of laryngeal elevation (due to involvement of the suprahyoid musculature). Whether altered function of the distal smooth muscle-containing esophagus (as may occur in PM and DM) occurs in IBM has not been specifically studied. As for the other inflammatory myopathies, controlled studies assessing the effects of treatment are unavailable. In general, however, IBM appears to be less responsive to corticosteroid and immunosuppressive therapy than are PM and DM [6, 138]. As in PM and DM, cricopharyngeal involvement causing severe dysphagia in IBM may be amenable to myotomy [51, 126, 212, 218].

## Systemic Lupus Erythematosis

Stevens and colleagues [199] performed manometry on 16 patients with systemic lupus erythematosis (SLE) and noted aperistalsis in four (25%). Ramirez-Mata and co-workers [175] performed manometric studies on 50 unselected SLE patients and found abnormalities in 16 (32%). Absent or diminished contractions were noted proximally (seven patients), distally (three patients), and diffusely (two patients). LES pressure was diminished in four patients. There was no relationship between the presence of esophageal dysfunction and activity, duration, or treatment of SLE. Gutierrez and co-workers [82] noted abnormal manometric studies in seven (50%) of 14 SLE patients. Although the SLE patients had diminished mean esophageal peristaltic amplitudes and LES pressures compared to a control population, these differences did not reach statistical significance. Three patients (21%) were noted to have aperistalsis. Lapadula and colleagues [117] studied 19 patients with SLE utilizing both esophageal radiographic and manometric examinations. Radiographic examinations were abnormal in only two (11%) patients, whereas manometric abnormalities were detected in 12 (63%) patients. Of the 12 patients with an abnormal manometric study, eight (67%) displayed abnormal motility of the esophageal body, including two patients with aperistalsis. None of the SLE patients in this study displayed severe LES impairment (defined as an LESP pressure of less than 5 mm Hg; normal, >10 mm Hg). On the basis of these findings, the authors of this investigation suggested that isolated impairment of esophageal body peristalsis in the setting of retained resting LES pressure was characteristic of SLE. Diffuse esophageal spasm in SLE has also been reported [165].

## Rheumatoid Arthritis

Sun and colleagues [200] reported manometric findings in a series of 66 patients with rheumatoid arthritis (RA). Findings included a significantly decreased mean amplitude of peristaltic contractions in the distal esophagus and a diminished mean LES pressure. There was no correlation between the manometric abnormalities and the duration or stage of disease. Lapadula and co-workers [117] performed esophageal radiographic and manometric testing in 24 RA patients. Ten patients (41%) had an abnormal esophagram and 14 patients (58%) demonstrated abnormal manometric testing. Similar to the findings in the SLE population studied in that investigation (see above), none of the patients with RA demonstrated severe impairment of the resting LES pressure, while 79% of patients with an abnormal manometric study had impaired peristalsis of the esophageal body. Aperistalsis of the distal esophagus has occasionally been noted in RA [117, 123, 207].

## Sjögren's Syndrome

Although dysphagia is a common symptom reported by patients with Sjögren's syndrome (SS), there is controversy as to whether esophageal motor dysfunction or xerostomia is the primary pathogenetic factor. A study by Ramirez-Mata and associates [174] found absent or decreased peristalsis in nine of ten patients with SS. These results are suspect as the manometric technique was suboptimal and use of dry swallows in conjunction with a brief interdeglutitive period may have contributed to the high frequency of manometric abnormalities noted. Kjellen and colleagues [110] studied 22 patients with SS and found only minor manometric abnormalities, which consisted of significantly shorter peristaltic contraction times and more rapid peristaltic velocity. Barium radiography revealed upper esophageal webs in two of the 20 patients studied by this technique. The majority of patients (73%) complained of dysphagia, which the authors suggested was a reflection of xerostomia rather than the motility abnormalities that were noted. Tsianos and colleagues [208] performed manometry on 27 patients with SS and found abnormalities in 11 (41%). The manometric abnormalities included aperistalsis (two patients), frequent triphasic or nonperistaltic contractions, low-amplitude peristaltic contractions, and hypotension of the LES. Clinical symptoms did not correlate with either manometric abnormalities or parotid flow rate. Although the data do not support their conclusions, the authors suggested that esophageal dysmotility was the most plausible explanation for dysphagia in these patients. Grande and colleagues [79] evaluated 20 patients with SS, 15 (75%) of whom complained of dysphagia. When comparing patients with and without dysphagia, there was no difference in esophageal motility pattern or parotid flow rate. The authors could not ascribe dysphagia to either esophageal dysmotility or xerostomia. Palma and co-workers [162] also found dysphagia to be present in the majority (81%) of the 21 patients studied with SS. Although aperistalsis was noted in 10% and a hypertensive LES in 19% of the patients studied, no correlation of abnormal motility with dysphagia could be found. The weight of evidence from the above studies appears to support the notion that although dysphagia is a common symptom in SS, it cannot at the present time be clearly attributed to either the esophageal dysmotility or the xerostomia which are frequently demonstrated in these patients.

## BEHÇET'S DISEASE

In 1937, a Turkish dermatologist, Hulushi Behçet, described two patients with recurrent oral and genital aphthous ulcerations and hypopyon iritis [15]. Since then, Behçet's disease (BD) has been recognized as a multisystem inflammatory disorder affecting the gastrointestinal tract in approximately 50% of patients [31]. Although cases have been reported worldwide, the distribution of disease is geographically concentrated in eastern Mediterranean countries and eastern Asia [157]. The pathogenesis is unclear, but viral or immunologic causes are suspected [16].

Diagnostic criteria are generally grouped into principal symptomatic features (such as oral and genital ulcerations, eye lesions, and skin lesions) and minor features, which include thrombophlebitis, cardiovascular lesions, arthritis, central nervous system lesions, gastrointestinal lesions, and a family history. BD is considered when three to four major criteria plus two minor criteria exist. The diagnosis may also be considered in the presence of only two or three major criteria if uveitis is present [119, 129].

Esophageal lesions of BD are rare and nonspecific. Ulcerations, erosions, diffuse esophagitis, dissection of the esophageal mucosa, perforation, hemorrhage, and esophageal varices (caused by thrombophlebitis of typical vascular BD) have all been described [8, 9, 23, 164, 221]. Levack and Hanson [121] reported an unusual case of BD-related tracheoesophageal fistulization. Bottomley and colleagues [22] performed upper gastrointestinal endoscopy on nine patients with well-documented BD and found esophageal involvement to be uncommon, being present in only one severely symptomatic patient (11%), in whom a proximal esophageal stricture with associated ulceration was noted. The authors concluded that endoscopic assessment is not routinely indicated in patients with BD who lack esophageal symptoms. Since esophageal involvement in BD is usually accompanied by other gastrointestinal lesions, (specifically, jejunal or ileocolonic ulcers), distinguishing BD from Crohn's disease may be particularly challenging [148].

The treatment of BD has been problematic and has recently been reviewed elsewhere in detail [113]. Corticosteroids have been widely used with a suppressive effect on most manifestations of BD, but such treatment does not prevent cerebral vasculitis or blindness. To date, two controlled investigations have shown similar efficacy for cyclosporin A [139] and azathioprine [222] for the treatment of eye disease. Given these results, either of these immunosuppressants combined with corticosteroids is now considered first-line therapy in the presence of posterior uveitis [113]. Kotter and co-workers [113] have extensive experience in treating BD and suggest utilizing either of these drug combinations with gastrointestinal tract involvement. These investigators reserve the use of triple-therapy with cyclosporin A, azathioprine, and corticosteroids for those with severe (manifested as retinal vasculitis, neurologic involvement, or vascular disease) or refractory disease. Given the rarity of this disease, controlled therapeutic trials specifically dealing with the treatment of esophageal involvement are unavailable; however, anecdotal instances of improvement with concomitant treatment of ileocolonic disease using a variety of agents, including sulfasalazine and cyclosporin A, have been reported [71, 139, 221]. A description of one patient with self-limited esophageal ulceration suggests that spontaneous remissions may occur [190].

## ENDOCRINE DISEASES

### Diabetes Mellitus

Diabetes mellitus can adversely involve every organ system in the body, and autonomic dysfunction can affect the gastrointestinal tract and cause gastroparesis and colonic dysmotility [13, 27]. Mandelstam and Lieber [130] were the first to investigate diabetics for evidence of esophageal dysfunction. In this study, all patients had evidence of autonomic neuropathy and exhibited delayed esophageal emptying during barium radiography. Radiographic esophageal abnormalities that have been noted in diabetics include delayed esophageal emptying, reduced frequency of primary peristalsis, failure of the peristaltic stripping wave, and the occurrence of nonpropulsive tertiary contractions [130, 131, 213]. Karayalcin and colleagues [104] studied 12 diabetics without esophageal symptoms and found a significantly prolonged mean esophageal transit time utilizing scintigraphic techniques.

Mandelstam and coauthors [131] reported the results of manometric studies on eight patients, which demonstrated decreases in peristaltic amplitude and diminished resting LES pressures. Hollis and colleagues [90] examined 50 unselected diabetic patients and an age-matched control population and found no difference in resting LES pressures. A prominent association between esophageal motor abnormalities and peripheral neuropathy was noted such that 80% of patients with peripheral neuropathy had dysmotility, whereas only 20% of patients without neuropathy had disordered esophageal motility. Furthermore, a correlation between the severity of esophageal motor dysfunction and peripheral neuropathy existed. In another study, esophageal motility abnormalities correlated with the presence of psychiatric disturbances but not with neuropathy [39]. The manometric abnormalities that have been noted in diabetics include decreases in peristaltic pressures, repetitive and spontaneous contractions, an increased frequency of nontransmitted peristaltic waves, and multiphasic peristaltic wave complexes [90, 124]. Decreased LES pressure and impaired LES relaxation also have been demonstrated [131, 211]. Manometric abnormalities in diabetes appear to occur more commonly in the smooth muscle-containing portion of the esophagus; however, a reduced frequency of primary peristaltic contractions has been noted in the cervical esophageal region [211]. Huppe and co-workers [95] prospectively investigated 33 diabetics utilizing esophageal manometry. Thirteen patients (40%) complained of dysphagia and 18 (55%) had reflux symptomatology. Mean resting UES and LES pressures and peristaltic amplitudes were statistically lower in the diabetic group; however, the values remained within the normal range. Mean peristaltic velocity and duration of contractions were similarly reduced. Diabetics also displayed a higher rate of nonprogressive esophageal contractions, and aperistalsis was noted in approximately 10% of the subjects. In contrast to other studies [124], Huppe and colleagues [95] found no increase in the frequency of multiphasic contractions. These authors also found no correlation between manometric abnormalities and the presence of neuropathy (peripheral or autonomic). Although over 60% of patients had esophageal symptoms, there was no relationship between these symptoms and esophageal dysmotility.

The pathogenesis of esophageal dysfunction in diabetics remains unclear. A direct relation to the metabolic disorder is lacking. Neuropathologic changes seen in the esophagus include preservation of the myenteric plexus, demyelination and Wallerian changes in the vagus, and Schwann cell loss in the parasympathetic fibers. Neural dysfunction appears to be the most tenable explanation for esophageal dysmotility.

Therapeutic trials utilizing promotility agents have been performed since esophageal dysmotility and impaired esophageal emptying are frequently noted in diabetic populations. Maddern and co-workers [127] found no improvement in esophageal transit when using the promotility agent domperidone. Although long-term data are lacking, one study has shown cisapride to be of benefit in improving esophageal transit time [92]. Recently, Fabiani and colleagues [66] investigated the use of Tolrestat (an aldolase-reductase inhibitor) in a long-term, placebo-controlled trial which included 66 noninsulin-dependent diabetics with asymptomatic peripheral and autonomic neuropathy. Prior to drug intervention, the treated group had a mean esophageal transit time of 29 seconds (upper limit of normal, 15 seconds). After 12 months of treatment with oral Tolrestat, the mean esophageal transit time improved significantly and decreased to 20 seconds.

**Thyroid Disease**

Patients with hypothyroidism may experience dysphagia. Christiansen and Clifton [34] reported manometric results in five patients with myxedema and dysphagia. Four subjects demonstrated a reduction in the amplitude and velocity of peristalsis and a prolonged duration of contraction. Serial studies have revealed an improvement of esophageal motor function during thyroid replacement therapy. Eastwood and colleagues [64] described a hypothyroid patient with a reduction in distal esophageal peristalsis, absent LES pressure, and GERD, in whom normalization of esophageal motility followed the institution of thyroid replacement. Wright and Penner [219] described a myxedematous patient who complained of cervical dysphagia to both liquids and solids. Baseline manometry revealed a hypertensive UES, which failed to relax appropriately upon deglutition. Thyroid replacement was prescribed, the dysphagia resolved, and repeat manometric assessment 8 months later revealed a normotensive UES, which relaxed normally. The authors postulated that myxedematous infiltration of the cricopharyngeus may have been responsible for the dysphagia and manometric findings described.

Less has been published regarding hyperthyroidism and esophageal dysfunction. Meshkinpour and co-workers [144] studied ten patients with Graves' disease and noted an increase in esophageal propagation velocity, which normalized with treatment. The clinical significance of these manometric findings in hyperthyroidism remains unclear as these abnormalities were not the cause of esophageal symptoms in the patients studied.

## AMYLOIDOSIS

Amyloidosis may involve the entire gastrointestinal tract, including the esophagus. Although the presence of amyloid in the esophagus is less frequently reported in pathologic studies, an investigation that employed endoscopic biopsies estimated the rate of esophageal involvement to be 72% [202]. The majority of patients examined by endoscopy have a normal-appearing esophagus; however, fine mucosal granularity (16%) and, less frequently, erosions, ulcerations, and mucosal friability may be noted.

Rubinaw and colleagues [180] reported that more than 60% of 30 patients with either primary or secondary amyloidosis had demonstrable esophageal manometric abnormalities. Manometric studies have demonstrated various abnormalities, including achalasia-like patterns (with aperistalsis and impaired LES relaxation); an incompletely relaxing, hypertensive LES; and decreased LES pressure with simultaneous, repetitive contractions [25, 43, 76, 118, 180]. Suris and colleagues [201] have reported an unusual case of secondary amyloidosis with esophageal involvement manifested by well-documented clinical, radiographic, and manometric features of idiopathic achalasia. Radiographically, a dilated, atonic esophagus may be seen in the presence or absence of distal narrowing [43, 146, 201].

The cause of esophageal motor dysfunction in amyloidosis remains unknown. An elegant study by Bjerle and colleagues [19] investigated 16 patients with familial amyloidosis and 14 healthy control subjects. The authors found esophageal distensibility by balloon inflation to be similar in both groups. The investigators also found that neostigmine (an acetylcholinesterase inhibitor) increased esophageal peristaltic amplitudes to a lesser extent in amyloidosis patients than in normal control subjects. This suggested that it was unlikely that amyloid deposition in the esophageal wall was responsible for the observed dysmotility that was documented in all 16 patients with esophageal amyloidosis. Autonomic denervation was considered a more plausible explanation for the observed esophageal dysfunction. Lefkowitz and colleagues [118] also found evidence of neurogenic dysfunction, with pharmacologic testing demonstrating evidence of impairment of the pathways responsible for normal LES relaxation.

Despite the frequent occurrence of pathologic and manometric abnormalities, consistent esophageal symptoms are uncommon and the clinical presentation of esophageal amyloidosis is variable. Dysphagia, an achalasia-like syndrome, hemorrhage, and perforation have all been reported [43, 84, 201]. Patients with esophageal amyloidosis and secondary achalasia may respond to pneumatic dilation of the LES [43, 201].

## ALCOHOLISM

Esophageal motor abnormalities have been described with both acute [89] and chronic [80, 217] ethanol ingestion. Acute ethanol ingestion causes transient esophageal dysmotility characterized by impaired esophageal body, LES, and UES functions, which regress within 24 hours [89]. Esophageal motor dysfunction may occur in chronic alcoholics, and although initially thought to occur only in association with secondary peripheral neuropathy [217], a recent investigation [204] has suggested that subclinical neuropathy is not related to the presence of esophageal dysmotility. Winship and co-workers [217] reported that patients with alcoholic neuropathy exhibited selective deterioration of esophageal body motility characterized by decreased frequency of peristalsis in the distal two-thirds of the esophagus, with preserved LES function. Secondary peristalsis in response to balloon distention was also diminished. These investigators found that patients without associated alcoholic neuropathy

displayed a less significant deterioration of peristaltic function. Grande and co-workers [80] studied 23 alcoholic patients and found elevated peristaltic pressures in the middle portion of the esophageal body in 13 (57%). The authors suggested that this manometric finding might be a marker of excessive alcohol consumption. There was also a hypertensive LES in 13 (57%) patients. Twelve patients (52%) exhibited increased distal esophageal acid exposure by pH monitoring; however, the presence of abnormal reflux parameters was not related to peristaltic dysfunction. Of perhaps most interest was the finding that dysmotility persisted at repeat testing performed 6 months later in all patients with ongoing alcoholism, whereas a reversion to normal motility was documented in all of those patients who remained abstinent from alcohol intake.

Although the mechanism of esophageal dysmotility in alcoholics remains unknown, vagus nerve degeneration in combination with alcoholic myopathic changes may be responsible. As in diabetes mellitus, the clinical significance of the abnormal manometric findings noted in alcoholics remains unclear since many patients offer no symptoms of an esophageal motility disorder.

## INFECTIOUS DISEASE

### American Trypanosomiasis (Chagas' Disease)

Chagas' disease, which was initially described in 1909 by the Brazilian Carlos Chagas, results from infection by the tropical hemoflagellate protozoan *Trypanosoma cruzi* [30]. Although the disease is endemic in South and Central America, rare cases have been identified in the United States [154]. Chagas' disease has a predilection to affect certain organs, including the heart and gastrointestinal tract. In patients surviving the acute infection and developing chronic disease, the overall prognosis is related to cardiac involvement. Although the esophagus and colon appear to be the most common segments of the gastrointestinal tract to be involved with longstanding infection, the stomach and small bowel also can be affected. The occurrence of gastrointestinal involvement in Chagas' disease appears to vary geographically and is considered extremely rare in Central America, Venezuela, and northeast Brazil, while it is more common in the remainder of South America [149]. These variations have been attributed to characteristics of different *T. cruzi* strains. Although chagasic megaesophagus is a major cause of morbidity in affected patients, the prevalence of esophageal disease is low, and autopsy series have reported the frequency of megaesophagus to range from 2.6% to 18.0% [7, 112]. There appears to be a 15- to 20-year latent phase between primary infection and the development of signs of megaesophagus, and men appear to be at higher risk of developing the disease than women. In the esophagus, the organism is responsible for denervation of the neural myenteric (Auerbach's) plexuses. There is evidence to suggest that denervation affects both inhibitory and cholinergic excitatory neurons [48, 49], but the mechanism of destruction of these intramural neurons is not understood. Production of a neural cytopathic toxin by the organism or autoimmune phenomena have been proposed as possible causal mechanisms.

Longstanding esophageal involvement in Chagas' disease may be clinically manifest by dysphagia, regurgitation, weight loss, and pulmonary aspiration. The evolution of esophageal symptomatology parallels the development of a dilated, atonic esophagus with an incompletely relaxing LES. With chagasic megaesophagus, the clinical history is indistinguishable from that of idiopathic achalasia. The diagnosis is based on the appropriate historical and epidemiologic evidence in a patient with megaesophagus. The usual immunologic criteria for diagnosis include a positive finding on enzyme-linked immunosorbent assay coupled with a positive result on either complement fixation or hemagglutination reaction.

Radiographic findings in Chagas' disease mimic those noted in idiopathic achalasia. Barium studies typically reveal a dilated, atonic esophagus with distal esophageal tapering reminiscent of a "bird's beak." An esophageal air-fluid level may be noted (Fig. 16–7). Features that distinguish

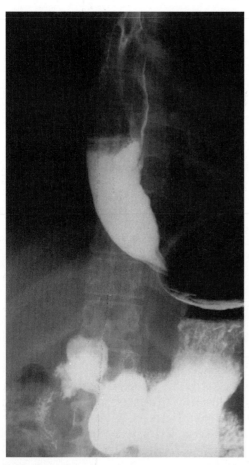

**FIG. 16–7.** Barium esophagogram from a patient with Chagas' disease, which demonstrates a dilated esophagus with tapering at the esophagogastric junction and an esophageal air-fluid level.

Chagas' disease from idiopathic achalasia include associated megaduodenum and megacolon.

Esophageal manometric findings are variable and often reflect the underlying pathologic process of acquired aganglionosis. de Oliveira and colleagues [56] investigated the esophageal manometric findings in a group of 53 subjects with positive serologic tests for Chagas' disease. Of the 43 patients with a nondilated esophagus, approximately half had no complaint of dysphagia. Sixteen patients (37%) displayed normal esophageal motility, three (7%) had multiphasic peristaltic contractions, nine (21%) demonstrated aperistalsis with a normally relaxing LES, and 15 (35%) showed aperistalsis with a nonrelaxing LES. Aperistalsis and a nonrelaxing LES were universally noted in the ten subjects with chagasic megaesophagus, all of whom had persistent dysphagia. Aperistalsis of the esophageal body and incomplete relaxation of the LES are typical features of advanced chagasic megaesophagus. Although these findings are similar to those noted in idiophatic achalasia, one study suggested that the resting LES pressures in patients with Chagas' disease tend to be lower than those in patients with achalasia [49]. This finding may reflect different impairments in the mechanisms of LES control in these patient populations [48].

Management of dysphagia and regurgitation in Chagas' disease is directed at diminishing the functional obstruction that is present at the esophagogastric junction. Dantas and co-workers [47] studied the effect of sublingual nifedipine in chagasic patients, and manometric evaluation revealed a 43% reduction in LES pressure after drug administration. A recent randomized, crossover study compared the effects of nifedipine (20 mg sublingually) with isosorbide dinitrate (5 mg sublingually) in 11 patients with chagasic achalasia [67]. Assessment by scintigraphic esophageal emptying studies revealed a statistically significant reduction in esophageal radioisotope retention after isosorbide dinitrate administration (median, 54% versus 78% $p < 0.001$). The clinical significance of such pharmacologic manipulations is as yet uncertain. Pneumatic dilation may be employed to mechanically disrupt the LES and alleviate functional obstruction at the esophagogastric junction. Surgical esophagomyotomy is preferred for those in whom this therapy fails. Pinotti and colleagues [167] have reviewed their experience acquired in the surgical management of 929 cases of chagasic megaesophagus. The surgical approach varied depending upon whether an excessively long and dilated esophagus (i.e., dolicomegaesophagus) was present. The 807 patients with "nonadvanced" megaesophagus underwent combined wide esophagocardiomyotomy and an antireflux procedure with no associated mortality. The other 122 patients with dolicomegaesophagus were subjected to esophageal resection, which carried a 4.1% mortality. Unfortunately, the above-mentioned therapies are suboptimal, and for advanced chagasic megaesophagus, no ideal treatment is presently available to predictably control symptoms on a long-term basis with acceptable recurrence, morbidity, and mortality rates [136].

Nifurtimox and benznidazole are the two drugs currently being used to treat Chagas' disease, and both agents are effective at decreasing the severity and duration of acute infection [109]. Unfortunately, these agents must be administered for prolonged periods and can cause serious adverse reactions, and parasitologic cure occurs in only half of patients [109, 133]. These drugs have not been shown to influence the clinical course of chronic *T. cruzi* infection. There is limited evidence from a recent open, nonrandomized trial to suggest that treatment with allopurinol may be useful in suppressing parasitemia in patients with chronic *T. cruzi* infection [74]. Suppression of parasitemia in the chronic stage of illness may not necessarily translate into clinical benefit if the pathogenesis of cardiac and gastrointestinal lesions has an immunologic basis.

## CHRONIC INTESTINAL PSEUDOOBSTRUCTION

Chronic intestinal pseudoobstruction (CIP) is a clinical syndrome caused by ineffective intestinal propulsion and is characterized by recurrent, episodic intestinal obstruction in the absence of a mechanical factor. The chronic form of the disease may be caused by a variety of disorders whose common feature is the ability to involve either gut smooth muscle or the myenteric plexus, with resultant impairment of smooth muscle contractility. The disease may be either primary and without an identifiable cause (e.g., chronic idiopathic intestinal pseudoobstruction) or secondary to a variety of inherited myopathic and neuropathic disorders, connective tissue diseases, neurologic diseases, and endocrinologic/metabolic disorders (Table 16–1).

Since CIP may involve all segments of the gastrointestinal tract, the clinical presentation will necessarily vary and may include dysphagia, abdominal pain and distention, vomiting, diarrhea (due to small bowel bacterial overgrowth), and constipation. Many patients with CIP have esophageal involvement, which may be asymptomatic or cause dysphagia, regurgitation, chest pain, or heartburn [186, 187]. Dysphagia occurs in approximately half of CIP patients, with other esophageal symptoms occurring less commonly [187].

Barium radiographs of the esophagus may reveal esophageal dilation. Schuffler and colleagues [187] suggested that myopathic processes tend to cause more prominent gut dilation and weaker contractility, while the neuropathic disorders are more often characterized by less apparent bowel dilation and uncoordinated, spastic contractions. As such, barium radiographs may reveal a dilated, atonic esophagus in those with myopathic processes (e.g., muscular dystrophy), while hyperactive, nonperistaltic contractions may suggest idiopathic achalasia or a spastic motility disorder in patients with neuropathic diseases. The first manometric study of five patients with idiopathic CIP revealed dysmotility in all, with findings including aperistalsis and incomplete LES relaxation [186]. Patients with myopathic diseases tend to exhibit low-amplitude or absent peristalsis and a relatively hypotensive LES, whereas those with neuropathic processes

are more likely to demonstrate manometric abnormalities reminiscent of achalasia or diffuse esophageal spasm. Although manometric findings may vary and many patients with CIP do not have dysphagia, the overwhelming majority have abnormal peristalsis, and normal manometric findings would therefore mitigate against the diagnosis.

Management of patients with esophageal involvement due to CIP should be individualized. GER should be treated vigorously, given the high frequency of altered peristalsis and presumed compromise of esophageal acid-clearing capacity. In patients in whom the esophageal disease mimics achalasia, pneumatic dilation [185] or surgical esophagomyotomy may be employed.

**TABLE 16–1.** *Etiologies of chronic intestinal pseudoobstruction*

Disorders of the myenteric plexus
  Familial visceral neuropathies
  Sporadic visceral neuropathies
    Paraneoplastic
    Infectious (Chagas' disease)
Disorders of the smooth muscle
  Primary
    Familial visceral myopathies
    Sporadic visceral myopathy
  Secondary
    Systemic sclerosis
    Idiopathic inflammatory myopathies
    Muscular dystrophy
    Amyloidosis
Neurologic disorders
  Multiple sclerosis
  Parkinson's disease
Endocrine and metabolic disorders
  Diabetes mellitus
  Hypothyroidism
  Hypoparathyroidism
  Pheochromocytoma
  Porphyria
  Hypocalcemia
  Hypomagnesemia
Drug-induced
  Anticholinergics
  Phenothiazines
  Tricyclic antidepressants
  Clonidine
  *Vinca* alkaloids
  Narcotics
Miscellaneous
  Jejunoileal bypass
  Eosinophilic gastroenteritis
  Celiac sprue
Idiopathic (chronic idiopathic intestinal pseudoobstruction)

## REFERENCES

1. Adamek RJ, et al. Long-term manometry of tubular esophagus in progressive systemic sclerosis. Clin Invest 1994;72:343
2. Akesson A, Wollheim FA. Organ manifestations in 100 patients with progressive systemic sclerosis: a comparison between the CREST syndrome and diffuse scleroderma. Br J Rheumatol 1989;28:281

3. Akesson A, et al. Esophageal dysfunction and radionuclide transit in progressive systemic sclerosis. Scand J Rheumatol 1987;16:291

4. Akesson A, et al. Visceral improvement following combined plasmapheresis and immunosuppressive drug therapy in progressive systemic sclerosis. Scand J Rheumatol 1988;17:313

5. Altman RD, Medsger TA, Bloch DA, Michel BA. Predictors of survival in systemic sclerosis (scleroderma). Arthritis Rheum 1991;34:403

6. Amato AA, Barohn RJ. Idiopathic inflammatory myopathies. Neurol Clin 1997;15:615

7. Andrade ZA, Andrade SG, Patolojia J. In Banerj H, Andrade ZA, eds, Trypanosoma cruzi e Doneca de Chagas. Rio de Janeiro: Guanabara Koogan, 1979

8. Anti M, et al. Ulcerative esophagitis in Behcet's syndrome [Letter]. Gastrointest Endosc 1985;31:289

9. Anti M, et al. Esophageal involvement in Behcet's syndrome. J Clin Gastroenterol 1986;8:514

10. Askanas V, Engel WK, Mirabella M. Idiopathic inflammatory myopathies: inclusion-body myositis, polymyositis and dermatomyositis. Curr Opin Neurol 1994;7:448

11. Atkinson M, Summerling MD. Oesophageal changes in systemic sclerosis. Gut 1966;7:402

12. Basilisco G, Barbera R, Molgora M, Vanoli M, Bianchi P. Acid clearance and oesophageal sensitivity in patients with progressive systemic sclerosis. Gut 1993;34:1487

13. Battle WM, et al. Colonic dysfunction in diabetes mellitus. Gastroenterology 1980;79:1217

14. Battle WM, et al. Abnormal colonic motility in progressive systemic sclerosis. Ann Intern Med 1981;94:749

15. Behcet H. Uber Rezidivierende, Apthose, durch ein Virus Verursachte Geschwure am Mund, am Auge und an den Genitalien. Dermatol Wochenschr 1937;105:1152

16. Behcet's disease. Lancet 1989;1:761

17. Belch JJ, et al. Decreased oesophageal blood flow in patients with Raynaud's phenomenon. Br J Rheumatol 1988;27:426

18. Bevans M. Pathology of scleroderma, with special reference to changes in the gastrointestinal tract. Am J Pathol 1945;21:25

19. Bjerle P, et al. Oesophageal dysfunction in familial amyloidosis with polyneuropathy. Clin Physiol 1993;13:57

20. Blackwell JN, et al. Radionuclide transit studies in the detection of oesophageal dysmotility. Gut 1983;24:421

21. Bohan A, et al. A computer-assisted analysis of 153 patients with polymyositis and dermatomyositis. Medicine 1977;56:255

22. Bottomley WW, et al. Esophageal involvement in Behcet's disease. Is endoscopy necessary? Dig Dis Sci 1992;37:594

23. Brodie TE, Oschner JL. Behcet's syndrome with ulcerative esophagitis: report of the first case. Thorax 1973;28:637

24. Brody J, Bellin DE. Calcinosis with scleroderma. Arch Dermatol Syph 1937;36:85

25. Burakoff R, et al. Esophageal manometry in primary and secondary amyloidosis: a study of 30 patients. Gastroenterology 1981;80:1118

26. Cameron AJ, Ott BJ, Payne WS. The incidence of adenocarcinoma in a columnar lined Barrett's oesophagus. N Engl J Med 1985;313:857

27. Campbell IW, et al. Gastric emptying in diabetic autonomic neuropathy. Gut 1977;18:462

28. Carette S, et al. Radionuclide esophageal transit in progressive systemic sclerosis. J Rheumatol 1985;12:478

29. Castell JA, Dalton CB, Castell DO. Pharyngeal and upper esophageal sphincter manometry in humans. Am J Physiol 1990;258:G173

30. Chagas C. Nova tripanozomiase humana. Estudos sobre a morfologia e o ciclo evolutivo do Eschizotrypanium cruzi n. ge. n. sp., agente etiologico de nova entidade morbida do homem. Mem Inst Oswaldo Cruz 1909;1:1

31. Chajek T, Fainaur M. Behcet's syndrome. Report of 41 cases and a review of the literature. Medicine 1975;54:179

32. Chapman PJ, Pascoe MD, van Zyl-Smith R. Successful use of captopril in the treatment of "scleroderma renal crisis." Clin Nephrol 1986;26:106

33. Chiou AW-H, Lin J-K, Wang F-M. Anorectal abnormalities in progressive systemic sclerosis. Dis Colon Rectum 1989;32:417

34. Christiansen J, Clifton J. Esophageal manometry in myxedema [Abstract]. Gastroenterology 1967;52:1130

35. Clements PJ, et al. Muscle disease in progressive systemic sclerosis: diagnostic and therapeutic considerations. Arthritis Rheum 1978;21:62

36. Clements PJ, et al. Esophageal motility in progressive systemic sclerosis (PSS). Comparison of cine-radiographic and manometric evaluation. Dig Dis Sci 1979;24:639

37. Clements PJ, et al. Cyclosporine in systemic sclerosis: results of a forty-eight-week open safety study in ten patients. Arthritis Rheum 1993;36:75

38. Clouse RE, Motor disorders. In Sleisinger MH, Fordtran JS, eds, Gastrointestinal Disease. Philadelphia: WB Saunders, 1993:370

39. Clouse RE, Lustman PJ, Reidel WL. Correlation of esophageal motility abnormalities with neuropsychiatric status in diabetes. Gastroenterology 1986;90:1146

40. Cohen MR, et al. Clinical heterogeneity and treatment response in inclusion body myositis. Arthritis Rheum 1989;32:734

41. Cohen S, et al. The pathogenesis of esophageal dysfunction in scleroderma and Raynaud's disease. J Clin Invest 1972;51:2663

42. Cohen S, et al. The gastrointestinal manifestations of scleroderma: pathogenesis and management. Gastroenterology 1980;79:155

43. Costigan DJ, Clouse RE. Achalasia-like esophagus from amyloidosis. Successful treatment with pneumatic bag dilatation. Dig Dis Sci 1983;28:763

44. Creamer B, Anderson HA, Code CF. Esophageal motility in patients with scleroderma and related diseases. Gastroenterology 1956;86:763

45. D'Angelo WA, et al. Pathologic observations in systemic sclerosis (scleroderma). Am J Med 1969;46:428

46. Dalakas MC. Polymyositis, dermatomyositis and inclusion body myositis. N Engl J Med 1991;325:1487

47. Dantas RO, et al. Effect of nifedipine on the lower esophageal sphincter pressure in Chagasic patients. Braz J Med Biol Res 1986;19:205

48. Dantas RO, et al. Cholinergic innervation of the lower esophageal sphincter in Chagas' disease. Braz J Med Biol Res 1987;20:527

49. Dantas RO, et al. Lower esophageal sphincter pressure in Chagas' disease. Dig Dis Sci 1990;35:508

50. Dantas RO, et al. Esophageal function does not always worsen in systemic sclerosis. J Clin Gastroenterol 1993;17:281

51. Darrow DH, et al. Management of dysphagia in inclusion body myositis. Arch Otolaryngol Head Neck Surg 1992;118:313

52. Davidson A, Russell C, Littlejohn GO. Assessment of esophageal abnormalities in progressive systemic sclerosis using radionuclide transit. J Rheumatol 1985;12:472

53. DeClerck LS, et al. D-Penicillamine therapy and interstitial lung disease in scleroderma. Arthritis Rheum 1987;30:643

54. DeMerieux P, et al. Esophageal abnormalities and dysphagia in polymyositis and dermatomyositis. Arthritis Rheum 1983;26:961

55. Denis P, et al. Esophageal motility and pulmonary function in progressive systemic sclerosis. Respiration 1981;42:21

56. de Oliveira RB, et al. The spectrum of esophageal motor disorders in Chagas' disease. Am J Gastroenterol 1995;90:1119

57. DeSchryver-Kecskemeti K, Clouse RE. Gastrointestinal neuropathic changes in a group of patients with systemic connective tissue disease. Dig Dis Sci 1984;29:549

58. Dietz F, et al. Cricopharyngeal muscle dysfunction in the differential diagnosis of dysphagia in polymyositis. Arthritis Rheum 1980;23:491

59. DiMarino AJ, et al. Duodenal myoelectrical activity in scleroderma. N Engl J Med 1973;289:1220

60. Dinsmore R, Goodman D, Dreyfuss JR. The air esophagram: a sign of scleroderma involving the esophagus. Radiology 1966;87:348

61. Doria A, et al. Esophageal involvement in mixed connective tissue disease. J Rheumatol 1991;18:685

62. Dornhorst AC, Pierce JW, Whimster LW. The esophageal lesion in scleroderma. Lancet 1954;1:698

63. Drane WE. Progressive systemic sclerosis: radionuclide esophageal scintigraphy and manometry. Radiology 1986;160:73

64. Eastwood GL, et al. Reversal of lower esophageal sphincter hypotension and esophageal aperistalsis after treatment for hypothyroidism. J Clin Gastroenterol 1982;4:307

65. Ehrmann S. Ueber die Beziehung der Sklerodermie Zu den Autotoxichen erythemen. Ubien Med Wochenschr 1903;53:1097

66. Fabiani F, DeVincentis N, Staffilano A. Effects of Tolrestat on oesophageal transit time and cholecystic motility in type 2 diabetic patients with asymptomatic diabetic neuropathy. Diabetes Metab 1995;21:360

67. Figueiredo MC, et al. Short report: comparison of the effects of sublin-

gual nifedipine and isosorbide dinitrate on oesophageal emptying in patients with chagasic achalasia. Aliment Pharmacol Ther 1992;6:507

68. Fiorucci S, et al. Effect of erythromycin administration on upper gastrointestinal motility in scleroderma patients. Scand J Gastroenterol 1994;29:807

69. Fitzgerald OM, et al. Esophageal motility studies in patients with Raynaud's phenomenon. J Rheumatol 1987;14:273

70. Flick JA, et al. Esophageal motor abnormalities in children and adolescents with scleroderma and mixed connective tissue disease. Pediatrics 1988;82:107

71. Foster GR. Behcet's colitis with oesophageal ulceration treated with sulphasalazine and cyclosporin. J R Soc Med 1988;81:545

72. Furst DE, Clements PJ. Hypothesis for the pathogenesis of systemic sclerosis. J Rheumatol 1997;(suppl 48)24:53

73. Furst DE, et al. Clinical and serological comparison of 17 chronic progressive systemic sclerosis (PSS) and 17 CREST syndrome patients matched for sex, age and disease duration. Ann Rheum Dis 1984;43:794

74. Gallerano RH, Marr JJ, Sosa RR. Therapeutic efficacy of allopurinol in patients with chronic Chagas' disease. Am J Trop Med Hyg 1990; 43:159

75. Garrett JM, Winkelmann RK, Schlegel JF, Code CF. Esophageal deterioration in scleroderma. Mayo Clin Proc 1971;46:92

76. Gilat T, Spiro HM. Amyloidosis and the gut. Am J Dig Dis 1968;13: 619

77. Gislinger H, et al. Efficacy of cyclosporine A in systemic sclerosis. Clin Exp Rheumatol 1991;9:383

78. Goetz RH. The pathology of progressive systemic sclerosis (generalized scleroderma). Clin Proc 1945;4:337

79. Grande L, et al. Esophageal motor function in primary Sjogren's syndrome. Am J Gastroenterol 1993;88:378

80. Grande L, et al. High amplitude contractions in the middle third of the esophagus: a manometric marker of chronic alcoholism? Gut 1996; 38:655

81. Greydanus MP, Camilleri M. Abnormal postcibal antral and small bowel motility due to neuropathy or myopathy in systemic sclerosis. Gastroenterology 1989;96:110

82. Gutierrez F, et al. Esophageal dysfunction in patients with mixed connective tissue diseases and systemic lupus erythematosus. Dig Dis Sci 1982;27:592

83. Hamel-Roy J, et al. Comparative esophageal and anorectal motility in scleroderma. Gastroenterology 1985;88:1

84. Heitzman EJ, Heitzman CC, Elliot CF. Primary esophageal amyloidosis. Arch Intern Med 1962;109:595

85. Hendel L, Stentoft P, Aggestrup S. The progress of oesophageal involvement in progressive systemic sclerosis during D-penicillamine treatment. Scand J Rheumatol 1989;18:149

86. Hendel L, Svejgaard E, Walsoe I, Kieffer M, Stenderup A. Esophageal candidosis in progressive systemic sclerosis: occurrence, significance, and treatment with fluconazole. Scand J Gastroenterol 1988;23:1182

87. Hendel L, et al. Omeprazole in the long-term treatment of severe gastro-oesophageal reflux disease in patients with systemic sclerosis. Aliment Pharmacol Ther 1992;6:565

88. Hochberg MC, Feldman D, Stevens MB. Adult onset polymyositis/ dermatomyositis: an analysis of clinical and laboratory features and survival in 76 patients with a review of the literature. Semin Arthritis Rheum 1986;15:168

89. Hogan WJ, et al. Ethanol-induced acute esophageal motor dysfunction. J Appl Physiol 1972;32:755

90. Hollis JB, Castell DO, Braddom RL. Esophageal function in diabetes mellitus and its relation to peripheral neuropathy. Gastroenterology 1977;73:1098

91. Horowitz M, et al. Abnormalities of gastric and esophageal emptying in polymyositis and dermatomyositis. Gastroenterology 1986;90:434

92. Horowitz M, et al. Effect of cisapride on gastric and esophageal emptying in insulin-dependent diabetes mellitus. Gastroenterology 1987; 92:1899

93. Horowitz M, et al. Effects of cisapride on gastric and esophageal emptying in progressive systemic sclerosis. Gastroenterology 1987; 93:311

94. House AJS, Griffiths GJ. The significance of an air oesophagram visualized on conventional chest radiographs. Clin Radiol 1977;28: 301

95. Huppe D, Tegenthoff M, Faig J. Esophageal dysfunction in diabetes mellitus: is there a relation to clinical manifestation of neuropathy? Clin Invest 1992;70:740

96. Jack CI, et al. Twenty-four-hour tracheal pH monitoring—a simple and non-hazardous investigation. Respir Med 1994;88:441

97. Jacob H, et al. The esophageal motility disorder of polymyositis. A prospective study. Arch Intern Med 1983;143:2262

98. Johnson DA, et al. Metoclopramide response in patients with progressive systemic sclerosis. Effect on esophageal and gastric motility abnormalities. Arch Intern Med 1987;147:1597

99. Johnson DA, et al. Pulmonary disease in progressive systemic sclerosis. A complication of gastroesophageal reflux and occult aspiration? Arch Intern Med 1989;149:589

100. Johnson RB, Monroe LS. Carcinoma of the esophagus developing in progressive systemic sclerosis. Gastrointest Endosc 1973;19:189

101. Kagen LJ, Hochman RB, Strong EW. Cricopharyngeal obstruction in inflammatory myopathy (polymyositis/dermatomyositis). Report of three cases and review of the literature. Arthritis Rheum 1985;28:630

102. Kahan A, Amor B, Menkes CJ. A randomized double-blind trial of diltiazem in the treatment of Raynaud's phenomenon. Ann Rheum Dis 1985;44:30

103. Kahan A, et al. The effect of cisapride on gastrooesophageal dysfunction in systemic sclerosis: a controlled manometric study. Br J Clin Pharmacol 1991;31:683

104. Karayalcin B, et al. Esophageal clearance scintigraphy in diabetic patients—a preliminary study. Ann Nucl Med 1992;6:89

105. Katzka DA, et al. Barrett's metaplasia and adenocarcinoma of the esophagus in scleroderma. Am J Med 1987;82:46

106. Kaufman HJ, Braverman IM, Spiro HM. Esophageal manometry in scleroderma. Scand J Gastroenterol 1968;3:246

107. Kilman WJ, Goyal RK. Disorders of pharyngeal and upper esophageal sphincter motor function. Arch Intern Med 1976;136:592

108. Kinder RR, Fleischman R. Systemic scleroderma: a review of organ systems. Int J Dermatol 1974;13:382

109. Kirchhoff LV. Chagas' disease. American trypanosomiasis. Infect Dis Clin North Am 1993;7:487

110. Kjellen G, et al. Esophageal function, radiography, and dysphagia in Sjogren's syndrome. Dig Dis Sci 1986;31:225

111. Klein H, et al. Comparative studies of esophageal function in systemic sclerosis. Gastroenterology 1992;102:1551

112. Koberle F. Pathogenesis of Chagas' disease. Ciba Found Symp 1974; 20:137

113. Kotter I, et al. Therapy of Behcet's disease. German J Ophthalmol 1996;5:92

114. Kramer P, Ingelfinger FJ. Motility of the human esophagus in control subjects and in patients with esophageal disorders. Am J Med 1949; 7:168

115. Kraus A, Alarcon-Segovia D. Air esophagogram and intestinal pseudoocclusion in a patient with scleroderma. J Rheumatol 1991;18:897

116. Lally EV, Jimenez SA, Kaplan SR. Progressive systemic sclerosis: mode of presentation, rapidly progressive disease course and mortality based on analysis of 91 patients. Semin Arthritis Rheum 1988;18:1

117. Lapadula G, et al. Esophageal motility disorders in the rheumatic diseases: a review of 150 patients. Clin Exp Rheumatol 1994;12:515

118. Lefkowitz JR, et al. Amyloidosis mimics achalasia's effect on lower esophageal sphincter. Dig Dis Sci 1989;34:630

119. Lehner T, Barnes CG. Criteria for diagnosis and classification of Behcet's syndrome. In Lehner T, Barnes CG, eds, Behcet's Syndrome. London: Academic, 1979:1

120. LeRoy EC, et al. Scleroderma (systemic sclerosis): classification, subsets and pathogenesis. J Rheumatol 1988;15:202

121. Levack B, Hanson D. Behcet's disease of the esophagus. J Laryngol Otol 1979;93:99

122. Limburg AJ, Smit AJ, Kleibeuker JH. The effect of cisapride on the esophageal motor function of patients with progressive systemic sclerosis or mixed connective tissue disease. Digestion 1991;49:156

123. Ljubich P, et al. Diffuse gastrointestinal dysmotility in a patient with rheumatoid arthritis. Am J Gastroenterol 1993;88:1443

124. Loo FD, et al. Multipeaked esophageal peristaltic pressure waves in patients with diabetic neuropathy. Gastroenterology 1985;88:485

125. Lopez-Orejero JA, et al. Reversal of vascular and renal crisis of scleroderma by oral angiotensin-converting enzyme blockage. N Engl J Med 1979;300:1417

126. Lotz BP, et al. Inclusion body myositis. Observations in 40 patients. Brain 1989;112:727

127. Maddern GJ, Horowitz M, Jamieson GG. The effect of domperidone

on oesophageal emptying in diabetic autonomic neuropathy. Br J Clin Pharmacol 1985;19:441

128. Maddern GJ, et al. Abnormalities of esophageal and gastric emptying in progressive systemic sclerosis. Gastroenterology 1984;87:922

129. Maeda K. Studies on Behcet's Disease. The Epidemiological Features and Examination of Manifestation, Patterns of Major and Minor Symptoms for Behcet's Disease Patients in University Hospitals. Tokyo: Behcet's Disease Research Committee of Japan, Ministry of Welfare, 1982:64

130. Mandelstam P, Lieber A. Esophageal dysfunction in diabetic neuropathy–gastroenteropathy. JAMA 1967;201:88

131. Mandelstam P, Siegel CI, Sieber A, Siegel M. The swallowing disorder in patients with diabetic neuropathy–gastroenteropathy. Gastroenterology 1969;56:1

132. Mansour KA, Malone CE. Surgery for scleroderma of the esophagus: a 12 year experience. Ann Thorac Surg 1988;46:513

133. Marr JJ, Docampo R. Chemotherapy for Chagas' disease: a perspective on current therapy and considerations for future research. Rev Infect Dis 1986;8:884

134. Marshall JB, et al. Gastrointestinal manifestations of mixed connective tissue disease. Gastroenterology 1990;98:1232

135. Martinez LO. Air in the esophagus as a sign of scleroderma. J Can Assoc Radiol 1974;25:234

136. Martins P, Morais BB, Cunha-Melo JR. Postoperative complications in the treatment of Chagasic megaesophagus. Int Surg 1993;78:99

137. Masi AT, et al. Preliminary criteria for the classification of systemic sclerosis (scleroderma). Arthritis Rheum 1980;23:581

138. Mastaglia FL, Phillips BA, Zilko P. Treatment of inflammatory myopathies. Muscle Nerve 1997;20:651

139. Masuda K, et al. Double-masked trial of cyclosporin versus colchicine and long-term open study of cyclosporin in Behcet's disease. Lancet 1989;1:1093

140. Matsui S. Uber die Pathologie und Pathogenese von Sklerodermia Universalis. Mitt Med Fakult Kaiseri Univ Tokyo 1924;31:55

141. McKinley M, Sherlock P. Barrett's esophagus with adenocarcinoma in scleroderma. Am J Gastroenterol 1984;79:438

142. Medsger TA Jr. Systemic sclerosis and malignancy—are they related? J Rheumatol 1985;12:1041

143. Medsger TA Jr, et al. Skeletal muscle involvement of progressive systemic sclerosis (PSS). Arthritis Rheum 1968;11:554

144. Meshkinpour H, Afrasiabi MA, Valenta LJ. Esophageal motor function in Graves' disease. Dig Dis Sci 1979;24:159

145. Miller LS, et al. Endoluminal ultrasonography of the distal esophagus in systemic sclerosis. Gastroenterology 1993;105:31

146. Miller RH. Amyloid disease: an unusual cause of megalo-oesophagus. S Afr Med J 1969;43:1202

147. Montesi A, et al. Oropharyngeal and esophageal function in scleroderma. Dysphagia 1991;6:219

148. Mori S, et al. Esophageal involvement in Behcet's disease. Am J Gastroenterol 1983;78:548

149. Mota E, et al. Mega esophagus and seroreactivity of *Trypanosoma cruzi* in a rural community in northeast Brazil. Am J Trop Med Hyg 1984;33:820

150. Muller-Ladner U, Benning K, Lang B. Current therapy of progressive systemic sclerosis (scleroderma). Clin Invest 1993;71:257

151. Murphy JR, et al. Prolonged clearance is the primary abnormal reflux parameter in patients with progressive systemic sclerosis and esophagitis. Dig Dis Sci 1992;37:833

152. Myers AR. Progressive systemic sclerosis. Gastrointestinal involvement. Clin Rheumatol Dis 1979;5:115

153. Naef AP, Savary M, Ozzello L. Columnar-lined lower esophagus: an acquired lesion with malignant predisposition: report on 140 cases of Barrett's esophagus with 12 adenocarcinomas. J Thorac Cardiovasc Surg 1975;70:826

154. Navin TR, et al. Human and sylvatic *Trypanosoma cruzi* infection in California. Am J Public Health 1985;75:366

155. Neschis M, Siegelmann SS, Rotstein J, Parker JG. The esophagus in progressive systemic sclerosis. A manometric and radiographic correlation. Am J Dig Dis 1970;15:443

156. Niv Y, et al. Barrett's epithelium and esophageal adenocarcinoma in scleroderma. Am J Gastroenterol 1988;83:792

157. O'Duffy JD. Behcet's syndrome. N Engl J Med 1990;322:326

158. Olive A, Juncosa S, Evison G, Maddison PJ. Air in the oesophagus: a sign of oesophageal involvement in systemic sclerosis. Clin Rheumatol 1995;14:319

159. Orringer MB. Surgical management of scleroderma reflux esophagitis. Surg Clin North Am 1983;63:859

160. Orringer MB, et al. Gastroesophageal reflux in esophageal scleroderma: diagnosis and implications. Ann Thorac Surg 1976;22:120

161. Orringer MB, et al. Combined Collis gastroplasty–fundoplication operations for scleroderma reflux esophagitis. Surgery 1981;90:624

162. Palma R, et al. Esophageal motility disorders in patients with Sjogren's syndrome. Dig Dis Sci 1994;39:758

163. Park RHR, McKillop JH, Belch JJF, Faichney A, MacKenzie JF. Achalasia-like syndrome in systemic sclerosis. Br J Surg 1990;77:46

164. Parkin JV, Wright DG. Behcet's disease and the alimentary tract. Postgrad Med J 1975;51:260

165. Peppercorn MA, Docken WP, Rosenberg S. Esophageal motor dysfunction in systemic lupus erythematosus: two cases with unusual features. JAMA 1979;242:1895

166. Pines A, et al. Corticosteroid induced remission of oesophageal involvement in mixed connective tissue disease. Postgrad Med J 1982;58:297

167. Pinotti HW, et al. The surgical treatment of megaesophagus and megacolon. Dig Dis 1993;11:206

168. Plotz PH, et al. Current concepts in the idiopathic inflammatory myopathies: polymyositis, dermatomyositis, and related disorders. Ann Intern Med 1989;111:143

169. Poirier NC, Taillefer R, Topart P, Duranceau A. Antireflux operations in patients with scleroderma. Ann Thorac Surg 1994;58:66

170. Poirier TJ, Rankin GB. Gastrointestinal manifestations of progressive systemic scleroderma based on a review of 364 cases. Am J Gastroentcrol 1972;58:30

171. Radigan LR, et al. Barrett esophagus. Arch Surg 1977;112:486

172. Rake G. On the pathology and pathogenesis of scleroderma. Bull Johns Hopkins Hosp 1931;48:212

173. Ramirez-Mata M, Ibanez G, Alarcon-Segovia D. Stimulatory effect of metoclopramide on the esophagus and lower esophageal sphincter of patients with PSS. Arthritis Rheum 1977;20:30

174. Ramirez-Mata M, Pena-Ancira FF, Alarcon-Segovia D. Abnormal esophageal motility in primary Sjogren's syndrome. J Rheumatol 1976;3:63

175. Ramirez-Mata M, Reyes PA, Alarcon-Segovia D, Garza R. Esophageal motility in systemic lupus erythematosus. Am J Dig Dis 1974;19:132

176. Riminton DS, et al. Inclusion-body myositis presenting soley as dysphagia. Neurology 1993;43:1241

177. Ringel SP, et al. Spectrum of inclusion body myositis. Arch Neurol 1987;44:1154

178. Rodnan GP, Benedek TG. An historical account of the study of progressive systemic sclerosis (diffuse scleroderma). Ann Intern Med 1962;57:305

179. Rosenow EC. Esophageal motility. Med Clin North Am 1970;54:863

180. Rubinaw A, et al. Esophageal manometry in systemic amyloidosis: a study of 30 patients. Am J Med 1983;75:951

181. Russell CO, et al. Radionuclide transit: a sensitive screening test for esophageal dysfunction. Gastroenterology 1981;80:887

182. Saladin TA, French AB, Zarafonetis CJ, Pollard HM. Esophageal motor abnormalities in scleroderma and related diseases. Am J Dig Dis 1966;11:522

183. Sattar MA, Guindi TR, Sugathan TN. Penicillamine in systemic sclerosis: a reappraisal. Clin Rheumatol 1990;9:517

184. Schneider HA, et al. Scleroderma esophagus: a nonspecific entity. Ann Intern Med 1984;100:848

185. Schuffler MD. Chronic intestinal pseudo-obstruction syndromes. Med Clin North Am 1981;65:1331

186. Schuffler M, Pope CE. Esophageal motor dysfunction in idiopathic intestinal pseudo-obstruction. Gastroenterology 1976;70:677

187. Schuffler M, et al. Chronic intestinal pseudo-obstruction: a report of 27 cases and review of the literature. Medicine 1981;60:173

188. Schuurkes JAJ, Akkermans LMA, VanNeuten JM. Stimulating effects of cisapride on antroduodenal motility in the conscious dog. In Roman C, ed, Gastrointestinal Motility. Lancaster: MTP Press, 1984:513

189. Segel MC, et al. Systemic sclerosis (scleroderma) and esophageal adenocarcinoma: is increased patient screening necessary? Gastroenterology 1985;89:485

190. Shapiro LS, Notis WM, Romanoff NR. Self-limited esophageal ulcerations in Behcet's syndrome. Arthritis Rheum 1983;26:690

191. Sharp GC, et al. Mixed connective tissue disease—an apparently dis-

tinct rheumatic disease associated with a specific antibody to an extractable nuclear antigen (ENA). Am J Med 1972;52:148

192. Shoenut JP, Wieler JA, Micflikier AB. The extent and pattern of gastro-esophageal reflux in patients with scleroderma esophagus: the effect of low-dose omeprazole. Aliment Pharmacol Ther 1993;7:509

193. Siebold JR. Scleroderma. In Kelly WN, et al., eds. Textbook of Rheumatology (3rd ed). Philadelphia: WB Saunders, 1989

194. Skinner DB, et al. Barrett's esophagus: comparison of benign and malignant cases. Ann Surg 1983;198:554

195. Spechler SJ, et al. Adenocarcinoma and Barrett's esophagus: an overrated risk. Gastroenterology 1984;87:927

196. Starnes VA, et al. Barrett's esophagus: a surgical entity. Arch Surg 1984;119:563

197. Steen VD. Treatment of systemic sclerosis. Curr Opin Rheumatol 1991;3:979

198. Stentoft P, Hendel L, Aggestrup S. Esophageal manometry and pH-probe monitoring in the evaluation of gastroesophageal reflux in patients with progressive systemic sclerosis. Scand J Gastroenterol 1987;22:499

199. Stevens MB, et al. Aperistalsis of the esophagus in patients with connective-tissue disorders and Raynaud's phenomenon. N Engl J Med 1964;270:1218

200. Sun DCH, et al. Upper gastrointestinal disease in rheumatoid arthritis. Am J Dig Dis 1974;19:405

201. Suris X, et al. Achalasia of the esophagus in secondary amyloidosis. Am J Gastroenterol 1993;88:1959

202. Tada S, Iida M, Iwashita A. Endoscopic and biopsy findings of the upper digestive tract in patients with amyloidosis. Gastrointest Endosc 1990;36:10

203. Takebayashi S, et al. Cervical esophageal motility: evaluation with US in progressive systemic sclerosis. Radiology 1991;179:389

204. Thompson JJ, Zinsser KR, Enterline HT. Barrett's metaplasia and adenocarcinoma of the esophagus and gastroesophageal junction. Hum Pathol 1983;145:42

205. Treacy WL, Baggenstoss AH, Slocumb CH, Code CF. Scleroderma of the esophagus. A correlation of histologic and physiologic findings. Ann Intern Med 1963;59:351

206. Troshinsky MB, et al. Pulmonary function and gastroesophageal reflux in systemic sclerosis. Ann Intern Med 1994;121:6

207. Tsianos EB, Drosos AA, Chiras CD, Moutsopoulos HM, Kitrido RC. Esophageal manometric findings in autoimmune rheumatic diseases: is scleroderma esophagus a specific entity? Rheumatol Int 1987;7:23

208. Tsianos EB, et al. The gastrointestinal involvement in primary Sjogren's syndrome. Scand J Rheumatol 1986;61:151

209. Tsianos EB, et al. The effects of peripheral cold exposure on oesophageal motility in patients with autoimmune rheumatic diseases and Raynaud's phenomenon. Clin Rheumatol 1991;10:311

210. Turner R, et al. Esophageal dysfunction in collagen disease. Am J Med Sci 1973;265:191

211. Vela AR, Balart LA. Esophageal motor manifestations in diabetes mellitus. Am J Surg 1970;119:21

212. Verma A, et al. Inclusion body myositis with cricopharyngeus muscle involvement and severe dysphagia. Muscle Nerve 1991;14:470

213. Vix V. Esophageal motility in diabetes mellitus. Radiology 1969;92:363

214. Wegener M, et al. Gastrointestinal transit through esophagus, stomach, small and large intestine in patients with progressive systemic sclerosis. Dig Dis Sci 1994;39:2209

215. Weihrauch TR, Korting GW. Manometric assessment of oesophageal involvement in progressive systemic sclerosis, morphoea and Raynaud's disease. Br J Dermatol 1982;107:325

216. Williamson WA, et al. Barrett's esophagus. Prevalence and incidence of adenocarcinoma. Arch Intern Med 1991;151:2212

217. Winship DH, et al. Deterioration of esophageal peristalsis in patients with alcoholic neuropathy. Gastroenterology 1968;55:173

218. Wintzen AR, et al. Dysphagia in inclusion body myositis. J Neurol Neurosurg Psychiatry 1988;51:1542

219. Wright RA, Penner DB. Myxedema and upper esophageal dysmotility. Dig Dis Sci 1981;26:376

220. Yarze JC, Varga J, Stampfl D, Castell DO, Jimenez SA. Esophageal function in systemic sclerosis: a prospective evaluation of motility and acid reflux in 36 patients. Am J Gastroenterol 1993;88:870

221. Yashiro K, et al. Esophageal lesions in intestinal Behcet's disease. Endoscopy 1986;18:57

222. Yazici H, et al. A controlled trial of azathioprine in Behcet's syndrome. N Engl J Med 1990;322:281

223. Zamost BJ, et al. Esophagitis in scleroderma. Prevalence and risk factors. Gastroenterology 1987;92:421

224. Zentilin P, et al. Improvement in esophageal motor abnormalities in systemic sclerosis patients treated with cyclosporine. Arthritis Rheum 1994;37:301

The Esophagus, Third Edition,
edited by D. O. Castell and J. E. Richter.
Lippincott Williams & Wilkins, Philadelphia © 1999.

# CHAPTER 17

# Foreign Bodies

Paul Yeaton and David A. Peura

Foreign-body ingestion represents a common problem faced by clinicians. Although it is difficult to estimate its true incidence, reports indicate that 1,500 [19] to 2,750 [16] individuals die annually in the United States as a result of ingested foreign objects. Eighty percent to 90% of swallowed objects that reach the stomach will pass uneventfully through the gastrointestinal tract and require no therapeutic intervention [84, 101]. Unfortunately, the remainder of ingested objects may become lodged in the esophagus, placing the patient at increased risk for development of complications, including bleeding due to mucosal damage, luminal obstruction, respiratory compromise, perforation, fistulization to surrounding structures, abscess formation, sepsis, and death. The physician must, therefore, be cognizant of appropriate management procedures including diagnostic modalities, therapeutic options and their proper applications and contraindications, and potential risk. In most instances, the goals of management will be relief of symptoms and prevention of complications. Several factors will influence decisions regarding management of impacted objects in the esophagus. These include (a) the type and nature of the object (e.g., blunt versus sharp or pointed, caustic versus nontoxic); (b) the location of the impaction (e.g., hypopharynx versus distal esophagus); (c) elapsed time since ingestion; (d) the presence of symptoms compatible with complete obstruction or other complications; and finally, (e) an assessment as to whether the patient can be safely managed with available physician skills, equipment, and facilities.

## ANATOMIC CONSIDERATIONS

Ingested foreign objects can lodge at any level of the gastrointestinal tract but most commonly become impacted in regions that are physiologically or pathologically narrowed

[7, 8]. This fact probably explains why the esophagus is the most frequent site of acute foreign-body obstruction [35]. The normal esophagus has four anatomic sites of narrowing: (a) the region of the cricopharyngeus muscle, (b) the level of the aortic arch, (c) the level of the left main stem bronchus, and (d) the lower esophageal sphincter. The location of esophageal impaction depends to some extent on the size and shape of the object, patient age, and the presence or absence of diseases that constrict the esophageal lumen. Large objects (e.g., coins) and angulated sharp objects (e.g., bones, aluminum pop tops, safety pins) are commonly trapped in the proximal esophagus [90]. The cervical portion is particularly prone to foreign-body impaction and has been reported to be the region of highest involvement in several series (Table 17–1) [31, 32, 43, 67, 84, 88].

Pathologic narrowing of the esophageal lumen is also an important predisposing factor for impaction. The etiology and frequency of pathologic constriction vary with patient age. For example, children who ingest objects such as coins or small toys that lodge in the esophagus will most frequently have no associated structural lesion. However, they may occasionally have a stricture due to prior caustic ingestion or a congenital abnormality such as esophageal stenosis, a web, or tracheoesophageal fistula [52]. In a series of 660 children admitted for foreign-body ingestion, eight developed impaction in the esophagus following surgery for esophageal atresia [88]. The cause in this group is believed to be altered motility and peristalsis around the anastomotic site.

In adults, the pathologic narrowing of the esophagus causing impaction is most often a peptic stricture or distal esophageal ring. Other causes include strictures due to caustics or pills and achalasia. Cancer rarely causes impaction. In 2,394 cases of esophageal foreign bodies over a 12-year period reviewed by Nandi and Ong [67] (343 pediatric and 2,051 adult), only nine patients with esophageal carcinoma presented with a foreign-body impaction. These data are particularly impressive since the authors' institution evaluates approximately 140 cases of esophageal carcinoma per year. Brooks [9] also noted that no patient with malignant disease

---

P. Yeaton: Digestive Health Center, University of Virginia Health Sciences Center, Charlottesville, Virginia 22906-0013.

D. A. Peura: Division of Gastroenterology and Hepatology, Department of Medicine, University of Virginia Health Sciences Center, Charlottesville, Virginia 22906.

**TABLE 17–1.** *Location of esophageal impactions*

| Study | Total no. of patients | No. in cervical esophagus (%) | No. in middle esophagus (%) | No. in distal esophagus (%) |
|---|---|---|---|---|
| Goff [32] | 180 | 152 (84) | 10 (6) | 18 (10) |
| Selivanov et al. [84] | 43 | 31 (72) | 11 (28)[a] | |
| Giordano et al. [31] | 159 | 79 (50) | 27 (17) | 46 (29)[b] |
| Nandi and Ong [67] | 844 | 710 (84) | 126 (15) | 8 (1) |
| Hollinger et al. [43] | 604 | 436 (73) | 118 (19) | 50 (8) |
| Spitz [88] | 231 | 153 (66) | 46 (20) | 32 (14) |

[a] Reported as lower two-thirds of esophagus.
[b] Site unknown in seven cases (4%).

of the esophagus had a retained foreign body during a 10-year period in which 200 esophageal foreign bodies were treated.

## CLINICAL SETTING

Foreign-body ingestions occur in all age groups, although 80% are seen in children [39, 98]. Natural curiosity during developmental years may compel a child to place nondigestible objects into his or her mouth, resulting in accidental swallowing. Coins are most commonly ingested by the pediatric population [14, 31, 73]; however, the diversity of objects that can be swallowed is limited only by one's imagination. Frequently swallowed objects include toys, crayons, stones, buttons, toothpicks, and safety pins. In one study involving 343 children, fish bones and coins were found in 146 and 134 children, respectively [67]. Crysdale and associates [18] evaluated 484 cases of esophageal foreign bodies in children. In their study, 63% of all patients were 3 years old or less at the time of ingestion. Chaikhouni and colleagues [14] observed that the highest percentage of esophageal foreign-body ingestion occurs in the months of July, August, and December during period of school vacation. A correlation between foreign-body type and age was also noted (Fig. 17–1).

In contrast to children, adults less often deliberately swallow nondigestible items, except for certain clearly defined high-risk groups. Among these are individuals who are mentally retarded or impaired due to psychiatric illnesses (e.g., schizophrenia, dementia), abusers of drugs and/or alcohol, and prisoners. Psychiatric patients present special problems in that they may be unable to relate a clear history of ingestion, they frequently ingest foreign objects repeatedly, they may take medications that alter bowel motility, and they are often uncooperative during attempted endoscopic extraction [78]. Numerous case reports have documented bizarre ingestions by psychiatric patients. Devanesan and co-workers [19] reported a schizophrenic patient operated on because of abdominal pain and an enlarging abdominal mass. Surgeons removed 648 metallic objects from the stomach, including coins, chains, keys, and broken thermometers.

Individuals who are incarcerated often deliberately ingest foreign objects for potential secondary gain from hospitalization. Unusual objects such as razor blades, cigarette lighters, bedsprings, wire, and toothpaste tubes are commonly removed from these patients. A recent epidemic of ingested hypodermic needles fashioned into "stars" was reported in a prison population. All six patients suffered esophageal perforation requiring emergent esophagotomy [95]. Prisoners

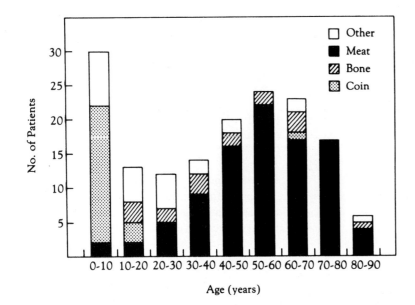

**FIG. 17–1.** Correlation between age and foreign-body type in 159 patients with esophageal foreign bodies. (From ref. 31, with permission. Copyright 1981, American Medical Association.)

are also more likely to reswallow an object once it has passed to prolong their hospitalization [47]. For this reason, they should be carefully observed.

Accidental swallowing of foreign bodies also occurs in adults. Occupationally related ingestion of objects such as sewing needles, buttons, screws, nails, washers, and paper clips has been reported. In addition, there are case reports of "iatrogenic" foreign-body ingestion of dental instruments, biopsy equipment, and nebulizers.

"True" foreign-body ingestion is less common in adults; however, food impaction is much more likely to occur. Food differs from other foreign bodies in that impaction (a) usually happens in the setting of intrinsic esophageal disease, (b) is more likely to involve the distal esophagus, and (c) generally occurs in older persons [34]. As previously mentioned, peptic strictures and B rings are the most common underlying pathologic findings. Webb and coauthors [101] reported a 97% incidence (39 of 40 patients) of an associated esophageal pathologic process in patients with meat impaction. Similarly, Vizcarrondo and colleagues [96] found a 78% incidence of associated esophageal disease in their patients with meat impaction. Any solid-food bolus is capable of obstructing a narrowed esophagus, but in clinical practice, impaction is due to raw fruits and vegetables and more commonly to red meat. The latter has prompted some authors to coin the phrase *steakhouse syndrome* [70]. As with "true" foreign-body ingestion, alcohol intoxication makes one vulnerable to food impaction. Denture wearers are also at risk due to a reduction of tactile sensation to the palate. This may impair awareness of food bolus size or the presence of bony fragments within meat. Poor vision, incomplete mastication due to ill-fitting dentures, and poor dentition may further predispose to food impaction in the elderly.

The term *cafe coronary* describes the emergency situation that occurs when a food bolus becomes impacted at or just below the cricopharyngeus and causes tracheal compression and acute airway compromise. Administration of emergency treatment, such as the Heimlich maneuver, from bystanders may be lifesaving.

A final category of esophageal foreign body capable of producing esophageal injury is pills. An extensive review by Kikendall and associates [48] revealed that antibiotics are the most common culprit, although many other drugs, including quinidine, nonsteroidal anti-inflammatory agents, ferrous sulfate, and potassium chloride, can cause esophagitis. The mechanism of pill-induced esophageal injury is usually chemical; however, recent unusual cases document esophageal obstruction after ingestion of a fiber-containing diet pill [83] and an extra-strength antacid tablet [105]. Chapter 31 is devoted to pill-induced esophageal injury.

## CLINICAL MANIFESTATIONS

Patients who have swallowed a foreign object can present with a wide array of symptoms and signs. Dysphagia, odynophagia, and increased salivation are the most common symptoms associated with esophageal impaction. Retching, emesis, and a persistent pain sensation in the neck or chest also characteristically occur. Sharp, pointed objects (e.g., fish bones) that abrade the mucosa may cause a persistent foreign-body sensation even after the object has passed or been extracted. Most adults with acute foreign-body obstruction will be able to relate a clear history of ingestion; however, mentally disturbed individuals and children may be unable to do so. The clinician should always consider the possibility of foreign-body obstruction in any infant or toddler who refuses feedings or who has unexplained gagging, coughing, or chronic pulmonary aspiration. Approximately 5% of patients with esophageal foreign bodies will present with airway obstruction [98]. Most adults will present within 12 hours of ingestion, whereas in up to 18% of children, the diagnosis may be delayed for a month or more [80]. Such unsuspected or prolonged impaction may lead to severe complications [36, 49, 89]. Factors resulting in delayed diagnosis include mild initial symptoms, radiolucency of the object, absence of a history of ingestion, and failure to consider foreign-body ingestion as a diagnostic possibility.

## DIAGNOSTIC EVALUATION

The goals of the diagnostic evaluation are to determine (a) the type and size of the object, (b) its precise location, (c) the presence of any associated complications, and (d) any underlying structural lesions of the esophagus.

The history in most patients will suggest the presence of a foreign body. In addition, the location of symptoms may be helpful in determining the site of obstruction. For example, when an object is impacted near the cricopharyngeus muscle, the patient would be expected to point lateral to the trachea and superior to the clavicle [39]. Objects lodged distally at the gastroesophageal junction may cause substernal chest pain. Esophageal pain is more likely to be referred proximally rather than distally to the site of impaction. Therefore, discomfort in the subxiphoid or epigastric region is more reliable for localizing the site of impaction than is discomfort in the suprasternal notch. One should always inquire about a prior history of dysphagia or impaction since these would suggest an underlying esophageal abnormality.

The physical examination is important primarily in detecting complications. Fever, tachycardia, and subcutaneous emphysema suggest perforation. Inability to swallow saliva and drooling indicate complete obstruction. In general, the physical examination should serve as a means for obtaining a global assessment of the individual's general medical condition and for identifying any problems that might interfere with subsequent diagnostic and therapeutic intervention.

Radiographic evaluation is helpful in many patients with symptomatic foreign-body ingestion. Plain films of the neck or chest can localize radiopaque objects lodged in the esophagus. Both anteroposterior and lateral views should be obtained since some radiopaque objects will be seen only in the lateral projection if they overlie the vertebral column.

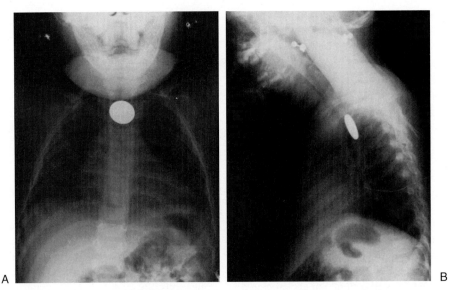

**FIG. 17–2.** Anteroposterior (**A**) and lateral (**B**) views of a coin lodged in the esophagus. Note that the flat surface is seen best on the anteroposterior view.

Combined views also help in distinguishing whether objects are in the esophagus or tracheobronchial tree. For example, coins lodged in the esophagus will usually lie in the coronal plane with the flat surface seen on anteroposterior view (Fig. 17–2). If located in the trachea, the flat surface is best seen on the lateral view, owing to sagittal orientation. Plain films can also demonstrate findings suggesting a complication such as subcutaneous emphysema, pneumomediastinum, pleural effusion, or pulmonary infiltrates due to aspiration. Although controversial because of radiation exposure, some authors believe that infants and children should have x-rays from the base of the head to the anus to determine whether multiple foreign objects are present [100]. Plain films are necessary in all children with a history of coin ingestion. Two recent reports [41, 82] demonstrated that 17% of children with a history of coin ingestion but no signs or symptoms at presentation had coins in the esophagus as shown by x-rays study. A review of 422 consecutive patients undergoing radiologic evaluation to exclude foreign-body ingestion found a radiopaque object in 249 (59%), of which 84% were ingested coins. One hundred twenty-three of these 208 coins (59%) were retained in the esophagus [38]. In the past, xeroradiography was believed to be useful to detect objects that are less radiodense [22]. Recent comparative studies, however, found that this soft tissue technique was less accessible, had higher radiation exposure, and was not superior to conventional radiography in the detection of foreign bodies [24]. In a group of 16 pediatric patients with radiographically proven metallic foreign bodies, 15 were successfully localized using a handheld metal detector; the only object not detected was an ingested needle. This has the potential to reduce radiation exposure in selected cases [79]. Objects such as wood, aluminum, glass, plastics, and meat may not be visible without the use of contrast solutions.

The choice of contrast agent is usually between barium sulfate and a water-soluble solution such as meglumine diatrizoate (Gastrografin). A contrast study may localize the site of impaction but makes subsequent endoscopy more difficult to perform. If barium is used, a minimal amount of thin solution is preferred. Barium-soaked cotton balls should be avoided since they are generally not helpful and may become lodged on an obstructing foreign body. Meglumine diatrizoate may be helpful in localizing a suspected perforation, but because of its hypertonicity (1,900 mOsm per liter), it may cause pulmonary edema if it enters the lungs [27]. For this reason, hypertonic contrast solutions should be avoided whenever aspiration or tracheoesophageal fistula is a possibility. A water-soluble, nonionic contrast agent such as metrizamide may have an advantage since it was shown in recent animal studies to cause no more histologic reaction than normal saline when introduced into the mediastinum and lungs [29, 30]. These nonionic agents are not routinely used in gastrointestinal studies, in part because they are costly. Computed tomography (CT) is seldom needed to diagnose foreign bodies, but occasionally, it can detect esophageal foreign bodies that are missed by all other modalities [26]. Despite the utility of x-ray techniques, failure to demonstrate a foreign body mandates endoscopy because some objects may escape radiographic detection.

Flexible esophagoscopy not only is of value diagnostically but also offers an opportunity for therapeutic intervention. The endoscopist should always be prepared to extract the foreign object at the time of initial endoscopy. The esophagus should be intubated using direct visualization, and if the suspected object is not found in the esophagus, complete examination of the stomach and duodenum should be performed.

## GENERAL APPROACH TO MANAGEMENT

Whenever therapeutic intervention is necessary, the physician must choose the modality that offers the highest likelihood of success without subjecting the patient to undue risk of complications.

The therapeutic modality of choice for esophageal foreign bodies is usually endoscopic extraction. Flexible fiberoptic endoscopy has been used with excellent results since the early 1970s and is the most significant advance in foreign-body management in recent decades. Berggreen and colleagues [4] evaluated the efficacy of esophageal foreign-body extraction in 76 adult and 116 pediatric patients. Flexible endoscopy and rigid esophagoscopy were equally successful (96.2% versus 100%, respectively); however, the risk of complications was significantly higher with rigid esophagoscopy (10% versus 5.1% for flexible endoscopy). Flexible endoscopy is therefore preferred due to its high success rate, low morbidity and mortality, and lower cost when compared to rigid esophagoscopy.

It is critical, when attempting foreign-body extraction from the upper gastrointestinal tract, to protect the patient's airway from inadvertent aspiration of saliva, retained esophageal or gastric contents, or the object itself. For this reason, intubation, general anesthesia, and rigid endoscopy are sometimes necessary. The endoscopist must always have equipment nearby for emergency airway management.

Timing of extraction is important and will depend on the location of the foreign body and its potential to cause complications if left untreated. Objects in the esophagus should always be managed expeditiously since prolonged delays lead to higher complication rates [14]. Objects reaching the stomach are unlikely to pass the pylorus if they are more than 5 to 6 cm long or 2 cm in diameter. Similarly, elongated objects are more likely to become impacted in the duodenum, making endoscopic extraction much more difficult. In the following sections, we review the management of specific types of foreign objects.

## Meat Impaction

The diagnosis of meat impaction is seldom a problem. Patients are usually able to relate the exact time symptoms began and the type of food ingested. They will frequently have a prior history of dysphagia, gastroesophageal reflux, or food impactions. When the esophagus is completely obstructed, they are unable to swallow and will often present to the emergency department holding a container for expectorated saliva. When a symptomatic patient presents with an appropriate history and characteristic symptoms of meat impaction, little is gained from further diagnostic studies to define the exact location or to look for bone fragments. A barium study may be used as a confirmatory test but is seldom necessary. If complete obstruction is observed with a barium study, residual contrast should be removed by suction with a nasogastric tube to avoid aspiration during bolus removal. Even if barium is not used, it may still be necessary to suction retained material from the esophagus prior to endoscopic intubation.

### Nonendoscopic Techniques

Several nonendoscopic techniques have been used successfully either to extract a food bolus or to promote its passage into the stomach. Although temptation may be great, the physician should not attempt to push the impacted bolus blindly into the stomach [72]. The high likelihood of an underlying stricture or other pathologic process creates an unacceptable risk of complication. Many patients will notice spontaneous passage of the impacted material with relief of symptoms prior to institution of any therapy. In such instances, they will still require complete evaluation, looking for underlying esophageal disease.

Pharmacologic agents such as glucagon have been used successfully for meat boluses lodged in the lower two-thirds of the esophagus. The initial report by Ferrucci and Long [23], using glucagon for esophageal food impaction, described success in three of six patients. Giordano [31] and Trenkner [93] and their colleagues reported success in relieving impactions in 37% and 43% of 19 and 14 patients, respectively. Presumably, glucagon works by decreasing lower esophageal sphincter pressure. Although glucagon can relax smooth muscle in the duodenum and small bowel, one manometric study showed no effect of pulsed intravenous glucagon on esophageal peristalsis [42]. The relatively low success rate of glucagon can be explained by its inability to affect the diameter of strictures or rings. A 1- to 2-mg, slow intravenous bolus of glucagon is generally safe but may cause nausea, vomiting, or ileus and hyperglycemia. This dose may be repeated after 5 to 10 minutes if necessary. Glucagon is contraindicated in individuals with insulinoma or pheochromocytoma and in those known to be hypersensitive to the drug. A multicenter, placebo-controlled, double-blind study of the ability of glucagon and diazepam to treat esophageal foreign bodies found no benefit over placebo [92]. Other agents such as nitroglycerin, diazepam, calcium channel blockers, and atropine have been used but seem to offer no significant advantage over glucagon.

Attempting to digest a meat bolus enzymatically with topical proteolytic agents was once popular but has recently fallen out of favor. This procedure, first described by Richardson [75] in 1945, involves placing an enzyme preparation in the esophagus. The patient drinks small amounts of the enzyme solution, or it is instilled directly into the esophagus by nasogastric tube. Enzyme preparations that have been employed contain either papain or chymotrypsin. Papain is a hydrolytic enzyme obtained from the latex of the tropical melon tree *Carica papaya*. Available commercially as unseasoned Adolph's Meat Tenderizer, it is claimed to digest approximately 55 times its weight of lean meat [77]. The usual therapeutic preparation contains 1 teaspoon of Adolph's Meat Tenderizer per 120 mL of water and is given every 15 minutes. Prior to each instillation, pooled saliva and residual solution should be aspirated from the esophagus with a nasogastric tube. This will lessen the risk of aspiration and permit direct application to the meat bolus. Caroid, a commercial preparation of papain, was once used as a 5% solution but is no longer readily available. The successful use of papain has been confirmed in several case reports and uncontrolled trials [9, 13, 37, 68, 77], including 16 of 17 patients reported by Richardson [75]. Despite reported success, two potentially life-threatening complications of papain cause most physicians, including us, to avoid its use. These are transmural digestion of the esophagus [2, 44] and hemorrhagic pulmonary edema if the compound is aspirated. Since, in theory, these enzymes act only on nonviable tissue, complications are more likely if esophageal ischemia or any condition that damages the integrity of the normal mucosa is present. Therefore, prolonged impaction (longer than 36 hours), bony fragments in the meat, and suspected perforation above the impaction are strong contraindications to the use of papain [68]. In addition, Goldner and Danley [33] showed that while Adolph's Meat Tenderizer does not damage normal esophageal mucosa (rabbit model), it may significantly increase preexisting esophageal inflammation. Failure of enzymatic digestion also presents a problem in that the meat bolus is soft and fragments easily, often necessitating piecemeal endoscopic removal.

There are several recent reports in the literature pertaining to the use of gas-forming agents to treat acute esophageal meat impaction [12, 45, 65, 74]. When ingested in sufficient quantities, these agents release carbon dioxide into the esophagus. Liberated carbon dioxide raises intraluminal pressure, distends the esophagus against a closed cricopharyngeal muscle, and in theory forces the bolus into the stomach. Barium swallows are done before and after treatment to document response. Rice and co-workers [74] reported 100% success in eight patients using a ''cocktail'' of tartaric acid and sodium bicarbonate. Other gas-forming agents successfully used include sodium bicarbonate, activated dimethicone, and citric acid (Carbex effervescent granules); carbonated beverages; and tonic water. Friedland [25] advocates using gas-forming agents as first-line therapy, followed by intravenous glucagon administration if results are not forthcoming. Perforation of the esophagus has occurred following use of this method and should be recognized as a potentially serious complication [87]. Robbins et al. [76] reports a combination of glucagon, an effervescent agent, and water for relief of acute esophageal food impaction. Using this technique, 33 of 48 episodes (69%) were relieved with one complication (2%), a mucosal laceration. We do not routinely employ gas-forming agents when managing patients with meat impactions and believe their use should be limited to settings in which other therapies are unavailable.

Another technique of nonendoscopic extraction of a meat bolus uses a modified gastric lavage tube [53]. With this procedure, the distal 8 cm of a 34 French lavage tube is cut off and the tip filed smooth. After localization of the bolus with barium, the modified tube is passed into the esophagus to the level of impaction. A 120-mL syringe is used to apply negative suction pressure during withdrawal of the bolus. The procedure can be performed through an overtube, if necessary, to protect the airway. Kozarek [52] reported successful removal of an impacted meat bolus in two-thirds of cases with the modified tube technique.

### Endoscopic Technique

Endoscopic removal is the best method of managing meat impaction. Endoscopy not only allows bolus removal but permits immediate evaluation of underlying obstructing anomalies. If endoscopy is performed early, it is often possible to remove the bolus in one piece with a single passage of the endoscope. For this reason, most authors prefer to attempt endoscopic extraction within the first 12 hours of food impaction. In the past, rigid endoscopy under general anesthesia was used, but now it is reserved for cases in which flexible fiberoptic endoscopy is not successful. Flexible endoscopic removal of a meat bolus can be accomplished in outpatients using only topical anesthesia and intravenous sedation. These advantages are especially important in this era of cost containment. Various commercially available accessories passed through the biopsy channel to effect bolus removal include the polypectomy snare, retrieval basket, polyp grabber, foreign-body forceps, and biopsy forceps (Fig. 17–3). If a large bolus cannot be removed in toto, then it can be carefully manipulated and broken up into smaller pieces. The smaller sections can then be extracted more easily or allowed to pass spontaneously.

When dealing with impacted meat (or food), we prefer using a standard flexible endoscope and polypectomy snare. After informed consent is obtained, the oropharynx is anesthetized with anesthetic spray and an appropriate dose of intravenous sedation is given slowly. If necessary, the esophagus is cleared of any excess saliva and secretions using a nasogastric tube. Once the bolus is visualized, a polypectomy snare is passed through the biopsy channel and the bolus is securely grasped with the snare wire. Under direct visualization, the bolus is slowly withdrawn with the endoscope to a level just below the cricopharyngeus muscle. At this point, the snare with the attached bolus is pulled snugly against the tip of the endoscope, the patient's neck is extended, and the entire device (endoscope, snare, and bolus) is quickly removed as a unit. The endoscopist must be careful to avoid dislodging the bolus in the hypopharyngeal region. Any portion of the bolus that is lost during removal must be immediately retrieved to prevent its aspiration. This is often possible using gloved fingers or forceps. Two cardinal rules to remember when extracting meat or any other object from the esophagus are (a) to protect the patient's airway and (b) to maintain control of the object at all times. It is advisable to minimize the number of endoscopic intubations since each manipulation increases the risk of aspiration. In cases where the meat is soft and fragmented, we have found

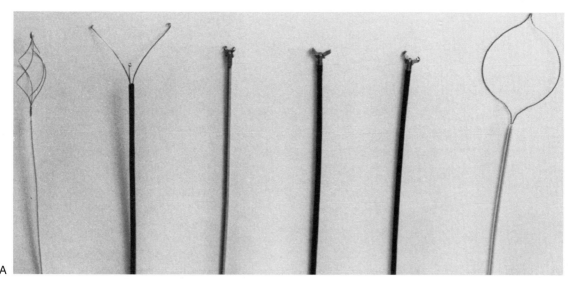

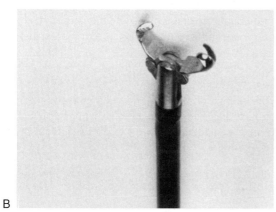

**FIG. 17–3. A:** Accessories available for foreign-body extraction. They include (**left to right**) retrieval basket, polyp grabber, biopsy forceps, foreign-body forceps, and polypectomy snare. **B:** Close-up of the foreign-body forceps, which are especially useful for coin extractions.

it helpful to use an overtube both to protect the airway and to facilitate intubations. After lubrication, a 44 French Maloney dilator is passed through the overtube, the entire unit is passed into the esophagus, and the dilator is removed. Subsequent manipulations are made through the indwelling overtube.

A recently reported, novel method of removing food impactions utilizes the Steigman-Goff Friction-Fit Adaptor, originally developed for band ligation of varices [103]. The endoscope is inserted through an overtube and is used as a direct-vision suction device to remove the food bolus. This approach is particularly useful with food that may fragment with standard snare or forceps removal.

Some authors have successfully used the flexible endoscope to push an obstructing bolus gently into the stomach, provided the area distal to the obstruction can be assessed beforehand [99]. With the push technique, a pediatric endoscope is used to bypass the bolus and assess the cause of the distal obstruction. The endoscope is then withdrawn proximal to the bolus and carefully pushed forward, guiding the impacted material into the stomach.

Finally, a recent report of an unconventional technique to manage meat impactions successfully illustrates the impor-

tance of physician ingenuity [51]. An elderly patient with multiple medical problems had meat impaction in the esophagus that proved refractory to all measures, including endoscopic extraction. A neodymium:yttrium-aluminum-garnet laser was used to cook the center of the meat bolus, causing it to shrink in size, thus making it possible to push the bolus into the stomach.

### Immediate Versus Delayed Dilation

Once a food bolus has been removed and a stricture identified, the issue of immediate versus delayed dilation must be addressed. If the impaction has been present for a short period and there is minimal esophagitis present, we prefer immediate dilation of the stricture. Alternatively, if the area cannot be adequately assessed, the patient may be placed on a liquid diet for 2 or 3 days, after which time reendoscopy and dilation can be performed.

### Coins

Coin ingestion most commonly occurs in children but occasionally occurs in adults, especially if they are intoxicated.

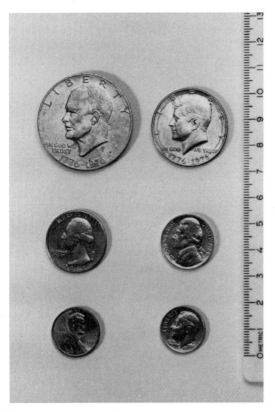

**FIG. 17–4.** Coin size and patient age determine whether a swallowed coin will lodge in the esophagus.

Size determines whether a swallowed coin will lodge in the esophagus (Fig. 17–4). In general, coins smaller than a quarter will not cause problems in adults but may in small children and infants, who have a narrower esophagus. X-ray magnification may cause coins to appear larger than their actual size. The mechanism of injury from esophageal coins is most often direct pressure necrosis, although aspiration and even perforation [66] are possible, especially if impaction is prolonged. For this reason, coins in the esophagus should be removed without delay. An exception to this rule is the coin lying in the distal third of the esophagus. Many coins in this location will pass spontaneously, so a period of observation not exceeding 12 hours is warranted [88]. In addition, because spontaneous coin passage is not uncommon, it is important to confirm the coin's position radiographically just prior to extraction. Coins that reach the stomach generally transit unevenfully and do not require extraction unless they fail to pass in 7 to 10 days. Pennies manufactured in the United States since 1982 are composed primarily of zinc (instead of copper) and tend to be more corrosive to the esophagus [100].

### Flexible Endoscopy

Flexible endoscopy is clearly the method of choice to extract coins from the esophagus. Gilger and co-workers [28] confirmed that conscious sedation is safe in children undergoing endoscopy; however, because oxygen desaturation occurred in 68%, they strongly advocate the routine use of continuous cardiac rhythm and pulse oximetry monitoring. Small children who are less likely to be cooperative, however, may require general anesthesia to expedite removal [4]. The various accessories useful for coin extraction are shown in Fig. 17–3. The foreign-body grasping forceps (rat tooth) are especially useful to grasp the elevated edge of a coin securely. These foreign-body forceps should be stored in a location separate from regular biopsy forceps to prevent their inadvertent use for purposes other than foreign-body extraction. Accidental use of this device to obtain a routine biopsy specimen can cause severe tissue injury and bleeding. A standard polypectomy snare is also very helpful and can be used if the foreign-body forceps is unavailable. Standard pinch biopsy forceps should not be used since they cannot predictably grip the edge of the coin.

With regard to technique of extraction, we perform a standard diagnostic endoscopy with the patient lying in the left lateral decubitus position. Once the coin is identified and grasped, the patient is placed in Trendelenburg's position to lessen the likelihood of aspiration. Using direct visualization, the coin is extracted while oriented in the frontal plane. This orientation is most likely to permit passage of the coin through the cricopharyngeus and hypopharyngeal region. A similar technique is used to extract other flat objects such as buttons.

### Extraction by Catheter

The use of balloon-tipped catheters to extract blunt objects such as coins from the esophagus is controversial. Standard Foley catheters as well as vascular-type catheters such as the Swan-Ganz and Fogarty have been used [21, 69]. The procedure is limited to individuals with an acute foreign-body impaction (less than 1 to 2 days) and objects that can definitely be identified as blunt and without sharp or pointed edges. Bigler [6] first reported Foley catheter foreign-body extraction in 1966. Subsequently, numerous other retrospective series have been published with success rates ranging from 55% to 100% [61]. Prior to attempting the procedure, the balloon should be checked to ensure that it inflates properly and the oropharynx should be sprayed with a local anesthetic. The use of sedation for balloon extraction is a matter of clinical preference [61]. A small amount of barium is given beforehand whenever there is any suspicion of an underlying esophageal pathologic process, especially in children with objects that lie below the thoracic inlet [11]. According to the method of Campbell and colleagues [11], a 14 or 16 French Foley catheter is passed orally, using fluoroscopic guidance, to a point just beyond the foreign body with the patient sitting upright. The patient is next placed in the oblique prone position, and the fluoroscopy table is turned into a steep head-down position. The balloon is inflated with contrast material and, under fluoroscopic observation, the catheter is withdrawn with moderate, steady traction. The catheter should not be passed nasally since it (a) may cause epistaxis, (b) may convert an esophageal foreign body to a nasopharyngeal foreign body, and (c) requires balloon deflation in the hypopharynx with the attendant risk of aspiration of the foreign body. Despite an overall success rate of 85% [61] and few reported complications, we do not use the Foley technique because it offers little control of the object or the airway during extraction. These violations of basic tenets of foreign-body management outweigh any potential cost savings of the procedure.

## Battery Ingestion

### Epidemiologic Features

The frequent occurrence of battery ingestion over the past several years reflects advances in electronic miniaturization. In 1983, it was estimated that 510 to 850 battery ingestions occurred annually in the United States [58]. This figure probably underestimates the true incidence since approximately 400 cases are reported annually to The National Button Battery Ingestion Hotline of the National Capital Poison Center at Georgetown University (T.L. Litovitz, *personal communication,* 1990). The majority of cases occur in children younger than 5 years and involve the small disc-type battery (so-called button battery) rather than the cylindric cell type [59]. Disc batteries are commonly the power source found in watches, clocks, calculators, games, toys, cameras, hearing aids, and most recently, musical greeting cards. Batteries intended for use in hearing aids constitute 44% of total ingestions [60]. The wide accessibility to these batteries undoubtedly contributes to the high incidence of accidental ingestion. Children will swallow batteries that have been discarded and are often able to enter the battery compartment of electronic devices easily and remove the battery directly. Battery ingestions in adults occur during suicide attempts, during replacement of used cells, after mistaking the battery for a tablet of medication, and after placing a battery on the tongue to test its potency [59].

### Pathophysiologic Features

As with coins, the risk of impaction of a disc battery in the esophagus relates mainly to size; most involve batteries longer than 21 mm in diameter [58]. Most ingested batteries are smaller than 12 mm [60] and have little potential to lodge in the esophagus. A battery that does lodge in the esophagus poses a serious problem owing to the severe caustic nature of its contents on esophageal mucosa. The typical button battery system is composed of anode and cathode that are separated by an electrolyte-soaked fabric (Fig. 17–5). The alkaline electrolyte is usually a 45% solution of potassium hydroxide but may be sodium hydroxide [58]. The amount and concentration of electrolyte base vary among different types and sizes of batteries. The batteries may also contain quantities of mercuric oxide, silver oxide, manganese diox-

ide, cadmium oxide, or lithium hydroxide [55]. Tissue destruction can occur rapidly, and the potential for perforation exists if mucosal contact is maintained at a specific site for several hours [62, 97]. Reported complications resulting from impacted esophageal button batteries include esophagotracheal fistulas, perforation into the aorta, mediastinitis, and death [90, 97].

The major mechanism of injury to the esophagus is leakage of the caustic alkaline solution from the battery, resulting in rapid liquefactive tissue necrosis. Experimental evidence shows that esophageal mucosal damage may occur within 1 hour and rapidly progress to involvement of all layers by 4 hours [62]. Alternative potentially pathogenic mechanisms include low-voltage electrical burns due to direct current between cathode and anode and local pressure necrosis, as seen with other embedded foreign bodies [54, 62, 91]. Urinary or blood mercury levels will sometimes be elevated following ingestion of mercury-containing batteries [55], but clinical evidence of mercury toxicity and requirement for chelation therapy are rare.

### Management

The first step in managing individuals with suspected button battery ingestion is prompt radiographic confirmation of the battery's presence and precise location. Both posteroanterior and lateral x-rays are helpful to distinguish a battery from a coin, which is similar in size and more commonly ingested. The posteroanterior view will often show a "double-density" shadow produced by a bilaminar disc battery [63]. On lateral view, the edges of a disc battery appear more rounded as opposed to the sharper image produced by a coin. If an ingested battery is lodged in the esophagus, then prompt endoscopic extraction is mandatory. Emetic agents are generally ineffective [60] and should not be given since they may cause further harm if caustic material is aspirated during induced emesis. Button batteries should not be removed with balloon-tipped catheters because extraction is not controlled and there is the potential for balloon-induced exacerbation of esophageal injury.

Endoscopic retrieval of disc batteries from the esophagus or stomach is challenging since they are difficult to grasp securely with foreign-body forceps or snares. A large review noted that only one of three attempted endoscopic extractions is successful [59]. An esophageal dilating balloon can be used to position the battery between the balloon and the endoscope tip, with subsequent removal under direct visualization. Alternatively, the battery can be manipulated into the stomach. Fortunately, disc batteries in the stomach will most often pass through the gastrointestinal tract without causing significant injury, although a single case of intestinal perforation has been reported when a battery lodged in a Meckel's diverticulum [104]. Thus, if initial x-rays show the battery location to be below the esophagus, the patient may be observed and follow-up films obtained in a few days if necessary. Operative intervention is appropriate if a battery

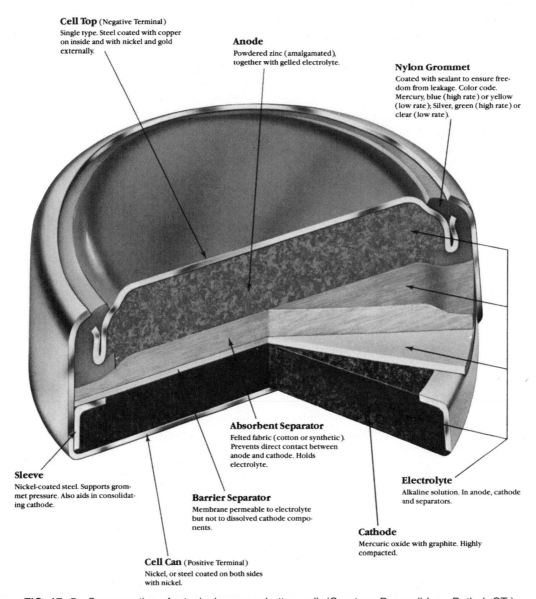

**Cell Top** (Negative Terminal)
Single type. Steel coated with copper on inside and with nickel and gold externally.

**Anode**
Powdered zinc (amalgamated), together with gelled electrolyte.

**Nylon Grommet**
Coated with sealant to ensure freedom from leakage. Color code. Mercury, blue (high rate) or yellow (low rate); Silver, green (high rate) or clear (low rate).

**Absorbent Separator**
Felted fabric (cotton or synthetic). Prevents direct contact between anode and cathode. Holds electrolyte.

**Sleeve**
Nickel-coated steel. Supports grommet pressure. Also aids in consolidating cathode.

**Barrier Separator**
Membrane permeable to electrolyte but not to dissolved cathode components.

**Electrolyte**
Alkaline solution. In anode, cathode and separators.

**Cathode**
Mercuric oxide with graphite. Highly compacted.

**Cell Can** (Positive Terminal)
Nickel, or steel coated on both sides with nickel.

**FIG. 17–5.** Cross section of a typical mercury button cell. (Courtesy Duracell Inc., Bethel, CT.)

cannot be endoscopically retrieved from the esophagus or manipulated into the stomach or whenever there are symptoms or signs of intestinal perforation. Once a battery has been removed from the esophagus, contrast radiographic studies should be performed as follow-up to exclude severe mucosal injury, fistulas, or strictures. To prevent recurrent problems after extraction, patients and caregivers should be counseled regarding proper use and disposal of batteries once removed from the original container.

### Dental Objects

Swallowed dentures or portions of dental prosthetic devices represent another category of frequently encountered esophageal foreign body [20, 40, 71]. Ingested dentures and prosthetic devices may become impacted in the pharynx or esophagus [15, 57]. Risk factors for denture ingestion include sedating drugs, certain medical conditions (e.g., epilepsy), and severe facial trauma with resultant swallowing of dentures. Contact sports and attempted cardiopulmonary resuscitation are other settings in which dental devices may slip into the esophagus or airway (Fig. 17–6) [85]. Most dental ingestions result from devices that are broken or loose and most often occur during sleep [71]. Partial dentures tend to become unretentive with time as a result of resorption of alveolar bone. Inadvertent iatrogenic problems due to ingestion of dental instruments such as orthodontic bands, drill bits, or rubber dam clamps sometimes occur. Devices such as retainers with sharp edges and bare wires can cause severe damage [40] and even fatal complications such as erosion into the aorta [86].

Management of denture ingestion is complicated by the

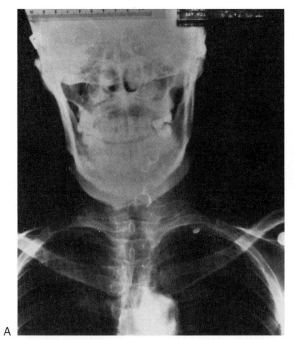

A

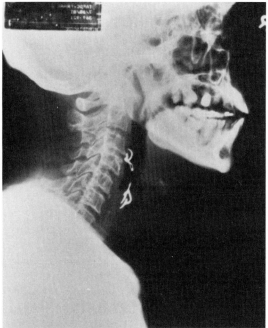

B

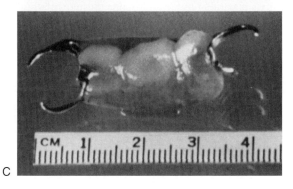

C

FIG. 17–6. **A, B:** Soft tissue radiographs showing a dental prosthetic device lodged in the hypopharynx after cardiopulmonary resuscitation. (From ref. 85, with permission.) **C:** Close-up of dental prosthetic device. (Courtesy Dr. C. Shih, Monterey Park, CA.)

fact that most of these devices are acrylic-based and thus are not visible on plain radiographs. Dental researchers have incorporated radiopaque materials such as barium sulfate and other inorganic salts into these devices, but most of these modified products have ultimately proved to be of inferior quality. The physician must be alert to the possibility of denture ingestion in a patient who has abrupt-onset dysphagia, especially if symptoms began during sleep and radiographs are negative. The same principles of endoscopic management apply with dental objects as with other noncaustic foreign bodies. Specifically, objects in the stomach should be managed based on their size, shape, likelihood of spontaneous passage, and risk of perforation. A novel approach to the management of an impacted denture was reported by Lam and co-workers [56] in which the denture was fractured with a holmium:yttrium-aluminum-garnet laser to permit extraction of the resulting smaller pieces. Objects lodged in the esophagus should be removed. Consultation with the patient's dentist may be helpful when planning removal, especially if the exact nature of the object is unclear.

A final type of dental object of interest to the endoscopist is the ordinary toothbrush. In a recent review, Kirk and co-workers [50] discovered 31 cases of accidental toothbrush swallowing in the literature. Importantly, some were lodged in the esophagus or pharynx, and no toothbrush reaching the stomach passed spontaneously. Thus, retrieval of an ingested toothbrush is always necessary and can often be accomplished endoscopically.

## Sharp and Pointed Objects

Objects that have sharp edges or pointed ends are particularly challenging to manage. Included in this category are razor blades, fragments of broken glass, toothpicks, nails, wire, animal bones, safety pins, sewing needles, curtain hooks, and many others. The major concern is their potential to cause lacerations or perforation of the intestine when swallowed or during attempted removal. Although the overall risk of intestinal tract perforation from a foreign body is less than 1%, the risk from sharp or pointed objects may be as high as 15% to 35% [100]. Cohen [17] noted that 12% of patients in his series who ingested sharp or pointed objects required laparotomy due to perforation. Even though deaths occur, it is intriguing that the majority of sharp or pointed objects will pass without causing significant damage.

The single best principle to follow when extracting a pointed object from the esophagus is that the pointed end should trail, not lead. This lessens the likelihood of perforation. Consider, for example, the situation of an open safety pin in the esophagus. If the pointed end is directed cephalad, it is best to try gently pushing it into the stomach before grasping the hinged region to pull it upward through the esophagus under direct visual guidance. Safety pin closure in the stomach using a snare has been described but is a difficult feat to accomplish [1]. In contrast, if the tip points distally, the safety pin may be withdrawn without reorientation (Fig. 17–7). Intubation of the endoscope should be done under direct vision to avoid striking a proximally located, sharp object and causing penetration into the esophageal wall. Extraction of sharp and pointed objects through an overtube is recommended to protect the esophagus from damage during withdrawal. Overtube diameter may be limiting for some patients and/or objects. An alternative device for the removal of sharp objects is a soft, latex protector hood that is designed to fit over the end of any endoscope [5]. Withdrawal through a rigid esophagoscope is also appropriate, especially for larger pins.

Razor blade ingestions are unusual but sometimes seen in prisoners and psychiatric patients [46, 102]. The razor blades are generally wrapped in tape or tissue paper or fragmented into several pieces to make swallowing easier. The smaller fragments are more likely to be found in the stomach or small intestine at the time of presentation [7]. When blades are found in the esophagus or stomach, they can often be managed using flexible endoscopy through an overtube or,

if required, rigid endoscopy. Once beyond the esophagus, fragmented blades will usually pass without causing significant damage [17, 46]. It is best to avoid using cathartics to assist the passage of these sharp objects since the presence of stool "coats" the object and facilitates passage through the remaining colon and anal canal.

Toothpick-related injuries occur in the United States each year at an estimated rate of 3.6 per 100,000 population [10]. Individuals between the ages of 25 and 44 have the highest rate of injury due to ingestion. Adults are at risk for accidental toothpick ingestion because toothpicks are commonly found in foods such as hors d'oeuvres, which are served with alcoholic beverages. Perforation of the esophagus or intestinal tract is possible because these seemingly innocuous objects are long, hard, sharp, and pointed. Moreover, diagnosis may be delayed owing to the inability to visualize toothpicks by plain x-rays. Late complications, including death, are possible if the diagnosis is delayed [3]. Flexible endoscopy is indicated for both diagnosis and retrieval whenever toothpick ingestion is a possibility. It is best to grasp the toothpick close to the tip so that its longitudinal axis is parallel to the endoscope during withdrawal. The use of an overtube also permits safer extraction.

### Narcotic-filled Balloons

An illegal, deliberate form of foreign-body ingestion involves swallowing narcotic-filled packages for the purpose of smuggling drugs. Prior to ingestion, packets of illicit drugs, typically cocaine [64] or heroin [94], are packaged in multiple layers of cellophane and latex (usually balloons or condoms). In the majority of cases, packets pass through the gastrointestinal tract without incident. However, this "body packer syndrome" is potentially lethal because damage to the packet can result in leakage of narcotic into the gastrointestinal tract with systemic absorption, intoxication, and even death. Endoscopy to remove the packets should be avoided since disruption can cause acute cocaine toxicity. Surgical removal should be considered when there are signs of intestinal obstruction or systemic toxicity, passage of packets is delayed, or packets appear to be fragile.

### Hypopharyngeal Objects

Objects lodged above the upper esophageal sphincter need special management. Removal of objects in this region requires familiarity with the anatomy and emergency airway management; thus, hypopharyngeal objects are often best referred to an otolaryngologist. Sometimes hypopharyngeal objects are easily visualized by indirect mirror examination or can be felt with the examiner's gloved finger. In such cases, the patient is placed in the supine position and the object extracted using an open laryngoscope and Kelly or McGill forceps. One must be careful to prevent dislodgment and subsequent airway compromise during extraction. Tracheal intubation and general anesthesia are necessary if the

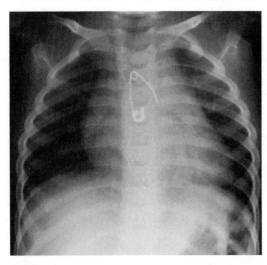

**FIG. 17–7.** Plain chest radiograph showing an open safety pin in the esophagus with the tip pointing distally. (From ref. 81, with permission.)

hypopharyngeal object cannot be easily identified and safely removed.

## PRECAUTIONARY MEASURES IN FOREIGN-BODY REMOVAL

Although many therapeutic options are available to remove foreign bodies from the esophagus, flexible endoscopic extraction is the procedure of choice. With operator ingenuity, a variety of endoscopic methods can be employed to extract many types of foreign bodies. The risks of removal are mainly those associated with diagnostic endoscopy as well as perforation, aspiration, and airway occlusion. To reduce the risk of potential complications, endoscopic extractions should be carried out only by individuals skilled in flexible endoscopy and experienced with the accessories used [72]. It is important to plan ahead by rehearsing the extraction procedure with a similar object and ensuring that good oral suction and emergency airway equipment are always available if needed. Following extraction of a foreign body, patients should be monitored for complications resulting from the foreign object or its removal. Adults also require thorough evaluation to exclude underlying structural esophageal lesions.

## REFERENCES

1. Altman AR, Gottfried EB. Intragastric closure of an ingested open safety pin. Gastrointest Endosc 1978;24:294
2. Andersen HA, Bernatz PE, Grindlay JH. Perforation of the esophagus after use of a digestant agent. Ann Otol Rhinol Laryngol 1959;68:890
3. Bee DM, et al. Delayed death from ingestion of a toothpick. N Engl J Med 1989;320:673
4. Berggreen PJ, et al. Techniques and complications of esophageal foreign body extraction in children and adults. Gastrointest Endosc 1993;39:626
5. Bertoni G, et al. A new protector device for safe endoscopic removal of sharp gastroesophageal foreign bodies in infants. J Pediatr Gastroenterol Nutr 1993;16:393
6. Bigler CF. The use of a Foley catheter for removal of blunt foreign bodies from the esophagus. J Thorac Cardiovasc Surg 1966;51:759
7. Brady PG. Endoscopic removal of foreign bodies. In Silvis SE, ed, Therapeutic Gastrointestinal Endoscopy. New York: Igaku-Shoin, 1990.
8. Brady PG. Esophageal foreign bodies. Gastroenterol Clin North Am 1991;20:691
9. Brooks JW. Foreign bodies in the air and food passages. Ann Surg 1972;175:720
10. Budnick LD. Toothpick-related injuries in the United States, 1979–1982. JAMA 1984;252:796
11. Campbell JB, Quattromani FL, Foley LC. Foley catheter removal of blunt esophageal foreign bodies. Experience with 100 consecutive children. Pediatr Radiol 1983;13:116
12. Campbell N, Sykes P. Non-endoscopic relief of oesophageal obstruction. Lancet 1986;2:1405
13. Cavo JW Jr, et al. Use of enzymes for meat impaction in the esophagus. Laryngoscope 1977;87:630
14. Chaikhouni A, Kratz JM, Crawford PA. Foreign bodies of the esophagus. Am Surg 1985;51:173
15. Cleater IG, Christie J. An unusual case of swallowed dental plate and perforation of the sigmoid colon. Br J Surg 1973;60:163
16. Clerf LH. Historical aspects of foreign bodies in the food and air passages. South Med J 1975;68:1449
17. Cohen H. Glass gluttony and gastrointestinal gouging. JAMA 1968;206:1582
18. Crysdale WS, Sendi KS, Yoo J. Esophageal foreign bodies in children. 15-year review of 484 cases. Ann Otol Rhinol Laryngol 1991;100:320
19. Devanesan J, et al. Metallic foreign bodies in the stomach. Arch Surg 1977;112:664
20. Devlin H. The inhalation and ingestion of dentures. Quintessence Int 1986;17:821
21. Dieter RA Jr, et al. Fogarty catheter removal of cervical esophageal meat bolus. Arch Surg 1972;105:790
22. Doust BD. Detection of aspirated foreign bodies with xero-radiography. Radiology 1974;111:725
23. Ferrucci JT Jr, Long JA. Radiologic treatment of esophageal food impaction using intravenous glucagon. Radiology 1977;125:25
24. Flom LL, Ellis GL. Radiologic evaluation of foreign bodies. Emerg Med Clin North Am 1992;10:163
25. Friedland GW. The treatment of acute esophageal food impaction. Radiology 1983;149:601
26. Gamba JL, et al. CT diagnosis of an esophageal foreign body. AJR Am J Roentgenol 1983;140:289
27. Gelfand DW. Complication of gastrointestinal radiology procedures: I. Complications of routine fluoroscopic studies. Gastrointest Radiol 1980;5:293
28. Gilger MA, et al. Oxygen desaturation and cardiac arrhythmias in children during esophagogastroduodenoscopy using conscious sedation. Gastrointest Endosc 1993;39:392
29. Ginai AZ, et al. Experimental evaluation of various available contrast agents for use in the upper gastrointestinal tract in case of suspected leakage. Effect on lungs. Br J Radiol 1984;57:895
30. Ginai AZ, et al. Experimental evaluation of various available contrast agents for use in the upper gastrointestinal tract in case of suspected leakage: effect on mediastinum. Br J Radiol 1985;58:585
31. Giordano A, et al. Current management of esophageal foreign bodies. Arch Otolaryngol 1981;107:249
32. Goff WF. What to do when foreign bodies are inhaled or ingested. Postgrad Med 1968;44:135
33. Goldner F, Danley D. Enzymatic digestion of esophageal meat impaction: a study of Adolph's Meat Tenderizer. Dig Dis Sci 1985;30:456
34. Hacker JF, Cattau EL. Management of gastrointestinal foreign bodies. Am Fam Physician 1986;34:101
35. Hamilton JK, Polter DE. Foreign bodies in the gut. In Sleisenger MH, Fordtran JS, eds, Gastrointestinal Disease: Pathophysiology, Diagnosis, Management (4th ed). Philadelphia: WB Saunders, 1989:210
36. Handler SD. Unsuspected esophageal foreign bodies in adults with upper airway obstruction. Chest 1981;80:234
37. Hargrove MD, Boyce HW. Meat impaction of the esophagus. Arch Intern Med 1970;125:277
38. Harned RK, et al. Esophageal foreign bodies: safety and efficacy of Foley catheter extraction of coins. AJR Am J Roentgenol 1997;168:443
39. Hess GP. An approach to throat complaints: foreign body sensation, difficulty swallowing and hoarseness. Emerg Med Clin North Am 1987;5:313
40. Hinkle FG. Ingested retainer: a case report. Am J Orthod Dentofacial Orthop 1987;92:46
41. Hodge D. Coin ingestion: does every child need an x-ray? Ann Emerg Med 1985;14:443
42. Hogan WJ, et al. Effect of glucagon on esophageal motor function. Gastroenterology 1975;69:160
43. Hollinger PH, et al. Congenital anomalies of the esophagus related to oesophageal foreign bodies. Am J Dis Child 1949;78:467
44. Holsinger JW, Fuson RL, Sealy WC. Esophageal perforation following meat impaction and papain ingestion. JAMA 1968;204:734
45. John DG, Lesser THJ, Thomas PL. Non-endoscopic relief of oesophageal obstruction. Lancet 1987;1:107
46. Johnson WE. On ingestion of razor blades. JAMA 1969;208:2163
47. Karp JG, Whitman L, Convit A. Intentional ingestion of foreign objects by male prison inmates. Hosp Community Psychiatry 1991;42:533
48. Kikendall JW, et al. Pill-induced esophageal injury. Dig Dis Sci 1983;28:1974
49. Kirberg AE. Long standing esophageal foreign body. Gastrointest Endosc 1986;32:304
50. Kirk AD, et al. Toothbrush swallowing. Arch Surg 1988;123:382
51. Klein I. Resourceful management of esophageal food impaction [Letter]. Gastrointest Endosc 1990;36:80

52. Kozarek RA. Esophageal foreign bodies and food impaction. In Hill LD, ed, The Esophagus. Philadelphia: WB Saunders, 1988:302
53. Kozarek RA, Sanowski RA. Esophageal food impaction: description of a new method for bolus removal. Dig Dis Sci 1980;25:100
54. Kuhns DW, Dire DJ. Button battery ingestions. Ann Emerg Med 1989;18:293
55. Kulig K, et al. Disk battery ingestion: elevated urine mercury levels and enema removal of battery fragments. JAMA 1983;249:2502
56. Lam YH, et al. Laser-assisted removal of a foreign body impacted in the esophagus. Lasers Surg Med 1997;20:480
57. Lavine MH, Stoopcock JC. An oesophageal foreign body of dental origin. J Am Dent Assoc 1968;76:1038
58. Litovitz TL. Button battery ingestions: a review of 56 cases. JAMA 1983;249:2495
59. Litovitz TL. Battery ingestions: product accessibility and clinical course. Pediatrics 1985;75:469
60. Litovitz T, Schmitz BF. Ingestion of cylindrical and button batteries: an analysis of 2382 cases. Pediatrics 1992;89:747
61. Mariani PJ, Wagner DK. Foley catheter extraction of blunt esophageal foreign bodies. J Emerg Med 1986;4:301
62. Maves MD, Carithers JS, Birck HG. Esophageal burns secondary to disc battery ingestions. Ann Otol Rhinol Laryngol 1984;93:364
63. Maves MD, Lloyd TV, Carithers JS. Radiographic identification of ingested disc batteries. Pediatr Radiol 1986;16:154
64. McCarron MM, Wood JD. The cocaine ''body packer'' syndrome. Diagnosis and treatment. JAMA 1983;250:1417
65. Mohammed SH, Hegedus V. Dislodgement of impacted oesophageal foreign bodies with carbonated beverages. Clin Radiol 1986;37:589
66. Nahman BJ, Mueller CF. Asymptomatic esophageal perforation by a coin in a child. Ann Emerg Med 1984;13:627
67. Nandi P, Ong GB. Foreign body in the oesophagus: review of 2394 cases. Br J Surg 1978;65:5
68. Nighbert E, Dorton H, Griffen WO. Enzymatic relief of the ''steakhouse syndrome.'' Am J Surg 1968;116:467
69. Nixon GW. Foley catheter method of esophageal foreign body removal: extension of applications. AJR Am J Roentgenol 1979;132:441
70. Norton RA, King GD. ''Steakhouse syndrome'': the symptomatic lower esophageal ring. Lahey Clin Found Bull 1963;13:55
71. Payne SDW, Henry M. Radiolucent dentures impacted in the oesophagus. Br J Surg 1984;71:318
72. Peura DA, Johnson LF. Treatment of esophageal obstruction. In Castell DO, Johnson LF, eds, Esophageal Function in Health and Disease. New York: Elsevier, 1983
73. Reilly JS, Walter MA. Consumer product aspiration and ingestion in children: analysis of emergency room reports to the national electronic injury surveillance system. Ann Otol Rhinol Laryngol 1992;101:739
74. Rice BT, Speigel PK, Dombrowski PJ. Acute esophageal food impaction treated by gas-forming agents. Radiology 1983;146:299
75. Richardson JR. New treatment for esophageal obstruction. Ann Otol Rhinol Laryngol 1945;54:328
76. Robbins MI, et al. Treatment of acute esophageal food impaction with glucagon, an effervescent agent, and water. AJR Am J Roentgenol 1994;162:325
77. Robinson AS. Meat impaction in the esophagus treated by enzymatic digestion. JAMA 1962;181:1142
78. Rourk GD, et al. Ingested foreign material in mentally disturbed patients. South Med J 1983;76:1125
79. Sacchetti A, et al. Hand held metal detector identification of ingested foreign bodies. Pediatr Emerg Care 1994;10:204
80. Sanowski RA. Foreign body extraction in the gastrointestinal tract. In Sivak MV Jr, ed, Gastroenterologic Endoscopy. Philadelphia: WB Saunders, 1987
81. Schmacher KJ, et al. Aortic pseudoaneurysm due to ingested foreign body. South Med J 1986;79:246
82. Schunk JE, Corneli H, Bolte R. Pediatric coin ingestions. Am J Dis Child 1989;143:546
83. Seidner DL, Rogerts IM, Smith MS. Esophageal obstruction after ingestion of a fiber-containing diet pill. Gastroenterology 1990;99:1820
84. Selivanov V, et al. Management of foreign body ingestion. Ann Surg 1984;199:187
85. Shih C, et al. Mishaps of CPR: the case of the missing dental bridge. N Engl J Med 1982;306:1057
86. Singh B. A fatal denture in the oesophagus. J Laryngol Otol 1978;92:829
87. Smith JC. Use of glucagon and gas-forming agents in acute esophageal food impaction. Radiology 1986;159:567
88. Spitz L. Management of ingested foreign bodies in childhood. BMJ 1971;4:469
89. Spitz L, Hirsig J. Prolonged foreign body impaction in the esophagus. Arch Dis Child 1982;257:551
90. Taylor RB. Esophageal foreign bodies. Emerg Med Clin North Am 1987;5:301
91. Temple DM, McNeese MC. Hazards of battery ingestion. Pediatrics 1983;71:100
92. Tibbling L, et al. Effect of spasmolytic drugs on esophageal foreign bodies. Dysphagia 1995;10:126
93. Trenkner SW, et al. Esophageal food impaction: treatment with glucagon. Radiology 1983;149:401
94. Utecht MJ, Stone AF, McCarron MM. Heroin body packers. J Emerg Med 1993;11:33
95. Vassilev BN, et al. Esophageal ''stars'': a sinister foreign body ingestion. South Med J 1997;90:211
96. Vizcarrondo FJ, Brady PG, Nord HJ. Foreign bodies in the upper gastrointestinal tract. Gastrointest Endosc 1983;29:208
97. Votteler TP, Nash JC, Rutledge JC. The hazard of ingested alkaline disk batteries in children. JAMA 1983;249:2504
98. Webb WA. Endoscopic management of foreign bodies of the upper gastrointestinal tract. Syllabus of the ASGE 1989 Postgraduate Course 1989:32–41
99. Webb WA. Current management of foreign bodies in the upper gastrointestinal tract. Hosp Physician 1989;25:21
100. Webb WA. Management of foreign bodies of the upper gastrointestinal tract: update. Gastroenterology 1995;41:39
101. Webb WA, et al. Foreign bodies of the upper gastrointestinal tract: current management. South Med J 1984;77:1083
102. Weisenberger JE. Hazards of eating razor blades. JAMA 1969;207:1719
103. Weiss D, Pouagare M, Mamel J. An improved method for removal of food impactions in the upper GI tract [Abstract]. Gastrointest Endosc 1993;39:254
104. Willis GA, Ho WC. Perforation of Meckel's diverticulum by an alkaline hearing aid battery. Can Med Assoc J 1982;126:497
105. Wisniewski RM, et al. An esophageal foreign body impaction from a Tums E-X tablet. Gastrointest Endosc 1997;45:518

*The Esophagus*, Third Edition,
edited by D. O. Castell and J. E. Richter.
Lippincott Williams & Wilkins, Philadelphia © 1999.

CHAPTER 18

# Surgery for Esophageal Motor Disorders

Thomas R. Eubanks and Carlos Pellegrini

## INTRODUCTION

Esophageal motor disorders may be divided into two simple categories: disorders of increased muscular activity and disorders of decreased muscular activity. Similarly, surgical intervention for motor disorders of the esophagus is based on two simple concepts: When the muscular activity is too great, the surgical treatment is based on transecting the appropriate muscle; if the muscular activity is insufficient, the only surgical treatment is esophageal resection.

Despite the limited surgical options available, a large body of literature has been generated on the surgical management of esophageal motor dysfunction. The controversies regarding motor disorders are rooted in areas such as indication, technique, and outcome of the various operations.

The motor disorders of the esophagus will be discussed in relation to their anatomic location, starting from the upper esophageal sphincter (UES) and working toward the gastroesophageal junction. A brief summary of each disease will be presented followed by the assessment and surgical treatment. The controversial issues for each topic will be discussed at the end of each section.

## UPPER ESOPHAGEAL SPHINCTER

Swallowing consists of oral, pharyngeal, and esophageal phases. The UES plays a role in the pharyngeal phase and in the transition from the pharyngeal to the esophageal phase. Pharyngoesophageal diverticulum (Zenker's diverticulum) and cricopharyngeal bar, also referred to as cricopharyngeal achalasia, have been identified as pathologic entities of the UES. Understanding the anatomy and function of the UES is essential to planning an operation to treat these maladies.

The pharynx meets the esophagus where the inferior pharyngeal constrictor joins the cricopharyngeus muscle. The inferior constrictor takes origin from the thyroid and cricoid

T. R. Eubanks: Department of Surgery, University of Washington, Seattle, Washington 98195-6410.

C. Pellegrini: Department of Surgery, University of Washington, and University of Washington Medical Center, Seattle, Washington 98195.

cartilage, and its fibers run obliquely and horizontally to insert on the median raphe (posterior aspect) of the pharynx. The cricopharyngeus muscle arises from the cricoid cartilage, passes posteriorly to the pharyngoesophageal junction, and inserts on the contralateral side of the cricoid cartilage. Some anatomists view the cricopharyngeal muscle as simply the most inferior segment of the inferior constrictor, differing from the other muscle fibers in that they do not insert into the median raphe [2]. However, the structures are seen as distinctly separate in the surgical approach to the UES. The interlacing of muscles fibers at the posterior aspect of the pharynx leaves areas of potential weakness where herniation of the mucosa may occur, especially when intraluminal pressures are elevated. The triangle of Killian is one of these areas and is found between the inferior constrictor and the cricopharyngeus muscle [41, 128]. Two additional areas where the relative paucity of muscle fibers creates a relative weakness in the pharyngeal wall are the Killian–Jamieson's area, between the fibers of the cricopharyngeus, and Laimer's triangle between the junction of the cricopharyngeus and the first circular fibers of the esophagus (Fig. 18–1) [121]. The purpose of the inferior constrictor is to compress the pharynx during swallowing, displacing the food bolus downward. The cricopharyngeus muscle maintains tonic contraction closing the inlet to the esophagus between swallows and relaxes during swallowing to allow bolus entry into the esophagus. The cricopharyngeus muscle generates most, but not all of the pressure at the manometrically identified UES, as the physiologic high-pressure zone is often found to be of greater length than the anatomically identified muscle fibers. The function of the UES is to prevent the entrance of air into the esophagus and more recently has been recognized for its role in preventing high gastroesophageal reflux from entering the larynx [18].

When a swallow is initiated, the UES relaxes while the oral and pharyngeal phases of deglutition proceed. As the tongue propels the bolus posteriorly, the larynx is elevated and compressed to prevent the bolus from entering the trachea. The bolus passes into the pharynx and the constrictors

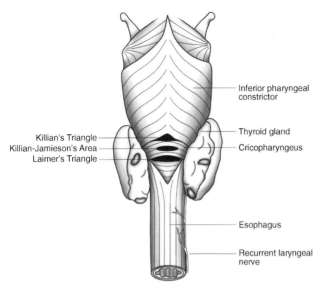

**FIG. 18–1.** Schematic drawing of the posterior aspect of the pharyngoesophageal junction with areas of weakness identified.

then contract to propel the bolus into the esophagus. The tonic contraction of the UES is inhibited and the bolus proceeds into the esophagus. This is a conceptually simple interpretation of deglutition. However, extensive study of the physiology of the UES and the pathophysiology of the diseases that affect the UES have revealed the complexity of the UES activity. A more concise description may be found elsewhere in the book.

## PHARYNGOESOPHAGEAL DIVERTICULUM (ZENKER'S)

Since all reported cases of pharyngoesophageal diverticulum have occurred in elderly patients, it is assumed to be an acquired disease. The diverticulum is not a true one, as it consists of only mucosa which escapes the pharynx between the areas of weakness in the muscle fibers described earlier. It is classified as a pulsion diverticulum because it is thought to arise from increased pressure within the pharynx. The reason for this increase in intraluminal pressure within the pharynx is not known, but at least four hypotheses have been advanced as an explanation [34]. The early explanation was that the UES was maintaining tonic contraction during swallowing in response to lower esophageal disease, such as gastroesophageal reflux. Then, the concept of achalasia of the UES, a failure to relax, was put forward as the explanation for the high resistance at the pharyngoesophageal junction. As manometric evaluation of the UES became available, it was found that the UES was capable of relaxing, but that lack of coordination between bolus propagation and sphincter relaxation was the primary cause of the increased pressure in the pharynx. Finally, there is evidence that suggests that the muscles of the cricopharyngeus and the proxi-

mal esophagus are fibrosed and therefore do not function as they normally would.

The last two theories have the greatest support, and both contribute conceptually to understanding the dysfunction of the UES. Manometry of the UES shows some degree of incoordination in more than two-thirds of patients [28]. The dysfunction occurs most frequently during the UES closure after relaxation and the initiation of the proximal esophageal peristalsis [74]. The precise nature of the dysfunction can be difficult to assess with stationary manometry because the UES is relatively narrow compared to the vertical distance it moves during normal deglutition. The combination of manometry with simultaneous fluoroscopy has helped resolve this problem. By ensuring proper placement of the manometry catheter at the UES, it was found that the sphincter was not relaxing completely, and that its baseline pressure was also decreased [71]. Further investigation of the sphincter muscles showed that they were replaced by fibrotic tissue, which explained the abnormal response of the sphincter to swallowing [63, 126, 131]. It is not known whether the fibrosis is a cause or effect of the disease.

### Clinical Evaluation

Pharyngoesophageal diverticulum usually occurs in the seventh or eighth decade of life. Cervical esophageal dysphagia and regurgitation are the most common complaints. Dysphagia may occur as a result of the dysfunctional UES. It may also be due to displacement or obstruction of the pharyngoesophageal junction caused by a large diverticulum and its contents. As the diverticulum enlarges, regurgitation of undigested food particularly during recumbency becomes more prevalent. Aspiration, halitosis, excessive salivation, and a fullness in the neck may also occur. The physical exam is usually not helpful but may reveal a palpable mass, most commonly on the left side of the neck, and a foul odor may be detected on the breath.

A contrast esophagogram should be obtained. It will usually reveal the diverticulum and will help to exclude a high esophageal tumor (Fig. 18–2). Although a videoesophagogram will also demonstrate abnormal movement of the contrast during deglutition, it is probably not necessary to obtain one. Other studies which can confirm the diagnosis include esophagoscopy and manometry. A 24-hour pH study has been used to determine if there is associated gastroesophageal reflux, which is believed by some to contribute to the pathogenesis of the disease. None of the last three tests is likely to alter the therapy, and they are probably not necessary in the average patient with a pharyngoesophageal diverticulum.

### Treatment

Prior to operative treatment of the diverticulum, the patient should be on a liquid diet for 1 or 2 days to minimize the amount of retained food particles in the diverticulum.

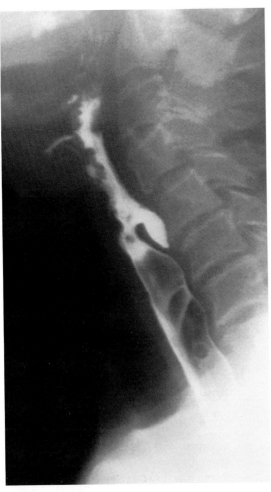

**FIG. 18–2.** Lateral view of an esophagogram demonstrating a Zenker's diverticulum projecting downward posterior to the cricopharyngeus muscle.

Although the preoperative contrast study will help to decide which side of the neck will provide the best exposure for the procedure, the left side is usually preferred. Most diverticula originate in the posterior aspect of the pharynx. As they grow, about 25% project to the left side and 10% project to the right side; thus the left side will be used in 90% of cases. The approach from the left is easier from an anatomic standpoint. The tracheoesophageal groove and the recurrent laryngeal nerve are more accessible due to the slight rightward shift of the trachea relative to the esophagus in the neck.

Access to the area is gained through a low cervical incision along the anterior border of the sternocleidomastoid muscle. The dissection proceeds along the avascular plane anterior to the sternocleidomastoid muscle, which is retracted laterally. The carotid sheath is retracted laterally as well, and the thyroid gland medially. Often, the middle thyroid vein is ligated and transected, as is the omohyoid muscle to improve exposure. As the tracheoesophageal groove is approached, care must be taken to avoid injuring the recurrent laryngeal nerve. With the posterolateral aspect of the

esophagus exposed, a bougie may be carefully passed into the esophagus. The surgeon should guide the bougie to prevent it from entering the diverticulum. With the bougie in place, a circumferential dissection of the esophagus is performed. The esophagus is then dissected cephalad along the posterior midline toward its junction with the pharynx. During this dissection, the diverticulum will be encountered (Fig. 18–3).

The diverticulum is grasped with a Babcock forceps, dissected free from adjacent structures, and elevated into the wound (Fig. 18–4). The neck of the diverticulum is cleared of the surrounding tissues. This should reveal the triangle of Killian. At this point, a myotomy is performed. The cricopharyngeus muscle and the proximal few centimeters of the longitudinal and circular muscle of the esophagus are also transected, so that the mucosa protrudes through the myotomy site (Fig. 18–5). The diverticulum should be excised whenever possible to reduce the amount of redundant mucosa at the pharyngoesophageal junction. To accomplish this, a linear stapler is placed across the neck of the diverticulum with a bougie inside the esophagus to prevent narrowing of the lumen (Fig. 18–6). The platysma is closed loosely and the skin is approximated. Drainage of the wound is not necessary. The patient is allowed a liquid diet on the first postoperative day, and if no evidence of a leak is present, the diet may be advanced.

### Outcome

Resolution of dysphagia and regurgitation may be expected and has been reported in 82% to 100% of patients

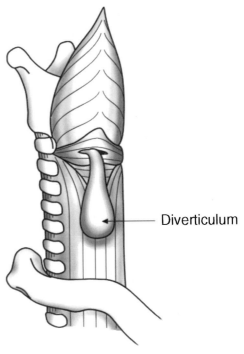

**FIG. 18–3.** Drawing of a diverticulum relative to the surgical landmarks of the posterior pharynx.

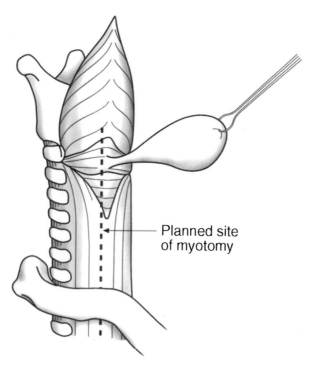

FIG. 18–4. Diverticulum elevated from the dissection site. The site of the planned myotomy is marked by the dotted line.

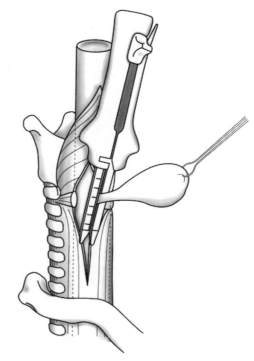

FIG. 18–6. The stapling and cutting device is placed across the neck of the diverticulum. Note that the bougie is in place prior to transecting the diverticulum.

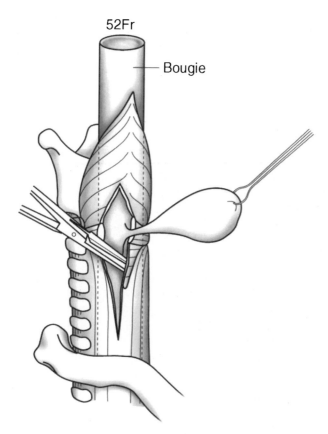

FIG. 18–5. The myotomy is extended onto the esophagus for several centimeters.

treated with this approach [7, 28, 61]. Despite the symptomatic improvement, the mechanism of deglutition is not entirely restored to normal. For example, postoperative video contrast studies show abnormalities in pharyngeal peristalsis, a visible cricopharyngeus, premature closure of the cricopharyngeus, and, occasionally, a residual diverticulum [127].

### Complications

Mortality from this procedure should be less than 1%. The most disturbing complication, esophagocutaneous fistula, occurs in 6% to 20% of cases but heals spontaneously [61]. Other potential complications include soft tissue infection, mediastinitis, recurrent laryngeal nerve injury, hematoma, and late stenosis. The frequency of these complications ranges between 1% and 6% [63]. Some authors feel that mucosal injury and recurrent laryngeal nerve injury may be reduced by operating with loupe magnification [60]. Recurrence rates are low, and if the diverticulum is excised while a bougie is in the esophagus, postoperative stenosis is rare.

### Controversies in Treatment

All patients with pharyngoesophageal diverticula who are able to tolerate an operation should probably be treated, as the natural history of the disease is one of progression leading to complications [34]. No medical therapy has been shown to be effective at treating these diverticula. Several elements of the surgical treatment have been topics of debate.

### Surgical Approach

The approach described previously has been the mainstay of surgical treatment in North America for several decades [45, 64, 82, 105, 112]. By contrast, many European surgeons prefer some variant of the peroral approach to treating pharyngoesophageal diverticula [9, 12, 16, 41, 54, 122, 123, 128, 129]. More recently, there has been some crossover in the approaches [7, 36, 48, 60, 62, 104, 132]. There have been no prospective, randomized trials comparing the transcervical and peroral approaches for treating pharyngoesophageal diverticula.

Most peroral methods of treating diverticula are variations of Dohlman's modification of Mosher's first description in 1917 [12]. Rigid endoscopy is used to gain exposure to the pharynx while the patient is under general anesthesia. The esophageal lumen and the diverticular neck are thus identified. The intervening muscle between the lumen of the esophagus and the pouch of the diverticulum is divided. The diverticulum is no longer a blind-ended pouch, as the anterior wall of the diverticulum communicates with the esophageal lumen. Most surgeons who use this technique employ cautery or laser technology to divide the muscles between the diverticulum and the esophagus. One of the problems with this technique is that it allows communication between the lumen of the esophagus and the deep tissue planes of the neck. Although the potential complications of deep tissue infection and mediastinitis are concerns, they occurred in only 12 of 544 patients treated in one of the largest studies [128]. Another method of transecting the tissue between the two structures is to employ a commercially available automatic stapling and cutting device [16]. One arm of the device is placed into the lumen of the esophagus and the other into the diverticulum. Four rows of staples are then fired into the tissue bridge, and a blade cuts between the inner two rows of staples. Thus, the tissue is stapled and divided, theoretically preventing the escape of esophageal contents from the cut edges. No large series have been reported using this technique to demonstrate a decrease in infection rate.

### Diverticulectomy versus Diverticulopexy

In an effort to decrease the incidence of soft tissue infection and mediastinitis, the diverticulum may be sutured to the precervical fascia so that the apex is cephalad to the neck (Fig. 18–7). By not breaching the esophageal mucosa, the incidence of infection would theoretically be decreased. In a nonrandomized study of 43 patients approached by a transcervical route, all patients had myotomies performed; 14 had diverticulectomy, and 29 had diverticulopexy [60]. Two patients in both groups developed neck infections, and one patient in the diverticulectomy group developed mediastinitis. There was no statistical difference in the incidence of

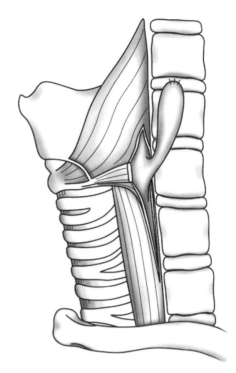

**FIG. 18–7.** Drawing of a diverticulopexy. The apex of the diverticulum is sutured to the precervical fascia.

wound infection or mediastinitis between the two groups. It may be argued that the study did not have enough patients to detect a difference in infectious complications. This may obscure the theoretical benefit of the diverticulopexy procedure. However, it should be noted that diverticulopexy was the procedure of choice in the most recent patients, as the authors discarded the use of diverticulectomy for treatment. Thus, no known difference exists between the two procedures with respect to outcome or complications.

Although in the past some advocated diverticulectomy alone, the incidence of recurrence was so high that it is now inadvisable to treat the diverticulum without performing a myotomy [45].

### Treating Associated Foregut Pathology

Other abnormalities of esophageal and gastric function may be found in up to 60% of patients with pharyngoesophageal diverticula [62]. The most common finding is gastroesophageal reflux disease. As with cricopharyngeal bar (discussed below), the association between the two is thought to stem from an attempt by the UES to prevent gastric contents from reaching the pharynx. The issue of addressing both entities simultaneously has waxed and waned for the past 30 years depending on the accepted explanation of the pathophysiology of pharyngoesophageal diverticulum [119]. Some surgeons believe that if abnormal gastroesophageal reflux is demonstrated preoperatively, it should be treated surgically during the same procedure as the pharyngoesophageal diverticulum. The rationale behind this approach is the assumption that once the cricopharyngeal myotomy is performed, the refluxed contents from the stomach may more easily enter the larynx causing laryngitis, hoarseness, and even aspiration. However, not all patients with Zenker's diverticulum have concomitant foregut pathology. The best approach is to address each pathologic entity based on its severity and the discomfort it creates for the patient. If heartburn, regurgitation of digested food, and esophagitis are the predominant findings in a patient who has a small Zenker's diverticulum on a contrast study, the reflux should be treated first, as some relief from both may be gained [18]. Similarly, if the patient has cervical dysphagia, regurgitation of undigested food, and a mildly abnormal 24-hour pH study, the pharyngoesophageal diverticulum should be treated alone.

### Conclusion

Zenker's diverticula are the result of a dysfunctional UES and a weakness in the posterior muscular fibers of the pharyngoesophageal junction. Regurgitation and cervical dysphagia are the most common symptoms. Diagnostic workup may be limited to a contrast study of the pharynx and the esophagus. Concurrent foregut pathology should be addressed on its own merit. No medical therapy is effective in the treatment of pharyngoesophageal diverticula. Surgical treatment, including resection of the diverticulum and cricopharyngeal myotomy, relieves symptoms and has excellent results.

## CRICOPHARYNGEAL BAR (UPPER ESOPHAGEAL SPHINCTER ACHALASIA)

A cricopharyngeal bar is identified radiographically by a persistent posterior indentation of contrast in the pharyngoesophageal segment. This is seen on a lateral view during a video esophagogram or a barium swallow (Fig. 18–8). In addition, residual contrast may be seen above the cricopharyngeus well after the UES has closed (Fig. 18–9). Despite the presence of such a finding, no consistent clinical symptoms have been identified in these patients. In fact, the etiology and the significance of a cricopharyngeal bar are unknown.

Based on the concept that the UES relaxes during swallowing, the persistent indentation has been described as either a failure to relax (thus the term UES achalasia) or incoordination of the constrictors and the cricopharyngeus muscle. Dantas et al. examined six patients with cricopharyngeal bars and eight controls without this finding on barium swallow [24]. The subjects were assessed using videofluoroscopy and UES manometry. The patients were found to have normal contraction of the pharynx, UES pressure, and bolus flow rate. When compared to the controls, the patients with cricopharyngeal bars had reduced UES relaxation during swallowing and increased upstream bolus pressures. From these data, it appears that cricopharyngeal bars arise as a result of failure of the muscle to completely relax.

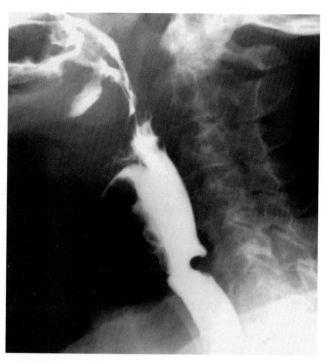

**FIG. 18–8.** Lateral view of an esophagogram showing a cricopharyngeal bar. The persistent indentation posteriorly is caused by the cricopharyngeus muscle.

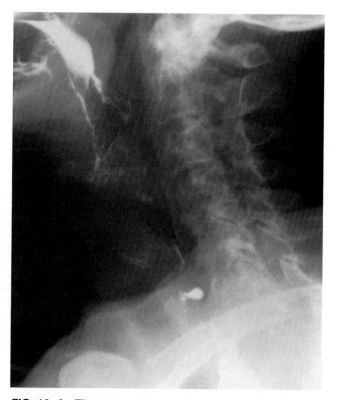

**FIG. 18–9.** The same patient at a later phase of swallowing, showing the persistent contrast above the cricopharyngeus muscle. Note how the relative position of the cricopharyngeus muscle has descended back toward the clavicle.

Others have found that resting, relaxation, and contraction pressures are normal in patients with cricopharyngeal bar [30]. In fact, these authors claim that the cricopharyngeal muscle is the only normal portion of the pharyngoesophageal segment, and that the inferior constrictor and the proximal esophagus are abnormally dilated.

Even when a cricopharyngeal bar can be demonstrated, the clinical significance of this finding is difficult to discern. Patients who are asymptomatic may have the same degree of narrowing as patients being evaluated for cervical esophageal dysphagia [24]. Furthermore, cricopharyngeal bar is seen in greater than 50% of patients with gastroesophageal reflux [13]. Because of the ambiguity of the finding and the lack of symptoms attributable to this dysfunction, surgical intervention for cricopharyngeal bar is only appropriate for very selected patients. The patients should not have a medical condition known to affect motility (myopathy, Parkinson's disease, or myasthenia gravis), neoplasia must be excluded, and gastroesophageal reflux should be eliminated as a cause of the cricopharyngeal bar [47]. If these requirements are satisfied, and the patient has symptoms referable to the cervical esophagus, a cricopharyngeal myotomy may provide some relief.

## ACHALASIA

Achalasia is the most common esophageal motor disorder that warrants surgical intervention. This disease is characterized by incomplete lower esophageal sphincter (LES) relaxation and absent esophageal peristalsis. As a consequence, esophageal emptying is impaired, which causes progressive dilation and lengthening of the organ. Both medical and surgical treatment are geared toward decreasing resistance to flow through the gastroesophageal junction. While this improves emptying and relieves symptoms of the disease, it does not directly affect the underlying etiology of the pathologic process.

Despite multiple attempts at defining the pathophysiology of achalasia, little is known about the etiology of the disease. Chagas disease does provide some insight into achalasia, as the symptoms, the anatomic findings, and the physiologic aspects of the two diseases are quite similar. In Chagas disease, *Trypanosoma cruzi* destroys the myenteric plexus of the esophagus, which is thought to be the cause of altered motor dysfunction and LES relaxation. Patients with achalasia also have a decreased number of neural cells in their myenteric plexus.

As the majority of cases occur between the fourth and sixth decades of life, there is little suspicion of a congenital cause. However, familial achalasia has been reported in up to six siblings in a single family [77]. Robertson et al. reported finding varicella zoster virus DNA in the esophageal muscular wall of 33% of patients with achalasia [103]. Other investigators have reported no correlation between viral infections and the incidence of achalasia [83].

The one pathologic finding that is agreed upon in achalasia is the relative paucity of the myenteric plexus in the esophageal wall. Whether this is a cause or an effect of achalasia is unknown. The lack of LES relaxation is thought to be related to impaired nonadrenergic, noncholinergic inhibitory control and the lack of nitric oxide synthase [73]. Despite the lack of nitric oxide, the LES is still sensitive to other enteric hormones such as secretin [76]. The etiology of achalasia, and therefore the chance to halt progression or prevent the disease, will require more investigation. For now, palliation of the symptoms is all physicians have to offer.

### Clinical Evaluation

Achalasia usually presents with symptoms of progressive dysphagia and regurgitation of undigested food. Other symptoms may include substernal chest pain, heartburn, and, rarely, abdominal pain. As the esophagus becomes more dilated, patients tend to complain less about dysphagia and more about regurgitation. Weight loss is common, and occasionally, patients are malnourished. Dysphagia is primarily related to the ingestion of solid food. Most patients relate a "need to push food down with liquids" and frequent episodes of complete occlusion of the esophagus leading to "vomiting." Because progression of the disease is insidious, most patients do not seek medical attention for quite some time. The average length of time between the onset of symptoms and operative intervention is 60 months [97].

Any time a patient presents with these complaints, other etiologies must be considered, such as tumors of the gastroesophageal junction, neurologic diseases, and connective tissue disorders. Pseudoachalasia, also called secondary achalasia, may be caused by neoplasms, paraneoplastic syndromes, pseudocysts, and postoperative obstruction of the gastroesophageal junction after a perihiatal operation [31, 88]. These patients present with manometric and radiologic signs of achalasia and may be difficult to distinguish from patients with achalasia. A careful history and physical exam will often aid in identifying patients with pseudoachalasia. Tumors generally occur in older patients, and the progression of dysphagia and weight loss is more rapid. Thus, the physician should be wary when the diagnosis of achalasia is entertained in a patient over the age of 70 years, particularly when the duration of symptoms has been less than 6 months and the weight loss is greater than 20 pounds. These patients should be carefully examined in search of palpable supraclavicular lymphadenopathy and other signs of a neoplastic process. In addition, their diagnostic evaluation should include an accurate assessment of the morphology of the esophageal wall. The test of choice is a transesophageal endoscopic ultrasound. If this is not available, a computed tomography scan may provide useful information as well.

Achalasia is rare in children, and a timely diagnosis is difficult. The time lapse between symptoms and correct diagnosis is between 6 months and 9 years. Children may manifest the disease by recurrent episodes of pneumonia, failure to thrive, coughing, and hoarseness [79]. Some teenagers have even been given a diagnosis of anorexia nervosa [53].

### Diagnostic Tests

Evaluation of patients suspected of having achalasia should include manometry, an esophagogram, and upper endoscopy. If possible, a 24-hour pH study should also be performed.

#### Manometry

Manometry is the gold standard for diagnosing achalasia. The criteria for diagnosis are (1) aperistalsis of the esophageal body, (2) incomplete relaxation of the LES, and (3) normal or hypertonic LES pressure (see chapter 10). Disorganized contractions of the esophageal body usually have normal or below-normal amplitudes. The waves are not propagated throughout the length of the esophagus and are often simultaneous. The LES pressure will fail to drop to the gastric baseline as it does in the normal state.

In some patients, chest pain is a predominant symptom. Many of them have high-amplitude contractions. In this variant of the disease, called vigorous achalasia, the high-amplitude waves are thought to cause pain. Thus, dilation or myotomy limited to the gastroesophageal junction, while enough to relieve dysphagia, may not be adequate to relieve pain in these patients. Parilla et al., however, reported excellent pain relief following a standard myotomy in patients with vigorous achalasia [89]. To help understand the origin of these high-amplitude contractions, Stuart et al. performed manometry on 13 patients with achalasia while they were consuming a standard meal. All patients developed elevated baseline esophageal pressures and peak contractile pressures that ranged from 65 to 120 mm Hg [116]. Although none of these patients had a diagnosis of vigorous achalasia on stationary manometry, all developed high contractile pressures when their esophagus became distended. The results of this study question the diagnosis of vigorous achalasia on stationary manometry alone.

The LES may also be assessed using vector volume analysis. This is performed with four or eight radially placed pressure transducers at the distal end of the probe. The probe is slowly pulled past the LES, and measurements are recorded from each transducer. A three-dimensional image is produced from the forces generated by the LES [115]. The benefit of this technique over routine manometry has not been established.

Assessment of the esophagus can also be performed with ambulatory 24-hour manometry. Two transducers are placed in the body of the esophagus, neither at the LES. It may be performed in patients when the stationary manometry is equivocal. The need for preoperative manometry when contemplating a functional procedure on the esophagus is unquestionable. It is necessary to prevent performing an improper operation, such as a total fundoplication on untreated achalasia [69].

#### Esophagogram

The esophagogram defines the anatomy of the esophageal body and may help to exclude tumor. The esophageal body will be dilated and the lumen will be smooth without evidence of peristaltic waves. Often an air–fluid level will be visible. A discrete narrowing at the gastroesophageal junction will be noted (Fig. 18–10). The tapering of the distal esophagus should be concentric, without evidence of a mass effect. Advanced disease will often reveal a tortuous esophagus or a "sigmoid esophagus" (Fig. 18–11). A diverticulum may be an associated finding.

Some have used contrast studies to evaluate the degree of esophageal dilation and the height of the contrast column before and after intervention [87]. Although improvement in these measures can be seen after treatment of achalasia, the correlation with clinical outcome is not clear.

#### Endoscopy

Upper endoscopy is essential in patients with dysphagia to exclude intraluminal esophageal neoplastic processes. It

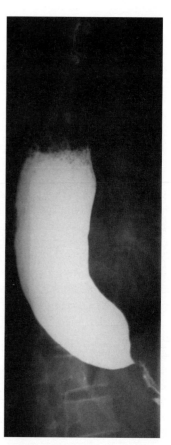

**FIG. 18–10.** Esophagogram demonstrating achalasia. The patient has a smooth, abrupt tapering of the distal esophagus and an air–fluid level proximally.

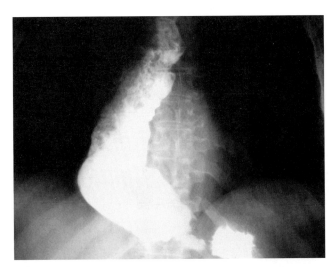

**FIG. 18–11.** A patient with more advanced achalasia demonstrating a sigmoid esophagus.

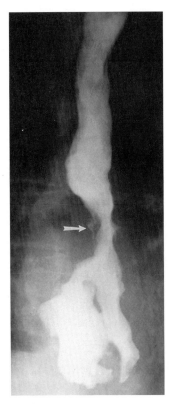

**FIG. 18–12.** This patient has a ragged tapering of the distal esophagus which is suspicious for malignancy.

may also identify other pathology in the stomach and duodenum. The expected findings in a patient with achalasia would be a dilated proximal esophagus, some retained food or liquid, and no evidence of esophagitis. The endoscope should pass the LES with minimal effort in patients with achalasia; if stubborn resistance is met, other causes of esophageal obstruction must be suspected. Endoscopic ultrasound is useful in these situations, as it provides a detailed view of the entire wall and may help identify tumors at the gastroesophageal junction (Figs. 18–12 and 18–13). It can also identify the proximal extent of hypertrophic muscle in the esophageal wall.

### 24-Hour pH Monitoring

The pH study will usually show little if any reflux in classic achalasia. The pH in both the proximal and distal channels should remain above 4. If, however, gastroesophageal reflux does occur, it cannot be cleared by the aperistaltic esophagus. For this reason, preoperative episodes of gastroesophageal reflux are important to document.

Interpreting the pH data may be difficult, and requires some degree of experience with achalasia. The data are often analyzed by a computer program which receives the data directly from a digital recording device. The automated analysis can be misleading because achalasia patients may have an acidic environment (pH < 4.0) without any reflux. This phenomenon has been demonstrated by Crookes et al., who showed that fermentation of bland food can generate a pH below 4.0 when mixed with saliva [19]. Careful inspection of the graphical tracing will reveal a gradual decrease in pH over several hours as opposed to the rapid decline in pH seen with episodes of reflux (Fig. 18–14). The distinction is important for clinical assessment in both preoperative and postoperative studies [109].

### Other Studies

Stationary manometry may not be possible in some patients as the gastroesophageal junction cannot be negotiated by the catheter. In this case, esophageal function may be determined using radionuclide transit and videofluoroscopic

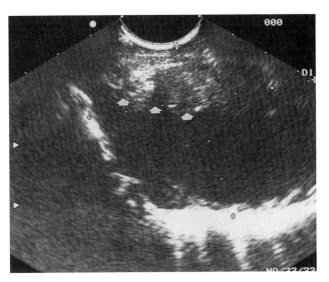

**FIG. 18–13.** Endoscopic ultrasound of the same patient as in Fig. 18–12. The arrows show that the tumor of the distal esophagus disrupting the normal tissue planes.

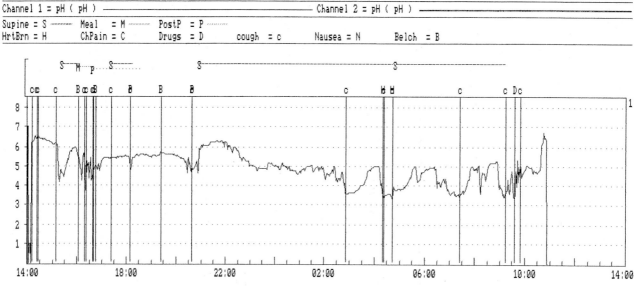

Channel 1 = pH ( pH )                                                    Channel 2 = pH ( pH )

Supine = S          Meal   = M          PostP  = P
HrtBrn = H          ChPain = C          Drugs  = D          cough  = c          Nausea = N          Belch  = B

**FIG. 18–14.** A 24-hour pH monitor tracing of a patient with achalasia. Between the times of 22:00 and 04:00, there is a gradual decrease in the pH consistent with fermentation.

studies. Using manometry as the standard, these studies have a sensitivity of 68% and 41%, respectively [113].

### Surgical Treatment

The aim of treatment is to decrease LES pressure and improve esophageal emptying. Both medical and surgical approaches are available. The decision to proceed with one or the other is discussed later. The standard surgical treatment is a myotomy with or without an antireflux procedure. The myotomy should be extended onto the cardia because 45% of the LES pressure is maintained by the stomach [68]. The principles of operative therapy are to transect completely the longitudinal and circular muscle fibers of the esophagus and the sling fibers of the cardia. The cut edges of the muscle must be separated widely and prevented from reapproximating. The length of the myotomy should be great enough to extend onto the stomach for 1 to 2 cm and to extend up the esophagus until normal muscle thickness is encountered.

Minimally invasive surgery techniques provide an excellent approach to this operation. Both laparoscopic and thoracoscopic approaches may be used [26, 96, 98, 101, 107]. For the average patient with achalasia, an abdominal approach is recommended as there is less pain, better access to the gastroesophageal junction, and no need to collapse the lung during the operation. The preparation and operation are carried out as described below.

### Preparation

The patient should be restricted to a liquid diet for at least 2 days prior to the operation. This helps clear solid material from the dilated body of the esophagus and prevents aspiration of food into the airway at the time of intubation. Use of a lighted bougie dilator and esophagoscopy should be available during the operation to facilitate transection of the muscle fibers and to determine the adequacy of the myotomy [95].

### Operation

The patient is placed in a low lithotomy position with the surgeon standing between the patient's legs and the assistant standing on the patient's left. A laparoscope holder may be used to secure the instrument which retracts the liver. Five trocars are used during the procedure. The assistant operates the laparoscope with the left hand and provides retraction with the right (Fig. 18–15).

After retracting the left lobe of the liver anteriorly, the peritoneum overlying the left crus is divided. The short gastric vessels are divided and the phrenoesophageal membrane is opened anteriorly. The right crus is then dissected so that the lateral and anterior attachments of the abdominal esophagus are freed. Posterior mobilization of the esophagus is not required unless a Toupet fundoplication is planned after completion of the myotomy. The anterior aspect of the esophagus should be dissected well into the mediastinum. At this time, the lighted bougie (no. 52 French) is introduced into the esophagus transorally. The fat overlying the gastroesophageal junction should be removed, and the anterior vagus dissected free from the esophageal wall. The cardiomyotomy site is marked with cautery in a straight line along the anterior portion of the esophagus and the stomach (Fig. 18–16). The distal esophageal muscle fibers are usually the most difficult to dissect, especially if previous dilation or botulinum toxin injection has been performed [51]. For this reason, the initial dissection is started on the stomach or an area of less-fibrosed esophagus. Cautery is used to divide the muscle fibers down to the submucosa (Fig. 18–17). When the proper plane is identified, the cardiomyotomy is extended cephalad until normal esophageal muscle is identified and caudad until the sling fibers of the cardia are divided (Fig. 18–18). Intraoperative endoscopy is performed to identify the gastroesophageal junction and to insure the myotomy is of sufficient length. This may be confirmed by adequate distention of the esophagus with insufflation.

Once the cardiomyotomy is sufficient, a partial anterior fundoplication (Dor) is performed (Fig. 18–19). With the bougie or the flexible endoscope in the esophagus, the fundus of the stomach is positioned anterior to the myotomy. Sutures are placed to anchor the fundus to the right and left crura as well as to the transected edges of the esophageal muscle. When the wrap is completed, the liver retractor is removed, and the incisions are closed.

A nasogastric tube is not used postoperatively. The patient is allowed a liquid diet on the night of the operation and begins a graduated solid diet the next morning. Most patients may be discharged from the hospital within 2 days. All patients are strongly encouraged to have manometry and pH studies 6 to 8 weeks after surgery.

Postoperative evaluation of the esophagus is important

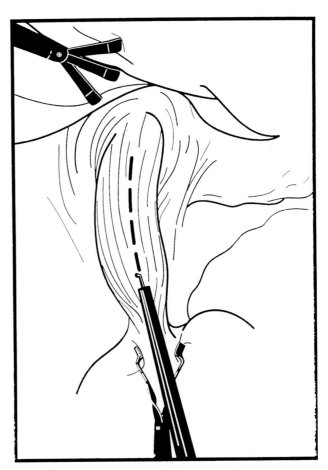

**FIG. 18–16.** The planned myotomy site is marked along the anterior surface of the esophagus with electrocautery.

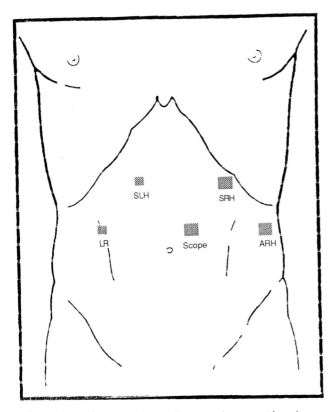

**FIG. 18–15.** Diagram showing the port placement for a laparoscopic Heller–Dor procedure. *SLH* and *SRH* mark the ports for the surgeon's left and right hands, respectively. *Scope* and *ARH* mark the ports for the assistant's left and right hands, respectively. *LR* marks the port for the liver retractor.

because the most common cause for late failure is likely to be gastroesophageal reflux disease. As discussed later in this section, it is often asymptomatic, so patients do not seek treatment. If pathologic reflux is present on the 24-hour pH study, the patients should be treated to help prevent peptic stricture formation at a later date.

### Outcome

At the University of Washington, 46 patients have undergone a laparoscopic Heller–Dor procedure for achalasia since 1992. The assessment of symptoms is based on a subjective score provided by the patients regarding the frequency of an event. Forty-two (91%) have had improvement in swallowing. The average frequency was several times per day prior to operative therapy and less than once per month after the operation. The same was true for the symptom of regurgitation—there was a 91% positive response to operative intervention. Of 11 patients who had chest pain more than once per week before the operation, eight patients responded to operative therapy favorably. The other three (27%) had persistent chest pain with the same frequency after the operation.

These results are similar to those reported by others. Relief from dysphagia is between 85% and 95% at 5 years, weight gain is common, and overall satisfaction with the operation is high [10, 21, 84]. Since the obstruction to flow is relieved, regurgitation is reduced. Relief from chest pain may occur in 60% to 75% of patients who had the symptom preoperatively.

Improved esophageal motility has been demonstrated after cardiomyotomy for achalasia [21]. Proximal peristalsis can be demonstrated in up to 50% of patients, midesophageal peristalsis in 25%, and distal in up to 9% [90]. This finding implies that LES contributes to the esophageal body dysfunction, but is not solely responsible for the disorganized peristalsis. Others argue that this finding does not represent an intrinsic change in the motility of the esophagus but is an artifact of manometry and that an apparent improvement in peristalsis is only a function of the decreased caliber of the esophagus after surgery [126].

### Complications

Early complications of the procedure are uncommon. In the 46 patients operated at the University of Washington,

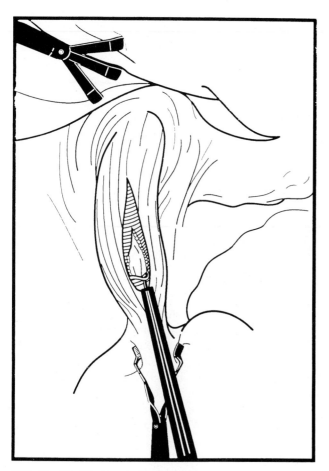

**FIG. 18–17.** The longitudinal and circular muscle fibers are transected with a combination of electrocautery and blunt dissection.

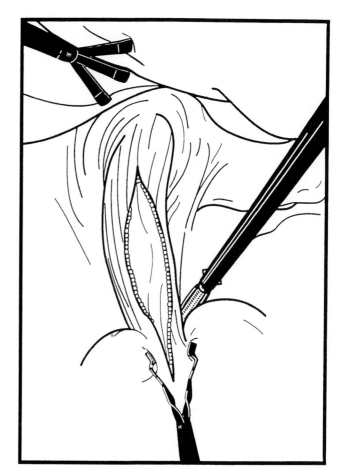

**FIG. 18–18.** Completed myotomy extending onto the stomach.

three had esophageal mucosal perforation during the procedure. Two of these patients had been treated with one or more botulinum toxin injections. The other perforation occurred early in the experience with laparoscopic myotomy. One patient developed a symptomatic left pleural effusion after the operation. The overall complication rate was 9%, and there was no mortality.

Esophageal perforation is repaired intraoperatively. The mucosa is closed primarily, then buttressed with the serosa of the stomach during the partial fundoplication. Initially, mucosal laceration was considered a reason for converting to an open procedure. However, if the surgeon is comfortable with videoendoscopic suturing, the procedure does not need to be converted.

Pneumothorax, bleeding, wound infection, and intraabdominal abscess are other complications that have been reported in less than 3% of cases [67]. Most early complications can be avoided by careful dissection. However, previous operations or botulinum toxin injections distort the natural tissue planes and thus increase the likelihood of one of these complications.

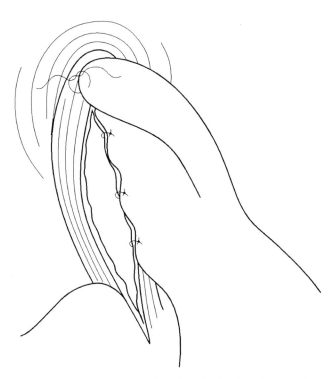

**FIG. 18–19.** The anterior hemifundoplication (Dor) is performed suturing the fundus to the cut edges of the myotomy site.

Late complications of myotomy are related mostly to the recurrence of the initial symptoms, particularly dysphagia.

Postoperative dysphagia may be caused by several discrete entities: incomplete myotomy, perihiatal scarring, progressive dysmotility of the esophagus, peptic stricture, and tumor. Some clinical clues may help distinguish among these, but physiologic and anatomic information must be obtained to confirm the diagnosis.

At the University of Washington, 4 of 46 patients operated for achalasia using a laparoscopic Heller–Dor procedure developed recurrent dysphagia. Two were found to have progressive dysmotility of the body of the esophagus, one had to have the fundoplication reversed because it was causing too much angulation of the gastroesophageal junction, and the last patient had obstructive symptoms caused by the crural fibers tethered across the gastroesophageal junction. The longest follow-up in these patients is 6 years.

In 129 patients followed for an average of 12 years, 40 were identified as having postoperative dysphagia [27]. Symptoms of incomplete myotomy occurred early and rarely caused dysphagia after 3 years. Postoperative scarring caused dysphagia 1 to 2 years after surgery. Gastroesophageal reflux caused dysphagia after 6 years. The authors were 100% accurate in diagnosing the cause of dysphagia using esophagogram, endoscopy, and manometry in the 12 patients whose diagnosis was confirmed by reoperation.

Incomplete myotomy may be prevented by extending the incision onto the stomach to insure transection of the sling fibers. The cut edges of the myotomy must be separated by at least 30% of the esophageal circumference. Perihiatal scarring may be prevented by minimizing the amount of electrocautery injury to the crura.

Pathologic gastroesophageal reflux may be detected in up to 40% of patients if 24-hour pH studies are performed [110]. This study assessed reflux after a limited thoracoscopic myotomy without the addition of an antireflux procedure. Most authors believe that the incidence of abnormal gastroesophageal reflux in a patient undergoing a myotomy and an antireflux procedure to be about 10% [10]. In the patients treated at the University of Washington, 4 of 46 patients had symptoms of heartburn more frequently than once per week after a laparoscopic Heller–Dor procedure. Of the patients who had postoperative 24-hour pH studies, 22% had abnormal acid exposure. Although it would seem that adding an antireflux procedure to the myotomy would help prevent abnormal gastroesophageal reflux, this has not been demonstrated in a randomized study.

The trade-off between relieving dysphagia and limiting reflux is clear—the greater the improvement of dysphagia, the higher is the incidence of reflux. This is clearly shown in a study by Pandolfo et al. [84]. In 11 patients, the authors used intraoperative manometry to assess the extent of LES relaxation during an open cardiomyotomy and anterior hemifundoplication via an abdominal approach. Manometric readings of the LES pressure were performed prior to and after the myotomy was completed. The myotomy was not considered complete until the LES pressure was less than 5 mm Hg. The results were compared to 16 patients who underwent the same procedure without the intraoperative study. Patients with intraoperative manometry had a 0% dysphagia rate but an 18.2% reflux rate. This compared to a 21.5% dysphagia rate and a 7.3% reflux rate in those who did not have intraoperative manometry. A more thorough myotomy leads to less dysphagia, but more reflux.

Besides peptic stricture, postoperative reflux may lead to other complications including esophagitis and Barrett's esophagus. Although some patients have pathologic reflux, many do not have symptoms. Jaakkola et al. found that four of 46 patients developed Barrett's esophagus after cardiomyotomy after an average follow-up of 13 years [55]. Others found dysplasia and intramucosal adenocarcinoma in patients with reflux after myotomy [27]. In a series of 100 patients undergoing myotomy, three developed cancer [21]. This stresses two points: the need to know which patients have reflux after the operation and the importance of following these patients with endoscopy.

The management of patients with postoperative dysphagia is not well defined. An attempt at conservative treatment using dilation is appropriate as long as no evidence of tumor is present. Parkman et al. successfully managed six patients with peptic stricture using multiple dilations (average 3.6 per patient) and acid suppression [86]. Conservative management is a reasonable strategy, as reoperation for dysphagia has a lower success rate than the initial operation [32].

### Recurrent Achalasia

Recurrence after operative treatment is reported to range from 8% to 13% [56, 75]. Late recurrence must be assessed carefully, as patients may develop dysphagia from other causes mentioned above. The diagnosis of recurrence must be confirmed by manometry, which should show a normal or elevated LES pressure and incomplete relaxation. Manometry may also reveal another motor disorder which may explain the symptoms and affect the treatment. Endoscopy and a contrast esophagogram should also be obtained to exclude other diseases such as a tumor or paraesphageal hernia. If recurrence is confirmed, there are several options available depending on the findings, the overall health of the patient, and the expertise that is available. Some patients may be treated with dilation. The endoscopist must be skilled in the use of pneumatic dilation because only the mucosa stands between the balloon and the mediastinum or the peritoneal cavity. If dilation is not available or if it fails to resolve the symptoms, a repeat myotomy may be considered. Between 70% and 80% of patients will respond to a repeat operation for recurrent or persistent achalasia [22, 43]. If the preoperative manometry reveals a diffuse esophageal abnormality, then a thoracic approach may be beneficial, especially if the first approach was via the abdomen. Otherwise, there is little evidence to support one approach over the other. If repeat myotomy is not helpful, then esophageal resection may be the only surgical alternative. The patient must be informed that this is a more extensive procedure and has a mortality rate between 2% and 8% [75, 124]. If esophageal resection is performed, the results can be expected to be good to excellent in 78% to 90% of patients [75, 99]. The choice of conduit for the operation is discussed later in this chapter.

### Emergent Operation after Perforation

Esophageal perforation may occur after pneumatic dilation in the treatment of achalasia. The management of the perforation depends on clinical assessment and the interpretation of the esophagogram. In a stable patient, a small contained perforation which does not communicate with other mediastinal structures or the pleural space may be treated with antibiotics and cessation of oral intake. If the patient has clinical manifestations or if radiographic studies show free communication with either the pleural cavity or the mediastinum (Fig. 18–20), then urgent operative intervention is indicated. Regardless of the initial management plan, a surgical evaluation should be obtained as soon as a perforation is expected.

The principles of operative intervention include debridement and irrigation to remove injured and necrotic tissue, closure of the perforation site, and myotomy. A posterolateral thoracic approach through the seventh intercostal space

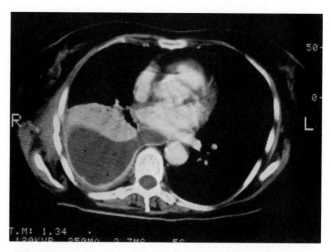

**FIG. 18–20.** Computed tomography scan showing communication of esophageal perforation with right pleural space.

is used. The mediastinum is exposed and cleansed of all esophageal contamination. After the perforation is debrided, a two-layered closure is used. The mucosa is sutured with an absorbable polygluconate-based 3-0 suture, and the muscularis is closed with a permanent suture. A myotomy should be performed on the opposite side of the perforation. Occasionally, the diaphragm may be enlarged and the cardia of the stomach used to place a serosal patch over the repair. In general, this is not feasible or advisable, as it creates a hiatal hernia. Two chest tubes are placed for drainage, and the incision is closed.

If the degree of soiling is extensive, or delay to operative intervention is prolonged, Schwartz et al. recommend diversion [106]. This would consist of esophagostomy, gastrostomy, and interruption of the gastroesophageal continuity. Rarely is it necessary to divert a patient, as esophageal resection or wide drainage of the perforated area can be safely performed in such situations [40].

Although a myotomy is usually performed during the emergent operation, one group has reported six patients in whom they simply repaired the perforation without performing a myotomy [100]. They found that none of their patients had recurrent symptoms of dysphagia after an average follow-up of 5 years. Others have approached perforation after dilation using minimally invasive surgery. These authors performed a primary repair using videoendoscopy and then drained the thorax with chest tubes [81].

The outcome of emergent surgery for perforation is often said to be the same as elective surgery. Ferguson et al. reported six patients treated emergently for perforation and compared them to 54 patients undergoing elective treatment for achalasia [38]. They found all six patients had good or excellent results based on symptoms scoring, whereas 88% of the elective cases had the same score. Postoperative endoscopy, pH studies, and manometry were not reported for either group. In another study, seven patients with perforation were compared to five elective procedures [106]. These authors found that the length of the operation, intensive care unit stay, and hospitalization were the same. Again, no postoperative studies were reported. Although there was no difference in the outcomes measured, these parameters may not be applicable today. For example, the average length of hospitalization was 11 days, and the intensive care unit stay was 1 day for the elective cases. Currently, the average length of stay is 2 days, and the patients rarely, if ever, go to the intensive care unit. Although it is often stated that the outcomes are no different in patients operated for perforation, the issue may need to be revisited with the advent of minimally invasive procedures.

## Controversies in Achalasia

The above approach to surgical management of achalasia may appear to be quite straightforward; however, many issues in the management of this disease process are topics of current debate. Several of these are discussed below.

### Medical Versus Surgical Treatment

Medical therapy with calcium channel blockers or nitrates is clinically ineffective and has been relegated to a role as a temporizing measure prior to or a supplemental treatment after definitive therapy [11, 29, 91, 118]. A more recent therapeutic modality involves injecting botulinum toxin into the LES. The effect of this treatment is also temporary, with only 66% of patients experiencing symptomatic relief at 6 months [91]. Although this may be appropriate therapy for patients who are at risk for operative intervention due to age or comorbid conditions, its long-term efficacy is unproved.

The two types of definitive therapy include pneumatic dilation and surgical transection of the esophageal muscle. Each approach has advantages and disadvantages. When the two are compared, the following issues arise: symptom resolution, immediate morbidity, degree of reflux as a result of therapy, and cost. Although several studies have been performed in an attempt to resolve the quandary, a consensus has not been reached. Retrospective studies comparing the results of surgery and forceful dilation are inconclusive because of selection bias, use of historical controls, and small sample size [1, 5, 65].

Only one study has prospectively randomized patients to either pneumatic dilation or surgery [20, 22]. In this study, 39 patients were treated by dilation and 42 by surgery. After 5 years of follow-up, excellent or good results were present in 65% of patients undergoing dilation and 95% of patients treated surgically. Interestingly, the authors of this paper performed both surgery and dilation on their study patients. The surgical procedure performed was an open abdominal cardiomyotomy extending onto the stomach for 5 to 10 mm and an anterior (Dor) fundoplication. Pneumatic dilation was accomplished using a Mosher bag inflated to 12 to 15 psi for 10 to 20 seconds. Two patients underwent emergency surgery for perforation of the esophagus after dilation. Postprocedure "acid reflux tests" were performed in both groups,

and reflux was documented in 8% of the dilation patients and 28% of the surgery patients. The authors concluded that surgery offered better clinical results than did dilation.

Their conclusion was questioned for several reasons [102]. The technical complaint was that the study only had a 65% response to pneumatic dilation because the duration and pressure of dilation were not sufficient. Others have reported a response rate of between 75% and 85% using more aggressive techniques [11, 72, 117, 118]. The degree of postoperative gastroesophageal reflux in the patients who underwent operation was criticized as being too high. Furthermore, since surgery required a longer inpatient and outpatient recovery, this facet of treatment should not have been ignored when assessing the appropriateness of the intervention. Indeed the cost of surgical treatment was found to be 2.4 times higher in a study comparing open operations to pneumatic dilations [85].

Gastroesophageal reflux has been thought to occur less frequently after dilation than surgical myotomy [1, 11]. However, studies which are cited to support this contention assess only symptoms of reflux. One study compared 24-hour pH monitoring on consecutive patients undergoing surgical and pneumatic dilation for achalasia [110]. Reflux was documented in 6 of 17 patients after dilation, and 6 of 15 after surgery. Only 33% of the patients with objective evidence of reflux had symptoms. The authors concluded that the amount of reflux is similar between the two modes of treatment and that the absence of symptoms does not exclude pathologic reflux.

The analysis of cost differences is valid, but the conclusions were drawn before minimally invasive approaches became employed by surgeons. The data that supports nonsurgical therapy were generated by comparing dilation to open operative procedures. Patients required 7 to 10 days of hospital care and several weeks of recuperation at home [1, 20, 85]. With minimally invasive techniques, the inpatient stay averages 2 days, and depending on lifestyle, patients may return to work in 1 week [49, 57, 101, 125]. Just as operative intervention evolved, so did pneumatic dilation. This procedure is now being performed on an outpatient basis and thus should lower the cost of this procedure as well [6, 15].

The question of the optimal initial treatment for achalasia remains unanswered. Aggressive pneumatic dilation may be able to attain similar results as operative therapy. However, since it is an uncontrolled disruption of the LES, the number of perforations will be proportional to the aggressiveness of the dilation technique. Furthermore, as greater success is obtained with dilation, the incidence of reflux will approach that of surgical intervention without an antireflux procedure. Further evaluation of the two interventions is needed to resolve the above issues. Certainly, young individuals with achalasia who are fit for an operation benefit from having a surgical myotomy as the first approach.

### Operative Approach

The first operative treatment of achalasia was described in 1913 by the procedure's namesake, Ernest Heller. His approach was via a laparotomy and consisted of a double myotomy. The open thoracic approach was championed in the United States by F. Henry Ellis in the 1950s. These two approaches were the only methods available to the surgeon until 1991, when Cuschieri and co-workers first described a successful laparoscopic myotomy [107]. Shortly after that, Pellegrini et al. described a thoracoscopic approach for achalasia and reported their experience with 17 patients [96]. Since that time, many authors have addressed the issues of open and videoendoscopic surgery.

The outcomes with the open and videoendoscopic abdominal approach appear to be similar [3, 17, 44, 78]. The benefits of minimally invasive surgery for the patient are to be found in the decreased hospital stay and recuperation.

Cuschieri and co-workers were the first to point out the potential advantages of reduced trauma and quicker recovery using a videoendoscopic technique [107]. Others supported their observation by demonstrating decreased recovery time, less pain, and improved aesthetic appearance of the incisions with laparoscopic myotomy [130]. In one study, the authors compared a matched group of laparotomy and laparoscopy Heller–Dor procedures [4]. Seventeen patients in each group were analyzed retrospectively for operative time, hospital stay, and return to normal activity. Although the operative time was greater for the minimally invasive group (178 vs. 125 minutes), the patients were discharged from the hospital earlier (4 vs. 10 days) and returned to normal activity earlier (14 vs. 30 days). Based on charges at the authors' institution, the cost of a laparoscopic myotomy compared to an open myotomy was about $400 lower. The largest component of cost in the laparoscopic procedure was the surgical supplies, and the largest component of cost in the open procedure was the length of stay. As experience has evolved, it has become clear that the use of an imaging system which allows for substantial magnification of the images and the excellent view of the field inherent in a videoendoscopic approach probably enhances the ability of surgeons to perform the operations with greater accuracy.

### Chest Versus Abdomen

As videoendoscopic procedures replaced the open techniques, the issue of whether the myotomy should be performed through the chest or the abdomen was raised. The same question existed during the era of open surgery, where the discussion focused on outcome—response to treatment, postoperative gastroesophageal reflux, and recurrence. Those who employ the thoracic approach point out that the esophagus and the gastroesophageal junction are more accessible from the chest. They also note that less mobilization of the structures which support the competency of the cardia is necessary, and therefore, an antireflux procedure is not needed [33, 42]. The laparoscopic approach, although requiring a larger mobilization of the cardioesophageal junction, allows instruments to be parallel to the axis of the esophagus, as opposed to being perpendicular during thoracoscopy.

Also, the majority of the LES is intra-abdominal and thus easier to approach laparoscopically [49]. The anesthetic management is simplified because there is no need to use single-lung ventilation and there is no need to use a chest tube postoperatively. Finally, another advantage of the abdominal approach is the ease of adding an antireflux procedure. Thus, most surgeons who treat achalasia using minimally invasive techniques use this approach [49, 52, 93, 101, 111].

### Adding an Antireflux Procedure

The issue of adding an antireflux procedure to a cardiomyotomy is controversial. It was reasoned in the past that if the cardiomyotomy extends too far onto the stomach, it may disrupt all the physiologic and anatomic contributions to the lower esophageal sphincter, thereby allowing gastroesophageal reflux to occur. If the cardiomyotomy does not extend too far onto the stomach, then no reflux will occur; however, the results of the operation may be inferior in terms of relieving dysphagia. In an attempt to solve both problems, the cardiomyotomy may be extended onto the stomach for a distance, and then the LES mechanism may be reconstructed with an antireflux procedure.

As previously noted, clinical assessment of reflux status underestimates the amount of reflux when compared to 24-hour pH studies in patients treated for achalasia. This holds true for patients treated operatively or by pneumatic dilation [110]. Therefore, all patients who undergo a myotomy should be evaluated postoperatively by 24-hour pH monitoring to determine objectively if pathologic reflux is occurring. Unfortunately, whether or not subclinical reflux causes late failure in the treatment of achalasia is not known.

If the myotomy is performed through the chest, a partial wrap can be constructed using the fundus of the stomach. Advocates of the thoracic approach believe that their procedure can usually be performed without the addition of an antireflux procedure, as they extend the myotomy onto the stomach for only a few millimeters [33, 35, 42]. The indications for adding an antireflux procedure would be the presence of a hiatal hernia, evidence of preoperative reflux, or gastric stasis. The reported rate of gastroesophageal reflux in patients undergoing myotomy via the thoracic approach without an antireflux procedure is between 5% and 62% [14, 32, 97]. The variability in the incidence of reflux is due to the manner in which reflux was measured. If the diagnosis is made clinically, then the rate is low (5% to 16%) [14, 32]; however if patients are subjected to pH studies, the rates are higher (35% to 62%) [97, 110]. Because gastroesophageal reflux was identified so frequently after thoracic myotomy, many surgeons moved to an abdominal approach where it is easier (and necessary) to perform some type of antireflux procedure.

Two types of fundal wraps are available to the surgeon using an abdominal approach to the esophagus: a complete wrap (Nissen) or some variation of a partial wrap (Dor,

Toupet, Thal). The most commonly used is the Dor fundoplication because it has several advantages. The first is that it is an anterior wrap, which eliminates the need to perform a posterior esophageal dissection. This preserves some attachment of the esophagus to the hiatus and will help to maintain an intraabdominal segment of distal esophagus. The second advantage of the Dor is that it allows the wall of the stomach to buttress the myotomy site. The cardia will help to seal any injury to the esophageal mucosa, prevent adhesion of the esophagus to the left lobe of the liver, and allow the myotomy edges to be sutured in an open position.

The amount of gastroesophageal reflux is less with the addition of an antireflux procedure. Peracchia et al. reported only an 8% pathologic gastroesophageal reflux rate based on pH studies after laparoscopic Heller–Dor procedures [98]. Similarly, Parilla et al. reported a 12% reflux rate after open Heller–Toupet procedures using 24-hour pH studies [87]. Another study reported no gastroesophageal reflux by pH studies in patients undergoing laparoscopic myotomies with partial fundoplications [101]. Although no randomized study has been performed comparing myotomy without fundoplication to myotomy with fundoplication, it appears that the addition of an antireflux procedure may reduce the likelihood of reflux, and thus may improve long-term results by avoiding complications associated with reflux.

### Conclusion

The symptoms of achalasia may be effectively treated by operative therapy. The principles of the operation include sufficient length of the myotomy, adequate separation of the transected muscle, and a plan to prevent postoperative gastroesophageal reflux. The operation may be performed using minimally invasive techniques. Postoperative assessment of gastroesophageal reflux should be performed in all patients to prevent late failure due to peptic stricture.

## SPASTIC DYSMOTILITY

The utilization of stationary and ambulatory esophageal manometry in the evaluation of patients with noncardiac chest pain has led to the identification of several uncommon esophageal dysmotility syndromes. Although criteria have been developed to aid in the diagnosis of these syndromes, the relative paucity of cases has hindered the development of standard treatment. All are considered together in this section because the experience with each is limited and the surgical treatments are similar.

*Diffuse esophageal spasm* (DES) is characterized by simultaneous contractions and intermittent normal peristalsis on manometry. Repetitive contractions, prolonged wave duration, high-amplitude contractions, spontaneous contractions, and an elevated LES pressure may also be observed

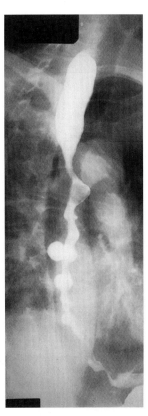

FIG. 18–21. Esophagogram showing diffuse esophageal spasm.

(Fig. 18–21). *Nutcracker esophagus* (NE) is diagnosed in patients who have a distal esophageal contraction amplitude greater than 180 mm Hg. An elevated LES pressure and prolonged wave duration may also be encountered but are not necessary for the diagnosis. In essence, this condition appears to be an "exaggeration" in the amplitude and duration of otherwise normal peristaltic waves. *Hypertensive lower esophageal sphincter* (HLES) is a condition diagnosed when the LES pressure is greater than 40 mm Hg, and there is an absence of any other disorders of the esophageal body which may account for the elevated sphincter pressure. More than 50% of patients with elevated LES pressures have other disorders of peristalsis [58]. *Nonspecific esophageal dysmotility* (NED) is a catchall category for patients with abnormal manometric findings that do not conform to the criteria of the other dysmotility syndromes. This category has been essentially replaced by *ineffective esophageal motility* (see chapter 11).

Epiphrenic diverticula are considered in this section because they are associated with some type of esophageal dysmotility in about 60% of patients [8]. When an operation is indicated, treatment of the disease is similar to the treatment of other motility disorders.

### Clinical Evaluation

Most patients present complaining of dysphagia and chest pain. Some may also complain of heartburn and regurgitation, especially if a diverticulum is present. Most often, the patients have undergone some form of cardiac evaluation for their chest pain. If this is not the case, the patient should be evaluated by the appropriate clinician to ensure this more common, life-threatening etiology is not the cause of the chest pain.

The clinical evaluation of a patient with noncardiac chest pain is similar to that of achalasia, which is described in the previous section. It should include manometry, a contrast study of the esophagus, and upper endoscopy. Manometry is necessary to define the type of motility disorder. The esophagogram and endoscopy are necessary to exclude other etiologies of abnormal motility such as benign and malignant neoplasms. A 24-hour pH study is also indicated to exclude gastroesophageal reflux, a much more common disease, as a cause for the dysmotility. Gastroesophageal reflux disease has been hypothesized to be a contributing factor to different esophageal dysmotility disorders, especially HLES [58]. Furthermore, surgical treatment is likely to disrupt the anatomic barriers to gastroesophageal reflux. If the patient has preexisting pathologic reflux, different operative strategies may be employed when surgical intervention is necessary.

Another consideration in the preoperative evaluation of patients with spastic dysmotility is the indication for 24-hour manometry. Although experience with this technique is limited to a few centers, the information gained may be very helpful in guiding therapy and predicting prognosis [37]. Ambulatory manometry is particularly useful in patients with daily symptoms who have been diagnosed with NE and NED on stationary manometry, as it may change the diagnosis in up to 30% of cases [114]. Ambulatory manometry allows the physician to correlate symptoms, as reported by the patient in an event diary, to the manometric measurements. Although the diagnosis may change with NE and NED, ambulatory manometry disagrees less often with stationary manometry when the diagnosis is DES. In this case, 24-hour manometry need not be performed. In difficult situations, endoscopic ultrasonography may define the area of the esophagus that is most affected, as the thickness of the muscularis can be accurately estimated by this study.

Occasionally, an epiphrenic diverticulum is found on a patient who has an upper gastrointestinal contrast study for an unrelated problem (Fig. 18–22). If the patient is clearly asymptomatic, then he or she may not need an operation. A follow-up esophagogram in 1 to 2 years will help gauge the progression of the diverticulum and reveal associated disease. Most of the asymptomatic diverticuli do not progress into clinical problems [8]. If, however, the patient has symptoms referable to the diverticulum, operative treatment is recommended. In this case, it is imperative to have a reliable manometric evaluation prior to operation as it will affect the surgical approach and the procedure.

## Treatment

Spastic dysmotility disorders of the esophagus have been infrequently treated by surgical therapy. The reason for this

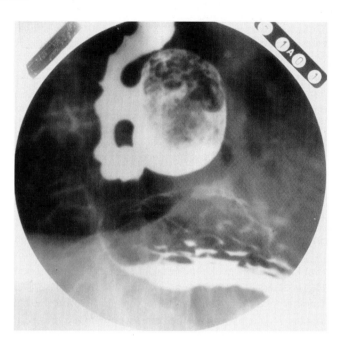

**FIG. 18–22.** Lateral view of an esophagogram revealing an anterior esophageal diverticulum.

is based partly on the fact that some reports have shown an 80% response to medical therapy [58] and partly on the reluctance of physicians to eliminate all peristaltic activity in the body of the esophagus with an operation. As with achalasia, spastic disorders are well suited to a minimally invasive operative approach. The procedure performed in most cases consists of a myotomy with or without an antireflux procedure. If a diverticulum is present, a diverticulectomy is also performed. Since the laparoscopic approach to a myotomy was described in the previous section, the thoracoscopic approach will be described here. This approach is usually employed when treating spastic motility disorders because a longer esophageal myotomy is needed to treat the symptoms of disease.

Two principles of operative therapy are important in treating spastic dysmotility. The first is that the site and extent of the myotomy must be directed by the findings of the manometry study. For example, if manometry shows the entire thoracic esophagus to be involved in the pathologic process, then the myotomy must span the length of the thoracic esophagus. The second issue is ablating the LES. Even if the LES pressure is normal, it should be transected. After an extensive myotomy of the esophageal body, the ability to transmit a bolus of food normally will be lost. Even a normal LES pressure would present a challenge to a myotomized esophagus.

The patient should be placed on a liquid diet for 2 days prior to the operation if esophageal emptying is inhibited. This will decrease the amount of solid debris in the lumen of the esophagus. A bougie, preferably lighted, is needed for the operation. The bougie should be placed under direct vision during the operation, especially if a diverticulum is present. This will prevent injury to the esophagus. A double-lumen endotracheal tube is necessary to allow single-lung ventilation.

A lateral decubitus position is used. Access to the lower esophagus, cardioesophageal junction, and upper stomach can only be achieved through a left-sided approach. Since most pathologic processes described above require ablation of the LES, the majority of myotomies will be performed from the left. The right-sided approach is best if the patient needs a myotomy of the entire esophagus, except its most inferior aspect. This approach is also useful for a midesophageal diverticulum located on the right side. An antireflux procedure cannot be performed easily from this approach. The working ports are placed to allow maximum vision of the inferior thoracic esophagus and the superior esophagus if needed. The ports are placed in an equilateral triangle, notably much closer than what is normally done in the abdomen, with the videoendoscope located in the fifth intercostal space, just inferior to the scapular tip. The working ports should be located in the posterior axillary line. A fourth port in the anterior axillary line is used by the assistant to retract the lung (Fig. 18–23). Both the surgeon and the assistant stand on the same side of the operating table, which is the ipsilateral side of chosen approach. Thus, both are standing at the patient's back, while the video cart monitor is in front of the patient. Carbon dioxide insufflation is not necessary for the procedure, as single-lung ventilation usually suffices.

The lung is retracted anteriorly after it is deflated (Fig. 18–24). The inferior pulmonary ligament is divided with cautery and blunt dissection, avoiding the inferior pulmonary vein. Once this is accomplished, the pleural reflection over the esophagus is taken down with cautery dissection so that the longitudinal muscle fibers of the esophagus may be identified (Fig. 18–25). At this point, the lighted bougie is passed into the esophagus by the anesthesiologist. By

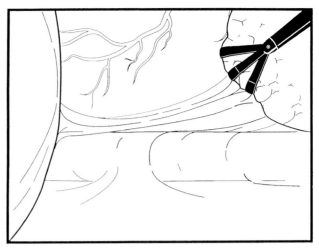

FIG. 18–24. The lung is retracted anteriorly, exposing the pleural reflection over the esophagus.

splaying the muscle fibers of the esophagus over the bougie with one instrument, cautery dissection down to the submucosa is performed. A combination of blunt dissection, spreading, and cauterization is used to divide the muscular layers of the esophagus for the length of the myotomy (Figs. 18–26 and 18–27). Flexible endoscopy should be used to verify the adequacy of the myotomy (Fig. 18–28). The vagus nerves should be avoided during this dissection. If a left-sided approach is used, a partial wrap (Dor or Belsey) may be added. If the right-sided approach is used, then the antireflux procedure is not possible. If a diverticulum is present, it may be dissected to its neck and transected by an automatic stapling and cutting device.

Two chest tubes are placed through trocar sites, and the remaining sites are closed. The patient is allowed to consume a liquid diet on the day of the operation, unless a diverticulum was resected, in which case the diet is started on the

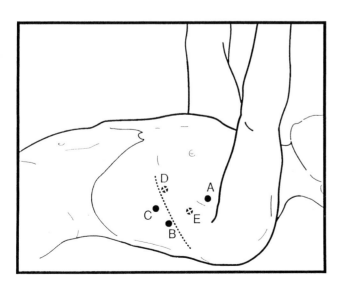

FIG. 18–23. Port placement for a thoracoscopic myotomy. (A) Optional lung retraction port, (B) scope port, (C, E) surgeon's left and right hands, respectively, (D) lung retractor.

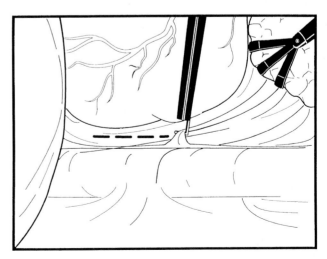

FIG. 18–25. The pleura is incised to expose the esophagus.

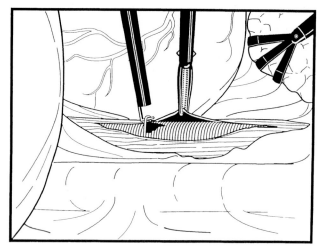

**FIG. 18–26.** The longitudinal and circular muscle fibers are transected.

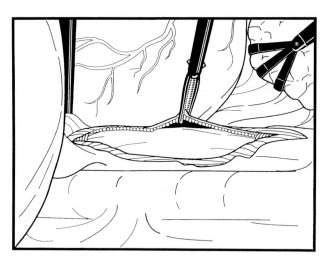

**FIG. 18–27.** Completed myotomy.

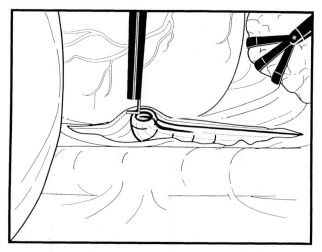

**FIG. 18–28.** Flexible endoscopy is performed to inspect the myotomy.

third postoperative day. Hospital stay varies, but patients are usually discharged within 2 days of starting a diet.

The length of the myotomy varies with each of the disease processes and with the findings of the preoperative evaluation. If HLES without concomitant esophageal body dysmotility is being treated, the myotomy is confined to the distal esophagus, LES, and cardia. If NE is being treated and preoperative manometry revealed high-amplitude contractions in the proximal esophagus, an extended myotomy should be performed, perhaps through a right thoracoscopic approach.

### Outcome

The surgical approach to patients with spastic motility disorders is based mostly on transferred principles from achalasia. Because the number of patients with these disorders is so small, and even fewer of them come to surgical therapy, only limited experience is available. Most information comes from case reports and technique articles [39, 70, 108]. Although no prospective, randomized studies are available comparing medical to surgical therapy, one article prospectively compared the outcome of the two treatments in patients with esophageal motility disorders [94]. In this study, patients with achalasia, DES, and NE were treated by medical therapy, including dilation, or operative therapy based on the request of the referring physician. The operation was performed via left thoracoscopy. Eight of 10 patients with DES or NE had good or excellent relief with surgical treatment. Only eight of 30 patients had the same level of relief with medical therapy. Although this study was not randomized, it did show the benefits of operative therapy over medical therapy. No long-term studies are available to assess the outcome of surgically treated patients.

### Complications

The operative complications are similar to those of myotomy performed for achalasia, except if a diverticulectomy is added. In this case, additional morbidity may be expected from opening the esophageal mucosa. Esophageal leak rates have been reported to be as high as 18% using an open technique [8]. Not enough data are available from videoendoscopic procedures to assess the incidence of esophageal leak.

### Conclusion

Operative intervention for spastic motility is not common. The myotomy should be tailored to the manometric findings. The thoracoscopic approach allows for a longer myotomy if necessary. Dysphagia improves more often than pain after surgical intervention.

## ESOPHAGEAL RESECTION

Resection of the esophagus is usually performed for malignant disease; however, this procedure is contemplated in esophageal motility disorders when certain conditions exist. If the esophagus is severely dilated and elongated after years of untreated disease, some authors have recommended resection as an initial therapy. Benign stricture, occurring as a result of previous intervention or as a natural sequelae of untreated disease, which cannot be treated by dilation is another indication for esophageal resection. Failure of previous operative therapy to relieve symptoms associated with motility disorders is another. Indeed after two or three operations on the esophagus to treat a stricture, esophagectomy is the best alternative. Some have used esophageal resection as treatment for a perforation occurring after dilation, particularly when the esophagus has other underlying pathology.

Patients must be aware of the technical challenge the operation poses. They should be aware of the significant morbidity (20% to 30%) and mortality (2% to 8%) accompanying the operation. Given the information, they may decide their symptoms are more acceptable than the risk of the procedure.

The principles of esophageal resection center on safe, effective removal of the esophagus and replacement using a conduit that allows for adequate nutritional intake. The most common approach to this procedure is a transhiatal approach from the abdomen, using the stomach as the conduit to anastomose to the cervical esophagus.

**Operative Approach**

Patients requiring esophagectomy for esophageal motor disorders are often nutritionally depleted. If preoperative nutritional supplementation is possible with high-calorie, high-protein liquids, some advantage in postoperative healing may be gained. The patients should be on a liquid diet 2 days before the operation to minimize the amount of solid debris present in the esophagus.

The patient is placed in the supine position on the operating table with the head turned to the right. A roll is usually placed across the lumbar area elevating the costal margin. This position facilitates exposure to the cervical esophagus, the abdomen, and the distal thoracic esophagus. The abdominal portion of the operation is performed first.

Generous mobilization of the duodenum is performed, elevating the second and third portions to the patient's left. The stomach is then mobilized along the greater curvature taking care to preserve the gastroepiploic artery. All short gastric vessels are ligated and transected to free the cardia. Division of the lesser omentum and the left gastric artery is performed next. The right gastric artery is carefully preserved. This will free the lesser curvature down to the previously mobilized duodenum. Any posterior attachments of the stomach are freed at this time.

Dissection of the lower esophagus requires a 2- to 3-cm opening of the hiatus. This is performed anteriorly after incising the phrenoesophageal ligament. After the anterior and lateral hiatal attachments are freed, circumferential dissection of the esophagus is completed. The gastroesophageal

junction and the distal 5 cm of the esophagus can be dissected sharply from the abdomen.

Posterior mediastinal dissection of the esophagus is performed bluntly. The plane of dissection is along the longitudinal muscle fibers of the esophagus. The pleura should not be violated. Blunt dissection can be performed to the thoracic outlet. During the blunt dissection of the esophagus, a second team (if available) may perform the neck dissection. Otherwise, the transhiatal dissection should proceed as far as possible prior to starting the neck dissection. Dissection of the esophagus is greatly facilitated if a bougie (no. 38 to 48 French) is placed and left in the lumen.

The approach to the cervical esophagus is similar to that of a pharyngoesophageal diverticulum. The longitudinal incision along the sternocleidomastoid muscle is extended to the suprasternal notch. The incision is developed through the avascular plane anterior to the sternocleidomastoid muscle. The carotid sheath is retracted laterally, the thyroid medially. Often, the middle thyroid vein is ligated and transected, as is the omohyoid muscle, to improve exposure. As the tracheoesophageal groove is approached, care must be taken to avoid injuring the recurrent laryngeal nerve. A bougie may be used to identify the extent of the esophageal diameter. Circumferential dissection of the esophagus is completed and a small Penrose drain is passed around the esophagus. The esophagus is then mobilized by a combination of blunt and sharp dissection toward the thoracic outlet. A sponge stick may be used to mobilize the inferior cervical esophagus. Simultaneous transhiatal and cervical dissection is done to facilitate esophageal mobilization. When the esophagus has been completely mobilized, a pyloroplasty is performed.

The stomach is then transected with an automatic stapling and cutting device so that a tube of stomach is created along the greater curvature. The stapler is placed at a point on the greater curvature 5 cm to the left of the gastroesophageal junction and angled toward the incisura on the lesser curvature. Two loads of the automatic stapling and cutting device may be necessary. The portion of stomach attached to the esophagus is then sutured to a short segment of surgical tubing. The tubing is sutured to the tubular stomach. The esophagus is then delivered from the cervical incision, carrying the replacement conduit behind. The stomach should be guided into the chest to prevent torsion and undue pressure on the sutures.

Once the stomach is in the neck, the surgical tubing is removed. The stomach should reach the planned site of the anastomosis easily. Any tension will increase the likelihood of an anastomotic leak postoperatively. If too much tension is present, the stomach must either be mobilized more, or an alternative conduit should be considered.

A point on the cervical esophagus is chosen for the anastomosis. A double-layered anastomosis is performed using interrupted nonabsorbable material on the outside and a running absorbable suture on the inside. The posterior outer layer should be placed prior to transecting the esophagus.

When the anastomosis is completed, the incisions are closed. The neck incision is drained with closed suction to allow egress of luminal contents in case a leak occurs.

Patients are admitted to the intensive care unit for cardiopulmonary support and monitoring for postoperative bleeding. If the patient progresses well after the first day, he or she may be transferred out of the intensive care unit. A liquid diet is started on the third postoperative day. If an anastomotic leak is suspected, a barium contrast study is performed prior to the initiation of a diet. Patients are instructed to eat small meals in an upright position to limit gastric distention in the chest and facilitate transit to the abdominal portion of the stomach.

### Outcome

Using the stomach as conduit, 78% of patients are able to swallow well and require no further intervention [80]. Although they will not have normal transit, they are able to maintain their weight and nutritional status. Less than 5% of patients have regurgitation that requires lifestyle modification consisting mostly of head elevation while supine. Overall, long-term follow-up 5 years after operative therapy shows good to excellent results in 68% of patients when all aspects of quality of life are considered [80]. Others have reported good results in 90% of patients undergoing esophageal resection for recurrent achalasia [75].

### Complications

Perioperative mortality ranges from 2% to 8% [23, 25, 80]. Intraoperative death usually occurs from bleeding which occurs during the blunt dissection in the mediastinum. Postoperative deaths occur as a result of nosocomial infections or an exacerbation of preexisting conditions [23].

In a review of 23 papers reporting transhiatal esophagectomy in 1,353 patients, the most common complications after surgery were found to be anastomotic leak (15%) and anastomotic stricture (14%) [59]. Most leaks may be treated without further operative intervention. Maintaining nutritional support and drainage of the wound via the closed suction catheter are all that is required. Anastomotic stricture is thought to occur as a result of a narrow anastomosis and the occurrence of a postoperative leak [50]. Other complications include hoarseness due to recurrent laryngeal nerve injury, symptomatic gastroesophageal reflux, and infection. Perioperative cardiac dysrhythmia has been reported in nearly 50% of patients but can be controlled medically [92].

### Controversies

The conduit used for esophageal replacement and the surgical approach to replacement are the main controversies in esophageal replacement. Of the conduits available, the stomach and the colon are the most common. The advantages of using the stomach are that only one anastomosis is performed as opposed to three, the blood supply to the stomach is better than that of the colon, and the plasticity of the stomach allows for easier lengthening [23, 25, 80]. Those who favor the colon as a conduit state that a longer segment may be replaced by the colon with less tension and long-term function is better [66, 120]. Furthermore, the likelihood of regurgitation and anastomotic stricture as a result of acid exposure is less with colonic interposition. Still, most gastrointestinal surgeons continue to use the stomach as the conduit of choice.

The surgical approach to a total esophagectomy for benign disease is accomplished efficiently through a transhiatal approach. The benefit is that the patient need not have a thoracotomy, with its inherent morbidity of the incision and single lung-ventilation. Although the procedure can be accomplished via a combined thoracoabdominal approach, this is generally not necessary for benign disease [25, 46]. A discussion of esophagectomy for malignancy can be found elsewhere in this book.

### Conclusion

The esophagus can be safely resected and replaced with the stomach. The patient should fully understand the risks of the operation, especially if it is being considered for benign disease. Operative principles include preservation of the blood supply of the stomach, careful mediastinal dissection, and a tension-free anastomosis. Patients will have a good functional outcome in 78% to 90% of cases. Benign stricture and anastomotic leak are the most common technical complications of the procedure.

## REFERENCES

1. Abid S, Champion G, Richter JE, McElvein R, Slaughter RL, Koehler RE. Treatment of achalasia: the best of both worlds. Am J Gastroenterol 1994;89:979
2. Agur A. Grant's Atlas of Anatomy. Baltimore: Williams & Wilkins, 1991:650
3. Ancona E, Peracchia A, Zaninotto G, Rossi M, Bonavina L, Segalin A. Heller laparoscopic cardiomyotomy with antireflux anterior fundoplication (Dor) in the treatment of esophageal achalasia. Surg Endosc 1993;7:459
4. Ancona E, et al. Esophageal achalasia: laparoscopic versus conventional open Heller–Dor operation. Am J Surg 1995;170:265
5. Anselmino M, et al. Heller myotomy is superior to dilatation for the treatment of early achalasia. Arch Surg 1997;132:233
6. Barkin JS, Guelrud M, Reiner DK, Goldberg RI, Phillips RS. Forceful balloon dilation: an outpatient procedure for achalasia. Gastrointest Endosc 1990;36:123
7. Barthlen W, Feussner H, Hannig C, Holscher AH, Siewert JR. Surgical therapy of Zenker's diverticulum: low risk and high efficiency. Dysphagia 1990;5:13
8. Benacci JC, Deschamps C, Trastek VF, Allen MS, Daly RC, Pairolero PC. Epiphrenic diverticulum: results of surgical treatment. Ann Thorac Surg 1993;55:1109; discussion 1114
9. Benjamin B, Innocenti M. Laser treatment of pharyngeal pouch. Aust N Z J Surg 1991;61:909
10. Bonavina L, Nosadini A, Bardini R, Baessato M, Peracchia A. Primary treatment of esophageal achalasia. Long-term results of myotomy and Dor fundoplication. Arch Surg 1992;127:222; discussion
11. Bourgeois N, Coffernils M, Sznajer Y, Panzer JM, Gelin M, Cremer

M. Non-surgical management of achalasia. Acta Gastroenterol Belg 1992;55:260

12. Bradwell RA, Bieger AK, Strachan DR, Homer JJ. Endoscopic laser myotomy in the treatment of pharyngeal diverticula. J Laryngol Otol 1997;111:627

13. Brady AP, Stevenson GW, Somers S, Hough DM, Di GE. Premature contraction of the cricopharyngeus: a new sign of gastroesophageal reflux disease. Abdom Imaging 1995;20:225

14. Cade RJ, Martin CJ. Thoracoscopic cardiomyotomy for achalasia. Aust N Z J Surg 1996;66:107

15. Ciarolla DA, Traube M. Achalasia. Short-term clinical monitoring after pneumatic dilation. Dig Dis Sci 1993;38:1905

16. Collard JM, Otte JB, Kestens PJ. Endoscopic stapling technique of esophagodiverticulostomy for Zenker's diverticulum. Ann Thorac Surg 1993;56:573

17. Collard JM, Romagnoli R, Lengele B, Salizzoni M, Kestens PJ. Heller–Dor procedure for achalasia: from conventional to video-endoscopic surgery. Acta Chir Belg 1996;96:62

18. Cote DN, Miller RH. The association of gastroesophageal reflux and otolaryngologic disorders. Comprehens Ther 1995;21:80

19. Crookes PF, Corkill S, DeMeester TR. Gastroesophageal reflux in achalasia. When is reflux really reflux? Dig Dis Sci 1997;42:1354

20. Csendes A, Velasco N, Braghetto I, Henriquez A. A prospective randomized study comparing forceful dilatation and esophagomyotomy in patients with achalasia of the esophagus. Gastroenterology 1981; 80:789

21. Csendes A, Braghetto I, Mascaro J, Henriquez A. Late subjective and objective evaluation of the results of esophagomyotomy in 100 patients with achalasia of the esophagus. Surgery 1988;104:469

22. Csendes A, Braghetto I, Henriquez A, Cortes C. Late results of a prospective randomised study comparing forceful dilatation and oesophagomyotomy in patients with achalasia. Gut 1989;30:299

23. Daniel TM, Fleischer KJ, Flanagan TL, Tribble CG, Kron IL. Transhiatal esophagectomy: a safe alternative for selected patients. Ann Thorac Surg 1992;54:686; discussion 689

24. Dantas RO, Cook IJ, Dodds WJ, Kern MK, Lang IM, Brasseur JG. Biomechanics of cricopharyngeal bars. Gastroenterology 1990;99: 1269

25. Davis EA, Heitmiller RF. Esophagectomy for benign disease: trends in surgical results and management. Ann Thorac Surg 1996;62:369

26. Delgado F, et al. Laparoscopic treatment of esophageal achalasia. Surg Laparosc Endosc 1996;6:83

27. Di SMP, et al. Onset timing of delayed complications and criteria of follow-up after operation for esophageal achalasia. Ann Thorac Surg 1996;61:1106; discussion 1110

28. D'Ugo D, Cardillo G, Granone P, Coppola R, Margaritora S, Picciocchi A. Esophageal diverticula. Physiopathological basis for surgical management. Eur J Card Thorac Surg 1992;6:330

29. Efrati Y, Horne T, Livshitz G, Broide E, Klin B, Vinograd I. Radionuclide esophageal emptying and long-acting nitrates (Nitroderm) in childhood achalasia. J Pediatr Gastroenterol Nutr 1996;23:312

30. Ekberg O. Cricopharyngeal bar: myth and reality. Abdom Imaging 1995;20:179

31. Ellingson TL, Kozarek RA, Gelfand MD, Botoman AV, Patterson DJ. Iatrogenic achalasia. A case series. J Clin Gastroenterol 1995;20: 96

32. Ellis FH. Esophagomyotomy by the thoracic approach for esophageal achalasia. Hepato-Gastroenterology 1991;38:498

33. Ellis FH Jr. Invited letter concerning: Technique for prevention of gastroesophageal reflux after transthoracic Heller's operation. J Thorac Cardiovasc Surg 1993;105:555

34. Ellis FH Jr. Pharyngoesophageal (Zenker's) diverticulum. Adv Surg 1995;28:171

35. Ellis FH Jr, Watkins E Jr, Gibb SP, Heatley GJ. Ten to 20-year clinical results after short esophagomyotomy without an antireflux procedure (modified Heller operation) for esophageal achalasia. Eur J Card Thorac Surg 1992;6:86; discussion 90

36. Engel JJ, Panje WR. Endoscopic laser Zenker's diverticulotomy. Gastrointest Endosc 1995;42:368

37. Eypasch EP, Stein HJ, DeMeester TR, Johansson KE, Barlow AP, Schneider GT. A new technique to define and clarify esophageal motor disorders. Am J Surg 1990;159:144; discussion 151

38. Ferguson MK, Reeder LB, Olak J. Results of myotomy and partial fundoplication after pneumatic dilation for achalasia. Ann Thorac Surg 1996;62:327

39. Filipi CJ, Hinder RA. Thoracoscopic esophageal myotomy—a surgical technique for achalasia diffuse esophageal spasm and "nutcracker esophagus." Surg Endosc 1994;8:921; discussion 925

40. Flynn AE, Verrier ED, Way LW, Thomas AN, Pellegrini CA. Esophageal perforation. Arch Surg 1989;124:1211; discussion 1214

41. Fremling C, Raivio M, Karppinen I. Endoscopic discision of Zenker's diverticulum. Ann Chir Gynaecol 1995;84:169

42. Gatzinsky P, Dernevik L, Bjork S, Sandberg N. Technique for prevention of gastroesophageal reflux after transthoracic Heller's operation. J Thorac Cardiovasc Surg 1993;105:553

43. Gayet B, Fekete F. Surgical management of failed esophagomyotomy (Heller's operation). Hepato-Gastroenterology 1991;38:488

44. Graham AJ, Finley RJ, Worsley DF, Dong SR, Clifton JC, Storseth C. Laparoscopic esophageal myotomy and anterior partial fundoplication for the treatment of achalasia. Ann Thorac Surg 1997;64:785

45. Gregoire J, Duranceau A. Surgical management of Zenker's diverticulum. Hepato-Gastroenterology 1992;39:132

46. Gupta NM, Goenka MK, Behera A, Bhasin DK. Transhiatal oesophagectomy for benign obstructive conditions of the oesophagus. Br J Surg 1997;84:262

47. Herberhold C, Walther EK. Endoscopic laser myotomy in cricopharyngeal achalasia. Adv Oto Rhino Laryngol 1995;49:144

48. Holinger PH, Johnston KC. Endoscopic surgery of Zenker's diverticula. Experience with the Dohlman technique. Ann Otol Rhinol Laryngol 1995;104:751

49. Holzman MD, Sharp KW, Ladipo JK, Eller RF, Holcomb GWR, Richards WO. Laparoscopic surgical treatment of achalasia. Am J Surg 1997;173:308

50. Honkoop P, et al. Benign anastomotic strictures after transhiatal esophagectomy and cervical esophagogastrostomy: risk factors and management. J Thorac Cardiovasc Surg 1996;111:1141; discussion 1147

51. Horgan S HK, Eubanks TR, Pellegrini CA. Does botox injection make esophagomyotomy a more difficult operation? Presented at SAGES Scientific Session, Seattle, WA, April 1–4, 1998

52. Hunter JG, Trus TL, Branum GD, Waring JP. Laparoscopic Heller myotomy and fundoplication for achalasia. Ann Surg 1997;225:655; discussion 664

53. Illi OE, Stauffer UG. Achalasia in childhood and adolescence. Eur J Pediatr Surg 1994;4:214

54. Ishioka S, Sakai P, Maluf FF, Melo JM. Endoscopic incision of Zenker's diverticula. Endoscopy 1995;27:433

55. Jaakkola A, Reinikainen P, Ovaska J, Isolauri J. Barrett's esophagus after cardiomyotomy for esophageal achalasia. Am J Gastroenterol 1994;89:165

56. Johnson O. Achalasia of the cardia: experience of extramucosal cardiomyotomy during a ten-year period. Ethiop Med J 1994;32:89

57. Jorgensen JO, Hunt DR. Laparoscopic management of pneumatic dilatation resistant achalasia. Aust N Z J Surg 1993;63:386

58. Katada N, et al. The hypertensive lower esophageal sphincter. Am J Surg 1996;172:439; discussion 442

59. Katariya K, Harvey JC, Pina E, Beattie EJ. Complications of transhiatal esophagectomy. J Surg Oncol 1994;57:157

60. Laccourreye O, et al. Esophageal diverticulum: diverticulopexy versus diverticulectomy. Laryngoscope 1994;104:889

61. Laing MR, Murthy P, Ah SKW, Cockburn JS. Surgery for pharyngeal pouch: audit of management with short- and long-term follow-up. J R Coll Surg Edinburgh 1995;40:315

62. Lerut T, et al. Pharyngo-oesophageal diverticulum (Zenker's). Clinical, therapeutic and morphological aspects. Acta Gastroenterol Belg 1990;53:330

63. Lerut T, van Raemdonck D, Guelinckx P, Dom R, Geboes K. Zenker's diverticulum: is a myotomy of the cricopharyngeus useful? How long should it be? Hepato-Gastroenterology 1992;39:127

64. Louie HW, Zuckerbraun L. Staged Zenker's diverticulectomy with cervical esophagostomy and secondary esophagostomy closure for treatment of massive diverticulum in severely debilitated patients. Am Surg 1993;59:842

65. Makela J, Kiviniemi H, Laitinen S. Heller's cardiomyotomy compared with pneumatic dilatation for treatment of oesophageal achalasia. Eur J Surg 1991;157:411

66. Mansour KA, Bryan FC, Carlson GW. Bowel interposition for esophageal replacement: twenty-five-year experience. Ann Thorac Surg 1997;64:752

67. Martins P, Morais BB, Cunha MJR. Postoperative complications in the treatment of chagasic megaesophagus. Int Surg 1993;78:99

68. Mattioli S, Pilotti V, Felice V, Di S-MP, D'Ovidio F, Gozzetti G. Intraoperative study on the relationship between the lower esophageal sphincter pressure and the muscular components of the gastro-esophageal junction in achalasic patients. Ann Surg 1993;218:635

69. Mattox HE, Albertson DA, Castell DO, Richter JE. Dysphagia following fundoplication: "slipped" fundoplication versus achalasia complicated by fundoplication. Am J Gastroenterol 1990;85:1468

70. McBride PJ, et al. Surgical treatment of spastic conditions of the esophagus. Int Surg 1997;82:113

71. McConnel FM, Hood D, Jackson K, O'Connor A. Analysis of intrabolus forces in patients with Zenker's diverticulum. Laryngoscope 1994;104:571

72. McJunkin B, McMillan WO Jr, Duncan HE Jr, Harman KM, White JJ Jr, McJunkin JE. Assessment of dilation methods in achalasia: large diameter mercury bougienage followed by pneumatic dilation as needed. Gastrointest Endosc 1991;37:18

73. Mearin F, et al. Patients with achalasia lack nitric oxide synthase in the gastro-oesophageal junction. Eur J Clin Inves 1993;23:724

74. Migliore M, Payne H, Jeyasingham K. Pathophysiologic basis for operation on Zenker's diverticulum. Ann Thorac Surg 1994;57:1616; discussion 1620

75. Miller DL, Allen MS, Trastek VF, Deschamps C, Pairolero PC. Esophageal resection for recurrent achalasia. Ann Thorac Surg 1995;60:922; discussion 925

76. Miyata M, Sakamoto T, Hashimoto T, Nakamura M, Sakaguchi H, Kawashima Y. Effect of secretin on lower esophageal sphincter pressure in patients with esophageal achalasia. Gastroenterol Japon 1991;26:712

77. Monnig PJ. Familial achalasia in children. Ann Thorac Surg 1990;49:1019

78. Morino M, Rebecchi F, Festa V, Garrone C. Laparoscopic Heller cardiomyotomy with intraoperative manometry in the management of oesophageal achalasia. Int Surg 1995;80:332

79. Myers NA, Jolley SG, Taylor R. Achalasia of the cardia in children: a worldwide survey. J Pediatr Surg 1994;29:1375

80. Orringer MB, Marshall B, Stirling MC. Transhiatal esophagectomy for benign and malignant disease. J Thorac Cardiovasc Surg 1993;105:265; disccusion 276

81. Nathanson LK, Gotley D, Smithers M, Branicki F. Videothoracoscopic primary repair of early distal oesophageal perforation. Aust N Z J Surg 1993;63:399

82. Nguyen HC, Urquhart AC. Zenker's diverticulum. Laryngoscope 1997;107:1436

83. Niwamoto H, Okamoto E, Fujimoto J, Takeuchi M, Furuyama J, Yamamoto Y. Are human herpes viruses or measles virus associated with esophageal achalasia? Dig Dis Sci 1995;40:859

84. Pandolfo N, Bortolotti M, Spigno L, Bozzano PL, Mattioli FP. Manometric assessment of Heller–Dor operation for esophageal achalasia. Hepato-Gastroenterology 1996;43:160

85. Parkman HP, Reynolds JC, Ouyang A, Rosato EF, Eisenberg JM, Cohen S. Pneumatic dilatation or esophagomyotomy treatment for idiopathic achalasia: clinical outcomes and cost analysis. Dig Dis Sci 1993;38:75

86. Parkman HP, Ogorek CP, Harris AD, Cohen S. Nonoperative management of esophageal strictures following esophagomyotomy for achalasia. Dig Dis Sci 1994;39:2102

87. Parrilla PP, Martinez DHL, Ortiz A, Aguayo JL. Achalasia of the cardia: long-term results of oesophagomyotomy and posterior partial fundoplication. Br J Surg 1990;77:1371

88. Parrilla P, Aguayo JL, Martinez DHL, Ortiz A, Martinez DA, Morales G. Reversible achalasia-like motor pattern of esophageal body secondary to postoperative stricture of gastroesophageal junction. Dig Dis Sci 1992;37:1781

89. Parrilla PP, Martinez DHLF, Ortiz EA, Morales CG, Molina MJ. Short myotomy for vigorous achalasia. Br J Surg 1993;80:1540

90. Parrilla P, Martinez DHLF, Ortiz A, Morales G, Garay V, Aguilar J. Factors involved in the return of peristalsis in patients with achalasia of the cardia after Heller's myotomy. Am J Gastroenterol 1995;90:713

91. Pasricha PJ, Kalloo AN. Recent advances in the treatment of achalasia. Gastrointest Endosc Clin North Am 1997;7:191

92. Patti MG, Wiener KJP, Way LW, Pellegrini CA. Impact of transhiatal esophagectomy on cardiac and respiratory function. Am J Surg 1991;162:563; discussion 566

93. Patti MG, Arcerito M, Pellegrini CA. Thoracoscopic and laparoscopic Heller's myotomy in the treatment of esophageal achalasia. Ann Chir Gynaecol 1995;84:159

94. Patti MG, et al. Comparison of medical and minimally invasive surgical therapy for primary esophageal motility disorders. Arch Surg 1995;130:609; discussion 615

95. Patti MG, Pellegrini CA. Endoscopic surgical treatment of primary oesophageal motility disorders. J R Coll Surg Edinburgh 1996;41:137

96. Pellegrini C, et al. Thoracoscopic esophagomyotomy. Initial experience with a new approach for the treatment of achalasia. Ann Surg 1992;216:291; discussion 296

97. Pellegrini CA, Leichter R, Patti M, Somberg K, Ostroff JW, Way L. Thoracoscopic esophageal myotomy in the treatment of achalasia. Ann Thorac Surg 1993;56:680

98. Peracchia A, Rosati R, Bona S, Fumagalli U, Bonavina L, Chella B. Laparoscopic treatment of functional diseases of the esophagus. Int Surg 1995;80:336

99. Peters JH, Kauer WK, Crookes PF, Ireland AP, Bremner CG, DeMeester TR. Esophageal resection with colon interposition for end-stage achalasia. Arch Surg 1995;130:632; discussion 636

100. Pricolo VE, Park CS, Thompson WR. Surgical repair of esophageal perforation due to pneumatic dilatation for achalasia. Is myotomy really necessary? Arch Surg 1993;128:540; discussion 543

101. Raiser F, et al. Heller myotomy via minimal-access surgery. An evaluation of antireflux procedures. Arch Surg 1996;131:593; discussion 597

102. Richter JE. Surgery or pneumatic dilatation for achalasia: a head-to-head comparison. Now are all the questions answered? Gastroenterology 1989;97:1340

103. Robertson CS, Martin BA, Atkinson M. Varicella-zoster virus DNA in the oesophageal myenteric plexus in achalasia. Gut 1993;34:299

104. Scher RL, Richtsmeier WJ. Endoscopic staple-assisted esophagodiverticulostomy for Zenker's diverticulum. Laryngoscope 1996;106:951

105. Schmit PJ, Zuckerbraun L. Treatment of Zenker's diverticula by cricopharyngeus myotomy under local anesthesia. Am Surg 1992;58:710

106. Schwartz HM, Cahow CE, Traube M. Outcome after perforation sustained during pneumatic dilatation for achalasia. Dig Dis Sci 1993;38:1409

107. Shimi S, Nathanson LK, Cuschieri A. Laparoscopic cardiomyotomy for achalasia. J R Coll Surg Edinburgh 1991;36:152

108. Shimi SM, Nathanson LK, Cuschieri A. Thoracoscopic long oesophageal myotomy for nutcracker oesophagus: initial experience of a new surgical approach. Br J Surg 1992;79:533

109. Shoenut JP, Micflikier AB, Yaffe CS, Den BB, Teskey JM. Reflux in untreated achalasia patients. J Clin Gastroenterol 1995;20:6

110. Shoenut JP, Duerksen D, Yaffe CS. A prospective assessment of gastroesophageal reflux before and after treatment of achalasia patients: pneumatic dilation versus transthoracic limited myotomy. Am J Gastroenterol 1997;92:1109

111. Slim K, Pezet D, Chipponi J, Boulant J, Mathieu S. Laparoscopic myotomy for primary esophageal achalasia: prospective evaluation. Hepato-Gastroenterology 1997;44:11

112. Spiro SA, Berg HM. Applying the endoscopic stapler in excision of Zenker's diverticulum: a solution for two intraoperative problems. Otolaryngol Head Neck Surg 1994;110:603

113. Stacher G, et al. Sensitivity of radionuclide bolus transport and videofluoroscopic studies compared with manometry in the detection of achalasia. Am J Gastroenterol 1994;89:1484

114. Stein HJ, DeMeester TR, Eypasch EP, Klingman RR. Ambulatory 24-hour esophageal manometry in the evaluation of esophageal motor disorders and noncardiac chest pain. Surgery 1991;110:753; discussion 761

115. Stein HJ, Korn O, Liebermann MD. Manometric vector volume analysis to assess lower esophageal sphincter function. Ann Chir Gynaecol 1995;84:151

116. Stuart RC, Byrne PJ, Lawlor P, O'Sullivan G, Hennessy TP. Meal area index: a new technique for quantitative assessment in achalasia by ambulatory manometry during eating. Br J Surg 1992;79:1162

117. Supe AN, Samsi AB, Bapat RD, Mathur SK, Ramakantan R. Pneumatic dilatation in achalasia cardia results and follow-up. J Postgrad Med 1990;36:181

118. Tack J, Janssens J, Vantrappen G. Non-surgical treatment of achalasia. Hepato-Gastroenterology 1991;38:493

119. Watemberg S, Landau O, Avrahami R. Zenker's diverticulum: reappraisal. Am J Gastroenter 1996;91:1494

120. Watson TJ, Peters JH, DeMeester TR. Esophageal replacement for end-stage benign esophageal disease. Surg Clin North Am 1997;77:1099

121. Westrin KM, Ergun S, Carlsoo B. Zenker's diverticulum—a historical review and trends in therapy. Acta Oto Laryngol 1996;116:351

122. Wouters B, van Overbeek JJ. Pathogenesis and endoscopic treatment of the hypopharyngeal (Zenker's) diverticulum. Acta Gastroenterol Belg 1990;53:323

123. Wouters B, van Overbeek JJ. Endoscopic treatment of the hypopharyngeal (Zenker's) diverticulum. Hepato-Gastroenterology 1992;39:105

124. Ximenes MR. Esophageal resection for recurrent achalasia. Ann Thorac Surg 1996;62:322

125. Xynos E, Tzovaras G, Petrakis I, Chrysos E, Vassilakis JS. Laparoscopic Heller's cardiomyotomy and Dor's fundoplication for esophageal achalasia. J Laparoendosc Surg 1996;6:253

126. Zaninotto G, Costantini M, Anselmino M, Boccu C, Ancona E. Onset of oesophageal peristalsis after surgery for idiopathic achalasia. Br J Surg 1995;82:1532

127. Zeitoun H, Widdowson D, Hammad Z, Osborne J. A video-fluoroscopic study of patients treated by diverticulectomy and cricopharyngeal myotomy. Clin Otolaryngol 1994;19:301

128. van Overbeek JJ. Meditation on the pathogenesis of hypopharyngeal (Zenker's) diverticulum and a report of endoscopic treatment in 545 patients. Ann Otol Rhinol Laryngol 1994;103:178

129. van Overbeek JJ. Microendoscopic $CO_2$ laser surgery of the hypopharyngeal (Zenker's) diverticulum. Adv Oto Rhino Laryngol 1995;49:140

130. Vara TC, Herrainz R. Esophageal achalasia: laparoscopic Heller cardiomyotomy. Int Surg 1995;80:376

131. Venturi M, et al. Biochemical markers of upper esophageal sphincter compliance in patients with Zenker's diverticulum. J Surg Research 1997;70:46

132. von Doersten PG, Byl FM. Endoscopic Zenker's diverticulotomy (Dohlman procedure): forty cases reviewed. Otolaryngol Head Neck Surg 1997;116:209

The Esophagus, Third Edition,
edited by D. O. Castell and J. E. Richter.
Lippincott Williams & Wilkins, Philadelphia © 1999.

CHAPTER 19

# Clinical Spectrum and Diagnosis of Gastroesophageal Reflux Disease

Elizabeth Klinkenberg-Knol and Donald O. Castell

## CLINICAL SPECTRUM

Thirty years ago, most reflux symptoms were attributed to hiatal hernia [29]. Twenty years ago, the diagnosis offered for the same symptoms would probably have been esophagitis. In recent times, use of the acronym *GERD* has become popular to describe the clinical manifestations of gastroesophageal reflux disease, including the variety of symptoms and forms of tissue damage secondary to the reflux of gastric contents. Presentations of GERD vary widely but can be logically placed into three different categories: typical symptoms, atypical symptoms, and complications. These comprise the spectrum of GERD (Fig. 19–1). In addition, reflux occurring in normal people that does not cause symptoms or esophageal mucosal injury is called *physiologic reflux*.

### Typical Symptoms

Heartburn and regurgitation are the typical symptoms of GERD. When present as predominant symptoms, they are usually quite specific, although not very sensitive [21]. Thus, GERD cannot be excluded in the absence of heartburn or regurgitation, including pathologic reflux leading to esophageal or extraesophageal manifestations with tissue injury. Less than half of patients with typical symptoms, however, will actually have endoscopic evidence of esophagitis, and in fact, neither the pattern nor the severity of these symptoms can be used to predict the presence or absence of esophagitis [29, 34, 40]. The patient with typical reflux symptoms but without endoscopic esophagitis presents a more difficult diagnostic problem. Heartburn and regurgitation during intercourse, referred to as *reflux dyspareunia,* are manifestations of reflux disease that are not commonly discussed. In one

series of 100 women with chronic reflux symptoms, 77% complained of troubling heartburn during intercourse [20]. The majority reported a favorable response to appropriate antireflux therapy, including avoidance of the ''missionary'' position.

### Atypical Symptoms

Angina-like chest pain, even with an exertional component, is one of the less typical symptoms of GERD. Ambulatory recording of intraesophageal pH has been used to document directly the relationship of chest pain episodes to reflux. Findings of such studies indicate that in approximately 50% of patients, noncardiac chest pain may be attributable to abnormal reflux [2, 4, 5, 10, 32].

Reflux also may be present as chronic hoarseness or other voice abnormalities associated with posterior inflammation of the larynx and vocal cords, a manifestation often referred to as *reflux laryngitis.* When studied with prolonged pH monitoring, more than 75% of such patients have been shown to have abnormal reflux, and acid exposure in the hypopharynx can be documented occasionally [18, 33, 39]. It has even been suggested that chronic reflux injury may eventually lead to malignant changes. Ward and Hanson [37] reported the diagnosis of laryngeal cancer in 19 of 138 patients with moderate or severe reflux during a 10-year period. None of these patients smoked or consumed alcohol, activities usually expected to be associated with laryngeal malignancies.

A variety of pulmonary symptoms may be associated with GERD. Nocturnal episodes of nonallergic asthma, particularly when preceded by a history of chronic reflux symptoms, are highly suggestive of reflux disease. Intraesophageal pH monitoring studies have demonstrated abnormal amounts of reflux in more than 20% of patients with chronic cough [12] and more than 80% of unselected patients with

E. Klinkenberg-Knol: Department of Gastroenterology, Free University Hospital, 1007 MB Amsterdam, The Netherlands.

D. O. Castell: Department of Medicine, Graduate Hospital, Philadelphia, Pennsylvania 19146.

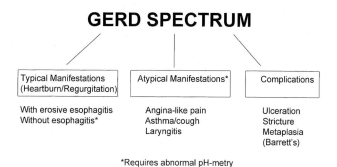

**FIG. 19–1.** Demonstration of the various manifestations comprising the clinical spectrum of gastroesophageal reflux disease (GERD).

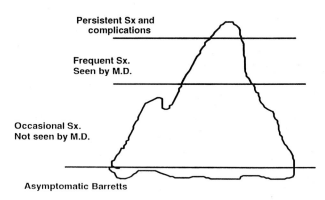

**FIG. 19–2.** The gastroesophageal reflux disease (GERD) iceberg displays the clinical presentations of typical manifestations. Details are provided in text. *Sx,* symptoms.

chronic asthma [35]. Although pH monitoring may show that pulmonary symptoms occur after a reflux episode, often they may occur during reflux or even before it, making it hard to ascertain whether reflux is causing coughing or coughing is causing reflux [9].

Protracted hiccups also have been observed in reflux patients. In one such case, hiccups resolved in response to treatment with cimetidine and recurred on esophageal exposure to acid during a Bernstein test [8]. A specific causal relationship has recently been questioned since changes in esophageal pressures during hiccups may actually be likely to cause reflux [24]. A variety of other atypical symptoms of GERD have been suggested. These include night sweats, loss of dental enamel, ear pain, and intermittent torticollis or peculiar posturing in children (Sandifer's syndrome).

## Complications

GERD can also present as severe, potentially life-threatening complications, such as erosive or ulcerative esophagitis and dysphagia secondary to peptic stricture. Such complications are frequently associated with the metaplastic changes of the epithelium referred to as Barrett's esophagus. In one study, 12% of unselected patients with chronic symptoms of heartburn and regurgitation had endoscopic and histologic changes in the esophageal epithelium consistent with Barrett's esophagus [40].

## PREVALENCE

Quantitative estimates of the actual prevalence of GERD in the United States are difficult to obtain because of the sparsity of epidemiologic studies and because many patients do not seek medical care for their symptoms. One often-cited study provided information on the prevalence of heartburn from a questionnaire survey of 1,004 individuals [27]. Included in the study population were 335 normal controls, 200 surgical inpatients, 246 medical inpatients, 121 patients attending a gastrointestinal clinic, and 102 pregnant patients attending an obstetrics clinic (Table 19–1). Overall, 11% of the entire study group reported daily heartburn, and an additional 12% and 15% described weekly or monthly heartburn, respectively, resulting in a total prevalence of 38% for heartburn in this sample of U.S. adults. The substantially higher prevalence of daily heartburn (25%) described by pregnant women in the obstetrics clinic as compared with subjects in the other four groups reflects the well-known association between heartburn and pregnancy. The popular concepts that heartburn occurs daily in approximately 10% of U.S. adults and that more than one-third have occasional heartburn had their genesis in these data.

The concept of the GERD iceberg, shown in Fig. 19–2, was developed to demonstrate the clinical presentation of typical GERD symptoms. The majority of patients with heartburn and regurgitation have intermittent symptoms for which they do not consult their physicians and for which

**TABLE 19–1.** *Estimated heartburn prevalence in the United States*

| Study group | No. of patients | Percentage experiencing heartburn | | | |
|---|---|---|---|---|---|
| | | Daily | Weekly | Monthly | Total |
| Controls | 335 | 7 | 14 | 15 | 36 |
| Surgical inpatients | 200 | 6 | 12 | 19 | 37 |
| Medical inpatients | 246 | 14 | 12 | 14 | 40 |
| Gastrointestinal clinic patients | 121 | 15 | 12 | 13 | 40 |
| Obstetrics clinic patients | 102 | 25 | 10 | 17 | 52 |
| Total | 1,004 | 11 | 12 | 15 | 38 |

From ref. 27, with permission.

they frequently take over-the-counter medications. Those with more persistent symptoms are more likely to see a physician for advice, with a small percentage of symptomatic individuals (probably 10% or less) represented by that group with complicated GERD seen by the gastroenterologist. One disturbing element in this clinical scenario is the group of patients who have Barrett's esophagus, even progressing to adenocarcinoma, who are "silent" refluxers and who do not present themselves for evaluation. In one study, 28% of patients presenting with symptomatic adenocarcinoma in a Barrett's esophagus had no preceding history of reflux symptoms [3].

## INFLUENCE OF FOOD ON REFLUX SYMPTOMS

Although the specific etiology of GERD has not been established, there appear to be definite relationships between symptoms and certain foods. An early study from our laboratory provided data from a detailed survey of intolerance to 39 different types of food in 50 patients, 25 with daily heartburn and 25 with only monthly symptoms [27]. Comparison of food intolerance with resting lower esophageal sphincter (LES) pressure measurements revealed interesting relationships, as shown in Fig. 19–3. A significant inverse correlation was found between the number of food intolerances and LES pressure. Patients with a normal LES pressure tended to experience heartburn only after consuming certain foods, including fried foods, spicy foods, and hot dogs, whereas those with a very low LES pressure experienced reflux symptoms with almost all types of food surveyed. Mean LES pressure was significantly lower for the 25 daily heartburn

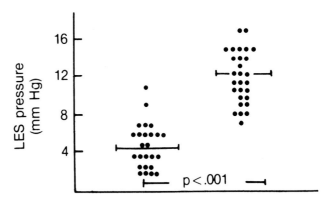

FIG. 19–4. Resting LES pressures for 25 patients with daily heartburn (**left**) and 25 patients with monthly heartburn (**right**).

patients than for the 25 patients with less frequent symptoms. In addition, all patients with daily symptoms had a resting LES pressure of less than 10 mm Hg (Fig. 19–4). These findings suggest that symptoms are likely to occur in patients with poor sphincter function regardless of the type of food consumed. The development of reflux symptoms in those with adequate sphincter function tends to be more clearly related to specific foods, particularly those with high fat content.

The potentially strong relationship between fat ingestion and chronic GERD has been emphasized by clinical studies. The initial report comparing the effect of various types of meals on LES pressure in healthy volunteers suggested that maintenance of LES competence may be particularly susceptible to fat [26]. In subjects with no reflux symptoms, the LES pressure decreased significantly in response to a corn oil meal. In contrast, an increase in LES pressure was associated with meals having a high protein content.

These findings were corroborated by a subsequent study that compared the effect of high-fat (61% by calorie) and low-fat (16%) meals on esophageal acid exposure, determined by pH monitoring [1]. Observations in normal subjects maintaining upright posture postprandially indicated a significant increase in acid exposure after the high-fat compared with the low-fat meal, particularly during the second and third hours after food ingestion. The fat content of the meal had little influence, however, on esophageal acid exposure in reflux patients in the upright positions. These patients experienced reflux after both the high-fat and the low-fat meals (Table 19–2). When normal subjects and reflux patients were studied in the recumbent position after eating, increased exposure of the esophagus to acid was noted in both groups after both high-fat and low-fat meals. Acid reflux was most pronounced during the second and third hours after consumption of these meals. Significantly decreased postprandial reflux was noted after a meal prepared in the fat substitute Olestra compared with an identical meal prepared in triglyceride [16]. The observations about the singular importance of dietary fat on reflux cited above are consis-

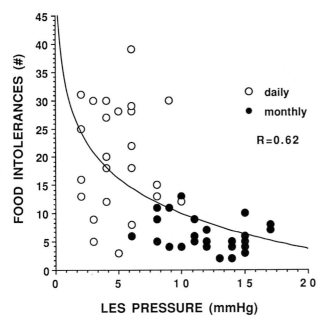

FIG. 19–3. Relationship between 39 foods causing heartburn and resting lower esophageal sphincter (*LES*) pressure in 25 patients with daily and 25 patients with monthly reflux symptoms.

**TABLE 19–2.** *Average upright esophageal acid exposure (% time) after high-fat versus low-fat meals in normals and reflux patients[a]*

|  | Low-fat meals | High-fat meals |
|---|---|---|
| Normals |  |  |
| First hour | 1.8 | 7.4 |
| Second hour | 2.1 | 8.1 |
| Third hour | 0.5 | 2.9 |
| Reflux patients |  |  |
| First hour | 19.5 | 25.8 |
| Second hour | 22.3 | 27.2 |
| Third hour | 26.1 | 9.8 |

[a] The fat content, by calories, of the low-fat and high-fat meals was 16% and 61%, respectively.

tent with modern concepts of pathophysiology of reflux. Recent observations that dietary fat will induce transient relaxations of the LES provide an attractive explanation for fat-induced reflux in individuals with normal resting LES pressure [11].

These studies support the concept that foods such as fat, which may decrease LES pressure, are more likely to precipitate symptoms in individuals having a sphincter that is usually competent to prevent reflux. Patients with persistently low LES pressures seem less likely to identify specific foods of this kind as symptom producers. Furthermore, the increased acid exposures seen in both normals and reflux patients for up to 3 hours after either meal when recumbent postprandially support the therapeutic recommendation to avoid lying down for 3 hours after eating.

The risk of developing GERD may well be related to habits of the Western world. As discussed in subsequent chapters, these include fatty and large meals, obesity, smoking, chocolate consumption, and possibly chronic use of certain drugs.

## DIAGNOSTIC EVALUATION

The diagnostic approach to the patient with possible GERD is multilayered, depending on the presentation. Since the symptoms are believed to be due to chronic reflux, the evaluation should attempt to document this abnormality. This patient who presents with typical heartburn and regurgitation with the usual positional and postprandial relationships requires little, if any, additional information to establish a presumptive diagnosis and initiate therapy. The patient whose symptoms are less clear or include atypical manifestations will usually need additional diagnostic testing. The variety of tests and procedures that are available to evaluate the patient with possible GERD can cause diagnostic confusion if not used appropriately. It is preferable to begin the diagnostic approach by defining the question to be answered in the individual patient. In Table 19–3, the variety of diagnostic tests that have been advocated for the patient with possible reflux are categorized according to the question being asked.

**TABLE 19–3.** *Diagnostic tests for gastroesophageal reflux disease categorized according to specific questions being asked*

Is abnormal reflux present?
  Barium upper gastrointestinal series
  Gastroesophageal scintiscan
  Standard acid reflux test
  pH monitoring
Is there mucosal injury?
  Barium upper gastrointestinal (air contrast) study
  Endoscopy
  Mucosal biopsy
Are symptoms due to reflux?
  Bernstein test
  pH monitoring (with symptom index)
  PPI treatment response[a]
Can prognostic or preoperative information be obtained?
  Esophageal motility evaluation
  pH monitoring

[a] PPI, proton pump inhibitor.

### Is Abnormal Reflux Present?

The critical question often is whether the patient has abnormal reflux, particularly in the patient with an atypical symptom pattern. Simply confirming that abnormal reflux is present is often satisfactory to support the clinical impression.

The first test usually performed to evaluate possible reflux, particularly by the primary-care physician, is an upper gastrointestinal series. This test is particularly helpful to rule out complications of GERD (ulcer, stricture) or other structural abnormalities of the esophagus, stomach, or duodenum. Radiographic reflux, the flow of barium from the stomach into the esophagus either spontaneously or induced by various maneuvers, has limited diagnostic value. It is, of course, dependent on the state of competence of the antireflux mechanism at a particular moment. Radiographic reflux has been demonstrated in as few as 60% of severely symptomatic patients or in as many as 25% of patients having no reflux symptoms. Thus, its reliability is questionable, with both poor specificity and sensitivity [15, 30]. Air contrast techniques provide more information (see Chapter 3). In recent years, it has become clear that most normal individuals have brief intermittent episodes of reflux (so-called physiologic reflux), particularly on those occasions when the LES will spontaneously relax or open [6].

Radioisotopic scintiscans have been advocated to document reflux and to provide quantitation of the amount of reflux. The gastroesophageal scintiscan employs a radioisotope (technetium 99m sulfur colloid) as a marker for reflux. Graded abdominal compression is used to unmask incompetence of the reflux barrier. Although originally proposed as a very sensitive test of reflux [7], its reliability has been questioned [14].

The use of an intraesophageal pH electrode to detect reflux was initially reported by Tuttle and Grossman in 1958 [36]. Subsequently, the standard acid reflux test was developed to stress the antireflux barrier in the laboratory while measuring reflux with a pH probe placed 5 cm above the LES. Following instillation of 300 mL of 0.1N hydrochloric acid into the stomach, the patient performs four maneuvers—deep breathing, Valsalva, Müller (inspiration against a closed glottis), and cough—repeated in the supine and right and left lateral decubitus positions and with the head down 20 degrees. Overall, 16 possibilities for acid reflux occur. A decrease in esophageal pH to less than 4 on at least three occasions is considered evidence of abnormal reflux. This test has relatively good overall sensitivity and specificity but is somewhat cumbersome and time-consuming in actual practice and is rarely used at present [30].

The current gold standard for the presence of abnormal reflux is ambulatory prolonged pH monitoring (see Chapter 6 for details). Patients record the time that they experience reflux symptoms during monitoring, thus allowing correlation of intraesophageal pH and subjective symptoms. A symptom index (SI) often helps clarify the association of specific symptoms with episodes of reflux, using the following equation [38]:

$$SI = \frac{\text{No. of symptoms occurring with pH} < 4.0}{\text{Total no. of symptoms}} \times 100$$

This test is of no value if the patient is incapable of gastric acid production. Clinical indications include patients presenting with difficult diagnostic problems or with atypical reflux symptoms (chest pain, cough, hoarseness), those not readily responding to therapy, or the preoperative and postoperative evaluation of antireflux surgery.

## Is There Evidence of Mucosal Injury?

Esophagitis is the *sine qua non* of GERD. This can occasionally be documented by careful air contrast barium esophagram showing mucosal lesions (erosions, ulcers) or stricture. Direct comparison of this technique with endoscopy has revealed that the finding of esophageal injury on air contrast esophagram is highly specific, although not very sensitive [28]. If the esophagram is negative, more sensitive testing is required.

Endoscopy is the diagnostic approach most frequently used to document esophageal injury. Erosions or ulcerations of the mucosa visualized through the endoscope are indications of reflux injury. The findings are definitive when clearly present but, unfortunately, may be subtle or absent, even in the presence of specific histologic abnormalities in mucosal biopsy specimens. Only 34% of patients with chronic heartburn evaluated in one study had esophagitis apparent on endoscopy [40].

Esophageal mucosal biopsy can be a more sensitive test of the presence of reflux injury since histologic abnormalities may be present even when careful endoscopic examination indicates a normal-appearing esophagus. The most reliable criterion for esophagitis on endoscopic biopsy is the presence of acute inflammatory cells (polymorphonuclear leukocytes or eosinophils). Since these are present in esopha-

geal biopsy specimens of only 20% of patients with reflux symptoms, other more sensitive epithelial changes have been proposed as being better diagnostic criteria. Increased papillary extension and basal zone hyperplasia are considered to be more sensitive findings occurring secondary to chronic gastroesophageal reflux [13].

## Are Symptoms Due to Gastroesophageal Reflux Disease?

The key question in many patients is whether their symptoms are clearly related to acid exposure and sensitivity of the esophageal mucosa to chronic reflux. The acid perfusion (Bernstein) test has been used for many years as a test of acid sensitivity, with a reported specificity and sensitivity of approximately 80% in GERD [30]. If the patient's symptoms are reproduced during perfusion of dilute hydrochloric acid and clear following saline perfusion, it is appropriate to conclude that chronic acid reflux is the cause of spontaneously occurring symptoms. This test, of course, is purely qualitative in character and provides no information on the degree of reflux.

If the SI is calculated as described earlier, 24-hour pH monitoring can define the relationship between specific symptoms and reflux. This test is limited by the requirement that the patient's symptoms must occur during the test period. It is not considered by many investigators to represent an endogenous Bernstein test [38].

The opposite approach to acid reflux testing is the use of proton pump inhibitor, (omeprazole, 20 mg b.i.d., or lansoprazole, 30 mg b.i.d.) as a diagnostic tool. The disappearance of symptoms by strong acid inhibition, given for at least 1 week, is a simple and inexpensive test for the diagnosis of GERD and has the advantage of ruling out the day-to-day variation of 24-hour pH monitoring [31].

## Can Prognostic Information Be Obtained?

Measurement of LES pressure was previously suggested as a possible means to diagnose reflux disease. The importance of the LES as a major barrier to reflux is well established. Although an LES pressure of less than 10 mm Hg has been considered an indication of an incompetent esophagogastric junction, there is much variation in this value. Many patients with well-documented esophagitis will have an LES pressure higher than 10 mm Hg, and some asymptomatic subjects with pressures below this value have been studied. Consequently, LES pressure in a given patient is often too imprecise to identify a potential for reflux, even though it is the most measurable part of the antireflux barrier and may distinguish populations of reflux patients from controls. LES pressure variability severely limits the sensitivity and specificity of this measurement as a diagnostic test. As a more useful clinical tool to diagnose an incompetent LES, a pressure of less than 6 mm Hg correlates well with abnormal reflux on pH testing. Extremely low LES pressures in this range may be valuable in predicting a more severe degree of reflux and a worse prognosis [23].

In addition to LES pressure measurements, careful assessment of peristaltic activity in the esophageal body may have greater importance in evaluating the severity of reflux disease and its prognosis [17, 22]. This test is particularly important as a preoperative assessment to inform the surgeon of potentially defective peristalsis prior to fundoplication.

Ambulatory pH monitoring can also provide important information about the severity of reflux disease and the reflux pattern present in a particular patient. That is, does the patient have reflux predominantly at night, or is upright, postprandial reflux more prevalent?

## WHAT IS THE IMPORTANCE OF A HIATAL HERNIA?

Although once considered to be of major importance in the production of GERD, the finding of a hiatal hernia either radiographically or endoscopically has limited accuracy in predicting whether a patient's symptoms are secondary to reflux. When carefully sought, a sliding hiatal hernia can be found in a high percentage of persons, most of whom will be asymptomatic. In a review of more than 1,000 patients in 1968, Palmer [29] estimated that only 9% of those with a radiographically demonstrated hiatal hernia had typical reflux symptoms. In addition, recent studies indicated no definite cause-and-effect relationship between the presence of symptomatic reflux and the finding of a hiatal hernia [19]. Since both heartburn and a sliding hiatal hernia are common phenomena, there is likely to be an association between the presence of these entities, although this should in no way imply cause and effect. Recent information indicates that hiatal hernias may contribute to the severity of GERD by "trapping" acid in the hernial sac, thus becoming more available to reflux during LES relaxation. This mechanism may prolong acid exposure and delay its clearance from the esophageal mucosa [25, 34]. Thus, although it may not primarily produce the reflux, the hernia may contribute to the esophageal injury. Most patients with severe esophagitis have a hiatal hernia found during endoscopic assessment [19].

## REFERENCES

1. Becker DJ, et al. A comparison of high and low fat meals on postprandial esophageal acid exposure. Am J Gastroenterol 1989;84:782
2. Breumelhohf R, et al. Analysis of 24-hour esophageal pressure and pH data in unselected patients with noncardiac chest pain. Gastroenterology 1990;99:1257
3. Cameron AJ, Ott BJ, Payne WS. The incidence of adenocarcinoma in columnar-lined (Barrett's) esophagus. N Engl J Med 1985;313:857
4. Cherian P, et al. Esophageal tests in the evaluation of non-cardiac chest pain. Dis Esophagus 1995;8:129
5. DeMeester TR, et al. Esophageal function in patients with angina-type chest pain and normal coronary angiograms. Ann Surg 1982;196:488
6. Dodds WJ, et al. Mechanisms of gastroesophageal reflux in patients with reflux esophagitis. N Engl J Med 1982;307:1547
7. Fisher RS, et al. Gastroesophageal (GE) scintiscanning to detect and quantitate GE reflux. Gastroenterology 1976;70:301
8. Gluck M, Pope CE. Chronic hiccups and gastroesophageal reflux disease. Ann Intern Med 1986;105:291
9. Hetzel DJ, Heddle R. Gastroesophageal reflux disease, pH monitoring, and treatment. Curr Opin Gastroenterol 1993;9:629
10. Hewson EG, et al. Twenty-four hour esophageal pH monitoring: the most useful test for evaluating noncardiac chest pain. Am J Med 1991; 90:576
11. Holloway RH, et al. Effect of intraduodenal fat on lower oesophageal sphincter function and gastro-oesophageal reflux. Gut 1997;40:449
12. Irwin RS, Curley FJ, French CL. Chronic cough. The spectrum and frequency of causes, key components of the diagnostic evaluation, and outcome of specific therapy. Am Rev Respir Dis 1990;141:640
13. Ismail-Beigi F, Horton PF, Pope CE. Histological consequences of gastroesophageal reflux in man. Gastroenterology 1970;58:163
14. Jenkins AF, Cowan RJ, Richter JE. Gastroesophageal scintigraphy: is it a sensitive test for gastroesophageal reflux disease? J Clin Gastroenterol 1985;7:127
15. Johnston BT, et al. Comparison of barium radiography with esophageal pH monitoring in the diagnosis of gastroesophageal reflux disease. Am J Gastroenterol 1996;91:1181
16. Just R, et al. A comparison of the effect of Olestra and triglyceride on postprandial esophageal acid exposure. Am J Gastroenterol 1993;88: 17334
17. Kahrilas PJ, et al. Esophageal peristaltic dysfunction in peptic esophagitis. Gastroenterology 1986;91:897
18. Katz PO. Ambulatory esophageal and hypopharyngeal pH monitoring in patients with hoarseness. Am J Gastroenterol 1989;85:38
19. Kaul B, et al. Hiatus hernia in gastroesophageal reflux disease. Scand J Gastroenterol 1986;21:31
20. Kirk AJ. Reflux dyspareunia. Thorax 1986;41:215
21. Klauser AG, Schindlbeck NE, Muller-Lissner SA. Symptoms in gastroesophageal reflux disease. Lancet 1990;335:205
22. Leite LP, et al. Ineffective esophageal motility (IEM): the primary finding in patients with non-specific esophageal motility disorder. Dig Dis Sci 1997;42:1853
23. Lieberman DA. Medical therapy for chronic reflux esophagitis: long-term follow-up. Arch Intern Med 1987;147:1717
24. Marshall JB, Landreneau RJ, Beyer KL. Hiccups: esophageal manometric features and relationship to gastroesophageal reflux. Am J Gastroenterol 1990;85:1172
25. Mittal RK, Lange RC, McCallum RW. Identification and mechanism of delayed esophageal acid clearance in subjects with hiatus hernia. Gastroenterology 1987;92:130
26. Nebel OT, Castell DO. Lower esophageal sphincter pressure changes after food ingestion. Gastroenterology 1972;63:778
27. Nebel OT, Fornes MF, Castell DO. Symptomatic gastroesophageal reflux: incidence and precipitating factors. Am J Dig Dis 1976;21:953
28. Ott DJ, Gelfand DW, Wu WC. Reflux esophagitis: radiographic and endoscopic correlation. Radiology 1979;130:583
29. Palmer ED. The hiatus hernia–esophagitis–esophageal stricture complex. Twenty year prospective study. Am J Med 1968;44:566
30. Richter JE, Castell DO. Gastroesophageal reflux. Pathogenesis, diagnosis, and therapy. Ann Intern Med 1982;97:93
31. Schenk BE, et al. Omeprazole as a diagnostic tool in gastroesophageal reflux disease. Am J Gastroenterol 1997;92:1997
32. Schofield PM, et al. Exertional gastroesophageal reflux: a mechanism for symptoms in patients with angina pectoris and normal coronary angiograms. BMJ 1987;294:1459
33. Shaker R, et al. Esophagopharyngeal distribution of refluxed gastric acid in patients with reflux laryngitis. Gastroenterology 1995;109:1575
34. Sloan S, Kahrilas PJ. Impairment of esophageal emptying with hiatal hernia. Gastroenterology 1991;100:596
35. Sontag SJ, et al. Most asthmatics have gastroesophageal reflux with or without bronchodilator therapy. Gastroenterology 1990;99:613
36. Tuttle SG, Grossman MI. Detection of gastroesophageal reflux by simultaneous measurements of intraluminal pressure and pH. Proc Soc Exp Biol Med 1958;93:225
37. Ward PH, Hanson DG. Reflux as an etiological factor of carcinoma of the laryngopharynx. Laryngoscope 1988;98:1195
38. Wiener GJ, et al. The symptom index: a clinically important parameter of ambulatory 24-hour esophageal pH monitoring. Am J Gastroenterol 1988;83:358
39. Wiener G, et al. Chronic hoarseness secondary to gastroesophageal reflux disease. Am J Gastroenterol 1989;12:1503
40. Winters C, Spurling TJ, Chobanian SJ. Barrett's esophagus. A prevalent, occult complication of gastroesophageal reflux disease. Gastroenterology 1987;92:118

*The Esophagus*, Third Edition,
edited by D. O. Castell and J. E. Richter.
Lippincott Williams & Wilkins, Philadelphia © 1999.

CHAPTER 20

# Hiatus Hernia

Peter J. Kahrilas and Anita E. Spiess

Although hiatus hernia was occasionally noted as a congenital anomaly or a consequence of abdominal trauma in the preradiographic literature, the prevalence of this condition was not appreciated until the evolution of imaging technology. Illustrative of this, Bowditch presented a treatise on diaphragmatic hernia to the Boston Society for Medical Observation in 1847 and commented, "the disease is so rare that no person would be likely to have more than one or two opportunities for operation during his whole lifetime" [9]. The irony of the following phrase in the introduction of a modern work by Skinner et al. is apparent, "surgical management of esophageal reflux and hiatus hernia, long-term results with 1030 patients" [54]. Also illustrating the dependence on radiography for the detection of hiatus hernia, the first description of a paraesophageal hernia was at postmortem examination in 1903 [5].

With the maturation of imaging technology, especially barium contrast radiography, it became reasonably easy to detect hiatus hernia antemortem. In 1926, Akerlund reported that hiatal hernia was found in 2.3% of all upper gastrointestinal x-ray studies [1]. With the improvement of radiographic techniques and a more systematic approach to their detection, more hernias were identified, such that by 1955 the reported incidence was 15% [52]. When provocative maneuvers were employed to accentuate herniation during fluoroscopy, the frequency increased more dramatically; of 955 patients subject to abdominal compression during an upper gastrointestinal x-ray series, hiatus hernia was diagnosed in 55% [61]. Coincident with this evolution in imaging, the clinical understanding of reflux disease also evolved. Our present concept of peptic esophagitis dates back to 1935 when Winkelstein first suggested that gastric secretions were the cause of the mucosal damage observed in peptic esopha-

gitis [62]. The term *reflux esophagitis* was later introduced in 1946 by Allison, thereby acknowledging that irritant gastric juices were refluxed from the stomach to the esophagus [2]. Since then, there has been considerable controversy regarding the relationship between esophagitis, heartburn, hiatal hernia, and the physiology of the lower esophagus. Recognizing this controversy and the fact that the main significance of hiatus hernia is in its relationship to reflux disease, it is impossible to discuss hiatus hernia without some discussion of reflux disease. Thus, this chapter will first focus on the relevant anatomy and classification of hiatus hernia and then examine our current understanding of the relationship between these anatomic variables and the pathophysiology of reflux disease.

## ANATOMY AND PHYSIOLOGY OF THE GASTROESOPHAGEAL JUNCTION

The hiatal orifice is an eliptically shaped opening through the diaphragm with its long axis in the sagittal plane through which the esophagus and vagus nerves gain access to the abdomen. Although there is some anatomic variability with partial contribution from the left crus, the most common anatomy is for the hiatus to be formed by elements of the right diaphragmatic crus [34]. The crura arise from tendinous fibers emerging from the anterior longitudinal ligament over the upper lumbar vertebrae; the left crus is usually attached to two lumbar vertebrae and the right to three. Additionally, accessory tendons may arise from the fascia over the psoas muscles and from the medial arcuate ligaments, but for the most part, these fibers eventually fan out laterally to insert into the central tendon of the diaphragm, away from the hiatal limbs. The crura pass upward in close contact with the vertebral bodies for most of their course and only incline forward as they arch around the esophagus [34].

Once muscle fibers emerge from the tendinous origin of the right crus, they form two overlying ribbonlike bundles separated from each other by connective tissue. The dorsal bundle forms the left limb of the right crus (thoracic aspect),

P. J. Kahrilas: Departments of Medicine and Communication Sciences and Disorders, Northwestern University Medical School, and, Division of Gastoenterology and Hepatology, Northwestern University Hospital, Chicago, Illinois 60611.

A. E. Spiess: Department of Gastroenterology, Northwestern University Medical School, Chicago, Illinois 60610.

and the ventral bundle becomes the right limb (abdominal aspect) of the right crus. As they approach the hiatus, the muscle bands diverge and cross each other in a scissorlike fashion with the ventral bundle passing upward and to the right and the dorsal bundle passing upward and to the left. The lateral fibers of each hiatal limb insert directly into the central tendon of the diaphragm, but the medial fibers, which form the hiatal margins, incline toward the midline and decussate with each other in a trellis like fashion in front of the esophagus [34]. Although there are variations of this standard pattern, the basic organization of two flattened muscle bundles first diverging like a scissor and then merging anterior to the esophagus is common to all arrangements (Fig. 20–1). Normally, there is about 1 cm of muscle separating the anterior rim of the hiatus from the central tendon of the diaphragm.

Under normal circumstances, the esophagus is anchored to the diaphragm, and the stomach cannot be displaced through the hiatus into the mediastinum. The main restraining structures are the phrenoesophageal ligaments, alternatively referred to as the phrenoesophageal membrane, and an aggregation of posterior structures including the vagus nerve and radicles of the left gastric vein and artery [7, 51]. The phrenoesophageal membrane is formed from the fascia transversalis on the under surface of the diaphragm and, to a lesser degree, fused elements of the endothoracic fascia. This elastic membrane inserts circumferentially into the esophageal musculature, close to the squamocolumnar junction, and extends for about 1 cm above the gastroesophageal junction, at which point it thins and merges with the perivis-

ceral fascia of the esophagus [12]. Thus, the axial position of the squamocolumnar junction is normally within or slightly distal to the diaphragmatic hiatus [27].

The anatomic relationship of the distal esophagus, hiatus, and stomach is transiently altered during swallow-initiated peristalsis. Physiologically, peristalsis is a sequenced contraction of both the longitudinal and circular muscle of the esophageal wall that is responsible for bolus propulsion through the esophagus [49]. In particular, with contraction of the esophageal longitudinal muscle, the esophagus shortens and the phrenoesophageal membrane is stretched; relaxation of the longitudinal muscle along with the elastic recoil of the phrenoesophageal membrane is then responsible for pulling the squamocolumnar junction back to its normal position at the termination of the peristaltic sequence. This is, in effect, *physiologic herniation,* since the gastric cardia tents through the diaphragmatic hiatus with each swallow (Fig. 20–2) [27]. This paradox has led to a confusing array of terminology, summarized in Fig. 20–3 [24]. The globular structure seen radiographically that forms above the diaphragm, beneath the tubular esophagus, during deglutition is termed the *phrenic ampulla,* which is bounded from above by the distal esophagus and from below by the crural diaphragm. Emptying of the ampulla occurs between inspirations in conjunction with relengthening of the esophagus [30]. As will become apparent in the discussion of sliding hiatus hernia, a type I hiatus hernia is an exaggeration of the normal phrenic ampulla, and the estimated prevalence of type I hernias varies widely at least in part because of inconsistent conventions of measurement. Not all of the structures illustrated in Fig. 20–3 are always evident radiographically. Commonly, only an A ring is evident (Fig. 20–4), in which case the limits of the measurement defining hiatus hernia becomes arbitrary. In such cases, the demonstration of rugal folds traversing the diaphragm is often used as a defining criterion. Alternatively, a B ring, but not an A ring may be evident radiographically, as in Fig. 20–5, in which case the B ring is of such prominence (luminal diameter less than 13 mm) as to be termed a *Schatzki ring.* In such a case, it is easy to apply the criterion of at least 2 cm between the B ring and the hiatus for defining a sliding hiatus hernia [44].

Aside from its antegrade propulsive function discussed above, the gastroesophageal junction also serves to minimize gastroesophageal reflux. This is accomplished by a complex valvular mechanism, the function of which is partly attributable to the esophagus, partly to the stomach, and partly to the crural diaphragm. The esophageal element has been extensively analyzed and consists of the lower esophageal sphincter (LES), a 2-cm segment of tonically contracted smooth muscle. The proximal margin of the LES extends up to and a short distance proximal to the squamocolumnar junction. The distal margin of the LES is more difficult to define, but careful anatomic studies suggest that it is composed of elements of the gastric musculature—the opposing clasp and sling fibers of the gastric cardia [29]. Finally, surrounding the LES at the level of the squamocolumnar junc-

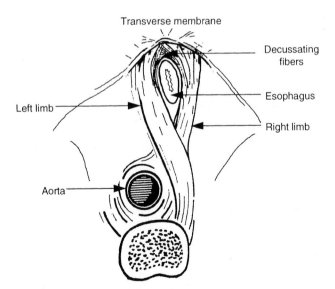

FIG. 20–1. The most common anatomy of the diaphragmatic hiatus, in which the muscular elements of the crural diaphragm derive from the right diaphragmatic crus. The right crus arises from the anterior longitudinal ligament overlying the lumbar vertebrae. Once muscular elements emerge from the tendon, two flat muscular bands, which cross each other in scissorlike fashion, form the walls of the hiatus and decussate with each other anterior to the esophagus. (Modified from ref. 34.)

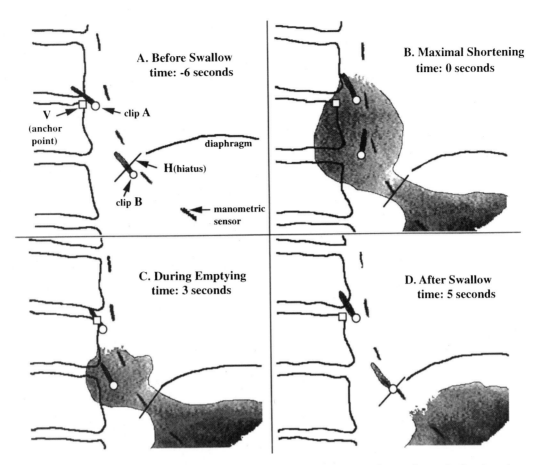

**FIG. 20–2.** Demonstration of *physiologic herniation* during swallow, using endoscopically placed mucosal clips. **A:** Before swallow. Clip B marks the position of the squamocolumnar junction 0.4 cm distal to the hiatus and 3.5 cm distal to the anchor point on the vertebral body (*V*). Clip A is affixed to the esophageal mucosa 3.1 cm proximally. Clip movements are referenced to point V on the vertebral column. **B:** At the time of maximal esophageal shortening, clip B is 1.8 cm proximal to the hiatus and 2.0 cm distal to point V. The distance between clips A and B is reduced to 2.2 cm, indicative of 29% shortening. **C:** As elongation proceeds, first both clips descend, after which clip B descends, stretching the A–B segment back to its initial length. **D:** After swallow, clip B is again at the level of the hiatus. (From ref. 27, with permission.)

tion is the crural diaphragm, composed mainly of the right diaphragmatic crus [53]. However, in other instances, the left crus is dominant, both crura provide equal contributions, or a band from the left crus crosses to the right (band of Low) [10, 32]. Elegant physiologic studies have clearly demonstrated that diaphragmatic contraction augments gastroesophageal junction pressure, in essence serving as an external sphincter [39]. Furthermore, if the esophagogastric junction is defined as either the end of the LES or the point at which the tubular esophagus joins the saccular stomach, there is normally about 2 cm of tubular esophagus distal to the squamocolumnar junction within the abdomen [27].

## TYPES OF HIATAL HERNIA

In general terms, hiatus hernia refers to herniation of elements of the abdominal cavity through the esophageal hiatus of the diaphragm. The most comprehensive classification scheme recognizes four types of hiatal hernia as enumerated below.

With *type I* or *sliding hiatal hernia,* there is a widening of the muscular hiatal tunnel and circumferential laxity of the phrenoesophageal membrane, allowing a portion of the gastric cardia to herniate upward. Largely because of the inherent subjectivity in defining type I hiatal hernia, estimates of prevalence vary enormously, from 10% to 80% of the adult population in North America [53]. In all probability, most type I hiatal hernias are asymptomatic, and even with larger type I hernias, the main clinical implication is the propensity to develop reflux disease, the likelihood of which increases with increasing hernia size. With a well-developed hernia, the esophageal hiatus abuts directly on the transverse membrane of the central tendon of the diaphragm, and the anterior hiatal muscles are absent or reduced to a few atrophic strands [34]. The hiatus itself is no longer a sagittal slit, but a rounded opening whose transverse diam-

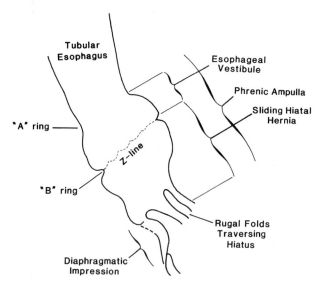

FIG. 20-3. Anatomic features of a sliding hiatus hernia viewed radiographically during swallowing. The A ring is a muscular ring visible during swallowing which demarcates the superior margin of the LES. The B ring at the squamocolumnar junction is present in only about 15% of individuals and allows for accurate division of the phrenic ampulla into the esophageal vestibule (A ring to B ring) and the sliding hiatus hernia (B ring to the subdiaphragmatic stomach). By convention, the distinction between normal and hiatus hernia is at least a 2-cm separation between the B ring and the hiatus. Rugal folds traversing the hiatus support the conviction that a portion of the stomach is supradiaphragmatic. (From ref. 24, with permission.)

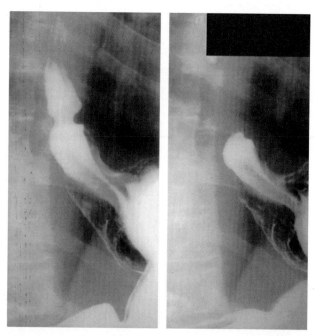

FIG. 20-4. Radiograph of a patient with a small axial hiatal hernia, a well developed A ring, and no B ring evident. In such cases, the criterion for defining hiatus hernia is the appearance of rugal folds traversing the diaphragmatic hiatus. The A ring has no anatomic correlate, but physiologically corresponds to the superior aspect of the lower esophageal sphincter.

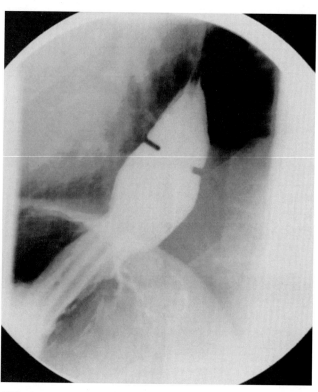

FIG. 20-5. Radiograph of a patient with a small axial hiatal hernia, a prominent B ring, and no A ring evident. The B ring occurs at the squamocolumnar junction and, when subtle, is referred to as the *transverse mucosal fold*. In instances such as this where there is marked compromise of the esophageal lumen, the B ring is referred to as a *Schatzki ring* and is a frequent cause of episodic solid-food dysphagia. When a B ring is evident, the criterion for defining hiatus hernia is a separation of at least 2 cm between the B ring and the diaphragmatic hiatus.

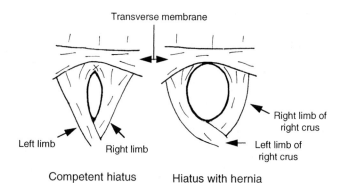

FIG. 20-6. Alteration of the hiatal anatomy associated with sliding hiatal hernia. Note that the main change is a widening of the hiatal canal. Associated with this, there can be substantial atrophy of the abutting muscular elements, thinning and elongation of the phrenoesophageal membrane, and axial displacement of the gastric cardia. (Modified from ref. 34.)

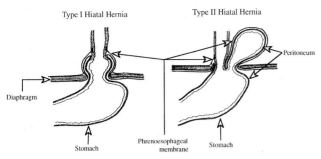

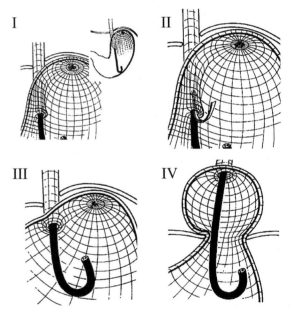

ing hiatal hernia enlarges further, such that more than 3 cm of gastric pouch is herniated upward, its presence is obvious regardless of technique because gastric folds are evident traversing the diaphragm both during swallow-induced shortening and at rest (Fig. 20–8). The progression from normal anatomy to obvious type I hernia is well illustrated in a recent analysis of the endoscopic appearance of the cardia, viewed in retroflexion (Fig. 20–9) [20].

Although there are instances in which trauma, congenital malformation, and iatrogeny can be clearly implicated, a variety of lines of evidence suggest that type I hiatus hernia is usually an acquired condition. Allison observed that the typical age of onset was in the fifth decade of life [23]. Pregnancy has long been suspected to be an inciting factor [16, 50]. Conceptually, Marchand argues that the compounded stresses of age-related degeneration, pregnancy, and obesity take their toll on a relatively weak point of the anatomy. The positive peritoneopleural pressure gradient acts to extrude the abdominal contents into the chest and,

**FIG. 20–7.** Sliding verses paraesophageal hiatal hernia. With sliding or axial hiatal hernia, there is thinning and elongation of the phrenoesophageal membrane leading to herniation of the stomach into the posterior mediastinum. As such, there is no potential for incarceration or strangulation. With paraesophageal herniation, visceral elements herniate through a focal weakness in the phrenoesophageal membrane with the potential to lead to the usual array of complications associated with visceral herniation through a constricted aperture. (Modified from ref. 53.)

eter approximates the sagittal diameter in size (Fig. 20–6). Associated with the widening of the hiatal orifice, the phrenoesophageal membrane becomes attenuated and inconspicuous in comparison to its normal prominence. However, although thinned, the phrenoesophageal membrane remains intact, and the associated herniated gastric cardia is contained within the posterior mediastinum (Fig. 20–7) [55]. In marginal instances, type I hiatal hernia is simply an exaggeration of the normal phrenic ampulla, making its identification dependent on measurement technique. However, when a slid-

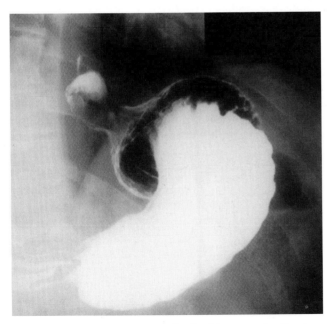

**FIG. 20–8.** Type I hiatal hernia. In this example, the herniated gastric cardia is evident at rest, after completion of esophageal emptying. Note the rugal folds traversing the diaphragmatic hiatus.

**FIG. 20–9.** Three-dimensional representation of the progressive anatomic disruption of the gastroesophageal junction as occurs with development of a type I hiatus hernia. In the grade I configuration (**upper left**), a ridge of muscular tissue is closely approximated to the shaft of the retroflexed endoscope. With a grade II configuration (**upper right**), the ridge of tissue is slightly less well defined, and there has been slight orad displacement of the squamocolumnar junction along with widening of the angle of His. In the grade III appearance (**lower left**), the ridge of tissue at the gastric entryway is barely present, and there is often incomplete luminal closure around the endoscope. Grade III deformity is nearly always accompanied by an obvious hiatal hernia. With grade IV deformity (**lower right**), no muscular ridge is present at the gastric entry. The gastroesophageal area stays open all the time, and squamous epithelium of the distal esophagus can be seen from the retroflexed endoscopic view. A hiatus hernia is always present. (Modified from Hill, LD, et al. Laparoscopic Hill repair. Contemp Surg 1994;44:1.)

although this extrusion is opposed by the entire surface of the diaphragm, of the openings through the diaphragm, only the esophageal hiatus is vulnerable to visceral herniation because it faces directly into the abdominal cavity. Furthermore, since the esophagus does not tightly fill the hiatus, the integrity of this opening depends upon its intrinsic structures, especially the phrenoesophageal membrane, which are designed to achieve a fine balance of mobility and stability [33]. Add to this vulnerability, the repetitive stresses of deep inspiration, Valsalva, vomiting, the physiologic herniation accompanying swallowing, and postural change, and then compound the stress by packing the abdominal cavity with adipose tissue or a gravid uterus, and eventually the integrity of the hiatus is gradually compromised. Another potential source of stress on the phrenoesophageal membrane is tonic contraction of the esophageal longitudinal muscle induced by gastroesophageal reflux and mucosal acidification [46].

The type I, or *sliding*, hiatal hernia described above accounts for the great majority of hiatal hernias. The less common types, *types II, III,* and *IV*, are varieties of *paraesophageal hernias*. Taken together, these account for at most 5% of all hiatal hernias [24, 47]. A type II hernia results from a localized defect in the phrenoesophageal membrane while the gastroesophageal junction remains fixed to the preaortic fascia and the median arcuate ligament (Fig. 20–7) [53]. The gastric fundus then serves as the leading point of herniation. The natural history of a type II hernia is progressive enlargement so that the entire stomach eventually herniates, with the pylorus juxtaposed to the gastric cardia, forming an upside-down, intrathoracic stomach (Fig. 20–10). Either as cause or effect, paraesophageal hernias are associated with abnormal laxity of structures normally preventing displacement of the stomach, the gastrosplenic and gastrocolic ligaments. As the hernia enlarges, the greater curvature of the stomach rolls up into the thorax. Because the stomach is fixed at the gastroesophageal junction, the herniated stomach tends to rotate around its longitudinal axis, resulting in an organoaxial volvulus (Fig. 20–11) [64]. Infrequently, rotation may alternatively occur around the transverse axis, resulting in a mesenteroaxial volvulus (Fig. 20–12) [47].

*Types III* and *IV hiatal hernias* are variants of the type II (purely paraesophageal) hernia described above. Type III hernias have elements of both types I and II hernias. With progressive enlargement of the hernia through the hiatus, the phrenoesophageal membrane stretches, displacing the gastroesophageal junction above the diaphragm, thereby adding a sliding element to the type II hernia (Fig. 20–13). Type IV hiatus hernia is associated with a large defect in the phrenoesophageal membrane, allowing other organs, such as colon, spleen, pancreas, and small intestine, to enter the hernia sac (Fig. 20–14).

Although their etiology is usually unclear, paraesophageal hernias are a recognized complication of surgical dissection of the hiatus as during antireflux procedures, esophagomyotomy, or partial gastrectomy. Many patients with a type II hernia are either asymptomatic or have only vague, intermit-

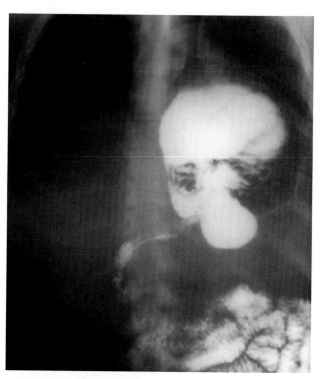

**FIG. 20–10.** Type II paraesophageal hiatal hernia. In this example, the entire stomach has herniated into the chest leading to an "upside-down stomach." Because the gastroesophageal junction remains within the hiatus, there is no element of type I herniation in this example. See also Fig. 20–23 to understand the resultant gastric configuration.

tent symptoms. The most common symptoms are epigastric or substernal pain, postprandial fullness, substernal fullness, nausea, and retching. An upright radiograph of the thorax may be diagnostic, revealing a retrocardiac air–fluid level within a paraesophageal hernia or intrathoracic stomach. Barium contrast studies are almost always diagnostic. Most complications of a type II hernia are reflective of the mechanical problem caused by the hernia. Gastric volvulus can cause dysphagia. Postcibal pain is usually related to gastric torsion. Bleeding, although infrequent, occurs from gastric ulceration or gastritis within the incarcerated hernia pouch

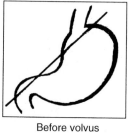
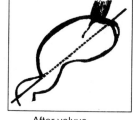

Before volvus          After volvus

**FIG. 20–11.** Organoaxial volvulus. The axis of rotation is the long axis of the stomach. (Modified from ref. 47.)

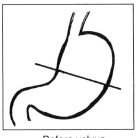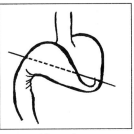

Before volvus          After volvus

**FIG. 20–12.** Mesenteroaxial volvulus. The axis of rotation is along the mesenteric attachment much the same as is seen with sigmoid colon volvulus. (Modified from ref. 47.)

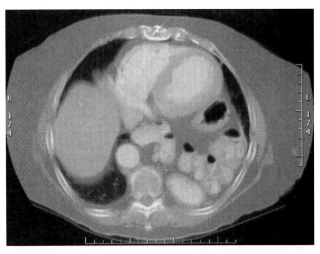

**FIG. 20–14.** Computerized tomography image through the chest showing a type IV paraesophageal hiatal hernia. In this example, the sigmoid colon (containing contrast) is clearly evident adjacent to the heart (also contrast enhanced). Lower cuts show the patient to be postsplenectomy, consistent with the observation that paraesophageal herniation occurs most commonly after surgical dissection in the area of the hiatus.

[53]. Respiratory complications result from mechanical compression of the lung by a large hernia or other organs herniating through the hiatus.

## THE ASSOCIATION OF TYPE I HIATUS HERNIA WITH REFLUX DISEASE

Endoscopic and radiographic studies suggest that 50% to 94% of patients with gastroesophageal reflux disease (GERD) have a type I hiatal hernia, while the corresponding prevalence in control subjects ranges from 13% to 59% [8, 45, 48, 64]. However, the importance of a type I hiatal hernia is obscured by the misconception that this is an all-or-none phenomenon. It is more useful to view type I hiatal hernia as a continuum of progressive disruption of the gastroesophageal junction, as illustrated in Fig. 20–9. Type I hiatus hernia impacts on reflux both by affecting the competence of the gastroesophageal junction in preventing reflux and in compromising the process of esophageal acid clearance once reflux has occurred.

### Pathogenesis of Gastroesophageal Reflux Disease

Symptomatic GERD results when the balance between aggressive forces (acid reflux, potency of refluxate) and defensive forces (esophageal acid clearance, mucosal resistance) tilts in favor of the aggressive forces. The intermittent nature of symptoms in some individuals with GERD suggests that the aggressive and defensive forces are part of a delicately balanced system. Significant aberration in any one of these pathophysiologic influences can result in tipping the balance of forces acting on the esophageal mucosa from

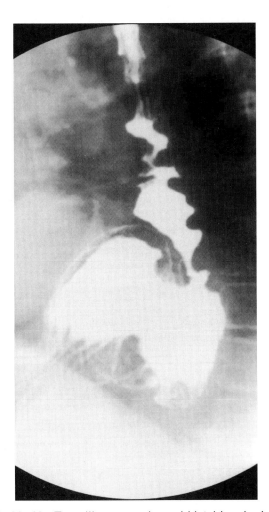

**FIG. 20–13.** Type III paraesophageal hiatal hernia. In this example, much of the stomach has herniated into the chest, but the leading edge of the herniating stomach has additionally herniated through a weakening of the phrenoesophageal membrane, contributing a paraesophageal component to the hernia. Because the gastroesophageal junction is well above the diaphragmatic hiatus, this is a mixed, or type III, paraesophageal hernia.

a compensated condition to a decompensated condition (i.e., heartburn, esophagitis). Although GERD is multifactorial in etiology with potentially important modifying roles played by mucosal defensive factors and differences in the potency of refluxate, the key events in the pathogenesis of GERD are reflux of acid and pepsin from the stomach into the esophagus and the decreased effectiveness of esophageal acid clearance.

The complexity of the gastroesophageal junction as an antireflux barrier has led to three dominant theories of pathogenesis of gastroesophageal junction incompetence: (a) transient LES relaxations, (b) hypotensive LES, and (c) anatomic disruption of the gastroesophageal junction associated with a hiatal hernia. Transient LES relaxations (tLESRs) account for the overwhelming majority of reflux events in normal individuals and in patients with normal LES pressure at the time of reflux [13, 14]. Transient LES relaxations appear without fixed temporal relation to an antecedent pharyngeal contraction, are unaccompanied by esophageal peristalsis, and persist for longer periods (greater than 10 seconds) than do swallow-induced LES relaxations [21]. The likelihood of reflux occurring during a tLESR is influenced by both the circumstances of the recording and the temporal proximity to a meal, with reflux during as many as 93% or as few as 9% [25, 41]. There has been no demonstration of an interplay between hiatus hernia and tLESRs. On the other hand, as summarized in the ensuing section, hiatus hernia has been shown to impact on reflux events attributable to mechanisms other than tLESR: (a) stress reflux (a relatively hypotensive LES that is overcome and "blown open" by an abrupt increase of intra-abdominal pressure) and (b) free reflux (a fall in intraesophageal pH without an identifiable change in either intragastric or LES pressure that can occur when the LES pressure is within 4 mm Hg of intragastric pressure).

Once the esophageal mucosa has been acidified by reflux of gastric juice across the gastroesophageal junction, the normal process of esophageal acid clearance (defined as restoration of esophageal pH to a value of 4) requires both effective esophageal emptying and normal salivation [18]. Esophageal emptying is defined as elimination of fluid from the esophagus. Thus, the two major potential causes of prolonged esophageal acid clearance are impaired esophageal emptying and impaired salivary function. Reduced salivary rate results in diminished salivary neutralizing capacity. Diminished salivation during sleep explains why reflux events during sleep or immediately before sleep are associated with markedly prolonged acid clearance times [43]. However, in the only large-scale analysis of salivary function in GERD, no difference was found between the resting salivary function of patients with esophagitis, young controls, or age-matched controls [58].

Impaired esophageal emptying in reflux disease was inferred by the observation that patients with abnormal acid clearance times were improved by an upright posture or by head-of-bed elevation, suggesting that gravity could improve abnormal clearing [59]. Two mechanisms of impaired volume clearance have been identified: (a) peristaltic dysfunction and (b) "rereflux" secondary to hiatal hernia. Significant findings of peristaltic dysfunction include the occurrence of failed peristaltic contractions and hypotensive (less than 30 mm Hg) peristaltic contractions that incompletely empty the esophagus [26]. Hiatal hernia and esophageal emptying are discussed in a following section.

## Hiatus Hernia and the Diaphragmatic Sphincter

Theories of the mechanism of gastroesophageal junction competence have seesawed between strictly anatomic explanations focusing on type I hiatus hernia, and physiologic explanations focusing on the vigor of LES contraction while ignoring the significance of anatomic factors. As detailed below, current thinking recognizes contributions from both sphincteric components. However, before discussing recent experimentation, it is instructive to look at the work of Allison, who, except for his not knowing of the existence of the intrinsic lower esophageal sphincter, exhibited masterful understanding of the gastroesophageal junction [3]: "the position of the stomach in relationship to the diaphragm is only important in so far as the diaphragm acts as a sphincter. . . . When the right crus of the diaphragm contracts, its action on the cardia is twofold: First, it compresses the walls of the esophagus from side to side, and second, it pulls down and increases the angulation of the esophagus." Allison also understood the analogy between the gastroesophageal junction and the anal sphincters:

> The alimentary canal passes through two diaphragms, the thoracoabdominal and the pelvic. In each of these nature has adopted the same device to achieve continence. In each the canal is made to take a fairly abrupt bend, and at the bend is supported by an intrinsic and an extrinsic muscular mechanism [Fig. 20–15]. At the anorectal junction the internal

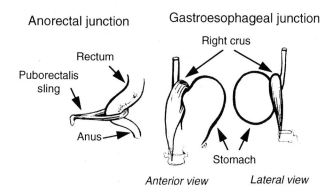

FIG. 20–15. The "pinchcock" action of the pelvic and crural diaphragms on the alimentary canal as it enters and exits the abdominal cavity. **Left:** The puborectalis sling around the anorectal junction. **Center:** Anterior view of the right crus of the diaphragm forming a sling around the gastroesophageal junction. **Right:** Lateral view of the crural sling. In each case, contraction of the diaphragm increases the angulation of the visceral tube, pinching it off and bolstering continence. (From ref. 3, with permission.)

sphincter is relatively well developed, but the main factor for continence is the puborectalis muscle which forms a lasso round the bend and hitches it forward to the back of the pubic bone. At the esophagogastric junction there is no thickening of the circular muscle fibers of the esophagus to form a sphincter, but the canal takes a bend forward and to the left, and this bend is lassoed and maintained by the right crus of the diaphragm which hitches it down to the lumbar spine.

Since the time of Allison's writings, the intrinsic sphincter of the gastroesophageal junction (the LES) has been described and much of his elegant conjecture forgotten. However, recent physiologic investigations have again advanced the ''two-sphincter hypothesis'' of gastroesophageal junction competence, suggesting that both the LES and the crural diaphragm encircling the LES serve a sphincteric function [11, 12, 38, 40]. The diaphragm augments the LES by a ''pinchcock effect'' of crural contraction as illustrated in Fig. 20–15. Evidence supporting a specialized sphincteric role of the crural diaphragm comes from the observation that the actions of the costal and crural parts of the diaphragm

function independently during certain gastrointestinal functions. During esophageal distension, vomiting, and eructation, electrical activity of the crural fibers was reportedly silent at the same time as the dome of the diaphragm was entirely active suggesting that the crural diaphragm participates in LES relaxation [4, 42]. This reflex inhibition of the crura disappears with vagotomy [15]. Thus, crural contraction augments the antireflux barrier during transient periods of increased intraabdominal pressure such as occur during inspiration, coughing, or abdominal straining. As evident by the data in Fig. 20–16, the susceptibility to reflux under these circumstances of abrupt increases of intra-abdominal pressure depends on both the instantaneous LES pressure and the integrity of the diaphragmatic sphincter [57]. Statistical modeling of the data in Fig. 20–16 suggests that the susceptibility to this mode of reflux is proportional to the size of a type I hernia (Fig. 20–17) [28]. The implication is that patients with hiatal hernia exhibit progressive disruption of the diaphragmatic sphincter proportional to the extent of axial herniation. Therefore, although neither hiatus hernia

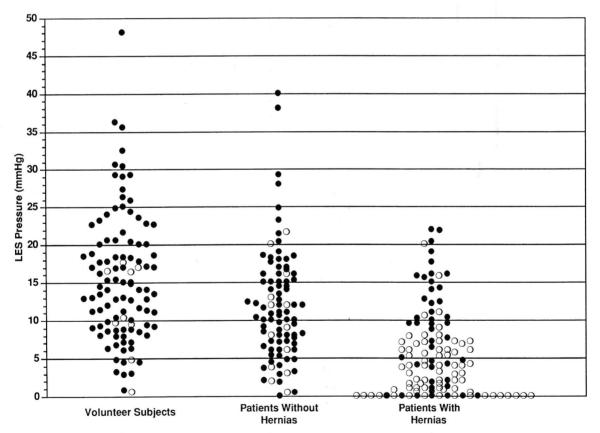

**FIG. 20–16.** Success or failure of individual provocative maneuvers (coughing, leg lifting, abdominal compression, Valsalva) at eliciting gastroesophageal reflux as a function of lower esophageal sphincter (LES) pressure among groups of normal controls, patients without hiatus hernia, and patients with radiographically defined hiatus hernia. LES pressure values were determined immediately prior to the onset of the maneuver. *Open circles* indicate individual trials of provocative maneuvers associated with gastroesophageal reflux, while *solid circles* indicate trials in which reflux did not occur. Reflux by the stress mechanism was much more easily elicited among the hiatus hernia patients. (From ref. 57, with permission.)

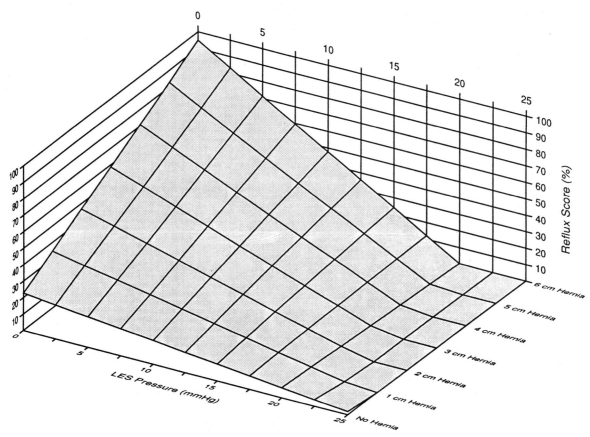

**FIG. 20–17.** Model of the relationship among LES pressure (x axis), size of hernia (y axis), and the susceptibility to gastroesophageal reflux induced by provocative maneuvers that increase abdominal pressure as reflected by the reflux score (z axis). The statistical model was created by stepwise regression analysis of the data in Fig. 20–16. The overall equation for the model is as follows: reflux score = 22.64 + 12.05 × (hernia size) − 0.83 × (LES pressure) − 0.65 × (LES pressure hernia size). The multiple correlation coefficient of this equation for the 50-subject data set was 0.86 ($R^2$ = 0.75), indicating that 75% of the observed variance in susceptibility to stress reflux among individuals was accounted for by the size of hiatus hernia and the instantaneous value of LES pressure. (From ref. 57, with permission.)

nor a hypotensive LES alone results in severe gastroesophageal junction incompetence, the two conditions interact with each other as evidenced by the statistical modeling in Fig. 20–17. This conclusion is consistent with the clinical experience that exercise, tight-fitting garments, and activities involving bending at the waist exacerbate heartburn in GERD patients (most of whom have hiatal hernias), especially after having consumed meals that reduce LES pressure.

Another hypothesis regarding the interrelationship between hiatal hernia and the LES is that type I hiatus hernia in and of itself may diminish LES pressure, a hypothesis consistent with observations made in both humans and nonhumans. Klein et al. studied the thoracoabdominal junction of ten patients after oncologically motivated resection of the gastroesophageal junction removed the entire intrinsic lower esophageal sphincter [28]. Subsequent manometric analysis revealed an end-expiratory intraluminal pressure of 6 ± 1 mm Hg within the ''sphincterless'' gastroesophageal junction, a value similar to the 3 ± 0.2 mm Hg observed

within the hiatal canal of hernia subjects [31]. Relevant animal data come from experimentally severing the phrenoesophageal ligament in dogs, analogous to the effect of axial hiatus hernia in which the ligament is stretched and its diaphragmatic attachments loosened [17, 49]. Severing the ligament substantially reduced peak gastroesophageal junction pressure, which was then restored with reanastomosis [36]. In the case of the hiatus hernia patients, reducing the hernia is the equivalent of reanastomosing the phrenoesophageal ligament, and doing so will in effect increase the LES pressure by causing the hiatal canal pressure to be superimposed on the intrinsic LES pressure [31]. Perhaps the only contradictory data are from diaphragmatic electromyographic (EMG) recordings, which strongly support the notion of a phasic, but not tonic, diaphragmatic contribution to gastroesophageal junction pressure [11, 12, 38, 40]. However, relying upon EMG recordings to completely represent the diaphragmatic contribution to gastroesophageal junction pressure ignores the possible contribution of passive forces such as diaphragmatic and arcuate ligament elasticity to intraluminal pressure. Certainly, in the case of the upper esophageal sphincter, such passive forces contribute an intraluminal pressure of similar magnitude after experimental abolition of the myogenic tone [6].

Another interesting observation pertains to the effect of hiatus hernia on the morphology of the LES high-pressure zone. Not only does the peak pressure within the LES high-pressure zone negatively correlate with the presence of hiatal hernia, but the overall length of the high-pressure zone can be significantly reduced in patients with large hiatal hernias, principally because of loss of the segment distal to the squamocolumnar junction (Fig. 20–18) [27]. This distal segment of the LES may be attributable to the sling fibers and clasp fibers of the gastric cardia, also referred to as the intraabdominal segment of the esophagus [29, 65]. This is probably the most confusing segment of esophageal anatomy, referred to by Inglefinger as an anatomic and functional no-man's-land [22]. Highlighting this confusion, Wolf remarked, "it is indeed strange that, when normally located below the hiatus, the 'submerged segment' resembles the esophagus while, when displaced above the hiatus, it resembles stomach. In fact, when a large hiatal hernia is present, the original submerged segment is incorporated into the hernia sac" [63]. Liebermann-Meffert et al. described a "fold transition line," evident in postmortem specimens, which appears analogous to the intragastric margin of the gastroesophageal

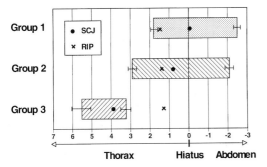

**FIG. 20–18.** Length and position of gastroesophageal junction high-pressure zone relative to the diaphragmatic hiatus among groups of normal subjects (group 1), subjects in whom the squamocolumnar junction (SCJ) was 0 to 2 cm above the diaphragm at rest (group 2), and subjects in whom the squamocolumnar junction was greater than 2 cm above the diaphragm at rest (group 3). Subject groups were defined by radiographically imaging an endoscopically placed metal mucosal clip. The horizontal bars depict the average limits of the high-pressure zone within each subject group (mean ± SE centimeters). The position of the respiratory inversion point (RIP) is constant among subject groups, while the position of the SCJ is progressively more cephalic in groups 2 and 3. Similar to the type IV patients in Fig. 20–9, the group 3 subjects in this investigation had a patulous hiatus and no detectable high-pressure zone at the diaphragmatic hiatus. Thus, the net effect was of shortening the high-pressure zone and positioning the SCJ relatively distally within the high-pressure zone such that it likely would be visible endoscopically from a retroflexed view. (From ref. 27, with permission.)

junction as imaged endoscopically and related to the angle of His as identified externally [29]. The squamocolumnar junction (SCJ) was 10.5 ± 4.4 mm proximal to the fold transition line when measured along the greater curvature. Although the relevance of this distal sphincter segment is controversial, Hill found the integrity of this "flap valve" (Fig. 20–9) to correlate with gastroesophageal junction competence against an antegrade pressure gradient in postmortem experiments [19]. With progressive proximal displacement of the SCJ above the hiatus, this distal segment eventually becomes disrupted and splays open, creating a radiographically evident saccular structure identifiable as a nonreducing hiatal hernia [28]. These observations suggest that the observed shortening of the LES high-pressure zone commented on by surgeons as indicative of a mechanically defective sphincter [60, 65] is probably largely a manometric correlate of a large nonreducing hiatal hernia.

## Compromise of Esophageal Emptying Related to Hiatus Hernia

The defining abnormality with esophagitis is excessive mucosal acid exposure, which, in turn, is dependent on both the frequency of reflux events and the time required to achieve acid clearance for each event. Prolongation of acid clearance among patients with reflux disease has long been recognized, especially with type I hiatus hernia while recumbent [23]. A series of investigations have demonstrated that hiatal hernias compromise fluid emptying from the distal esophagus [37, 56]. Sloan and Kahrilas analyzed the impact of hiatal hernia on esophageal emptying using simultaneous videofluoroscopy and manometry in patients with axial hiatal hernias compared to normal subjects [56]. Subjects were divided into three groups: (a) volunteers with a phrenic ampulla less than 2 cm in length, (b) patients or volunteers with maximal ampullary or hiatal hernia length greater than 2 cm that reduced between swallows (reducing hernia group), and (c) patients with hernias that did not reduce between swallows (nonreducing hiatus hernia). Each subject performed ten barium swallows and the outcome of each in terms of esophageal emptying was noted. Possible outcomes were complete clearance, minimal clearance because of failed peristalsis, late retrograde flow of barium from the ampulla back up the tubular esophagus (Fig. 20–19), or early retrograde flow from the ampulla occurring coincident with LES relaxation (Fig. 20–20). As shown in Fig. 20–21, the overall efficacy of esophageal emptying was significantly impaired in both hiatus hernia groups, but it was especially poor in the group with nonreducing hernias. The group with nonreducing hernias had complete emptying in only one-third of test swallows and exhibited early retrograde flow, a phenomenon unique to this group, in almost half.

This work corroborated findings by Mittal and co-workers, who used concurrent pH recording and scintiscanning to examine the efficacy of fluid emptying and acid clearance in patients with hiatal hernia and compared them to a group

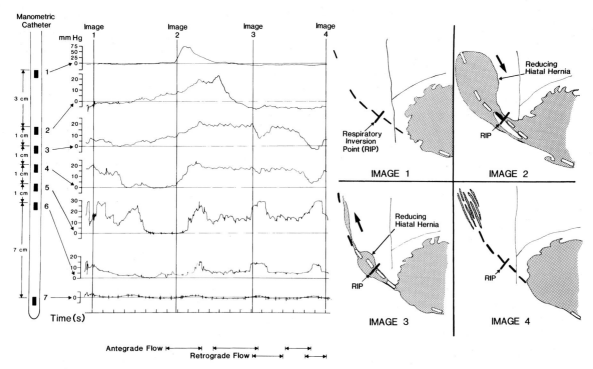

**FIG. 20–19.** Concurrent manometric and videofluorographic recording of a 10-ml barium swallow in a subject with a reducing hiatal hernia characterized by late retrograde flow. The tracings from the video images on the right correspond to the four selected times from the swallowing sequence indicated by the numbers at the top of the vertical lines intersecting the manometric record. The schematic diagram to the left indicates the relative spacing of the pressure-sensing ports (side holes located proximal to the markers in the fluoroscopic images). The lines at the bottom of the tracing indicate the timing and direction of barium flow. **Image 1** depicts the instant of swallowing when barium was visible only in the stomach. **Image 2** depicts the instant the stripping wave was at the level of the most proximal sensor; the hiatal hernia had formed and sensors 2–4 were in a common cavity within the hernia. **Image 3** depicts when retrograde flow began, at which point sensors 2 and 3 were above the hernia, sensor 4 was measuring intrahernial pressure, sensors 5 and 6 were at the level of the diaphragm, and sensor 7 remained within the stomach. **Image 4** shows residual barium in the distal esophagus and no hiatal hernia, with sensors 3–6 now straddling the high-pressure zone comprised of the lower esophageal sphincter and diaphragm. (From ref. 56, with permission.)

of esophagitis patients without hernias. Regardless of the presence of esophagitis, the hernia groups had impaired acid clearance because there was *reflux* from the hernia sac during swallowing (Fig. 20–22) [37]. *Rereflux* occurs predominantly during inspiration and can be attributed to loss of the normal one-way valve function of the crural diaphragm. By pinching off the distal esophagus, the crural diaphragm prevents backward flow from the stomach during each inspiration when it would be favored by a positive abdominal–thoracic pressure gradient. This one-way valve function of the crural diaphragm is grossly impaired with large type I hernias because a gastric pouch persists above the diaphragm as seen in Sloan's patients with nonreducing hernias [56].

### Conclusions

The gastroesophageal junction is anatomically and physiologically complex, making it vulnerable to dysfunction by several mechanisms. GERD has several potential causes, the unifying theme being increased esophageal acid exposure.

A variety of lines of evidence suggest that hiatal hernia is a significant pathophysiologic factor in approximately 50% of instances. The importance of hiatal hernia is obscured by imprecise usage of the term and the misconception that hiatal hernia is an all-or-none phenomenon. It is more accurate to view hiatal hernia as a continuum of progressive disruption of the gastroesophageal junction, with larger hernias being of greater significance. The dynamic anatomy of the gastroesophageal junction outlined herein highlights the difficulty of defining hiatal hernia and elucidating the relationship between hiatal hernia, the diaphragmatic hiatus, the lower esophageal sphincter, and gastroesophageal reflux disease. Hence, although it is clear that hiatal hernia is a contributing factor in the pathogenesis of gastroesophageal reflux disease, it is equally clear that GERD is a multifactorial process that defies overly reductionist explanation.

### TREATMENT

Repair of an isolated, asymptomatic type I hiatal hernia is rarely indicated. If symptoms of GERD occur in associa-

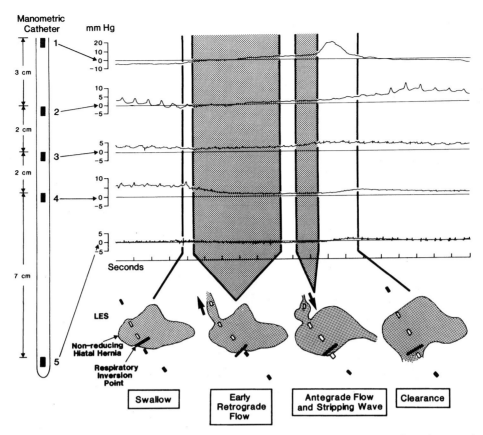

**FIG. 20–20.** Concurrent manometric and video recording of a 10-ml barium swallow characterized by early retrograde flow in a subject with a nonreducing hiatal hernia. Tracings from the video images are below the manometric record and correspond to the times on the manometric tracings intersected by the vertical lines. The schematic diagram to the left depicts the relative spacing of the pressure sensors whose tracings are depicted. The arrows next to the video image indicate the direction of barium flow. The first video image to the far left shows a barium-filled hiatal hernia at the time the swallow is initiated with sensor 1 in the distal esophagus, sensor 2 in the lower esophageal sphincter (LES), sensor 3 within the hernia, sensor 4 measuring crural contractile activity, and sensor 5 within the abdominal stomach. The second image was about 1 second after the swallow and depicts the onset of retrograde flow; intrahernial pressure was 2 mm Hg and LES pressure was 0 mm Hg. Retrograde flow continued for 5 seconds until the peristaltic contraction reached the distal esophagus. The third image depicts antegrade flow with the stripping wave progressing down the esophagus and LES pressure increasing to equal the intrahernia pressure (~4 mm Hg). The final image to the far right shows barium cleared from the esophagus with the LES pressure now exceeding the intrahernial pressure. (From ref. 56, with permission.)

tion with a large hiatus hernia, either medical or surgical treatment is indicated to control the reflux as discussed extensively elsewhere in this volume. Conversely, enlarging type II, III, and IV hernias pose a constant risk of serious complications similar to complications of a viscus herniated through an aperture elsewhere in the body: incarceration, obstruction, torsion, gangrene, and perforation [54]. These hernias never regress and progressively enlarge. If left untreated, the paraesophageal hernia eventually reaches the stage of the giant intrathoracic stomach. At this point, the patient may have substernal pain and pressure, or a gastric ulcer may develop in the poorly draining stomach [19]. More problematic, when the fundus becomes distended and prolapses out of the posterior mediastinum through the esophageal opening into the abdomen, obstruction occurs at the

esophageal, mid gastric, and duodenal levels (Fig. 20–23). If this is not relieved promptly, incarceration may become irreducible. Among a group of 10 such patients with strangulated and incarcerated hiatal hernias, Hill reported a 50% mortality. Conversely, among 19 patients in whom preoperative preparation and decompression was possible, there was no mortality [19]. Thus, once a paraesophageal hernia is identified, it should be treated surgically even in the absence of symptoms. Surgical approaches to type II hiatal hernias can be divided into five components, not all of which are required in each case [35]: (a) reduction of the herniated stomach into the abdomen, (b) herniotomy (excision of the hernia sac), (c) herniorrhaphy (closure of the hiatal defect), (d) antireflux procedure, and (e) gastropexy (attachment of the stomach subdiaphragmatically to prevent reherniation.

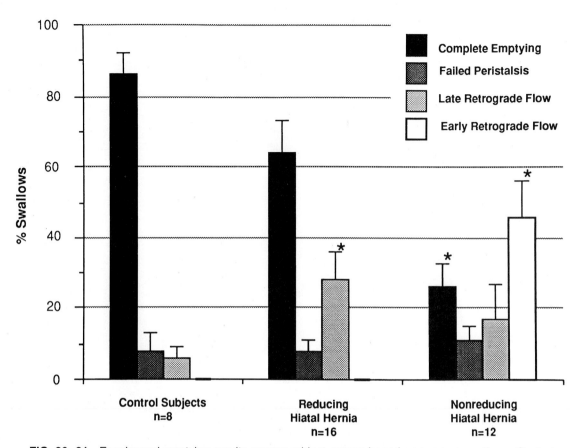

**FIG. 20–21.** Esophageal emptying results among subject groups based on ten test swallows. Control subjects had complete esophageal emptying without retrograde flow in 86 ± 6% of test swallows compared to 61 ± 9% in the reducing hernia group and 31 ± 8% in the nonreducing hernia group ($p <$ 0.05 vs. controls). The distinction between reducing hernia and nonreducing hernia was the radiographic observation of persistent rugal folds traversing the diaphragmatic hiatus in the nonreducing hernia group. The reducing hernia group exhibited significantly more instances of late retrograde flow (Fig. 20–19) ($p <$ 0.05 vs. controls), and the nonreducing hernia group were the only individuals to exhibit early retrograde flow (Fig. 20–20) ($p <$ 0.05 vs. other groups). (From ref. 56, with permission.)

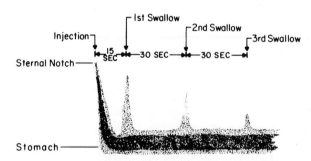

**FIG. 20–22.** Graphical depiction of a radionuclide acid clearance study in a subject with a hiatus hernia. Fifteen seconds after the injection of a 15-ml bolus of 0.1 N HCl labeled with 200 $\mu$Ci of $^{99m}$Tc-sulfur colloid, subjects swallowed every 30 seconds. The vertical axis represents the region from the sternal notch to the stomach. The horizontal axis is the time scale. The radioactivity is represented by the black area and absence of radioactivity is represented by the absence of black color. Soon after injection, the radioactivity appears in the stomach. However, note the biphasic response, i.e., an initial reflux of isotope into the esophagus followed by clearance of the isotope during the first three swallows. (From ref. 37, with permission.)

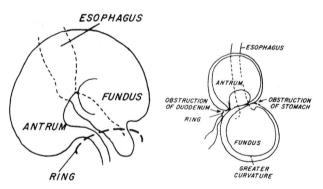

**FIG. 20–23.** Obstruction and entrapment as a complication of type II paraesophageal hernia with an upside-down stomach. The drawing on the left shows the hernia prior to obstruction with the gastroesophageal junction still fixed at the hiatus. This drawing is analogous to the radiograph in Fig. 20–10. With distention and filling of the fundus, it has the potential to form an organoaxial volvulus (Fig. 20–11) and reherniate through the hiatus. Obstruction then develops at the duodenum and at the mid portion of the stomach. Mortality of this condition is substantial. (From ref. 19, with permission.)

Opinion varies as to whether or not an antireflux procedure is necessary if concomitant pathologic reflux has not been demonstrated. The most common procedure done is a Nissen fundoplication. Gastropexy is employed if the stomach is unusually mobile after reduction. Following surgical repair of a type II hiatal hernia, the prognosis is excellent. The recurrence rate for type II hernias is higher than that for type I hernias presumably because the tissues of the hiatus are more compromised [53].

# REFERENCES

1. Akerlund A. Hernia diaphragmatica hernia oesophagei, vom anatomischen unt rontgenologischen Gesichtspunct. Acta Radiol 1926;6:3
2. Allison PR. Peptic ulcer of the esophagus. J Thorac Surg 1946;15:308
3. Allison PR. Reflux esophagitis, sliding hiatal hernia, and the anatomy of repair. Surg Gynecol Obstet 1951;92:419
4. Altschuler SM, Boyle JT, Nixon TE, Pack AI, Cohen S. Simultaneous reflex inhibition of lower esophageal sphincter and crural diaphragm in cats. Am J Physiol 1985;249:G586
5. Andrew LT. The height of the diaphragm in relation to the position of certain abdominal viscera. Lancet 1903;1:790
6. Asoh R, Goyal RK. Manometry and electromyography of the upper esophageal sphincter in the opossum. Gastroenterology 1978;74:514
7. Barrett NR. Discussion on hiatus hernia. Proc R Soc Med 1932;122:736
8. Berstad A, Weberg R, Frøyshov Larsen I, Hoel B, Hauer-Jensen M. Relationship of hiatus hernia to reflux oesophagitis. A prospective study of coincidence, using endoscopy. Scand J Gastroenterol 1986;21:55
9. Bowditch HI. Treatise on Diaphragmatic Hernia. Buffalo, NY: Hewett, Thomas & Co, 1853
10. Boyd DP. Surgery in hiatus hernia. Surg Clin North Am 1964;44:597
11. Boyle JT, Altschuler SM, Nixon TE, Tuchman DN, Pack AI, Cohen S. Role of the diaphragm in the genesis of lower esophageal sphincter pressure in the cat. Gastroenterology 1985;88:723
12. Boyle JT, Altschuler SM, Nixon TE, Pack AI, Cohen S. Responses of feline gastroesophageal junction to changes in abdominal pressure. Am J Physiol 1987;253:G315
13. Dent J, et al. Mechanism of gastroesophageal reflux in recumbent asymptomatic human subjects. J Clin Invest 1980;65:256
14. Dodds WJ, Dent J, Hogan WJ, Arndorfer RC. Effect of atropine on esophageal motor function in humans. Am J Physiol 1981;240:G290
15. De Troyer A, Rosso J. Reflex inhibition of the diaphragm by esophageal afferents. Neurosci Lett 1982;30:43
16. Evans JR, Bouslog JS. Hiatus hernia. Radiology 1940;34:530
17. Friedland GW. Historical review of the changing concepts of lower esophageal anatomy: 430B.C.–1977. Am J Roentgenol 1978;131:373
18. Helm JF, Dodds WJ, Pelc LR, Palmer DW, Hogan WJ, Teeter BC. Effect of esophageal emptying and saliva on clearance of acid from the esophagus. N Engl J Med 1984;310:284
19. Hill LD. Incarcerated paraesophagal hernia. A surgical emergency. Am J Surg 1973;126:286
20. Hill LD, et al. The gastroesophageal flap valve: in vitro and in vivo observations. Gastrointest Endosc 1996;44:541
21. Holloway RH, Penagini R, Ireland AC. Criteria for objective definition of transient lower esophageal sphincter relaxation. Am J Physiol 1995;268:G128
22. Inglefinger FJ. Esophageal motility. Physiol Rev 1958;38:533
23. Johnson, LF. 24-hour pH monitoring in the study of gastroesophageal reflux. J Clin Gastroenterol 1980;2:387
24. Kahrilas PJ. Hiatus hernia causes reflux: fact or fiction? Gullet 1993;3(Suppl):21
25. Kahrilas PJ, Gupta RR. Mechanisms of acid reflux associated with cigarette smoking. Gut 1990;31:4
26. Kahrilas PJ, Dodds WJ, Hogan WJ. Effect of peristaltic dysfunction on esophageal volume clearance. Gastroenterology 1988;4:73
27. Kahrilas PJ, et al. Attenuation of esophageal shortening during peristalsis with hiatus hernia. Gastroenterology 1995;109:1818
28. Klein WA, Parkman HP, Dempsey DT, Fisher RS. Sphincterlike thoracoabdominal high pressure zone after esophagogastrectomy. Gastroenterology 1993;105:1362
29. Liebermann-Meffert D, Allgöwer M, Schmid P, Blum AL. Muscular equivalent of the lower esophageal sphincter. Gastroenterology 1979;76:32
30. Lin S, et al. The phrenic ampulla: distal esophagus or potential hiatal hernia? Am J Physiol 1995;268:G320
31. Lin S, Chen J, Manka M, Kahrilas PJ. The LES and the hiatal sphincter: in unity there is strength. Gastroenterology 1997;112:A199
32. Low A. A note on the crura of the diaphragm and the muscle of Treitsz. J Anat Lond 1907;42:93
33. Marchand P. A study of the forces productive of gastro-oesophageal regurgitation through the diaphragmatic hiatus. Thorax 1957;12:189
34. Marchand P. The anatomy of esophageal hiatus of the diaphragm and the pathogenesis of hiatus herniation. Thorac Surg 1959;37:81
35. Menguy, R. Surgical management of large paraesophageal hernia with complete intrathoracic stomach. World J Surg 1988;12:415
36. Michelson E, Siegel CI. The role of the phrenico-esophageal ligament in the lower esophageal sphincter. Surg Gynecol Obstet 1964;118:1291
37. Mittal RK, Lange RC, McCallum RW. Identification and mechanism of delayed esophageal acid clearance in subjects with hiatus hernia. Gastroenterology 1987;92:130
38. Mittal RK, Rochester DF, McCallum RW. Electrical and mechanical activity in the human lower esophageal sphincter during diaphragmatic contraction. J Clin Invest 1988;81:1182
39. Mittal RK, Rochester DF, McCallum RW. Sphincteric action of the diaphragm during a relaxed lower esophageal sphincter in humans. Am J Physiol 1989;256:G139
40. Mittal RK, et al. Human lower esophageal sphincter pressure response to increased intra-abdominal pressure. Am J Physiol 1990;258:G624
41. Mittal RK, Holloway RH, Penagini R, Blackshaw LA, Dent J. Transient lower esophageal sphincter relaxation. Gastroenterology 1995;109:601
42. Monges H, Salducci J, Naudy B. Dissociation between the electrical activity of the diaphragmatic dome and crura muscular fibers during esophageal distension, vomiting, and eructation. An electromyographic study in the dog. J Physiol (Paris) 1978;74:541
43. Orr WC, Robinson MG, Johnson LF. Acid clearance during sleep in the pathogenesis of reflux esophagitis. Dig Dis Sci 1981;26:423
44. Ott DJ, et al. Esophagogastric region and its rings. Am J Roentgenol 1984;142:281
45. Ott DJ, et al. Predictive relationship of hiatal hernia to reflux esophagitis. Gastrointest Radiol 1985;10:317
46. Paterson WG, Kolyn DM. Esophageal shortening induced by short-term intraluminal acid perfusion in opossum: a cause of hiatus hernia? Gastroenterology 1994;107:1736
47. Peridikis G, Hinder RA. Paraesophageal hiatal hernia. In Nyhus LM, Condon RE, eds, Hernia. Philadelphia: JB Lippincott Co, 1995:544
48. Petersen H, et al. Relationship between endoscopic hiatus hernia and gastroesophageal reflux symptoms. Scand J Gastroenterol 1991;26:921
49. Pouderoux P, Lin S, Kahrilas PJ. Timing, propagation, coordination, and effect of esophageal shortening during esophageal peristalsis. Gastroenterology 1997;112:1147
50. Rigler LG, Eneboe JB. Incidence of hiatus hernia in pregnant women and its significance. J Thorac Surg 1935;4:262
51. Schatzki R. Die hernien des hiatus oesophageus. Deutsches Arch Klin Med 1932;173:85
52. Serpanti M. The results of systematic search for hiatal hernia in the course of 480 upper gastrointestinal x-ray series. J Radiol 1955;36:919
53. Skinner DB. Hernias (hiatal, traumatic, and congenital). In Berk JE, ed, Gastroenterology (4th ed). Philadelphia: WB Saunders, 1985:705
54. Skinner DB, Belsey RHR, Russel PS. Surgical management of esophageal reflux and hiatus hernia. Long term results with 1030 patients. J Thorac Cardiovasc Surg 1967;53:33
55. Skinner DB, Roth JLA, Sullivan BH, Stein GN, Levine M. Reflux esophagitis. In Berk JE, ed. Gastroenterology (4th ed). Philadelphia: WB Saunders, 1985:717
56. Sloan S, Kahrilas PJ. Impairment of esophageal emptying with hiatal hernia. Gastroenterology 1991;100:596
57. Sloan S, Rademaker AW, Kahrilas PJ. Determinants of gastroesophageal junction incompetence: hiatal hernia, lower esophageal sphincter, or both? Ann Intern Med 1992;117:977

58. Sonnenberg A, et al. Salivary secretion in reflux esophagitis. Gastroenterology 1982;83:889
59. Stanciu C, Bennett JR. Esophageal acid clearing: one factor in production of reflux esophagitis. Gut 1974;15:852
60. Stein HJ, DeMeester TR, Naspetti R, Jamieson J, Perry RE. Three-dimensional imaging of the lower esophageal sphincter in gastroesophageal reflux disease. Ann Surg 1991;214:374
61. Stilson WL, et al. Hiatal hernia and gastroesophageal reflux. A clinical analysis of more than 1000 cases. Radiology 1969;93:1323
62. Winkelstein A. Peptic esophagitis. A new clinical entity. JAMA 1935;104:906
63. Wolf BS. Sliding hiatal hernia: the need for redefinition. Am J Roentgenol 1973;117:231
64. Wright RA, Hurwitz AL. Relationship of hiatal hernia in endoscopically proved reflux esophagitis. Dig Dis Sci 1979;24:311
65. Zaninotto G, DeMeester TR, Schwizer W, Johansson KE, Cheng SC. The lower esophageal sphincter in health and disease. Am J Surg 1988;155:104

*The Esophagus*, Third Edition,
edited by D. O. Castell and J. E. Richter.
Lippincott Williams & Wilkins, Philadelphia © 1999.

# CHAPTER 21

# Pathophysiology of Gastroesophageal Reflux Disease

## Motility Factors

Ravinder K. Mittal

## INTRODUCTION

Is gastroesophageal reflux disease an acid or motility disorder of the esophagus? Indeed, gastric acid is the major offender and is primarily responsible for the esophageal mucosal damage in reflux diseases. However, the gastric acid secretion in the majority of patients with reflux disease is normal. The reason that gastric acid reaches the esophagus is due to the motility abnormality of the lower esophageal sphincter (LES). Deranged esophageal peristalsis, when present, allows acid and possibly other noxious agents to remain in the esophagus for extended periods of time and induce esophageal mucosal damage. Therefore, even though the major noxious agent in reflux disease is gastric acid, the motility abnormalities of the LES and esophagus are primary etiologic factors and fundamental to the understanding of reflux disease.

## LOWER ESOPHAGEAL SPHINCTER

### Historical Perspective

A person can stand upside down after eating a large hearty meal, yet no food refluxes into the mouth or the esophagus. It is intuitively clear that there must be a valvular or sphincter mechanism at the lower end of the esophagus. In a 1958 review article, Ingelfinger stated that the pinchcock action of the diaphragm was important in the prevention of gastroesophageal reflux [41]. Fyke and Code were the first to record an intraluminal high-pressure zone between the esophagus

R. K. Mittal: Department of Gastroenterology, School of Medicine University of California, San Diego, and Gastroenterology Section, Medical Service, Department of Veterans Affairs Medical Center, La Jolla, California 92123.

and the stomach [31]; they suggested that intrinsic muscles of the lower end of the esophagus were entirely responsible for maintaining this pressure. It was not until 1985 that the diaphragmatic hiatus was proven to play a role in the valvular mechanism at the esophagogastric junction (EGJ) [10]. Studies conducted during the last several years convincingly show that there is not one, but two LESs. The dual-sphincter mechanism at the EGJ is composed of intrinsic smooth muscles of the LES and extrinsic skeletal muscles of the diaphragmatic hiatus. In humans, under normal conditions, the LES is approximately 4 cm in length and the crural diaphragm, which forms the esophageal hiatus, is about 2 cm in length. The crural diaphragm encircles the proximal 2 cm of the LES [33]. Therefore, a portion of the LES is intra-abdominal and a portion is located in the hiatus itself (Fig. 21–1). The intra-abdominal portion of the LES is frequently termed the submerged segment of the esophagus [73]. The lower end of the esophagus has also been referred to as the phrenic ampulla by radiologists because it has a bulbar shape on barium swallow [87]. The anatomic structure of the phrenic ampulla is poorly characterized.

Recent studies using ultrasound techniques [54] demonstrate that the muscles of the LES are thicker than those of the adjacent esophagus. However, the muscle thickness in the LES region is not fixed; there is a direct relationship between the LES pressure and its thickness [55]. The LES has a rich nerve supply. However, the location of the neurons in the LES differs from the rest of the esophagus [86]. Within the LES, the myenteric plexus lies in several muscle planes, in contrast to the body of the esophagus, where the major plexus lies between the longitudinal and the circular muscle layers.

Intrinsic muscles of the stomach may also contribute to the antireflux barrier. The sling or oblique fibers of the stomach are located below the high-pressure zone. These fibers

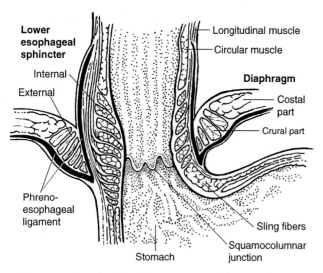

**FIG. 21–1.** Schematic of the anatomy of the esophagogastric junction. The smooth muscles of the lower end of the esophagus and the crural diaphragm are the two sphincteric mechanisms at the esophagogastric junction. The two sphincters are anatomically superimposed and anchored to each other by the phrenoesophageal ligament. (From Mittal RK, Balaban DH. Mechanisms of disease: the esophagogastric junction. N Engl Med 1997;336:924, with permission.)

are arranged in a C-shaped fashion with the closed end of the C located on the greater curvature and the open end oriented toward the lesser curvature [52]. The exact function of these fibers is not clear; they may be responsible for the flap valve mechanism considered to be important in the prevention of gastroesophageal reflux [92].

The respiratory diaphragm, which is the major organ for the ventilatory function of the lung, also has a LES function. The diaphragm is composed of a costal part, arising from the ribs, and a crural part, which originates from the vertebral column. The two parts of the diaphragm have separate embryologic origins. The crural diaphragm develops from the dorsal mesentery of the esophagus, and the costal diaphragm from myoblasts originating in the lateral body wall [51]. The crural diaphragm, which forms the esophageal hiatus and constitutes the "extrinsic sphincter mechanism," is actually shaped like a canal. In humans, this canal is formed primarily by the right crus of the diaphragm [17]. The fibers in this canal are oriented in a cranial to caudal direction toward the outer aspect and obliquely toward the inner aspect. The LES and crural diaphragm are anchored to each other by the phrenoesophageal ligament, a condensation of loose areolar tissue. This ligament extends from the undersurface of the diaphragm and attaches to the esophagus approximately at the upper border of the LES.

### Esophagogastric Junction Pressure under Various Physiologic Conditions

The intraluminal pressure at the EGJ is a measure of the strength of the antireflux barrier. There are convincing data

in both animals and humans that the two anatomic structures, i.e., the LES and crural diaphragm, contribute to the EGJ pressure. Electrical stimulation of the crural diaphragm increases the EGJ pressure in cats [2]. Furthermore, the crural diaphragm is capable of maintaining a high-pressure zone at the abdominothoracic junction in patients who have undergone surgical resection of the LES [50].

To avoid confusion, the intraluminal pressure at the lower end of the esophagus shall be referred to as the EGJ pressure. The pressure generated from the contraction of LES smooth muscle is called the LES pressure, and pressure due to contraction of the crural diaphragm is termed the crural diaphragm pressure. Distinguishing these two pressures is important because it emphasizes the individual contributions of each structure to the EGJ pressure.

The LES or EGJ pressure is measured in reference to the intragastric pressure. Prolonged continuous pressure monitoring reveals that the EGJ pressure varies over time. These variations are either due to LES or crural diaphragm contractions. The LES pressure varies from minute to minute, and these pressure fluctuations are usually of small amplitude, ranging from 5 to 10 mm Hg. However, large LES pressure fluctuations coupled with the migrating motor complex (MMC) activity of the stomach may also occur. The frequency of these phasic pressure fluctuations is the same as that of MMC, usually 3/minute. The LES pressure may exceed 80 mm Hg during phase III of the MMC and typically peaks prior to the onset of gastric contraction [19].

The second type of variation in the EGJ pressure is related to the crural diaphragm contraction, which is linked with respiration. With each inspiration, as the crural diaphragm contracts, there is an increase in the EGJ pressure [65]. The amplitude of the inspiratory pressure increase is directly proportional to the force of crural diaphragmatic contraction. During tidal inspiration, the EGJ pressure increase is 10 to 20 mm Hg, and with deep inspiration the pressure increase ranges from 100 to 150 mm Hg. The crural diaphragm also contributes to the EGJ pressure during nonrespiratory physical activities such as straight leg raising and abdominal compression. These activities can induce sustained or tonic contractions of the crural diaphragm [66]. The crural diaphragm reflexively contracts during coughing, Valsalva maneuver, and any physical condition which increases intraabdominal pressure.

### Neural Control of the Lower Esophageal Sphincter and Crural Diaphragm

The tone in the LES muscle is the result of myogenic and neurogenic mechanisms. The relative contribution of these two mechanisms varies among different species. In humans, the LES tone is comprised of both neurogenic and myogenic components. A significant percentage of the LES tone in humans is due to cholinergic innervation [22]. Myogenic tone is due to shifts of intracellular calcium stores within the LES muscle [7].

There is a large number of excitatory and inhibitory neuro-transmitters within LES muscle; however, their physiologic significance remains unclear. The modulation of LES tone that occurs with MMC activity is largely mediated through the vagus nerve [12, 13]. The swallow-associated LES relaxation is mediated through the central nervous system (dorso-motor nucleus of the vagus nerve). The efferents travel to the LES via the vagus nerve and the myenteric plexus. The synapse between the vagal fibers and myenteric neurons employs a cholinergic mechanism, and the postsynaptic neuro-transmitter is noncholinergic, nonadrenergic [32]. Several studies confirm that nitric oxide is the noncholinergic, non-adrenergic neurotransmitter [93], but vasoactive intestinal peptide may also play a role.

The crural diaphragm, like the remainder of the diaphragm, is controlled through the phrenic nerves. Although the diaphragmatic hiatus is composed of muscles mainly from the right crus, it is innervated bilaterally through the left and right phrenic nerves. Spontaneous inspiratory activity of the crural diaphragm is due to the activity of inspiratory neurons located in the syncytium of the brain stem [82]. This activity is transmitted to the phrenic nerve nucleus located in the cervical spinal cord. Voluntary control of the diaphragm originates within the cortical neurons. The crural diaphragm contracts a fraction of a second earlier than the costal diaphragm, and this may have physiologic significance in relationship to its antireflux barrier function [16].

Esophageal sensory mechanisms can mediate reflex relaxation of the crural diaphragm. Esophageal distension and a swallow induce selective inhibition of the crural diaphragm muscle [3]. Transient relaxation of the LES, a major mechanism of gastroesophageal reflux, belching, and vomiting, is also accompanied by simultaneous relaxation of the LES and crural diaphragm [57, 72].

## Physiologic Significance of the Two Lower Esophageal Sphincters

Why do we need two lower esophageal sphincters? The answer to this question rests on the physical principle that the intraluminal EGJ pressure determines the strength of the antireflux barrier, and the pressure gradient between the esophagus and stomach (PGES) is the driving force for gastroesophageal reflux. Under normal situations, the EGJ pressure is constantly adapting to changes in the PGES that occur during various physiologic circumstances. The changes in PGES are related either to muscular contractions of the esophagus and stomach or to pressure changes within the intrathoracic and intrabdominal cavities. Contraction of the esophagus is protective with respect to reflux. On the other hand, gastric contraction increases the pressure gradient in favor of reflux. Therefore, LES contraction is coupled with gastric contraction during MMC activity of the stomach, thus preventing reflux. Contraction of the inspiratory muscles of respiration produces negative intrathoracic and intraesophageal pressure, thus increasing the PGES. Similarly, contrac-

tion of the abdominal wall and diaphragm increases the stomach pressure and PGES. All of the maneuvers accompanied by contraction of inspiratory and abdominal wall muscles that increase PGES are accompanied by contraction of the crural diaphragm and a protective increase in EGJ pressure. The rapid changes in PGES caused by skeletal muscle contraction of the chest and abdomen are thus counteracted by rapidly contracting skeletal sphincter muscle of the crural diaphragm.

## Mechanisms of Reflux

Based upon an understanding of the two lower esophageal sphincters, one would intuitively think that weakness of either the LES or crural diaphragm is the cause of gastro-esophageal reflux. Indeed, some patients with reflux disease have a weak LES, some have a weak crural diaphragm, and some have both. However, in mild to moderate nonerosive reflux disease, the LES [20] and crural diaphragm pressures [68] are normal. In fact a number of patients with mild to moderate disease have a hypertensive LES [48]. The incidence of low LES pressure increases with the severity of esophagitis [20], and spontaneous inspiratory crural diaphragm pressure is low in 50% of patients with endoscopic reflux disease [68]. A large body of information indicates that transient relaxation of the LES and crural diaphragm (TLESR) is the major mechanism of reflux in normal subjects and patients with reflux disease [70].

## TRANSIENT LOWER ESOPHAGEAL SPHINCTER RELAXATION

McNally et al. first observed non-swallow-related LES relaxation as a mechanism of belching in 1964 [58]. However, it was not until 1980 that the phenomenon of TLESR and its relationship to gastroesophageal reflux was described in detail [18]. Overall, TLESR is the single most common mechanism underlying gastroesophageal reflux. In normal subjects, the majority of reflux episodes occur during TLESRs, with almost all the remainder occurring during swallow-induced LES relaxation associated with failed or incomplete primary peristalsis. This pattern of reflux mechanism is remarkably consistent among subjects, both supine and ambulant [84]. Most studies have shown that TLESR is also the most common mechanism of reflux in patients with reflux disease and accounts for between 63% and 74% of reflux episodes [23, 63, 78]. Similar findings have also been reported in children with reflux disease [15, 94].

Mechanisms of reflux in patients with reflux disease are less homogeneous than in normal subjects. While more than 50% of patients, usually those without endoscopic evidence of esophagitis, reflux exclusively through TLESR, many patients have a mixed picture in which a significant minority of reflux episodes occur during swallow-induced LES relaxation, persistently absent basal LES pressure, and straining by deep inspiration or increased intra-abdominal pressure.

The proportion of reflux episodes that can be ascribed to TLESRs varies inversely with the severity of reflux disease [57], presumably because of the increasing prevalence of defective basal LES pressure as the severity of esophagitis increases [20]. The presence or absence of esophagitis does not seem to influences the rate of TLESRs [5, 24].

## Characteristics of Transient Lower Esophageal Sphincter Relaxation

Transient LES relaxations are abrupt falls in LES pressure to the level of intragastric pressure that are not triggered by swallowing, as manifested by the distinctive pattern of pharyngeal or mylohyoid muscle contraction (Fig. 21–2). In most studies, a fall in LES pressure of 5 mm Hg has been regarded as minimum. Transient LES relaxations are typically of longer duration than swallow-induced LES relaxation, lasting from 10 to 45 seconds. The criteria that have proved optimal for the definition of TLESRs are (a) the absence of a pharyngeal swallow signal for 4 seconds before to 2 seconds after the onset of LES relaxation, or a mylohyoid EMG complex for 3 seconds before the onset of LES relaxation; (b) LES pressure fall of $\geq 1$ mm Hg/second; (c) a time from the onset to complete relaxation of $\leq 10$ seconds; and (d) a nadir pressure of $\leq 2$ mm Hg. Excluding LES relaxations associated with multiple rapid swallows, LES pressure drops to 2 mm Hg which have a duration of greater than 10 sec can also be classified as TLESRs [37]. A number of events in the esophagus, stomach, and crural diaphragm have been identified that accompany TLESRs. Contractions in the pharynx and mylohyoid muscle have been reported to occur at the onset of 20% to 45% of TLESRs, respectively [62], although these pharyngeal and mylohyoid complexes are much smaller (approximately 50%) than those associated with swallowing and can be interpreted as partial or incomplete swallows. Distal esophageal pressure waves, clearly unrelated to swallowing, often occur at the onset of TLESRs and, when recorded at more than one site, usually have a synchronous onset. During the period of LES inhibition, there

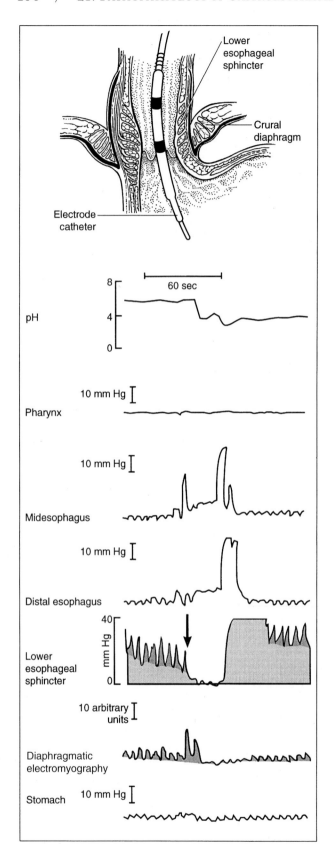

FIG. 21–2. A spontaneous, transient lower esophageal sphincter relaxation (TLESR). The onset of TLESR is indicated by the vertical arrow. Relaxation occurs in the absence of a swallow as manifested by the absence of a pharyngeal pressure wave. The LES relaxation is complete to the level of the intragastric pressure (horizontal line at the bottom of the LES tracing) and is sustained for more than 20 seconds. TLESR is associated with inhibition of the crural diaphragm as indicated by the loss of inspiratory LES pressure oscillations and inspiratory diaphragmatic electromyography (DEMG). Reflux (drop in esophageal pH) occurs following complete LES and crural diaphragm relaxation and is associated with an increase in intraesophageal pressure. (From Mittal RK, Balaban DH. Mechanisms of disease: the esophagogastric junction. N Engl J Med 1997;336:924, with permission.)

is also inhibition of the esophageal body, which is manifested by inhibition of primary peristalsis during prolonged relaxations [88]. The gastric fundus also shows changes consistent with active inhibition during TLESRs. A small drop in intragastric pressure, usually in the range of 2 to 4 mm Hg, occurs during TLESRs. In addition to the events in upper gastrointestinal smooth muscle, there is also selective and complete inhibition of the crural diaphragm despite continued activity of the costal diaphragm during TLESRs [61]. Thus, TLESR is not a response localized to the LES. Rather, it appears to be part of a more generalized inhibition of a number of structures within and outside of the upper gastrointestinal tract which influence flow across the gastroesophageal junction. These structures are either innervated by the vagus nerve or are linked to the brain stem, or both. This pattern of inhibition is consistent with a coordinated pattern of activity designed to facilitate the retrograde flow of gastric contents during belching.

## Stimuli that Trigger Transient Lower Esophageal Sphincter Relaxations

### Gastric Distension

Gastric distension is a potent stimulus for TLESR. This is not surprising given the fact that TLESR is the mechanism by which gas is vented from the stomach during belching. Approximately 15 ml of air is delivered to the stomach with each swallow [26] and without an in-built venting mechanism, uncontrolled gastrointestinal bloating would occur. Studies in which the stomach has been partitioned surgically have revealed that the subcardiac region of the stomach is primarily responsible for triggering TLESR [28]. Reduction of the compliance of this region by buttressing it with mesh reinforcement substantially reduces TLESR in dogs. Although distension of other parts of the stomach can increase the rate of TLESR, the thresholds for distension is substantially higher in these regions and the response less marked. In humans, a volume of 750 to 1,000 ml causes a fourfold increase in the rate of TLESRs within the first 10 minutes. In some studies, a similar effect has been reported after meals [40, 77]. Meals are also associated with a significant increase in the proportion of TLESRs associated with reflux, and it is possible that this effect rather than an increase in the rate of TLESRs is responsible for the postprandial increase in reflux.

### Pharyngeal Mechanisms

Pharyngeal intubation increases the rate of TLESRs. In fasted patients in whom LES pressure was monitored via a gastrostomy tube, pharyngeal intubation for 1 hour increased the rate of TLESRs threefold, from 2 to 6/hour during the period of intubation [67]. Pharyngeal stimulation is usually associated with full expression of the oral, pharyngeal, and esophageal phases of deglutition [59]. LES relaxation without swallowing can be induced by instillation of minute amounts of liquid into the hypopharynx in humans [71] and light stroking of the pharynx or low-frequency stimulation of the superior laryngeal nerve in the opossum [74]. This reflex depends on the afferent nerve fibers from the pharynx or larynx [90] traveling in the superior laryngeal branch of the vagus and the glossopharyngeal nerves; both nerves project to the nucleus tractus solitarii (NTS). The occurrence of small mylohyoid and pharyngeal complexes at the onset of some TLESRs may be an evidence of subthreshold or incomplete swallowing. A recent study did show that LES relaxation caused by stimulation of pharynx with small amounts of water can last up to 60 seconds or longer. Interaction among stimuli is a real possibility; thus, pharyngeal stimulation may either trigger TLESRs directly or lower the threshold for triggering by gastric distension.

### Factors Modulating the Rate of Transient Lower Esophageal Sphincter Relaxations Are Posture, Sleep, Anesthesia, and Stress

In both healthy humans and dogs, the stimulation of TLESRs produced by gaseous gastric distension is almost totally suppressed in the supine posture [42, 43, 53]. In patients with reflux disease, TLESRs occur significantly less frequently in the supine [30] and lateral recumbent positions compared to sitting. TLESRs do not occur during stable sleep [29]; reflux episodes that do occur during the nighttime sleep periods are totally confined to periods of arousal during sleep that may last for only 10 seconds.

Spontaneous TLESRs are also completely suppressed in dogs by even light general anesthesia [14]. Cold stress has also been shown to reduce the frequency of TLESRs [76].

### Neural Pathways Mediating Transient Lower Esophageal Sphincter Relaxation: Vagal Control Mechanisms

The vagus mediates swallow-induced LES relaxation [80, 83] and inhibition of gastric tone or receptive relaxation during swallowing [11] (Fig. 21–3). The efferent pathway for TLESRs is also presumably in the vagus nerve; in dogs, TLESRs are completely abolished by cooling of the cervical vagus [56], and eructation is substantially inhibited by truncal vagotomy 5 cm above the diaphragm [91]. The absence of TLESRs in patients with achalasia suggests that TLESRs share a final common pathway with swallow-induced LES relaxation [39]. Gastric distension probably triggers TLESRs through stimulation of tension receptors in the proximal stomach [1, 8]; particularly the gastric cardia. Afferent fibers which signal gastric distension are known to project to the NTS [81] and to the dorsal motor nucleus of the vagus (DMV), either directly or via interneurons [47]. The DMV contains the cell bodies of vagal efferent neurons which project to the LES [13]. Gastric mechanoreceptors have been

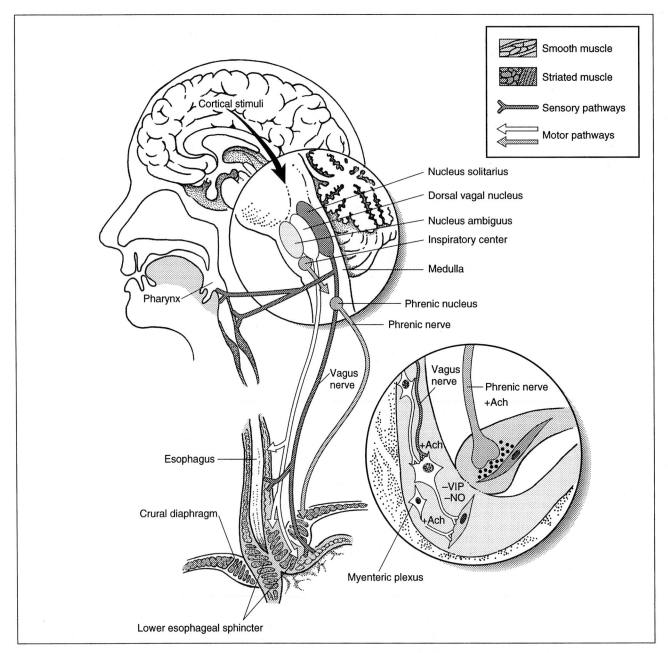

**FIG. 21–3.** Schematic of the neural pathway to the LES and crural diaphragm. Swallow-induced esophageal peristalsis and LES relaxation result from excitation of receptors located in the pharynx. The afferent stimulus travels to the sensory nucleus (*NTS,* nucleus tractus solita rius). A programmed set of events from the dorsomotor nucleus of the vagus (DMV) and nucleus ambiguus (NA) mediate esophageal peristalsis and LES relaxation. The vagal fibers communicate with myenteric neurons, which in turn mediate LES relaxation. The postganglionic transmitter is nitric oxide (*NO*) and vasoactive intestinal peptide (*VIP*). Transient LES relaxation (TLESR), (the major mechanism of reflux), appears to share the same neural pathway. The afferent signals for TLESR may originate in the pharynx, larynx, and stomach. The efferent pathway is in the vagus nerve, and nitric oxide is the postganglionic neurotransmitter. Crural diaphragm contraction is controlled by the inspiratory center in the brain stem, which communicates with the phrenic nerve nucleus. The crural diaphragm is innervated by right and left phrenic nerves through motor end plates and nicotinic cholinergic receptors. *Ach,* Acetylcholine; +, excitatory; −, inhibitory. (From Mittal RK, Balaban DH. Mechanisms of disease: the esophagogastric junction. N Engl J Med 1997;336:924, with permission.)

postulated to serve as the afferent pathway for a number of vagal reflexes including reflex relaxation of the gastric corpus. Such a neural pathway could therefore potentially mediate TLESRs. In the opossum, LES relaxation can also be induced by intrinsic gastric nerves independently of extrinsic nerves [85]. Whether or not such a pathway mediates TLESRs is not known, but it cannot be involved in the associated inhibition of the crural diaphragm during TLESRs. The complete abolition of TLESRs by cervical vagal cooling [56] also argues against a dominant role for a local intramural pathway in mediating TLESRs.

The selective inhibition of the crural diaphragm that is characteristic of TLESRs also occurs during vomiting [72] and esophageal distension [3] and to a partial degree during swallowing. Presumably, this inhibition is coordinated in the brain stem, although the precise site at which this occurs is unclear. Rhythmic respiration is controlled mainly by premotor neurons in the dorsal respiratory group within the NTS and the adjacent reticular formation [6], which in turn activate diaphragmatic motor neurons in the ventral horn of the cervical spinal cord. The NTS is also the destination for afferent input from the vagus and glossopharyngeal nerves and has been suggested as a potential site for the integrated neural control of inhibition of respiration during swallowing. However, inhibition of the crural diaphragm by esophageal distension and, by implication, during TLESRs does not appear to be through inhibition of the medullary premotor inspiratory neurons of the respiratory center, but via a separate, as-yet-unidentified pathway [4]. TLESR is a long period (10 to 60 seconds) of simultaneous LES and crural diaphragm relaxation. Relaxations of both the LES and crural diaphragm during TLESR are essential for the occurrence of reflux in normal subjects [69].

Based on the evidence, it is possible to construct a hypothetical pathway for the triggering of TLESRs (Fig. 21–3). The basic element is a vagal reflex pathway triggered by gastric distension or pharyngeal stimulation and integrated in the brain stem. The threshold for triggering is lowered by concurrent stimulation of the pharynx (and possibly larynx) and increased potentially by the supine posture, sleep, and anesthesia. The efferent vagal output is controlled by a pattern generator in the brain stem and mediates the esophageal, LES, gastric, and diaphragmatic events during TLESR. Under usual circumstances, the pharyngeal components of deglutition are bypassed, but these can be partly activated on occasion causing the small pharyngeal and mylohyoid complexes that occur with some TLESRs.

Gastroesophageal reflux disease is characterized by a higher frequency of reflux episodes. This has been attributed in different studies to both a higher frequency of TLESRs and a higher incidence of reflux during TLESRs. Probably the unresolved discrepancy in the frequency of TLESRs is due to the use of differing definitions of TLESR in different studies. An early study reported that TLESRs occurred at a frequency of about 3/hour in patients with reflux disease compared with 2/hour in normal subjects, although this study

included swallow-associated LES relaxations associated with failed primary peristalsis in the definition of TLESR [21]. Since then, several other studies have reported frequencies of TLESRs of 3 to 8/hour in patients with reflux disease and 2 to 6/hour in normal subjects. The size of the meal, posture, and sleep status are some of the variables that influence the frequency of TLESRs and may vary among studies. The nature of afferent and/or efferent dysfunction that leads to more frequent episodes of TLESR in patients with reflux disease is not clear.

More agreement exists about the higher incidence of reflux during TLESRs in patients compared to normal subjects. In normal subjects about 40% to 50% of TLESRs are accompanied by acid reflux compared with 60% to 70% in patients with reflux disease [23, 63, 71]. The factors that determine whether reflux occurs during TLESRs have not been studied systematically. Possibilities include abdominal straining, the presence of hiatus hernia, the degree of esophageal shortening, and duration of TLESRs. Abdominal straining occurs with 15% to 20% of TLESRs and increases the likelihood of reflux from 30% to 60%. However, the prevalence of straining during reflux episodes does not seem to be different between normal subjects and patients with reflux disease. Hiatus hernia is associated with an increased prevalence of reflux during swallow-induced LES relaxation presumably because of pooling of acid in the herniated gastric pouch [64]. A similar mechanism could increase the likelihood of reflux during TLESRs, although this has not been formally examined.

Although not available for clinical use, pharmacologic suppression of TLESR is possible and a desirable form of therapy in reflux disease. Triggering of TLESRs by gastric distension can be inhibited by cholecystokinin (CCK)-A receptor and nitric oxide antagonists [9]. This effect of CCK-A antagonist appears to be mediated through a peripheral rather than a central mechanism. Infusion of CCK-A increases the frequency of TLESRs and this increase can be abolished by administration of a nitric oxide antagonist. These observations suggest that CCK-A released after meals may contribute to the provocation of TLESRs by meals, and that nitric oxide is the neurotransmitter released at the postganglionic site in the vagal pathway that is responsible for mediating TLESRs. Atropine also reduces the frequency of TLESRs and reflux after a meal, and the mechanism of its action appears to be at the level of the central nervous system [27, 69]. Whether these or other pharmacologic agents will prove to be useful in the treatment of reflux disease remains to be studied. TLESR is a normal physiologic event required for belching. TLESR can be blocked by nitric oxide antagonists. However, nitric oxide is also important in swallow-induced LES relaxation, and its blockade can result in dysphagia and an "achalasia-like" condition. Morphine has recently been found to decrease the TLESR frequency in normal subjects through an unknown mechanism [79]. Whether these agents or their derivatives can be effective in the treatment of reflux disease remains to be seen.

## EFFECT OF ANTIREFLUX THERAPY ON TRANSIENT LOWER ESOPHAGEAL SPHINCTER RELAXATION

The effect of medical therapy for reflux disease on TLESRs has received little attention. In patients with reflux disease, the presence or absence of endoscopically visible esophagitis does not influence the rate of TLESRs after meals. However, the effect of healing of esophagitis with acid suppressants on the rate of TLESRs is controversial; omeprazole has been reported to have no effect [24], while H2 antagonists have been reported to decrease the rate of TLESRs [5]. At standard doses, cisapride does not appear to influence the rate of TLESRs up to 3 hours after a meal [38]. The failure of therapy to influence the cause of reflux presumably explains why reflux disease relapses so promptly when medical therapy is ceased. Although a plethora of studies have investigated the effect of antireflux surgery on LES function, only one has examined the effect on TLESRs [44]. This study showed that fundoplication has two major effects: a 50% reduction in the rate of TLESRs and a reduction in the proportion of TLESRs that were accompanied by reflux from 47% to 17%. The mechanisms underlying these effects include the creation of an artificial high-pressure zone around the LES by fundoplication that persists during both transient and swallow-induced LES

relaxation [49], and possibly a reduction in the degree of distension of the gastric cardia by the gastric wrap, which may reduce the gastric distension-induced stimulation of TLESRs.

## LOWER ESOPHAGEAL SPHINCTER HYPOTENSION IN REFLUX DISEASE

Even though TLESR is the major mechanism of reflux, a low LES pressure is an important mechanism of reflux in patients with reflux disease [36]. In the presence of a low LES pressure, reflux is thought to occur either freely from the stomach into the esophagus (free reflux) or during periods of abdominal strain (contraction of abdominal wall, which increases intragastric pressure). Swallow-induced reflux and reflux episodes in which the mechanism cannot be clearly determined also occur in the setting of a low LES pressure [63]. However, it is interesting that a low LES pressure induced by atropine in normal subjects does not cause reflux episode [69]. All the straining maneuvers i.e., coughing, abdominal straining, straight leg raising, etc., do not induce reflux during LES hypotension induced by atropine. The contraction of the crural diaphragm during these maneuvers is a protective antireflux barrier and is probably sufficient to guard against the occurrence of reflux during periods of increased intraabdominal pressure. How a low LES pressure then causes reflux is not entirely clear. One possibility is that a combination of a low pressure and hiatus hernia is required for the occurrence of erosive esophagitis. A low

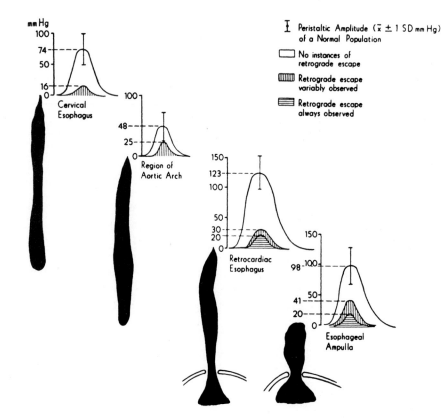

**FIG. 21–4.** Data on impaired esophageal volume clearance categorized by esophageal region. The necessary peristaltic amplitude increases progressively with increasingly distal esophageal locations. Upper curves indicate the mean peristaltic amplitude of normal subjects in each esophageal region. Vertically hatched areas indicate peristaltic amplitudes variably associated with impaired esophageal bolus clearance, and horizontal hatched areas indicate amplitudes invariably associated with impaired volume clearance. (From Kahrilas PJ. The anatomy and physiology of dysphagia. In Gelfand DW, Richter JE, eds, Dysphagia, Diagnosis and Treatment. New York: Igaku-shoin, 1989.)

LES pressure may allow movement of acid from the herniated pouch into the esophagus across hypotensive LES. Alternatively, in the presence of a hernia, the diaphragmatic hiatus is incompetent and allows the stomach contents to move freely from the stomach pouch below the diaphragm into the herniated sac and then into the esophagus. Along those lines, a study found that the severity of esophagitis appears to correlate directly with the size of hiatus hernia and indirectly with the magnitude of the LES pressure [36]. The larger the hernia, the wider is the esophageal hiatus, and the more likely it is that the crural diaphragm component of the sphincter is incompetent. The role of hiatus hernia in reflux disease is discussed in detail in chapter 20.

Patients with erosive esophagitis usually have a low LES pressure. The degree of endoscopic esophagitis seems to correspond directly with the LES pressure. A low LES pressure is the hallmark in patients with scleroderma of the esophagus and is considered to be the primary etiologic factor. Patients with scleroderma have the most severe form of the reflux esophagitis. A low LES pressure in scleroderma is due to the replacement of the LES muscle by connective tissue [60]. The reason for a low LES pressure in the more common variety of reflux disease is not entirely clear. It is possible that a low LES pressure is due to primary myogenic or neurogenic failure of the LES muscle. Even though there are no data to prove the matter one way or the other, it is entirely possible that a low LES pressure is secondary to acid-induced damage to the LES muscle. Animal experiments reveal that instillation of acid into the cat esophagus results in the reduction of LES pressure [25]. However, healing of esophagitis with omeprazole does not improve LES pressure in patients with erosive disease. The reason for the latter may be that acid-induced damage causes permanent and irreversible alterations in the contractile apparatus of the LES muscle.

It is possible to propose a unifying hypothesis that incorporates TLESR, a low LES pressure, and hiatus hernia in the pathogenesis of reflux disease [89]. The initial pathologic event in reflux disease is most likely the frequent TLESRs and acid reflux episodes. Acid in the esophagus causes esophagitis, which leads to a low LES pressure and esophageal hypotension [25]. Furthermore, esophagitis induces esophageal shortening through acid-induced contraction of the longitudinal muscles [75]. Subsequently fibrosis develops, resulting in a hiatus hernia. The hiatus hernia, in turn, enlarges the esophageal hiatus, thus impairing the sphincter function of the crural diaphragm. The appearance of a hiatus hernia and a weak diaphragmatic sphincter introduces additional mechanisms of reflux, thus exacerbating the esophagitis. Although plausible, definite proof of this hypothesis awaits further investigation.

## ROLE OF ESOPHAGEAL PERISTALSIS IN REFLUX DISEASE

Esophageal peristalsis plays a key role in the clearance of refluxed material from the esophagus. Esophageal acid clearance is a two-step process, bolus clearance and acid neutralization [34, 35]. If a 15-ml or smaller bolus of acid is instilled into the esophagus, the majority of the acid can be cleared from the esophagus into the stomach by a peristaltic contraction of the esophagus. The remainder of the acid lining the esophageal mucosa is neutralized by saliva traversing the esophagus during subsequent swallow-induced peristaltic contractions. It takes seven to ten swallows following esophageal acidification for the restoration of the normal esophageal pH of 5 to 7.

How strong of an esophageal peristaltic contraction does one need for an efficient bolus clearance? An esophageal contraction of greater than 30 mm Hg is usually sufficient in the supine position for bolus clearance (Fig. 21–4) [46]. A subgroup of patients, usually with severe reflux disease, have low esophageal contraction amplitude (termed ineffective esophageal motility; see chapter 11), which could result in an impaired ability to clear an acid bolus from the esophagus following a reflux episode [45]. The prevalence of peristaltic dysfunction increases with the increasing severity of esophagitis. A study by Kahrilas et al. reported that 25% of individuals with mild and 50% of patients with severe esophagitis had severe peristaltic dysfunction [46]. The definition of abnormal peristalsis, based on studies in normal subjects, was that 50% of tested peristaltic sequences had to have a demonstrable abnormality (Fig. 21–5). Whether esophageal peristaltic dysfunction is a primary defect or results secondarily from acid-induced esophagitis is not clear. There is good experimental evidence to indicate that acid injury to the esophagus can impair esophageal contractions [25]. However, healing of esophagitis in patients with low contraction amplitudes does not revert the contraction amplitudes back to normal. Patients with scleroderma and mixed connective disorders have a similar defect in peristalsis due to the replacement of the esophageal muscles with fibrous connective tissue [60].

## SUMMARY

The smooth muscle lower esophageal sphincter and crural diaphragm are two main components of the antireflux barrier. Gastroesophageal reflux occurs primarily due to an incompetent lower esophageal sphincter. Transient relaxation of the lower esophageal sphincter and crural diaphragm is the major mechanism of reflux in patients with reflux disease. The nature of afferent dysfunction that causes frequent TLESRs is not known. Other mechanisms of reflux are a hypotensive lower esophageal sphincter and the presence of hiatus hernia. Severity of esophagitis correlates directly with the size of hernia and indirectly with the LES pressure. Ineffective esophageal motility found in patients with moderate to severe reflux disease impairs bolus clearance of the acid and thus increases acid contact time with the esophageal mucosa. Future studies need to address the nature of neural dysfunction that leads to frequent TLESRs and the mechanism by which hiatus hernia develops and contributes to the pathogenesis of reflux disease.

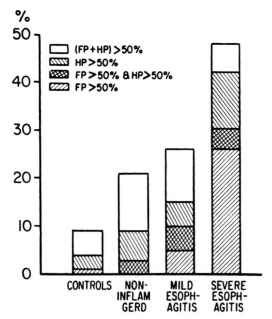

**FIG. 21–5.** Bar graph indicating the prevalence of peristaltic dysfunction in patient and control groups. The control group was composed of 31 normal volunteers and 48 patients who were having manometry for reasons other than reflux disease and major motor disorders. Patients with reflux disease ($n$ = 33) had a positive Bernstein test, but no demonstrable esophagitis by endoscopy or histology. Patients with mild esophagitis ($n$ = 38) had either histologically demonstrable esophagitis or endoscopically evident exudative esophagitis. Patients with severe esophagitis ($n$ = 27) had either esophageal ulcerations or strictures. The criteria for abnormality was the occurrence of either failed primary (*FP*) or regional hypotensive peristalsis (27 mm Hg) in the distal esophagus (*HP*) with more than half of the test swallows. Overall 9% of the controls, 21% of patients with mild esophagitis, and 48% of patients with severe esophagitis had abnormal peristaltic function by these criteria. (From ref. 45.)

# REFERENCES

1. Andrews PLR, Grundy D, Scratcherd T. Vagal afferent discharge from mechanoreceptors in different regions of the ferret stomach. J Physiol (Lond) 1980;298:513
2. Altschuler SM, Boyle JT, Nixon TE, Pack AI, Cohen S. Disassociation of costal and crural contractile effects on the gastroesophageal high pressure zone. Gastroenterology 1985;88:1305
3. Altschuler SM, Boyle JT, Nixon TE, Pack AI, Cohen S. Simultaneous reflex inhibition of lower esophageal sphincter and crural diaphragm in cats. Am J Physiol 1985;249:G586
4. Altschuler SM, Davies RO, Pack AI. Role of medullary inspiratory neurones in the control of the diaphragm during oesophageal stimulation in the cats. J Physiol (Lond) 1987;391:289
5. Baldi F, Longanesi A, Frrarini F, Michieletti G, Morselli-Labate A. Oesophageal motor function and outcome of treatment with H2-blockers in erosive oesophagitis. J Gastrointest Motil 1992;4:165
6. Berger AJ, Mitchell RA, Severingham SW. Regulation of respiration I. N Engl J Med 1977;297:134
7. Biancani P, Hillemeier C, Bitar KN, Makhlouf GM. Contraction mediated by $Ca^{2+}$ influx in esophageal muscle and by $Ca^{2+}$ release in the LES. Am J Physiol 1987;253:G760
8. Blackshaw L, Grundy D, Scratcherd T. Vagal afferent discharge from gastric mechanoreceptors during contraction and relaxation of the ferret corpus. J Autonom Nerv Syst 1987;18:19
9. Boulant J, Fioramonti J, Dpoigny M, Bommelaer G, Bueno L. Cholecystokinin and nitric oxide in transient lower esophageal sphincter relaxation to gastric distension in dogs. Gastroenterology 1994;107:1059
10. Boyle JT, Altschuler SM, Nixon TE, Tuchman DN, Pack AI, Cohen S. Role of the diaphragm in the genesis of lower esophageal sphincter pressure in the cat. Gastroenterology 1985;88:723
11. Cannon WB, Lieb CW. The receptive relaxation of the stomach. Am J Physiol 1912;29:267
12. Chung SA, Diamant NE. Small intestinal motility in fasted and postprandial states: effects of transient vagosympathetic blockade. Am J Physiol 1987;252:G301
13. Collman PI, Tremblay L, Diamant NE. The central vagal efferent supply to the esophagus and lower esophageal sphincter of the cat. Gastroenterology 1993;104:1430
14. Cox M, Martin C, Dent J, Westmore M. Effect of general anaesthesia on transient lower oesophageal sphincter relaxations in the dog. Aust NZ J Surg 1988;58:825
15. Cucchiara S, Staiano A, Di Lorenzo C, De Luca G, della Rocca A, Auricchio S. Pathophysiology of gastroesophageal reflux and distal esophageal motility in children with gastroesophageal reflux disease. J Pediatr Gastroenterol Nuttr 1988;7:830
16. Darian GB, DiMarco AF, Kelsen SG, Supinski GS, Gottfried SB. Effects of progressive hypoxia on parasternal, costal and crural diaphragm activation. J Appl. Physiol 1989;66:2579
17. Delattre JF, Palot JP, Ducasse A, Flament JB, Hureau J. The crura of the diaphragm and diaphragmatic passage. Anat Clin 1985;4:271
18. Dent J, et al. Mechanism of gastroesophageal reflux in recumbent asymptomatic human subjects. J Clin Invest 1980;65:256
19. Dent J, Wylie J, Dodds J, Sekiguchi T, Hogan W, Arndorfer RC. Interdigestive phasic contractions of the human lower esophageal sphincter. Gastroenterology 1983;84:453
20. Dent J, Holloway RH, Toouli J, Dodds WJ. Mechanisms of lower esophageal sphincter incompetence in patients with symptomatic gastroesophageal reflux. Gut 1988;29:1020
21. Dodds WJ, et al. Mechanism of gastroesophageal reflux in patients with reflux disease. N Engl J Med 1982;307:1547
22. Dodds WJ, Dent J, Hogan WF, Arndorfer RC. Effect of atropine on esophageal motor function in humans. Am J Physiol 1989;240:G290
23. Dodds WJ, Kahrilas PJ, Dent J, Hogan WJ, Kern MK, Arndorfer RC. Analysis of spontaneous gastroesophageal reflux and esophageal acid clearance in patients with reflux esophagitis. J Gastrointest Motil 1990; 2:79
24. Downton J, Dent J, Heddle R, Toouli J, Buckle PJ, MacKinnon AM, Wyman JB. Elevation of gastric pH heals peptic oesophagitis—a role for omeprazole. J Gastroenterol Hepatol 1987;2:317
25. Eastwood GL, Castell DO, Higgs RH. Experimental esophagitis in cats impairs lower esophageal sphincter pressure. Gastroenterology 1975; 69:14
26. Ergun G, Kahrilas P, Lin S, Logemann J, Harig J. Shape, volume, and content of the deglutitive pharyngeal chamber imaged by ultrafast computerised tomography. Gastroenterology 1993;105:1396
27. Fang JC, Sarosiek I, Arora T, Yamamoto Y, Liu J, Mittal RK. Cholinergic blockade inhibits gastroesophageal reflux and transient lower esophageal sphincter relaxation through a central mechanism. Am J Gastroenterol 1997;9:1590
28. Franzi S, Martin C, Cox M, Dent J. Response of canine lower esophageal sphincter to gastric distension. Am J Physiol 1990;259:G380
29. Freidin N, et al. Sleep and nocturnal acid reflux in normal subjects and patients with reflux esophagitis. Gut 1991;32:1275
30. Freidin N, Mittal RK, McCallum RW. Does body posture affect the incidence and mechanism of gastro-oesophageal reflux? Gut 1991;32: 133
31. Fyke FE, Code CF. Gastroesophageal sphincter in healthy human beings. Gastroenterologia (Basel) 1956;86:135
32. Goyal RK, Rattan S. Nature of vagal inhibitory innervation to the lower esophageal sphincter. J Clin Invest 1975;55:1119
33. Heine KJ, Dent J, Mittal RK. Anatomical relationship between the crural diaphragm and the lower esophageal sphincter: an electrophysiologic study. J Gastrointest Motil 1993;5:89
34. Helm JF, et al. Determinants of esophageal acid clearance in normal subjects. Gastroenterology 1983;85:607
35. Helm JF, et al. Effect of esophageal emptying and saliva on clearance of acid from the esophagus. N Engl J Med 1984;310:284

36. Holloway RH, Dent J. Pathophysiology of gastroesophageal reflux: lower esophageal dysfunction in reflux disease. Gastorenterol Clin North Am 1990;19:517

37. Holloway RH, Penagini R. Criteria for the objective definition of transient lower esophageal sphincter relaxation. Am J Physiol 1994;268:G183

38. Holloway RH, Downton J, Mitchell BE, Dent J. Effect of cisapride on postprandial gastrooesophageal reflux. Gut 1989;30:1187

39. Holloway RH, Wyman JB, Dent J. Failure of transient lower oesphageal sphincter relaxation in response to gastric distention in patients with achalasia: evidence for neural mediation of transient lower oesphageal sphincter relaxations. Gut 1989;30:762

40. Holloway RH, Kocyan P, Dent J. Provocation of transient lower esophageal sphincter relaxations by meals in patients with symptomatic gastroesophageal reflux. Dig Dis Sci 1991;36:1034

41. Ingelfinger FJ. Esophageal motility, Physiol Rev 1958;38:533

42. Ireland AC, Dent J, Holloway RH. Preservation of postural suppression of belching in patients with reflux esophagitis (abstract). Gastroenterology 1992;102:A87

43. Ireland AC, Dent J, Holloway RH. The role of head position in the postural control of transient lower oesophageal sphincter relaxations and belching. Gullet 1992;2:81

44. Ireland AC, Holloway RH, Toouli J, Dent J. Mechanisms underlying the antireflux action of fundoplication. Gut 1993;34:303

45. Kahrilas PJ, et al. Esophageal peristaltic dysfunction in peptic esophagitis. Gastroenterology 1986;91:897

46. Kahrilas PJ, Dodds WJ, Hogan WJ. Effect of peristaltic dysfunction on esophageal volume clearance. Gastroenterology 1988;94:73

47. Kalia M, Mesulam MM. Brainstem projections of sensory and motor components of the vagus complex in the cat. II. Laryngeal, tracheobronchial, pulmonary, cardiac, and gastrointestinal branches. J Comp Neurol 1980;193:467

48. Katzka DA, Sidhu M, Castell DO. Hypertensive lower esophageal sphincter pressures and gastroesophageal reflux disease: an apparent paradox that is not unusual. Am J Gastroenterol 1995;90:280

49. Kiroff GK, Maddern GJ, Jamieson GG. A study of factors responsible for the efficacy of fundoplication in the treatment of gastro-oesophageal reflux. Aust NZ J Surg 1984;54:109

50. Klein WA, Parkman HP, Williams L, Fisher RS. Sphincter-like thoraco-abdominal high pressure zone after esophagogastrectomy. Gastroenterology 1993;105:1362

51. Langman J, Medical Embryology. Baltimore: William & Wilkins, 1975:305

52. Liebermann-Meffert M, Allgower M, Schmidt P, Blum A. Muscular equivalent of the lower esophageal sphincter. Gastroenterology 1979;76:31

53. Little A, Cox M, Martin C, Dent J, Franzi S, Lavelle R. Influence of posture on transient lower oesophageal sphincter relaxation and gastro-oesophageal reflux in dogs. J Gastroenterol Hepatol 1989;4:49

54. Liu JB, et al. Transnasal ultrasound of the esophagus: preliminary morphologic and function studies. Radiology 1992;184:721

55. Liu J, Parashar V, Mittal RK. Asymmetry of the lower esophageal sphincter: is it related to the muscle thickness or shape of the lower esophageal sphincter? Am J Physiol 1997;272:G1509

56. Martin CJ, Patrikios J, Dent J. Abolition of gas reflux and transient lower esophageal sphincter relaxation by vagal blockage in the dog. Gastroenterology 1986;91:890

57. Martin C, Dodds W, Liem H, Dantas R, Layman R, Dent J. Diaphragmatic contribution to gastroesophageal competence and reflux in dogs. Am J Physiol 1992;263:G551

58. McNally EF, Kelly JE, Ingelfinger FJ. Mechanism of belching: effects of gastric distention with air. Gastroenterology 1964;46:254

59. Miller AJ. Neurophysiological basis of swallowing. Dysphagia 1986;1:91

60. Miller LS, et al. Endoluminal ultrasonography of the distal esophagus in systemic sclerosis. Gastroenterology 1993;105:31

61. Mittal RK, Fisher MJ. Electrical and mechanical inhibition of the crural diaphragm during transient relaxation of the lower esophageal sphincter. Gastroenterology 1990;99:1265

62. Mittal RK, McCallum RW. Characteristics of transient lower esophageal sphincter relaxation in humans. Am J Physiol 1987;252:G636

63. Mittal RK, McCallum RW. Characteristics and frequency of transient relaxations of the lower esophageal sphincter on patients with reflux esophagitis. Gastroenterology 1988;95:593

64. Mittal RK, Lange RC, McCallum RW. Identification and mechanism of delayed esophageal acid clearance in subjects with hiatus hernia. Gastroenterology 1987;92:130

65. Mittal RK, Rochester DF, McCallum RW. Electrical and mechanical activity in the human lower esophageal sphincter during diaphragmatic contraction. J Clin Invest 1988;81:1182

66. Mittal RK, Fisher M, Rochester DF, Dent J, McCallum RW, Sluss J. Human lower esophageal sphincter response to increased abdominal pressure. Am J Physiol 1990;258:624

67. Mittal RK, Stewart WR, Schirmer BD. Effect of a catheter in the pharynx on the frequency of transient lower esophageal relaxations. Gastroenterology 1992;103:1236

68. Mittal RK, Chowdhry NK, Liu J. Is the sphincter function of crural diaphragm impaired in patients with reflux esophagitis. Gastroenterology 1995;108:A169

69. Mittal RK, Holloway R, Dent J. Effect of atropine on the frequency of transient lower esophageal sphincter relaxation and acid reflux in normal subjects. Gastroenterology 1995;109:1547

70. Mittal RK, Holloway RH, Penagini R, Blackshaw LA, Dent J. Transient lower esophageal sphincter relaxation. Gastroenterology 1995;109:601

71. Mittal RK, Chiareli C, Liu J, Shakeer R. Characteristics of LES relaxation induced stimulation of the pharynx with minute amounts of water. Gastroenterology 1996;111:378

72. Monges H. Dissociation between the electrical activity of the diaphragmatic dome and crura muscular fibers during esophageal distension, vomiting and eructation. An electromyographic study in the dog. J Physiol (Paris) 1978;74:541

73. Ott DJ, Gelfand DW, Wu WC, Castell DO. Esophagogastric region and its rings. Am J Roentgend 1984;142:281

74. Paterson WG, Rattan S, Goyal RK. Experimental induction of isolated lower esophageal sphincter relaxation in anesthetized opossums. J Clin Invest 1986;77:1187

75. Paterson WG, Kolyn DM. Esophageal shortening induced by short-term intraluminal acid perfusion in opossum: a cause for hiatus hernia? Gastroenterology 1994;107:1738

76. Penagini R, Bartesaghi B, Bianchi PA. Effect of cold stress on postprandial lower esophageal sphincter competence and gastroesophageal reflux in healthy subjects. Dig Dis Sci 1992;37:1200

77. Penagini R, Bartesaghi B, Conte D, Bianchi P. Rate of transient lower oesophageal sphincter relaxations of healthy humans after eating a mixed nutrient meal: time course and comparison with fasting. Eur J Gastroenterol Hepatol 1992;4:35

78. Penagini R, Schoeman M, Holloway R, Dent J, Tippett M. Mechanisms of reflux in ambulant patients with reflux esophagitis (abstract). Gastroenterology 1994;A159:106

79. Penagini R, Picone A, Bianchi P. Morphine reduces gastroesophageal reflux in reflux disease though a decrease in the rate of transient lower esophageal sphincter relaxation. Gastroenterology 1996;110:A227

80. Reynolds RPE, El-Sharkawy TY, Diamant NE. Lower esophageal sphincter function in the cat: role of central innervation assessed by transient vagal blockade. Am J Physiol 1984;246:G666

81. Rinaman L, Card JP, Schwaber JS, Miselis RR. Ultrastructural demonstration of a gastric monosynaptic vagal circuit in the nucleus of the solitary tract in rat. J Neurosci 1989;9:1985

82. Roussos C, Macklem PT. The respiratory muscle. N Engl J Med 1982;307:786

83. Ryan JP, Snape WJ, Cohen S. Influence of vagal cooling on esophageal function. Am J Physiol 1977;232:E159

84. Schoeman MN, Akkermans LMA, Tippett MD, Dent J, Holloway RH. Mechanisms of gastroesophageal reflux in ambulant healthy human subjects. Gastroenterology 1995;109:1315

85. Schulze-Delrieu K, Percy WH, Ren J, Shirazi SS, Von Derau K. Evidence for inhibition of opossum LES through intrinsic gastric nerves. Am J Physiol 1989;256:G198

86. Sengupta A, Paterson WG, Goyal RK. Atypical localization of myenteric neurons in the opossum lower esophageal sphincter. Am J Anat 1987;180:352

87. Shezhang L, Brasseur JG, Pouderoux P, Kahrilas PK. The phrenic ampulla: distal esophagus or potential hiatal hernia. Am J Physiol 1995;268:G320

88. Sifrim D, Janssens J, Vantrappen G, Tokuhara T. Is the esophageal body inhibited during inappropriate LES relaxations? (abstract). Gastroenterology 1992;102:A514

89. Sloan S, Rademaker AW, Kahrilas PJ. Determinants of gastroesophageal junction incompetence: hiatal hernia, lower esophageal sphincter, or both? Ann Intern Med 1992;117:977

90. Storey AT. Laryngeal initiation of swallowing. Exp Neurol 1968;20:
359

91. Strombeck D, Harrold D, Ferrier W. Eructation of gas through the
gastroesophageal sphincter before and after truncal vagotomy in dogs.
Am J Vetin Res 1987;48:207

92. Thor K, Hill LD, Mercer CD, Kozarek RA. Reappraisal of the flap
valve mechanism: a study of a new valvuloplasty procedure in cadavers.
Acta Chir Scand 1987;153:25

93. Yamato S, Saha JK, Goyal RK. Role of nitric oxide in lower esophageal
sphincter relaxation to swallowing. Life Sci 1992;50:1263

94. Werlin SL, Dodds WJ, Hogan WJ, Arndorfer RC. Mechanisms of gastroesophageal reflux in children. J Pediatr 1980;97:244

*The Esophagus*, Third Edition,
edited by D. O. Castell and J. E. Richter.
Lippincott Williams & Wilkins, Philadelphia © 1999.

CHAPTER 22

# Pathophysiology of Gastroesophageal Reflux Disease

## Esophageal Epithelial Resistance

Roy C. Orlando

Gastroesophageal (acid) reflux is an almost universal and daily occurrence, even in asymptomatic healthy subjects [17, 52]. Nevertheless, only a small percentage of the population at risk develops reflux esophagitis, and even fewer demonstrate evidence of severe (macroscopic) disease. Clearly, mechanisms other than the antireflux barriers, such as the lower esophageal sphincter, diaphragmatic pinchcock, and acute angle of His, are important determinants of reflux disease. In effect, the antireflux barriers are the first line of defense, designed only to limit the frequency and volume of contact between gastric contents and the esophageal epithelium. When these barriers fail, a second line of defense, known as esophageal clearance, comes into play. Esophageal clearance consists of esophageal peristalsis and gravity, for volume removal, and swallowed salivary secretions and secretions from esophageal submucosal glands, for acid neutralization. It limits the duration of contact between gastric contents and the esophageal epithelium. However, esophageal clearance is not instantaneous and, perhaps more importantly, almost all of its components (except submucosal gland secretion, which has not been studied) are inoperable when subjects are asleep [18, 64, 116]. Thus, the total daily dwelling time for acid contact with the esophagus may be considerable, so that a third line of defense is needed to avoid significant injury to the epithelium. This third line of defense is commonly referred to as tissue resistance [81, 83, 103].

Tissue resistance reflects intrinsic processes within mucosa that serve to minimize damage during the time of con-

tact between acid (and other injurious luminal agents) and epithelium. That tissue resistance is, in fact, an effective means for protecting esophageal epithelium against acid damage is best illustrated by experimental studies in animals and humans (Bernstein test) in which the antireflux barriers and esophageal clearance mechanisms are bypassed. In such studies, the healthy esophageal epithelium may be continuously exposed to acid for substantial periods of time (e.g., hydrochloric (HCL), pH 2, for up to $3\frac{1}{2}$ hours in animals and HCl, pH 1.1, for 25 to 30 minutes in humans), yet it is observed to exhibit little or no evidence of damage [5, 54, 65, 85, 101, 110, 112, 113].

This chapter describes a number of established and potential preepithelial, epithelial, and postepithelial defenses that may contribute to tissue resistance in the esophagus (Table 22–1). Its goal is to provide a greater appreciation of tissue resistance as a dynamic and complex group of processes with an important and perhaps crucial role in the prevention of reflux esophagitis. The approach taken is based on three premises: (a) that gastroesophageal reflux leads to an attack by acid and pepsin on the esophageal epithelium from the luminal surface; (b) that the hydrogen ion ($H^+$) is the major ion responsible for epithelial necrosis; and (c) that, for significant epithelial injury to result from this attack, $H^+$ must enter and acidify the esophageal cells.

### PREEPITHELIAL DEFENSES

When gastroesophageal reflux occurs, gastric juice is introduced into the esophageal lumen. However, this alone does not ensure epithelial contact with noxious gastric contents, because preepithelial defenses such as mucus, the unstirred water layer, and surface bicarbonate ions ($HCO_3^-$)

R. C. Orlando: Department of Gastroenterology and Hepatology, Tulane University Medical Center, New Orleans, Louisiana 70112-2699.

**TABLE 22–1.** *Factors contributing to esophageal mucosal resistance against injury by luminal acid*[a]

Preepithelial defense
  Mucous layer
  Unstirred water layer
  Surface bicarbonate ion concentration
Epithelial defense
  Structures
    Cell membranes
    Intercellular junctional complexes
      (tight junctions, glycoconjugates/lipid)
  Functions
    Epithelial transport (e.g., $Na^+/H^+$ exchanger, $Na^+$-dependent $Cl^-/HCO_3^-$ exchanger)
    Intracellular and extracellular buffers
    Cell replication
Postepithelial Defense
  Blood flow
  Tissue acid–base status

[a] From Orlando RC. Esophageal epithelial defenses against acid injury. Am J Gastroenterology 1994;89:S48, with permission.

could potentially act, as they do in stomach and duodenum, as physicochemical barriers to such contact (Fig. 22–1).

## Mucus

The epithelium of stomach and duodenum has a surface layer of mucus that serves as both a lubricant and a protective barrier against mechanical and, to some extent, chemical injury. Due to its composition of high-molecular-weight glycoproteins, mucus has both viscoelastic and gel properties. These properties enable it to prevent large protein molecules, such as pepsin, from gaining access to the underlying epithelium [2]. Mucus is not an effective barrier to $H^+$ [42, 135],

although at least one report suggests that it may slow the rate of $H^+$ diffusion toward the tissue [92]. More importantly, mucus probably participates in epithelial protection against $H^+$ by expanding the unstirred water layer, that is, the area of low turbulence adjacent to the tissue [73, 125, 126].

In stomach and duodenum, mucus is derived from mucus-secreting surface cells or from mucus-secreting cells within the submucosal glands. A mucous layer is also to be expected in the esophagus. This layer could potentially be derived from salivary secretions and the secretions of esophageal submucosal glands. However, submucosal glands with secretary ducts that open directly onto the surface of the epithelium are reportedly limited to the proximal esophagus, near the upper esophageal sphincter, and the distal esophagus, near the esophagogastric junction [3, 39]. Thus, for a complete layer of mucus, the secretions of the salivary and proximal esophageal glands would need to coat the upper and, by virtue of the peristaltic activity sweeping mucus distally, the middle and lower esophagus. The distal esophageal glands, on the other hand, appear strategically located to ensure an adequate mucous coat near the esophagogastric junction, the region most susceptible to reflux injury. Nonetheless and despite the existence of these secretary structures, a well-defined layer of surface mucus has not been described in the human esophagus. Perhaps less surprising is that a well-defined surface mucous layer has also not been identified in the rabbit esophagus, given that the rabbit is a species whose esophagus is essentially devoid of submucosal glands [9, 40].

## Unstirred Water Layer and Bicarbonate Ions

The unstirred water layer is significant because of its capacity to act as a sink for $HCO_3^-$. This sink establishes an alkaline microenvironment close to the epithelial surface

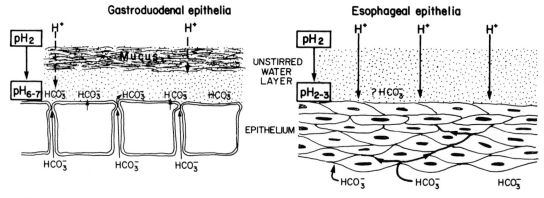

PREEPITHELIAL DEFENSES

**FIG. 22–1.** Preepithelial defense. In gastric and duodenal epithelia, $H^+$ must cross the mucus-unstirred water layer–bicarbonate barrier before contact can be made with the surface of the epithelium. Diffusion of pepsin, but not $H^+$ is blocked by mucus; however, $H^+$ can be neutralized by $HCO_3^-$ residing in the unstirred water layer. In contrast to gastric and duodenal epithelia, the preepithelial defense in the esophagus is poorly developed, having an ineffective mucus–$HCO_3^-$ barrier to buffer backdiffusing $H^+$. (From ref. 83, with permission.)

[21, 135] in which $HCO_3^-$ serves as an effective barrier to $H^+$, neutralizing it as it penetrates the mucous layer en route to the epithelium. The capacity of $HCO_3^-$ to sustain a significant pH gradient across the mucus-unstirred water layer has been demonstrated for stomach and duodenum in animals and humans [58, 99, 136]. In these studies, the passage of pH-sensitive electrodes from lumen to epithelium shows that at a luminal pH of 2 the mucus and unstirred water layers are capable of supporting a pH of 5 to 7 at the epithelial surface. However, Quigley and Turnberg [99] found that reduction of luminal pH to 2 in human esophagus resulted in a pH at the epithelial cell surface of 2 or 3 (Fig. 22–1). This apparent lack of protection by preepithelial factors in human esophagus may be due to the absence of a mucus-expanded unstirred water layer or the lack of $HCO_3^-$ within the unstirred layer. The lack of $HCO_3^-$ may reflect (a) the inability of stratified squamous epithelium to secrete $HCO_3^-$ [40]; (b) the electrical "tightness" of stratified squamous epithelium, indicating a limited capacity for blood-to-lumen $HCO_3^-$ diffusion [95]; or (c) a paucity of submucosal $HCO_3^-$-secreting glands [40]. Regardless of cause, however, the lack of protection by the preepithelial factors in esophagus places the major burden for mounting a defense against luminal acid squarely on factors within the epithelium proper.

## EPITHELIAL DEFENSES

The epithelial defenses come into play when prolonged contact of acid with epithelium permits excess $H^+$ to penetrate beyond the limited preepithelial defenses in the esophagus. The epithelial defenses are composed of both structural and functional elements. Some of the more prominent and best studied of these elements are listed in Table 22–1.

### Esophageal Epithelial Structure

The lining of the esophagus is a partially or nonkeratinized stratified squamous epithelium [3, 10] that more or less resembles in structure and function the epithelia of skin, rumen, oral cavity, and cervix. In most species, esophageal stratified squamous epithelium is divided into three layers: stratum corneum, stratum spinosum, and stratum germinativum. Less frequently, a fourth layer, the stratum granulosum, is identified by the presence of keratohyalin granules in the cytoplasm of its cells. Depending on the species, the stratum corneum may consist of one or more layers of flattened cells lining the luminal surface. The cells in the most luminal layer are the oldest within the epithelium and are in varying stages of degeneration [10]. Therefore, this layer may provide some mechanical protection, but little or no effective barrier to $H^+$ penetration. It is the more viable, deeper layers of the stratum corneum that together constitute the major structural barrier to the permeation of ions and molecules into the epithelium [28, 61, 75]. Therefore, when $H^+$ has successfully eluded the limited preepithelial defenses in the

esophagus, the stratum corneum provides the next line of defense against its advance into the tissue.

Morphologically, the two structural components of the stratum corneum that serve as a barrier to $H^+$ are the lipid bilayers constituting the plasma membrane of the cells and a series of intercellular junctional elements (to be discussed below). These structures combine to produce an electrical resistance in the range of 1,000 to 2,500 ohms·cm² for human and rabbit esophageal epithelium [9, 85, 97, 98]. Electrical resistances in this range characterize the esophagus as a "tight" epithelium with a low capacity for the intercellular diffusion of ions from blood to lumen or lumen to blood. This contrasts with the more ion-permeable "leaky" epithelia, such as gallbladder and small intestine, with electrical resistances of less than 500 ohms·cm² [19, 95]. Therefore, for esophagus the intercellular junctional complex appears to govern overall tissue permeability and electrical resistance.

Knowledge about the nature of the intercellular junctional complex in esophageal epithelium is limited, though there are data to suggest that it is composed of both tight junctions and an intercellular "cement," the latter depending on species comprised of either lipid or mucinous material [28, 61] (Fig. 22–2). The presence of tight junctions is reminiscent of frog skin, another moist, stratified squamous epithelium in which tight junctions (zonulae occludentes) are the major intercellular barriers [32, 75, 95]. Tight junctions formed by the interaction of integral membrane proteins from adjacent cell membranes encircle the cells of the layer and seal off the lumen from the intercellular space, much as the plastic wrapping around a six-pack of canned beverages seals off the space above and below the plane of the cans' surface [19]. Thus, tight junctions act as a barrier to molecules passing between the cells from lumen to blood and vice versa. Tight junctions, however, are neither impermeable nor equally permeable to all ions; that is, the junction exhibits permselectivity in the rates at which different ionic species pass through it [19, 95]. Since most tissues have negatively charged ions (e.g., carboxyl, phosphate, and sulfate groups) lining the junctions, they are usually more permeable to cations than to anions. However, as $H^+$ enters the junction, it can titrate the negatively charged ions and so change its permselectivity from cation-selective to anion-selective [19, 79, 95]. This change in permselectivity may, at least in theory, act to slow the rate of $H^+$ entry into the tissue via this pathway.

The esophageal epithelium of the mouse and rabbit, unlike frog skin, contains an intercellular material that appears to contribute to its barrier function. In this regard, the esophageal epithelium more closely resembles human skin, a dry, stratified squamous epithelium in which spot welds (maculae occludentes) are supported in their function by the presence of an intercellular lamellar-lipid material. This material is apparently secreted into the intercellular space from membrane-coating granules localized within the lower layers of epidermis [26–28]. Notably, it is this lamellar-lipid material that appears to create the barrier to diffusion through the

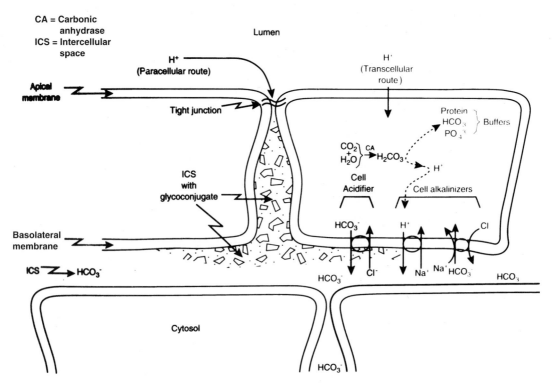

**FIG. 22–2.** Epithelial defense. Some of the recognized epithelial defenses against acid injury are illustrated. Structural barriers to H$^+$ diffusion include the cell membrane and intercellular junctional complex. Functional components include intracellular buffering by negatively charged proteins and HCO$_3^-$ and H$^+$ extrusion processes (Na$^+$/H$^+$ exchange and Na$^+$-dependent Cl$^-$/HCO$_3^-$ exchange) for regulation of intracellular pH. (Modified from ref. 81.)

intercellular space of human skin and mouse esophagus [28]. However, an intercellular mucin, rather than lipid, appears to subserve a similar barrier function in the esophageal epithelium of the rabbit [61], and, by virtue of its presence, may also do so in human esophagus [49].

Before describing those esophageal epithelial functions that participate in protection against acid injury, it is helpful to review what is known about esophageal epithelial transport, because the sequence and mechanisms of acid injury are better appreciated from this perspective.

**Esophageal Epithelial Transport**

The stratified squamous epithelium of the esophagus exhibits *in vivo* a lumen negative potential difference (PD) of approximately $-30$ mV in rabbit and $-15$ mV in humans [132]. *In vitro* studies in the Ussing chamber have established that this PD for both humans [85] and rabbits [97] results primarily from the active transport of Na$^+$ from lumen to blood. Net Na$^+$ transport is reduced by either mucosal application of amiloride or serosal application of ouabain [97]. This suggests that the transport characteristics of the esophageal epithelium closely resemble those of the more extensively studied stratified squamous epithelium of frog skin. Based on the frog skin model [78], transport in esopha-

geal epithelium can be summarized as follows. Initially, luminal Na$^+$ passively enters the cells by passing down a concentration gradient through Na$^+$ channels in the apical cell membrane. After entering these cells, Na$^+$ diffuses to adjacent cells through cell-to-cell connections called gap junctions. The sodium pump NaK, ATPase located on the basolateral cell membranes then pumps Na$^+$ into the intercellular space below the level of the junctional barriers. Because the permeability barrier effectively limits Na$^+$ movement toward the lumen, its net movement is toward the serosal surface of the tissue and into blood.

Whereas the net movement of Na$^+$ from luminal to serosal surface is accomplished relatively rapidly by the expenditure of cellular energy, the accompanying anion, usually Cl$^-$, moves passively and more slowly in the same direction along its electrical gradient. Thus, the active movement of Na$^+$ from luminal to serosal surface, the slower passive movement of Cl$^-$ in the same direction, and the limited back diffusion of ions due to structural barriers combine to separate charges in space. This process creates a measurable PD. Understanding, the factors that determine PD are of more than theoretical interest, since the transmural PD has been used to study the pathogenesis of acid injury to the esophageal epithelium [10, 87, 89] and to identify patients with esophagitis and Barrett's esophagus [46, 88].

Since the *in vivo* measurement of esophageal PD in healthy animals reflects the structural and functional integrity of the tissue, it is not surprising that acid-injured epithelia have an altered PD [24, 55, 88, 133]. However, changes in PD may reflect not only epithelial injury, but also physiologic changes in epithelial permeability and transport. In addition, the PD may be altered by nonepithelial factors, such as liquid junction potentials that develop when the ion compositions of the luminal solution and the recording electrode are different [88, 89, 100]. Thus, *in vivo*, PD changes need to be interpreted cautiously and validated with *in vitro* techniques, where variables can be better controlled.

## Rabbit Model of Acid Injury to Esophageal Epithelium

The effects of acid on the rabbit esophageal epithelial structure and function have been studied by using the *in vivo* measurement of esophageal PD to monitor damage and by correlating the change in PD with changes in esophageal transport and morphology [10, 87, 89]. During acid perfusion, the esophageal epithelium exhibits a biphasic PD response. Initially, there is a transient increase in PD, followed by a gradual, progressive fall in PD toward zero (Fig. 22–3). Notably, a similar biphasic PD pattern can be discerned in human subjects during acid-perfusion (Bernstein) tests [85] and an abolition of PD demonstrated in those with severe esophagitis [88]. From studies of rabbit esophageal epithelium exposed to acid in the Ussing chamber, it is evident that the initial increase in esophageal PD in the presence of luminal acid results from $H^+$ diffusion from lumen to blood

[89]. When $H^+$ diffuses across the tissue, it also disappears from the lumen, prompting some investigators to utilize $H^+$ disappearance as a marker of altered epithelial permeability or of epithelial injury [13, 24, 41, 55, 60, 112].

The path that $H^+$ takes across the tissue may be via the cell membranes (transcellular route), the intercellular junctions (paracellular route), or both [89, 96]. That $H^+$ may travel through the $Na^+$ channel, and thereby possibly alter its function, was reported by Palmer [91] in toad bladders. Data from our laboratory indicated that brief periods of acid exposure do alter the $Na^+$ channel, in that $Na^+$ absorption is stimulated through an electrogenic amiloride-sensitive apical membrane pathway [89]. However, data in the Ussing chamber using the irreversible $Na^+$ channel blocker phenamil and data from surface cells impaled with double-barreled, pH-sensitive intracellular microelectrodes indicate that the apical cell membrane of these cells is highly impermeant to $H^+$ (little to no cytosolic acidification occurs even at luminal pH 2) and that the $Na^+$ channel, though altered functionally, is not the major route by which $H^+$ enters and destroys the esophageal epithelium [54, 90]. There is also evidence that acute exposure to $H^+$ materially alters the intercellular junctional complexes in the esophagus. After the esophageal PD had fallen to 50% of initial value in acid-exposed rabbit esophageal epithelium, the decline in PD correlated with a reduction in electrical resistance, and the latter was paralleled by an increase in transepithelial mannitol flux [87]. These findings are consistent with an increase in epithelial permeability through the paracellular pathway. Morphologic studies corroborate this interpretation of the data by showing no cell necrosis in acid-exposed rabbit tissues, but marked dilatation of the intercellular spaces, and in acid-exposed frog skins, there is a separation of the epithelial tight junctions [34]. Notably, dilated intercellular spaces have been noted in humans with both nonerosive and erosive forms of (acid) reflux-induced esophagitis [50, 94, 129] (Fig. 22–4). The implication of this observation is that patients with reflux disease have an increase in paracellular permeability in the esophageal epithelium. Since it is reported that the sen-

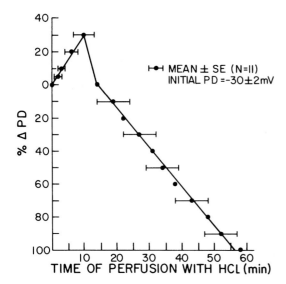

**FIG. 22–3.** The percent change in rabbit esophageal transmural potential difference (delta PD) plotted against the time of exposure to 80 mmol HCl–80 mmol NaCl. A transient increase in PD occurs during the first 10 minutes. This is followed by a progressive decline in PD until it reaches zero at 1 hour. Values are means ± standard error, *n* = 11. PD = –30 mV ± 2 mV. (From ref. 87, with permission.)

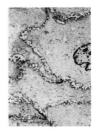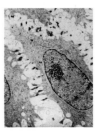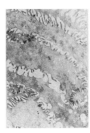

**FIG. 22–4.** Transmission electron photomicrographs of an esophageal mucosal biopsy from a (control) subject without esophageal disease (**left**), a subject with heartburn and erosive esophagitis (**center**), and a subject with heartburn and nonerosive esophagitis on endoscopy (**right**). Note the widened intercellular spaces in the two subjects with heartburn. Original magnification ×3,000. (Modified and reprinted from ref. 129, with permission.)

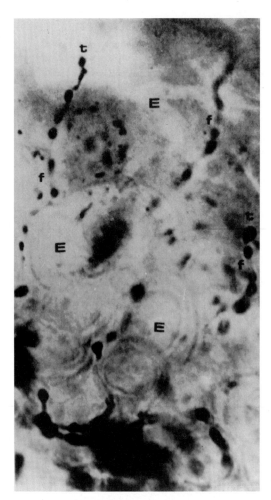

**FIG. 22–5.** Photomicrograph showing the nerve fibers (*f*) traversing the intercellular spaces of esophageal epithelium. Macaque. $OsO_4$–$ZnI_2$ solution. ×320. (From ref. 106, with permission.)

sory neurons in esophageal epithelium reside within the intercellular spaces and may extend to within three cell layers of the lumen, this increase in paracellular permeability may explain their propensity to develop symptoms (heartburn) when acid is refluxed into the esophageal lumen [105, 106] (Fig. 22–5). Moreover, it is interesting to note that these early effects of acid exposure on the $Na^+$ channel and the permeability of the intercellular junctions are reversible and unassociated with cell necrosis [87]. This latter observation highlights the fact that, even when $H^+$ penetrates across the structural barriers (and precipitates the symptom of heartburn), additional mechanisms are available within the epithelium to prevent cell necrosis.

### Esophageal Epithelial Functions

The functional elements comprising the epithelial defense against luminal HCl include intracellular and extracellular buffers for $H^+$, intracellular pH ($pH_i$) regulatory processes, and the cell reparative mechanisms, the latter discussed in

the next section. The buffers within the esophageal epithelium include phosphates, proteins, and $HCO_3^-$. All are available for the buffering or neutralization of backdiffusing $H^+$ both within the cell cytosol and the intercellular space. Bicarbonate, which is the critical element in the buffering system, is derived from two sources, one intrinsic, produced by the action of the enzyme carbonic anhydrase [14], and the other extrinsic, a product of passive diffusion from blood [84] (Fig. 22–6). These systems, though effective, are limited in capacity (estimated at 60 mmol of $H^+$ at pH 7.4 (N. A. Tobey and R. C. Orlando, *unpublished observations*). When this capacity is exceeded by $H^+$ entry, $pH_i$ falls to acidic levels. Acidification of the cytosol, however, is not accepted passively, for it triggers the activity of other protective mechanisms, including two basolateral membrane exchangers designed for acid extrusion, an amiloride-sensitive $Na^+/H^+$ exchanger (NHE-1 isotype), and a DIDS-sensitive, $Na^+$-dependent $Cl^-/HCO_3^-$ exchanger [15–17] (Fig. 22–2). These mechanisms are driven by the gradient for $Na^+$ entry created by the sodium pump and act to rapidly remove excess $H^+$ from the cell. The end result is the restoration of $pH_i$ to neutrality within minutes, assuming that the rate of $H^+$ entry into the tissue has diminished due to effective luminal acid clearance. Notably, the $H^+$ removed from the cell and into the intercellular space by the $Na^+/H^+$ exchanger or the $H^+$ diffusing across the junctions is buffered by extracellular $HCO_3^-$ derived from blood. The presence of sufficient buffer within the intercellular space is crucial since failure to neutralize intercellular acidity results in rapid cell acidification and cell necrosis [127]. Of note is that there is a second basolateral membrane $Cl^-/HCO_3^-$ exchanger within the esophageal cells; this one, too, is DIDS-sensitive, but $Na^+$-independent. It is designed to ensure that $pH_i$ does not rise to alkaline levels either by too exuberant $H^+$ removal by the acid-extruding mechanisms or from an exogenous alkaline challenge from the lumen [15]. The $Cl^-/HCO_3^-$ exchanger in these instances operates by extruding $HCO_3^-$ in exchange for extracellular $Cl^-$, thereby reducing an elevated $pH_i$ to neutrality.

### POSTEPITHELIAL DEFENSES

The postepithelial factors that contribute to esophageal protection against acid injury are products of the blood supply (Fig. 22–6). The blood supply delivers nutrients and oxygen for normal cell functions, including cell repair and replication, and removes potentially noxious metabolic byproducts, including $CO_2$ and acids. In regard to the latter, it is important to recognize that the blood supply is critical for preservation of normal tissue acid–base balance, especially because it supplies $HCO_3^-$ to the intercellular space for the buffering of extracellular $H^+$. The importance of tissue acid–base balance in protecting gastric mucosa against injury has been documented [57, 59, 115]. However, the mechanism for this protection appears less well defined, and in one report, it was suggested that the mechanism for $HCO_3^-$

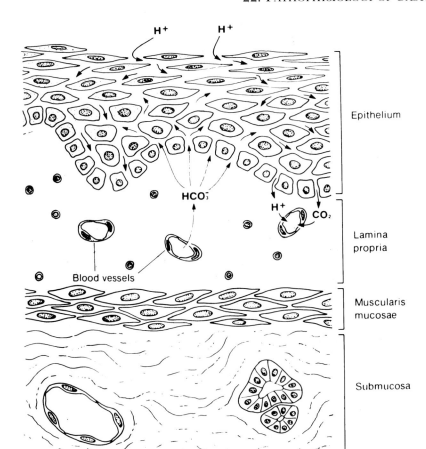

**FIG. 22–6.** Postepithelial defense. The major postepithelial defense against acid injury is an adequate blood supply. In addition to providing essential nutrients and oxygen for cell metabolism, the blood supply maintains tissue acid–base balance, a defense dependent upon blood delivery of $HCO_3^-$ and removal of $H^+$ and $CO_2$. (From Orlando RC. Reflux esophagitis. In Yamada, T, Alpers, DH, Owyang, C, Powell DW, Silverstein FE, eds, Textbook of Gastroenterology. Philadelphia: JB Lippincott Co, 1991: 1123, with permission.)

protection against acid injury was by the buffering of $H^+$ intracellularly rather than within the intercellular space [59].

Notably, as shown by Bass and colleagues [4] and Hollwarth and co-workers [48], the blood supply of the esophagus is not a fixed function, in that it can increase in response to the threat of tissue injury from exposure to luminal acid. However, irreversible injury (cell necrosis) eventually results when the rate at which the blood-derived $HCO_3^-$ can diffuse from interstitial fluid to upper layers of epithelium is exceeded by the rate of $H^+$ entry; this results in profound tissue and cellular acidification. From this, it should be clear that, while defenses within the epithelium provide much of the protection against acid injury, it is the blood supply that supports, orchestrates, and sustains the protective process. This is, to a degree, self-evident, in as much as the deprivation of blood to living tissues invariably leads to cell necrosis.

## EPITHELIAL REGENERATION

When acid exposure is prolonged, the preepithelial, epithelial, and postepithelial defense mechanisms can be overwhelmed, leading to a decline in epithelial pH and irreversible cell injury. This is evident *in vivo* when acid perfusion in rabbit esophagus has reduced the PD by 80% to 100% of initial value (i.e., approaches zero) (Fig. 22–3). Function-

ally, net $Na^+$ transport and NaK, ATPase activity are inhibited [87, 89], and morphologically, cell edema and cell necrosis are evident. It is tempting to attribute cell injury and death to the observed $H^+$ inhibition of NaK, ATPase activity, with its consequent ability to impair both cellular pH and volume regulation. However, this appears not to be the case, since cell necrosis does not accompany inhibition of NaK ATPase activity by ouabain [72, 86]. This lack of cell injury by ouabain may reflect the presence of feedback mechanisms that reduce $Na^+$ entry across the apical cell membranes in response to decreased $Na^+$ exit [15, 123]. One such mechanism may involve stimulation of a $Na^+/Ca^{2+}$ exchanger, with the resultant increase in intracellular $Ca^{2+}$ reducing the permeability of the apical membrane $Na^+$ channels [3, 13]. An increase in intracellular $Ca^{2+}$, however, may be a two-edged sword since acidification appears to activate via a calcium-dependent mechanism, a membrane NaK2Cl cotransporter. This protein then transports large numbers of ions into the cell, and at a time when the cell has little ability to extrude ions. Consequently, an osmotic gradient is created that favors excessive water entry and so cell edema [128, 130]. Since one effect of cell edema is to reduce the concentration of $H^+$ and raise $pH_i$, one might speculate that under such circumstances the cell sacrifices volume regulation in favor of pH regulation. Finally, whether the cell dies a volume-regulatory death is unclear since cell acidity may produce necrosis by other, unexplored processes working in parallel with those that produce cell edema.

Esophageal ulceration eventually develops when repeated bouts of cell necrosis from acid exposure are not offset by epithelial reparative attempts. For epithelial repair to take place normally, there must be preservation of the stratum germinativum, the latter being the only cells within the tissue capable of replication [22, 63, 74, 77]. Although not experimentally proved, the destruction of the stratum germinativum or its basement membrane appears to be a necessary prelude to the development of such serious complications of reflux esophagitis as esophageal strictures and Barrett's esophagus [82].

Although the mechanisms controlling the rate of cell replication in the esophagus are unknown, there is experimental evidence that cell replication increases after acute acid exposure and clinical evidence that it increases during prolonged acid injury. Thus, DeBacker and colleagues [16] reported that a single, 30-minute exposure to HCl stimulates cell replication in dog esophagus within 20 to 34 hours of exposure, and Livstone and co-workers [67] found an increase in tritiated-thymidine uptake, a marker of epithelial turnover, in esophageal biopsies from patients with severe esophagitis. Basal cell hyperplasia, which is considered one of the biopsy hallmarks of reflux esophagitis, represents the morphologic correlate of this increased rate of cell replication (Fig. 22–7) [51]. Based on studies in mice and humans, a normal turnover rate for the esophageal epithelium appears to be 5 to 8 days [6, 63]. Since the rate of replication increases with HCl injury, it would seem possible for the epithelium to regenerate in as little as 2 to 4 days. From a therapeutic standpoint, this suggests that complete epithelial protection from H+ for even short periods of time might be sufficient for recovery, though clinically this does not appear to be entirely borne out. In gastric and duodenal epithelium, there is another epithelial reparative defense, known as epithelial

restitution [120]. Epithelial restitution is of importance because it can occur rapidly (as little as 30 minutes). The rapid nature of the repair is a consequence of its not requiring DNA synthesis and cell replication, only the migration of adjacent viable cells over areas denuded by the loss of injured and necrotic cells. Although studies are limited, data suggest that, in esophagus, epithelial restitution either does not occur or occurs at a much slower rate than in other upper gastrointestinal epithelia [128].

## EFFECTS OF BILE SALTS AND OTHER NOXIOUS AGENTS ON THE ESOPHAGEAL EPITHELIUM

The major focus of this chapter has been on injury to the esophageal epithelium from H+. In addition, other agents and factors may contribute to the injury in reflux esophagitis. Indeed, many investigations indicate that the addition of conjugated bile salts, alcohol, or pepsin to an acid solution or exposure to heat or hypertonicity prior to exposure to an acid solution produces greater injury in a shorter time than does the acid solution alone [7, 12, 65, 66, 71, 101, 111–113, 119]. However, it is also important to recognize that when acid is absent, these agents and environments, in clinically relevant amounts, are relatively innocuous in the esophagus. For this reason, their ability to damage reflects their ability to act as "barrier breakers" that enhance epithelial permeability to H+. The mechanism(s) by which each agent alters barrier function is highly variable. For example, bile salts enhance transcellular H+ entry in both gastric and esophageal mucosa by micellar dissolution of cell membrane lipids [21, 113], whereas the proteolytic enzyme pepsin appears to enhance paracellular H+ entry by digestion of intercellular proteins in esophagus [113]. Further, alcohol can act by enhancing H+ entry through both transcellular and paracellular pathways [7, 111, 118], the former by increasing cell membrane fluidity and the latter through its junctional

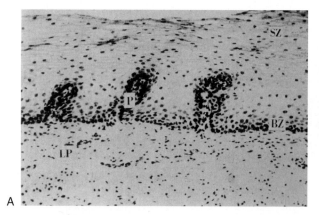
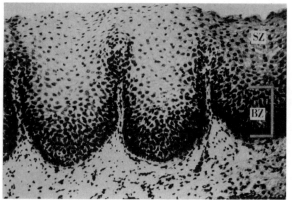

FIG. 22–7. **A:** Normal esophageal suction biopsy from a healthy subject without esophagitis. Basal zone thickness is approximately 10% of total epithelial thickness; papillae extend approximately one-half the distance to the epithelial surface. **B:** Abnormal suction biopsy from a subject with symptomatic reflux. Basal zone thickness is approximately 35% of total epithelial thickness; papillae extend over two-thirds of the distance to the epithelial surface. *BZ,* basal zone, *SZ,* stratified zone; *P,* papillae; *LP,* lamina propria. Hematoxylin and eosin ×170. (From ref. 51, with permission.)

damaging effects. Hypertonic solutions have also been shown to increase paracellular permeability in stratified squamous epithelium including that of the esophagus [31, 35]. Moreover, experimentally, esophageal sensitivity to acid injury occurs in rabbit esophagus that has been pretreated with a hypertonic solution even for as little as 10 minutes and with otherwise innocuous levels of acidity, e.g., pH 2 [70]. A parallel of this in humans is that hypertonic solutions can induce heartburn in subjects known to have an acid-sensitive esophagus [68]. It is unknown, however, whether the symptoms result from stimulation of nerve endings by the hypertonic environment or by concomitant exposure to refluxed acid during the procedure. Nonetheless, regardless of specific mechanism, the common denominator by which these agents operate is through enhancement of $H^+$ entry. $H^+$ entry is the factor that ultimately transforms what would be a minor insult to the tissue into one that is clinically significant. Such a crucial role for acid has recently been supported by the dramatic success of the proton pump inhibitors in reflux esophagitis, the drugs acting by potent and selective inhibition of the gastric parietal cell's acid-secretory mechanism [47, 117].

## REFERENCES AND SELECTED READINGS

1. Allen A, Garner A. Mucus and bicarbonate secretion in the stomach and their possible role in mucosal protection. Gut 1980;21:249
2. Allen A, Phil D. The structure and function of gastrointestinal mucus. In Harmon JW, ed, Basic Mechanisms of Gastrointestinal Mucosal Cell Injury and Protection. Baltimore: Williams & Wilkins, 1981:351
3. Al Yassin T, Toner PG. Fine structure of squamous epithelium and submucosal glands of human esophagus. J Anat 1977;123:705
4. Bass BL, et al. HCl back diffusion interferes with intrinsic reactive regulation of esophageal mucosal blood flow. Surgery 1984;96:404
5. Bateson MC, et al. Oesophageal epithelial ultrastructure after incubation with gastrointestinal fluids and their components. J Pathol 1981; 133:33
6. Bell B, Almy TP, Lipkin M. Cell proliferation kinetics in the gastrointestinal tract of man: III. Cell renewal in esophagus, stomach and jejunum of a patient with treated pernicious anemia. J Natl Cancer Inst 1967;38:615
7. Bor S, Tobey NA, Abdulnour-Nakhoul S, Marten E. Ethanol predisposes to acid damage in rabbit esophagus. Gastroenterology 1997; 112:A77
8. Bowen JC, Fairchild RB. Oxygen in gastric mucosal protection. In Harmon JW, ed, Basic Mechanisms of Gastrointestinal Mucosal Cell Injury and Protection. Baltimore: Williams & Wilkins, 1981:259
9. Boyd DD, Carney CN, Powell DW. Neurohumoral control of esophageal epithelial electrolyte transport. Am J Physiol 1980;239:G5
10. Carney CN, Orlando RC, Powell DW, Dotson MM. Morphologic alterations in early acid-induced epithelial injury of the rabbit esophagus. Lab Invest 1981;45:198
11. Carter MJ. Carbonic anhydrase: isoenzymes, properties, distribution, and functional significance. Biol Rev 1972;47:465
12. Chung RSK, Johnson GM, DenBesten L. Effect of Na taurocholate and ethanol on hydrogen ion absorption in rabbit esophagus. Am J Dig Dis 1975;20:582
13. Chung RSK, Magri J, DenBesten L. Hydrogen ion transport in the rabbit esophagus. Am J Physiol 1975;229:496
14. Civan MM, Cragoe EJ Jr, Peterson-Yantorno K. Intracellular pH in frog skin: effects of $Na^+$, volume and cAMP. Am J Physiol 1988; 225:FI26
15. Cuthbert AW, Shum WK. Does intracellular sodium modify membrane permeability to sodium ions? Nature 1977;266:468
16. DeBacker A, Haentjens P, Willems G. Hydrochloric acid: a trigger of cell proliferation in the esophagus of dogs. Dig Dis Sci 1985;30: 884
17. DeMeester TR, et al. Patterns of gastroesophageal reflux in health and disease. Ann Surg 1976;184:459
18. Dent J, Dodds WJ, Friedman RH, Sekiguci T, Hogan WJ, Arndorfer RC, Petrie DJ. Mechanism of gastroesophageal reflux in recumbent asymptomatic subjects. J Clin Invest 1980;65:256
19. Diamond JM. Channels in epithelial cell membranes and junctions. Fed Proc 1978;37:2639
20. Dodds WJ, Hogan WJ, Helm JF, Dent J. Pathogenesis of reflux esophagitis. Gastroenterology 1981;81:376
21. Duane WC, Weigand DM. Mechanism by which bile salt disrupts the gastric mucosal barrier in the dog. J Clin Invest 1980;66:1044
22. Eastwood GL. Gastrointestinal epithelial renewal. Gastroenterology 1977;72:962
23. Eastwood GL, et al. Beneficial effect of indomethacin on acid-induced esophagitis in cats. Dig Dis Sci 1981;26:601
24. Eckardt VF, Adami B. Esophageal transmural potential difference in patients with symptomatic gastroesophageal reflux. Klin Wochenschr 1980;58:293
25. Elias PM, Brown BE. The mammalian cutaneous permeability barrier: defective barrier function in essential fatty acid deficiency correlates with abnormal intercellular lipid deposition. Lab Invest 1978;39:574
26. Elias PM, Friend DS. The permeability barrier in mammalian epidermis. J Cell Biol 1975;65:180
27. Elias PM, Goerke J, Friend DS. Mammalian epidermal barrier layer lipids: composition and influence on structure. J Invest Dermatol 1977;69:535
28. Elias PM, McNutt NS, Friend DS. Membrane alterations during codification of mammalian squamous epithelia: a freeze-fracture, tracer and thin-section study. Anat Rec 1977;189:577
29. Emilio MG, Machado MM, Menano HP. The production of a hydrogen ion gradient across the isolated frog skin. Biochem Biophys Acta 1970;203:394
30. Emmelin N. Nervous control of salivary glands. In Code CF, ed, Handbook of Physiology, Alimentary Canal, section 6, vol 2. Washington, DC: American Physiological Society, 1967:595
31. Erlij D, Martinez-Palomo A. Opening of tight junctions in frog skin by hypertonic urea solutions. J Membr Biol 1972;9:229
32. Farquhar MG, Palade GE. Functional organization of amphibian skin. Proc Natl Acad Sci 1964;51:569
33. Farrell RL, Roling GT, Castell DO. Cholinergic therapy of chronic heartburn. Ann Intern Med 1974;80:573
34. Ferreira KG, Hill BS. The effect of low external pH on properties of the paracellular pathway and junctional structure in frog skin. J Physiol 1982;332:59
35. Fischbarg J, Whittembury G. The effect of external pH on osmotic permeability, ion and fluid transport across isolated frog skin. J Physiol 1978;275:403
36. Geboes K, et al. Vascular changes in the esophageal mucosa: an early histologic sign of esophagitis. Gastrointest Endosc 1980;26:29
37. Grayson S, Johnson-Winegar AD, Elias PM. Isolation of lamellar bodies from neonatal mouse epidermis by selective sequential filtration. Science 1983;221:962
38. Guth PH. Local metabolism and circulation in mucosal defense. In Harmon JW, ed, Basic Mechanisms of Gastrointestinal Mucosal Cell Injury and Protection. Baltimore: Williams & Wilkins, 1981;253
39. Hafez ESE. Functional anatomy of mucus-secreting cells. In Elstein M, Parke DV, eds, Mucus in Health and Disease. New York: Plenum Publishing, 1977:19
40. Hamilton BH, Orlando RC. In vivo alkaline secretion by mammalian esophagus. Gastroenterology 1989;97:640
41. Harmon JW, Johnson LF, Maydonovitch CL. Effects of acid and bile salts on the rabbit esophageal mucosa. Dig Dis Sci 1981;87:280
42. Heatley NG. Mucosubstance as a barrier to diffusion. Gastroenterology 1959;37:313
43. Helm JF, Dodds WJ, Hogan WJ, Soergel KH, Egide MS, Wood CM. Acid neutralizing capacity of human saliva. Gastroenterology 1982; 83:69
44. Helm JF, Dodds WJ, Riedel DR, Teeter BC, Hogan WJ, Arndorfer RC. Determinants of esophageal acid clearance in normal subjects. Gastroenterology 1983;85:607
45. Helm JF, Dodds WJ, Pelc LR, Palmer DW, Hogan WJ, Teeter BC. Effect of esophageal emptying and saliva on clearance of acid from the esophagus. N Engl J Med 1984;310:284
46. Herlihy KJ, Orlando RC, Bryson JC, Bozymski EM, Carney CN, Powell DW. Barrett's esophagus: clinical, endoscopic, histologic,

manometric and electrical potential difference characteristics. Gastroenterology 1984;86:436

47. Hetzel DI, Dent J, Reed WD, Narielvala FM, Mackinnon M, McCarthy JH. Healing and relapse of severe peptic esophagitis after treatment with omeprazole. Gastroenterology 1988;95:903

48. Hollwarth ME, Smith M, Kvietys PR, Granger DN. Esophageal blood flow in the cat. Gastroenterology 1986;90:622

49. Hopwood D, Logan KR, Coghill G, Bouchier IAD. Histochemical studies of mucosubstances and lipids in normal human oesophageal epithelium. Histochem J 1977;9:153

50. Hopwood D, Milne G, Logan KR. Electron microscopic changes in human oesophageal epithelium in oesophagitis. J Pathol 1979;129:161

51. Ismail-Beigi F, Horton PF, Pope CE II. Histological consequences of gastroesophageal reflux in man. Gastroenterology 1970;58:163

52. Johnson LF, DeMeester TR. Twenty-four hour pH monitoring of the distal esophagus. Am J Gastroenterol 1974;62:325

53. Kent PW, Allen A. The biosynthesis of intestinal mucins: effect of salicylate on glycoprotein biosynthesis by sheep colonic and human gastric mucosal tissues *in vitro*. Biochem J 1967;106:645

54. Khalbuss WE, Marousis CG, Subramanyam M, Orlando RC. Effect of HCl on transmembrane potentials and intracellular pH in rabbit esophageal epithelium. Gastroenterology 1995;108:662

55. Khamis B, Kennedy C, Finucane J, Doyle JS. Transmural potential difference: diagnostic value in gastro-oesophageal reflux. Gut 1978;19:396

56. Kiriluk LB, Merendino KA. The comparative sensitivity of the mucosa of the various segments of the alimentary tract in the dog to acid-peptic action. Surgery 1954;35:547

57. Kivilaakso E. High plasma $HCO_3^-$ protects gastric mucosa against acute ulceration in the rat. Gastroenterology 1981;81:921

58. Kivilaakso E, Flemstrom G. $HCO_3^-$ secretion and pH gradient across the surface mucus gel in rat duodenum. Gastroenterology 1982;82:1101A

59. Kivilaakso E, Barzilai A, Schiessel R, Crass R, Silen W. Ulceration of isolated amphibian gastric mucosa. Gastroenterology 1979;77:31

60. Kivilaakso E, Fromm D, Silen W. Effect of bile salts and related compounds on isolated esophageal mucosa. Surgery 1980;87:280

61. Lacy ER, Tobey NA, Cowart K, Orlando RC. The esophageal mucosal barrier: structural correlates. Gastroenterology 1989;96:A281

62. Layden TJ, Schmidt L, Agnone L, Lisitza P, Brewer J, Goldstein JL. Rabbit esophageal cell cytoplasmic pH regulation: role of $Na^+-H^+$ antiport and $Na^+$-dependent $HCO_3^-$ transport systems. Am J Physiol 1992;263(3 Pt 1):G407

63. Leblond CP, Greuiich RC, Pereira JPM. Relationship of cell formation and cell migration in the renewal of stratified squamous epithelia. In Montagna W, Billingham RE, eds, Advances in Biology of Skin, vol 5. Wound Healing. New York: Pergamon Press, 1974:39

64. Lichter I, Muir RC. The pattern of swallowing during sleep. Electroencephalogr Clin Neurophysiol 1975;38:427

65. Lillemoe KD, Johnson LF, Harmon JW. Role of the components of the gastroduodenal contents in experimental acid esophagitis. Surgery 1982;92:276

66. Lillemoe KD, Johnson LF, Harmon JW. Alkaline esophagitis: a comparison of the ability of components of gastroduodenal contents to injure the rabbit esophagus. Gastroenterology 1983;85:621

67. Livstone EM, Sheahan DG, Behar J. Studies of esophageal epithelial cell proliferation in patients with reflux esophagitis. Gastroenterology 1977;73:1315

68. Lloyd DA, Borda IT. Food-induced heartburn: effect of osmolality. Gastroenterology 1981;80:740

69. Logan K, Hopwood D, Milne G. Ultrastructural demonstration of cell coat on the surface of normal oesophageal epithelium. Histochem J 1977;9:495

70. Long JD, Marten E, Tobey NA, Orlando RC. The relationship between esophageal epithelial paracellular permeability and susceptibility to injury by luminal HCl. Gastroenterology 1996;110:A179

71. Long JD, Marten E, Tobey NA, Orlando, RC. Effects of luminal hypertonicity on rabbit esophageal epithelium. Am J Physiol 1997;273:G647

72. MacKnight ADC, Leaf A. Regulation of cellular volume. Physiol Rev 1977;57:510

73. Mantle M, Mantle D, Allen A. Polymeric structure of pig small-intestinal mucus glycoprotein. Biochem J 1981;195:277

74. Marques-Pereira JP, Leblond CP. Mitosis and differentiation in the stratified-squamous epithelium of the rat esophagus. Am J Anat 1965;117:73

75. Martinez-Palomo A, Erlij D, Bracho H. Localization of permeability barriers in the frog skin epithelium. J Cell Biol 1971;50:277

76. Menguy R, Masters YF. The effects of aspirin on gastric mucus production. Surg Gynecol Obstet 1965;92:1

77. Messier B, Leblond CP. Cell proliferation and migration as revealed by radioautography after injection of thymidine-$H^3$ into rats and mice. Am Anat 1960;106:247

78. Mills JW, Ernst SA, DiBona DR. Localization of Na-pump sites in frog skin. J Cell Biol 1977;73:88

79. Moreno JH, Diamond JM. Discrimination of monovalent inorganic cations by ''tight'' junctions of gallbladder epithelium. J Membr Biol 1974;15:277

80. Northway MG, et al. Radiation esophagitis in the opossum: radioprotection with indomethacin. Gastroenterology 1980;78:883

81. Orlando RC. Esophageal epithelial resistance. In Castell DO, Wu WC, Ott DJ, eds, Gastroesophageal Reflux Disease: Pathogenesis, Diagnosis, Therapy. Mount Kisco, NY: Futura, 1985:55

82. Orlando RC. Pathology of reflux oesophagitis and its complications. In Jamieson GG, ed, Surgery of the Oesophagus. New York: Churchill-Livingstone, 1988:189

83. Orlando RC. Esophageal epithelial defense against acid injury. J Clin Gastroenterol 1991;13(Suppl 2):S1

84. Orlando RC. Reflux esophagitis. In Yamada T, Alpers DH, Owyang C, Powell DW, Silverstein FE, eds, Textbook of Gastroenterology. New York: Lippincott–Raven, 1998

85. Orlando RC, Powell DW. Studies of esophageal epithelial electrolyte transport and potential difference in man. In Allen A, et al., eds, Mechanisms of Mucosal Protection in the Upper Gastrointestinal Tract. New York: Raven Press, 1984:75

86. Orlando RC, Tobey NA. Comparative sensitivity of rabbit esophageal epithelium to serosal versus mucosal acid. Gastroenterology 1989;96:A512

87. Orlando RC, Powell DW, Carney CN. Pathophysiology of acute acid injury in rabbit esophageal epithelium. J Clin Invest 1981;68:286

88. Orlando RC, et al. Esophageal potential difference measurements in esophageal disease. Gastroenterology 1982;83:1026

89. Orlando RC, Bryson JC, Powell DW. Mechanisms of HCl injury in rabbit esophageal epithelium. Am J Physiol 1984;246:G718

90. Orlando RC, Tobey NA, Cragoe EJ. Is there a role for transcellular (apical membrane) diffusion of hydrogen ions in acute acid injury to rabbit esophageal epithelium? In O'Brien P, Garner A, eds, Mechanisms of Injury, Protection, and Repair of the Upper Gastrointestinal Tract. New York: Wiley, 1991:199

91. Palmer LG. Ion selectivity of the apical membrane Na channel in the toad urinary bladder. J Membr Biol 1982;67:91

92. Pfeiffer CJ. Experimental analysis of hydrogen ion diffusion in gastrointestinal mucus glycoprotein. Am J Physiol 1981;240:G176

93. Pope CE II. Pathophysiology and diagnosis of reflux esophagitis. Gastroenterology 1976;70:445

94. Pope CE II. Gastroesophageal reflux disease (reflux esophagitis) In: Sleisenger MH, Fordtran JS, eds. Gastrointestinal Disease: Pathophysiology, Diagnosis, Management, vol 1, 2nd ed. Philadelphia: WB Saunders, 1978:541

95. Powell DW. Barrier function of epithelia. Am J Physiol 1981;241:G275

96. Powell DW. Physiological concept of epithelial barriers. In Allen A, et al., eds, Mechanisms of Mucosal Protection in the Upper Gastrointestinal Tract. New York: Raven Press, 1984:1

97. Powell DW, Morris SM, Boyd DD. Water and electrolyte transport by rabbit esophagus. Am J Physiol 1975;229:438

98. Powell DW, Orlando RC, Carney CN. Acid injury of the esophageal epithelium. In Harmon JW, ed, Basic Mechanisms of Gastrointestinal Mucosal Cell Injury and Protection. Baltimore: Williams & Wilkins, 1981:155

99. Quigley EMM, Turnberg LA. pH of the microclimate lining the human gastric and duodenal mucosa *in vivo*—studies in control subjects and in duodenal ulcer patients. Gastroenterology 1987;92:1876

100. Read NW, Fordtran JS. The role of intraluminal junction potentials in the generation of the gastric potential difference in man. Gastroenterology 1979;76:932

101. Redo SF, Bames WA, de la Sierra CA. Perfusion of the canine esophagus with secretions of upper gastrointestinal tract. Ann Surg 1959;149:556

102. Reed PI, Davies WA. Controlled trial of a new dosage form of carbenoxolone (pyrogastrone) in the treatment of reflux esophagitis. Dig Dis 1978;23:161

103. Richter JE, Castell DO. Gastroesophageal reflux: pathogenesis, diagnosis, therapy. Ann Intern Med 1982;97:93

104. Rick R, et al. Electron microprobe analysis of frog skin epithelium: evidence for a syncytial sodium transport compartment. J Membr Biol 1978;39:313

105. Robles-Chillida EM, Rodrigo J, Mayo I, Arnedo A, Gomez A. Ultrastructure of free-ending nerve fibers in oesophageal epithelium. J Anat 1981;133:227

106. Rodrigo J, Hernandez DJ, Vidal MA, Pedrosa JA. Vegetative innervation of the esophagus III. Intraepithelial endings. Acta Anat 1975;92:242

107. Rose B, Rick R. Intracellular pH, intracellular Ca and junctional cell to cell coupling. J Membr Biol 1978;44:377

108. Russel JM, Boron WF. Role of chloride transport in regulation of intracellular pH. Nature 1976;264:73

109. Sachs G. $H^+$ pathways and pH changes in gastric tissue. Gastroenterology 1978;75:750

110. Safaie-Schirazi S. Effect of pepsin on ionic permeability of canine esophageal mucosa. J Surg Res 1977;22:5

111. Safaie-Shirazi S, DenBesten L, Zike WL. Effect of bile salts on the ionic permeability of the esophageal mucosa and their role in the production of esophagitis. Gastroenterology 1975;68:728

112. Salo J, Kivilaakso E. Role of luminal $H^+$ in the pathogenesis of experimental esophagitis. Surgery 1982;92:61

113. Salo JA, Lehto VP, Kivilaakso E. Morphologic alterations in experimental esophagitis: light microscopic and scanning and transmission electron microscopic study. Dig Dis Sci 1983;28:440

114. Schiesset R, et al. PGE2 stimulates gastric chloride transport: possible key to cytoprotection. Nature 1980;283:671

115. Schiessel R, Merhav A, Matthews J, Barzilai AM, Silen W. Role of nutrient $HCO_3^-$ in the protection of amphibian gastric mucosa. Am J Physiol 1980;239:G536

116. Schneyer LH, et al. Rate of flow of human parotid, sublingual and submaxillary secretions during steep. J Dent Res 1956;35:109

117. Schulman MI, Orlando RC. Treatment of gastroesophageal reflux: the role of proton pump inhibitors. In Schrier RW, Baxter JD, Abboud F, Fauci AS, eds, Advances in Internal Medicine, vol. 40. St. Louis: Mosby–Year Book, 1995:273

118. Shirazi SS, Platz CD. Effect of alcohol on canine esophageal mucosa. J Surg Res 1978;25:373

119. Sikka D, Marten E, Tobey NA, Orlando RC. Effect of heat on the barrier and transport functions of rabbit esophageal epithelium. Gastroenterology 1996;110:A258

120. Silen W. Gastric mucosal defense and repair. In Johnson LR, et al., eds, Physiology of the Gastrointestinal Tract, vol 2, 2nd ed. New York: Raven Press, 1987:1055

121. Sinar DR, Fletcher JR, Castell DO. The beneficial effect of methyl $PGE_2$ to diminish caustic esophageal injury. Clin Res 1982;30:498A

122. Spring KR, Ericson AC. Epithelial cell volume modulation and regulation. J Membr Biol 1982;69:167

123. Taylor A, Windhager EE. Possible role of cytosolic calcium and Na–Ca exchange in regulation of transepithelial sodium transport. Am J Physiol 1979;236:F505

124. Thanik KD, Chey WY, Shah AN, Gutierrez JG. Reflux esophagitis: effect of oral bethanechol on symptoms and endoscopic findings. Ann Intem Med 1980;93:805

125. Thomson ABR. Unstirred water layers: a basic mechanism of gastrointestinal mucosal cell cytoprotection. In Harmon JW, ed, Basic Mechanisms of Gastrointestinal Mucosal Cell Injury and Protection. Baltimore: Williams & Wilkins, 1981:327

126. Thomson ABR. Unstirred water layers: possible adaptive and cytoprotective function. In Allen A, et al., eds, Mechanisms of Mucosal Protection in the Upper Gastrointestinal Tract. New York: Raven Press, 1984:233

127. Tobey NA, Powell DW, Schreiner VJ, Orlando RC. Serosal bicarbonate protects against acid injury to rabbit esophagus. Gastroenterology 1989;96:1466

128. Tobey NA, Cragoe, EJ Jr, Orlando RC. HCl-induced cell edema in rabbit esophageal epithelium: a bumetanide-sensitive process. Gastroenterology 1995;109:414

129. Tobey NA, Carson JL, Alkiek RA, Orlando RC. Dilated intercellular spaces: a morphological feature of acid reflux-damaged human esophageal epithelium. Gastroenterology 1996;111:1200

130. Tobey NA, Koves G, Orlando RC. HCl-induced cell edema in primary cultured rabbit esophageal epithelium. Gastroenterology 1997;112:847

131. Turin L, Warner A. Carbon dioxide reversibly abolishes ionic communication between cells of early amphibian embryo. Nature 1977;270:56

132. Turner KS, Powell DW, Carney CN, Orlando RC, Bozymski EM. Transmural electrical potential difference in the mammalian esophagus in vivo. Gastroenterology 1978;75:286

133. Vidins EI, Fox JEF, Beck IT. Transmural potential difference (PD) in the body of the esophagus in patients with esophagitis, Barrett's epithelium and carcinoma of the esophagus. Am J Dig Dis 1971;16:991

134. Wertz PW, Downing DT. Glycolipids in mammalian epidermis: structure and function in the water barrier. Science 1982;217:1261

135. Williams SE, Turnberg LA. Studies of the ''protective'' properties of gastric mucus: evidence for mucus bicarbonate barrier. Gut 1979;20:A922

136. Williams SE, Turnberg LA. The demonstration of a pH gradient across mucus adherent to rabbit gastric mucosa: evidence for a mucus–bicarbonate barrier. Gut 1981;22:94

The Esophagus, Third Edition,
edited by D. O. Castell and J. E. Richter.
Lippincott Williams & Wilkins, Philadelphia © 1999.

CHAPTER 23

# Duodenogastroesophageal Reflux

Michael F. Vaezi

Gastroesophageal reflux disease (GERD) represents retrograde flow of gastric contents into the esophagus with or without associated histologic changes. Most healthy individuals intermittently reflux gastric contents into the esophagus. These episodes occur most commonly postprandially, are short lived, and rarely cause symptoms or esophageal mucosal injury. However, excessive gastroesophageal reflux may produce symptoms, and nearly 50% of these patients have complications of GERD, including esophagitis, strictures, or Barrett's esophagus at endoscopy [15].

The noxious agents responsible for injuring the esophageal mucosa originate from both gastric and duodenal sources. Hydrochloric acid (HCL) and pepsin are the important gastric agents predisposing to the development of esophageal symptoms and mucosal injury [22, 27, 47, 77]. Additionally, gastric juice may intermix with duodenal contents by transpyloric reflux of bile and pancreatic secretions. Regurgitation of duodenal contents into the stomach is normal, occurring most commonly at night and postprandially [48, 58, 67, 82]. However, when excessive, it may be associated with gastritis, gastric ulcers, postcholecystectomy syndrome, dyspepsia, and esophageal mucosal damage [11, 17, 20, 28, 29, 34, 36, 38, 43, 68, 69, 78, 79]. The term duodenogastroesophageal reflux (DGER) refers to regurgitation of duodenal contents through the pylorus into the stomach, with subsequent reflux into the esophagus. Previously, the term *bile reflux* and *alkaline reflux* were used to describe this process. However, duodenal contents contain more than just bile, and recent studies show that the term *alkaline reflux* is a misnomer since pH > 7 does not correlate with reflux of duodenal contents [13].

The importance of DGER relates to findings in both animal and human studies that factors other than acid, namely bile and pancreatic enzymes, may play a significant role in mucosal injury and symptoms in patients with GERD. However, the relative importance of acid or DGER to the development of esophageal mucosal injury is controversial.

Until recently, the main difficulty has been extrapolating the findings in animal studies to humans. However, recent studies using state-of-the-art methods for detecting esophageal reflux of both acid and duodenal contents are helping unravel the role of these potentially injurious agents in producing esophageal mucosal injury. This chapter reviews the important animal and human studies that clarify the role of gastric and duodenal contents in causing esophageal symptoms and mucosal damage. Then, the available tests for identifying DGER are discussed and their advantages and disadvantages reviewed. Finally, the medical and surgical therapies for DGER are discussed.

## IMPORTANCE OF ACID AND PEPSIN

### Animal Studies

Substantial experimental and clinical evidence strongly supports the importance of acid and pepsin in causing esophageal mucosal injury. Using the canine esophagus, Redo et al. [77] investigated the role of acid alone and in combination with various pepsin concentrations by infusing pepsin at concentrations up to 10% and at pH values of less than and greater than 2. They reported no esophageal damage with HCl infusion alone, while acid in combination with low concentrations of pepsin at pH less than 2 caused the most severe esophagitis. Meanwhile, Goldberg et al. [27] demonstrated esophageal mucosal damage in the intact feline esophagus with either very high concentrations of acid (pH 1.0 to 1.3) or lower acid concentrations (pH 1.6 to 2.0) in the presence of pepsin. Using a perfused rabbit esophagus model, Lillemoe et al. [51] confirmed that acid infusion alone did not produce mucosal damage or increase esophageal mucosal permeability as measured by the net flux of $H^+$, K, glucose, and hemoglobin. However, the addition of pepsin to the infusate in a dose-dependent manner was associated with increased degrees of gross esophageal mucosal injury and changes in esophageal mucosal permeability. Thus, animal studies suggest that the esophageal mucosa is relatively resistant to reflux of acid alone unless it occurs at very high concentrations (pH 1.0 to 1.3). On the other hand, the combi-

M. F. Vaezi: Department of Gastroenterology, The Cleveland Clinic Foundation, Cleveland, Ohio 44195.

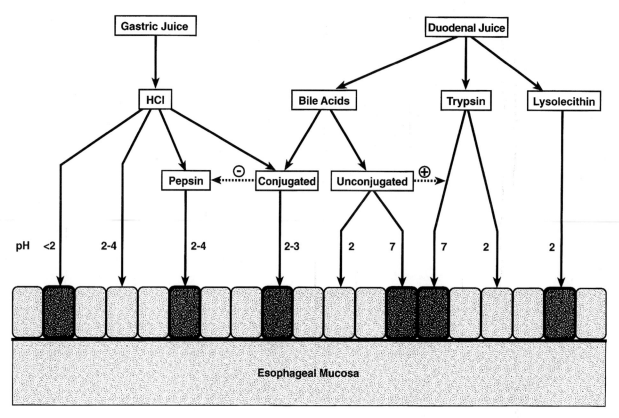

**FIG. 23–1.** Proposed agents responsible for esophageal mucosal injury.

nation of acid and even small concentrations of pepsin results in macroscopic as well as microscopic esophageal mucosal injury (Fig. 23–1).

## Human Studies

Studies by Aylwin et al. [1] gave the first scientific evidence identifying the importance of acid and pepsin in the development of heartburn and esophageal mucosal injury. Using continuous esophageal aspiration in patients with hiatal hernia and esophagitis, they found that patients with esophagitis had aspirates of lower pH and higher pepsin concentration than those without esophagitis. Later, Tuttle et al. [103, 104] measured the pH of the distal esophagus, finding that the reflux of pH < 4 material coincided with the onset of heartburn, while a rise to a more neutral pH coincided with relief of symptoms.

Subsequently, a series of studies showed that patients with various grades of esophagitis, including Barrett's esophagus, have increased frequency and duration of esophageal exposure to pH < 4 refluxate [24, 35, 92, 94, 111]. Iascone et al. [39] reported a direct relationship between the severity of esophageal mucosal injury and the degree and frequency of mucosal exposure to acid reflux. Later, studies by De-Meester et al. [15] found that 90% of patients with esophagitis had increased amounts of acid reflux by 24-hour pH monitoring. The same group [95] reported that patients with

Barrett's esophagus had significantly higher exposure times to pH < 4 than patients with esophagitis, who had higher exposure times than healthy controls. Later, Stein et al. [97] reported that patients with Barrett's esophagus had greater exposure times to more caustic gastric acid concentrations (pH < 3 or 2), suggesting a significant role for acid reflux in the development of esophagitis and Barrett's esophagus.

Separating the role of pepsin from acid in the production of esophagitis is difficult, since the optimum pH for the enzymatic activity of pepsin is below 3. Studies show a positive correlation between the degree of abnormal acid and pepsin exposure and the severity of esophagitis. Bremner et al. [9] observed that patients with increased esophageal exposure to pH 1 to 2, corresponding to the known pKa of pepsin, had the most significant degrees of esophagitis. In a recent study, Gotley et al. [29] found that esophageal aspirates from patients with esophagitis had significantly higher concentrations of acid and pepsin than the aspirates from healthy controls. Furthermore, patients with Zollinger-Ellison syndrome, where the basal acid output is high and gastric pH favors optimum acidity for pepsin activity, have a 40% to 60% incidence of esophagitis despite normal or increased lower esophageal sphincter pressures [64].

It is important to note that the frequency and duration of esophageal acid exposure are not always predictive of the degree of esophageal mucosal injury. This suggests the importance of other factors including DGER, the inherent resistance of esophageal mucosa to acid injury, and the role of saliva- and bicarbonate-producing submucosal glands in the distal esophagus to neutralize refluxed acid [16, 32, 62, 89].

## ROLE OF DUODENAL CONTENTS

### Animal Studies

The role of duodenal contents, specifically bile acids and the pancreatic enzyme trypsin, in the development of esophageal mucosal injury is controversial and the subject of many *in vitro* animal studies [14, 26, 33, 49, 66]. Early studies by Cross and Wangensteen [14] suggested a role for bile and its constituents, namely bile acids, in esophageal mucosal damage. Using a dog model with biliary diversion and a jejunal conduit anastomosing directly to the esophagus, Moffat and Berkas [66] showed that canine bile was capable of producing various degrees of erosive esophagitis, thereby confirming earlier studies by Cross and Wangensteen [14].

More recent studies show that esophageal mucosal damage by bile acids is dependent on the conjugation state of the bile acids and the pH of the refluxate (Fig 23–1). Using net acid flux (NAF) across the esophageal lumen as an index of mucosal injury, Harmon et al. [33] showed that taurine-conjugated bile salts taurodeoxycholate and taurocholate (both with pKa of 1.9) increased NAF at pH 2, while the unconjugated forms increased NAF at pH 7, but not at pH 2. Hence, conjugated bile acids are more injurious to the esophageal mucosa at acidic pH, while unconjugated bile acids are more harmful at pH 5 to 8. Using rabbit esophageal perfusion studies, Kivilaakso et al. [49] confirmed the pH-dependent damage caused by conjugated and unconjugated bile acids, and additionally showed the injurious effect of trypsin on the esophageal mucosa at pH 7.0. They concluded that ''alkaline'' reflux esophagitis was caused by both unconjugated bile acids and trypsin at neutral pH values.

Since the reflux of gastroduodenal contents usually occurs intermixed with the acidic contents of the stomach, several investigators have studied the synergistic and inhibitory interactions of HCl with pepsin, trypsin, and bile acids [51, 52, 79, 80]. Lillemoe et al. [51] compared the injurious effects of the various duodenal components on rabbit esophageal mucosa at pH 2. At this acidic pH, trypsin had no effect on net flux of ions across the esophageal mucosa, since the enzyme is inactive at pH values below 4. Meanwhile, taurocholate produced no esophageal mucosal damage at a neutral pH, but in an acidic medium (pH 1.2), there was esophageal mucosal disruption as measured by net ion permeability. Similarly, Salo and Kivilaakso [79] found that both taurocholate and lysolecithin, the latter a normal constituent of duodenal juice formed by pancreatic phospholipase, a hydrolysis of lecithin in bile causes histologic damage and alteration of the rabbit esophageal transmucosal potential difference in the presence of HCl, but there was no effect in the absence of HCl.

Bile acids, depending on their conjugated states, also have both synergistic and inhibitory interactions with trypsin and pepsin. In perfusion studies of the rabbit esophagus, Salo and Kivilaakso [80] found that the unconjugated bile acid cholate significantly increased mucosal damage caused by trypsin at pH 7.0. On the other hand, Lillemoe et al. [52] found that the degree of esophageal mucosal injury and permeability decreased in a dose-dependent manner when increasing concentrations of the conjugated bile acid taurodeoxycholate were added to pepsin.

Therefore, as shown in Fig. 23–1, there is evidence in the animal model for synergism between HCl and pepsin as well as HCl and conjugated bile acids and lysolecithin in causing esophageal mucosal damage. Similarly, unconjugated bile acids seem to augment the damaging effect of trypsin at pH 7. HCl is inhibitory to the damaging effects of trypsin and unconjugated bile acids, whereas conjugated bile acids decrease the damaging effect of pepsin at acidic pH.

### Mechanism of Injury

The mechanisms of esophageal mucosal damage by pepsin and trypsin are clearly related to the proteolytic properties of these enzymes. Both promote detachment of the surface cells from the epithelium, presumably by digesting the intercellular substances and surface structures that contribute to the maintenance of cohesion between cells [81, 88]. Each agent causes the most damage at its optimal pH activity range, pH 2 to 3 for pepsin and pH 5 to 8 for trypsin.

The mechanism for mucosal damage by HCl is more complicated and depends upon a series of events. Experimental work by Orlando, Powell, and co-workers [12, 72, 73, 76] in the rabbit esophagus indicates that $H^+$ impairs cell volume regulation, causing cell death by inactivation of the $Na^+/K^+$-ATPase pump located in the basolateral cell wall in the stratum spinosum of the mucosa. Inhibition of $Na^+/K^+$-ATPase occurs at the same time that an amiloride-sensitive $Na^+$ pump is activated, causing increased entry and accumulation of $Na^+$ intracellularly and resulting in excess intracellular volume and subsequent cell death. Snow et al. [91] proposed an alternative mechanism by which acid-induced esophageal mucosal injury may inhibit normal cell volume regulatory mechanisms. Using isolated rabbit esophageal mucosal basal cells, these investigators found pH-dependent alteration in $K^+$ and/or $Cl^-$ conductance.

The mechanism by which bile acids cause mucosal damage is not fully understood. Studies suggest two hypotheses. The first is that bile acids damage mucosal cells by their detergent property and solubilization of the mucosal lipid membranes. This theory is supported by studies in gastric mucosa where bile acid-induced mucosal injury was correlated with the release of phospholipids and cholesterol into the lumen [19, 100, 101]. However, studies with rabbit esophageal mucosa [84, 86] show significant mucosal barrier disruption occurring at bile acid concentrations below the level where phospholipids are solubilized. Therefore, this mechanism is less likely to explain the esophageal mucosal disruption caused by bile acids.

Alternatively, the second and more favored hypothesis suggests that bile acids gain entrance across the mucosa because of their lipophilic state, causing intramucosal damage primarily by disorganizing membrane structure or interfering with cellular function. Support for this model comes from several experimental studies. Batzri et al. [7] found that bile acids, once penetrating the mucosal barrier, are trapped inside the cells by intracellular ionization, explaining the several fold increase in intracellular concentrations of bile acids [85]. Furthermore, studies by Schweitzer et al. [7, 86] correlated bile acid entry and mucosal accumulation with bile acid-mediated mucosal damage. These findings explain the previous observations of increased mucosal injury by conjugated bile acids at pH 2 and unconjugated bile acids at pH 7. The un-ionized forms predominate at more acidic pH for conjugated bile acids (pKa 1.9), and at more neutral pH for unconjugated bile acids (pKa 5.1). The un-ionized forms of the bile acids are more lipophilic, allowing access through the esophageal mucosal barrier into the intracellular compartment, where they are trapped by ionization and subsequently cause mucosal damage.

### Human Studies

The clinical evidence for the possible damaging effects of DGER on the esophageal mucosa remains controversial. This may be because there is no "gold standard" for detecting DGER. Various direct and indirect methodologies are employed for measuring DGER including endoscopy, aspiration studies (both gastric and esophageal), scintigraphy, ambulatory pH monitoring, and, most recently, ambulatory bilirubin monitoring. As summarized in Table 23–1, these tests have their strengths and shortcomings; however, reviewing the human studies using these tests can help us better appreciate the role of DGER in causing esophageal symptoms and mucosal injury.

## TESTS FOR DUODENOESOPHAGEAL REFLUX

### Endoscopy

Bile is frequently seen in the esophagus and stomach of patients during endoscopy; however, the clinical significance of these observations is unclear. Recently, Nasrallah et al. [70] evaluated 110 patients with bile-stained gastric mucosa at endoscopy by measuring gastric bile acids and scintigraphic quantitation of bile reflux. They found no correlation between the gastric bile acid concentrations, degree of histologic injury, or severity of endoscopic changes, suggesting that there was little clinical importance to bile-stained mucosa at endoscopy. Similarly, using scintigraphy and gastric pH monitoring to assess DGER, Stein et al. [96] found poor sensitivity (37%), specificity (70%), and positive predictive value (55%) for endoscopy in the diagnosis of excessive DGER.

### Aspiration Studies

#### Stomach

One of the earliest methods used for evaluating DGER was the aspiration of gastric contents with fluid analysis for bile acids. Using this technique, Kaye and Showalter [46] found no significant difference between *fasting* gastric bile acid concentrations of patients with esophagitis (0.057 mg/ml) compared to controls (0.039 mg/ml), while *postprandially* esophagitis patients had higher gastric bile acid concen-

**TABLE 23–1.** *Advantages and disadvantages of methods for detecting duodenogastroesophageal reflux*[a]

| Method | Advantages | Disadvantages |
|---|---|---|
| Endoscopy | Easy visualization of bile | Poor sensitivity, specificity, or positive predictive value<br>Requires sedation<br>High cost |
| Aspiration studies | Less invasive than endoscopy<br>No sedation<br>Low cost | Short duration of study<br>Requires familiarity with enzymatic assay for BA |
| Scintigraphy | Noninvasive | Semiquantitative at best<br>Radiation exposure<br>High cost |
| pH monitoring | Easy to perform<br>Relatively noninvasive<br>Prolonged monitoring<br>Ambulatory | pH > 7 not a marker for DGER<br>Not specific for DGER |
| Bilirubin monitoring (Bilitec) | Easy to perform<br>Relatively noninvasive<br>Prolonged monitoring<br>Ambulatory<br>Good correlation with gastric BA concentrations | Current design underestimates DGER by about 30% in acidic medium (pH < 3.5)<br>Requires modified diet |

[a] BA, Bile acid; DGER, duodenogastroesophageal reflux.

trations (0.89 mg/ml vs. 0.21 mg/ml). Similarly, Gillen et al. [25] found no difference in the *fasting* bile acid concentrations of patients with complicated (strictures, ulcers, dysplasia, adenocarcinoma) (0.025 mM) or uncomplicated (0 mM) Barrett's esophagus compared to patients with esophagitis (0 mM) or normal controls (0 mM). However, they reported significantly higher *postprandial* bile acid concentrations in patients with complicated Barrett's esophagus (0.19 mM) compared to the other groups (0.017 mM to 0.040 mM). The studies finding increased postprandial bile acid concentrations have been criticized because they all employed the 3-$\alpha$-hydroxysteroid dehydrogenase enzymatic assay, which has recently been reported to have low specificity and accuracy in detecting bile acids in the postprandial, but not the fasting state [65].

Recent studies by Vaezi et al. [105] of patients with complicated and uncomplicated Barrett's esophagus found that the mean *fasting* bile acid concentrations were higher in complicated (0.5 mM) compared to uncomplicated (0.24 mM) Barrett's patients, with both concentrations being higher than controls (0.02 mM) (Fig. 23–2). These investigators also found that the increased fasting bile acid concentrations in Barrett's patients was accompanied by greater amounts of acid and bile reflux, suggesting that both components may be synergistically involved in producing esophageal mucosal damage.

A limitation of gastric aspiration studies is the presumption that the presence of bile acids in the stomach is a good indicator of esophageal exposure to duodenal contents and therefore DGER. This is supported by the observations that

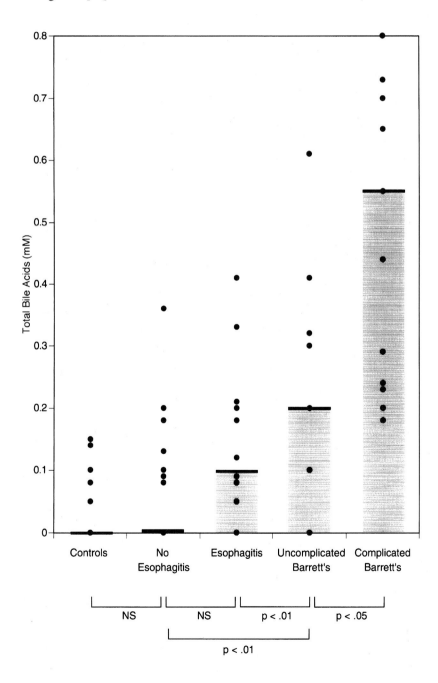

**FIG. 23–2.** Individual and median fasting gastric bile acid concentration for five study populations: controls, acid reflux patients with and without esophagitis, and patients with uncomplicated and complicated Barrett's esophagus. (From ref. 106, with permission.)

only one-half of DGER episodes into the antrum reach the fundus of the stomach, and then, all that is present in the fundus may not reflux into the esophagus [16].

### *Esophagus*

Continuous and intermittent esophageal aspiration studies have assessed the role of bile acids in esophageal mucosal damage. Unlike studies of gastric aspirates, studies with esophageal aspiration technique are quite variable and are technique dependent. Two independent groups of investigators, Smith et al. [90] and Johnsson et al. [41] found only small concentrations of bile acids (2.5 $\mu$M to 64 $\mu$M) in the esophageal aspirate of patients with GERD. Mittal et al. [65], in a 3-hour postprandial bile aspiration study, found no bile acids in either the fasting or postprandial esophageal aspirates of patients with GERD. The above studies differed with respect to esophageal aspiration period, ranging from 3 hours in the study by Mittal et al. [65] to 15 hours in the study by Smith et al. [70] and 24 hours in the study by Johnsson et al. [41].

On the other hand, Gotley et al. [28], studying 45 patients with esophagitis and 10 controls, using continuous collection of esophageal aspiration over 16 hours, found increased amounts of conjugated bile acids, measured by high-performance liquid chromatography, in the majority (87%) of aspirates. Most bile acid reflux occurred at night, with only 7% of samples having bile acids concentrations above 1.0 mM, the toxic concentration producing esophageal mucosal damage. Interestingly, acid reflux episodes measured by 24-hour pH monitoring occurred concomitantly with reflux of conjugated bile acids. Similarly, a recent study by Kauer et al. [45] using 17-hour continuous esophageal aspiration in 43 normal subjects and 37 patients with reflux disease found significantly ($p < 0.003$) higher bile acids in reflux patients (86%) than controls (58%). Furthermore, they found that the mean bile salt concentration was higher in patients during the postprandial and supine periods. However, they did not report the pH of the collected esophageal refluxate.

### Scintigraphy

Radionuclide techniques offer a noninvasive method for studying DGER. Tolin et al. [102] compared DGER measured by phenol red aspiration and external scintigraphy measuring $^{99m}$Tc-HIDA [N-(2,6-dimethylphenylcarbamoylmethyl) iminodiacetic acid], finding a good correlation between DGER and scintigraphy. Similarly, other investigators [21, 37] have compared intragastric bile acid concentrations and scintigraphy and found a significant correlation between both free and total gastric bile acids and the degree of bile reflux.

Scintigraphic studies find that DGER is a common phenomenon in normal individuals postprandially [58, 67], requiring that the evaluation of abnormal DGER be quantitative. Matikainen et al. [61] found no difference in the scintigraphic amount of DGER into the esophagus between 40 patients with esophagitis (10% scintigraphic reflux) and 150 healthy controls (14% scintigraphic reflux). Likewise,

Krog et al. [50] found no evidence of DGER in 15 patients with hiatal hernia and esophagitis. However, Waring et al. [110] reported that patients with Barrett's esophagus, especially those with complicated Barrett's, had more frequent DGER detected by $^{99m}$Tc-DISIDA (o-diisopropyl iminodiacetic acid) scintigraphy than healthy volunteers. A more recent study by Liron et al. [56] using $^{99m}$Tc-HIDA scanning confirms the above results, finding higher DGER in patients with Barrett's esophagus than GERD patients without Barrett's or healthy controls.

Although less invasive than other methods for detecting DGER, the reliability and accuracy of scintigraphy has been challenged. Drane et al. [18] observed that scintigraphy was at best a semiquantitative measure of bile reflux, finding that several technical problems may compromise the accuracy of this technique for measuring DGER. The most common problem was the overlap of small bowel and stomach occurring in 36% of patients, which is not correctable. Other problems included overlap of the left lobe of the liver and stomach, patient movement, and the intermittent nature of bile reflux.

### Ambulatory pH Monitoring

Prolonged pH monitoring offers a unique opportunity for studying acid and possibly DGER in the ambulatory state throughout the circadian cycle. Stein et al. [93] reported that gastric monitoring of pH > 7 was superior to DISIDA radionucleotide scintigraphy in detecting DGER in patient with foregut symptoms. Similarly, Brown et al. [10] observed a good correlation ($R = 0.36$, $p < 0.001$) between gastric bile acid concentrations and ambulatory gastric pH monitoring.

Using 24-hour esophageal pH monitoring, Pellegrini et al. [74] were the first to study the relationship between acid and "alkaline" reflux in patients with gastroesophageal reflux disease. Acid reflux was defined as pH < 4 in the lower esophagus, while "alkaline" reflux, an indirect marker of DGER, was defined as pH > 7. Normal values were defined as the mean and two standard deviation of values obtained during 24-hour pH studies in 15 healthy volunteers. Compared to patients with acid reflux, alkaline-refluxers had less heartburn, but more frequent and severe regurgitation and higher rate of esophageal strictures. Additionally, there were no pure "alkaline"-refluxers, as all patient without prior gastric surgery also had episodes of acid reflux. Later, the same group [54, 55] found that patients with esophagitis had less "alkaline" reflux and more acid reflux than patients without esophagitis. In contrast, Schmid et al. [83], studying patients with various degrees of esophagitis, reported significantly higher amounts of both acid and "alkaline" reflux in patients with complicated esophagitis compared to healthy subjects. Their results, similar to the findings in gastric aspiration studies, suggested a synergistic role for acid and bile in esophagitis.

At the same time, Attwood et al. [2–4, 6] reported that "alkaline" reflux was greater in patients with Barrett's esophagus when compared to patients with esophagitis or normal controls. Furthermore, they found that pH > 7 was significantly higher in complicated Barrett's patients (stricture, ulcer, dysplasia) than Barrett's patients without complications, while pH < 4 did not distinguish the two groups. These authors went on to suggest that prolonged exposure to duodenal contents alone may promote the development of complicated Barrett's esophagus and even adenocarcinoma. However, the investigators did not attempt to resolve the physiological paradox of patients with marked amount of acid reflux also refluxing independently large amounts of "alkaline" material.

The measurement of esophageal pH > 7 as a marker of DGER is confounded by several problems. Precautions must be taken to use only glass electrodes, dietary restriction of foods with pH < 7, inspection of patients for periodontal disease, and dilation of strictures to avoid pooling of saliva. Therefore, it is not surprising that several authors [16, 30, 62, 89] have questioned the accuracy of "alkaline" pH as a parameter for monitoring duodenal reflux into the esophagus. Gotley et al. [30] found no relationship between "alka-

line" exposure time and esophageal bile acids or trypsin. Similarly, Mattioli et al. [62], using a triple-probe pH monitor placed in the distal esophagus, fundus, and antrum, found that "alkaline" reflux, defined as a rise in pH > 7 from the antrum to esophagus, was extremely uncommon (0.75%) in 279 patients. Therefore, these authors suggested that increases of esophageal pH above 7 were most likely due to other reasons (saliva, food, oral infection, obstructed esophagus) rather than reflux of duodenal contents. This speculation was substantiated by studies from Singh et al. [89] and DeVault et al. [16], who found that increased saliva production or bicarbonate production by the esophageal submucosal glands was the most common cause of esophageal pH > 7, while DGER was rare in patients with intact stomach. Using an ambulatory bilirubin-monitoring device combined with pH monitoring, Vaezi et al. [106] reported no difference in the percentage of total time pH was greater than 7 between controls, patients with GERD, and those with Barrett's esophagus (Fig. 23–3). Furthermore, Champion et al. [13],

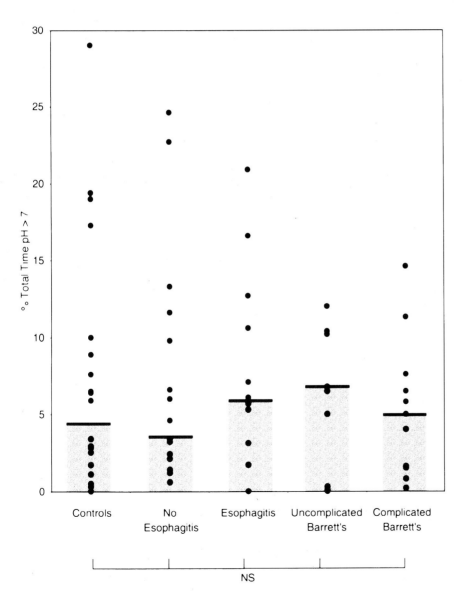

**FIG. 23–3.** "Alkaline" reflux (percentage of the total time pH is greater than 7) for five study populations: controls, acid reflux patients with and without esophagitis, and patients with uncomplicated and complicated Barrett's esophagus. Individual data and group median shown. (From ref. 106, with permission.)

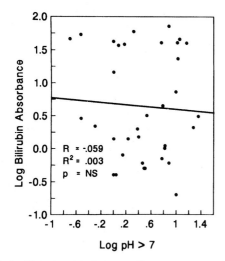

**FIG. 23–4.** Relationship between the percentage of the time bilirubin absorbance is equal to or greater than 0.14 as a marker of bile reflux and esophageal pH greater than 7 in a group of healthy controls, patients with gastroesophageal reflux disease (GERD), and those with Barrett's esophagus. (From ref. 13, with permission.)

as well as other several recent studies [40, 60], found no correlation between pH $> 7$ and bile reflux into the esophageal lumen (Fig. 23–4), suggesting that the term "alkaline" reflux was a misnomer and should not be used when referring to DGER. Finally, Just et al. [42] found a poor correlation ($R = 0.26$) between intragastric pH ("alkaline shift") and intragastric bilirubin absorbance, concluding that the measurement of "alkaline reflux" in the esophagus or stomach with ambulatory pH monitoring alone is "an outdated technique."

## Ambulatory Bilirubin Monitoring (Bilitec 2000)

Recently, a new fiberoptic spectrophotometer (Bilitec 2000, Synectics, Stockholm, Sweden) was developed which detects DGER in an ambulatory setting, independent of pH [8]. This instrument utilizes the optical properties of biliru-

bin, the most common bile pigment. Bilirubin has a characteristic spectrophotometric absorption band at 450 nm. The basic working principle of this instrument is that an absorption near this wavelength implies the presence of bilirubin and therefore represents DGER (Fig. 23–5).

This system, resembling a standard ambulatory pH unit, consists of a miniaturized fiberoptic probe, which carries light signals into the tip and back to the optoelectronic system via plastic fiberoptic bundle. The Teflon probe head is 9.5 mm in length and 4 mm in diameter. There is a 2.0-mm open groove in the probe across which two wavelengths of light are emitted and material sampled. Two light-emitting diodes at 470 and 565 nm represent the sources for the measurement of bilirubin and the reference signals, respectively. The portable photodiode system converts the light into an electrical signal. After amplification, the signals are processed by an integrated microcomputer, and the difference in absorption between the two diodes is calculated, representing absorption in the samples of DGER (Fig. 23–5). The period between two successive pulses from the same source, representing sampling time, is 8 seconds. In addition, the software averages between the absorbances calculated over two successive samplings in order to decrease the noise of the measurements. A total of 5,400 sample recordings may be stored during a 24-hour period.

DGER data are usually measured as the percentage of the time bilirubin absorbance is equal to or greater than 0.14 and can be analyzed separately for total, upright, and supine periods (Fig. 23–6). Percentage of the time bilirubin absorbance is equal to or greater than 0.14 is commonly chosen as a cutoff because studies show that values below this number represent scatter due to suspended particles and mucus present in the gastric contents [8]. In a recent study [106] using 20 healthy controls, the 95th percentile values for the percentage of total, upright, and supine times that bilirubin was equal to or greater than 0.14 were 1.8, 2.2, and 1.6, respectively (Fig. 23–7).

Several reports have indicated a good correlation between Bilitec readings and bile acid concentration measured by duodenogastric aspiration studies: $R = 0.71$, $p < 0.01$ [8] and $R = 0.82$, $p < 0.001$ [108]. Furthermore, our studies

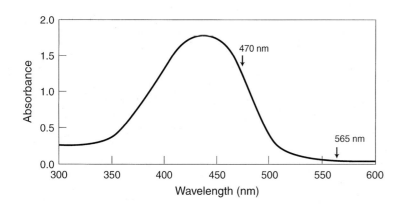

**FIG. 23–5.** Spectrophotometric absorbance property of bilirubin. The arrows indicate the two wavelengths used by the Bilitec for detecting duodenogastroesophageal reflux (DGER). Detection of DGER depends on the difference in absorbance between 470 and 565 nm, suggesting reflux of bilirubin.

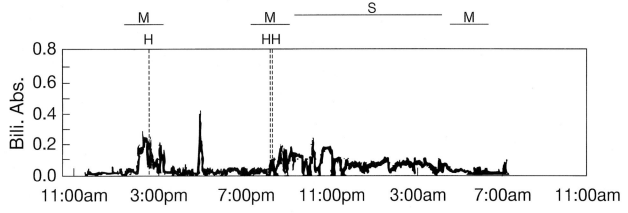

| HIGH EPISODE | | Total | Upright | Supine | Meal | PostP | Heartburn |
|---|---|---|---|---|---|---|---|
| Duration | (HH:MM) | 19:54 | 12:54 | 07:00 | 00:20 | 06:00 | 00:12 |
| Number of episodes | (#) | 30 | 28 | 2 | 0 | 21 | 1 |
| Number of episodes longer than 30.0 min | (#) | 0 | 0 | 0 | 0 | 0 | 0 |
| Longest episode | (min) | 28 | 23 | 28 | 0 | 23 | 4 |
| Total time Absorbance above 0.14 | (min) | 181 | 128 | 53 | 0 | 97 | 4 |
| Fraction time Absorbance above 0.14 | (%) | 15.2 | 16.2 | 12.7 | 0.0 | 26.8 | 33.3 |
| Median Absorbance value | | --- | --- | --- | | --- | --- |

S = Supine    C = Chest pain .    M = Meal
H = Heartburn    P = PostP

**FIG. 23–6.** A typical tracing and data generated by the Bilitec in measuring DGER. Data are typically reported as percentage of the time bilirubin absorbance is equal to or greater than 0.14 (total, upright, or supine).

show that Bilitec readings correspond to bile acid concentrations in the range of 0.01 to 0.60 mM, which are more representative of bile acid concentrations found in the human stomach (0.1 to 1.0 mM). Additionally, a recent study by Stipa et al. [98] found a good correlation ($R = 0.7$) between Bilitec readings and concentrations of pancreatic enzymes in aspirated esophageal fluid samples from patients with esophagitis. Therefore, this spectrophotometric technique is

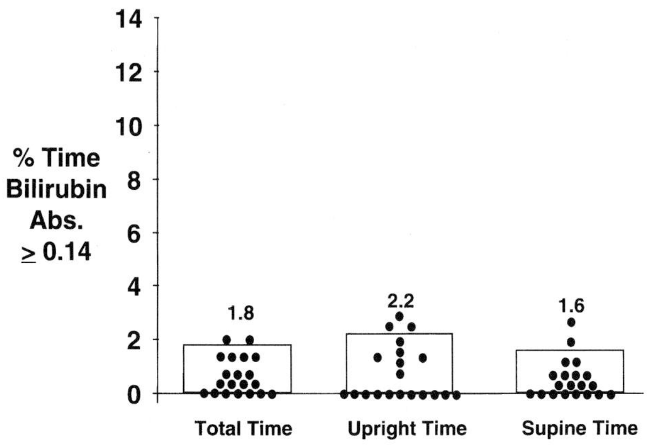

an important advance in the assessment of DGER permitting more accurate studies of patients with syndromes associated with DGER. Additionally, it should be used concomitantly with pH monitoring to measure the esophageal exposure to both acid and DGER, since both are usually refluxed together in patients with no prior gastric surgery.

Due to limitations in the current Bilitec model, it is only a semiquantitative means of detecting DGER. Validation studies by Vaezi et al. [108] found that this instrument underestimates bile reflux by least 30% in an acidic medium (pH < 3.5). In solutions with pH < 3.5, bilirubin undergoes monomer-to-dimer isomerization, which is reflected by a shift in the absorption wavelength from 453 to 400 nm. Since Bilitec readings are based on the detection of absorption at 470 nm, this shift results in underestimation of the degree of DGER. Therefore, Bilitec measurements of DGER must always be accompanied by the simultaneous measurement of esophageal acid exposure using prolonged pH monitoring. Furthermore, a variety of substances may result in false-positive readings by the Bilitec, since it indiscriminately records any substance absorbing around 470 nm. This necessitates use of a modified diet to avoid interference and false readings [8, 108]. Also, it is important to remember that Bilitec measures reflux of bilirubin and not bile acids or pancreatic enzymes, thereby presuming that the presence of bilirubin in the refluxate is accompanied by other duodenal contents. Although this is true in most cases, a few medical conditions (Gilbert and Dubin-Johnson syndromes) may re-

**FIG. 23–7.** Percentage of the time bilirubin absorbance is equal to or greater than 0.14 in 20 normal subjects: total, upright, supine. Values within the boxed-in area represent the 95th percentile of the normal range.

sult in disproportionate secretion of bilirubin as compared to other duodenal contents, especially bile acids [57].

Despite its limitations, Bilitec is an important advance in the assessment of DGER in the clinical arena. Several studies using this new device are providing important insight into the role of DGER in causing esophageal mucosal injury in humans. In a preliminary report, DeMeester's group [44] found no significant difference in esophageal bilirubin exposure in patients with esophagitis compared to healthy controls; however, patients with Barrett's esophagus had significantly more bilirubin and acid reflux than controls. On the other hand, Vaezi et al. [106] found a significant, but graded increase in *both* acid and DGER from controls to esophagitis patients, with the highest values observed in patients with Barrett's esophagus (Fig. 23–8). Furthermore,

DGER had a strong correlation with acid reflux ($R = 0.78$), but had a poor association with pH $> 7$ ($R = 0.06$). Further support for the graduated increase in *both* acid and DGER comes from recent studies by Vaezi et al. [105] of patients with and without complications of Barrett's esophagus. They found that both groups of Barrett's patients refluxed significantly greater quantities of bile and acid into their lower esophagus than controls. More importantly, reflux of acid paralleled DGER and both were significantly higher in patients with complicated Barrett's than the uncomplicated group. The results of these studies were recently confirmed by other investigators [45, 60, 106]. Marshall et al. [60] studied 55 patients with GERD and found a good correlation between the degree of acid and DGER ($R = 0.55$). Furthermore, expanded studies by Vaezi and Richter [106] found

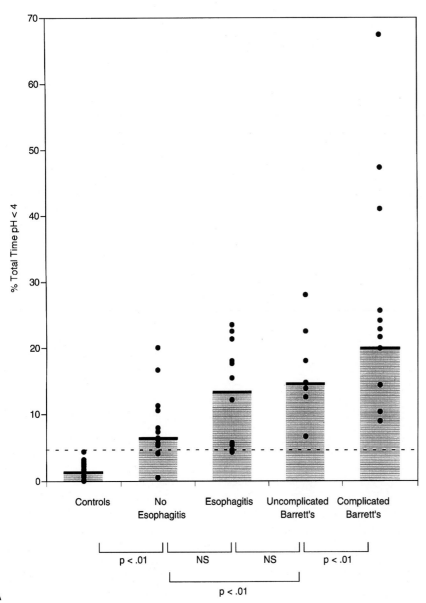

**FIG. 23–8.** Group median values for (**A**) acid reflux and (**B**) duodenogastroesophageal reflux DGER for five study populations: controls, acid reflux patients with and without esophagitis, and patients with uncomplicated and complicated Barrett's esophagus. (From ref. 106, with permission.)

A

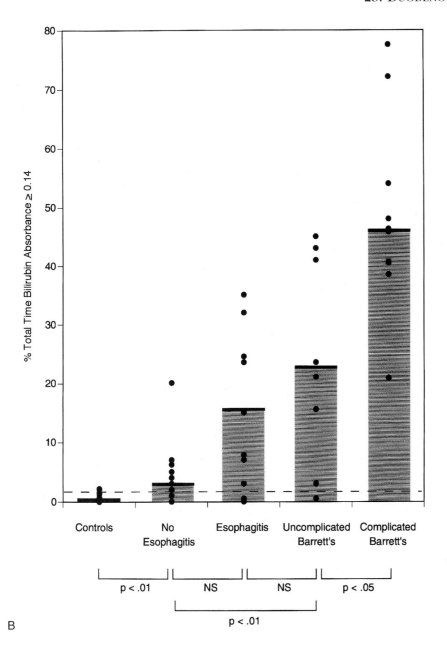

B

**FIG. 23–8.** *(continued)*

that simultaneous esophageal exposure to both acid and DGER was the most prevalent reflux pattern occurring in 95% of patients with Barrett's esophagus and 79% of GERD patients (Fig. 23–9). In fact, they found a strong correlation ($R = 0.73$) between acid and DGER in controls, reflux patients, and those with Barrett's esophagus (Fig. 23–10). Thus, these studies support the earlier findings in animals that suggested a possible synergy between acid and DGER in the development of esophagitis and Barrett's esophagus.

The role of DGER in producing esophageal mucosal injury in the absence of acid reflux was not clarified until recently. Studies by Marshall et al. [60], using prolonged pH and bilirubin monitoring in 38 patients with GERD, found that DGER in the absence of acid reflux was a rare event (7%) in patients without prior gastric surgery. Additionally, Sears and colleagues [87] studied 13 partial gastrectomy patients with reflux symptoms and found increased DGER by Bilitec monitoring in 77% of patients. This patient population represents an excellent human model for increased DGER because of the incompetent pylorus and free regurgitation of duodenal contents into the stomach, resulting in gastric bile acids concentrations (0.5 mM to 3.0 mM) known to cause esophageal mucosal injury in the animal model (>1 mM). Endoscopic esophagitis, however, was present only in those who had concomitant acid reflux. Subsequently, Vaezi et al. [107] confirmed these observations and found that only 24% of upper gastrointestinal symptoms reported by partial gastrectomy patients were due to DGER

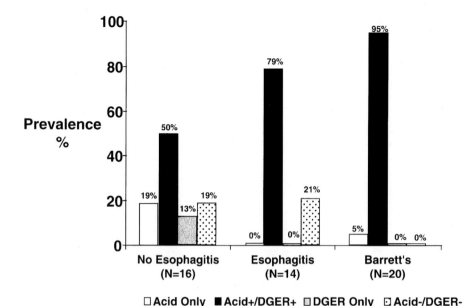

**FIG. 23–9.** Prevalence of esophageal exposure to acid and DGER in the gastroesophageal reflux disease (GERD) subgroups. Esophageal exposure to acid and DGER occurred in 50% of patients without esophagitis, 79% of patients with esophagitis, and 95% of patients with Barrett's esophagus. *Open bar,* Acid only; *solid bar,* acid+/DGER+; *shaded bar,* DGER only; *dotted bar,* acid−/DGER−. (From ref. 106, with permission.)

in the absence of acid reflux. These studies show that DGER without excessive acid reflux can cause reflux symptoms but does not usually produce esophagitis.

## MEDICAL AND SURGICAL TREATMENT OF DUODENOGASTROESOPHAGEAL REFLUX

It is well known that aggressive medical therapy to suppress acid secretion will heal most cases of esophagitis. Recently, some groups [2–4, 6, 35] have suggested that prolonged acid suppression in patients with severe esophagitis or Barrett's esophagus may promote DGER causing further mucosal injury with progression to Barrett's esophagus or even adenocarcinoma. This claim is based upon isolated animal studies [5, 75] and a handful of clinical reports, mainly from the same laboratory [2–4, 6, 94]. The clinical relevance of these reports is questionable, since the association between DGER and complicated Barrett's esophagus or adenocarcinoma was defined by esophageal pH monitoring (i.e., pH > 7), which has since been shown to be an unreliable parameter for detecting DGER. More importantly, a careful review of the literature shows that the overwhelming majority of studies do not support this concept.

Both animal and human studies indicate that DGER in the absence of acid reflux is usually not damaging to the esophageal mucosa. Furthermore, recent studies by Champion et al. [13] in nine patients with severe GERD (esophagitis-3, Barrett's esophagus-6) found that aggressive acid suppression with omeprazole (20 mg twice daily) dramatically decreased *both* acid and DGER (Fig. 23–11). The above findings have recently been reproduced by two other independent groups of investigators. Gut et al. [31] found that esophageal acid and DGER were both significantly (*p* < 0.02) reduced after 28 days of treatment with pantoprazole (40 mg four times daily) compared to pretreatment values

in 7 patients with endoscopic evidence of GERD. Similarly, Marshall et al. [59] studied esophageal and gastric bile reflux in 23 patients with Barrett's esophagus and found a significant (*p* < 0.005) reduction in both esophageal and gastric acid (pH monitoring) and bile (Bilitec) reflux after 6 to 10 weeks of treatment with omeprazole (20 mg twice daily). The studies by Champion et al. [13] and Marshall et al. [59] suggest that the decrease in DGER measured after proton-pump inhibitors may be due to their inhibition of both gastric acidity and volume, making less gastric contents available to reflux into the esophagus despite even a low lower esophageal sphincter pressure. In support of this proposed mechanism are previous studies showing about 40% reduction in gastric volume by 40 mg of omeprazole [23, 53]. Therefore, medical therapy with aggressive acid suppression may not only protect the esophageal mucosa from the damaging effects of acid and eliminate the synergy between acid, pepsin, and bile, but it may also decrease the volume of both acid and bile refluxing into the esophagus.

Several agents have been used to treat bile gastritis and symptoms associated with DGER. These included antacids, namely aluminum hydroxide, sucralfate, prostaglandin E2, cimetidine and ranitidine, cholestyramine, metoclopramide, and ursodeoxycholic acid [71]. Although, these agents showed efficacy for mild to moderate "bile gastritis," the results were less than promising for "alkaline reflux esophagitis," limiting their use in DGER. Prior to the findings by Champion et al. [13], the best therapy for decreasing DGER into the esophagus was thought to be an antireflux operation correcting the defective lower esophageal sphincter. Therefore, the findings by Champion et al. [13] have important implications for treating patients with both acid and bile reflux. This study suggests that medical therapy with proton-pump inhibitors may decrease both acid and DGER to a similar degree as antireflux surgery. Medical therapy has the

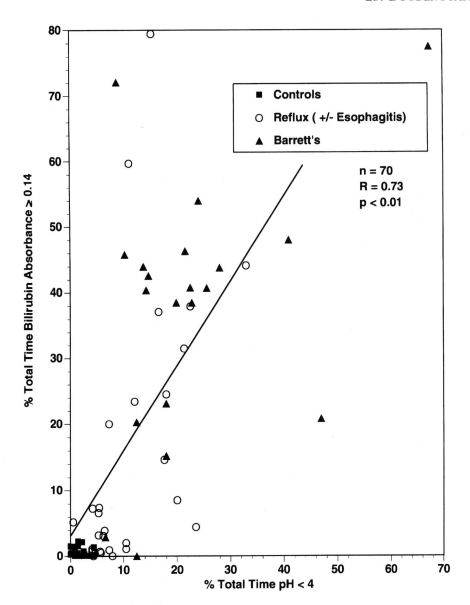

FIG. 23–10. Relationship between acid reflux (percentage of the time pH is greater than 4) and DGER (percentage of the time bilirubin absorbance is equal to or greater than 0.14) in normal healthy controls, patients with gastroesophageal reflux disease (GERD), and patients with Barrett's esophagus. (From ref. 106, with permission.)

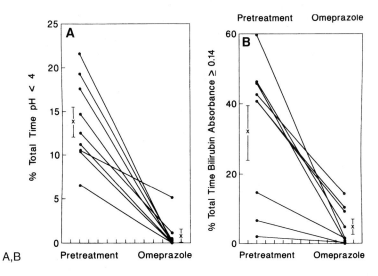

FIG. 23–11. Influence of marked acid suppression with omeprazole (20 mg twice daily) on acid reflux (A) and DGER (B) in nine patients with GERD. (From ref. 13, with permission.)

advantage of avoiding a surgical procedure and its associated complications, an important consideration in the elderly and those with contraindications to surgery. However, in younger patients in whom long-term medical therapy is anticipated, antireflux surgery may be a more suitable and cost-effective alternative.

In partial-gastrectomy patients having mild upper gastrointestinal symptoms due to nonacidic DGER, previous older studies found that administration of aluminum hydroxide-containing antacids (30 cc four times daily), cholestyramine (1.0 g four times daily), or ursodeoxycholic acid may improve symptoms [71]. In a recent randomized double-blind crossover study [109], cisparide (20 mg four times daily) was found to significantly reduce both DGER measured by the Bilitec and associated upper gastrointestinal symptoms (i.e., abdominal pain, bloating, belching, regurgitation, nausea, and vomiting) in patients after vagotomy and antrectomy or pyloromyotomy for chronic ulcer disease. Thus, medical therapy with promotility drugs is an alternative to surgical Roux-en-Y diversion. Medical options are important since a recent study by McAlhany et al. [63] found that up to 36% of patients who underwent Roux-en-Y diversion for bile reflux were unsatisfied with the results of surgery within 6 months of the operation. Nevertheless, patients unresponsive to aggressive medical therapy for well-documented non-acid DGER should be considered for bile diversion operations such as Roux-en-Y or Henley isoperistaltic jejunal interposition as the best surgical options for this difficult-to-manage problem.

# REFERENCES

1. Aylwin JA. The physiological basis of reflux esophagitis in sliding distal diaphragmatic hernia. Thorax 1953;8:38
2. Attwood SEA. New advances in the understanding of Barrett's esophagus. Surg Ann 1993;25:151
3. Attwood SEA, DeMeester TR, Bemner CG, Barlow AP, Hinder RA. Alkaline gastroesophageal reflux: implications in the development of complications in Barrett's columnar-lined lower esophagus. Surgery 1989;106:764
4. Attwood SEA, Barlow AP, Norris TL, Watson A. Barrett's esophagus: effect of antireflux surgery on symptom control and development of complications. Br J Surg 1992;79:1050
5. Attwood SEA, Smyrk TC, DeMeester TR, Mirvish SS, Stein HJ, Hinder RA. Duodenoesophageal reflux and the development of esophageal adeno-carcinoma in rats. Surgery 1992;111:503
6. Attwood SEA, Ball CS, Barlow AP, Jenkinson L, Norris TL, Watson A. Role of intragastric and intraoesophageal alkalinization in the genesis of complications in Barrett's columnar lined lower oesophagus. Gut 1993;34:11
7. Batzri S, Harmon JW, Schweitzer EJ, Toles R. Bile acid accumulation in gastric mucosal cells. Proc Soc Exp Biol Med 1991;197:393
8. Bechi P, et al. Long-term ambulatory enterogastric reflux monitoring. Validation of a new fiberoptic technique. Dig Dis Sci 1993;38:1297
9. Bremner RM, Crookes PF, DeMeester TR, Peters JH, Stein H. Concentration of refluxed acid and esophageal mucosal injury. Am J Surg 1992;164:522
10. Brown TH, Holbrook I, King RFG, Ibrahim K. 24-hour intragastric pH measurement in the assessment of duodenogastric reflux. World J Surg 1992;16:995
11. Burden WR, Hodges RP, Hsu M, O'Leary JP. Alkaline reflux gastritis. Surg Clin North Am 1991;71:33
12. Carney CN, Orlando RC, Powell DW. Morphologic alterations in early acid induced epithelial injury of the rabbit esophagus. Lab Invest 1981;45:198
13. Champion G, Richter JE, Vaezi MF, Singh S, Alexander R. Duodenogastroesophageal reflux: relationship to pH and importance in Barrett's esophagus. Gastroenterology 1994;107:747
14. Cross FS, Wangensteen OH. Role of bile and pancreatic juice in the production of esophageal erosions and anemia. Proc Soc Exp Biol Med 1961;77:862
15. DeMeester TR, Wernly JA, Little AG, Bermudez G, Skinner DB. Technique, indications, and clinical use of 24 hour esophageal pH monitoring. J Thorac Cardiovasc Surg 1980;79:656
16. DeVault KR, Georgeson S, Castell DO. Salivary stimulation mimics esophageal exposure to refluxed duodenal contents. Am J Gastroenterol 1993;88:1040
17. Dixon MF. Progress in pathology of gastritis and duodenitis. In Williams GT, ed. Current Topics in Pathology. Berlin: Springer-Verlag, 1990:1
18. Drane WE, Karvelis K, Johnson DA, Silverman ED. Scintigraphic evaluation of duodenogastric reflux. Problems, pitfalls, and technical review. Clin Nucl Med 1987;12:377
19. Duane WC, Wiegand DM. Mechanism by which bile salt disrupts the gastric mucosal barrier in the dog. J Clin Invest 1980;66:10
20. DuPlessis DJ. Pathogenesis of gastric ulceration. Lancet 1965;1:974
21. Eriksson B, Emas S, Jacobsson H, Larsson SA, Samuelsson K. Comparison of gastric aspiration and HIDA scintigraphy in detecting fasting duodenogastric bile reflux. Scand J Gastroenterol 1988;23:607
22. Ferguson DJ, Sanchez-Palomera E, Sako Y, Caltworthy HW, Toon RW, Wangensteen OH. Studies on experimental esophagitis. Surgery 1950;28:1022
23. Festen HPN, Tuynman HARE, Defize J, Pals G, Frants RR, Straub JP. Effect of single and repeated doses of oral omeprazole on gastric acid and pepsin secretion and fasting serum pepsinogen I levels. Dig Dis Sci 1986;31:561
24. Gillen P, Keeling P, Byrne PJ, Hennessy TPJ. Barrett's esophagus: pH profile. Br J Surg 1987;74:774
25. Gillen P, Keeling P, Byrne PJ, Healy M, O'Moore RR, Hennessy TPJ. Importance of duodenogastric reflux in the pathogenesis of Barrett's oesophagus. Br J Surg 1988;75:540
26. Gillison EW, DeCastro VAM, Nyhus LM, Kusakari K, Bombeck CT. The significance of bile in reflux esophagitis. Surg Gynecol Obstet 1972;134:419
27. Goldberg HI, Dodds WJ, Gee S, Montgomery C, Zboralske FF. Role of acid and pepsin in acute experimental esophagitis. Gastroenterology 1969;56:223
28. Gotley DC, Morgan AP, Cooper MJ. Bile acid concentrations in the refluxate of patients with reflux oesophagitis. Br J Surg 1988;75:587
29. Gotley DC, Morgan AP, Ball D, Owens RW, Cooper MJ. Composition of gastrooesophageal refluxate. Gut 1991;32:1093
30. Gotley DC, Appleton GVN, Cooper MJ. Bile acids and trypsin are unimportant in alkaline esophageal reflux. J Clin Gastroenterol 1992;14:2
31. Gut A, Gaia C, Netzer P, Halter F, Inauen W. Reduction of esophageal bile and acid reflux by pantoprazole in patients with reflux esophagitis. Gastroenterology 1997;112:A135
32. Hamilton BH, Orlado RC. In vivo alkaline secretion by mammalian esophagus. Gastroenterology 1989;97:640
33. Harmon JW, Johnson LF, Maydonovitch CL. Effects of acid and bile salts on the rabbit esophageal mucosa. Dig Dis Sci 1981;26:65
34. Harmon JW, Bass BL, Batzri S. Alkaline reflux gastritis. In Nyhus LL, ed, Problems in General surgery. Philadelphia: JB Lippincott Co: 1993:201
35. Hennessy TPJ. Barrett's esophagus. Br J Surg 1985;72:336
36. Hopcwood D, Bateson MC, Milner G, Bouchier IAD. Effects of bile acids and hydrogen ion on the fine structure of oesophageal epithelium. Gut 1981;22:306
37. Houghton PWJ, McC Mortensen NJ, Thomas WEG, Cooper MJ, Morgan AP, Davies ER. Intragastric bile acids and scintigraphy in the assessment of duodenogastric reflux. Br J Surg 1986;73:292
38. Hubens A, Van de Kelft E, Roland J. The influence of cholecystectomy on the duodenogastric reflux of bile. Hepato-Gastroenterology 1989;38:384
39. Iascone C, DeMeester TR, Little AG, Skinner DB. Barrett's esophagus: functional assessment, proposed pathogenesis, and surgical therapy. Arch Surg 1983;118:543
40. Iftikhar SY, et al. Alkaline gastroesophageal reflux: dual probe pH monitoring. Gut 1995;37:465

41. Johnsson F, Joelsson B, Floren CH, Nilsson A. Bile salts in the esophagus of patients with esophagitis. Scand J Gastroenterol 1988;6:712

42. Just RJ, Leite LP, Castell DO. Changes in overnight fasting intragastric pH show poor correlation with duodenogastric bile reflux in normal subjects. Am J Gastroenterol 1996;91:1567

43. Kalima TV. Reflux gastritis unrelated to gastric surgery. Scand J Gastroenterol 1982;17(suppl 79):66

44. Kauer WK, Ireland AP, Burdiles P, Clark GWB, Peters JH, DeMeester TR. The correlation between bile and acid reflux in Barrett's esophagus. Gastroenterology 1994;106:A104

45. Kauer WKH, et al. Composition and concentration of bile acid reflux into the esophagus of patients with gastroesophageal reflux disease. Surgery 1997;122:874

46. Kaye MD, Showalter JP. Pyloric incompetence in patients with symptomatic gastroesophageal reflux. J Lab Clin Med 1974;83:198

47. Kiriluk LB, Merendino KA. Comparative sensitivity of mucosa of various segments of alimentary tract in dog to acid-peptic action. Surgery 1954;35:547

48. King PM, Pryde A, Heading RC. Transpyloric fluid movement and antroduodenal motility in patients with gastroesophageal reflux. Gut 1987;28:545

49. Kivilaakso E, Fromm D, Silen W. Effect of bile salts and related compounds on isolated esophageal mucosa. Surgery 1980;87:280

50. Krog M, Gustavsson S, Jung B. Studies on oesophagitis—no evidence for pyloric incompetence as a primary etiological factor. A scintigraphic study with $^{99}$Tc$^m$-Solco-HIDA. Acta Chir Scand 1982;148:439

51. Lillemoe KD, Johnson LF, Harmon JW. Role of the components of the gastroduodenal contents in experimental acid esophagitis. Surgery 1982;92:276

52. Lillemoe KD, Johnson LF, Harmon JW. Taurodeoxycholate modulates the effects of pepsin and trypsin in experimental esophagitis. Surgery 1985;97:662

53. Lind T, Cederberg C, Ekenved G, Haglund U, Olbe L. Effect of omeprazole—a gastric proton pump inhibitor—on pentagastrin stimulated acid secretion in man. Gut 1983;24:270

54. Little AG, DeMeester TR, Kirchner PT, O'Sullivan GC, Skinner DB. Pathogenesis of esophagitis in patients with gastroesophageal reflux. Surgery 1980;88:101

55. Little AG, Martinez EI, DeMeester TR, Blough RM, Skinner DB. Duodenogastric reflux and reflux esophagitis. Surgery 1984;96:447

56. Liron R, Parrilla P, de Haro M, Ortiz A, Robles R, Lujan JA, Fuente T, Andres B. Quantification of duodenogastric reflux in Barrett's esophagus. Am J Gastroenterol 1997;92:32

57. Lumeng L, O'Connor KW. Differential diagnosis of jaundice. In Ostrow JD, ed, Bile Pigments and Jaundice. New York: Marcel Dekker Inc: 1986:475

58. Mackie C, Hulks G, Cuschieri A. Enterogastric reflux and gastric clearance of refluxate in patients with and without bile vomiting following peptic ulcer surgery. Ann Surg 1986;204:537

59. Marshall REK, Anggiansah A, Owen WA, Owen WJ. Reduction of gastroesophageal bile reflux by omeprazole in Barrett's esophagus: an initial experience. Gut 1996;39:T115

60. Marshall REK, Anggiansah A, Owen WA, Owen WJ. The relationship between acid and bile reflux and symptoms in gastroesophageal reflux disease. Gut 1997;40:182

61. Matikainen M, Taavitsainen M, Kalima TV. Duodenogastric reflux in patients with heartburn and esophagitis. Scand J Gastroenterol 1981;16:253

62. Mattioli S, et al. Ambulatory 24 hour pH monitoring of the esophagus, fundus and antrum. Dig Dis Sci 1990;35:929

63. McAlhany JC, Hanover TM, Taylor SM, Sticca RP, Ashmore JD. Long-term follow-up of patients with Roux-en-Y gastrojejunostomy for gastric disease. Ann Surg 1994;219:451

64. Miller LS, et al. Esophageal involvement in the Zollinger Ellison syndrome (ZES). Gastroenterology 1990;98:341

65. Mittal RK, Reuben A, Whitney JO, McCallum RW. Do bile acids reflux into the esophagus? A study in normal subject and patients with GERD. Gastroenterology 1987;92:371

66. Moffat RC, Berkas EM. Bile esophagitis. Arch Surg 1965;91:963

67. Muller-Lissner SA, Fimmel CJ, Sonnenberg A. Novel approach to quantify duodenogastric reflux in healthy volunteers and in patients with type I gastric ulcer. Gut 1983;24:510

68. Muller-Lissner SA, Schindlbeck NE, Heinrich C. Bile salt reflux after cholecystectomy. Scand J Gastroenerol 1987;22(suppl 139):20

69. Nano M, et al. Biliary reflux after cholecystectomy: a prospective study. Hepato-Gastroenterology 1990;37:233

70. Nasrallah SM, Johnston GS, Gadacz TR, Kim KM. The significance of gastric bile reflux seen at endoscopy. J Clin Gastroenterol 1987;9:514

71. Nath BJ, Warshaw AL. Alkaline reflux gastritis and esophagitis. Annu Rev Med 1984;35:383

72. Orlando RC, Powell DW, Carney CN. Pathophysiology of acute acid injury in rabbit esophageal epithelium. J Clin Invest 1981;68:286

73. Orlando RC, Bryson JC, Powell DW. Mechanism of H$^+$ injury in rabbit esophageal epithelium. Am J Physiol 1984;9:G718

74. Pellegrini CA, DeMeester TR, Wernly JA, Johnson LF, Skinner DB. Alkaline gastroesophageal reflux. Am J Surg 1978;75:177

75. Pera M, et al. Influence of pancreatic and biliary reflux on the development of esophageal carcinoma. Ann Thorac Surg 1993;55:1386

76. Powell DW, Orlando RC, Carney CN. Acid injury of the esophageal epithelium. In Harmon JW, ed, Basic Mechanism of Gastrointestinal Mucosal Cell Injury and Protection. Baltimore: Williams & Wilkins, 1981:55

77. Redo SF, Barnes WA, de la Sierra AO. Perfusion of the canine esophagus with secretions of the upper gastro-intestinal tract. Ann Surg 1959;149:556

78. Ritchie WP. Alkaline reflux gastritis: a critical reappraisal. Gut 1984;25:975

79. Salo J, Kivilaakso E. Role of luminal H$^+$ in the pathogenesis of experimental esophagitis. Surgery 1982;92:61

80. Salo JA, Kivilaakso E. Contribution of trypsin and cholate to the pathogenesis of experimental alkaline reflux esophagitis. Scand J Gastroenterol 1984;19:875

81. Salo JA, Lehto VP, Kivilaakso E. Morphological alteration in experimental esophagitis. Dig Dis Sci 1983;28:440

82. Schidlbeck NE, Heinrich C, Stellard F, Paumgartner G, Muller-Lissner SA. Healthy controls have as much bile reflux as gastric ulcer patients. Gut 1987;28:1577

83. Schmid B, DeTarnowsky G, Layden T. Alkaline gastroesophageal reflux—role in esophageal injury. Gastroenterology 1981;80:A1275

84. Schweitzer EJ, Harmon JW, Bass BL, Batzri S. Bile acid efflux precedes mucosal barrier disruption in the rabbit esophagus. Am J Physiol 1984;10:G480

85. Schweitzer EJ, Bass BL, Batzri S, Harmon JW. Bile acid accumulation by rabbit esophageal mucosa. Dig Dis Sci 1986;31:1105

86. Schweitzer EJ, Bass BL, Batzri S, Young PM, Huesken J, Harmon JW. Lipid solubilization during bile salt-induced esophageal mucosal barrier disruption in the rabbit. J Lab Clin Med 1987;110:172

87. Sears RJ, Champion G, Richter JE. Characteristics of partial gastrectomy (PG) patients with esophageal symptoms of duodenogastric reflux. Am J Gastroenterol 1995;90:211

88. Shimono M, Clementi F. Intercellular junction of oral epithelium. J Ultrastruct Res 1977;59:101

89. Singh S, Bradley LA, Richter JE. Determinants of oesophageal "alkaline" pH environment in controls and patients with gastro-oesophageal reflux disease. Gut 1993;34:309

90. Smith MR, Buckton GK, Bennett JR. Bile acid levels in stomach and esophagus of patients with acid gastroesophageal reflux. Gut 1984;25:A556

91. Snow JC, Goldstein JL, Schmidt LN, Lisitza P, Layden TJ. Rabbit esophageal cells show regulatory volume decrease: ionic basis and effect of pH. Gastroenterology 1993;105:102

92. Stein HJ, Siewert JR. Barrett's esophagus: pathogenesis, epidemiology, functional abnormalities, malignant degeneration, and surgical management. Dysphagia 1993;8:276

93. Stein HJ, et al. Clinical use of 24-hour gastric monitoring vs o-diisopropyl iminodiacetic acid (DISIDA) scanning in the diagnosis of pathologic duodenogastric reflux. Arch Surg 1990;125:966

94. Stein HJ, Barlow AP, DeMeester TR, Hinder RA. Complications of gastroesophageal reflux disease. Ann Surg 1992;216:35

95. Stein HJ, Hoeft S, DeMeester TR. Reflux and motility pattern in Barrett's esophagus. Dis Esophagus 1992;5:21

96. Stein HJ, Smyrk TC, DeMeester TR, Rouse J, Hinder RA. Clinical value of endoscopy and histology in the diagnosis of duodenogastric reflux disease. Surgery 1992;112:796

97. Stein HJ, Hoeft S, DeMeester TR. Functional foregut abnormalities in Barrett's esophagus. J Thorac Cardiovasc Surg 1993;105:107

98. Stipa F, Stein HJ, Feussner H, Kraemer S, Siewert JR. Assessment of non-acid esophageal reflux: comparison between long-term reflux

aspiration test and fiberoptic bilirubin monitoring. Dis Esophagus 1997;10:24

99. Stoker DL, Williams JG. Alkaline reflux oesophagitis. Gut 1991;32: 1090

100. Tanaka K, Fromm F. Effect of bile acid and salicylate on isolated surface and glandular cells of rabbit stomach. Surgery 1983;93:660

101. Thomas AJ, Nahrwold DL, Rose RC. Detergent action of sodium taurocholate on rat gastric mucosa. Biochim Biophys Acta 1972;282: 210

102. Tolin RD, et al. Enterogastric reflux in normal subjects and patients with Bilroth II gastroenterostomy. Measurement of enterogastric reflux. Gastroenterology 1979;77:1027

103. Tuttle SG, Bettarello A, Gossman MI. Esophageal acid perfusion test and a gastroesophageal reflux in patients with esophagitis. Gastroenterology 1960;38:861

104. Tuttle SG, Rufin F, Bettarello A. The physiology of heartburn. Ann Intern Med 1961;55:292

105. Vaezi MF, Richter JE. Synergism of acid and duodenogastroesopha-geal reflux in complicated Barrett's esophagus. Surgery 1995;117: 699

106. Vaezi MF, Richter JE. Role of acid and duodenogastroesophageal reflux in gastroesophageal reflux disease. Gastroenterology 1996;111: 1192

107. Vaezi MF, Richter JE. Contribution of acid and duodenogastroesophageal reflux to esophageal mucosal injury and symptoms in partial gastrectomy patients. Gut 1997;41:297

108. Vaezi MF, LaCamera RG, Richter JE. Bilitec 2000 ambulatory duodenogastric reflux monitoring system. Studies on its validation and limitations. Am J Physiol 1994;267:G1050

109. Vaezi MF, Sears R, Richter JE. Double-blind placebo-controlled cross-over trial of cisapride in postgastrectomy patients with duodenogastric reflux. Dig Dis Sci 1996;41:754

110. Warring JP, Legrand J, Chinichian A, Sanowski RA. Duodenogastric reflux in patients with Barrett's esophagus. Dig Dis Sci 1990;35:759

111. Zamost BJ, Hirschberg J, Ippoliti AF. Esophagitis in scleroderma: prevalence and risk factors. Gastroenterology 1987;92:421

*The Esophagus*, Third Edition,
edited by D. O. Castell and J. E. Richter.
Lippincott Williams & Wilkins, Philadelphia © 1999.

CHAPTER 24

# Conservative Therapy (Phase 1) for Gastroesophageal Reflux Disease (Lifestyle Modifications)

David A. Katzka and Donald O. Castell

The past few years have seen the advent of new approaches to the diagnosis and treatment of gastroesophageal reflux disease (GERD). Better understanding of the pathophysiology of the disease has afforded a number of new therapeutic options, particularly potent and effective acid-suppressing medications. With these alternatives, less emphasis is now placed on simplistic traditional modes of therapy such as diet modifications, antacid use, postural measures, and drug restriction. Perhaps this tendency to forget the older conservative therapies is a mistake. In this chapter, we discuss the rationale for and evidence of efficacy of a conservative approach to the management of GERD.

Medical management of GERD has evolved as we have come to a better understanding of the pathogenesis of this disorder. Prior to the late 1970s, therapy consisted primarily of efforts at lifestyle modification in conjunction with use of antacids or alginic acid. The modifications included elevation of the head of the bed, avoidance of tight-fitting garments, restriction of alcohol and smoking, dietary therapy, weight loss, and avoidance of meals before bedtime [10, 83]. The introduction of histamine $H_2$-receptor antagonists and prokinetic agents pushed these conservative measures to the background while the efficacy of newer pharmacologic regimens was evaluated. The continued influx of new drugs effective at treating reflux has prompted a stepwise approach to these patients, as outlined in Table 24–1. Phase 1 therapy consists of lifestyle modifications and the use of antacids or alginate, over-the-counter (OTC) doses of histamine $H_2$-receptor antagonists, and possible agents that increase salivary flow.

D. A. Katzka: Division of Gastroenterology, Graduate Hospital, Philadelphia, Pennsylvania 19146.

D. O. Castell: Department of Medicine, Graduate Hospital, Philadelphia, Pennsylvania 19146.

Despite continued pharmacologic advancements in medical therapy of GERD, a high percentage of these patients require continuous acid-suppressive therapy, and approximately 10% will require antireflux surgery for control of their symptoms or complications [17, 18]. The expense and potential side effects of chronic pharmacologic therapy underscore the importance of phase 1 treatment modalities as components in the medical approach to this disorder. Unfortunately, these potentially effective primary forms of therapy are often neglected in an age of exciting and efficient acid-suppressive regimens. It is our opinion that phase 1 therapy should not be viewed as a poorly understood empiric strategy to a complex problem. Rather, it is founded on well-studied therapeutic manipulations of simple physiologic determinants of reflux.

## MODIFIABLE FACTORS ASSOCIATED WITH GASTROESOPHAGEAL REFLUX DISEASE

### Body Position

Postural therapy of gastroesophageal reflux is based on concomitant changes in reflux parameters with changes in body position. In normal subjects, physiologic reflux occurs less frequently in the supine than the upright position [49]. This may be related to a protective increase in lower esophageal sphincter (LES) pressure while supine [3]. In chronic reflux sufferers, different patterns have been identified with 24-hour pH monitoring. In one study of 100 patients, nine were shown to reflux only in the upright position, 37 only in the supine position, and 54 in both positions. In those patients who refluxed while supine and in those who did so in both positions, the frequency of supine reflux episodes, duration of acid clearance times, and incidence of esophagitis were all increased compared with controls [27]. These

**TABLE 24–1.** *Stepwise approach to the management of gastroesophageal reflux disease*

Phase 1
  Diet modification (smaller meals, decrease fat content)
  Elevation of head of bed
  Avoidance of recumbency for 3 hours after eating
  Avoidance of adverse medications
  Restriction of smoking and alcohol
  Antacids and alginic acid
  Histamine receptor antagonists (over-the-counter) dose
  Saliva-stimulating agents
Phase 2A
  Histamine receptor antagonists (prescription dose)
  Prokinetic agents
Phase 2B
  Proton pump inhibitors
Phase 3
  Antireflux surgery

observations suggest that for a substantial fraction of reflux patients the frequency and duration of reflux episodes are influenced by posture.

The manipulation of body position produces physiologic benefits on a number of reflux parameters. In normal subjects, improvement in acid clearance results from changing position from supine to upright [55]. Initial studies with intraesophageal pH monitoring in reflux patients demonstrated that elevation of the head of the bed with blocks reduced the number of reflux episodes as well as the amount of time necessary for acid clearance [99]. A subsequent evaluation of postural therapy showed that head-of-the-bed elevation on 6-inch blocks caused only a modest and not significant decrease in reflux episodes but a dramatic and significant decrease in esophageal clearance time and total nocturnal acid exposure [50]. Improvements in acid clearance and decreases in total reflux duration have also been demonstrated with the use of a 10-inch-high foam rubber wedge under the shoulders [3]. Lying recumbent postprandially on the right side has been shown to result in significantly greater reflux than lying on the left side [54]. In a brief letter to the editor of *JAMA,* the use of waterbeds was retrospectively associated with esophagitis, an effect possibly related to a lack of head support [56]. A recent crossover study, however, failed to demonstrate greater recumbent acid exposure in reflux patients sleeping flat on a waterbed compared to sleeping flat on a regular bed [105]. This observation does not absolutely refute the possibility of an association between esophagitis and regular waterbed use because of the mechanical inability to elevate the head of the waterbed.

## Foods

Patients and clinicians alike have long been aware of a relationship between reflux symptoms and the consumption of various foods. The role of dietary factors in gastroesophageal reflux focuses on either their effects on LES pressure or their direct irritative effects on the esophageal mucosa.

Dietary manipulations may be expected to have a predictable influence, either advantageous or deleterious, on the quantity and character of subsequent reflux episodes.

A variety of foods are known to decrease LES pressure [2, 15, 21, 72]. Among those substances having adverse effects on the LES are chocolate, carminatives, and foods rich in fat. Chocolate is believed to exert this effect through the percent of methylxanthines (particularly theobromine) and their influences on cyclic adenosine monophosphate [112]. Ambulatory intraesophageal pH monitoring has documented increased esophageal acid exposure after chocolate ingestion [71]. Carminatives, such as spearmint and peppermint, are oil extracts of plants used as food seasoners or flavorings. Evidence for sphincter relaxation has been demonstrated after ingestion of these substances [93]. The ability of peppermint to decrease LES pressure may be mediated through inhibition of calcium channels in smooth muscle [47]. Although LES pressures were not measured, a recent study showed that onions can produce increased symptoms of heartburn and belching in association with increased acid exposure [1].

Ingestion of a high-fat meal has been shown to decrease LES pressure and to cause increased esophageal acid exposure for up to 3 hours after eating [6, 72]. This increased postprandial reflux was particularly striking in healthy volunteers without a history of chronic heartburn, underscoring the potential for fat to augment so-called physiologic reflux. The combined effects of fat both to decrease sphincter pressure and to delay gastric emptying greatly increase its potential as a major factor in the pathogenesis of GERD. In fact, fat-induced reflux is probably the primary cause of fatty food intolerance.

Coffee is commonly implicated as a cause for reflux symptoms, although its influence on LES control is disputed. One study showed that coffee actually increases sphincter pressure in healthy volunteers but changed it only minimally in reflux patients more likely to have coffee-related dyspepsia [24]. A conflicting study showed evidence for a coffee-related decrease in LES pressure [100]. More recent data argue against any effect of coffee on LES pressure [85].

A recent study evaluating the effect of coffee on reflux as measured through ambulatory pH studies reported a marked increase in esophageal acid exposure occurring in patients with known reflux disease (abnormal pH study or esophagitis) [77]. More compelling evidence in this study shows that when decaffeinated coffee is given in these same patients, the level of acid reflux is reduced by approximately 85%. It may be then that caffeine unmasks or worsens underlying reflux in those patients who are predisposed as opposed to normal volunteers, in whom there may be little effect. It seems more likely that any effect of coffee on reflux-associated symptoms is related to direct mucosal irritation and effects on acid production [66, 78].

A number of poorly tolerated foods provoke symptoms in reflux patients by mechanisms other than inhibition of LES pressure. Many commonly consumed beverages, including cola, beer, and milk, are potent stimuli of gastric acid secretion and will increase the quantity of acid available [66]. Evidence of esophageal mucosal sensitivity to some foods can be elicited from reflux patients by the intraesophageal infusion of acidic (pH 3.5 to 5.0) foods, including coffee, orange juice, or spicy tomato drink, suggesting that these substances exert their effects by direct esophageal irritation [78]. This irritative capacity may be related primarily to the high osmolarity of the ingested substances [64] since esophageal sensitivity persisted after these foods were brought to a neutral pH by addition of alkali [100].

### Alcohol

Alcohol, when given intravenously to normal volunteers, decreased LES pressure and adversely affected esophageal peristalsis [48]. Intraesophageal pH studies in supine, healthy subjects after alcohol ingestion demonstrated significant impairment of normal acid clearance with resultant prolonged nocturnal acid exposure [104]. These effects suggest that alcohol use may have definite deleterious effects on defenses against pathologic acid reflux [101].

### Smoking

Cigarette smoking has been shown to decrease LES pressure and increase the frequency of reflux episodes [28, 52, 97]. There is evidence as well for deleterious effects of smoking on esophageal clearance and salivary function [51, 55]. Despite these findings, conflicting data have emerged regarding the influence of smoking on the rate of healing and recurrence of reflux esophagitis [11, 57]. Smokers have more episodes of reflux during 24-hour esophageal pH monitoring compared to nonsmokers, but the total time of esophageal acid exposure is similar in both groups [88]. Although cessation of smoking results in an improvement in the frequency of reflux episodes, the total time of acid exposure is not immediately affected [106]. An adverse effect of cigarettes on the antireflux barrier is well documented, but further studies are needed to define the relationship between smoking and chronic GERD.

### Stress

Stress is a factor that historically has been associated with GERD, yet there are few data to support this association. One study in normal volunteers did not demonstrate increased gastroesophageal reflux during times when subjects were administered difficult tasks [25]. This study did not answer the question, however, of whether stress exacerbates reflux in patients with underlying GERD. In a recent study, patients with symptomatic reflux were administered difficult tasks. The result did not demonstrate a change in reflux parameters in relation to stress but, in fact, showed an increase in symptom reporting during stress, suggesting increased symptom sensitivity [13].

### Medications

A number of commonly used medications decrease LES pressure, thus potentiating gastroesophageal reflux in susceptible individuals. Because of the higher-than-expected incidence of reflux among asthmatics, theophylline has been investigated and shown to have a detrimental effect on LES pressure as well as a tendency to increase gastric acid secretion [12, 31]. Twenty-four-hour esophageal pH monitoring of symptomatic asthmatics demonstrated an increase in duration of acid exposure and symptoms with the use of theophylline [30]. There are some preliminary data suggesting that these effects might be minimized with low-dose or slow-release oral preparations [40]. In a recent study of 104 asthmatics, 80% demonstrated abnormal gastroesophageal reflux and many had decreased LES pressures compared to controls. There were, however, no differences in reflux parameters measured with ambulatory pH recording between asthmatics who required bronchodilators and those who did not [96]. Beta$_2$-adrenergic drugs, some of which are also used in asthma therapy, have inhibitory effects on sphincter pressure when taken orally, but an inhaled preparation may minimize this influence [89]. Other frequently used medications that have the ability to decrease LES pressure include alpha-adrenergic antagonists; prostaglandins E$_1$, E$_2$, and A$_2$; anticholinergic agents; dopamine; nitrates; meperidine; diazepam; morphine; a variety of anesthetics; and calcium channel blockers [16]. Calcium channel blockers may also exacerbate reflux by adverse effects on esophageal acid clearance [81].

Oral contraceptives have been implicated in potentially decreasing LES pressures, an effect postulated to be related to the progesterone content of these substances [102]. Heartburn occurs in more than 50% of women during pregnancy, and reflux-related symptoms tend to get worse as the pregnancy progresses [73]. This well-known clinical observation is believed to be produced by a hormonally induced (progesterone?) decrease of LES pressure superimposed on increases in intragastric pressure in the latter stages of gestation [4, 103].

### Obesity

Most physicians advocate weight loss for obese patients with gastroesophageal reflux, although supporting data are not very convincing. One study of 25 morbidly obese individuals failed to show an association between excessive weight and decreased LES pressure [74]. A later study showed a correlation of morbid obesity with reflux, as well as lower-than-expected sphincter pressures, among many overweight patients [38]. In these heavy individuals, the gastroesophageal pressure gradient may be a more important determinant of reflux than the actual LES pressure [68]. It has been suggested that obesity, like tight-fitting garments, may potentiate reflux by its continuous augmentation of the gastroesophageal pressure gradient, which encourages reflux during sphincter relaxations, regardless of the cause [29]. A more likely explanation for the observed clinical relation between weight gain or weight loss and increased or decreased reflux symptoms may be associated changes in dietary fat intake [19].

## Exercise

In a subset of patients, physical exertion plays an integral role in the genesis of gastroesophageal reflux. This may be particularly important to evaluate in individuals with angina-like chest pain and normal coronary angiograms. In one such population of 52 patients, 23 were demonstrated to have reflux with pH monitoring during exercise treadmill testing. In all but one of these 23, the typical exertional chest pain occurred simultaneously with the reflux [90]. Jogging has been shown to induce reflux in otherwise healthy individuals [23] and to be significantly decreased by taking ranitidine (300 mg) prior to exercise [59]. This finding suggests that exercise may prove to be an important contributor to the pathogenesis of GERD.

## Efficacy of Conservative Medical Therapy

A lack of well-controlled trials has prevented definitive evaluation of the efficacy of conservative medical therapy in patients with GERD [18]. In an early randomized study comparing the medical and surgical managements of reflux esophagitis, patients were followed for 20 to 46 months after either surgical (fundoplication) or chronic medical therapy. Because it comprised standard medical therapy at the time, the latter consisted only of phase 1 therapy, including elevation of the head of the bed, antacids, bland diet, and weight loss. Only 19% of patients managed medically were judged to have a good to excellent response to therapy compared to 73% of surgical patients [9]. As more pharmacologic options became available, a later study including phase 2 medications (cimetidine, metoclopramide) showed a similar result; 20% of patients had long-lasting remission with phase 1 medical management, and all were managed without surgery [63]. Inferences from either of these studies about the conservative management of GERD should be guarded. Both studies selected patients with poorly responsive severe GERD, clearly those at the tip of the iceberg. For the vast majority of reflux sufferers, well-designed studies of phase 1 therapy remain scarce.

By changing patients from supine to upright, measurable improvements in many indices of gastroesophageal reflux can be seen, including acid clearance, frequency of reflux episodes, and quantity of refluxed material [55, 65, 99]. These data support the long-standing recommendations of avoiding lying down after meals and of sleeping with the head of the bed on blocks. Whether postural manipulations translate to clear therapeutic benefit in reflux patients is rarely addressed. The use of 24-hour pH monitoring has allowed the demonstration of improved acid clearance in

reflux patients sleeping with the head of the bed raised or on a foam wedge [39, 50]. Similar monitoring in infants showed a clear benefit of positioning for the prevention of gastroesophageal reflux [76, 110]. In a double-blind study of 71 patients with reflux esophagitis treated with either placebo or ranitidine, 50% were instructed to raise the head of the bed on 8-inch blocks during 6 weeks of therapy. This maneuver significantly improved heartburn compared to sleeping flat during placebo treatment, and the effect of both therapies (ranitidine and bed blocks) together was better than that of either alone. Elevation of the head of the bed was also of particular benefit to smokers and alcohol consumers compared to ranitidine [41].

In the largest multicenter study designed to assess the efficacy of ranitidine in the treatment of GERD, 284 reflux patients were randomized to treatment with the $H_2$-receptor antagonist or a placebo. Therapy in both groups included elevation of the head of the bed and antacid consumption as needed. Clear evidence of the beneficial effects of ranitidine was demonstrated after 6 weeks, but 41% of the endoscopically abnormal patients randomized to the placebo group had healed during that period as well. A substantial improvement in the frequency and duration of heartburn was also shown [95]. An unusually high placebo response rate is noted in many drug trials of reflux therapy. This phenomenon is unlikely to be related completely to the natural history of the disorder and perhaps is more attributable to patient education and the reinforcement of reflux-modifying behavior such as elevation of the head of the bed combined with regular antacid use.

As low-dose $H_2$ antagonists are now available OTC, they are considered "conservative" therapy and fall under the purview of this chapter heading. Despite the fact that these OTC $H_2$ antagonists have become one of the dominant (if not the dominant) forms of OTC therapy for GERD, little objective data are available as regards their efficacy. Most data with $H_2$ antagonists as given above are with higher (i.e., prescription) doses of these medications. Nevertheless, several recent studies have focused on the ability of these medications in OTC doses to alter gastric acid secretion. For example, in normal volunteers, 10 mg of famotidine has been shown to significantly reduce titratable gastric acid in response to both a meal [58] and pentagastrin [35]. Both low-dose famotidine and ranitidine also reduce postprandial gastric acidity as measured by continuous monitoring of intragastric pH [80].

Other studies have focused on the ability of OTC $H_2$ antagonists to prevent or treat heartburn and dyspepsia. For example, in two large controlled, randomized trials, 10 mg famotidine was shown to be superior to placebo and antacid in reducing several dyspeptic symptoms [32, 94].

Thus, there is some objective basis for the use of OTC $H_2$ antagonists in the treatment of GERD but certainly not in proportion to the number of current users. Furthermore, given the lack of efficacy of prescription-strength $H_2$ antagonists in more serious forms of GERD, these drugs when used in OTC dosages are likely to be useful only in patients with symptoms of GERD but without pathologic esophageal injury.

Until the introduction of $H_2$-receptor blockers in the mid-1970s, antacids were the mainstays of the pharmacologic therapy of GERD. Their popularity was based on the ability of these substances to buffer the acid content of gastric secretions. This neutralizing capacity varies from one preparation to another and may influence the total acid load disproportionately more than the pH of gastric secretions [69]. In doses adequate to increase gastric pH, an inactivation of pepsin may result [87]. Antacids have also been shown to increase LES pressure, an effect most likely related to gastric alkalinization [46].

Compounds containing alginic acid with or without antacid are frequently recommended for reflux patients. The potential benefit of alginic acid is related to its ability to create a foamy raft on the surface of the gastric pool, which has been shown to enhance the antireflux barrier, minimizing direct contact of gastric secretions with vulnerable esophageal mucosa [7]. The recent observations by Moss and colleagues [70] on the flotation ability of alginic acid suggest a strong potential for an antireflux action primarily in the upright position. This would support observations of the symptomatic relief obtained in patients during the daytime hours. Recent studies from our laboratory indicated that Gaviscon, an alginic acid–antacid combination, has an active effect that is preferentially found in the upright position [20]. We used the technique of promoting reflux in healthy volunteers with a high-fat (61% fat calories) meal, a method previously reported from our laboratory to promote increased reflux in both the upright and supine positions [6]. Following the ingestion of an identical meal on four occa-

sions, the subjects were given either extra-strength Gaviscon or active placebo (antacid with equal neutralizing ability) in random sequence as they were also randomly assigned to the upright or supine position for 3 hours postprandially. These studies revealed that Gaviscon ingestion resulted in significantly ($p < 0.01$) fewer total minutes of reflux and total numbers of reflux episodes compared to antacids ingested in the upright position (Fig. 24–1). No significant differences were noted when Gaviscon was compared to placebo with the patients in the supine position postprandially. These studies support prior observations of the potential effectiveness of Gaviscon to relieve daytime symptoms, particularly those occurring after meals in the upright position. They also suggest a potential role for Gaviscon in the treatment of patients having breakthrough symptoms during the day while receiving therapy with acid-suppressing medications.

Indirect support for the use of antacids and alginic acid in the management of GERD can be obtained from a number of recent studies. In one pediatric trial, antacids were as effective as cimetidine in the management of reflux, although no placebo group was studied [26]. Two studies designed to assess the efficacy of bethanechol with respect to antacids showed a substantial and comparable response with both therapies [62, 84]. A trial of antacids versus antacids with dimethicone in reflux esophagitis showed similar good response rates in both groups [75].

Symptomatic improvement with the use of the antacid–alginate combination in reflux patients was reported to be approximately 80% in two open-label studies without placebo groups [42, 111]. In a trial designed to assess the efficacy of sucralfate compared to an alginate–antacid compound in the treatment of reflux esophagitis, significant symptomatic

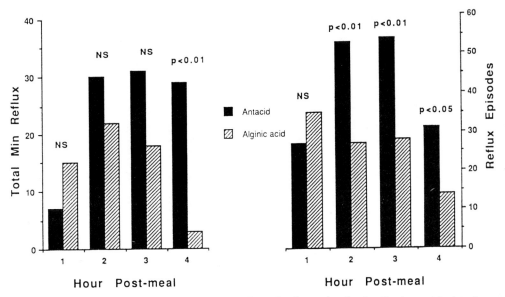

**FIG. 24–1.** Total minutes of reflux and total number of reflux episodes for the ten subjects after each of the 4 hours following the high-fat meal in the upright position, showing decreased reflux with alginic acid compared to antacid with equal neutralizing ability.

improvement was noted in approximately 70% of the alginate-treated group, a result not improved with sucralfate [60]. When used with metoclopramide, alginate–antacid was as effective as ranitidine in the management of esophagitis among dyspeptic alcoholics [101]. In two studies designed to evaluate the effectiveness of a carbenoxolone–alginate–antacid combination for reflux esophagitis, alginate–antacid alone proved to be very effective in the symptomatic control of this disorder [79, 113]. It should be noted that despite the several trials that showed reasonable efficacy of the alginic acid–antacid combination, one recent study showed that this combination may be inferior to alginic acid alone [107]. The authors showed, by both pH monitoring and a new portable scintigraphic method of measuring gastroesophageal reflux, that Gaviscon is more effective than an alginic acid–antacid combination in suppressing reflux of both acid and stomach content. These results are compatible with data suggesting that the metal ions from the antacids may bind to the alginic acid, causing a defect in raft formation as well as making less antacid available for neutralizing activity [108].

Several studies have compared the effectiveness of alginate–antacid to that of antacids alone. One nonblinded trial showed equal effectiveness for these two agents in the symptomatic control of reflux esophagitis, whereas a similar study demonstrated a clear superiority for alginate–antacid [22, 36]. Three double-blind studies showed alginate–antacid and antacids to have significant and comparable effectiveness in the control of reflux symptoms compared to prestudy symptom levels [33, 67, 92], whereas one such study favored alginate–antacid [5]. All of these studies were limited, however, by the absence of a true placebo treatment group.

Definitive validation of a therapeutic benefit from the use of antacids in GERD is limited by the scarcity of well-designed, blinded, placebo-controlled trials (Table 24–2). Graham and Patterson [34] compared antacids with placebo for the short-term treatment of reflux and included an initial 1-week placebo trial for all patients in an effort to eliminate the expected placebo responders from the study group. In this trial, no significant difference could be demonstrated between antacids and placebo for the symptomatic management of this disease. Favorable evidence for the usefulness of antacids is found in a blinded study comparing antacids with ranitidine and placebo in patients with reflux esophagitis [37]. This study showed comparable efficacy of antacids and ranitidine in the short-term therapy of esophagitis, with a clear benefit of both of these agents over a placebo with regard to symptomatic relief. A more recent double-blind comparison of antacids and placebo in reflux esophagitis patients showed a statistically significant benefit in symptom response in the antacid-treated group [109].

Several placebo-controlled, double-blind studies showed favorable evidence for a therapeutic benefit of alginate–antacid [8]. In one such study of symptomatic reflux patients, alginate–antacid-treated patients reported subjective improvement compared to a placebo group, and this medication influenced favorably a number of measurable reflux parameters [98]. A similar study showed a beneficial effect of alginate in the pediatric population [14]. In a recent comparison of alginate–antacid versus placebo for acute heartburn induced by a symptom-provoking meal, significant superiority in symptomatic improvement was demonstrated for alginate–antacid [61].

Finally, a new conservative agent for esophageal reflux that has been recently examined is a pectin-based formulation that may also act by the "raft-forming" mechanism similar to alginic acid. In one study, this agent was superior to placebo in improvement of symptoms and esophagitis scores in patients with gross esophagitis. Interestingly, however, there was no difference from placebo when patients were studied with ambulatory pH monitoring [43].

## Agents that Increase Salivary Flow

Saliva has been shown to be an important defense mechanism of the esophagus in preventing reflux damage by virtue of its ability to (a) decrease local acidity by both dilution and neutralization with bicarbonate [44], (b) initiate primary

**TABLE 24–2.** *Placebo-controlled, blinded trials of antacids or alginate for gastroesophageal reflux*

| Study | No. of patients | Drug studied | Effect on symptoms | Other effects |
|---|---|---|---|---|
| Beeley and Warner [8] | 28 | Alginate–antacid vs. placebo vs. alginate | Alginate–antacid superior to placebo | — |
| Stanciu and Bennett [97] | 60 | Alginate–antacid vs. placebo vs. alginate | Alginate–antacid superior to both | Alginate–antacid superior by pH monitoring |
| Graham et al. [33] | 32 | Antacid vs. placebo | Antacid comparable to placebo | Comparable by endoscopy |
| Grove et al. [37] | 37 | Antacid vs. placebo vs. ranitidine | Antacid superior to placebo | Comparable by endoscopy |
| Lanza et al. [61] | 60 | Alginate–antacid vs. placebo | Alginate–antacid superior to placebo | — |
| Buts et al. [14] | 20 | Alginate vs. placebo | Alginate superior to placebo | Alginate superior by pH monitoring |
| Weberg and Berstad [109] | 47 | Antacid vs. placebo | Antacid superior to placebo | — |

peristalsis and subsequent acid clearance [53], and (c) possibly facilitate esophageal healing through epidermal growth factors [86]. A reflexive increase in salivary flow may occur during acid reflux (water brash), also suggesting its importance in preventing reflux injury. Interestingly, there are little objective data evaluating agents that increase salivary flow as therapy for GERD, despite the fact that chewing gum and sucking hard candy have been used for years on an empiric basis in patients with reflux symptoms. In a recent experiment, volunteers given chewing gum were shown to have significantly shorter clearance times of acid infused into the esophagus [91]. Similarly, it has been shown in the past that oral lozenges may also accelerate esophageal acid clearance times and produce saliva in quantities capable of neutralizing physiologic amounts of hydrochloric acid [45]. Thus, although not extensively proven, agents that increase salivary flow may well be useful for GERD.

## CONCLUSIONS

The last twenty years have seen an evolution of improved strategies in the diagnosis and treatment of GERD. Effective acid-suppressive and LES-enhancing drugs have relegated more conservative modes of therapy to the background. Despite this trend, simple lifestyle modifications and the use of antacids with or without alginic acid remain the backbone of treatment for the vast majority of reflux sufferers, many of whom are never seen by a physician. Although well founded on the current understanding of the physiologic determinants of reflux, the therapeutic benefit of these measures lacks unanimity of support in the literature. It is likely that large-scale studies in this area will remain scarce owing to the inherent difficulties of satisfactorily controlling for such elusive variables as dietary restriction. Most available data support the limited efficacy of phase 1 therapy of GERD, particularly for symptom control. The simplicity and cost of such interventions further justify their continued consideration for all patients suffering from this disorder. It is our belief that no long-term therapeutic program for chronic GERD is complete without instructing the patients on the phase 1 components of treatment, thus allowing the patient to be actively involved in managing his or her disease. This is particularly emphasized by the recognition that gastroesophageal reflux is frequently a persistent, recurring, lifelong problem and that expensive acid-suppressive therapies are commonly required for continuous maintenance.

## REFERENCES

1. Allen ML, et al. The effect of raw onions on acid reflux and reflux symptoms. Am J Gastroenterol 1990;85:377
2. Babka JC, Castell DO. On the genesis of heartburn: the effects of specific foods on the lower esophagus sphincter. Dig Dis 1973;18:391
3. Babka JC, Hager GW, Castell DO. The effect of body position on lower esophagus sphincter pressure [Letter]. Dig Dis 1973;18:391
4. Bainbridge ET, et al. Gastro-oesophageal reflux in pregnancy: altered function of the barrier to reflux in asymptomatic women during early pregnancy. Scand J Gastroenterol 1984;19:85
5. Barnardo DE, et al. A double-blind controlled trial of Gaviscon in patients with symptomatic gastro-oesophageal reflux. Curr Med Res Opin 1975;3:388
6. Becker DJ, et al. A comparison of high and low fat meals on postprandial esophageal acid exposure. Am J Gastroenterol 1989;84:782
7. Beckloff GL, Chapman JH, Shiverdecker P. Objective evaluation of an antacid with unusual properties. J Clin Pharmacol 1972;12:11
8. Beeley M, Warner JO. Medical treatment of symptomatic hiatus hernia with low-density compounds. Curr Med Res Opin 1972;1:63
9. Behar J, et al. Medical and surgical management of reflux esophagitis: A 38-month report on a prospective clinical trial. N Engl J Med 1975;293:263
10. Bennett JR. Medical management of gastro-oesophageal reflux. Clin Gastroenterol 1976;5:175
11. Berenson MM, et al. Effect of smoking in a controlled study of ranitidine treatment in gastroesophageal reflux disease. J Clin Gastroenterol 1987;9:499
12. Berquist WE, Rachelefsky GS, Kadden M. Effect of theophylline on gastroesophageal reflux in normal adults. J Allergy Clin Immunol 1981;67:407
13. Bradley LA, et al. The relationship between stress and symptoms of gastroesophageal reflux: the influence of psychological factors. Am J Gastroenterol 1993;88:11
14. Buts JP, Barudi C, Otte JB. Double-blind controlled study on the efficacy of sodium alginate (Gaviscon) in reducing gastroesophageal reflux assessed by 24H continuous pH monitoring in infants and children. Eur J Pediatr 1987;146:156
15. Castell DO. Diet and the lower esophageal sphincter. Am J Clin Nutr 1975;28:1296
16. Castell DO. The lower esophageal sphincter: physiologic and clinical aspects. Ann Intern Med 1975;83:390
17. Castell DO. Future medical therapy of reflux esophagitis. J Clin Gastroenterol 1986;8(suppl 1):81
18. Castell DO. Medical therapy for reflux esophagitis: 1986 and beyond. Ann Intern Med 1986;104:112
19. Castell DO. Obesity and gastroesophageal reflux: is there a relationship? Eur J Gastroenterol Hepatol 1996;8:625
20. Castell DO, et al. Alginic acid decreases postprandial upright gastroesophageal reflux. Comparison with equal-strength antacid. Dig Dis Sci 1992;37:589
21. Chernow B, Castell DO. Diet and heartburn. JAMA 1979;241:2307
22. Chevrel B. A comparative crossover study on the treatment of heartburn and epigastric pain: liquid Gaviscon and a magnesium-aluminum antacid gel. J Int Med Res 1980;8:300
23. Clark CS, et al. Gastroesophageal reflux induced by exercise in healthy volunteers. JAMA 1989;261:3599
24. Cohen S. Pathogenesis of coffee-induced gastrointestinal symptoms. N Engl J Med 1980;303:122
25. Cook IJ, Collins SM. Does acute emotional stress influence frequency or duration of gastroesophageal reflux in human subjects? Gastroenterology 1986;90:1380(abstr)
26. Cucchiara S, et al. Antacids and cimetidine treatment for gastro-oesophageal reflux and peptic oesophagitis. Arch Dis Child 1984;59:842
27. DeMeester TR, et al. Patterns of gastroesophageal reflux in health and disease. Ann Surg 1976;184:459
28. Dennish GW, Castell DO. Inhibitory effect of smoking on the lower esophageal sphincter. N Engl J Med 1971;284:1136
29. Dent J. Recent views on the pathogenesis of gastro-oesophageal reflux disease. Baillieres Clin Gastroenterol 1987;1:727
30. Ekstrom T, Tibbing L. Influence of theophylline on gastroesophageal reflux and asthma. Eur J Clin Pharmacol 1988;35:353
31. Foster LJ, Trudeau WL, Goldman AL. Bronchodilator effects on gastric acid secretion. JAMA 1979;241:2613
32. Gottlieb S, et al. Efficacy and tolerability of famotidine in preventing heartburn and related symptoms of upper gastrointestinal discomfort. Am J Ther 1995;2:314
33. Graham DY, Lanza F, Dorsch ER. Symptomatic reflux esophagitis: a double-blind controlled comparison of antacids and alginate. Curr Ther Res 1977;22:653
34. Graham DY, Patterson DJ. Double-blind comparison of liquid antacid and placebo in the treatment of symptomatic reflux esophagitis. Dig Dis Sci 1983;28:559

35. Grimley CE, et al. Early and late effects of low-dose famotidine, ranitidine, or placebo on pentagastrin-stimulated gastric acid secretion in man. Aliment Pharmacol Ther 1996;10:743

36. Grossman AE, et al. Reflux esophagitis: a comparison of old and new medical management. J Kans Med Soc 1973;74:423

37. Grove O, et al. Ranitidine and high-dose antacid in reflux oesophagitis: a randomized, placebo-controlled trial. Scand J Gastroenterol 1985;20:457

38. Hagen J, et al. Gastroesophageal reflux in the massively obese. Int Surg 1987;72:1

39. Hamilton JW, et al. Sleeping on a wedge diminishes exposure of the esophagus to refluxed acid. Dig Dis Sci 1988;33:518

40. Haringsma J, Bartelsman JFWM, Tytgat GNJ. Chronic low-dose theophylline has no significant effect on lower esophageal sphincter pressure in healthy volunteers. Gastroenterology 1989;96:A197(abstr)

41. Harvey RJ, et al. Effects of sleeping with the bed-head raised and of ranitidine in patients with severe peptic oesophagitis. Lancet 1987;2:1200

42. Hassan SS. Treatment of moderate to severe gastro-oesophageal reflux with an alginate/antacid combination. Curr Med Res Opin 1980;6:645

43. Havelund T, Aalykke C, Rasmussen L. Efficacy of a pectin-based anti-reflux agent on acid reflux and recurrence of symptoms and esophagitis in gastroesophageal reflux disease. Eur J Gastroenterol Hepatol 1997;9:509

44. Helm JF, et al. Acid neutralizing capacity of human saliva. Gastroenterology 1982;83:69

45. Helm JF, et al. Effect of esophageal emptying and saliva on clearance of acid from the esophagus. N Engl J Med 1984;310:284

46. Higgs RH, Smith RD, Castell DO. Gastric alkalinization: effect of lower-esophageal sphincter pressure and serum gastrin. N Engl J Med 1974;291:486

47. Hills JM, Aaronson PI. The mechanism of action of peppermint oil on gastrointestinal smooth muscle. An analysis using patch clamp electrophysiology and isolated tissue pharmacology in rabbit and guinea pig. Gastroenterology 1991;101:55

48. Hogan WJ, Viegas de Andrade SR, Winship DH. Ethanol-induced acute esophageal motor dysfunction. J Appl Physiol 1972;32:755

49. Johnson LF, DeMeester TR. Twenty-four hour pH monitoring of the distal esophagus. Am J Gastroenterol 1974;62:325

50. Johnson LF, DeMeester TR. Evaluation of the head of the bed, bethanechol, and antacid foam tablets on gastroesophageal reflux. Dig Dis Sci 1981;26:673

51. Kahrilas PJ, Gupta RR. The effect of smoking on salivation and esophageal acid clearance. J Lab Clin Med 1989;114:431

52. Kahrilas PJ, Gupta RR. Mechanisms of acid reflux associated with cigarette smoking. Gut 1990;31:4

53. Kapila YV, et al. Relationship between swallow rate and salivary flow. Dig Dis Sci 1984;29:528

54. Katz LC, Just R, Castell DO. Body position affects recumbent postprandial reflux. J Clin Gastroenterol 1994;18:280

55. Kjellen G, Tibbling L. Influence of body position, dry and water swallows, smoking and alcohol on esophageal acid clearing. Scand J Gastroenterol 1978;13:283

56. Kleinman M, Plain G. Reflux esophagitis and the waterbed [Letter]. JAMA 1987;257:2033

57. Koelz JR, et al. Healing and relapse of reflux esophagitis during treatment with ranitidine. Gastroenterology 1986;91:1198

58. Kovacs TOG, et al. The action of low-dose famotidine vs. prescription doses of cimetidine and ranitidine on human gastric acid secretion as titrated by sodium hydroxide: a placebo-controlled study. Pract Gastroenterol 1996;20(suppl):S5

59. Kraus BB, Sinclair J, Castell DO. Gastroesophageal reflux in runners. Characteristics and treatment. Ann Intern Med 1990;112:429

60. Laitinen S, et al. Sucralfate and alginate/antacid in reflux esophagitis. Scand J Gastroenterol 1985;20:229

61. Lanza FL, et al. Effectiveness of foaming antacid in relieving induced heartburn. South Med J 1986;79:327

62. Levi P, et al. Bethanechol versus antacids in the treatment of gastroesophageal reflux. Helv Paediatr Acta 1985;40:349

63. Lieberman DA. Medical therapy for chronic reflux esophagitis: long-term follow-up. Arch Intern Med 1987;147:1717

64. Lloyd DA, Borda IT. Food-induced heartburn: effect of osmolality. Gastroenterology 1981;80:740

65. Malmud LS, Fisher RS. Quantitation of gastroesophageal reflux be-

fore and after therapy using the gastroesophageal scintiscan. South Med J 1978;71(suppl 1):10

66. McArthur K, Hogan D, Isenberg JI. Relative stimulatory effects of commonly ingested beverages on gastric acid secretion in humans. Gastroenterology 1982;83:199

67. McHardy G. A multicentric randomized clinical trial of Gaviscon in reflux esophagitis. South Med J 1978;71(suppl 1):16

68. Mercer CD, et al. Gastroesophageal pressure gradients and lower esophageal sphincter pressures in severely obese patients. Gastroenterology 1982;82:1129 (abstr)

69. Morrissey JF, Barreras RF. Antacid therapy. N Engl J Med 1974;290:550

70. Moss HA, et al. Anti-reflux agents: stratification or flotation? Eur J Gastroenterol Hepatol 1990;2:45

71. Murphy DW, Castell DO. Chocolate and heartburn: evidence of increased esophageal acid exposure after chocolate ingestion. Am J Gastroenterol 1988;83:633

72. Nebel OT, Castell DO. Lower esophageal sphincter pressure changes after food ingestion. Gastroenterology 1972;63:778

73. Nebel OT, Fornes MF, Castell DO. Symptomatic gastroesophageal reflux: incidence and precipitating factors. Am J Dig Dis 1976;21:953

74. O'Brien TF. Lower esophageal sphincter pressure and esophageal function in obese humans. J Clin Gastroenterol 1980;2:145

75. Ogilvie AL, Atkinson M. Does dimethicone increase the efficacy of antacids in the treatment of reflux oesophagitis? J R Soc Med 1986;79:584

76. Orenstein SR, Whitington PF. Positioning for prevention of infant gastroesophageal reflux. J Pediatr 1983;103:534

77. Pehl C, et al. The effect of decaffeination of coffee on gastro-esophageal reflux in patients with reflux disease. Aliment Pharmacol Ther 1997;11:483

78. Price SF, Smithson KW, Castell DO. Food sensitivity in reflux esophagitis. Gastroenterology 1981;80:740

79. Reed PI, Davies WA. Controlled trial of a new dosage form of carbenoxolone (Pyrogastrone) in the treatment of reflux esophagitis. Dig Dis 1978;23:161

80. Reilly TG, et al. Low dose famotidine and ranitidine as single postprandial doses: a three-period placebo-controlled comparative trial. Aliment Pharmacol Ther 1996;10:749

81. Richter JE. A critical review of current medical therapy for gastroesophageal reflux disease. J Clin Gastroenterol 1986;8(suppl 1):72

82. Richter JE, Castell DO. Drugs, foods, and other substances in the cause and treatment of reflux esophagitis. Med Clin North Am 1981;65:1223

83. Roufail WM. Medical management of patients with reflux esophagitis. South Med J 1978;71(suppl 1):43

84. Saco LS, et al. Double-blind controlled trial of bethanechol and antacid versus placebo and antacid in the treatment of erosive esophagitis. Gastroenterology 1982;82:1369

85. Salmon PR, et al. Effect of coffee on human lower esophageal function. Digestion 1981;21:69

86. Sarosiek J, et al. Enhancement of salivary esophagoprotection: rationale for a physiologic approach to gastroesophageal reflux disease. Gastroenterology 1996;110:675

87. Scarpignato C. Pharmacological bases of the medical treatment of gastroesophageal reflux disease. Dig Dis 1988;6:117

88. Schindbeck NE, et al. Influence of smoking and esophageal intubation on esophageal pH-metry. Gastroenterology 1987;92:1994

89. Schindbeck NE, et al. Effects of albuterol on esophageal motility and gastroesophageal reflux in healthy volunteers. JAMA 1989;260:3156

90. Schofield PM, et al. Exertional gastroesophageal reflux: a mechanism for symptoms in patients with angina pectoris and normal coronary angiograms. BMJ 1987;294:1459

91. Schonfeld J, et al. Esophageal acid and salivary secretion: is chewing gum a treatment option for gastro-esophageal injury? Digestion 1997;59:111

92. Scobie BA. Endoscopically controlled trial of alginate and antacid in reflux oesophagitis. Med J Aust 1976;1:627

93. Sigmund CJ, McNally EF. The action of a carminative on the lower esophageal sphincter. Gastroenterology 1969;56:13

94. Simon TJ, et al. Self-directed treatment of intermittent heartburn: a randomized, multicenter, double-blind, placebo-controlled evaluation of antacid and low doses of an $H_2$-receptor antagonist (famotidine). Am J Ther 1995;2:304

95. Sontag S, et al. Ranitidine therapy for gastroesophageal reflux disease: results of a large double-blind trial. Arch Intern med 1987;147: 1485

96. Sontag SJ, et al. Most asthmatics have gastroesophageal reflux with or without bronchodilator therapy. Gastroenterology 1990;99:613

97. Stanciu C, Bennett JR. Smoking and gastro-oesophageal reflux. BMJ 1972;3:793

98. Stanciu C, Bennett JR. Alginate/antacid in the reduction of gastro-oesophageal reflux. Lancet 1974;1:109

99. Stanciu C, Bennett JR. Effects of posture on gastro-oesophageal reflux. Digestion 1977;15:104

100. Thomas FB, et al. Inhibitory effect of coffee on lower esophageal sphincter pressure. Gastroenterology 1980;79:1262

101. Tonnesen H, et al. Reflux oesophagitis in heavy drinkers: effect of ranitidine and alginate/metoclopramide. Digestion 1987;38:69

102. Van Thiel DH, Gavaler JS, Sternple J. Lower esophageal sphincter pressure in women using sequential oral contraceptives. Gastroenterology 1976;71:232

103. Van Thiel DH, et al. Heartburn of pregnancy. Gastroenterology 1977; 72:666

104. Vitale GC, et al. The effect of alcohol on nocturnal gastroesophageal reflux. JAMA 1987;258:2077

105. Wang JC, et al. Does sleeping on a waterbed promote gastroesophageal reflux? Dig Dis Sci 1989;34:1585

106. Waring JP, et al. The immediate effects of cessation of cigarette smoking on gastroesophageal reflux. Am J Gastroenterol 1989;84:1076

107. Washington N, Greaves JL, Iftikhari SY. A comparison of gastro-oesophageal reflux in volunteers assessed by ambulatory pH and gamma monitoring after treatment with either liquid Gaviscon or Algicon suspension. Aliment Pharmacol Ther 1992;6:579

108. Washington N, et al. The effect of inclusion of aluminum hydroxide in alginate-containing raft-forming antacids. Int J Pharmacol 1986; 28:139

109. Weberg R, Berstad A. Symptomatic effect of a low dose antacid regimen in reflux oesophagitis. Scand J Gastroenterol 1989;24:401

110. Weihrauch TR. Gatsro-oesophageal reflux: pathogenesis and clinical implications. Eur J Pediatr 1985;144:215

111. Williams DL, Haigh GG, Redfern JN. The symptomatic treatment of heartburn and dyspepsia with liquid Gaviscon: a multicentre general practitioner study. J Int Med Res 1979;7:551

112. Wright LE, Castell DO. The adverse effect of chocolate on lower esophageal sphincter pressure. Dig Dis 1975;20:703

113. Yong GP, et al. Treatment of reflux oesophagitis with a carbenoxolone/antacid/alginate preparation: a double-blind controlled trial. Scand J Gastroenterol 1986;21:1098

*The Esophagus*, Third Edition,
edited by D. O. Castell and J. E. Richter.
Lippincott Williams & Wilkins, Philadelphia © 1999.

CHAPTER 25

# Medical Management of Gastroesophageal Reflux Disease

Malcolm Robinson

When the last edition of this text was prepared, this chapter described a decade of relative constancy in the treatment of gastroesophageal reflux disease (GERD). Since GERD affects up to 10% of the general population, its treatment is an important medical issue. Accepted antireflux therapy has certainly changed recently, and there have been a number of important advances in our understanding of GERD and its treatment. Nevertheless, GERD can still be considered as a continuum, ranging from mild heartburn to serious complications, such as severe erosive esophagitis, stricture, and Barrett's esophagus. Most authorities recommend a stepwise approach to the management of GERD, beginning with simple therapeutic modalities and graduating to more potent or more aggressive modalities as required [28]. Conservative therapy for mild GERD remains appropriate, including lifestyle modifications (elevated head of bed, no late heavy meals, as well as avoidance of those specific foods and medications that may worsen reflux) along with antacids and over-the-counter (OTC) histamine $H_2$-receptor antagonists (H2RAs). A few years ago, H2RAs were the "gold standard" of antireflux therapy. Although these medications remain extremely useful for GERD symptoms and for milder forms of this disease complex, they have been largely superseded by the proton pump inhibitors (PPIs), or $H^+,K^+$-adenosine triphosphatase (ATPase), inhibitors for treatment of more serious forms of reflux disease. Prokinetic therapy with agents such as cisapride and domperidone has an expanded role, most useful in mild GERD. Prokinetics seem most appropriate when associated symptoms suggest dysmotility and when gastroparesis is present. In rare instances of PPI resistance or in young patients with GERD who prefer not to continue long-term medical management, antireflux surgery has assumed a more prominent role. Enthusiasm for surgical intervention in GERD has also grown as a result of the lowered morbidity and mortality associated with laparoscopic procedures.

Therapeutic options for GERD include a number of antacids. Chewed tablet antacids appear to be particularly effective for maintaining elevated esophageal pH for up to 90 minutes [26]. Despite the "low-tech" professional view of antacids, they are quite popular with heartburn sufferers, and they should be recommended for symptom relief in individuals who have not already utilized them on their own.

There are four H2RAs marketed in the United States, several PPIs, and a growing roster of prokinetic agents. A strong argument can be made for eliciting the specific pathophysiology in individual patients and adjusting therapy to meet the requirements of the variable presentations of reflux disease. There has been a regrettable tendency to assume that the most potent and newest treatment for any disorder will always be the best option since most patients will respond admirably to more modest therapeutic modalities. Despite commercial promotions, physicians should exercise good judgment in the selection of conservative therapies and available medications for their patients. The rationale for conservative measures such as lifestyle changes for the treatment of GERD has been outlined by Kitchin and Castell [59].

Since GERD is chronic in most instances, it can be considered along with other longstanding disorders, such as atherosclerotic cardiovascular disease, diabetes mellitus, and hypertension. Maintenance therapy is therefore an important issue. Cost-benefit ratios must be carefully considered for acute and maintenance therapy, and better data are needed to guide selection of treatment, particularly chronic medical therapy versus surgery. Unfortunately, many studies addressing cost containment entail the participation of companies and/or authors with strong commercial biases. Therefore, proposed regimens and cost-benefit data may be unreliable and not necessarily reflect the effects of treatment

M. Robinson: Division of Gastroenterology, Department of Medicine, University of Oklahoma Teaching Hospitals, Oklahoma City, Oklahoma 73104.

on quality of life (QOL) or be consistent with rigorous assumptions regarding the natural history of GERD.

Although changes in available agents and the rapidly evolving literature guarantee that the discussion which follows will be incomplete, this chapter will attempt to provide an update on GERD treatment which is as current as possible.

## PRINCIPLES OF TREATMENT

The objectives of treatment are continued relief of symptoms, avoidance of complications, and, with far less certainty, healing of the esophageal mucosa [50]. Esophageal mucosal damage has been demonstrated in 40% to 65% of symptomatic GERD patients [8, 105, 114, 129], with abnormal esophageal histology in 94% [8]. Microscopic changes range from neutrophilic or eosinophilic infiltrates to clear-cut erosions, ulcerations, strictures, and metaplastic columnar epithelium. Recent studies have focused on symptomatic patients with normal or erythematous but otherwise intact esophageal mucosa. For such "endoscopy-negative" patients, the sole therapeutic objective is alleviation of symptoms.

All authorities agree that GERD results from disturbances in esophageal motility [93], involving abnormalities in the coordinated gastrointestinal (GI) neuromuscular activity which ordinarily prevents pathologic reflux. If abnormal motility underlies GERD, prokinetic therapy seems imminently rational to correct such reflux-provoking pathophysiologies as decreased lower esophageal sphincter (LES) pressure and impaired esophageal clearance mechanisms. Impaired gastric emptying may also merit correction in the relatively infrequent instances when it contributes to GERD. Unfortunately, although useful for some dysmotility, usual prokinetic drugs do not improve the transient lower esophageal sphincter relaxations (tLESRs) that produce most reflux episodes.

The central role of motility abnormalities in the pathogenesis of GERD has been universally accepted, but it is equally clear that prolonged esophageal mucosal exposure to acid and pepsin ultimately causes both reflux symptoms and esophageal mucosal injury. Symptoms and pathology worsen with increasing esophageal acid contact time (percentage exposure to esophageal pH less than 4 over a 24-hour period) [9, 57, 106]. Antisecretory agents such as H2RAs and $H^+,K^+$-ATPase inhibitors act by suppressing gastric acid secretion, thereby reducing the acidity and volume of potential refluxate.

When esophageal acid contact time is normalized, symptoms remit and damaged mucosa heals. Complete clinical success often requires control of both daytime and nocturnal acidity, particularly in more severe disease [9, 17].

Future research will further elucidate details of factors that may produce or exacerbate GERD. Duodenogastric reflux remains a subject of controversy [136]. Other GERD-related abnormalities might include increased esophageal mucosal permeability and such impaired defense mechanisms as deficient production of bicarbonate-rich esophageal submucosal gland secretions and epidermal growth factor [54, 86].

*Helicobacter pylori* appears to have no pathogenic role in reflux disease [93, 138]. However, recent controversial studies suggest that reflux symptoms may be exacerbated by the eradication of *H. pylori* [65].

## H₂-RECEPTOR ANTAGONISTS

H2RAs were once the cornerstone of the pharmacologic treatment of GERD and were the standards against which newer compounds were compared. They remain useful for the treatment of GERD symptoms and can help heal mild-to-moderate erosive esophagitis. Four H2RAs are currently available for clinical use: cimetidine (Tagamet), famotidine (Pepcid), ranitidine (Zantac), and nizatidine (Axid). By binding competitively to $H_2$ receptors in the gastric parietal cell, these agents inhibit basal and stimulated acid secretion and, consequently, peptic activity. Conventional doses reduce acid secretion by 60% to 70% [58].

### Standard-Dose Therapy

Of the available H2RAs, cimetidine and ranitidine have been the most extensively studied in GERD. Early (1978 to 1983) trials of cimetidine 1,000 to 1,600 mg per day in divided doses for 6 to 8 weeks confirmed rapid symptom relief in five of ten trials, decreased antacid consumption in five of eight studies, and improved esophagitis in three of ten trials [10]. Trials (1982 to 1987) of ranitidine 150 mg b.i.d. for 6 to 8 weeks demonstrated more consistent symptom relief, decreased antacid consumption, and endoscopically verified improvement or healing of esophagitis [10, 124]. Improved results compared with cimetidine were consistent with the greater potency and more prolonged acid suppression of ranitidine. In a trial involving 284 patients (62% with erosive esophagitis), ranitidine 150 mg b.i.d. decreased nocturnal and daytime heartburn and improved endoscopic findings compared with placebo [122]. Ranitidine healed erosive esophagitis in 56% of patients compared with 41% for placebo. Ranitidine has been very successful from the commercial standpoint, probably because of its wide acceptance as effective in GERD, clearly the most important indication for H2RA use.

Although famotidine is the most potent available H2RA, routine famotidine doses in GERD have comparable antisecretory effects to usual doses of ranitidine and nizatidine. Clinical studies of famotidine in GERD are fewer than studies of its competitors [102, 111]. Famotidine 20 mg b.i.d. for 12 weeks reduced symptoms and healed esophagitis better than placebo in 338 patients with grades 0 to 4 esophagitis [111]; famotidine 40 mg at bedtime surpassed placebo but was less effective numerically than the 20 mg b.i.d. dose.

Nizatidine was effective in a controlled trial of 466 esophagitis patients [21]. Nizatidine 150 mg b.i.d. reduced heartburn severity and led to modestly improved healing compared with placebo at 6 and 12 weeks. In contrast, nizatidine 300 mg hs was ineffective at healing esophagitis.

There have been relatively few trials comparing H2RAs in GERD. Symptomatic and endoscopic responses were similar in a comparison in 22 patients taking cimetidine 400 mg b.i.d. or ranitidine 150 mg b.i.d. for 8 weeks [32].

In general, when administered in equivalent antisecretory doses, H2RAs are equally efficacious. Short-term therapy usually alleviates reflux symptoms, decreases antacid consumption, and promotes healing of mild-to-moderate esophagitis. In a large review [124], H2RA therapy for 6 to 12 weeks relieved reflux symptoms in about half of patients. Endoscopic improvement was documented in 31% to 88% of patients by meta-analysis [10]. Esophagitis healed completely in 27% to 45% of patients, primarily those with grade 1 or 2 lesions [10].

Healing rates in individual studies differ substantially, presumably correlating with esophagitis severity in various patient populations. Other factors confounding clinical trial interpretation include lack of uniform endoscopy grading systems. Standard ulcer-healing doses of H2RAs may not completely heal acid-injured esophageal mucosa in all patients, particularly those with severe esophagitis. In particular, once-nightly regimens are unlikely to be effective. In contrast to peptic ulcer disease, therapeutic efficacy in GERD depends on almost complete acid inhibition over the full 24-hour period. Single nocturnal dosing of H2RAs does not adequately control pH, nor will a single nighttime dose abolish daytime symptoms, which often occur postprandially and in the early evening [9]. While standard doses of H2RAs may be effective for mild-to-moderate GERD, many patients with moderate-to-severe (grades 2 to 4) esophagitis may not heal, and some will remain symptomatic.

### High-Dose Therapy

With recognition of the benefits of profound acid suppression for relief of symptoms and healing of erosive esophagitis, higher doses or more frequently administered H2RAs, or both, have been evaluated in clinical trials (Table 25–1). Limited data from such studies seem to support improved symptom control and mucosal healing with cimetidine 800 mg b.i.d.; ranitidine 150 or 300 mg q.i.d., famotidine 40 mg b.i.d., and nizatidine 300 mg b.i.d.

Trials in Europe and the United States using ranitidine 150 and 300 mg q.i.d. have demonstrated endoscopic healing rates of 62% to 70% at 8 weeks and 74% to 83% at 12 weeks [29, 75, 108, 118]. In addition, higher-dose H2RA regimens led to better symptom control and decreased antacid use. Although expensive, the "double" dose of ranitidine 150 mg q.i.d. is more affordable than the similarly efficacious quadruple regimen of 300 mg q.i.d. Double doses famotidine and nizatidine as well as cimetidine 800 mg b.i.d. have 12-week healing rates of 67% to 76% versus 36% for placebo [20, 75, 89, 119, 141].

Esophagitis healing correlates with decreased esophageal acid exposure and duration of antisecretory therapy [10].

**TABLE 25–1.** *Effect of high-dose H$_2$-receptor antagonists on healing of reflux esophagitis*

| Author | Grade of pretreatment esophagitis | n | Regimens | Duration (wk) | Endoscopic healing rates | | | | Comments |
|---|---|---|---|---|---|---|---|---|---|
| | | | | | Week 4 | Week 6 | Week 8 | Week 12 | |
| McCarty-Dawson et al., 1996 [75] | 2–4 (adapted Hetzel; 94% grades 2–4) | 229 | RAN 150 mg q.i.d. | 12 | 49%* | — | 67%* | 77%* | *p < 0.02 vs. CIM |
| | | 236 | RAN 150 mg b.i.d. | | 38% | — | 56% | 71% | |
| | | 231 | CIM 800 mg b.i.d. | | 37% | — | 52% | 68% | |
| Silver et al., 1996 [118] | Erosive esophagitis | 772$^a$ | RAN 300 mg b.i.d. | 12 | NA | — | 51%*† | 66%*† | *p ≤ 0.004 vs. PLA |
| | | | RAN 150 mg q.i.d. | | 37%‡ | — | 62%‡ | 77%‡ | †p ≤ 0.041 vs. RAN 150 |
| | | | PLA | | 21% | — | 36% | 52% | ‡p < 0.001 vs. PLA |
| Euler et al., 1993 [29] | 2–4 (adapted Hetzel; 89% grades 2–3) | 106 | RAN 300 mg q.i.d. | 12 | 47%* | — | 62%* | 74%* | *p < 0.001 vs. PLA |
| | | 106 | RAN 150 mg q.i.d. | | 45%* | — | 69%* | 79%* | |
| | | 116 | PLA | | 19% | — | 28% | 40% | |
| Simon et al., 1993 [119] | 2–4 (95% grades 2–3); strictures in 4%, 9%, 6% | 175 | FAM 40 mg b.i.d. | 12 | — | 48% | — | 71%* | *p ≤ 0.05 vs. RAN |
| | | 93 | FAM 20 mg b.i.d. | | — | 52% | — | 68% | |
| | | 172 | RAN 150 mg b.i.d. | | — | 42% | — | 60% | |
| Wesdorp et al., 1993 [141] | 1–4 (77% grades 1–2) | 223 | FAM 40 mg b.i.d. | 12 | — | 58%* | — | 76%* | *p < 0.05 |
| | | 220 | FAM 20 mg b.i.d. | | — | 43% | — | 67% | |
| Cloud and Offen, 1992 [20] | 1–4 (59% grades 2–3) | 169 | NIZ 300 mg b.i.d. | 6 | 17% | 39%† | — | — | *p ≤ 0.05 vs. PLA$^b$ |
| | | 168 | NIZ 150 mg b.i.d. | | 20%* | 41%† | — | — | †p < 0.001 vs. PLA$^b$ |
| | | 178 | PLA | | 12% | 26% | — | — | |
| Roufail et al., 1992 [108] | 2–4 (adapted Hetzel; 87% grades 2–3) | 120 | RAN 300 mg q.i.d. | 12 | 46%* | — | 70%* | 81%* | *p ≤ 0.001 vs. PLA |
| | | 109 | RAN 150 mg q.i.d. | | 45%* | — | 68%* | 83%* | |
| | | 113 | PLA | | 20% | — | 33% | 58% | |
| Palmer et al., 1990 [89] | Erosive or ulcerative esophagitis (not graded; ulcers in 49% and 42%) | 93 | CIM 800 mg b.i.d. | 12 | — | 50%* | — | 67%* | *p < 0.01 |
| | | 86 | PLA | | — | 20% | — | 36% | |

CIM, cimetidine; FAM, famotidine; NA, not available; NIZ, nizatidine; PLA, placebo; RAN, ranitidine.
$^a$ Number of patients entered into study.
$^b$ Three-week healing rates were calculated, not 4-week rates.

Clinical trials and metaanalyses confirm dose-response relationships between acid suppression by famotidine and ranitidine and total esophageal acid contact time [55, 87, 109]. One multicenter study demonstrated enhanced healing of grade 3 or 4 esophagitis after 12 weeks versus 8 weeks, although more than 80% of patients with less severe (grade 2) esophagitis healed in 8 weeks [108]. Prolonged high-dose H2RA treatment for 24 weeks failed to heal erosive esophagitis unhealed after 12 weeks [141].

Since some patients with GERD have increased gastric acid secretion, an argument can be made for more aggressive antisecretory therapy in such individuals. Graduated therapy designed to attain normal acid secretion and normal esophageal acid exposure is a reasonable therapeutic goal. Hypersecretion was prospectively demonstrated in a subset of a large group of patients with heartburn (19%) and/or erosive esophagitis (28%) and Barrett's esophagus (35%) [22]. Basal acid output exceeding 10 mEq per hour correlated with the need for increased H2RA doses to control GERD.

Nevertheless, most patients attain symptom relief and relevant healing with conventional H2RA doses. Standard b.i.d. doses are still appropriate for GERD. Higher or more frequent doses have been used with more severe grades of esophagitis resistant to standard regimens. In the late 1990s, most gastroenterologists use PPI therapy when standard doses of H2RAs fail.

## Safety Profile

As a class, H2RAs have been among the most frequently used and safest drugs. The overall incidence of adverse reactions is low and similar to placebo, totaling about 4%. Potential drug–drug interactions have been a source of concern [30, 72]. Cimetidine, an imidazole compound, can inhibit hepatic metabolism of coadministered drugs via reversible binding to mixed-function oxidases of the cytochrome P450 (CYP) system. Potential adverse clinical effects seem most likely to occur with coadministration of drugs with a narrow therapeutic index, such as phenytoin, theophylline, and warfarin. Compared with cimetidine, ranitidine binds less avidly to CYP enzymes, while famotidine and nizatidine do not bind to this enzyme system. The dangers of drug–drug interactions have probably been overemphasized. Despite some concerns to the contrary, H2RAs do not alter serum ethanol levels after moderate alcohol intake [95].

There are fewer data on the safety experience with high-dose H2RAs. Adverse events in efficacy trials were similar to those with placebo [20, 29, 89, 108, 118]. High doses of cimetidine and, to a lesser extent, ranitidine have been associated with elevated serum prolactin levels, which rarely result in gynecomastia [30].

## H$^+$,K$^+$-ATPASE INHIBITORS/PROTON PUMP INHIBITORS

Hydrochloric acid secretion by gastric parietal cells ultimately depends on the proton pump, an enzyme called H$^+$,K$^+$-ATPase, the final common step in the acid secretory pathway. H$^+$,K$^+$-ATPase inhibitors bind to the proton pump and profoundly suppress basal and stimulated acid secretion. A single dose of omeprazole may inhibit 24-hour acid secretion by more than 90% [116].

Large numbers of clinical reports deal with omeprazole (Prilosec) and lansoprazole (Prevacid), a substituted benzimidazole similar to omeprazole (Table 25–2). Results with a third H$^+$,K$^+$-ATPase inhibitor, pantoprazole, have also been released. Rabeprazole may well emerge as an important new PPI [99]. Rabeprazole appears to have a particularly rapid onset of action and enhanced potency. Based on a metaanalysis of GERD studies from 1984 to 1996, PPIs heal endoscopically confirmed esophagitis in more patients than other antireflux agents do (84% vs. 52% for H2RAs, 39% for sucralfate, and 28% for placebo), regardless of drug dose or treatment duration (for up to 12 weeks) [17]. Esophagitis healed faster with PPIs than with H2RAs. PPIs also provided faster, more complete relief of heartburn.

## Omeprazole

A U.S. study evaluated omeprazole in 230 symptomatic patients with grades 2 to 4 esophagitis (56% with grade 3 or 4) [125]. Omeprazole 20 or 40 mg daily for up to 8 weeks was superior to placebo for complete symptom relief as well as esophagitis healing at 4 and 8 weeks. Antacid use was greatly reduced in both groups. Although the study failed to demonstrate significantly greater efficacy with 40 mg than with 20 mg, this finding may be related to study size or sampling error. Similarly, prolonged esophageal pH studies performed in our laboratory did not differentiate the acid-lowering effects of 20 and 40 mg [101]. This result also may have been related to small sample size. Differing from the U.S. study, an international study showed that omeprazole 40 mg per day was more effective than 20 mg per day in healing esophagitis [46]. An international pH study, conducted in a population similar to the one in the U.S. study, demonstrated a statistically significant reduction in 24-hour esophageal acid exposure with 40 versus 20 mg [90]. These findings seem most consistent with our current understanding of PPI pharmacology.

As is true for the H2RAs, cumulative omeprazole healing rates were lower with higher grades of esophagitis [43, 46]. For example, after 4, 8, and 12 weeks of treatment with omeprazole 40 mg per day, grade 1 esophagitis healed in 90%, 90%, and 100% of patients, respectively. In grades 2 and 3 esophagitis, the proportions healed were 70%, 85%, and 91% [43].

Results of five double-blind trials demonstrated improved symptom relief and esophageal histology with omeprazole 20 and 40 mg per day compared with ranitidine 150 mg b.i.d. [106].

In 98 patients with unhealed erosive esophagitis after 3 months of treatment with cimetidine (>1,200 mg per day)

**TABLE 25-2.** *Effect of proton pump inhibitors on healing of reflux esophagitis*

| Author | Grade of pretreatment esophagitis | n | Regimens | Duration (wk) | Endoscopic healing rates | | | | | Comments |
|--------|-----------------------------------|---|----------|---------------|-------|-------|-------|-------|-------|----------|
| | | | | | Week 2 | Week 4 | Week 6 | Week 8 | Week 12 | |
| Sontag et al., 1997 [128] | ≥2; H2RA-resistant | 105 | LAN 30 mg q.AM[a] | 8 | 63%* | 75%* | — | 84%* | — | *p < 0.001 vs. RAN |
| | | 54 | RAN 150 mg b.i.d. | | 27% | 43% | — | 32% | — | |
| Castell et al., 1996 [16] | Erosive esophagitis | 422 | LAN 30 mg once daily | 8 | 65%*† | 83%*† | 89%*† | 90%*† | — | *p < 0.001 vs. PLA |
| | | 218 | LAN 15 mg once daily | | 56%* | 75%* | 80%* | 79%* | — | †p < 0.05 vs. LAN 15 |
| | | 431 | OME 20 mg once daily | | 61%* | 82%*‡ | 90%*‡ | 91%*‡ | — | ‡SS vs. LAN 15 |
| | | 213 | PLA | | 24% | 33% | 37% | 40% | — | |
| Bardhan et al., 1995 [6] | Reflux esophagitis | 229[b] | LAN 60 mg once daily | 8 | — | 72%* | — | 91%* | — | *p < 0.01 vs. RAN |
| | | | LAN 30 mg once daily | | — | 84%* | — | 92%* | — | |
| | | | RAN 150 mg b.i.d. | | — | 39% | — | 53% | — | |
| Corinaldesi et al., 1995 [23] | 2–3 (82% grade 2) | 120 | PAN 40 mg once daily | 8 | — | 79% | — | 94% | — | NS |
| | | 121 | OME 20 mg once daily | | — | 79% | — | 91% | — | |
| Koop et al., 1995 [63] | 2–3 (80% and 81% grade 2) | 166 | PAN 40 mg once daily | 8 | — | 69% | — | 82%* | — | *p < 0.01 vs. PLA (per protocol)[c] |
| | | 83 | RAN 150 mg b.i.d. | | — | 57% | — | 67% | — | |
| Robinson et al., 1995 [100] | 1–4 (62% grades 3–4); H2RA-resistant | 27[d] | LAN 60 mg q.AM | 12 | 62% | 77% | 89% | 89% | 89% | NS |
| | | 23[d] | LAN 30 mg q.AM | | 57% | 87% | 91% | 96% | 100% | |
| Feldman et al., 1993 [31] | ≥2; H2RA-resistant | 62 | LAN 30 mg q.AM | 8 | 71%* | 80%* | 88%* | 89%* | — | *p < 0.001 |
| | | 33 | RAN 300 mg b.i.d. | | 21% | 33% | 45% | 38% | — | |
| Sontag et al., 1992 [125] | ≥2 | 91 | OME 40 mg q.AM | 8 | — | 45%* | — | 75%* | — | *p ≤ 0.01 vs. PLA |
| | | 93 | OME 20 mg q.AM | | — | 39%* | — | 74%* | — | |
| | | 46 | PLA | | — | 7% | — | 14% | — | |
| Lundell et al., 1990 [73] | ≥2 (22% and 15% had Barrett's or stricture); H2RA-resistant | 51 | OME 40 mg q.AM | 12 | — | 63%* | — | 86%* | 90%† | *p < 0.05 |
| | | 47 | RAN 300 mg b.i.d. | | — | 17% | — | 38% | 47% | †p < 0.0001 |
| Hetzel et al., 1988 [46] | ≥2 (48% and 37% had columnar esophageal mucosa or stricture) | 82 | OME 40 mg q.AM | 8 | — | 82%* | — | 85% | — | *p = 0.05 |
| | | 82 | OME 20 mg q.AM | | — | 70% | — | 79% | — | |

H2RA, H₂-receptor antagonist; LAN, lansoprazole; NS, not statistically significant; OME, omeprazole; PAN, pantoprazole; PLA, placebo; RAN, ranitidine; SS, statistically significant.

[a] After 4 weeks, patients received LAN 30 mg q.AM or LAN 60 mg q.AM for another 4 weeks.

[b] Number of patients entered into study.

[c] Intent-to-treat healing rates of 62% (PAN) and 47% (RAN) at 4 weeks ($p < 0.05$) and 74% (PAN) and 55% (RAN) at 8 weeks.

[d] Number of evaluable patients.

or ranitidine (>300 mg per day), omeprazole 40 mg q.AM improved healing compared with ranitidine 300 mg b.i.d. at 4, 8, and 12 weeks (63% versus 17%, 86% versus 38%, and 90% versus 47%, respectively) [73]. Complete heartburn relief occurred earlier with omeprazole (86% versus 32% at 4 weeks). Omeprazole 40 mg per day for 8 weeks has been shown to heal severe esophagitis in more than 80% of patients resistant to high-dose H2RAs [79]. In 61 patients with grade 3 or 4 esophagitis, 30% did not heal with omeprazole 20 mg, while 15% did not heal with 40 mg [49]. Refractory patients had documented persistence of nocturnal reflux, and nonhealing correlated with inadequate acid suppression. Hendel et al. [44] healed esophagitis in all patients by increasing PPI doses to completely control esophageal acid exposure (<3.4%).

At least 10% of patients are refractory even to multiple daily doses of omeprazole [60]. Omeprazole resistance varies by study and is totally unpredictable in individual patients. Lack of response may be due to a variable combination of inadequate gastric acid suppression, LES incompetence, and esophageal dysmotility. In 19 patients with such severely refractory esophagitis, complications such as hemorrhage and stricture, Barrett's esophagus, and failed antireflux surgery were common [60].

The effect of various dosing schedules of omeprazole 40 mg per day on gastric acid exposure was studied in 19 healthy volunteers [64]. Omeprazole 40 mg was administered for 7 days with breakfast, at dinner, or in 20-mg twice-daily regimens. Twice-daily dosing prolonged intragastric pH of greater than 4.0 (77% of 24 hours) compared with either single-dose schedule (67% of 24 hours). The 40-mg once-daily schedules did not differ in effect on 24-hour intragastric acidity. Omeprazole 20 mg b.i.d. is the optimal dosing for patients unresponsive to a single morning dose [64].

## Safety Profile

Omeprazole is well tolerated in the short term. The incidence of adverse events with omeprazole resembles the incidences with H2RAs (about 1%) and placebo (0.8% to 1.4%) [79]. Serum gastrin elevations persisted 2 weeks after treatment with omeprazole 20 and 40 mg [125]. No clinically significant adverse events or laboratory abnormalities have been attributed to omeprazole. Omeprazole is a potent inhibitor of a specific CYP enzyme. While drug interactions have been reported with diazepam, phenytoin, antipyrine, aminopyrine, and coumarin, significant pharmacologic inhibition appears unlikely with dosages of less than 30 mg per day. Indeed, drug–drug interactions with the whole class of PPIs are clinically insignificant at any dose utilized in benign disease.

Longer-term safety experience with omeprazole 20 to 40 mg per day resembles the short-term data [74]. Nevertheless, there are some lingering concerns regarding PPI therapy, including possible intragastric bacterial overgrowth and susceptibility to GI infections. The clinical significance of hypergastrinemia remains unclear. Marked hypochlorhydria could result in bacteria-mediated nitrosamine production, a potential risk factor for gastric cancer. Sharma et al. [117] found elevated total bacterial cell counts, nitrate concentrations, and N-nitrosamine concentrations in gastric juice but no change in the proportion of bacterial species after administration of omeprazole 30 mg per day. Similarly high bacterial counts have been documented recently in elderly patients with drug-induced hypochlorhydria [92]. Rodent studies demonstrated gastric enterochromaffin-like (ECL) cell hyperplasia and carcinoid formation after lifelong high-dose omeprazole. Evaluation of gastric endocrine cells in patients on long-term omeprazole revealed no increased volume density of ECL cells or dysplastic or neoplastic lesions [24, 121]. As yet, no PPI has been found to be responsible for carcinoid development in humans.

Omeprazole seems safe for long-term treatment of GERD, and safety concerns thus far remain entirely theoretical. Data confirm the bioavailability and effectiveness of omeprazole granules administered via nasogastric tube, an important issue in critically ill patients who may require antisecretory therapy [4, 67].

### Lansoprazole

Lansoprazole 15 to 60 mg per day has been evaluated in placebo- and ranitidine-controlled trials. Lansoprazole 30 mg per day produced 4-week healing rates of 80% to 84% and 8-week rates of 89% to 92% compared with 39% to 52% at 4 weeks and 53% to 70% at 8 weeks. For ranitidine 150 mg b.i.d. Greater symptom improvement also was attained with lansoprazole [6, 66, 100]. Lansoprazole also healed esophagitis refractory to 12 weeks of standard-dose H2RAs. In one trial [31], 95 H2RA-resistant patients with grades 2 to 4 esophagitis (47% with grade 3 or 4) received lansoprazole 30 mg per day or ranitidine 150 mg b.i.d. Lansoprazole healed 89% of patients at 8 weeks (versus 38%), achieved impressive early healing (by week 2), and was more effective at reducing heartburn and antacid use. Com-

plete mucosal healing was achieved in 18 of 22 patients with severe (grade 3 or 4) esophagitis and 16 of 17 patients with Barrett's esophagus. In another U.S. trial [128], 159 patients with at least grade 2 esophagitis resistant to 3 or more months of standard-dose H2RAs received ranitidine 150 mg b.i.d. for 8 weeks or lansoprazole 30 mg for 4 weeks followed by lansoprazole 30 or 60 mg for another 4 weeks. Healing rates with lansoprazole were significantly higher after 2, 4, and 8 weeks. In addition, lansoprazole was superior in terms of symptom relief.

In a study involving 1,284 patients [16], omeprazole 20 mg per day and lansoprazole 30 mg per day produced similar esophagitis healing rates at 4 and 8 weeks but earlier symptom relief was associated with use of lansoprazole. Effects of lansoprazole on acid suppression corroborate its apparent clinical superiority over omeprazole [131]. Antisecretory superiority has been reconfirmed, along with more rapid onset of acid control with lansoprazole [133]. A European study suggested that lansoprazole 30 mg seems comparable to omeprazole 40 mg in erosive esophagitis [84]. Lansoprazole dosing seems unaffected by coadministration of food, although early morning ante cibum dosing is recommended. Like omeprazole, lansoprazole can be administered as granules through a nasogastric tube [18].

### Safety Profile

Lansoprazole is well tolerated in short-term and long-term clinical trials. The number of adverse side effects with lansoprazole is comparable to those observed with placebo, ranitidine, and omeprazole [66]. In one U.S. trial, higher than normal fasting serum gastrin levels (>100 pg per mL) occurred in five of 54 patients pretreatment and in 14 of 54 after 8 weeks of lansoprazole 30 mg per day [31]. After lansoprazole 10 to 60 mg per day for 7 days, healthy volunteers had elevated postprandial serum gastrin levels compared with placebo; fasting gastrin levels normalized 7 days posttherapy [112]. No safety issues have developed with extensive additional clinical trials and a large lansoprazole post-marketing experience.

### Pantoprazole

Pantoprazole 40 mg per day effectively reduces gastric acid secretion. GERD studies have established an equivalence to omeprazole [23, 82] and superiority to ranitidine [63]. Pantoprazole is well tolerated with a benign side-effect profile and exhibits no clinically relevant drug–drug interactions due to its lower affinity for hepatic CYP [33]. Pantoprazole is said to have greater acid stability than other PPIs as well as more selective affinity for the "proton pumping" part of ATPase [51]. The properties of pantoprazole, relative to lansoprazole and rabeprazole in particular, require further investigation.

### Rabeprazole

Rabeprazole is similar to the other three PPIs described. Like lansoprazole, it seems to have a significantly faster onset of antisecretory activity than omeprazole [143]. In European and U.S. trials in GERD, rabeprazole has resembled ranitidine and omeprazole [19]. Early data suggest that low-dose rabeprazole may be particularly satisfactory in maintenance therapy. Additional trials will be important to fully delineate the niche for this PPI among its counterparts.

### Perprazole

Perprazole is an optical isomer of omeprazole currently under investigation for the full range of acid-peptic disorders. Its metabolism is different from that of omeprazole, and initial studies suggest more predictable antisecretory activity. There are important marketing issues in the development of this compound, and it is intended that perprazole may eventually replace omeprazole.

## PROKINETIC AGENTS

A prokinetic approach to antireflux treatment is supported by the knowledge that conservative measures, such as head-of-bed elevation and avoidance of "refluxogenic" foods or drugs, are effective because they partially correct impaired motility factors that also should respond to prokinetic drugs. Normalizing underlying dysmotility is a reasonable goal of antireflux treatment. However, while bethanechol and metoclopramide may relieve mild reflux symptoms, they have inconsistently healed esophagitis. The absence of clear-cut efficacy plus the potential for central nervous system and other adverse reactions seen with earlier prokinetic agents have limited their use. The introduction of cisapride, a prokinetic drug specifically approved for the relief of nocturnal heartburn, has generated renewed interest in this class of agents for the treatment of GERD.

The mechanisms by which prokinetic drugs exert their effects on GI smooth muscle are incompletely elucidated, but each current agent seems to have a unique pharmacology, accounting for variations in clinical efficacy and safety.

### Bethanechol

Bethanechol (Urecholine) acts on cholinergic receptors. This choline derivative increases LES pressure and esophageal peristaltic contractions but seems not to affect gastric emptying. A potential detriment of bethanechol is stimulation of gastric acid secretion.

Although bethanechol was better than placebo for reflux symptoms, definitive evidence is lacking for healing of esophagitis [94]. At 25 mg q.i.d., as suggested for the treatment of GERD, bethanechol can cause abdominal cramping, blurred vision, fatigue, and other cholinergic symptoms.

### Metoclopramide

Metoclopramide (Reglan and others) stimulates GI smooth muscle by a number of mechanisms. In addition to inhibiting dopamine receptors, this *p*-aminobenzoic acid derivative may stimulate acetylcholine release from intramural nerves. Metoclopramide increases LES pressure, enhances gastric emptying, and may coordinate GI motor activity. It appears not to affect esophageal contractions. Some, but not all, studies with metoclopramide showed improvement in reflux symptoms and modest degrees of endoscopic healing.

Metoclopramide inhibits dopamine receptors in the CNS and peripherally. Metoclopramide-induced hyperprolactinemia can produce galactorrhea and menstrual dysfunction in many patients. Antidopaminergic side effects, including lethargy, extrapyramidal motor effects, and even tardive dyskinesia, occur in up to 20% of patients [2]. Most gastroenterologists have abandoned metoclopramide due to its side effects. A prospective comparison of 51 patients on metoclopramide (average, 31 mg per day for 2.6 years) with 51 control subjects demonstrated tardive dyskinesia in 29% of metoclopramide recipients and 17.6% of nonusers [36]. The frequency and severity of metoclopramide-related extrapyramidal symptoms may have been considerably underestimated in the past, and these newer data suggest that such reactions may occur at much lower doses of metoclopramide than previously believed.

### Cisapride

Cisapride (Propulsid) appears to stimulate acetylcholine release by specific enteric nerves or may directly trigger neuromuscular activity in GI smooth muscle. This benzamide compound increases LES pressure in patients with hypotensive LES tone, heightens amplitude of esophageal peristaltic contractions, enhances gastric emptying, and improves antroduodenal coordination. Prokinetic actions may be mediated by an agonist effect on serotonin [specifically 5-hydroxytryptamine$_4$ (5-HT$_4$)] receptors [145].

Cisapride 10 or 20 mg q.i.d., before meals and at bedtime, and 20 mg b.i.d. has been evaluated in patients with moderate to severe heartburn and predominantly grades 1 to 2 esophagitis (Table 25–3). In one trial [96], cisapride consistently relieved reflux symptoms, with the 10 mg q.i.d. regimen producing significant improvements in daytime and nocturnal heartburn at 4 weeks compared with placebo. The higher-dosage regimen improved symptoms throughout the 12-week study. Antacid consumption fell with 20 mg q.i.d. After 12 weeks, cisapride 20 mg q.i.d., but not 10 mg q.i.d., significantly improved esophagitis compared with placebo. In retrospect, the selection of esophagitis patients for U.S. cisapride studies may have been unwise since subsequent experience has found this agent most useful in less severe GERD. European studies [5] have always seemed to provide better results for erosive esophagitis than U.S. trials.

The severity of daytime and nocturnal heartburn and other reflux symptoms (regurgitation, eructation, and early satiety) improved with cisapride 20 mg b.i.d. in a 4-week U.S. placebo-controlled study [14]. European studies demonstrated that cisapride 20 mg b.i.d. for 8 to 12 weeks is comparable to 10 mg q.i.d. for controlling reflux symptoms and healing

**TABLE 25–3.** *Effect of cisapride on healing of reflux esophagitis*

| Author | Grade of pretreatment esophagitis | n | Regimens | Duration (wk) | 12-Week endoscopic healing rates | Comments |
|---|---|---|---|---|---|---|
| Schutze et al., 1997 [115] | 1–2 | 205 | CIS 20 mg b.i.d. | 8–12 | 73%[a] | NS |
| | | 202 | CIS 10 mg q.i.d. | | 73%[a] | |
| Richter and Long, 1995 [96] | 1–4 (70% grades 1–2) | 61 | CIS 20 mg q.i.d. | 12 | 51%* | *p ≤ 0.044 vs. PLA |
| | | 56 | CIS 10 mg q.i.d. | | 41% | |
| | | 60 | PLA | | 36% | |
| Geldof et al., 1993 [37] | 1–3 (81% grades 1–2) | 55 | CIS 20 mg b.i.d. | 8–12 | 71%[a,b] | NS |
| | | 49 | CIS 10 mg q.i.d. | | 52%[a,b] | |
| | | 51 | RAN 150 mg b.i.d. | | 80%[a,b] | |
| Baldi et al., 1988 [5] | 1–2 | 21 | CIS 10 mg q.i.d. | 12 | 63%* | *p = 0.005 |
| | | 19 | PLA | | 12% | |
| Janisch et al., 1988 [53] | 1–2 | 28 | CIS 10 mg q.i.d. | 6–12 | 89%[a] | NS |
| | | 28 | RAN 150 mg b.i.d. | | 79%[a] | |

CIS, cisapride; PLA, placebo; RAN, ranitidine; NS, not statistically significant.

[a] Healing rate at study end point.

[b] Healing rates in patients with pretreatment grades 1–2.

grades 1 to 2 esophagitis [115]. Cisapride 10 mg q.i.d. and 20 mg b.i.d. is comparable to ranitidine 150 mg b.i.d. in improving mild-to-moderate (grade 1 or 2) esophagitis [37, 53].

Cisapride appears to be safe and well tolerated. International experience suggests that the overall incidence of adverse events is similar to that with placebo (13.7% versus 11.2%, respectively) [145]. Notably absent are the CNS side effects associated with metoclopramide. Cisapride is metabolized in the liver by the isoenzyme CYP3A4. There has been recent concern about development of potentially serious tachyarrhythmias when cisapride is coadministered with drugs that inhibit CYP3A4, such as certain antifungal drugs (fluconazole, itraconazole, ketoconazole) and macrolide antibiotics (clarithromycin, erythromycin) [25]. Cisapride is contraindicated in patients who are taking drugs that are metabolized by CYP3A4 or that prolong the QT interval on the electrocardiogram. Cisapride should also be given with extreme caution to patients known to have unstable ischemic heart diseases, hypokalemia, hypomagnesemia, and other disorders predisposing them to cardiac arrhythmias.

### Investigational Prokinetic Agents

#### Domperidone

Like metoclopramide, domperidone (Motilium) blocks dopamine receptors. However, this benzimidazole derivative does not easily or completely cross the blood–brain barrier and is primarily a peripheral dopamine antagonist. Oral domperidone at clinical doses produces variable effects on LES pressure and esophageal peristalsis but does enhance gastric emptying in a dose-dependent manner. This agent is thought to be particularly helpful in patients who complain of nausea.

Studies in GERD with domperidone 60 to 80 mg daily in t.i.d. or q.i.d. regimens have produced equivocal results, with a few reports of symptom improvement and esophagitis healing [94]. Some comparative trials showed similar efficacy between domperidone and famotidine or ranitidine.

Domperidone is associated with few significant side effects and is relatively free of extrapyramidal and other CNS side effects. However, hyperprolactinemia may occur in 10% to 15% of patients, giving rise to breast enlargement, galactorrhea, and amenorrhea.

#### Erythromycin

The macrolide antibiotic erythromycin stimulates GI muscle activity, probably due to motilin agonist properties. Erythromycin 250 mg t.i.d. orally increases postprandial LES pressure and strikingly improves gastric emptying but shows no effect on esophageal peristalsis.

Use of oral erythromycin in GERD has led to variable and somewhat disappointing results. Limiting factors include a significant incidence of side effects, such as nausea, vomiting, and abdominal cramping; the potential for drug–drug interactions; and the possible development of drug tolerance.

Several new motilides are under development. They are intended to have prokinetic effects without any antibiotic properties, and it is hoped that they will lack the propensity for tolerance sometimes associated with erythromycin.

#### Mosapride

Mosapride is an investigational prokinetic agent with 5-$HT_4$ receptor agonist activity and some properties of 5-$HT_3$ antagonism. Recent studies have shown that mosapride effectively decreases total esophageal acid exposure and the number of reflux episodes [110].

### MUCOSAL PROTECTIVE AND OTHER AGENTS

#### Sucralfate

Sucralfate (Carafate), a sulfated disaccharide complex with aluminum, has been infrequently studied in GERD. A nonsystemic agent, sucralfate might act by adhering to the esophageal mucosal surface, providing a physical barrier against the injurious effects of refluxed gastric contents. It has minimal gastric buffering action, does not modify gastric acid or pepsin secretion, and does not affect LES pressure or other motor functions.

In European trials, acute therapy with liquid sucralfate 1 g q.i.d. was superior to placebo and comparable to antacids and standard-dose H2RAs (cimetidine 400 mg q.i.d. and ranitidine 150 mg b.i.d.) for control of symptoms and healing of low-grade esophagitis [40]. Sucralfate achieved esophagitis healing rates of 54% to 72% at 12 weeks, compared with 40% to 41% for placebo [40]. In a pilot study, sucralfate 4 g per day for 4 to 6 months healed esophagitis in six of eight patients with complicated GERD previously unhealed with H2RAs [107].

If supported by additional trials, these findings would indicate that esophageal epithelial resistance is important in refractory GERD and that sucralfate might enhance esophageal mucosal defenses. However, a large, well-designed U.S. multicenter trial showed no symptomatic improvement or healing after 8 weeks of sucralfate suspension [144]. Further investigation is needed to delineate the role, if any, of sucralfate and similar coating agents in GERD. Interest in this agent has decreased in recent years.

## Other Agents

While anticholinergic drugs reduce gastric acid secretion, they also can depress LES and upper GI motor function and, thus, at least theoretically should be avoided in patients with GERD. However, a selective cholinergic antagonist, pirenzepine, which binds specifically to $M_1$ muscarinic receptors of the parietal cell, has no adverse effects on esophageal motility [142]. In a 24-hour esophageal pH study, pirenzipine reduced reflux time and reflux episodes lasting longer than 5 minutes [113]. In 47 patients with GERD, pirenzepine 50 mg b.i.d. for 12 weeks significantly improved symptoms and reduced antacid use compared with placebo [85]. Few anticholinergic side effects occur with antisecretory doses. Pirenzepine has been used outside the United States to treat peptic ulcer disease. Newer data show that atropine and other anticholinergic agents can reduce tLESRs [80]; this could presage a new outlook on nonselective anticholinergic therapy for GERD [62].

Bismuth formulations have not been extensively evaluated for GERD, although bismuth subsalicylate (Pepto-Bismol) is widely used for dyspepsia, including symptoms that may reflect GERD. Prostaglandin analogs appear to be ineffective for treating GERD.

## COMBINATION THERAPY

In patients refractory to acid suppression alone who have motility abnormalities defined by esophageal manometry or nuclear emptying techniques, synergistic therapy might consist of a prokinetic agent with an antisecretory agent. This approach is not uncommon among clinical gastroenterologists. The addition of sucralfate slurry q.i.d. to an H2RA has occasionally been considered in patients unresponsive to single-agent therapy, but the efficacy and safety of this combination have not been established.

Some studies have shown synergism between cimetidine and metoclopramide [70], while others have refuted this [132]. For grade 2 or 3 esophagitis, cimetidine 1 g per day plus cisapride 10 mg q.i.d. for 12 weeks produced greater symptomatic and endoscopic improvements than cimetidine alone [35]. Ranitidine 150 mg b.i.d. plus cisapride 20 mg b.i.d. healed grades 2 and 3 esophagitis better than ranitidine alone; symptom relief in the two treatment arms was similar [78]. Prolonged pH studies have shown that the combination of cisapride and ranitidine reduced total reflux, supine reflux, and postprandial reflux compared with ranitidine alone [52]. Cisapride plus ranitidine was more effective at reducing GERD relapse than ranitidine alone but not when compared to cisapride alone [139], suggesting that the prokinetic agent provides the clinical benefit.

Ranitidine 150 mg b.i.d. plus metoclopramide 10 mg q.i.d. was compared with omeprazole 20 mg q.AM in 184 erosive esophagitis patients (grade 2 or 3 in about 86% of patients) [103]. Single-agent omeprazole was more effective at improving daytime and nocturnal heartburn. Mucosal healing also was superior with omeprazole at 4 and 8 weeks (68% and 82% healing, respectively, versus 30% and 46% with the combination). Principally because of metoclopramide, the combined regimen had significantly more adverse events and treatment-related withdrawals. Similar findings were reported with the same regimens in a recent study in patients with persistent reflux symptoms after ranitidine therapy [97]: omeprazole monotherapy improved symptoms and healed esophagitis more effectively than ranitidine monotherapy or combined ranitidine plus metoclopramide. Regardless of esophagitis grade, more patients receiving the PPI experienced complete symptom relief.

There are no studies of combination therapy with bethanechol. The combination of domperidone plus an antisecretory drug has not been shown to be more effective than treatment with either agent alone [94].

The addition of sucralfate to an H2RA regimen did not result in enhanced esophageal mucosal healing [45]. Indeed, endoscopic improvement was reported in fewer than 50% of patients receiving either cimetidine 300 mg q.i.d. plus sucralfate (1 g after meals and 2 g hs) or cimetidine alone [45].

Adjunctive use of colloidal bismuth in GERD has been reported to be effective in a small study [12]: While ten patients with severe (grade 3 or 4) esophagitis did not heal with cimetidine 800 mg hs, seven of the ten healed on the combination of colloidal bismuth subcitrate 120 mg q.i.d. and cimetidine 800 mg hs.

Peghini et al. [91] showed that the addition of ranitidine to b.i.d. omeprazole was more effective than a third dose of the PPI for control of nocturnal acid breakthrough. A newer study [104] suggests that h.s. ranitidine might be as useful as a second dose of omeprazole for acid breakthrough on a single dose of omeprazole 20 mg daily.

## EFFICACY IN SYMPTOMATIC PATIENTS WITH NORMAL ESOPHAGEAL MUCOSA

Pharmacotherapy in patients with reflux symptoms and normal esophageal mucosa has provoked considerable current interest. Most antacid users have endoscopy-negative GERD with mild recurring symptoms, and the popularity of antacids attests to their success in controlling esophageal acid contact time in these individuals. In an Italian retrospective analysis [88], however, 19 to 33 endoscopy-negative GERD patients remained symptomatic after 3 to 6 months of treatment with either antacid or antacid plus domperidone 10 mg t.i.d. This suggests that a subset of antacid users has more severe GERD, findings that have been confirmed by a recent epidemiologic study of frequent antacid users in the United States [105].

Three trials have compared acid-suppressive agents with placebo in endoscopy-negative GERD. In 389 patients with frequent heartburn and normal endoscopic findings, famotidine 20 mg b.i.d. for 6 weeks was more effective than famotidine 40 mg hs or placebo for relief of symptoms and reduction of antacid consumption [102]. In 509 endoscopy-negative heartburn patients, symptoms resolved in 46% receiving omeprazole 20 mg per day for 4 weeks compared with 31% receiving omeprazole 10 mg per day and 13% receiving placebo [71]. Omeprazole 20 mg b.i.d. for 4 weeks decreased the frequency and severity of reflux symptoms in 11 of 18 GERD patients with normal acid exposure and endoscopic findings [140]. Symptom improvement was particularly notable when heartburn correlated with reflux episodes at least half the time. This positive symptom index suggests that such individuals have acid-sensitive esophageal mucosa, part of the GERD spectrum.

Recent large-scale trials compared omeprazole with H2RAs and cisapride in a combined population of patients with esophagitis and those with endoscopy-negative GERD. In 994 patients from a primary-care setting, Venables et al. [137] found that omeprazole 20 mg per day for 4 weeks was superior in terms of symptom control to omeprazole 10 mg per day or ranitidine 150 mg b.i.d. (61%, 49% and 40%, respectively). This study also demonstrated comparable QOL variables in patients with and without esophagitis. Galmiche et al. [34] reported greater heartburn resolution in 424 patients receiving omeprazole 10 or 20 mg daily for 4 weeks compared with cisapride 10 mg q.i.d. (56%, 65%, and 41%, respectively). QOL improved in all groups. A reviewer [68] of the data of Galmiche and Venables and their associates noted that patients with and without esophagitis responded similarly to cisapride, ranitidine, and omeprazole 10 mg qd, but esophagitis patients responded best to omeprazole 20 mg once daily. Another study [7], involving 221 patients,

also reported no difference in heartburn relief between patients with grade 2 or 3 esophagitis and those with normal endoscopic findings or grade 1 lesions.

## SELECTION OF APPROPRIATE THERAPY

Given the vast array of therapeutic options, clinicians should tailor treatment to the individual patient, based on specific factors that contribute to pathologic reflux, such as gastric acid hypersecretion or impaired esophageal or gastric motility. At least theoretically, such "designer" therapy is highly attractive and should achieve better results than approaches mismatched with pathophysiology. In any case, the reality of clinical practice demands individualization of therapy, mostly according to symptomatic response (Table 25–4).

A safe, effective prokinetic agent should be considered as initial single-agent therapy in selected GERD patients with documented motor disturbances or with suggestive accompanying symptoms. For example, an otherwise unexplained symptom complex including heartburn, epigastric pain, early satiety, postprandial abdominal distention, sour eructations, nausea, and vomiting suggests a variant of gastroparesis. Systemic diseases that could impair GI neuromuscular function, such as diabetes mellitus, also favor the use of prokinetic agents. Since cisapride is efficacious for many GERD patients, it certainly could be an alternative primary therapy for usual heartburn even in the absence of any specific suggestion of dysmotility [1].

**TABLE 25–4.** *Pharmacologic treatment of gastroesophageal reflux disease (GERD)*

Initial empiric therapy for uncomplicated GERD[a]
- H$_2$ antagonist at standard doses
  Cimetidine, up to 800 mg b.i.d. or 400 mg q.i.d.
  Famotidine, 20 mg b.i.d.
  Nizatidine, 150 mg b.i.d.
  Ranitidine, 150 mg b.i.d.
- Prokinetic agent
  Cisapride, 10 mg q.i.d. or 20 mg b.i.d.
- PPI
  Omeprazole, 20 mg once daily
  Lansoprazole, 30 mg once daily

Aggressive medical therapy for complicated or refractory disease[a]
- Famotidine, nizatidine, or ranitidine at double the dosing frequency using the standard dose or more
- Combination therapy of H$_2$ antagonist plus prokinetic agent
  Cisapride, 10–20 mg q.i.d. or 20 mg b.i.d. or 10–20 mg h.s.
  Metoclopramide, up to 10 or 15 mg q.i.d.
- PPI, one to four times daily

Next step in aggressive medical therapy[a]
- Combination therapy of PPI plus prokinetic agent
  Cisapride, 10–20 mg q.i.d.
  Metoclopramide, up to 10 mg or 15 mg q.i.d.

[a] Concomitant nonpharmacologic measures (lifestyle modifications) recommended.

In patients with erosive esophagitis unresponsive to standard-dose H2RAs, options include increased dose frequency, an added prokinetic drug, and a switch to a PPI. Similarly, failure of empiric primary prokinetic therapy should lead to combination treatment or consideration of PPI use. A subset of patients are unresponsive to standard-dose H2RA therapy and require omeprazole or lansoprazole (or their successors). However, such patients should be treated with the knowledge that PPIs may be difficult to discontinue following long-term use. Step-down therapy, beginning with PPI administration, has many philosophical adherents, but this approach may not be practical due to the somewhat "addictive" nature of aggressive acid suppression. Step-up therapy, initially with an H2RA or cisapride, seems preferable since many patients with erosive esophagitis will heal and even more will attain substantial symptom relief with moderate acid suppression and/or an effective prokinetic agent. In most individuals with mild-to-moderate disease, H2RAs and empiric prokinetic therapy offer long-term safety and possibly lower cost.

An incomplete response to omeprazole 20 mg once daily may mandate 20 mg b.i.d., which is more effective for 24-hour control of gastric acid than a single 40-mg omeprazole dose [64]. An insufficient response to omeprazole b.i.d. should lead to physiologic studies (ambulatory pH monitoring), which might support combination therapy with a prokinetic agent or further escalation of PPI dosage. The addition of h.s. H2RA dosing to PPI therapy has already been mentioned. H2RA efficacy in this setting may relate to the sensitivity of nocturnal acid secretion to histamine stimulation.

Surgical consultation is appropriate for patients unresponsive to aggressive medical therapy. Some clinicians believe that surgical intervention should be considered at an early stage for esophagitis in the setting of Barrett's esophagus, although esophagitis associated with Barrett's esophagus usually responds to antisecretory therapy.

## LONG-TERM THERAPY

GERD should be viewed as a chronic and relapsing disorder. Healing of erosive esophagitis with acid-suppressive therapy does not appear to alter the natural history. After successful healing and discontinuation of antisecretory treatment, reflux symptoms recur rather promptly in most patients (50% to 80% within 6 to 9 months) [46, 69, 123]. Asymptomatic recurrences of esophagitis appear to be uncommon, reported in 8.6% of patients in one study [13].

In a prospective Swiss study [81] of 750 patients with grades 1 to 3 esophagitis treated empirically, 46% had an isolated episode and required no further therapy, while 32% had recurrent episodes without progression of severity and 23% progressed to a more severe grade. McDougall et al. [76] assessed GERD patients with a retrospective questionnaire: 75% still had GERD-related morbidity more than 10 years after the diagnosis was made. Almost one-third had

daily heartburn, 19% had weekly heartburn, and similar fractions required daily acid suppression. Fortunately, complications were infrequent, with only 2% developing strictures and 1% evolving to recognizable Barrett's esophagus.

Limited data on maintenance therapy with H2RAs have not been uniformly encouraging, with relapses generally occurring in at least half of patients on low doses [15]. Ranitidine and famotidine b.i.d. appear to prevent relapse [120, 123]. On the other hand, even high-dose H2RA regimens (ranitidine or nizatidine 300 mg b.i.d.) did not prevent relapse in refractory patients with erosive esophagitis healed with lansoprazole [3]: at 4 weeks, 12 of 14 patients had increased reflux symptoms and 11 of 14 had endoscopic relapse. The efficacy of long-term H2RA therapy needs careful reevaluation, including the issue of development of tolerance.

Maintenance therapy with PPIs has been extensively studied (Table 25–5). Omeprazole 20 mg per day was more effective than ranitidine 150 mg b.i.d. for remission (12-month relapse rates of 11% to 23% versus 54% to 75%) [27, 39]. Weekend therapy generally has not been effective [27, 127]. Klinkenberg-Knol et al. [61] reported a 5-year relapse rate of 47% in H2RA-resistant patients healed with omeprazole 40 mg daily. Most relapses occurred within 12 months of dose reduction (to the maintenance regimen of omeprazole 20 mg daily), and esophagitis in all patients rehealed with up to 60 to 80 mg of omeprazole daily.

Lansoprazole 15 mg q.AM maintained remission better than ranitidine 150 mg b.i.d. and placebo (12-month relapse rates of 21% to 33%, 68% and 76% to 87%, respectively) [38, 98, 126]. Lansoprazole 30 mg did not differ from 15 mg in these studies [98, 126].

Pantoprazole seems effective, based on data from a 1-year open-labeled trial in 222 patients healed with omeprazole or pantoprazole [83]. No published data are yet available on rabeprazole for maintenance therapy. In 30 patients with grade 4 esophagitis (stricture), omeprazole 20 mg b.i.d. was more effective than lansoprazole 30 mg b.i.d. and pantoprazole 40 mg b.i.d. in preventing relapse (4-week rates of 10%, 80%, and 70%, respectively) [56]. These results are inconsistent with the known pharmacology of these agents despite the authors' suggestion that omeprazole might afford better dose-dependent acid-inhibitory titration.

In a 26-month follow-up of 20 GERD patients treated with cimetidine and metoclopramide, Lieberman [69] found that relapse was associated with lower LES pressures than occurred with sustained remission (4.9 versus 13.1 mm Hg). Such underlying dysmotility supports long-term prokinetic treatment, and European trials have shown that cisapride once or twice daily can prevent relapse, particularly in patients with mild erosive esophagitis [11, 134, 135]. In 443 patients healed with antisecretory agents, cisapride 20 mg hs and 10 mg b.i.d. was significantly more effective than placebo for symptomatic and mucosal remission over 12 months [11]. In 298 patients healed with an H2RA or ome-

**TABLE 25–5.** *Prevention of relapse of reflux esophagitis*

| Author | Acute treatment regimens | n | Maintenance regimens | Duration (mo) | Endoscopic relapse rates 6 Mo | Endoscopic relapse rates 12 Mo | Comments |
|---|---|---|---|---|---|---|---|
| Gough et al., 1996 [38] | LAN, 30 mg once daily, 8 wk | 75 | LAN, 30 mg/day | 12 | — | 20%* | *p < 0.001 vs. RAN |
| | | 86 | LAN, 15 mg/day | | — | 31%* | |
| | | 74 | RAN, 300 mg b.i.d. | | — | 68% | |
| Robinson et al., 1996 [98] | LAN, 30 mg/day or RAN, 150 mg b.i.d., 8 wk | 56 | LAN, 30 mg q.AM | 12 | — | 10%* | *p < 0.001 vs. PLA |
| | | 60 | LAN, 15 mg q.AM | | — | 21%* | |
| | | 57 | PLA | | — | 76% | |
| Sontag et al., 1996 [126] | LAN, 30 mg once daily (n = 133), or RAN, 150 mg b.i.d. (n = 13), 8 wk | 54 | LAN, 30 mg q.AM | 12 | — | 45%* | *p < 0.001 vs. PLA |
| | | 53 | LAN, 15 mg q.AM | | — | 33%* | |
| | | 56 | PLA | | — | 87% | |
| Simon et al., 1995 [120] | FAM, 20–40 mg b.i.d. | 72 | FAM, 40 mg b.i.d. | 6 | 11%* | — | *p < 0.001 vs. PLA |
| | | 69 | FAM, 20 mg b.i.d. | | 22%* | — | |
| | | 31 | PLA | | 62% | — | |
| Vigneri et al., 1995 [139] | OME, 40 mg once daily, 4–8 wk | 35 | CIS, 10 mg t.i.d. | 12 | — | 46% | *p ≤ 0.02 vs. CIS and RAN |
| | | 35 | RAN, 150 mg t.i.d. | | — | 51% | †p = 0.05 vs. RAN |
| | | 35 | OME, 20 mg once daily | | — | 20%* | ‡p ≤ 0.03 vs. CIS, RAN, and RAN + CIS |
| | | 35 | RAN, + CIS | | — | 34%† | |
| | | 35 | OME, + CIS | | — | 11%‡ | |
| Dent et al., 1994 [27] | OME, 20 mg q.AM, 4–8 wk | 53 | OME, 20 mg q.AM | 12 | — | 11%* | *p < 0.001 vs. OME wkend and RAN |
| | | 55 | OME, 20 mg wkend[a] | | — | 68% | |
| | | 51 | RAN, 150 mg b.i.d. | | — | 75% | |
| Hallerback et al., 1994 [39] | OME, 20–40 mg/day, 8–12 wk | 131 | OME, 20 mg q.AM | 12 | — | 23%* | *p < 0.005 vs. RAN |
| | | 133 | OME, 10 mg q.AM | | — | 42%† | †p < 0.001 vs. RAN |
| | | 128 | RAN, 150 mg b.i.d. | | — | 54% | |
| Blum et al., 1993 [11] | CIM, 1,600 mg/day RAN, 300 mg/day, or OME, 40 mg/day | 151 | CIS, 20 mg hs | 12 | — | 32%* | *p = 0.005 vs. PLA |
| | | 149 | CIS, 10 mg b.i.d. | | — | 34%† | †p = 0.02 vs. PLA |
| | | 143 | PLA | | — | 51% | |
| Tytgat et al., 1992 [135] | H2RA (67%) or OME (33%) | 147 | CIS, 20 mg b.i.d. | 6 | 27%*/51%/47% | — | Relapses of grades 1/2/3, respectively; *p = 0.02 vs. PLA |
| | | 151 | PLA | | 48%/55%/56% | — | |

CIS, cisapride; FAM, famotidine; LAN, lansoprazole; OME, omeprazole; PLA, placebo; RAN, ranitidine.
All study participants had pretreatment esophagitis of grade ≥2, except for Blum et al. (all grades under MUSE classification), Gough et al. (not known), Tytgat et al. (grades 1–3, with 67% grades 2–3), Vigneri et al. (grades 1–3, with 84% grades 1–2).
[a] Weekend therapy: OME 20 mg q.AM on Fridays, Saturdays, and Sundays only.

prazole, cisapride 20 mg b.i.d. for 6 months prolonged remission of grade 1 esophagitis [135]; earlier relapses occurred in patients healed acutely with omeprazole (4 to 6 weeks) than with H2RAs (about 6 months). If one assumes that patients treated with omeprazole had more severe esophagitis (40% received PPI therapy due to H2RA-refractory status), relapse occurs earlier and more frequently in severe esophagitis. Cisapride 20 mg h.s. was ineffective long-term in grades 2 to 3 esophagitis healed with omeprazole [77], but the use of omeprazole could have rendered these individuals more refractory. Hatlebakk et al. [42] found no prevention of relapse after 6 months of cisapride 20 mg h.s. or b.i.d. compared with placebo in 535 patients healed with H2RA or PPI, including 118 without esophagitis who had demonstrable pathologic reflux by pH-metry.

Vigneri et al. [139] compared five maintenance therapies in esophagitis. Highest remission rates were found with omeprazole 20 mg per day plus cisapride 10 mg t.i.d. (89%), followed by omeprazole 20 mg per day alone (80%). Lower remission rates were seen with ranitidine 150 mg t.i.d. plus cisapride 10 mg t.i.d. (66%), cisapride 10 mg t.i.d. alone (54%), and ranitidine 150 mg t.i.d. alone (49%).

Full-dose H2RAs and low-dose prokinetic agents for maintenance therapy still seem rational for many patients.

For some, PPI maintenance therapy will be required. Maintenance therapy needs to be individualized, depending on the initial presentation and disease severity. During long-term therapy, conservative antireflux measures, as discussed in chapter 24, should be encouraged for all GERD patients. Unresolved concerns with PPIs, including the potential consequences of prolonged hypergastrinemia, bacterial overgrowth in the stomach, and impaired vitamin $B_{12}$ absorption, suggest that chronic PPIs probably should be used only in more severe or refractory GERD.

## COST-BENEFIT CONSIDERATIONS

In many countries, including Australia and Canada, any new drug must demonstrate cost-effectiveness before it is eligible for reimbursement in government programs [130]. Thus, there is a strong incentive for cost-effectiveness analysis of therapeutic options beyond helping clinicians predict outcomes.

Based on patient charges from retail pharmacies, the cost of omeprazole 20 mg can be 18.2% to 23.7% higher than the cost of standard H2RAs [48], and prices of the latter continue to decline after patent expirations for cimetidine and ranitidine. When generic omeprazole becomes available, the equation will change further.

In a study considering QOL [41], three long-term esophagitis treatments were compared. High-dose H2RAs were thought more costly but less effective than PPIs. PPIs were more cost-effective than standard-dose H2RAs in cases in which esophagitis symptoms significantly impaired QOL and in settings where differences in drug-acquisition cost were small. Long-term omeprazole therapy was deemed equivalent to laparoscopic Nissen fundoplication for middle-aged patients with grade 3 or 4 esophagitis for up to 5 years [47]. However, cost differences favored PPIs over 10 years, subject to price issues and surgical morbidity concerns. Such studies do not consider the extreme unlikelihood of a federal agency such as the Food and Drug Administration approving a "treatment" for benign disease with even a small definite mortality and the morbidity associated with surgery.

## CONCLUSIONS

Antisecretory therapy for GERD differs from that for peptic ulcer disease, perhaps due to the esophageal and gastric motility abnormalities contributing to acid reflux. Acid-suppressing agents are the most popular forms of antireflux therapy, with H2RAs and PPIs being highly effective for symptom relief and mucosal healing. Although the motility abnormalities associated with GERD do not fully respond to any current treatment option, newer prokinetic agents may be very effective as primary or adjunctive therapy. The availability of increasingly sophisticated medical therapy has lowered the incidence of truly refractory GERD. Future therapeutic considerations will continue to focus on long-term safety and efficacy, along with better assessments of cost-effectiveness. Well-designed clinical trials with more precisely defined patient populations, uniform assessment of esophagitis, and consensus on end points will lead to an evolution in antireflux pharmacotherapy. As this chapter is written, it is already possible to individualize therapy for many patients based on the presence of specific physiologic abnormalities and the availability of a widening variety of medical and surgical therapeutic alternatives.

## REFERENCES

1. Achem SR, Robinson M. A prokinetic approach to treatment of gastroesophageal reflux disease. Dig Dis 1998;16:38
2. Albibi R, McCallum RW. Metoclopramide: pharmacology and clinical application. Ann Intern Med 1983;98:86
3. Antonson CW, Robinson MG, Hawkins TM, McIntosh DL, Campbell DR. High doses of histamine antagonists do not prevent relapses of peptic esophagitis following therapy with a proton pump inhibitor. Gastroenterology 1990;98:A16
4. Balaban DH, Duckworth CW, Peura DA. Nasogastric omeprazole: effects on gastric pH in critically ill patients. Am J Gastroenterol 1997;92:79
5. Baldi F, et al. Cisapride versus placebo in reflux esophagitis: a multicenter double-blind trial. J Clin Gastroenterol 1988;10:614
6. Bardhan KD, et al. Lansoprazole versus ranitidine for the treatment of reflux oesophagitis. Aliment Pharmacol Ther 1995;9:145
7. Bate CM, et al. Omeprazole is more effective than cimetidine for the relief of all grades of gastro-oesophageal reflux disease-associated heartburn, irrespective of the presence or absence of endoscopic oesophagitis. Ailment Pharmacol Ther 1997;11:755
8. Behar J, Biancani P, Sheahan DG. Evaluation of esophageal tests in the diagnosis of reflux esophagitis. Gastroenterology 1976;71:9
9. Bell NJV, Burget D, Howden CW, Wilkinson J, Hunt RH. Appropriate acid suppression for the management of gastro-oesophageal reflux disease. Digestion 1992;51(suppl 1):59
10. Bell NJV, Hunt RH. Role of gastric acid suppression in the treatment of gastro-oesophageal reflux disease. Gut 1992;33:118
11. Blum AL, et al. Effect of cisapride on relapse of esophagitis: a multinational, placebo-controlled trial in patients healed with an antisecretory drug. Dig Dis Sci 1993;38:551
12. Borkent MV, Beker JA. Treatment of ulcerative reflux oesophagitis with colloidal bismuth subcitrate in combination with cimetidine. Gut 1988;29:385
13. Carlsson R, Galmiche JP, Dent J, Lundell L, Frison L. Prognostic factors influencing relapse of oesophagitis during maintenance therapy with antisecretory drugs: a meta-analysis of long-term omeprazole trials. Aliment Pharmacol Ther 1997;11:473
14. Castell D, et al. Cisapride 20 mg b.i.d. provides effective daytime and nighttime relief in patients with symptoms of chronic gastroesophageal reflux disease. Gastroenterology 1997;112:A84
15. Castell DO. Long-term therapy for chronic gastroesophageal reflux. Arch Intern Med 1987;147:1701
16. Castell DO, Richter JE, Robinson M, Sontag SJ, Haber MM. Efficacy and safety of lansoprazole in the treatment of erosive reflux esophagitis. Am J Gastroenterol 1996;91:1749
17. Chiba N, De Gara CJ, Wilkinson JM, Hunt RH. Speed of healing and symptom relief in grade II to IV gastroesophageal reflux disease: a meta-analysis. Gastroenterology 1997;112:1798
18. Chun AH, Shi HH, Achari R, Dennis S, Cavanaugh JH. Lansoprazole: administration of the contents of a capsule dosage formulation through a nasogastric tube. Clin Ther 1996;18:833
19. Cloud ML, Enas N, Humphries TJ, Bassion S. Rabeprazole in treatment of acid peptic diseases: results of three placebo-controlled trials in duodenal ulcer, gastric ulcer, and gastroesophageal reflux disease (GERD). Dig Dis Sci 1998;43:993
20. Cloud ML, Offen WW. Nizatidine versus placebo in gastroesophageal reflux disease: a six-week, multicenter, randomized, double-blind comparison. Dig Dis Sci 1992;37:865
21. Cloud ML, Offen WW, Robinson M. Nizatidine versus placebo in gastroesophageal reflux disease: a 12-week, multicenter, randomized, double-blind study. Am J Gastroenterol 1991;86:1735
22. Collen MJ, Johnson DA, Sheridan MJ. Basal acid output and gastric acid hypersecretion in gastroesophageal reflux disease: correlation with ranitidine therapy. Dig Dis Sci 1994;39:410
23. Corinaldesi R, Valentini M, Belaiche J, Colin R, Geldof H, Maier C. Pantoprazole and omeprazole in the treatment of reflux oesophagitis: a European multicentre study. Aliment Pharmacol Ther 1995;9:667
24. Creutzfeldt W, Lamberts R, Stockmann F, Brunner G. Quantitative studies of gastric endocrine cells in patients receiving long-term treatment with omeprazole. Scand J Gastroenterol 1989;24(suppl 166):122
25. Cupp MJ, Tracy TS. Cytochrome P450: new nomenclature and clinical implications. Am Family Physician 1998;57:107
26. Decktor DL, Robinson M, Maton PN, Lanza FL. Effects of aluminum/magnesium hydroxide and calcium carbonate on esophageal and gastric pH in subjects with heartburn. Am J Ther 1995;40:546
27. Dent J, et al. Omeprazole v ranitidine for prevention of relapse in reflux oesophagitis: a controlled double blind trial of their efficacy and safety. Gut 1994;35:590
28. DeVault KR, Castell DO. Guidelines for the diagnosis and treatment of gastroesophageal reflux disease. Arch Intern Med 1995;155:2165
29. Euler AR, Murdock RH Jr, Wilson TH, Silver MT, Parker SE, Powers L. Ranitidine is effective therapy for erosive esophagitis. Am J Gastroenterol 1993;88:520
30. Feldman M, Burton ME. Histamine$_2$-receptor antagonists: standard therapy for acid-peptic diseases. N Engl J Med 1990;323:1672–1680, 1749–1755
31. Feldman M, et al. Treatment of reflux esophagitis resistant to H$_2$-receptor antagonists with lansoprazole, a new H$^+$/K$^+$-ATPase inhibitor: a controlled, double-blind study. Am J Gastroenterol 1993;88:1212

32. Fielding JF, Doyle GD. Comparison between ranitidine and cimetidine in the treatment of reflux oesophagitis. Ir Med J 1984;77:356

33. Fitton A, Wiseman L. Pantoprazole: a review of its pharmacological properties and therapeutic use in acid-related disorders. Drugs 1996; 51:460

34. Galmiche JP, Barthelemy P, Hamelin B. Treating the symptoms of gastro-oesophageal reflux disease: a double-blind comparison of omeprazole and cisapride. Aliment Pharmacol Ther 1997;11:765

35. Galmiche JP, et al. Combined therapy with cisapride and cimetidine in severe reflux oesophagitis: a double blind controlled trial. Gut 1988; 29:675

36. Ganzini L, Casey DE, Hoffman WF, McCall AL. The prevalence of metoclopramide-induced tardive dyskinesia and acute extrapyramidal movement disorders. Arch Intern Med 1993;153:1469

37. Geldof H, Hazelhoff B, Otten MH. Two different dose regimens of cisapride in the treatment of reflux oesophagitis: a double-blind comparison with ranitidine. Aliment Pharmacol Ther 1993;7:409

38. Gough AL, Long RG, Cooper BT, Fosters CS, Garrett AD, Langworthy CH. Lansoprazole versus ranitidine in the maintenance treatment of reflux oesophagitis. Aliment Pharmacol Ther 1996;10:529

39. Hallerback B, et al. Omeprazole or ranitidine in long-term treatment of reflux esophagitis. Gastroenterology 1994;107:1305

40. Hameeteman W. Clinical studies of sucralfate in reflux esophagitis: the European experience. J Clin Gastroenterol 1991;13(suppl 2):S16

41. Harris RA, Kuppermann M, Richter JE. Proton pump inhibitors or histamine-2 receptor antagonists for the prevention of recurrences of erosive reflux esophagitis: a cost-effectiveness analysis. Am J Gastroenterol 1997;92:2179

42. Hatlebakk JG, Johnsson F, Vilien M, Carling L, Wetterhus S, Thogersen T. The effect of cisapride in maintaining symptomatic remission in patients with gastro-oesophageal reflux disease. Scand J Gastroenterol 1997;32:1100

43. Havelund T, et al. Omeprazole and ranitidine in treatment of reflux oesophagitis: double blind comparative trial. BMJ 1988;296:89

44. Hendel J, Hendel L, Hage E, Hendel J, Aggestrup S, Nielsen OH. Monitoring of omeprazole treatment in gastro-oesophageal reflux disease. Eur J Gastroenterol Hepatol 1996;8:417

45. Herrera JL, Shay SS, McCabe M, Peura DA, Johnson LF. Sucralfate used as adjunctive therapy in patients with severe erosive peptic esophagitis resulting from gastroesophageal reflux. Am J Gastroenterol 1990;85:1335

46. Hetzel DJ, et al. Healing and relapse of severe peptic esophagitis after treatment with omeprazole. Gastroenterology 1988;95:903

47. Heudebert GR, Marks R, Wilcox CM, Centor RM. Choice of long-term strategy for the management of patients with severe esophagitis: a cost-utility analysis. Gastroenterology 1997;112:1078

48. Hixson LJ, Kelley CL, Jones WN, Tuohy CD. Current trends in the pharmacotherapy for gastroesophageal reflux disease. Arch Intern Med 1992;152:717

49. Holloway RH, Dent J, Narielvala F, Mackinnon AM. Relation between oesophageal acid exposure and healing of oesophagitis with omeprazole in patients with severe reflux oesophagitis. Gut 1996;38:649

50. Howden CW, Castell DO, Cohen S, Freston JW, Orlando RC, Robinson M. The rationale for continuous maintenance treatment of reflux esophagitis. Arch Intern Med 1995;155:1465

51. Huber R, Kohl B, Sachs G, Senn-Bilfinger J, Simon WA, Sturm E. Review article: the continuing development of proton pump inhibitors with particular reference to pantoprazole. Aliment Pharmacol Ther 1995;9:363

52. Inauen W, et al. Effects of ranitidine and cisapride on acid reflux and oesophageal motility in patients with reflux oesophagitis: a 24 hour ambulatory combined pH and manometry study. Gut 1993;34:1025

53. Janisch HD, Huttemann W, Bouzo MH. Cisapride versus ranitidine in the treatment of reflux esophagitis. Hepatogastroenterology 1988; 35:125

54. Jankowski J, Coghill G, Tregaskis B, Hopwood D, Wormsley KG. Epidermal growth factor in the oesophagus. Gut 1992;33:1448

55. Jansen JBN, Baak LC, Lamers CB. Effect of increasing doses of ranitidine on exposure of the oesophagus to gastric acid in patients with gastroesophageal reflux disease. Scand J Gastroenterol 1988; 23(suppl 154):2

56. Jaspersen D, Diehl KL, Schoeppner H, Geyer P, Martens E. A comparison of omeprazole, lansoprazole and pantoprazole in the maintenance treatment of severe reflux oesophagitis. Aliment Pharmacol Ther 1998;12:49

57. Joelsson B, Johnsson F. Heartburn: the acid test. Gut 1989;30:1523

58. Jones DB, Howden CW, Burget DW, Kerr GD, Hunt RH. Acid suppression in duodenal ulcer: a meta-analysis to define optimal dosing with antisecretory drugs. Gut 1987;28:1120

59. Kitchin LI, Castell DO. Rationale and efficacy of conservative therapy for gastroesophageal reflux disease. Arch Intern Med 1991;151:448

60. Klinkenberg-Knol EC, Meuwissen SGM. Combined gastric and oesophageal 24-hour pH monitoring and oesophageal manometry in patients with reflux disease, resistant to treatment with omeprazole. Aliment Pharmacol Ther 1990;4:485

61. Klinkenberg-Knol EC, et al. Long-term treatment with omeprazole for refractory reflux esophagitis: efficacy and safety. Ann Intern Med 1994;121:161

62. Koerselman J, Pursnani KG, Peghini P, Mohiuddin MA, Katzka D, Castell DO. Oral anticholinergic therapy with dicyclomine results in decreased gastroesophageal reflux. Gastroenterology 1997;112:A178

63. Koop H, Schepp W, Dammann HG, Schneider A, Luhmann R, Classen M. Comparative trial of pantoprazole and ranitidine in the treatment of reflux esophagitis: results of a German multicenter study. J Clin Gastroenterol 1995;20:192

64. Kuo B, Castell DO. Optimal dosing of omeprazole 40 mg daily: effects on gastric and esophageal pH and serum gastrin in healthy controls. Am J Gastroenterol 1996;91:1532

65. Labenz J, Blum AL, Bayerdorffer E, Meining A, Stolte M, Borsch G. Curing *Helicobacter pylori* infection in patients with duodenal ulcer may provoke reflux esophagitis. Gastroenterology 1997;112:1442

66. Langtry HD, Wilde MI. Lansoprazole: an update of its pharmacological properties and clinical efficacy in the management of acid-related disorders. Drugs 1997;54:473

67. Larson C, Cavuto NJ, Flockhart DA, Weinberg RB. Bioavailability and efficacy of omeprazole given orally and by nasogastric tube. Dig Dis Sci 1996;41:475

68. Lauritsen K. Management of endoscopy-negative reflux disease: progress with short-term treatment. Aliment Pharmacol Ther 1997; 11(suppl 2):87

69. Lieberman DA. Medical therapy for chronic reflux esophagitis: long-term follow-up. Arch Intern Med 1987;147:1717

70. Lieberman DA, Keeffe EB. Treatment of severe reflux esophagitis with cimetidine and metoclopramide. Ann Intern Med 1986;104:21

71. Lind T, et al. Heartburn without oesophagitis: efficacy of omeprazole therapy and features determining therapeutic response. Scand J Gastroenterol 1997;32:974

72. Lipsy RJ, Fennerty B, Fagan TC. Clinical review of histamine$_2$ receptor antagonists. Arch Intern Med 1990;150:745

73. Lundell L, et al. Omeprazole or high-dose ranitidine in the treatment of patients with reflux oesophagitis not responding to "standard doses" of H$_2$-receptor antagonists. Aliment Pharmacol Ther 1990;4:145

74. Maton PN, et al. Long-term efficacy and safety of omeprazole in patients with Zollinger-Ellison syndrome: a prospective study. Gastroenterology 1989;97:827

75. McCarty-Dawson D, Sue SO, Morrill B, Murdock RH Jr. Ranitidine versus cimetidine in the healing of erosive esophagitis. Clin Ther 1996;18:1150

76. McDougall NI, Johnson BT, Kee F, Collins JS, McFarland RJ, Love AH. Natural history of reflux oesophagitis: a 10 year follow up of its effect on patient symptomatology and quality of life. Gut 1996;38:481

77. McDougall NI, Watson RG, Collins JS, McFarland RJ, Love AH. Maintenance therapy with cisapride after healing of erosive oesophagitis: a double-blind placebo-controlled trial. Aliment Pharmacol Ther 1997;11:487

78. McKenna CJ, Mills JG, Goodwin C, Wood JR. Combination of ranitidine and cisapride in the treatment of reflux oesophagitis. Eur J Gastroenterol Hepatol 1995;7:817

79. McTavish D, Buckley MMT, Heel RC. Omeprazole: an updated review of its pharmacology and therapeutic use in acid-related disorders. Drugs 1991;42:138

80. Mittal RK, Holloway R, Dent J. Effect of atropine on the frequency of reflux and transient lower esophageal sphincter relaxation in normal subjects. Gastroenterology 1995;109:1547

81. Monnier P, Ollyo JB, Fontolliet C, Savary M. Epidemiology and natural history of reflux esophagitis. Semin Laparosc Surg 1995;2:2

82. Mossner J, Holscher AH, Herz R, Schneider A. A double-blind study of pantoprazole and omeprazole in the treatment of reflux oesophagitis: a multicentre trial. Aliment Pharmacol Ther 1995;9:321

83. Mossner J, Koop H, Porst H, Wubbolding H, Schneider A, Maier C. One-year prophylactic efficacy and safety of pantoprazole in controlling gastro-oesophageal reflux symptoms in patients with healed reflux oesophagitis. Aliment Pharmacol Ther 1997;11:1087

84. Mulder CJ, Dekker W, Gerretsen M. Lansoprazole 30 mg versus omeprazole 40 mg in the treatment of reflux oesophagitis grade II, III, and IVa (a Dutch multicentre trial). Eur J Gastroenterol Hepatol 1996; 8:1101

85. Niemela S, et al. Pirenzepine in the treatment of reflux oesophagitis: a placebo-controlled, double-blind study. Scand J Gastroenterol 1986; 21:1193

86. Orlando RC. The pathogenesis of gastroesophageal reflux disease: the relationship between epithelial defense, dysmotility, and acid exposure. Am J Gastroenterol 1997;92:3S

87. Orr WE, Robinson MG, Humphries TJ, Antonello J, Cagliola A. Dose-response effects of famotidine on patterns of gastro-oesophageal reflux. Aliment Pharmacol Ther 1988;2:229

88. Pace F, Santalucia F, Bianchi Porro G. Natural history of gastro-oesophageal reflux disease without oesophagitis. Gut 1991;32:845

89. Palmer RH, Frank WO, Rockhold FW, Wetherington JD, Young MD. Cimetidine 800 mg twice daily for healing erosions and ulcers in gastroesophageal reflux disease. J Clin Gastroenterol 1990;12(suppl 2):S29

90. Pasqual JC, Hemery P, Bruley S, Galmiche JP. Comparison of the effects of two doses of omeprazole on 24-hour esophageal pH in gastroesophageal reflux disease. Gastroenterology 1987;92: 1567(abstr)

91. Peghini P, Katz P, Gilbert J, Castell D. Ranitidine controls nocturnal gastric acid breakthrough during b.i.d. proton pump inhibitor (PPI) treatment. Am J Gastroenterol 1997;92:1600 (abstr)

92. Pereira SP, Gainsborough N, Dowling RH. Drug-induced hypochlorhydria causes high bacterial counts in the elderly. Aliment Pharmacol Ther 1998;12:99

93. Quigley EMM. Gastroesophageal reflux disease: the roles of motility in pathophysiology and therapy. Am J Gastroenterol 1993;88:1649

94. Ramirez B, Richter JE. Promotility drugs in the treatment of gastro-oesophageal reflux disease. Aliment Pharmacol Ther 1993;7:5

95. Raufman JP, Notar-Francesco V, Raffaniello RD, Straus EW. Histamine-2 receptor antagonists do not alter serum ethanol levels in fed, nonalcoholic men. Ann Intern Med 1993;118:488

96. Richter JE, Long JF. Cisapride for gastroesophageal reflux disease: a placebo-controlled, double-blind study. Am J Gastroenterol 1995; 90:423

97. Richter JE, Sabesin SM, Kogut DG, Kerr RM, Wruble LD, Collen MJ. Omeprazole versus ranitidine or ranitidine/metoclopramide in poorly responsive symptomatic gastroesophageal reflux disease. Am J Gastroenterol 1996;91:1766

98. Robinson M, Lanza F, Avner D, Haber M. Effective maintenance treatment of reflux esophagitis with low-dose lansoprazole: a randomized, double-blind, placebo-controlled trial. Ann Intern Med 1996; 124:859

99. Robinson M, Maton PN, Rodriguez S, Greenwood B, Humphries TJ. Effects of oral rabeprazole on oesophageal and gastric pH in patients with gastro-oesophageal reflux disease. Aliment Pharmacol Ther 1997;11:973

100. Robinson M, Sahba B, Avner D, Jhala N, Greski-Rose PA, Jennings DE. A comparison of lansoprazole and ranitidine in the treatment of erosive oesophagitis. Aliment Pharmacol Ther 1995;9:25

101. Robinson M, et al. Effect of different doses of omeprazole on 24-hour oesophageal acid exposure in patients with gastro-oesophageal reflux. Aliment Pharmacol Ther 1991;5:645

102. Robinson M, et al. Famotidine (20 mg) b.d. relieves gastro-oesophageal reflux symptoms in patients without erosive oesophagitis. Aliment Pharmacol Ther 1991;5:631

103. Robinson M, et al. Omeprazole is superior to ranitidine plus metoclopramide in the short-term treatment of erosive oesophagitis. Aliment Pharmacol Ther 1993;7:67

104. Robinson M, et al. Bedtime ranitidine vs. omeprazole for control of nocturnal acid. Gastroenterology 1998 (in press)

105. Robinson M, et al. Heartburn requiring frequent antacid use may indicate significant illness. Arch Intern Med 1998;158

106. Robinson MG, Decktor DL. Experience with omeprazole in erosive esophagitis. Aliment Pharmacol Ther 1991;5(suppl 1):69

107. Ros E, Pujol A, Bordas JM, Grande L. Efficacy of sucralfate in refractory reflux esophagitis: results of a pilot study. Scand J Gastroenterol 1989;24(suppl 156):49

108. Roufail W, Belsito A, Robinson M, Barish C, Rubin A. Ranitidine for erosive esophagitis: a double-blind, placebo-controlled study. Aliment Pharmacol Ther 1992;6:597

109. Russell J, Orr WC, Wilson T, Finn AL. Effects of ranitidine, given t.d.s., on intragastric and oesophageal pH in patients with gastrooesophageal reflux. Aliment Pharmacol Ther 1991;5:621

110. Ruth M, Hamelin B, Rohss K, Lundell L. The effect of mosapride, a novel prokinetic, on acid reflux variables in patients with gastro-oesophageal reflux disease. Aliment Pharmacol Ther 1998;12:35

111. Sabesin SM, Berlin RG, Humphries TJ, Bradstreet DC, Walton-Bowen KL, Zaidi S. Famotidine relieves symptoms of gastroesophageal reflux disease and heals erosions and ulcerations: results of a multicenter, placebo-controlled, dose-ranging study. Arch Intern Med 1991;151:2394

112. Sanders SW, Tolman KG, Greski PA, Jennings DE, Hoyos PA, Page JG. The effects of lansoprazole, a new $H^+,K^{(+)}$-ATPase inhibitor, on gastric pH and serum gastrin. Aliment Pharmacol Ther 1992;6:359

113. Sato TL, Wu WC, Castell DO. Randomized, double-blind, placebo-controlled crossover trial of pirenzepine in patients with gastroesophageal reflux. Dig Dis Sci 1992;37:297

114. Schnell T, et al. Endoscopic screening for Barrett's esophagus, esophageal adenocarcinoma and other mucosal changes in ambulatory subjects with symptomatic gastroesophageal reflux. Gastroenterology 1985;88:1576(abstr)

115. Schutze K, Bigard MA, Van Waes L, Hinojosa J, Bedogni G, Hentschel E. Comparison of two dosing regimens of cisapride in the treatment of reflux oesophagitis. Aliment Pharmacol Ther 1997;11: 497

116. Sharma BK, Walt RP, Pounder RE, Gomes MD, Wood EC, Logan LH. Optimal dose of oral omeprazole for maximal 24 hour decrease of intragastric acidity. Gut 1984;25:957

117. Sharma BK, et al. Intragastric bacterial activity and nitrosation before, during, and after treatment with omeprazole. BMJ 1984;289:717

118. Silver MT, Murdock RH Jr, Morrill BB, Sue SO. Ranitidine 300 mg twice daily and 150 mg four times daily are effective in healing erosive oesophagitis. Aliment Pharmacol Ther 1996;10:373

119. Simon TJ, Berlin RG, Tipping R, Gilde L. Efficacy of twice daily doses of 40 or 20 milligrams famotidine or 150 milligrams ranitidine for treatment of patients with moderate to severe erosive esophagitis. Scand J Gastroenterol 1993;28:375

120. Simon TJ, Roberts WG, Berlin RG, Hayden LJ, Berman RS, Reagan JE. Acid suppression by famotidine 20 mg twice daily or 40 mg twice daily in preventing relapse of endoscopic recurrence of erosive esophagitis. Clin Ther 1995;17:1142

121. Solcia E, Rindi G, Havu N, Elm G. Qualitative studies of gastric endocrine cells in patients treated long-term with omeprazole. Scand J Gastroenterol 1989;24(suppl 166):129

122. Sontag S, Robinson M, McCallum RW, Barwick KW, Nardi R. Ranitidine therapy for gastroesophageal reflux disease: results of a large double-blind trial. Arch Intern Med 1987;147:1485

123. Sontag S, et al. Ranitidine versus placebo in long-term treatment of gastroesophageal reflux (GERD). Gastroenterology 1985;88: 1595(abstr)

124. Sontag SJ. Rolling review: gastro-oesophageal reflux disease. Aliment Pharmacol Ther 1993;7:293

125. Sontag SJ, et al. Two doses of omeprazole versus placebo in symptomatic erosive esophagitis: the U.S. multicenter study. Gastroenterology 1992;102:109

126. Sontag SJ, Kogut DG, Fleischmann R, Campbell DR, Richter J, Haber M. Lansoprazole prevents recurrence of erosive reflux esophagitis previously resistant to H2-RA therapy. Am J Gastroenterol 1996;91: 1758

127. Sontag SJ, et al. Daily omeprazole surpasses intermittent dosing in preventing relapse of oesophagitis: a US multi-centre double-blind study. Aliment Pharmacol Ther 1997;11:373

128. Sontag SJ, et al. Lansoprazole heals erosive reflux esophagitis resistant to histamine $H_2$-receptor antagonist therapy. Am J Gastroenterol 1997;92:429

129. Spechler SJ. Epidemiology and natural history of gastro-oesophageal reflux disease. Digestion 1992;51(suppl 1):24

130. Sridhar S, Huang J, O'Brien BJ, Hunt RH. Clinical economics review: cost-effectiveness of treatment alternatives for gastro-oesophageal reflux disease. Aliment Pharmacol Ther 1996;10:865

131. Takeda H, Hokari K, Asaka M. Evaluation of the effect of lansoprazole in suppressing acid secretion using 24-hour intragastric pH monitoring. J Clin Gastroenterol 1995;20(suppl 1):S7

132. Temple JG, et al. Cimetidine and metoclopramide in oesophageal reflux disease. BMJ 1983;286:1863

133. Tolman KG, Sanders SW, Buchi KN, Karol MD, Jennings DE, Ringham GL. The effects of oral doses of lansoprazole and omeprazole on gastric pH. J Clin Gastroenterol 1997;24:65

134. Toussaint J, Gossuin A, Deruyttere M, Huble F, Devis G. Healing and prevention of relapse of reflux oesophagitis by cisapride. Gut 1991;32:1280

135. Tytgat GNJ, et al. Effect of cisapride on relapse of reflux oesophagitis, healed with an antisecretory drug. Scand J Gastroenterol 1992;27:175

136. Vaezi MF, Singh S, Richter JE. Role of acid and duodenogastric reflux in esophageal mucosal injury: a review of animal and human studies. Gastroenterology 1995;108:1897

137. Venables TL, Newland RD, Patel AC, Hole J, Wilcock C, Turbitt ML. Omeprazole 10 milligrams once daily, omeprazole 20 milligrams once daily, or ranitidine 150 milligrams twice daily, evaluated as initial therapy for the relief of the symptoms of gastro-oesophageal reflux disease in general practice. Scand J Gastroenterol 1997;32:965

138. Vicari J, Falk GW, Richter JE. *Helicobacter pylori* and acid peptic disorders of the esophagus: is it conceivable? Am J Gastroenterol 1997;92:1097

139. Vigneri S, et al. A comparison of five maintenance therapies for reflux esophagitis. N Engl J Med 1995;333:1106

140. Watson RG, Tham TC, Johnston BT, McDougall NI. Double blind cross-over placebo controlled study of omeprazole in the treatment of patients with reflux symptoms and physiological levels of acid reflux—the "sensitive oesophagus." Gut 1997;40:587

141. Wesdorp ICE, Dekker W, Festen HPM. Efficacy of famotidine 20 mg twice a day versus 40 mg twice a day in the treatment of erosive or ulcerative reflux esophagitis. Dig Dis Sci 1993;38:2287

142. Williams JG, Deakin M, Ramage JK. Effect of cimetidine and pirenzepine in combination on 24 hour intragastric acidity in subjects with previous duodenal ulceration. Gut 1986;27:428

143. Williams M, Sercombe J, Pounder RE. Comparison of the effects of rabeprazole and omeprazole on 24-hour intragastric acidity and plasma gastrin concentration in healthy subjects. Am J Gastroenterol 1997;92:1627(abstr)

144. Williams RM, et al. Multicenter trial of sucralfate suspension for the treatment of reflux esophagitis. Am J Med 1987;83(suppl 3B):61

145. Wiseman LR, Faulds D. Cisapride: an updated review of its pharmacology and therapeutic efficacy as a prokinetic agent in gastrointestinal motility disorders. Drugs 1994;47:116

*The Esophagus*, Third Edition,
edited by D. O. Castell and J. E. Richter.
Lippincott Williams & Wilkins, Philadelphia © 1999.

CHAPTER 26

# Barrett's Esophagus

Alan J. Cameron

In Barrett's esophagus, the squamous epithelium of the distal esophagus is replaced by columnar epithelium. This epithelium resembles that of the intestine, contains goblet cells, and is different from the normal lining of the gastric cardia. Barrett's esophagus is an acquired disorder, associated with gastroesophageal reflux. It is thought that reflux damages the normal squamous epithelium, which is then replaced by more acid-resistant columnar epithelium. Patients with Barrett's esophagus have an increased risk of developing esophageal adenocarcinoma.

## DEFINITIONS

This is a controversial area. For the sake of clarity, the following definitions are suggested:

*Long-segment Barrett's esophagus.* Usually, the diagnosis of Barrett's esophagus is straightforward. Endoscopy shows a long segment of the lower esophagus to have a salmon red color, which contrasts with the pink squamous epithelium proximally. Biopsies from the red mucosa show goblet cell intestinal metaplasia (also referred to as specialized columnar epithelium). One definition of a Barrett's esophagus required at least 3 cm of esophagus to be lined with columnar epithelium [66].

*Short-segment Barrett's esophagus.* This refers to shorter lengths, or tongues, of columnar epithelium, less than 3 cm, seen by the endoscopist in the distal esophagus, with intestinal metaplasia on biopsy.

*Intestinal metaplasia at the esophagogastric junction.* This refers to patients with this microscopic finding on biopsy but no visible columnar epithelium in the esophagus on endoscopy.

## PATHOGENESIS

Incompetence of the lower esophageal sphincter (LES) is a major factor in causing gastroesophageal reflux. Patients

with Barrett's esophagus usually have low resting pressures in the LES. Mean LES pressure in a group of patients with Barrett's esophagus was 5 mm Hg, compared to 9 mm Hg in patients with uncomplicated reflux esophagitis and 17 mm Hg in controls [33] (Fig. 26–1). Also, esophageal body motility is often impaired in Barrett's esophagus, with low amplitude and failed peristaltic waves on swallowing being common [38]. Impaired motility results in impaired clearance of refluxed gastric juice.

Hiatal hernia is an additional factor in allowing reflux to occur. Most patients with severe reflux have a hiatal hernia [41]. Barrett's esophagus is especially associated with hiatal hernia, as was recognized on barium x-rays in early descriptions of the condition [1, 43]. In an endoscopic study, the writer found a 3 cm or larger hiatal hernia in 76% of patients with Barrett's esophagus, 50% of patients with reflux esophagitis, and 17% of patients with no esophagitis [11].

Esophageal motor abnormalities and the presence of a hernia are the principal causes of reflux. Patients with Barrett's esophagus have severe reflux, as shown by 24-hour esophageal pH monitoring (Fig. 26–2). The mean proportion of total recording time that esophageal pH was under 4 in Barrett's patients was 28% compared to 14% in esophagitis and 3% in controls in one study [33] and 33% in Barrett's versus 11% in esophagitis in another [25]. Reflux of bile into the esophagus has been similarly monitored over 24-hour studies using a bilirubin spectrophotometric probe, the Bilitec 2000. Bile reflux was found (mean values) 43% of the recording time in Barrett's, 12% in uncomplicated gastroesophageal reflux disease (GERD), and 2% in controls [19]. Acid and bile reflux were generally simultaneous, and suppression of acid secretion and subsequent acid reflux with omeprazole also reduced bile reflux, probably by reducing the volume of gastric content available for reflux [19]. Bile acids may increase the harmful effect of acid and pepsin on the esophageal squamous epithelium.

Animal experiments showed that, if the lining of the distal esophagus was excised and a cardioplasty performed to allow free reflux, columnar epithelium could regenerate in

A. J. Cameron: Department of Gastroenterology, Mayo Clinic, Rochester, Minnesota 55905.

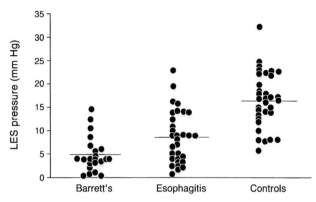

**FIG. 26–1.** Patients with Barrett's esophagus have lower resting pressure in the lower esophageal sphincter (LES) than controls or patients with reflux esophagitis. (From ref. 33, with permission. Copyright 1983, American Medical Association.)

the area previously occupied by squamous epithelium [9]. This did not occur without continuing acid reflux. Absent reflux, squamous epithelium returned. Further experiments using a similar model showed that columnar epithelium could regenerate even if a distal cuff of squamous epithelium was left intact [26]. Therefore, the columnar cells could not have migrated into the esophagus from the proximal stomach. The principal histological type in a Barrett's esophagus is an intestinal metaplasia [48], which again would not suggest migration from the stomach. It has been proposed that the columnar epithelium in Barrett's esophagus may originate in undifferentiated cells in the esophageal gland ducts [26]. Little is known about the development stage of Barrett's esophagus in humans. The prevalence is low in children and rises with age, but the length of columnar epithelium does not change with age [14]. This is consistent with a relatively rapid development of a Barrett's esophagus to its full length, rather than gradual upward creep of columnar epithelium over a number of years.

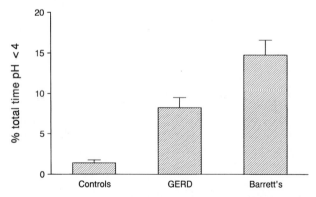

**FIG. 26–2.** In Barrett's esophagus, 24-hour esophageal pH monitoring shows more prolonged acid exposure than in controls or reflux esophagitis. (From ref. 19, with permission.)

# EPIDEMIOLOGY

Most information on the epidemiology of Barrett's esophagus relates to cases with long (3 cm or more) segments of columnar epithelium [10].

Population-based studies show that about 7% of adults experience heartburn every day and that a further 10% to 15% have heartburn at least once a week [44, 70]. Prospective studies in patients with frequent heartburn have shown that 11% to 12% had a Barrett's esophagus [39, 74]. These studies were in male populations, and some patients did not have intestinal metaplasia on biopsy. In a more recent study, we found a Barrett's esophagus in 3.5% of patients with reflux symptoms at least weekly [13]. Taking both sexes, the estimated prevalence of long-segment Barrett's esophagus in persons with reflux symptoms is 3.5% to 7%. The prevalence of Barrett's esophagus is very low in childhood and rises with age [14]. The condition is at least twice as prevalent in men compared to women.

Most patients with Barrett's esophagus have reflux symptoms, but a few do not. In patients having endoscopy for any indication, the estimated prevalence of Barrett's esophagus is around 1% in different series [10]. We estimated the prevalence in the general population of Olmsted County, Minnesota, by two different methods [18]. The clinically diagnosed prevalence was 22.6 per 100,000. Seven Barrett's were found in 733 consecutive autopsies. The estimated ("true") prevalence based on findings at autopsy (corrected for age and sex distribution) was 376 per 100,000. This data showed that most cases of Barrett's esophagus in the general population had not been detected and so are not accessible for cancer surveillance programs. However, with the increasing use of endoscopy, the number of clinically diagnosed cases is increasing.

## Other Motility Disorders

Barrett's esophagus may be associated with motility disorders that allow gastroesophageal reflux to occur. It has been reported with scleroderma [17, 38] and in patients with achalasia who have reflux following previous surgical myotomy [38].

## Incidence of Adenocarcinoma

Most adenocarcinomas of the esophagus and many adenocarcinomas of the esophagogastric junction arise in a Barrett's esophagus. The incidence of these adenocarcinomas has greatly increased in recent decades. Data from the National Cancer Institute's Surveillance, Epidemiology, and End Results program showed a threefold increase comparing the years 1976–1987 with 1988–1990 [8]. We found in Olmsted County that the incidence of adenocarcinoma in both locations rose more than fivefold between 1935–1971

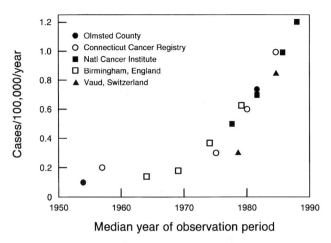

**FIG. 26–3.** The incidence of adenocarcinoma of the esophagus in population-based studies has shown a marked rise since about 1970. (From ref. 50, with permission.)

and 1974–1989 [50] (Fig. 26–3). The reasons for the increase are unknown. These adenocarcinomas occur more frequently in men than in women and in whites than in blacks.

## Genetic Association

Families have been reported in which multiple members had Barrett's esophagus, sometimes with adenocarcinoma, affecting more than one generation [20, 35]. Relatives of patients with Barrett's esophagus and adenocarcinoma have an increased prevalence of reflux symptoms compared to control relatives [60]. An inherited predisposition to reflux, perhaps autosomal dominant, seems likely in some families.

## Occurrence in Children

Barrett's esophagus with goblet cell metaplasia can occur in children as an acquired disorder [32]. It is rare compared to the prevalence in adults. The youngest report was at age 5. Many cases were found in children with severe neurological disease, such as mental retardation and cerebral palsy. Most have a diaphragmatic hernia. In the review by Hassall [32], ten cases of esophageal adenocarcinoma had been reported in the literature in young persons, aged 11 to 25.

## DIAGNOSIS

### Symptoms

Common presenting complaints of patients with Barrett's esophagus are heartburn and acid regurgitation. Reflux symptoms are similar in patients with Barrett's esophagus and in patients with uncomplicated reflux esophagitis, and these two groups cannot be distinguished by the history [74], although Barrett's esophagus patients may have had symptoms for a larger number of years on average. Dysphagia

due to stricture or inflammation, often at the level of the proximally displaced squamocolumnar junction, may occur. Pain or bleeding may result from esophagitis or, occasionally, from the development of an ulcer crater within the columnar-lined esophagus. Some patients with Barrett's esophagus are not recognized until an adenocarcinoma develops, for example, when progressive dysphagia results in investigation that reveals both the tumor mass and the Barrett's esophagus.

### X-ray

Barium x-ray is an insensitive diagnostic method in Barrett's esophagus. In most cases, there are no specific findings for the disorder [74]. Most cases have a hiatal hernia. Free gastroesophageal reflux may be seen on fluroscopy. More suggestive are the presence of a benign-appearing midesophageal stricture (Fig. 26–4) or a peptic ulcer crater resembling

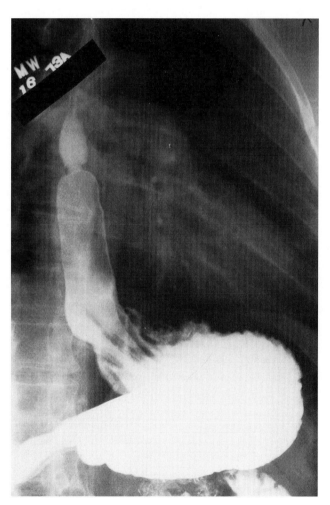

**FIG. 26–4.** Barium x-ray sometimes suggests a Barrett's esophagus. Note the benign mid-esophageal stricture, incompetent LES, and hiatal hernia. On endoscopy, columnar epithelium extended up as far as the stricture.

a gastric ulcer found in the body of the esophagus. A reticular mucosal pattern has been reported.

### Endoscopy

Endoscopy is the principal method for making a diagnosis of Barrett's esophagus (see chapter 4). The normal squamous epithelium is a pale pink color. The columnar epithelium of the stomach is red, and the junction between squamous and columnar epithelium is normally found at the lower end of the esophagus. In Barrett's esophagus, the distal esophagus is lined with red columnar epithelium, extending upward for a variable distance, often 3 to 10 cm but occasionally involving most of the esophagus. Care has to be taken not to confuse the columnar lining of a sliding hiatal hernia with the columnar lining of a true Barrett's esophagus. It is sometimes difficult to determine the precise location of the lower end of the esophagus at endoscopy, especially when a hiatal hernia is present. Endoscopic markers of the esophagogastric junction include the widening from the tubular esophagus to the saccular stomach, the upper margin of the gastric mucosal folds, and the level at which esophageal contractions are no longer seen. The proximal margin of the Barrett's esophagus may be horizontal, or there may be irregular, often tongue-shaped, upward extensions of columnar epithelium. The upper limit of the Barrett's esophagus usually has a clearly defined border separating it from pink squamous epithelium. If there is active reflux esophagitis, there may be superficial erosions with intense erythema at the margins and white or yellow central zones in the squamous epithelium immediately above the columnar area. Especially in patients without active inflammation or who have had antireflux treatment, pale islands of regenerative or residual squamous epithelium can be seen in the columnar area. Punched-out benign ulcer craters may be seen in the columnar area also. A stricture may be seen. The endoscopist should especially look for any evidence of adenocarcinoma, such as nodularity or mass.

### Inlet Patches

Islands of heterotopic gastric epithelium should not be confused with Barrett's esophagus. These occur at the upper end of the esophagus, where one or more round or oval, flat, sharply defined patches of red epithelium are often seen by the endoscopist who examines this area carefully. The prevalence at endoscopy is 2% to 10% [7, 34]. Unlike Barrett's esophagus, these lesions are congenital and not acquired, being also common in children. Biopsy shows gastric epithelium, which may contain acid-secreting parietal cells. Most are found incidentally and cause no symptoms. Rare cases have been reported in which upper esophageal strictures or ulcers occurred, perhaps related to acid secretion from the patch. Adenocarcinoma has also been reported in a few instances [7], but there is no evidence that the risk of esophageal cancer is higher than in the general population. Surveil-

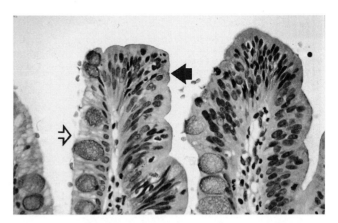

**FIG. 26–5.** Barrett's esophagus. Note the numerous goblet cells, an essential diagnostic feature in Barrett's esophagus. The area next to the *white arrow* is nondysplastic. The nuclei are regularly aligned at the base of the columnar cells. The area next to the *black arrow* shows low-grade dysplasia, with nuclear stratification and crowding. Similar changes are seen in the villus-like structure on the **right.** (From ref. 12, with permission.)

lance is not indicated for patients with the incidental finding of an inlet patch.

### Histological Confirmation

Biopsy is required to confirm the diagnosis of Barrett's esophagus (Fig. 26–5). Especially for shorter lengths of red epithelium seen in the lower esophagus on endoscopy, the gross appearance of Barrett's can be mimicked by superficial ulceration in squamous epithelium. When biopsies from the lower esophagus show only gastric fundic or cardiac-type epithelium, the diagnosis of Barrett's esophagus is probably incorrect. The characteristic histological finding in a Barrett's esophagus is a distinctive metaplastic intestinal-type epithelium. This type of epithelium occupies much or all of the columnar-lined area in most cases of Barrett's esophagus [3]. Also, this is the type of epithelium in which adenocarcinoma arises [15]. Barrett's is a glandular epithelium, with mucin-type cells, and the most distinguishing feature is the presence of goblet cells. These are readily seen in ordinary hematoxylin and eosin-stained sections and can be demonstrated more prominently in sections stained with alcian blue. In resection cases of Barrett's esophagus, the muscularis mucosa is often thickened, duplicated, or fibrotic [12].

### TREATMENT FOR REFLUX

The treatment of symptomatic gastroesophageal reflux is similar whether a Barrett's esophagus is present or not. In those few patients with Barrett's esophagus and no symptoms or esophagitis, no treatment may be necessary. In some patients, weight reduction; avoidance of late-evening, large, and fatty meals; and elevation of the head of the bed may suffice. A twice-daily dose of an $H_2$-receptor antagonist drug (cimetidine, ranitidine, nizatidine, or famotidine) can be used, the nonprescription preparations available in the United States being less expensive than when obtained on prescription. The most effective drugs for controlling gastric acid output and thus reducing esophageal acid reflux are the proton pump inhibitors (PPIs), such as omeprazole and lansoprazole. In practice, many patients with Barrett's esophagus require long-term use of a PPI drug to control symptoms of esophagitis.

Long-term treatment with a PPI drug does not result in any significant regression of the length of columnar epithelium, as shown in several treatment trials lasting over a few years [61]. Pale-colored islands of squamous epithelium often appear in the columnar area during treatment, but most of the columnar area remains. Of more importance, there is no evidence that treatment reduces cancer risk.

Patients with Barrett's esophagus and reflux, especially younger subjects requiring long-term PPI medication to control symptoms, may benefit from an antireflux surgical procedure. The usual procedure is a laparoscopic Nissen or Toupet operation. This normally controls symptoms and esophagitis, but again, the Barrett's esophagitis does not regress and the risk of developing adenocarcinoma is not reduced.

Benign ulcers in a Barrett's esophagus usually heal with antireflux treatment. Esophageal strictures are treated by dilatation and measures to deal with reflux.

## RISK OF CANCER

Patients with a long segment (over 2 to 3 cm) of Barrett's esophagus have an estimated 30 to 125 times increased risk of developing esophageal cancer compared to the general population [16, 68]. In a review of 18 previous reports in which patients with Barrett's esophagus were followed up, the median cancer incidence was about 1 per 100 patient-years [71]. In many of these reports, follow-up was short, with the risk that prevalent cancers were found after entry and classified as incidence cases. In recent series with longer follow-up, a lower cancer rate of 1 per 180 to 200 patient-years was found [21]. Most patients with Barrett's esophagus die of unrelated causes and not from esophageal cancer; in one report, only two of 79 deaths were due to esophageal adenocarcinoma [72]. Most patients developing cancer present with symptoms caused by the tumor itself, and in these individuals, the length of time that Barrett's has preceded the cancer is usually unknown. Epidemiological data suggest that the mean interval from developing a Barrett's esophagus to developing cancer may be 20 to 30 years [14].

## PROGRESSION TO ADENOCARCINOMA

It is believed that adenocarcinoma in Barrett's esophagus evolves in stages, from indefinite or low-grade dysplasia, followed by high-grade dysplasia, and finally invasive cancer [29, 30]. Non-dysplastic columnar epithelium is referred

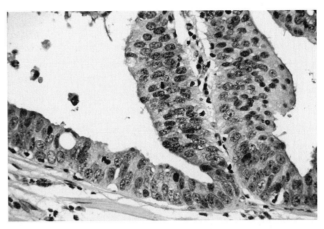

**FIG. 26–6.** High-grade dysplasia. Dysplastic nuclei are stratified and extend to the luminal surface of the cells. Residual goblets are rare. The neoplastic-appearing cells have not invaded the basement membrane. (From ref. 12, with permission.)

to as metaplasia. The term *dysplasia* indicates that the epithelium shows evidence of developing neoplastic change, with cellular and sometimes glandular architectural changes but without invasion through the basement membrane. In dysplasia (Figs. 26–5, 26–6), the cell nuclei may be enlarged, hyperchromatic, and variable in size and shape, with increased mitotic figures [12]. The nuclei show loss of polarity and stratification; that is, they are no longer located in a uniform pattern at the bases of the cells but are stacked above each other and, in high-grade dysplasia, may extend to the luminal surfaces of the cells. Cytoplasm and the number of goblet cells are reduced. In intramucosal adenocarcinoma, the dysplastic cells have invaded through the basement membrane but not through the muscularis mucosae. Evaluation of the degree of dysplasia is subject to observer variation, and experts may differ in their interpretations [57]. Apparent regression of dysplasia on subsequent endoscopic biopsies may be due to sampling error; studies on esophageal resection specimens show that metaplasia and different grades of dysplasia usually coexist in a random distribution [12, 40]. In esophageal specimens resected for adenocarcinoma, high-grade dysplasia is frequently found in the areas of Barrett's esophagus not involved by gross tumor [15, 28].

## SURVEILLANCE METHODS

Because of the cancer risk, it is usual practice to follow patients with known Barrett's esophagus with periodic endoscopy and biopsy for early cancer detection. Adenocarcinoma in Barrett's esophagus has a better prognosis when surgical resection is performed at an early stage, before an obstructing mass has developed [69]. High-grade dysplasia usually cannot be recognized by the endoscopist, and early invasive adenocarcinoma may be detectable only by biopsy [56]. Areas of invasive cancer and high-grade dysplasia are often small [12]. It is suggested that the endoscopist examining a Barrett's esophagus should take biopsies from any unusual appearing area, such as nodularity, ulceration, or stricture, and from all four quadrants at 2-cm intervals throughout the columnar-lined segment of the esophagus [36]. Standard [12] or jumbo [36] biopsies may be used. Surgical resection is usually advised if invasive adenocarcinoma is found.

Balloon cytology has been compared with endoscopy as a less expensive surveillance technique [23]. Cytology had a specificity of 80% for high-grade dysplasia or carcinoma; it is not yet recommended as a substitute for endoscopy and biopsy. Endoscopic ultrasound is an accepted technique for staging of known esophageal malignancy but is not helpful in detecting the presence of small intramucosal carcinomas in a Barrett's esophagus [22].

More specific markers of developing malignancy in Barrett's esophagus have been a subject of intensive research. Neoplasia develops in a series of steps with genomic instability and the development of aneuploid cell populations [55]. Ramel et al. [54] used flow cytometry to evaluate DNA abnormalities in cells obtained on biopsy sampling. Nine of 13 patients with Barrett's esophagus who had aneuploid or increased $G_2$/tetraploid fractions developed high-grade dysplasia on follow-up compared to 0 of 49 patients with normal flow cytometry. The same group [54] found overexpression of the p53 tumor-suppressor gene in biopsies from 5% of patients with no dysplasia, 15% with indefinite/low-grade dysplasia, 45% with high-grade dysplasia, and 53% with adenocarcinoma in the Barrett's esophagus. A number of other molecular genetic abnormalities have been found in the development of Barrett's adenocarcinomas [46]. While these are of fundamental importance in understanding the biology of these cancers, at the present time none has replaced histological interpretation of dysplasia as the primary clinical means of predicting the development of adenocarcinoma in patients with Barrett's esophagus.

## MANAGEMENT OF DYSPLASIA

When high-grade dysplasia is reported on endoscopic biopsy, it is suggested that a second pathologist expert in this area be asked to review the microscopic slides to ensure that the dysplasia is indeed of high grade. If the diagnosis of high-grade dysplasia is confirmed but no tumor mass is seen on endoscopy, there may actually be a cancer present. In patients having resection for a preoperative diagnosis of high-grade dysplasia, an invasive adenocarcinoma was found by the pathologist in the resected specimen in 33% [47], 38% [2], and 50% [51] of cases. Later prospective reports showed a missed cancer in 0% to 10.5% [12, 36], but in these series there were also patients with a preoperative biopsy diagnosis of early adenocarcinoma in whom only high-grade dysplasia was found by the pathologist after resection. In another report [58], 38% of patients having resection for high-grade dysplasia had an intramucosal carcinoma in the resected esophagus; none had deeper invasion or lymph node metastases.

The patient with high-grade dysplasia is at increased risk for developing an invasive adenocarcinoma in subsequent years if one is not already present. Information on this risk is rather limited. In one report [37], a carcinoma was found in 26% of patients in the next 1 to 6 years but 47% still had only high-grade dysplasia and in 27% high-grade dysplasia could no longer be found. In another follow-up report, only 19% of patients with high-grade dysplasia developed adenocarcinoma over a mean 7.5-year follow-up [64].

When a pathological report of high-grade dysplasia is made, the endoscopic findings should be reviewed carefully. Some patients will have a flat and endoscopically benign-appearing esophagus. Others may have areas of nodularity, stricture, irregular ulceration, or other indication that adenocarcinoma is already present. Further investigation, such as repeat endoscopy with multiple biopsies of the suspicious area, computed tomographic scan, and endoscopic ultrasound, should be considered.

For the patient with high-grade dysplasia and no apparent invasive cancer who is fit enough to undergo a major surgical procedure, resection has been recommended by a majority of authors [2, 30, 47, 51, 59, 65]. Close endoscopic follow-up, with surgery if adenocarcinoma is detected later, has been advised by others [29, 36, 64]. There are no controlled trials comparing these different approaches. More recently, photodynamic therapy (PDT) has been used for high-grade dysplasia [45].

Surgical resection of the esophagus is a major procedure with significant morbidity and a mortality rate of some 3% in special centers, higher in units where it is performed less often [12, 52, 58]. Postoperative sequelae such as weight loss, regurgitation, dumping, and anastomotic strictures have to be balanced against the benefit of preventing potential cancer deaths.

Low-grade dysplasia is more common and less significant than high-grade. In 270 consecutive patients with Barrett's esophagus at the Mayo Clinic, high-grade was found in 5%, low-grade in 34%, indefinite for dysplasia in 17%, and no dysplasia in 44%. In one report [49], 50 patients with low-grade dysplasia were followed for a mean of about 4 years; one progressed to high-grade, and none developed esophageal cancer. Resection is not advised for low-grade dysplasia.

## SHORT-SEGMENT BARRETT'S ESOPHAGUS AND INTESTINAL METAPLASIA

Adenocarcinoma of the esophagogastric junction is about twice as common as adenocarcinoma of the esophagus [50]. Tumors in both locations are associated with reflux symptoms, most often occur in white men, are increasing in incidence, and have similar histological features [15]. They may represent the same disease process; however, long-segment Barrett's esophagus is found with most esophageal adenocarcinomas but with fewer junction cancers. Junction adenocarcinomas (tumor midpoint within 2 cm of the esophagogastric junction) may be associated with short segments or tongues of intestinal metaplasia in the lower esophagus [31, 63]. Junction adenocarcinomas may originate in a small area of metaplasia, later overgrown and concealed by the enlarging tumor mass [15].

Tongues and short segments (under 3 cm) of columnar-appearing epithelium can be seen on endoscopy in patients without cancer. Provided that biopsy confirms intestinal metaplasia, it seems reasonable to diagnose a short Barrett's esophagus in such cases. At present, the risk that such a patient will later develop an adenocarcinoma of the esophagogastric junction is unknown. With a smaller area of abnormal epithelium at risk, the chance of cancer developing might be less than in a long Barrett's esophagus.

Biopsies taken just below a normally located squamocolumnar junction at the lower end of the esophagus show intestinal metaplasia in some 20% of subjects having endoscopy [13, 42, 67]. This microscopic finding was noted in patients with or without gastroesophageal reflux. This is a controversial area [66], with a recent study suggesting that these changes are secondary to *Helicobacter pylori* infection rather than acid reflux [27]. It is suggested that patients with only microscopic findings and no visible columnar epithelium in the esophagus should not be given a diagnosis of Barrett's esophagus. They may be classified as having intestinal metaplasia at the esophagogastric junction. Their cancer risk is probably minimal since one-fifth of the population have this finding.

## FREQUENCY OF SURVEILLANCE

Endoscopy and biopsy are expensive and cause some patient discomfort. Occasionally, complications occur. Detecting one case of high-grade dysplasia or early cancer does not equate with saving one cancer death. Although the benefit of early diagnosis and treatment at first seems obvious, patients could die of complications from endoscopy or surgery some time, possibly years, before they would have died of their cancer. A decision analysis study using a Markov model took these and other factors into account [52, 53]. The greatest quality-adjusted increase in life expectancy was found with surveillance every 2 to 5 years, with resection for high-grade dysplasia. Surveillance every year was very expensive and had little effect on life expectancy. Regardless of these statistics, patients and their physicians worry about the presence of a disorder with an increased cancer risk and are often reluctant to let years pass between examinations.

My current practice is as follows:

1. For the patient with a clearly visible Barrett's esophagus, either longer or somewhat shorter than 3 cm, and no dysplasia, the first follow-up at 1 year, then every 2 to 3 years.
2. When a biopsy shows intestinal metaplasia with no visible Barrett's on endoscopy, follow-up is of unproven value and probably not needed. We cannot follow up one-fifth of the population.
3. If biopsy shows low-grade dysplasia, follow up at 6 to 12 months.
4. For high-grade dysplasia, after confirmation, discuss resection, with endoscopic ablation therapy as a less proven alternative. If the patient declines these, repeat endoscopy at 3-month intervals for the next year then, if still no cancer is found, at 6-month intervals.

## ENDOSCOPIC MUCOSAL ABLATION

Removal of the abnormal epithelium (mucosa) is a new and attractive alternative therapy for Barrett's esophagus with dysplasia, which is being intensively investigated at the time of this writing. For the patient with high-grade dysplasia especially, the standard alternatives of a major surgical resection with its attendant risks and frequent digestive sequelae versus observation and frequent surveillance with the anxiety that a cancer may be missed are not ideal. It is now possible to remove the esophageal columnar epithelium by endoscopic means, allowing regeneration of squamous epithelium in an anacid environment. Potential advantages include less risk than a major surgical procedure, with the preservation of a relatively normally functioning esophagus.

In mucosal ablation techniques, prevention of continued acid esophageal reflux is needed. Usually, long-term PPI drug therapy in adequate doses to suppress acid secretion is given, for example, omeprazole 20 mg twice daily or more. A surgical fundoplication has sometimes been used as an alternative.

Several different modalities have been used to destroy the Barrett's columnar epithelium [61]. The ideal method would produce a widespread mucosal injury but avoid deeper damage involving the esophageal muscular wall, with the risks of perforation and stricture. Early studies used argon, yttrium-aluminum-garnet (YAG) or potassium titanyl phosphate (KTP) laser light beamed down the endoscope to achieve heat coagulation [6]; regeneration of squamous epithelium was confirmed. Sampliner et al. [61, 62] treated 13 patients with endoscopic multipolar electrocoagulation, which is readily available and does not require expensive equipment. After an average six sessions per patient, ten of 13 patients had complete reversal of the Barrett's to squamous epithelium and five had minor complications from treatment.

PDT uses a different principle. A photosensitizing drug is given, usually intravenously, and then light is used to produce superficial necrosis of tissue by a photochemical reaction. Wang et al. [73] treated 40 patients using a hematoporphyrin derivative followed by phototherapy with a 630-nm tunable dye laser. The mean length of columnar epithelium declined from 7 to 4.5 cm after therapy. Two patients treated with superficial carcinoma had no evidence of disease on follow-up; two with high-grade dysplasia that was not completely ablated developed carcinoma on follow-up. Overholt and Panjehpour [45] used porfimer sodium and a centering balloon. They treated 36 patients, all with Barrett's esophagus, 14 also having a superficial cancer. The columnar epithelium was completely eliminated in ten patients. The authors stated that all 15 malignancies were ablated, with no recurrence on follow-up of 6 to 62 months. With these long-acting drugs, the patient must avoid sun exposure for a month to prevent sunburn. Barr et al. [5] used a shorter-acting drug, 5-aminolevulinic acid, again with a 630-nm laser. In all five cases, areas of high-grade dysplasia were eliminated.

Argon beam plasma coagulation is a new technique for mucosal ablation. An electric spark is passed down an endoscopically delivered jet of inert argon gas. Early results are encouraging [4]. A squamous lining was restored in all 35 patients, but in 31% biopsies showed residual columnar lining underneath.

These endoscopic treatment methods are promising but still experimental. There are drawbacks. At present, treatments are time-consuming and expensive. Repeated therapeutic endoscopies are needed. Severe pain sometimes results from destruction of the epithelium, and perforation and bleeding are possible. Sun sensitivity was discussed above. After successful reversal, the esophagus becomes more sensitive to acid [24], and patients will likely need long-term PPI medication. In one series, 21 of 36 treated patients later required dilatation for strictures [45]. Sometimes, squamous epithelium has regenerated, but biopsies show remaining columnar metaplasia underneath the squamous lining [4]. Treatment can greatly reduce and sometimes eliminate the squamous epithelium, but whether this results in a corresponding reduction in the esophageal cancer risk is not yet known. Patients currently treated will still need endoscopic surveillance. Continuing improvement in methodology and controlled studies to demonstrate the effect on prevention of deaths from cancer are anticipated.

## REFERENCES

1. Allison PR, Johnstone AS. The esophagus lined with gastric mucous membrane. Thorax 1953;8:87
2. Altorki NK, et al. High-grade dysplasia in the columnar-lined esophagus. Am J Surg 1991;161:97
3. Antonioli DA, Wang HH. Morphology of Barrett's esophagus and Barrett's associated dysplasia and adenocarcinoma. Gastroenterol Clin North Am 1997;26:495
4. Attwood SEA, Byrne JP, Armstrong GR. A detailed analysis of the pattern of neo-squamous epithelium following endoscopic argon beam plasma coagulation of Barrett's esophagus. Gastroenterology 1998; 114:A60 (abst.)
5. Barr H, Shepherd NA, Dix A, Roberts DJH, Tan WC, Krasner N. Eradication of high-grade dysplasia in columnar-lined (Barrett's) esophagus by photodynamic therapy with endogenously generated protoporphyrin IX. Lancet 1996;348:584
6. Berenson MM, Johnson TD, Markowitz NR, Buchi KN, Samowitz WS. Restoration of squamous mucosa after ablation of Barrett's esophageal epithilium. Gastroenterology 1993;104:1686
7. Berkelhammer C, Bhavagan M, Templeton A, Raines R, Walloch J. Gastric inlet patch containing submucosally infiltrating adenocarcinoma. J Clin Gastroenterol 1997;25:678
8. Blot WJ, Devesa SS, Fraumeni JF. Continued climb in rates of esophageal adenocarcinoma: an update. JAMA 270;1320:1993
9. Bremner CG, Lynch VP, Ellis FH. Barrett's esophagus: congenital or acquired? An experimental study of esophageal mucosal regeneration in the dog. Surgery 1970;68:209
10. Cameron AJ. Epidemiology of columnar-lined esophagus and adenocarcinoma. Gastroenterol Clin North Am 1997;26:487
11. Cameron AJ. Barrett's esophagus. Prevalence and size of hiatal hernia. Gastroenterology 1998;114:A83 (abst.)
12. Cameron AJ, Carpenter HA. Barrett's esophagus, high-grade dysplasia and early adenocarcinoma: a pathologic study. Am J Gastroenterol 1997;92:586
13. Cameron AJ, Kamath PS, Carpenter HA. Prevalence of Barrett's esophagus and intestinal metaplasia at the esophagogastric junction. Gastroenterology 1997;112:A82(abst)
14. Cameron AJ, Lomboy CT. Barrett's esophagus: age, prevalence and extent of columnar epithelium. Gastroenterology 1992;103:1241
15. Cameron AJ, Lomboy CT, Pera M, Carpenter HA. Adenocarcinoma of the esophagogastric junction and Barrett's esophagus. Gastroenterology 1995;109:1541
16. Cameron AJ, Ott BJ, Payne WS. The incidence of adenocarcinoma in columnar-lined (Barrett's) esophagus. N Engl J Med 1985;313:857
17. Cameron AJ, Payne WS. Barrett's esophagus occurring as a complication of scleroderma. Mayo Clin Proc 1978;53:612
18. Cameron AJ, Zinsmeister AR, Ballard DJ, Carney JA. Prevalence of columnar-lined (Barrett's) esophagus. Comparison of population-based clinical and autopsy findings. Gastroenterology 1990;99:918
19. Champion G, Richter JL, Vaeze MF, Singh S, Alexander R. Duodenogastric reflux: relationship to pH and importance in Barrett's esophagus. Gastroenterology 1994;107:747
20. Crabb DW, Berk MA, Hall TR, Conneally PM, Biegel AA, Lehman GA. Familial gastroesophageal reflux and development of Barrett's esophagus. Ann Intern Med 1985;103:52
21. Drewitz DJ, Sampliner RE, Garewal HS. The incidence of adenocarcinoma in Barrett's esophagus: a prospective study of 170 patients followed 4.8 years. Am J Gastroenterol 1997;92:212
22. Falk GW, Catalano MF, Sivak MF, Rice TW, Van Dam JV. Endosonography in the evaluation of patients with Barrett's esophagus and high-grade dysplasia. Gastrointest Endosc 1994;40:207
23. Falk GW, et al. Surveillance of patients with Barrett's esophagus for dysplasia and cancer with balloon cytology. Gastroenterology 1997; 112:1787
24. Fass R, Yalam JM, Camargo L, Johnson C, Garewal HS, Sampliner RE. Increased esophageal chemoreceptor sensitivity to acid in patients after successful reversal of Barrett's esophagus. Dig Dis Sci 1997;42: 1853
25. Gillen P, Keeling P, Byrne PJ, Hennessy TPJ. Barrett's esophagus: pH profile. Br J Surg 1987;74:774
26. Gillen P, Keeling P, Byrne PJ, West AB, Hennessy TPJ. Experimental columnar metaplasia in the canine esophagus. Br J Surg 1988;75:113
27. Goldblum JR, et al. Inflammation and intestinal metaplasia of the gastric cardia: the role of gastroesophageal reflux and H. pylori infection. Gastroenterology 1998;114:633
28. Haggitt RC, Tryzelaar J, Ellis FH, Colcher H. Adenocarcinoma complicating columnar epithelium-lined (Barrett's) esophagus. Am J Clin Pathol 1978;70:1
29. Hameeteman W, Tytgat GNJ, Houthoff HJ, van den Tweel JG. Barrett's esophagus: development of dysplasia and adenocarcinoma. Gastroenterology 1989;96:1249
30. Hamilton SR, Smith RRL. The relationship between columnar epithelial dysplasia and invasive adenocarcinoma arising in Barrett's esophagus. Am J Clin Pathol 1987;87:301
31. Hamilton SR, Smith RRL, Cameron JL. Prevalence and characteristics of Barrett esophagus in patients with adenocarcinoma of the esophagus or esophagogastric junction. Hum Pathol 1988;19:942
32. Hassall E. Columnar-lined esophagus in children. Gastroenterol Clin North Am 1997;26:533
33. Iascone C, DeMeester TR, Little AG, Skinner DB. Barrett's esophagus. Functional assessment, proposed pathogenesis, and surgical therapy. Arch Surg 1983;118:543
34. Jabbari M, et al. The inlet patch: heterotopic gastric mucosa in the upper esophagus. Gastroenterology 1985;89:352
35. Jochem VJ, Fuerst PA, Fromkes JJ. Familial Barrett's esophagus associated with adenocarcinoma. Gastroenterology 1992;102:1400
36. Levine DS, Haggitt RC, Blount PL, Rabinovitch PS, Rusch VW, Reid BR. An endoscopic biopsy protocol can differentiate high-grade dysplasia from early adenocarcinoma in Barrett's esophagus. Gastroenterology 1993;105:40
37. Levine DS, Haggitt RC, Irvine S, Reid BJ. Natural history of high-

grade dysplasia in Barrett's esophagus. Gastroenterology 1996;110:A550(abst)

38. Lidums I, Holloway R. Motility abnormalities in the columnar lined esophagus. Gastroenterol Clin North Am 1997;26:519

39. Mann NS, Tsai MF, Nair PK. Barrett's esophagus in patients with symptomatic reflux esophagitis. Am J Gastroenterol 1989;84:1494

40. McArdle JE, Lewin KJ, Randall G, Weinstein W. Distribution of dysplasias and early invasive carcinoma in Barrett's esophagus. Hum Pathol 1992;23:479

41. Mittal RK, Balaban DH. The esophagogastric junction. N Engl J Med 1997;336:924

42. Morales TG, Sampliner RE, Bhattacharyya A. Intestinal metaplasia of the gastric cardia. Am J Gastroenterol 1997;92:414

43. Naef AP, Savary M, Ozzello L. Columnar-lined lower esophagus: an acquired lesion with malignant predisposition: report on 140 cases of Barrett's esophagus with 12 adenocarcinomas. J Thorac Cardiovasc Surg 1975;70:826

44. Nebel OT, Fornes MF, Castell DO. Symptomatic gastroesophageal reflux: incidence and precipitating factors. Am J Dig Dis 1976;21:953

45. Overholt BF, Panjehpour M. Photodynamic therapy for Barrett's esophagus: clinical update. Am J Gastroenterol 1996;91:1719

46. Palanca-Wessels MC, Barrett MT, Galipeau PC, Rohrer KL, Reid BJ, Rabinovitch PS. Genetic analysis of long-term Barrett's esophagus epithelial cultures exhibiting cytogenetic and ploidy abnormalities. Gastroenterology 1998;114:295

47. Palley SL, Sampliner RE, Garewal HS. Management of high-grade dysplasia in Barrett's esophagus. J Clin Gastroenterol 1989;11:369

48. Paull A, Trier JS, Dalton MD, Camp RC, Loeb P, Goyal RK. The histologic spectrum of Barrett's esophagus. N Engl J Med 1976;295:476

49. Pedrosa MC, Klein MA, Sostek MB, Clark KM, Schimmel EM. Follow up of low grade dysplasia in Barrett's esophagus. Gastroenterology 1996;110:A225(abst)

50. Pera M, Cameron AJ, Trastek VF, Carpenter HA, Zinsmeister AR. Increasing incidence of adenocarcinoma of the esophagus and esophagogastric junction. Gastroenterology 1993;104:510

51. Pera M, et al. Barrett's esophagus with high-grade dysplasia. An indication for esophagectomy? Ann Thorac Surg 1992;54:199

52. Provenzale D, Kemp AJ, Arora S, Wong JB. A guide for surveillance of patients with Barrett's esophagus. Am J Gastroenterol 1994;89:670

53. Provenzale D, Schmitt CM. Surveillance of patients with Barrett's esophagus—a cost-utility analysis based on new estimates of cancer risk. Gastroenterology 1997;112:A36

54. Ramel S, et al. Evaluation of p53 protein expression in Barrett's esophagus by two-parameter flow cytometry. Gastroenterology 1992;102:1220

55. Reid BJ, Blount PL, Rubin CE, Levine DS, Haggitt RC, Rabinovitch PS. Flow-cytometric and histological progression to malignancy in Barrett's esophagus: prospective endoscopic surveillance of a cohort. Gastroenterology 1992;102:1212

56. Reid BJ, Weinstein WM, Lewin KJ. Endoscopic biopsy can detect high-grade dysplasia or early adenocarcinoma in Barrett's esophagus without grossly recognizable neoplastic lesions. Gastroenterology 1988;94:81

57. Reid BJ, et al. Observer variation in the diagnosis of dysplasia in Barrett's esophagus. Hum Pathol 1988;19:166

58. Rice TW, Falk GW, Achkar E, Petras RE. Surgical management of high-grade dysplasia in Barrett's esophagus. Am J Gastroenterol 1993;88:1832

59. Robertson CS, Mayberry JF, Nicholson DA, James PD, Atkinson M. Value of endoscopic surveillance in the detection of neoplastic change in Barrett's esophagus. Br J Surg 1988;75:760

60. Romero Y, et al. Familial aggregation of gastroesophageal reflux in patients with Barrett's esophagus and esophageal adenocarcinoma. Gastroenterology 1997;113:1449

61. Sampliner RE. Ablative therapies for the columnar-lined esophagus. Gastroenterol Clin North Am 1997;26:685

62. Sampliner RE, Fennerty RE, Garewal HS. Reversal of Barrett's esophagus with acid suppression and multipolar electrocoagulation: preliminary results. Gastrointest Endosc 1996;44:532

63. Schnell TG, Sontag SJ, Chejfec G. Adenocarcinomas arising in tongues or short segments of Barrett's esophagus. Dig Dis Sci 1992;37:137

64. Schnell T, et al. High grade dysplasia is not an indication for surgery in patients with Barrett's esophagus. Gastroenterology 1996;110:A590(abst)

65. Spechler SJ, Goyal RK. Cancer surveillance in Barrett's esophagus: what is the end point? Gastroenterology 1994;106:275

66. Spechler SJ, Goyal RK. The columnar lined esophagus, intestinal metaplasia and Norman Barrett. Gastroenterology 1996;110:614

67. Spechler SJ, Zeroogian JM, Antonioli DA, Wang HH, Goyal RK. Prevalence of metaplasia at the gastro-oesophageal junction. Lancet 1994;344:1533

68. Spechler SJ, et al. Adenocarcinoma and Barrett's esophagus: an overrated risk? Gastroenterology 1984;87:927

69. Streitz JM, Ellis FH, Gibb PS, Balogh K, Watkins E. Adenocarcinoma in Barrett's esophagus. A clinicopathological study of 65 cases. Ann Surg 1991;213:122

70. Thompson WG, Heaton KW. Heartburn and globus in apparently healthy people. Can Med Assoc J 1982;126:46

71. Tytgat GNJ. Does endoscopic surveillance in esophageal columnar metaplasia have any real value? Endoscopy 1995;27:19

72. Van der Burgh A, et al. Oesophageal cancer is an uncommon cause of death in patients with Barrett's esophagus. Gut 1996;39:5

73. Wang KK, Geller A, Gutta K, Laukka M, Wong Kee Song M. Photodynamic therapy in the treatment of Barrett's esophagus. Gastroenterology 1996;110:A290(abst)

74. Winters C, et al. Barrett's esophagus. A prevalent, occult complication of gastroesophageal reflux disease. Gastroenterology 1987;92:118

*The Esophagus*, Third Edition,
edited by D. O. Castell and J. E. Richter.
Lippincott Williams & Wilkins, Philadelphia © 1999.

# CHAPTER 27

# Esophageal Strictures

## J. Barry O'Connor and Joel E. Richter

The clinical spectrum of gastroesophageal reflux disease (GERD) is diverse. The majority of patients follow a benign course characterized by intermittent symptoms of heartburn and acid regurgitation. However, nearly 40% develop esophagitis, which may be severe in half of these cases. One of the most frequent sequelae of long-standing severe esophagitis is the formation of a peptic esophageal stricture, occurring in 10% of patients with reflux esophagitis seeking medical evaluation. The morbidity faced by patients with peptic strictures is significant and derives from their potential to have a chronic relapsing course, increased risk of food impaction, propensity for pulmonary aspiration, frequently coexistent Barrett's esophagus, and need for esophageal dilation occasionally complicated by perforation. In this chapter, we review the pathophysiology, predisposing factors, clinical presentation, diagnosis, and treatment of peptic strictures.

## PATHOPHYSIOLOGY

The presence of GERD is a *sine qua non* for the development of a peptic esophageal stricture. Contact between acid and the esophageal mucosa is required to injure the mucosa, leading to nonerosive or erosive esophagitis and, at the most severe end of the spectrum, esophageal stricture with or without Barrett's esophagus. The mechanisms predisposing to stricture development are similar to other forms of GERD but are usually more severe and exaggerated, thereby increasing acid contact time.

### Lower Esophageal Sphincter

Lower esophageal sphincter (LES) dysfunction can be of three types: (a) spontaneous transient relaxations (tLESRs), (b) transient "stress reflux" resulting from increased intra-abdominal pressure, and (c) free reflux [20]. Stress reflux

J. B. O'Connor: Center for Swallowing and Esophageal Disorders, Department of Gastroenterology, The Cleveland Clinic Foundation, Cleveland, Ohio 44195.
J. E. Richter: Center for Swallowing and Esophageal Disorders, Department of Gastroenterology, The Cleveland Clinic Foundation, and Department of Medicine, The Cleveland Clinic Foundation Health Science Center of the Ohio State University, Cleveland, Ohio 44195.

and free reflux are associated with low basal LES pressures. Irrespective of the mechanism of LES relaxation, equalization of gastric and intraesophageal pressures occurs, the "common cavity" phenomenon, facilitating the reflux of gastric contents. In patients with peptic strictures, low basal LES pressures are more important than TLESRs. Several studies have shown that mean LES pressures are lower in patients with peptic strictures compared with healthy controls or patients with milder degrees of reflux disease [32, 43]. For example, Ahtardis et al. [1] studied 25 consecutive patients with heartburn and no strictures and 25 consecutive patients with peptic strictures. As shown in Fig. 27–1, there was a wide range of LES pressures in the healthy control and reflux groups. However, patients in the stricture group had a mean LES pressure of 4.9 mm Hg, none had LES pressures greater than 8 mm Hg, and there was no overlap with control subjects (mean LES pressure of 20 mm Hg). Additional evidence supporting the role of a competent LES in preventing reflux is provided by a surgical study by Larrain et al. [42], in which benign strictures improved following restoration of LES pressure, without further need for acid-suppressing medications or dilation.

### Esophageal Clearance Mechanisms

Once acid enters the esophagus, it is cleared by three mechanisms. First, peristaltic contractions move the largest volume of acidic fluid into the stomach, saliva neutralizes the remaining acid, and in the upright position, gravity assists drainage of residual acid from the esophagus. Many patients with peptic strictures have associated esophageal motility disorders, further prolonging abnormal acid contact time. Ahtardis et al. [1] found that 64% of stricture patients had motility disorders compared to 32% of patients without stricture. Simultaneous or repetitive contractions were the most commonly identified manometric abnormalities. The prevailing concept is that the dysmotility is irreversible and secondary to chronic acid damage. However, a case report found a patient with peptic stricture whose peristaltic abnor-

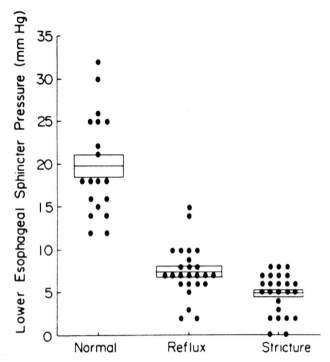

**FIG. 27–1.** Lower esophageal sphincter pressures in normal subjects, in patients with symptomatic gastroesophageal reflux with a positive Bernstein test, and in patients with a peptic stricture of the esophagus. The mean ± SEM is shown for each group. From ref. 1, with permission.

malities reverted to normal following Nissen fundoplication, suggesting the occasional reversibility of these motility abnormalities with control of acid reflux [53]. Studies of salivary function in patients with peptic strictures are not available. The effect of gravity on acid clearance in peptic strictures was examined by Harvey and colleagues [31]. They studied 71 patients with peptic stricture, randomizing them to ranitidine or placebo and separately to raising the head of the bed to a 10% slope or not. Patients were assessed by symptom scores and endoscopy before and after 6 weeks of treatment. Among those patients not receiving $H_2$ blockers, 58% improved with head-of-bed elevation compared to only 28% who slept flat in bed. Of those receiving $H_2$ blockers, more patients improved when the head of the bed was elevated versus flat (86% versus 76%).

### Gastric Factors

Gastric factors, particularly the acid concentration of the gastric refluxate, play an important role in the development of peptic strictures. For example, patients with Zollinger-Ellison syndrome (ZES) have a 10% to 13% incidence of peptic strictures, slightly increased over the general reflux population [50, 67]. Although the esophagitis in ZES patients was easily controlled when basal acid output was decreased to less than 10 mEq per hour, the frequency of peptic stricture dilation only decreased when acid output was re-

duced to very low values (less than 1 mEq per hour). Acid combined with bile or duodenal contents may be more injurious to the esophageal mucosa than acid alone [79]. Using ambulatory pH monitoring, Atwood et al. [4] noted significant amounts of alkaline reflux (pH greater than 7) in Barrett's patients (92% of whom had peptic strictures) compared to patients with uncomplicated esophagitis or controls. There is no good evidence that delayed gastric emptying promotes the development of peptic strictures.

### Hiatal Hernia

Hiatal hernias are common incidental findings, occurring in 10% to 15% of the general population. The incidence of hernias increases across the spectrum of GERD, being found in 42% of patients with reflux symptoms without esophagitis, 63% of patients with endoscopic esophagitis, and 85% of patients with peptic strictures [6, 35]. Potential mechanisms whereby the hiatal hernia can induce or promote reflux include (a) by acting as a fluid trap to limit the effectiveness of lower esophageal clearance of refluxed material, (b) by promoting transient nondeglutitive relaxation, (c) by mechanically reducing basal LES pressure, and (d) by causing a reduction in the length of the high-pressure zone [51].

### Esophageal Epithelial Defense Mechanisms

Changes in preepithelial and epithelial defense mechanisms may play a role in the development of peptic strictures. Preepithelial defenses include mucus, bicarbonate ions, and the surface unstirred water layer. Epithelial defenses consist of the stratified squamous epithelial cells and their tight intercellular junctions, which are relatively impermeable to hydrogen ions. The precise role of these factors and epithelial growth factors in the pathogenesis of peptic strictures is unknown.

### HISTOPATHOLOGY

Early histological findings of reflux esophagitis include thickening of the basal zone (>15% of epithelial thickness), elongated dermal papillae (>67% of epithelial thickness) [8, 15], mucosal infiltration by neutrophils and eosinophils, congested venules at the top of the papillae [27], and focal epithelial necrosis. In more severe esophagitis, inflammation extends through the muscularis mucosa into the submucosa or even into the surrounding mediastinal soft tissue. When esophagitis progresses to involve all layers of the esophagus (panmural inflammation), stricture formation results.

Peptic strictures are usually located in the distal esophagus because the stricturing process begins at the squamocolumnar junction. However, in patients with Barrett's esophagus, the squamocolumnar junction is located more proximally and peptic strictures are found at this higher level rather than at the gastroesophageal junction. Peptic strictures are usually less than 1 cm long, only occasionally extending to 8 cm in length. When evaluating patients with strictures longer than 3 to 4 cm, the clinician should took for predisposing conditions such as ZES, superimposed pill esophagitis, or prolonged nasogastric intubation.

## CONDITIONS PREDISPOSING TO PEPTIC STRICTURES

### Scleroderma

Esophageal disease is reported in 70% to 95% of patients with scleroderma, and nearly all patients have associated Raynaud's phenomenon. Scleroderma involvement of the esophagus is characterized by aperistalsis of the esophageal body and low or absent LES pressure, resulting in marked impairment of acid clearance [54]. Zamost et al. [85] found that esophageal symptoms were present in more than 70% of patients with scleroderma, while 60% had esophagitis at endoscopy. Of the 53 esophagitis patients, 13 (24%) had peptic strictures by barium esophagram or endoscopy. Other series report a 2% to 48% rate of peptic strictures in scleroderma patients [34, 39, 57]. In a recent study based on the administrative discharge database of more than 14,201 Veterans Administration patients, El-Serag and Sonnenberg [23] determined that patients with a discharge diagnosis of scleroderma were 12.3 times more likely to have peptic esophageal strictures compared to other patients. Peptic strictures are more troublesome in patients with scleroderma because they present a major obstruction which the atrophied, aperistaltic esophageal muscle is unable to overcome.

### Zollinger-Ellison Syndrome

Zollinger-Ellison syndrome (ZES) is characterized by hypersecretion of acid, increased volume of gastric secretions, and the propensity to develop diffuse gastric and small bowel ulcerations. Initially, it was felt that the esophagus was spared secondary to augmentation of LES pressures by the elevated levels of serum gastrin. However, Richter et al. [67] found that 60% of ZES patients had classic reflux symptoms or esophagitis. Later, Miller et al. [50] reported on the frequency of esophageal involvement in 122 patients with ZES, observing that 45% had reflux symptoms, 43% had endoscopic esophagitis, and 8% had peptic strictures. Their strictures were difficult to manage with $H_2$ blockers, and all required aggressive treatment with omeprazole. Similar rates of peptic stricture formation were recently reported by Bondeson et al. [11] in 24 consecutive patients with ZES.

### Nasogastric Tube Placement

Prolonged nasogastric intubation predisposes to GERD by interfering with LES function and prolonging contact time between acid and the esophageal mucosa [55]. Buchin and Spiro [12] found that 9/84 patients (11%) developed stricture from 4 days to 2 months after nasogastric intubation.

### After Treatment for Achalasia

The treatment of achalasia with esophagomyotomy or pneumatic dilation either cuts or ruptures the LES, in some cases rendering it incompetent. As a result, these patients are prone to severe reflux disease because the absence of peristaltic esophageal contractions prolongs acid contact time. Several surgical series report symptomatic rates of GERD between 0% and 60% following Heller myotomy [18, 63, 65], with a mean of 10% to 20%. GERD is more common following an esophagomyotomy without an antireflux procedure. In contrast to the high rate following surgery, GERD occurs in only 2% to 8% of patients following pneumatic dilation because basal LES pressures are reduced by 39% to 68% while esophagomyotomy usually reduces sphincter pressure by at least 75% [78]. Complicated strictures following esophagomyotomy and pneumatic dilation are reported [64], but the exact incidence is unknown.

### Lower Esophageal Rings

Although some have suggested a congenital origin, recent studies suggest that GERD may play an important role in the pathology of the lower esophageal (Schatzki's) rings, an association being found in 26% to 73% of patients with rings [3, 22]. A longitudinal study of the natural history of lower esophageal rings and their relationship to esophageal strictures was reported by Chen et al. in 1987 [14]. They identified 22 patients who had radiographically diagnosed rings on more than one esophagram at least 1 year apart along with upper endoscopy within 2 weeks of radiological examination. In two patients, rings developed in a previously normal esophagus over a follow-up period of 4 years. Among the 20 patients with a ring present on the first examination, the diameter of the ring decreased in 15%, an esophageal stricture developed in 40%, and no change in the caliber of the rings occurred in the remaining 45% after a mean follow-up period of 3.6 years. Among the nine patients in whom there was no progression in the ring, only one had esophagitis at endoscopy. In contrast, among the eight patients who developed strictures, seven had endoscopic findings of esophagitis. These findings confirm that some rings may evolve into strictures, representing a progressive form of GERD.

### Nonsteroidal Anti-inflammatory Drugs

The relationship between peptic strictures and nonsteroidal anti-inflammatory drugs (NSAIDs) has been elucidated in several studies. Heller et al. [33] studied 76 patients undergoing dilation for benign peptic strictures. Six patients had taken medications known to cause esophagitis, such as potassium chloride or emepronium bromide. Of the remaining 70 patients, 22 (31%) had regularly taken NSAIDs before the onset of dysphagia compared to only ten (14%) in a hospital control group ($p < 0.02$). In a similarly designed study using community controls, Wilkins et al. [83] reported that 49% of patients with benign strictures compared to 12% of controls were prescribed NSAIDs for at least 6 weeks in the previous year. El-Serag et al. [23] used a Veterans Administration hospital discharge database to compare the prevalence of peptic strictures in patients prone to taking NSAIDs. Because this database does not contain data on medication use, the authors used conditions associated with frequent ingestion of NSAIDs, such as osteoarthritis, back pain, and femur fracture as surrogate markers. Using a case-control design to analyze 14,201 patients discharged with a diagnosis of peptic esophageal stricture, the authors found that the incidence of peptic strictures was greater in men than women [odds ratio (OR) = 1.55], in white than non-white (OR = 2.45), and in a variety of conditions treated with NSAIDs (OR = 1.16 to 1.78). The mechanisms whereby NSAIDs may cause esophagitis and peptic strictures include depletion of esophageal mucosal protective prostaglandins, direct mechanical effects of or pH changes induced by the pill, and stimulation of collagen synthesis.

## CLINICAL PRESENTATION

Dysphagia is the most common presenting symptom in patients with benign esophageal strictures. Dysphagia is usually for solids but may progress to include liquids. The presence of dysphagia for liquids early in the disease should suggest a motility disorder, such as achalasia, rather than a simple peptic stricture. The severity of dysphagia is difficult to accurately measure. Many patients with chronic peptic strictures will alter their diet and, although not eating a "regular" diet, no longer complain of dysphagia because they avoid foods which precipitate this symptom. Standard dysphagia scales, which measure only the frequency of dysphagia, underestimate these patients' symptoms. Therefore, it is important to inquire about the types of foods which precipitate dysphagia. Diet scales score dysphagia according to those foods that are most difficult to swallow for stricture patients, such as meat and bread, to those easiest to swallow, like mashed potatoes and liquids.

A history of typical heartburn symptoms is present in 75% of peptic stricture patients [61]. However, some patients will describe a decrease in heartburn as their stricture disease becomes more severe as a result of decreased acid refluxate into the esophagus through the obstructed lumen. A careful clinical history to differentiate other causes of stricture, particularly pill esophagitis, is important in this group of patients.

Atypical presentations of peptic strictures, which may delay the correct diagnosis, include chronic cough and asthma [30]. These symptoms are due to aspiration of food into the lung, microaspiration of acid into the tracheobronchial tree, or reflex bronchoconstriction following esophageal acid reflux [46]. Chest pain may be caused by esophagitis, esophageal spasm, or food impaction at the level of the stricture. Weight loss is uncommon because patients with peptic strictures have a good appetite and maintain their caloric intake by adopting a soft or liquid diet. Significant weight loss should suggest carcinoma or achalasia.

## DIAGNOSIS

### Radiology

Although endoscopy and barium esophagography are complementary studies in the diagnosis of patients with suspected peptic strictures, barium is usually recommended as the initial study of choice. The barium study provides information on the location, diameter, and length of the stricture, while guiding the endoscopist in the choice of dilation technique and need for fluoroscopy. The sensitivity of the barium esophagram in identifying peptic strictures is much better than that of endoscopy in most studies. Proper radiographic techniques required to demonstrate strictures include rapid swallowing or Valsalva maneuver to adequately distend the esophagus and the use of marshmallow, 13-mm tablets, or food to identify the site of obstruction. Using these techniques, over 95% of peptic strictures can be identified. For example, Ott et al. [59] found the sensitivity of the barium esophagram to be 100% for strictures less than 9 mm in diameter and to decrease only to 90% for strictures greater than 10 mm in diameter. Most strictures were short in length: 14% were less then 0.6 cm in length, 75% were 0.6 to 2.5 cm, and 11% were longer than 2.5 cm. Another interesting finding in this study was the ability of the barium esophagram to detect esophagitis close to the stricture on the basis of mucosal irregularity at the stricture margin. A smooth margin predicted the absence of esophagitis at endoscopy with 85% accuracy, while irregular margins predicted esophagitis with 74% accuracy. Only half of the patients with strictures had active esophagitis.

Another useful radiographic technique in peptic stricture patients is measuring the ability to swallow a barium tablet of known size within a specified time period. Goldschmid et al. [29] developed a system to objectively measure esophageal lumen patency. They studied 35 consecutive patients with mechanical dysphagia. (Eighteen had peptic strictures.) Subjective measures of patency were assessed by dysphagia scores (scale 0 = unable to swallow through 5 = no dysphagia) and diet scales (from nothing by mouth through able to swallow unrestricted diet). All patients had endoscopy with measurement of the esophageal lumen, using biopsy forceps as the "gold standard." Patients were given barium pills, sequentially increasing in size from 5 to 25 mm, until a pill failed to traverse the esophagus within 20 seconds. Pill size correlated best with the endoscopic estimate of the stricture ($r = 0.85$), while the weakest correlation was between the dysphagia scale and the endoscopic estimates ($r = 0.48$). The reason for this rather poor correlation likely was the change in diet adopted by many patients with strictures, effectively eliminating foods that cause dysphagia. Timed measurement to pass a barium tablet can be useful as an objective assessment of esophageal strictures in research studies and as a means of objectively documenting response to specific treatment.

### Endoscopy

Endoscopy is essential in evaluating all esophageal strictures. Esophagoscopy can define the extent and etiology of the stricture. It is important to remember that the use of smaller endoscopes and minimal conscious sedation (both sometimes prevent adequate esophageal distension) predisposes the endoscopist to miss subtle strictures, i.e., greater than 13 mm [59]. Peptic strictures are located in the distal esophagus and always involve the squamocolumnar junction. Strictures located elsewhere should raise the suspicion of other etiologies. The endoscopic appearance of a peptic stricture is usually a smooth stenosis in the distal esophagus which fails to open after air insufflation. Esophagitis may be seen above the stricture in about half of cases. Other sequelae of severe acid reflux disease, such as Barrett's esophagus, pseudodiverticula, and fibrous bands, may also be identified by endoscopy. Spechler et al. [73] studied 25 selected patients with chronic peptic strictures and no evidence of Barrett's esophagus on prior endoscopy. Biopsies of the distal esophagus revealed intestinal metaplasia in 11 of 25 (44%) patients. The authors speculated that the high prevalence of Barrett's esophagus in these patients was due to GERD predisposing to both conditions and/or stricture-induced stasis favoring development. Biopsies should be taken from the proximal edge as well as blindly from the depths of the stricture if there is any suspicion of malignancy. Even when initial investigations do not reveal a malignancy, cancer will be discovered in some patients on follow-up examinations [16]. Most patients requiring esophageal dilation can have this done at the time of initial endoscopy, regardless of whether biopsies are taken, as long as the stricture can be well evaluated for length and tortuosity either by a previous barium esophagram or during the diagnostic portion of the endoscopy.

## DIFFERENTIAL DIAGNOSIS

A careful history can determine the etiology of strictures in about 85% of cases [13]. Peptic strictures comprise 60% to 70% of benign strictures in the United States [60]. Other causes include radiation therapy, caustic injury, pill esophagitis, infectious esophagitis, esophageal rings, sclerotherapy, idiopathic eosinophilic esophagitis, and anastomotic (esophagogastric) strictures (Table 27–1).

Patients with peptic stricture are at risk for superimposed pill esophagitis because of partial mechanical obstruction or associated poor esophageal motility. Drugs especially known to cause or aggravate esophageal strictures include doxycycline, potassium chloride, quinidine, NSAIDs, ascorbic acid, ferrous sulfate, and alendronate. Delayed-release preparations are prone to induce strictures as their dis-

**TABLE 27–1.** *Differential diagnosis of peptic strictures*

Caustic ingestion
Crohn's disease
Eosinophilic esophagitis
Epidermolysis bullosa
Esophageal atresia
Infections
   Monilia
   Tuberculosis
   Typhoid
Medications
   Alendronate
   Ferrous sulfate
   NSAIDs
   Phenytoin
   Potassium chloride
   Quinidine
   Tetracycline
   Vitamin C
Postoperative
Radiation
Rings or webs
Sclerotherapy

solution time is markedly prolonged, extending the contact time with esophageal mucosa [9]. Other drugs, such as tetracyclines, acetylsalicylic acid, and ascorbic acid, reduce the pH of their surroundings to less than 4 after complete dissolution, thereby causing injury based on acid damage. Emphasizing this point, Bonavina et al. [9] in a retrospective study found that 11/55 (20%) patients with benign esophageal strictures were also taking medications which could cause or aggravate a previously existing acid-induced stricture. More importantly, the authors noted that five of these 11 strictures would have been ascribed to GERD if normal 24-hour pH studies had not been obtained. Pill-induced strictures are preventable by avoiding potentially toxic drugs in susceptible patients and instructing all patients to ingest pills while in an upright position, with at least 6 to 8 oz of liquids and at least 30 minutes before lying down.

## TREATMENT

The clinical course of peptic strictures is chronic and progressive. At first presentation, dysphagia is usually present for 4 to 6 years [1]. To treat peptic esophageal strictures effectively, it is important to understand the pathophysiology and natural history of strictures and to have well-defined treatment goals (relief of dysphagia, healing of esophagitis). Knowledge of the therapeutic options and an understanding of the importance of controlling acid reflux are essential to successful treatment.

### Lifestyle Modifications

Lifestyle modifications should be recommended to all patients with esophageal strictures, although they are usually insufficient as sole treatment. Because patients with peptic strictures have low LES pressures, they are prone to reflux when recumbent. Therefore, they should avoid eating before lying down and elevate the head of the bed. Smoking must be discouraged and alcohol and caffeine intake moderated. Patients should chew their food well to avoid food impaction. In addition, a careful review of medications is essential to avoid those drugs implicated in pill-induced injury as well as medications which can lower LES pressure and promote reflux, such as theophyllines, nitrates, and calcium channel blockers.

## Acid Suppression and Outcome of Peptic Strictures

Traditionally, the mainstay of treating peptic strictures has been mechanical dilation. In recent years, however, the importance of ongoing esophagitis in the natural history of peptic strictures has been clarified. In a study of 64 stricture patients, Dakkak et al. [19] compared dysphagia scores based on a test meal with esophageal stricture diameter, measured by barium wax spheres. Stricture diameter alone explained only 29% of the variance in dysphagia scores. However, 66% of the dysphagia variance was explained when both stricture diameter and severity of esophagitis were included. Thus, esophagitis in stricture patients aggravates dysphagia independent of the degree of stenosis.

Treatment of peptic strictures with $H_2$-receptor antagonists or promotility agents does not decrease the need for subsequent stricture dilations [25]. However, recent studies with proton pump inhibitors show that aggressive acid suppression not only heals esophagitis but decreases the need for peptic stricture dilation (Table 27–2). In the largest study, Smith et al. [72] randomized 366 patients with peptic stricture to either omeprazole 20 mg per day or ranitidine 300 mg b.i.d., following them for 12 months. Both investigators and patients were blind to treatment assignment, and dilation was performed when clinically indicated. At 12 months, 30% of patients on omeprazole required redilation compared to 46% of patients on ranitidine ($p < 0.01$). In addition, 76% of the omeprazole-treated patients were free of dysphagia compared to 64% of the ranitidine group. In a similar study, Marks et al. [47] compared stricture patients being treated with omeprazole 20 mg per day versus ranitidine 150 mg b.i.d. after initial dilation. They found a decreased need for redilation in the omeprazole group (41% versus 73%), the difference being very close to statistical significance ($p = 0.07$). Esophagitis healing and dysphagia relief were superior in those patients randomized to omeprazole. As part of the study, a cost analysis was performed comparing proton pump inhibitors with $H_2$-receptor antagonists. Over the 6-month period, the average cost to render a patient free of dysphagia with omeprazole was $1,744 compared to $2,957 with $H_2$-receptor antagonists, a cost savings of 50%. Jaspersen et al. [37] randomized patients with peptic strictures to higher-dose omeprazole (40 mg per day) or ranitidine 150 mg b.i.d. for 12 months. Patients in the omeprazole group required a mean of two redilations compared to four and a half redilations in the ranitidine group ($p < 0.0001$). In a smaller trial, Silvis et al. [20] compared 14 patients randomized to omeprazole 20 mg per day versus 17 patients randomized to ranitidine 150 mg b.i.d. Patients assigned to omeprazole were less likely to require redilation, 21% versus 23% in the ranitidine group. The insignificant difference was likely due to lack of power related to the small study size. Finally, Swarbrick et al. [74] compared lansoprazole 30 mg per day to ranitidine 300 mg b.i.d. in 141 evaluable patients. Overall, 36% in the lansoprazole group compared to 51% of the ranitidine group required redilation over the follow-up period of 12 months.

## Intralesional Steroids

Intralesional steroid injection may reduce inflammation and delay or prevent fibrosis, thereby improving peptic strictures. Case series of patients treated with intralesional steroids provide preliminary evidence of the efficacy and safety

**TABLE 27–2.** *Randomized trials comparing proton pump inhibitors and $H_2$-receptor antagonists in the management of peptic esophageal strictures*

| Author | Design[a] | No. of patients | Therapy[b] (mg) | F/U (mo) | % needing repeat dilation | % free of dysphagia | No. of redilations |
|---|---|---|---|---|---|---|---|
| Smith et al. [72] | RCT, DB | 180 | OME20/day | 12 | 30% | 76% | — |
| | | 185 | RAN300 b.i.d. | | 46% ($p < 0.01$) | 64% | — |
| Swarbrick et al. [74] | RCT, DB | 70 | LAN30/d | 12 | 36% | — | — |
| | | 71 | RAN300 b.i.d. | | 51% ($p =$ NS) | — | — |
| Jaspersen et al. [37] | RCT | 20 | OME40/d | 12 | — | — | 2 |
| | | 18 | RAN150 b.i.d. | | — | — | 4.5 ($p < 0.0001$) |
| Marks et al. [47] | RCT, DB | 18 | OME20/day | 6 | 41% | — | — |
| | | 16 | RAN150 b.i.d. | | 73% ($p = 0.07$) | — | — |
| Silvis et al. [70] | RCT, DB | 14 | OME20/day | 10 | 21% | — | — |
| | | 17 | RAN150 b.i.d. | | 23% ($p =$ NS) | — | — |

[a] RCT, randomized controlled trial; DB, double-blind.
[b] RAN150, ranitidine 150 mg or equivalent; OME, omeprazole; LAN, lansoprazole.

of this procedure. Kirsch et al. [40] reported on two patients with peptic strictures who were refractory to dilation therapy, i.e., received only transient relief after multiple dilations. They were treated with intralesional injection of triamcinolone (10 mg per mL in 0.5-mL aliquots) into four quadrants of the narrowest region of the stricture. Both patients had dramatic subjective improvement after steroid injection. On follow-up, one patient remained asymptomatic at 3 weeks, but the other had recurrence of symptoms at 2 months. No adverse events occurred. Zein et al. [87] treated three young stricture patients (aged 7 to 14) with two sessions of triamcinolone injections, followed by Savary or balloon dilation. The patients needed between one and six dilations prior to steroid injection but no dilations after injection. None of the patients' strictures recurred after a mean follow-up of 2 years. However, two of the patients had antireflux surgery at the same time as the injections, which may be an important confounding factor. Therefore, we believe, based on these few case studies, that a definitive statement on the efficacy of intralesional steroids is not possible.

### Bougienage

Per oral dilation of peptic strictures has been performed for more than 400 years. Dilators slowly evolved from relatively stiff, crude instruments, such as whale bone, to modern flexible thermoplastic bougies and balloons. Currently, there are three types of dilators commonly in use in the United States: (a) mercury-filled, rubber Maloney, or Hurst dilators; (b) wire-guided Savary-Gilliard or American dilators; and (c) balloon dilators which are passed through-the-scope (TTS) or over a guide wire (Fig. 27–2).

Maloney dilators are mercury-filled, flexible, tapered dilators with a contour similar to that of the Savary-Gilliard but without the central lumen for passage over a guide wire. Hurst dilators are similar to Maloney bougies but have a

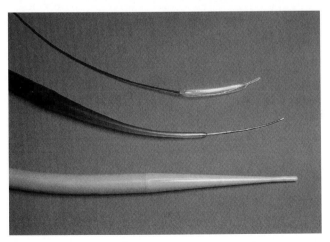

**FIG. 27–2.** Esophageal dilators. From the top down are the through-the-scope (TTS) balloon, the Savary-Gilliard polyvinyl bougie with guide wire, and the mercury-filled Maloney bougie.

blunt rather than a tapered leading end. These dilators are indicated in uncomplicated, short strictures which are not angulated or tortuous. Although these dilations are usually performed in the outpatient setting, some patients may self-dilate at home [52]. Dilation with mercury bougies is usually done in the sitting position, allowing gravity to assist passage of the dilator. The dilator is passed through the mouth and kept in position across the stricture for an arbitrary length of time (about 1 minute) before removal. The dilators are passed in gradually increasing sizes, and generally, no more than three dilators are passed in any one session. In general, fluoroscopy is not required for passage of mercury-weighted Maloney dilators in uncomplicated peptic strictures.

In 1985, Dumon et al. [21] reported on the Savary-Gilliard system of dilators. They found that these wire-guided, thermoplastic bougies were more flexible, were easier to introduce through the mouth, and traversed the pharynx more easily than the older Eder-Puestow dilators. The authors also preferred the "feel" of the Savary-Gilliard dilators. The Savary-Gilliard dilators have replaced the Eder-Puestow dilators in most, if not all, institutions. Savary-Gilliard dilators have a tapered tip, a central channel for passage over a guide wire, and radiopaque markings on the bougie for use with fluoroscopy. They range in size from 15F to 60F (5 to 20 mm). American dilators are similar to Savary-Gilliard dilators but are impregnated with barium and the tapered tip is shorter. Guide wire dilators are particularly suited to long, tight, or angulated strictures. When using these dilators, the initial step is placing the guide wire. This can be performed by fluoroscopy or at the time of endoscopy. The wire, which has a flexible tip, is passed into the gastric antrum as confirmed by fluoroscopy or endoscopy. The dilators are then passed serially over the wire, while maintaining the position of the wire with respect to the patient's mouth. This can be safely done now without fluoroscopy as the wire has graduated markings helping to ensure proper position and lack of migration.

Through-the-scope (TTS) balloons are passed through the biopsy channel of the endoscope under direct visualization. They have the advantages of being easy to use and not requiring fluoroscopy, but they are not reusable and are expensive.

In general, one should follow the "rule of threes" when dilating peptic strictures. That is, pass no more than three consecutive dilators that meet moderate resistance during a single dilating session. Although there is no objective evidence supporting this approach, it makes good sense not to overstretch a fibrotic stricture at one sitting. These patients have a chronic problem, and this cautious approach will minimize the chances of esophageal perforation.

The question "Is fluoroscopy necessary for bougienage?" has been addressed by three studies [36, 48, 75]. These studies evaluated the efficacy and safety of passing dilators without fluoroscopic guidance, while comparing blind Maloney dilation to dilation with fluoroscopy. Overall, the success rates for Maloney dilation with fluoroscopy varied from 76% to 96%, compared to 80% to 97.6% for "blind" Maloney dilation. The procedure-related complication rates for blind Maloney dilation ranged from 11.3% to 24% and reflect non-life-threatening events such as passage of a dilator into the trachea or curling of the dilator tip in the esophagus. No esophageal perforations occurred in either group. Current practice in the gastroenterology community favors mercury-filled bougie dilation without fluoroscopy. Two studies have examined the need for fluoroscopy when using wire-guided dilators [26, 38]. These uncontrolled studies were done to determine whether the addition of fluoroscopy to a marked guide wire technique improved the safety of dilation. When the dilation was performed without fluoroscopy, the guide wire moved no more than 30 cm in either direction and was easily repositioned. Dilations were judged successful in all cases, and there were no serious complications. Therefore, most strictures in which the endoscope can be passed into the stomach can be dilated without fluoroscopic guidance. All tight, complicated strictures which do not permit passage of the endoscope should be dilated with fluoroscopic positioning of the guide wire or by using TTS balloons.

## Choosing Among Types of Dilators

The choice of dilator depends on many factors, but the anatomy of the stricture is the most important consideration. The stricture anatomy and the esophageal contour above and below the stricture must be clearly defined by endoscopy and/or barium esophagram prior to initial dilation. Most simple strictures can be dilated with rubber, mercury-filled dilators. Maloney and Hurst dilators are therefore indicated in straight, less tight strictures (>1.2 to 1.4 cm diameter) and are usually passed blindly, without fluoroscopy. Mercury-filled dilators tend to curl up when passed in patients with tight strictures (less than 36F) and also may curl up in esophageal diverticula or large hernias above or below the stricture, increasing the risk of perforation. Wire-guided or TTS dilators are stiffer and better suited to longer, tighter, and more irregular strictures. They also have a lower risk of

perforation in patients with large hiatal hernias or esophageal diverticula. In addition, they may be passed with minimal or no sedation.

Several randomized controlled trials have compared polyvinyl bougies to TTS balloons in the dilation of peptic strictures (Table 27–3) [17, 68, 69, 84]. In all, 200 patients were randomized to bougie versus balloon dilation with a mean follow-up period of 2 years (12 to 36 months). Most patients were treated with $H_2$-receptor blockers. The need for repeat dilation for patients assigned to dilation with polyvinyl bougies was 36% to 74% compared to 39% to 58% for the Rigiflex balloon group, with no consistent evidence of one type of balloon being superior to the other. No perforations were noted among 200 patients. Since polyvinyl dilators are reusable, the costs associated with them are less than those for TTS balloon dilators. This cost differential must be balanced against the convenience of balloons and the fact that fluoroscopic guidance is not necessary when dilating with TTS balloons.

The outcome of benign esophageal strictures treated with dilation is illustrated in Table 27–4. Several general observations can be made regarding long-term outcome: (a) one-third to one-half of patients will require long-term, repeat dilations, (b) the need for dilation is highest in the first year, (c) concurrent potent acid suppression and healing of esophagitis reduce the need for repeat dilation, and (d) the length and diameter of the stricture have little bearing on the need for repeat dilation. Consideration of these factors will facilitate long-term planning of dilations.

## Complications of Endoscopic Dilations

Esophageal perforation is the most important complication of stricture dilation. The perforation rate following dilation is about 0.25% per procedure; however, the risk is higher in complex (longer, narrower, more angulated) strictures. This increased risk is reflected by wire-guided dilators being associated with higher perforation rates than Maloney

**TABLE 27–3.** *Controlled trials comparing bougie and balloon dilators*

| Author | Design[a] | Number | Dilator type[b] | Medical therapy[c] | Dilator diameter (max) | Mean f/u (mo) | % improvement | Need repeat dilation | Perforation per patient |
|---|---|---|---|---|---|---|---|---|---|
| Cox et al. [17][d] | RCT | 39 | C, EP | H2RA | 58F | ≤12 | NS | 15% | 0% |
| | | 46 | RB | H2RA | 20 mm | ≤12 | NS | 39% | 0% |
| Shemesh and Czerniak [69][e] | RCT | 30 | PVB | H2RA, M, C | 6–17 mm | 13 | 100% | 36% | 0% |
| | | 30 | RB | H2RA, M, C | 6–18 mm | 15 | 100% | 58% | 0% |
| Saeed et al. [68] | RCT | 17 | PVB | H2RA | 45F | 24 | 100% | 74% | 0% |
| | | 17 | RB | H2RA | 15 mm | 24 | 100% | 52% | 0% |
| Yamamoto et al. [84] | RCT | 16 | EP | NS | 45F | ≤36 | 100% | 38% | 0% |
| | | 15 | MTB | NS | 20 mm | ≤36 | 100% | 27% | 0% |

[a] RCT, randomized controlled trial.
[b] PVB, polyvinyl bougie; EP, Eder-Puestow; C, Celestin; RB, Rigiflex balloon; MTB, MediTech balloon.
[c] H2RA, $H_2$-receptor antagonist; M, metoclopramide; C, cisapride; NS, not specified.
[d] Etiology of strictures: 81% peptic, 13% postoperative.
[e] Etiology of strictures: 65% peptic, 18% caustic, 17% postoperative.

**TABLE 27–4.** *Long-term efficacy of dilation for esophageal strictures*

| Author | Design[a] | Number | Dilator type[b] | Dil diameter (max) | Mean f/u (mo) | Need repeat dilation | Perforation per patient |
|---|---|---|---|---|---|---|---|
| Lanza and Graham [41] | R | 92 | MB, EP | ≥41F | 21 | 54% | 0% |
| Ogilvie et al. [56] | P | 50 | EP | 45F | 9–48 | 60% | 2% |
| Wesdorp et al. [82] | P | 100 | MB, EP | ≥54F | 41 | 12% | 8% |
| Patterson et al. [61] | R | 154 | MB, EP | ≥40F | 26 | 57% | 3.2% |
| Fellows et al. [24] | R | 100 | C | 54F | 25 | 58% | 1% |
| Glick [28] | R | 76 | MB, EP | ≥44F | 21 | 65% | 1.3% |
| Saeed et al. [68] | RCT | 17 | PVB | ≥45F | 24 | 74% | 0% |
| Saeed et al. [68] | RCT | 17 | TTS | 15 mm | 24 | 52% | 0% |

[a] R, retrospective review; P, prospective trial; RCT, randomized controlled trial.
[b] PVB, polyvinyl bougie; MB, mercury bougie; EP, Eder-Puestow; C, Celestin; TTS, "through-the-scope" balloon.

dilators; 0.6% versus 0.4% in one study [71]. It is unclear from reported studies whether using fluoroscopy reduces perforation rates. The following recommendations may reduce the risk of esophageal perforation: (a) check the anatomy of the esophagus and the stricture, by endoscopy and barium esophagram, prior to dilation; (b) dilate slowly, especially in chronic strictures; and (c) use fluoroscopy, particularly in initial dilations and when dilating complex strictures [76].

Bacteremia is more common following esophageal dilation (up to 40%) than most other gastrointestinal procedures; therefore, antibiotic prophylaxis should be used where clinically appropriate [2, 49]. Other less common complications of stricture dilation include pulmonary aspiration, bleeding, intubation of the trachea, and chest pain.

## Surgery for Peptic Strictures

Surgical therapy for peptic strictures is indicated in those who fail or are not suitable candidates for aggressive medical therapy. Specific indications for surgery include nondilatable stricture, frequent stricture recurrence after dilation, failure of esophagitis to heal on maximal medical therapy, and the requirement for long-term acid-suppressing medications (e.g., in a young person). Some of these indications are rare today with the availability of proton pump inhibitors. In fact, all patients with difficult to manage strictures, despite aggressive acid suppression, need evaluation for other complicating factors, especially pill-induced damage [9].

Several operations are available for patients with severe GERD and peptic strictures. The standard Nissen fundoplication is the most commonly performed operation. The choice between partial or complete fundoplication depends primarily on the adequacy of the "esophageal pump." In patients with impaired motility and poor esophageal clearance, partial fundoplication is preferred to avoid postoperative dysphagia. Contraindications to performing a fundoplication include a nondilatable stricture, a prior partial gastrectomy, and severe esophageal shortening. Gastroplasty (Collis procedure) and fundoplication and indicated when inadequate esophageal mobilization does not allow sufficient length to form a tension-free intra-abdominal fundoplication. This is the preferred operation in patients with severe esophageal shortening. Esophagoplasty (Thal procedure) involves making a longitudinal, full-thickness incision in the stricture and covering the defect with a gastric serosal patch. The limitations of this procedure are that it does not prevent recurrent reflux and that it has higher mortality than fundoplication. Given the possible role of bile reflux in peptic strictures, acid-reducing and alkaline-diversion procedures sometimes are performed for peptic strictures. Acid is reduced by an antrectomy, while a Roux-en-Y loop diverts bile away from the stomach. The operation is used in patients with prior gastric resection but may be complicated by gastroparesis. The most radical surgery for peptic strictures is resection of the esophagus with reconstruction. This procedure is usually reserved for patients with an irreversibly damaged esophagus with transmural fibrosis. Suggestive clinical features include inability to adequately dilate a stricture, rapid recurrence of a stricture after dilation, and aperistalsis, as determined by manometry [86]. Total esophagectomy with gastric pull-up or a jejunal or colonic interposition is required in these intractable cases.

The outcome following antireflux surgery depends on many factors, the experience of the surgeon being most important. Table 27–5 summarizes a representative series of patients treated surgically for peptic strictures. The results of partial or complete fundoplication are good or excellent in about 77% of cases (range, 43% to 90%). Anywhere from 1% to 43% of patients require repeat dilation after surgery, but this is usually confined to one or two dilation sessions. Mortality rates should be less than 0.5%, with the morbidity less than 20% [77]. As a general rule, results are better in major medical centers, where the volume of operations is sufficient to provide surgeons with a large experience. There are no randomized, controlled trials comparing antireflux surgery to conservative management ($H_2$ antagonists and bougienage). However, one study compared a group of patients treated by antireflux surgery with a control group treated medically over a 3-year period [81]. Of the 78 patients in the medically treated group, 41% needed only one additional dilation whereas the remainder required an average of 3.1 subsequent dilations. In contrast, 71% of the 42 patients undergoing antireflux surgery needed only a single

**TABLE 27–5.** *Sample studies of antireflux surgery for peptic strictures*

| Author | Number patients | Operation[a] | Success | Mortality |
|---|---|---|---|---|
| Rees [66] | 27 | ARP | 82% | 3.7% |
| Orringer and Orringer [58] | 58 | ARP | NS | 0% |
| Bonavina et al. [10] | 36 | ARP | 78% | 2.7% |
| Vollan et al. [80] | 43 | ARP | 79% | 0% |
| Maher et al. [45] | 68 | ARP | 65% | 4% |
| Little et al. [44] | 34 | ARP | 82% | 0% |
| Payne [62] | 84 | ARP | 85% | 0% |
| Payne [62] | 17 | ER | 76% | 0% |
| Bischof et al. [7] | 11 | ER | 43% | Not stated |
| Bender and Walbaum [5] | 89 | ER | 62% | 8.9% |
| Little et al. [44] | 18 | ER | 67% | 16.7% |

[a] ARP, antireflux procedure; ER, esophagectomy and reconstruction.

dilation, with the remainder requiring an average of 1.6 subsequent dilations. With the widespread use of proton pump inhibitors and the safety of bougienage, we anticipate a decreasing need for antireflux surgery for peptic strictures in the future.

# REFERENCES

1. Ahtardis G, et al. Clinical and manometric findings in benign peptic stricture of the esophagus. Dig Dis Sci 1979;24:858
2. Antibiotic prophylaxis for gastrointestinal endoscopy. ASGE guidelines. Gastrointest Endosc 1995;42:630
3. Arvanitakis C. Lower esophageal ring: endoscopic and therapeutic aspects. Gastrointest Endosc 1977;24:17
4. Attwood SE, et al. Alkaline gastroesophageal reflux: implications in the development of complications in Barrett's columnar lined lower esophagus. Surgery 1989;106:764
5. Bender EM, Walbaum PR. Esophagogastrectomy for benign esophageal stricture. Ann Surg 1987;205:385
6. Bergstad A, et al. Relationship of hiatal hernia to reflux esophagitis. A prospective study of the incidence using endoscopy. Scand J Gastroenterol 1986;21:55
7. Bischoff G, et al. Surgery versus conservative bougienage in the treatment of peptic esophageal strictures: long term results of 200 patients. Gastroenterology 1992;102:A42
8. Black DD, Haggitt RC, Orenstein SR, Whitington PF. Esophagitis in infants. Morphometric histological diagnosis and correlations with measures of gastroesophageal reflux. Gastroenterology 1990;98:1408
9. Bonavina L, DeMeester TR, McChesney L, Schwizner W, Albertucci M, Bailey RT. Drug-induced esophageal strictures. Ann Surg 1987;2:173
10. Bonavina L, et al. Surgical treatment of reflux stricture of the oesophagus. Br J Surg 1993;80:317
11. Bondeson AG, Bondeson L, Thompson NW. Stricture and perforation of the esophagus: overlooked threats in the Zollinger-Ellison syndrome. World J Surg 1990;14:361
12. Buchin PJ, Spiro HM. Therapy of esophageal stricture: a review of 84 patients. J Clin Gastroenterol 1981;3:121
13. Castell DO, Donner MW. Evaluation of dysphagia: a careful history is crucial. Dysphagia 1987;2:65
14. Chen YM, Gelfand DW, Ott DJ, Munitz HA. Natural progression of the lower esophageal mucosal ring. Gastrointest Radiol 1987;12:93
15. Collins BJ, Elliott H, Sloan JM, McFarland RJ, Love AHG. Oesophageal histology in reflux esophagitis. J Clin Pathol 1985;38:1265
16. Cox JGC, et al. Balloon or bougie for dilation of benign oesophageal stricture? An interim report of a randomized controlled trial. Gut 1988;29:1741
17. Cox JGC, et al. Balloon or bougie for dilation of esophageal stricture? Dig Dis Sci 1994;39:776
18. Csendes A, Larrain A, Strauzner R, Ayala M. Long-term clinical, radiographic and manometric follow-up of patients with achalasia of the esophagus treated with esophagomyotomy. Digestion 1975;13:27
19. Dakkak M, Hoare RC, Maslin SC, Bennett JR. Oesophagitis is as important as oesophageal stricture diameter in determining dysphagia. Gut 1993;34:152
20. Dodds WJ, et al. Mechanisms of gastroesophageal reflux in patients with reflux esophagitis. N Engl J Med 1982;307:1547
21. Dumon J, Meric B, Sivak M, Fleicher D. A new method of esophageal dilation using Savary-Gilliard bougies. Gastrointest Endosc 1985;31:379
22. Eastridge CE, Pate JW, Mann KA. Lower esophageal ring: experiences in treatment of 88 patients. Ann Thorac Surg 1984;37:103
23. El-Serag HB, Sonnenberg A. Association of esophagitis and esophageal strictures with diseases treated with non-steroidal anti-inflammatory drugs. Am J Gastroenterol 1997;92:52
24. Fellows IW, Raina S, Holmes GKT. Celestin dilatation of benign esophageal strictures: a review of 100 patients. Am J Gastroenterol 1986;81:1052
25. Ferguson R, Dronfield MW, Atkinson M. Cimetidine in treatment of reflux esophagitis with peptic stricture. BMJ 1979;2:472
26. Fleischer DE, et al. A marked guide wire facilitates esophageal dilation. Am J Gastroenterol 1989;84:359
27. Geboes K, Desmet V, Vantrappen G, Mebis J. Vascular changes in the esophageal mucosa. An early histologic sign of esophagitis. Gastrointest Endosc 1980;26:29
28. Glick ME. Course of esophageal stricture managed by bougienage. Dig Dis Sci 1982;27:884
29. Goldschmid S, Boyce HW, Brown JI, Brady PG, Nord HJ, Lyman GH. A new objective measurement of esophageal lumen patency. Am J Gastroenterol 1989;10:1255
30. Harding SM. Pulmonary abnormalities in gastroesophageal reflux disease. In Richter JE, ed, Ambulatory esophageal pH monitoring (2nd ed). Baltimore: Williams & Wilkins, 1997
31. Harvey RF, et al. Effects of sleeping with the bead-head raised and of ranitidine in patients with severe peptic esophagitis. Lancet 1987;2:1200
32. Heitman P, Csendes A, Strauszer T. Esophageal strictures and lower esophagus lined with columnar epithelium. Functional and morphologic studies. Am J Dig Dis 1971;16:307
33. Heller SR, Fellows IW, Ogilvie AL, Atkinson M. Non-steroidal anti-inflammatory drugs and benign oesophageal strictures. BMJ 1982;285:167
34. Henderson RD, Pearson FC. Surgical management of esophageal scleroderma. J Thorac Cardiovasc Surg 1973;66:686
35. Hiatt GA. The roles of esophagoscopy vs radiograph in diagnosing benign peptic esophageal strictures. Gastrointest Endosc 1977;23:194
36. Ho SB, et al. Fluoroscopy is not necessary for Maloney dilation of chronic esophageal strictures. Gastrointest Endosc 1994;41:11
37. Jaspersen D, Schwacha H, Schorr W, Brennenstuhl M, Raschka C, Hammar CH. Omeprazole in the treatment of patients with complicated gastro-oesophageal reflux disease. J Gastroenterol Hepatol 1996;11:900
38. Kadakia SC, Parker A, Carrougher JG, Shaffer RT. Esophageal dilation with polyvinyl bougies, using a marked guidewire without the aid of fluoroscopy: an update. Am J Gastroenterol 1993;88:1381
39. Kemp Harper JA, Jackson DC. Progressive systemic sclerosis. Br J Radiol 1964;38:825

40. Kirsch M, Blue M, Desai RK, Sivak MV. Intralesional steroid injections for peptic strictures. Gastrointest Endosc 1991;37:180
41. Lanza FL, Graham DY. Bougienage is effective therapy for most benign esophageal strictures. JAMA 1978;240:844
42. Larrain A, Csendes A, Pope CE. Surgical correction of reflux: an effective therapy for esophageal strictures. Gastroenterology 1975;69:578
43. Larrain A, et al. Manometric evaluation after posterior gastropexy for the treatment of strictures of the esophagus secondary to reflux. Surg Gynecol Obstet 1973;136:564
44. Little AG, et al. Surgical management of esophageal strictures. Ann Thorac Surg 1988;45:144
45. Maher JW, Hocking MP, Woodward ER. Long-term follow up of the combined fundic patch fundoplication for treatment of longitudinal peptic strictures of the esophagus. Ann Surg 1981;194:64
46. Mansfield LE, Stein MR. Gastroesophageal reflux and asthma: a possible reflex mechanism. Ann Allergy 1978;41:224
47. Marks RD, et al. Omeprazole versus H2-receptor antagonists in treating patients with peptic stricture and esophagitis. Gastroenterology 1994;108:907
48. McClave SA, Wright RA, Brady PG. Prospective randomized study of Maloney esophageal dilation—blinded versus fluoroscopic guidance. Gastrointest Endosc 1990;36:272
49. Meyer GW. Endocarditis prophylaxis and esophageal dilation. Gastrointest Endosc 1989;35:129
50. Miller LS, Vinayek R, Frucht H, Gardner JD, Jensen RT, Maton PN. Reflux esophagitis in patients with Zollinger-Ellison syndrome. Gastroenterology 1990;98:341
51. Mittal RK, Lange RC, McCallum RW. Identification and mechanism of delayed esophageal acid clearance in subjects with hiatus hernia. Gastroenterology 1987;92:130
52. Moody GA, Probert CS. Mercury bougie self-dilation of the esophagus in the 1990s. J Clin Gastroenterol 1992;15:264
53. Moses F. Reversible aperistalsis as a complication of gastroesophageal reflux disease. Am J Gastroenterol 1987;82:272
54. Murphy JR, McInally P, Peller P. Prolonged clearance is the primary abnormal reflux parameter in patients with progressive systemic sclerosis and esophagitis. Dig Dis Sci 1992;37:833
55. Nagler R, Spiro HM. Persistent GER induced during prolonged gastric intubation. N Engl J Med 1963;269:495
56. Ogilvie AL, Ferguson R, Atkinson M. Outlook with conservative treatment of peptic oesophageal strictures. Gut 1980;20:23
57. Orringer MB, Dabich L, Zarafonetis CJD. Gastroesophageal reflux in esophageal scleroderma: diagnosis and implications. Ann Thorac Surg 1976;22:120
58. Orringer MB, Orringer JS. The combined Collis-Nissen operation: early assessment of reflux control. Ann Thorac Surg 1982;33:534
59. Ott DJ, Gelfand DW, Lane TG, Wu WC. Radiological detection and spectrum of appearance of peptic esophageal strictures. J Clin Gastroenterol 1982;4:11
60. Palmer ED. The hiatus hernia–esophagitis–esophageal stricture complex: twenty year prospective study. Am J Med 1968;44:566
61. Patterson DJ, et al. Natural history of benign esophageal stricture treated by dilation. Gastroenterology 1983;85:346
62. Payne WS. Surgical management of reflux induced esophageal stenoses: results in 101 patients. Br J Surg 1984;71:971
63. Pellegrini CA, Leichter R, Patti M, Somberg K, Ostroff JW, Way L. Thoracoscopic esophageal myotomy in the treatment of achalasia. Ann Thorac Surg 1993;56:680
64. Picchio M, et al. Jejunal interposition for peptic stenosis of the esophagus following esophagomyotomy for achalasia. Int Surg 1997;82:198
65. Raiser F, et al. Heller myotomy via minimal access surgery. An evaluation of antireflux procedures. Arch Surg 1996;131:593
66. Rees JR. The surgical treatment of complicated peptic esophagitis. Am Surg 1987;53:497
67. Richter JE, Pandol SJ, Castell DO, McCarthy DM. Gastroesophageal reflux disease in the Zollinger-Ellison syndrome. Ann Intern Med 1981;95:37
68. Saeed ZA, Winchester CB, Ferro PS, Michaletz PA, Schwartz JT, Graham DY. Prospective randomized comparison of polyvinyl bougies and through-the-scope balloons for dilation of peptic strictures of the esophagus. Gastrointest Endosc 1995;41:189
69. Shemesh E, Czerniak A. Comparison between Savary-Gilliard and balloon dilation of benign esophageal strictures. World J Surg 1990;14:518
70. Silvis SE, Farahmand M, Johnson JA, Ansel HJ, Ho SB. A randomized blinded comparison of omeprazole and ranitidine in the treatment of chronic esophageal stricture secondary to acid peptic esophagitis. Gastrointest Endosc 1996;43:216
71. Silvis SE, Nebel O, Rogers G, Sugawa C, Mandelstam P. Endoscopic complications: results of the 1974 American Society for Gastrointestinal Endoscopy survey. JAMA 1976;235:928
72. Smith PM, et al. A comparison of omeprazole and ranitidine in the prevention of recurrence of benign esophageal stricture. Gastroenterology 1994;107:1312
73. Spechler SJ, Sperber H, Doos WG, Schimmel EM. The prevalence of Barrett's esophagus in patients with chronic peptic esophageal stricture. Dig Dis Sci 1983;28:769
74. Swarbrick ET, Gough AL, Foster CS, Christian J, Garrett AD, Langworthy CH. Prevention of recurrence of esophageal stricture, a comparison of lansoprazole and high-dose ranitidine. Eur J Gastroenterol Hepatol 1996;8:431
75. Tucker LF. The importance of fluoroscopic guidance for Maloney dilation. Am J Gastroenterol 1992;87:1709
76. Tulman AB, Boyce HW. Complications of esophageal dilation and guidelines for their prevention. Gastrointest Endosc 1981;27:229
77. Tytgat GN, et al. Long term strategy for the treatment of gastroesophageal reflux disease. Gastroenterol Int 1991;4:21
78. Vaezi MF, Richter JE. Current therapies for achalasia: comparison and efficacy. Am J Gastroenterol 1998;27:21
79. Vaezi M, Singh S, Richter JE. Role of acid and duodenogastric reflux in esophageal mucosal injury: a review of animal and human studies. Gastroenterology 1995;108:1897
80. Vollan G, et al. Long term results after Nissen fundoplication and Belsey Mark IV operation in patients with reflux esophagitis and peptic stricture. Eur J Surg 1992;158:357
81. Watson A. Reflux stricture of the esophagus. Br J Surg 1987;74:443
82. Wesdorp ICE, Bartelsman JF, den Hartog Jager FC, Huibregtse K, Tytgat GN. Results of conservative treatment of benign esophageal strictures: a follow up study in 100 patients. Gastroenterology 1982;82:487
83. Wilkins WE, Ridley MG, Ponziak AL. Benign stricture of the oesophagus: role of nonsteroidal anti-inflammatory drugs. Gut 1984;25:478
84. Yamamoto H, Hughes RW, Schroeder KW, Viggiano TR, DiMagno EP. Treatment of benign esophageal stricture by Eder-Puestow or balloon dilators: a comparison between randomized and prospective non-randomized trials. Mayo Clin Proc 1992;67:228
85. Zamost BJ, Hirschberg J, Ippoliti AF, Furst DE, Clements PJ, Weinstein WM. Esophagitis in scleroderma. Prevalence and risk factors. Gastroenterology 1987;92:421
86. Zaninotto G, DeMeester GR, Bremner CG. Esophageal function in patients with reflux-induced strictures and its relevance to surgical treatment. Ann Thorac Surg 1989;47:362
87. Zein NN, Greseth JM, Perrault J. Endoscopic intralesional steroid injections in the management of refractory esophageal strictures. Gastrointest Endosc 1995;41:596

*The Esophagus*, Third Edition,
edited by D. O. Castell and J. E. Richter.
Lippincott Williams & Wilkins, Philadelphia © 1999.

CHAPTER 28

# Gastroesophageal Reflux Laryngitis

Robert Thayer Sataloff and Joseph R. Spiegel

Occult chronic gastroesophageal reflux (GER) is an etiologic factor in a high percentage of patients with laryngologic complaints. When gastric contents rise above the level of the upper esophageal sphincter, the condition may be called laryngopharyngeal reflux (LPR). Although it is seen in otolaryngologic patients of all ages, the problem has been documented particularly in professional voice users. In 1991, Sataloff and coauthors [37] reported reflux laryngitis (RL) in 265 (45%) of the 583 consecutive professional voice users, including singers and others, who sought medical care during a 12-month period, although RL was often diagnosed incidentally and was not always responsible for the patient's primary voice complaint. The incidence may be lower in patients with other vocations, but it is interesting to note that Koufman and co-workers [22] found increased GER in 78% of patients with hoarseness. Additional studies of the epidemiology and prevalence of RL are needed.

## ANATOMY AND PHYSIOLOGY OF PHONATION

To appreciate the importance of RL, it is helpful to understand basic concepts about the delicate mechanism of phonation. A detailed discussion of the subject is beyond the scope of this chapter, and only a brief review is presented. For a more thorough understanding of current concepts in phonation, the reader is referred to recent reviews [13, 35–38, 40].

The anatomy of the voice is not limited to the larynx. The vocal mechanism also includes the abdominal and back musculature, rib cage, lungs, the pharynx, oral cavity, and nose. Each component performs an important function in voice production. Although the larynx is essential to normal voice production, it is possible to produce voice even without a larynx, for example, in patients who have undergone laryngectomy. In addition, virtually all parts of the body play

some role in voice production and may be responsible for voice dysfunction. Even something as remote as a sprained ankle may alter posture, thereby impairing abdominal, back, and thoracic muscle function and resulting in vocal inefficiency, weakness, and hoarseness.

The larynx is composed of four basic anatomic units: skeleton, intrinsic muscles, extrinsic muscles, and mucosa. The most important parts of the laryngeal skeleton are the thyroid cartilage, cricoid cartilage, and two arytenoid cartilages (Fig. 28–1). Intrinsic muscles of the larynx are connected to these cartilages. One of the intrinsic muscles, the *thyroarytenoid* or *vocalis muscle,* extends on each side from the arytenoid cartilage to the inside of the thyroid cartilage just below the thyroid prominence ("Adam's apple"), forming the body of the vocal folds (formerly called the vocal cords). The vocal folds act as the oscillator, or voice source, of the vocal tract. The space between the vocal folds is called the *glottis* and is used as an anatomic reference point.

The soft tissues lining the larynx are much more complex than originally thought. The mucosa forms the thin, lubricated surface of the vocal folds that makes contact when the glottis is closed. It is similar to the mucosa lining the inside of the mouth. Throughout most of the larynx, there are goblet cells and pseudostratified, ciliated columnar epithelium designed for handling mucous secretions, similar to mucosa found throughout the respiratory tract. However, the mucosa overlying the vocal folds themselves is different. First, it is stratified squamous epithelium, better suited to withstand the trauma of vocal fold contact. Second, the vocal fold is not simply muscle covered with mucosa. Rather, it consists of five layers (Fig. 28–2). Mechanically, the vocal folds act more like three layers, consisting of the *cover* (epithelium and superficial layer of the lamina propria), *transition* (intermediate and deep layers of the lamina propria), and *body* (the vocalis muscle). It is essential for surgeons to understand this anatomy and the importance of preserving it during surgical intervention. It is also essential to recognize that even minor changes in this structure, such as edema in the superficial layer of the lamina propria (Reinke's space), may alter phon-

R. T. Sataloff and J. R. Spiegel: Department of Otolaryngology—Head and Neck Surgery, Graduate Hospital, Philadelphia, Pennsylvania 19146, and Department of Otolaryngology—Head and Neck Surgery, Thomas Jefferson University, Philadelphia, Pennsylvania 19107.

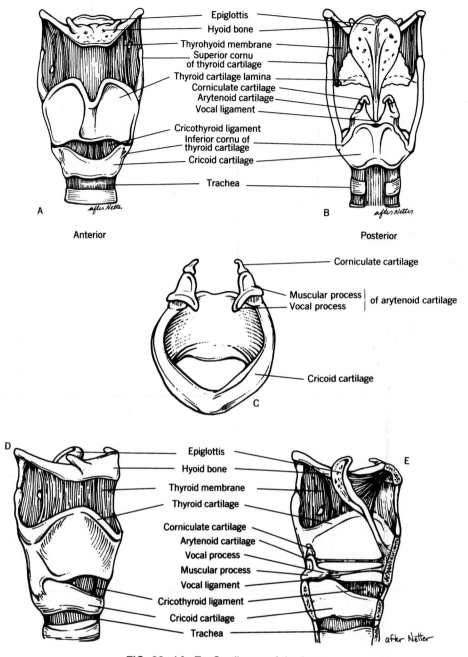

**FIG. 28–1A–E.** Cartilages of the larynx.

ation substantially. This layer is most prone to edema when exposed to irritants, such as gastric juice.

The *supraglottic vocal tract* includes the pharynx, tongue, palate, oral cavity, nose, and other structures. Together, they act as a *resonator* and are largely responsible for vocal quality, or timbre, and the perceived character of all speech sounds. The vocal folds themselves produce only a "buzzing" sound. During the course of vocal training for singing, acting, or healthy speaking, changes occur not only in the larynx but also in the muscle motion, muscle control, and shape of the supraglottic vocal tract. The *infraglottic vocal*

*tract* serves as the power source for the voice. Singers and actors refer to the entire power source complex as their "support" or "diaphragm."

The physiology of voice production is exceedingly complex. Volitional production of voice begins in the cerebral cortex. Vocalization involves complex interaction among centers for speech, the precentral gyrus in the motor cortex, motor nuclei in the brain stem and spinal cord, the larynx, thoracic and abdominal musculature, vocal tract articulators, the auditory system (for feedback and fine adjustments), and other areas. Phonation requires interaction among the power

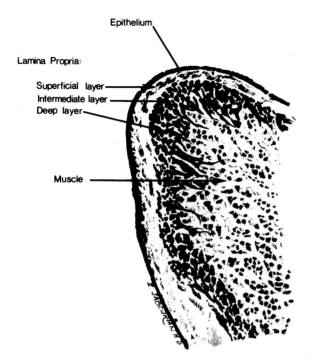

**FIG. 28–2.** The structure of the vocal fold. (From ref. 15, with permission.)

source, oscillator, and resonator. The voice may be likened to a brass instrument, such as a trumpet. Power is generated by the chest, abdomen, and back musculature producing a high-pressure air stream. The trumpeter's lips open and close against the mouthpiece, producing a buzz similar to the sound produced by the vocal folds. This sound then passes through the trumpet, which has resonant characteristics that shape the sound we associate with trumpet music. The non-mouthpiece portion of a brass instrument is analogous to the supraglottic vocal tract. During phonation, rapid, complex adjustments of the infraglottic musculature are necessary because the resistance changes almost continuously as the glottis closes, opens, and changes shape. At the beginning of each phonatory cycle, the vocal folds are approximated. Subglottic pressure builds up, opening the vocal folds from bottom to top and back to front. They close in the same order due to a combination of forces, including tissue elasticity, Bernoulli effect, and the aerodynamics of the glottic slit configuration. This series of events results in a complex, traveling mucosal wave and sophisticated cross-sectional vertical phase differences in wave motion along the vocal folds. This complexity is necessary for normal phonation. Anything that interferes with it may result in voice dysfunction. Hence, it should be clear that acid irritation of the vocal folds is capable not only of producing annoying irritative symptoms (burning, lump in the throat) but, moreover, of actually interfering with phonation by causing edema and inflammation of the vibratory margin and lamina propria that truly alter voice.

## HISTORICAL PERSPECTIVES ON REFLUX LARYNGITIS

In addition to erythema and edema, more serious vocal fold pathology may be caused by RL. In 1968, Cherry and Margulies [5] recognized that RL might be a causative factor in contact ulcers and granulomas of the posterior portion of the vocal folds. They also observed that treatment of peptic esophagitis resulted in resolution of vocal process granulomas. Delahunty and Cherry [9] followed up on this observation by applying gastric juice to the vocal processes of two dogs and saliva to the vocal processes of a third dog, used as a control. The control dog's vocal folds remained normal; the other dogs developed granulomas at the sites of repeated acid application. The experiment by Delahunty and Cherry is particularly interesting. The posterior portion of the left vocal fold of two dogs was exposed to gastric acid for a total of only 20 minutes per day, 5 days out of every 7, for a total of 29 days of exposure in a 39-day period. A total of 20 minutes out of 24 hours may not seem like an extensive exposure period. However, erythema and edema were apparent in both dogs by the fourth day of the first week. At the beginning of the second week, the larynges appeared normal after the 2-day rest period. However, visible reaction was provoked within 2 days after application was resumed, and the vocal folds never regained normal appearance. Marked inflammation, thickening, and irregularities were apparent in both dogs by the fourth week, and epithelial slough at the site of acid contact occurred on day 29 in one dog and day 32 in the other. Granulation tissue appeared shortly thereafter. A similar procedure on a control animal was performed, applying saliva to the vocal fold instead of gastric juice, and the vocal fold remained normal. This research suggests that even relatively short periods of acid exposure may cause substantial abnormalities in laryngeal mucosa. Since then, numerous authors have recognized the importance of RL as a causative factor in laryngeal ulcers and granulomas, including intubation granuloma [5, 6, 12, 13, 17, 26, 28, 29, 34, 41, 43]. In addition to its etiologic involvement in intubation granuloma, RL has long been recognized as a contributing factor to posterior glottic stenosis, especially following intubation [3]. Olson [29] has suggested that it may also be a causative factor in cricoarytenoid joint arthritis through chronic inflammation and ulceration, beginning on the mucosa and involving the synovial cricoarytenoid joint. In addition to posterior glottic and supraglottic stenosis, subglottic stenosis has been reported as a complication of reflux [1, 10].

It appears likely that acid RL may also be causally related to laryngeal carcinoma. The association of gastroesophageal RL disease with Barrett's esophagus and esophageal carcinoma has been well established. Delahunty [8] biopsied the posterior laryngeal mucosa in a patient with RL and reported epithelial hyperplasia with parakeratosis and papillary downgrowth. Olson [29] reported five patients (young, nonsmokers, nondrinkers) with posterior laryngeal carcinoma in whom he believed reflux to be a cofactor. This issue was also addressed by Morrison [27]. Although the causal relationship between reflux and laryngeal cancer has not been established with absolute certainty, it appears probable.

In addition to its possible carcinogenic potential, the chronic irritation of RL may be responsible for failure of wound healing. Reflux appears to delay the resolution not only of vocal process ulcers and granulomas but also of healing following vocal fold surgery. For this reason, otolaryngologists are becoming increasingly aggressive about diagnosing and treating reflux before subjecting patients to vocal fold surgery, even for conditions unrelated to the reflux.

Evidence suggests that sudden infant death syndrome (SIDS) may also be causally related to acid reflux into the larynx [45]. Hence, SIDS must join laryngeal and esophageal cancer at the top of the list of important otolaryngologic consequences of RL. Wetmore [45] investigated the effects of acid on the larynges of maturing rabbits by applying solutions of acid or saline at 15-day intervals up to 60 days of age. Since the larynx not only is a site of resistance in the airway but also contains the afferent limb for reflexes that regulate respiration, he discovered that acid exposure resulted in significant obstructive, central, and mixed apnea. Gasping respirations and frequent swallowing were observed as associated symptoms. Central apnea occurred in all age groups but had a peak incidence at 45 days. Acid-induced obstructive apnea in rabbits is similar to the obstructive apnea previously recognized in human infants with gastroesophageal disease [39, 45]. However, the demonstration of acid-induced central apnea produced by acid stimulation of the larynx is more ominous. Central apnea has been demonstrated in other animal models as a result of different forms of laryngeal stimulation. Central apnea resulting in fatal asphyxia has also been described in several animal models. Wetmore's study [45] suggests that GER alone is capable of triggering fatal central apnea. This is particularly compelling when one recognizes that the peak incidence of central apnea, occurring at 45 days in the rabbit, corresponds well with the peak incidence of SIDS in humans, which occurs between 2 and 4 months of age.

## PATHOPHYSIOLOGY

LPR can affect anyone, but it appears particularly common and symptomatic in professional voice users, especially singers. This is true for several reasons. First, the technique of singing utilizes "support," which involves forceful compression of the abdominal muscles designed to push the abdominal contents superiorly and pull the sternum down. This action compresses the air in the thorax and generates a force for the stream of expired air, but it also compresses the stomach and works against the lower esophageal sphincter. Singing is an athletic endeavor, and the mechanism responsible for reflux in singers is similar to that associated with reflux following other athletic activities, lifting, and other conditions that alter abdominal pressures, such as pregnancy (which is also influenced by hormonal factors). Second, many singers do not eat before performing because a full stomach interferes with abdominal support and promotes reflux. Performances usually take place at night. Consequently, the singer returns home hungry and eats a large meal before bed. Third, performance careers are particularly stressful, and this factor may be associated with increased acid production. Fourth, many singers pay little attention to good nutrition, frequently consuming caffeine, fatty foods (including fast foods), spicy foods, citrus products (especially lemons), and tomatoes (including pizza and spaghetti). In addition, because of the great demands singers place upon their voices, even slight alterations caused by peptic mucositis of the larynx produce symptoms that may impair performance. Thus, singers are certainly more likely to seek care because of reflux symptoms than are people in professions with fewer vocal demands. However, careful inquiry and physical examination reveal similar problems among all patients. Most of the voice problems associated with RL appear to be due to direct mucosal damage from proximal reflux. The effects of distal reflux alone on laryngeal function have not been studied.

Voice abnormalities and vocal fold pathology due to reflux of gastric juice onto the vocal folds may occur. Severe coughing may cause vocal fold hemorrhage or mucosal tears, sometimes leading to permanent dysphonia by causing scarring that obliterates the layers of the lamina propria and fixes the epithelium to deeper layers. Aspiration also makes reactive airway disease difficult to control. Even mild pulmonary obstruction impairs voice support. Consequently, afflicted patients subconsciously strain to compensate with muscles in the neck and throat, which are designed for delicate control, not for power source functions [9]. This behavior is typically responsible for vocal nodules and other lesions related to voice abuse. It also appears likely that some extraesophageal symptoms of reflux are due to stimulation of the vagus nerve rather than (or in addition to) topical irritation. The role of vagal reflexes in RL remains to be clarified.

## PATIENT HISTORY

For patients with voice complaints, an extensive and complex history is required to assess not only the possibility of head and neck disorders but also the numerous systemic problems that may be responsible for voice disorders [34]. These include endocrinologic, neurologic, musculoskeletal, pulmonary, gastroenterologic, and other types of disorder. Patients with RL frequently have characteristic histories and physical findings that lead the astute clinician to the diagnosis. It is important to determine whether the patient is a professional voice user, especially if he or she is a singer. Not only is reflux seen frequently in singers, but also its symptoms are more troublesome in this population.

Common symptoms of RL include morning hoarseness, prolonged voice warm-up time (greater than 20 to 30 minutes), halitosis, excessive phlegm, frequent throat clearing, dry mouth, coated tongue, sensation of a lump in the throat (globus sensation, although recent observations raise questions about this association), throat tickle, dysphagia, regurgitation of food, chronic sore throat, possibly geographic tongue, nocturnal cough, chronic or recurrent cough, difficulty breathing (especially at night), aspiration, closing off of the airway (laryngospasm), poorly controlled asthma (which causes dysphonia by interfering with the support mechanism), pneumonia, recurrent airway problems in infants, and occasionally dyspepsia (epigastric discomfort) or pyrosis (heartburn). However, dyspepsia and pyrosis are frequently absent. Interestingly, if patients stop reflux treatment after a few months, classic dyspepsia and pyrosis seem to be present commonly when symptoms recur, although this clinically observed phenomenon has not been studied formally.

In addition to prolonged vocal warm-up time, professional singers and actors may complain of voice practice intolerance, which may involve frequent throat clearing and excessive phlegm, especially during the first 10 to 20 minutes of vocal exercises or songs. Although the majority of otolaryngologists have only begun to acknowledge the importance of reflux in causing otolaryngologic disease, many authors have recognized the association for more than two decades [1, 2, 7, 8, 11, 14, 16–19, 21, 23–25, 30–33, 35, 36, 42–44, 46, 47]. Otolaryngologists are becoming increasingly diligent about looking for arytenoid erythema and edema, suspecting LPR as the underlying problem, and treating it as the primary approach to therapy for these conditions.

## PHYSICAL EXAMINATION

Physical examination of patients with throat and voice complaints must be comprehensive. Of course, a thorough head and neck examination is always included, with attention to the ears and hearing, nasal patency, the oral cavity and temporomandibular joints, allergic appearance, the larynx, and the neck. At least a limited general physical examination is included to look for signs of systemic dysfunction that may present as throat or voice complaints. More comprehensive specialized physical examinations by medical consultants should be sought when indicated.

Laryngoscopic examination typically reveals erythema and edema of the mucosa overlying the arytenoid cartilages, the posterior aspect of the larynx, and often the posterior portion of the true vocal folds (Color Plates 48 and 49). In severe cases, the erythema and edema may be more extensive. Mild, diffuse, nonspecific laryngitis and halitosis are also commonly present. In some patients with LPR severe enough to involve the oral cavity, there is also loss of dental enamel. Hence, transparency of the lower portion of the central incisors may be seen occasionally in reflux patients, although it may be more common in patients with bulimia and those who habitually eat lemons. When the patient has complaints of vocal difficulties, laryngeal examination may also include formal assessment of the speaking and singing voice and strobovideolaryngoscopy for slow-motion evaluation of the vibratory margin of the vocal folds. Objective voice analysis quantifies voice quality, pulmonary function, valvular efficiency of the vocal folds, harmonic spectral characteristics, neuromuscular function on electromyography, and other factors [36].

## TESTS

Tests to confirm the presence of RL are discussed elsewhere in this book and will not be reviewed in this chapter. However, a couple of points are worth special emphasis. At present, 24-hour pH monitoring is considered the most definitive study. Several interesting studies have highlighted the association between reflux and otolaryngologic symptomatology. For example, Wiener and colleagues [46] performed 24-hour pH monitoring on 33 patients who had chronic hoarseness not attributable to other causes and laryngeal findings suggestive of acid irritation. Twenty-six (78.8%) of the patients had severe GER, with pH findings at least three times greater than the upper limit of normal. Reflux in the upright position was greater in patients with chronic hoarseness than in patients with proven esophagitis. Katz [19] performed 24-hour pH monitoring on ten patients suspected of having RL. Hypopharyngeal reflux (2 cm above the upper esophageal sphincter) was demonstrated conclusively in seven of the ten patients. The frequency and duration of distal esophageal reflux episodes in three of these patients would have been classified as normal, and the abnormal reflux would have been missed if the hypopharyngeal sensors had not been used. Most of these patients demonstrated high-frequency, short-duration, upright reflux. Jacob and associates [16] studied 40 patients with GER, 25 of whom had symptoms of RL. Their 24-hour pH monitoring studies revealed that patients with laryngeal symptoms show significantly more proximal esophageal acid exposure, especially at night. Studies performed in our laboratory in conjunction with Castell showed that dual-electrode pH recording can document abnormal distal and proximal esophageal reflux induced by singing (Fig. 28–3). The singing challenge shown in Fig. 28–3 can also unmask meaningful reflux in patients with otherwise normal pH on 24-hour monitoring studies.

Occasionally, patients will show abnormalities on barium swallow with water siphonage but normal pH on 24-hour monitoring studies. Although in this situation, the barium study finding is usually interpreted as a "false-positive," this assumption may require further investigation, especially in professional singers and actors, in whom barium swallow studies with water siphonage provide a good clinical approximation of daily activities. To optimize mucosal function, it is essential for singers and actors to remain well hydrated. Consequently, they drink large amounts of water, routinely carry water bottles with them, and drink substantial quan-

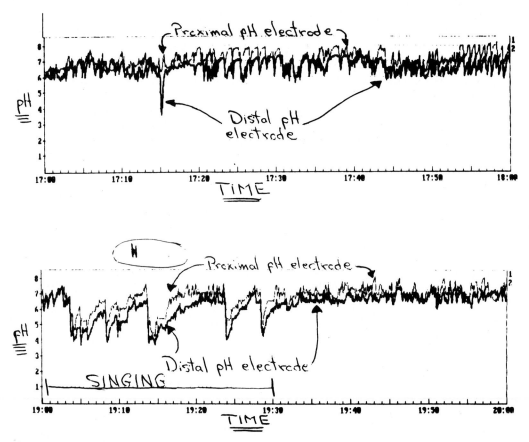

**FIG. 28–3.** Dual-electrode pH probe monitoring while singing for a 30-minute period of the 1 hour shown. The patient experienced typical heartburn, and increased proximal and distal acid exposure was prominent during singing.

tities shortly before they sing. This routine behavior is similar to the water siphon portion of the barium swallow, and this raises the question of whether positive results on water siphonage tests may provide useful information at least in professional voice users, even when 24-hour pH monitoring demonstrates normal pH.

## TREATMENT

Treatment considerations in reflux patients are discussed elsewhere. However, it should be emphasized that patients with RL frequently require more intensive therapy with higher doses of $H_2$ blockers or earlier use of omeprazole than patients with dyspepsia in the absence of laryngeal symptoms and signs. In addition to monitoring symptoms and signs of RL, response to treatment is best judged by combined intraesophageal and intragastric pH monitoring of patients while they are receiving treatment. Such studies are worthwhile even when patients are taking proton pump inhibitors since some patients are omeprazole-resistant [4, 20]. Our recent observations suggest that omeprazole resistance also can develop in patients who initially respond well to the medication. Moreover, it must be recognized that a normal pH 24-hour monitoring study does not indicate the ab-

sence of reflux. Rather, it demonstrates the absence of *acid* reflux. Reflux of pH-neutral liquid may still be present and may produce symptoms, especially in singers and actors. Study of this phenomenon and its optimal management is badly needed. At the present time, it seems likely that we may conclude that surgical correction of reflux is appropriate in a higher percentage of patients, especially considering the efficacy and decreased morbidity associated with laparoscopic fundoplication and the potential costs associated with the use of $H_2$ blockers or omeprazole for periods of many years. Research into appropriate treatment regimens is ongoing, and extensive additional investigation on the consequences of reflux upon the larynx and on all of the other mucosal surfaces above the cricopharyngeus muscle is needed.

## REFERENCES

1. Bain WM, et al. Head and neck manifestations of gastroesophageal reflux. Laryngoscope 1983;93:175
2. Barkin RL, Stein ZL. GE reflux and vocal pitch [Letter]. Hosp Pract 1989;24:20
3. Bogdassarian RS, Olson NR. Posterior glottic laryngeal stenosis. Otolaryngol Head Neck Surg 1980;88:765
4. Bough ID, Castell DO, Sataloff RT, Hills JR. Gastroesophageal reflux disease resistant to omeprazole therapy. J Voice 1995;9:205

5. Cherry J, Margulies S. Contact ulcer of the larynx. Laryngoscope 1968; 78:1937
6. Cherry J, et al. Pharyngeal localization of symptoms of gastroesophageal reflux. Ann Otol Rhinol Laryngol 1970;79:912
7. Chodosh P. Gastro-esophago-pharyngeal reflux. Laryngoscope 1977; 87:1418
8. Delahunty JE. Acid laryngitis. J Laryngol Otol 1972;86:335
9. Delahunty JE, Cherry J. Experimentally produced vocal cord granulomas. Laryngoscope 1968;78:1941
10. Fligny I, Francois M, Algrain Y, Polonovski JM, Contencin P, Narcy P. Stenoses sous-glottiquee et refluxgastro-oesophagien. Ann Otolaryngol Chir Cervicofac 1989;106:193
11. Freeland AP, Ardran GM, Emrys-Roberts E. Globus hystericus and reflux oesophagitis. J Laryngol Otol 1974;88:1025
12. Goldberg M, Noyek A, Pritzker KPH. Laryngeal granuloma secondary to gastroesophageal reflux. J Otolaryngol 1978;7:196
13. Gould WJ, Sataloff RT, Spiegel JR. Voice Surgery. St. Louis: Mosby, 1993
14. Hallewell JD, Cole TB. Isolated head and neck symptoms due to hiatus hernia. Arch Otolaryngol 1970;92:499
15. Hirano M. Clinical Examination of the Voice. New York: Springer-Verlag, 1981
16. Jacob P, Kahrilas PJ, Herzon G. Proximal esophageal pH-metry in patients with reflux laryngitis. Gastroenterology 1991;100:305
17. Johnson LF. New concepts and methods in the study and treatment of gastroesophageal reflux disease. Med Clin North Am 1981;65:1195
18. Kambic V, Radsel Z. Acid posterior laryngitis. Aetiology, histology, diagnosis and treatment. J Laryngol Otol 1984;98:1237
19. Katz PO. Ambulatory esophageal and hypopharyngeal pH monitoring in patients with hoarseness. Am J Gastroenterol 1990;85:38
20. Klinkenberg-Knol EC, Meuwissen GSM. Combined gastric and oesophageal 24 hour pH monitoring and oesophageal manometry in patients with reflux disease, resistant to treatment with omeprazole. Aliment Pharmacol Ther 1990;4:485
21. Koufman JA. Otolaryngologic manifestations of gastroesophageal reflux disease (GERD): a clinical investigation of 225 patients using ambulatory 24 hr pH monitoring and an experimental investigation of the role of acid and pepsin in the development of laryngeal injury. Laryngoscope 1991;101(suppl 53, part 2)
22. Koufman JA, Wiener GJ, Wu WC, Castell DO. Reflux laryngitis and its sequelae: the diagnostic role of ambulatory 24-hour pH monitoring. J Voice 1988;2:78
23. Kuriloff DB, Chodosh P, Goldfarb R, Ongseng F. Detection of gastroesophageal reflux in the head and neck: the role of scintigraphy. Ann Otol Rhinol Laryngol 1989;98:74
24. Lumpkin SMM, Bishop SG, Katz PO. Chronic dysphonia secondary to gastroesophageal reflux disease (GERD): diagnosis using simultaneous dual-probe prolonged pH monitoring. J Voice 1989;3:351
25. McNally PR, Maydonovitch CL, Prosek RA, Collette RP, Wong RKH. Evaluation of gastroesophageal reflux as a cause of idiopathic hoarseness. Dig Dis Sci 1989;34:1900
26. Miko TL. Peptic (contact ulcer) granuloma of the larynx. J Clin Pathol 1989;42:800
27. Morrison M. Is chronic gastroesophageal reflux a causative factor in glottic carcinoma? Otolaryngol Head Neck Surg 1988;99:370
28. Ohman L, et al. Esophageal dysfunction in patients with contact ulcer of the larynx. Ann Otol Rhinol Laryngol 1983;92:228
29. Olson NR. Effects of stomach acid on the larynx. Proc Am Laryngol Assoc 1983;104:108
30. Olson NR. The problem of gastroesophageal reflux. Otolaryngol Clin North Am 1986;19:119
31. Ossakow SJ, Elta G, Colturi T, Bogdassarian R, Nostrant TT. Esophageal reflux and dysmotility as the basis for persistent cervical symptoms. Ann Otol Rhinol Laryngol 1987;96:387
32. Pesce G, Caligaris F. Le laringiti posteriori nella pathologia dell'apparato digerente. Arch Ital Laringol 1966;74:77
33. Sataloff RT. Professional singers: the science and art of clinical care. Am J Otolaryngol 1981;8:251
34. Sataloff RT. Professional Voice: The Science and Art of Clinical Care. New York: Raven Press, 1991
35. Sataloff RT. The human voice. Sci Am 1993;267:108
36. Sataloff RT. Professional Voice: The Science and Art of Clinical Care (2nd ed.). San Diego: Singular Publishing Group, 1997;319–330, 735–753, 765–774
37. Sataloff RT, Spiegel JR, Hawkshaw MJ. Strobovideolaryngoscopy: results and clinical value. Ann Otol Rhinol Laryngol 1991;100:725
38. Scherer RS. Physiology of phonation: a review of basic mechanics. In Ford CN, Bless DM, eds, Phonosurgery. New York: Raven Press, 1991: 77
39. Spitzer GR, et al. Awake apnea associated with gastroesophageal reflux: a specific clinical syndrome. J Pediatr 1984;104:200
40. Sundberg J. The Science of the Singing Voice. DeKalb: Northern Illinois University Press, 1987
41. Teisanu E, Hecioia D, Dimitriu T, Calarasu R, Marinescu A. Tulburari Faringolaringiene la Bolnavii cu Reflux Gastroesofagian. Otorinolaringologia 1978;23:279
42. Vaughan CW, Strong MS. Medical management of organic laryngeal disorders. Otolaryngol Clin North Am 1984;17:705
43. Ward PH, Berci G. Observations on the pathogenesis of chronic nonspecific pharyngitis and laryngitis. Laryngoscope 1982;92:1377
44. Ward PH. Contact ulcers and granulomas of the larynx: new insights into their etiology as a basis for more rational treatment. Otolaryngol Head Neck Surg 1980;88:262
45. Wetmore RP. The effects of acid upon the larynx of the maturing rabbit and their possible significance to sudden infant death syndrome. Laryngoscope 1993;103:1242
46. Wiener GJ, Koufman JA, Wu WC, Cooper JB, Richter JE, Castell DO. Chronic hoarseness secondary to gastroesophageal reflux disease: documentation with 24-h ambulatory pH monitoring. Am J Gastroenterol 1989;84:1503
47. Wilson JA, et al. Gastroesophageal reflux and posterior laryngitis. Ann Otol Rhinol Laryngol 1989;98:405

*The Esophagus*, Third Edition,
edited by D. O. Castell and J. E. Richter.
Lippincott Williams & Wilkins, Philadelphia © 1999.

CHAPTER 29

# Pulmonary Complications of Gastroesophageal Reflux

Susan M. Harding

Gastroesophageal reflux disease (GERD) may trigger, cause, or exacerbate many common adult pulmonary diseases. The tracheobronchial tree and the esophagus have common embryonic foregut origins and share autonomic innervation through the vagus nerve [5]. The physiologic link between GERD and pulmonary disease has been extensively studied in chronic cough and asthma; however, there are still many unanswered questions. Both GERD and pulmonary disease are common in the human population and could coexist without a direct interaction. Recently, a population-based study performed in Olmstead County, Minnesota, found that 20% of residents aged 25 to 74 years reported weekly reflux symptoms, and almost 60% had heartburn or regurgitation within the previous year [50]. Likewise, pulmonary symptoms are common. Cough represents one of the most common complaints of patients in the ambulatory care setting, and asthma prevalence in the United States approximates 20 million [60, 78].

To solidify the association between GERD and pulmonary disease, three criteria should be met. First, patients with GERD should have a higher prevalence of pulmonary disease than patients without GERD. Second, pathophysiologic mechanisms between GERD and pulmonary disease should explain how the disease processes interact. Esophageal acid should exacerbate the pulmonary process. Third, if GERD is a contributor to the pulmonary process, then antireflux therapy should improve or even resolve the pulmonary process in many patients. Since the cause and exacerbating factors of many pulmonary diseases may be multifactorial, predictive variables should identify subsets of patients who respond dramatically to antireflux therapy.

Pulmonary disease and GERD do coexist. Urschel and

Paulson [96] examined respiratory symptoms in 636 patients referred for antireflux surgery. Sixty-one percent of patients had respiratory symptoms, including cough (47%), bronchitis (35%), asthma and wheezing (16%), pneumonitis (16%), and hemoptysis (13%). One of the best studies to date examining the coexistence of GERD and pulmonary disease was performed by El-Serag and Sonnenberg [13]. In a case-control study involving inpatients treated in 172 Veterans Administration hospitals in the United States, they compared the frequency of asthma, chronic bronchitis, chronic obstructive pulmonary disease, pulmonary fibrosis, bronchiectasis, pulmonary collapse, and pneumonia in 101,366 patients having erosive esophagitis or esophageal stricture to the frequency of the same conditions in a control population of 101,366 random subjects without GERD admitted during the same time period [13]. Table 29–1 shows that veterans with erosive esophagitis or stricture had a higher risk of having pulmonary disease, including asthma, with an odds ratio of 1.51 [13]. This chapter reviews the prevalence, pathogenesis, diagnosis, and treatment of GERD-related chronic cough and asthma and pertinent data in other pulmonary disorders where the association is not as well characterized.

## GASTROESOPHAGEAL REFLUX DISEASE-RELATED CHRONIC COUGH

### Prevalence

Using a systematic protocol evaluating the anatomy of the cough reflex prospectively, Irwin et al. [35] found the cause of cough in all patients, and specific therapy directed toward the cause resulted in cough resolution in 98% of patients. Further developing this protocol, they found that postnasal drip, asthma, and GERD caused cough in 99.4% of patients if they were not receiving angiotensin-converting enzyme inhibitors, were nonsmokers, and had a normal chest radiograph [36]. Irwin et al. also found that cough was due to a

S. M. Harding: Department of Medicine, UAB Sleep/Wake Disorders Center, Division of Pulmonary, Allergy, and Critical Care Medicine, University of Alabama at Birmingham, Birmingham, Alabama 35294.

**TABLE 29–1.** *Pulmonary disorders associated with esophagitis or stricture[a]*

| Pulmonary variable | Odds ratio | Cases (n = 101,366) | Controls (n = 101,366) |
|---|---|---|---|
| Asthma | 1.51 | 4,314 | 2,602 |
| Pulmonary fibrosis | 1.36 | 1,511 | 952 |
| Pulmonary collapse | 1.31 | 2,463 | 1,595 |
| Chronic bronchitis | 1.28 | 8,659 | 4,931 |
| Bronchiectasis | 1.26 | 522 | 280 |
| COPD[b] | 1.22 | 8,557 | 4,920 |
| Pneumonia | 1.15 | 17,283 | 12,794 |

[a] All *p* values <0.002.
[b] COPD, chronic obstructive pulmonary disease.
From ref. 13, with permission.

single condition in 73%, to multiple disorders in 26%, and to unknown causes in 1%. The prevalence of GERD in patients with chronic cough is 10% if the diagnosis was made by history, endoscopy, or barium esophagogram [35]. Adding 24-hour esophageal pH testing to the diagnostic protocol, GERD was the cause of cough in 40% of patients [62]. Cough may be the sole manifestation of GERD, with patients denying heartburn and other esophageal symptoms. Utilizing 24-hour esophageal pH testing, Irwin et al. [36] found that 43% of patients with GERD-related cough denied heartburn or a sour taste in the mouth. Ing et al. [30] found significant episodes of reflux in ten patients who denied GERD symptoms. In yet another patient population, Irwin et al. [39] reconfirmed that chronic cough can be the only manifestation of GERD, finding that GERD was clinically silent in 75% of patients. Clinically silent GERD-related cough may also be prevalent in the elderly [75]. GERD-related cough is common not only in the tertiary care setting of Irwin et al. but also in community-based practices [73].

### Pathogenesis

There are two pathophysiologic mechanisms of GERD-related cough: first, acid in the distal esophagus simulates an esophagotracheobronchial cough reflex and, second, microaspiration. Irwin et al. [38], using dual-probe esophageal pH monitoring, noted that cough occurred simultaneously with acid in the distal esophagus 28% of the time versus 6% of the time in the proximal esophagus. Also, endoscopy showed evidence of distal, but not proximal, esophagitis. They hypothesized that acid stimulated inflamed distal esophageal mucosal receptors, resulting in reflex-mediated cough. Ing et al. [30] also examined the reflex mechanism. Distal reflux occurred simultaneously with coughing in 78% of cough episodes. They found no evidence of aspiration based on chest radiographs and laryngeal examinations. Ing et al. [32] also examined esophageal acid clearance and found that patients with cough had more reflux episodes

than control subjects (88.3 versus 5.7) and had prolonged esophageal acid clearance times (3 versus 0.7 minutes). All patients who underwent endoscopy had evidence of distal esophagitis. They hypothesized that patients with chronic cough have impaired esophageal acid clearance, resulting in prolonged esophageal acid contact times, increasing the likelihood of mucosal injury at the distal esophageal mucosa [32]. Irwin et al. [39] also found that bronchoscopy was normal, failing to reveal evidence of microaspiration.

Ing et al. [33] examined the afferent pathway of the cough reflex in 22 patients with GERD-related cough. Patients had a significant increase in cough frequency with acid (n = 36) versus saline (n = 8) infusion. Blocking the afferent pathway of the cough reflex with esophageal lidocaine inhibited acid-induced coughs. Blocking the efferent cough reflex with inhaled ipratropium (an anticholinergic agent) also inhibited cough, but esophageal ipratropium did not, further supporting the presence of a vagally mediated cough reflex [33].

In summary, multiple observations point toward an esophagotracheobronchial reflex mechanism: (a) most reflux-induced coughs were recorded at the distal and not the proximal esophageal pH probe and correlated with distal and not proximal esophageal acid events; (b) endoscopic evidence of distal esophagitis was often present; (c) laryngoscopy and bronchoscopy failed to reveal evidence of acid-induced injury from aspiration; (d) acid-induced coughs were inhibited by esophageal lidocaine, which inhibits the afferent limb of the reflex pathway, as well as by inhaled ipratropium bromide, which inhibits the efferent limb of the reflex pathway. Microaspiration may still play a role in selected patients, especially since Paterson and Murat [69] observed rare episodes of gastrohypopharyngeal reflux in nine of 15 cough patients.

Multiple investigators have proposed a self-perpetuating positive feedback cycle between cough and GERD, where cough precipitates reflux [33]. Ing et al. [29] postulated that chronic cough may worsen GERD by triggering swallow-related transient lower esophageal sphincter (LES) relaxation on a background of raised transdiaphragmatic pressure.

### Treatment Outcome

If reflux plays a key role in cough, then aggressive treatment of reflux should result in cough resolution. Table 29–2 outlines clinical trials evaluating the outcome of antireflux therapy for GERD-related cough. Most of the studies were not double-blind, placebo-controlled. Trials used conservative treatment, $H_2$ antagonists, and prokinetic agents; two trials included proton pump inhibitors. Combining the trials reported in the adult population, 106 of 118 (approximately 90%) patients had cough resolution. Effective treatment regimens may require vigorous acid suppression over a prolonged time period. The time between initiating antireflux therapy and cough resolution was more than 50 days in all trials.

**TABLE 29–2.** *Outcome of antireflux therapy for gastroesophageal reflux disease-related cough in adults*[a]

| Study | Study design | Patient number | Intervention[b] | Response rate (%) | Cough resolution (days) |
|---|---|---|---|---|---|
| Irwin et al. [35] | Prospective | 5 | Conservative, AA or $H_2$ | 100 | — |
| Irwin et al. [38] | Prospective | 9 | Conservative, $H_2$, and/or PK | 100 | 161 |
| Fitzgerald et al. [16] | Prospective | 20 | Conservative, AA, $H_2$, and PK | 70 | 90 |
| Irwin et al. [36] | Prospective | 28 | Conservative, $H_2$, and/or PK | 100 | 179 |
| Waring et al. [100] | Prospective | 25 | Conservative, $H_2$, PPI | 80 | — |
| Smyrnios et al. [81] | Prospective | 20 | Conservative, $H_2$ with/without PK | 97 | — |
| Vaezi et al. [97] | Retrospective | 11 | $H_2$ or PPI | 100 | 53 |

[a] All studies were uncontrolled and unblinded.
[b] AA, antacid; $H_2$, $H_2$ antagonist; PK, prokinetic agent; PPI, proton pump inhibitor.

Ing et al. [31] reported a randomized, double-blind, placebo-controlled crossover trial using ranitidine 150 mg twice a day for 2 weeks, finding that cough scores fell significantly with ranitidine treatment. Nevertheless, 2 weeks of therapy is not adequate to measure a therapeutic response. Fitzgerald et al. [16] reported a 70% response rate in 20 patients using a 3-month treatment regimen that included conservative therapy, $H_2$ antagonists, and a prokinetic agent. Of the cough nonresponders, four underwent surgical fundoplication, with all experiencing cough resolution within 3 months postoperatively. This study suggests that $H_2$ antagonists and prokinetic agents may not adequately control reflux in selected patients and that these patients may require more aggressive therapy with proton pump inhibitors or surgery [16].

Two studies used proton pump inhibitors. Pratter et al. [74] treated patients with conservative therapy and ranitidine 150 mg twice daily for 2 weeks. If esophageal pH testing showed inadequate acid suppression, then omeprazole 20 mg was initiated, with all patients responding to this treatment. Vaezi and Richter [97] retrospectively reviewed cough outcome in 11 patients, with six patients receiving omeprazole 20 mg b.i.d., and all had cough resolution.

In studies using primarily conservative measures, $H_2$ antagonists, or prokinetic agents, the time period for cough resolution was between 90 and 179 days [16, 36, 38]. There are no prospective double-blind, placebo-controlled trials utilizing proton pump inhibitors to see if the time required for cough resolution is shortened. Antireflux surgery is reserved for patients with proven GERD who fail aggressive medical treatment, including proton pump inhibitors [16]. Although an optimal therapeutic regimen has not been investigated, Irwin [34] recommends that all patients be educated on conservative therapy (high-protein/low-fat diet, avoiding substances which lower LES pressure, eating and drinking limited to 2 hours before bedtime, and elevation of the bed). Medical therapy should include a prokinetic agent and a gastric acid-secretion inhibitor ($H_2$ antagonist or proton pump inhibitor) [34]. Therapy should be prolonged, continued an additional 3 months after cough resolution, and then gradually tapered and discontinued. Since GERD is a chronic disease, cough may return when treatment or medication is stopped, so episodic and prolonged therapy may be required [34].

### Clinical Presentation and Diagnostic Evaluation

All patients with chronic cough should have a history, physical examination targeted toward the most common causes of cough, and a chest radiograph. They should be questioned for symptoms of GERD, including heartburn, acid regurgitation, and worsening cough with foods which decrease LES pressure. Mello et al. [62], using a prospective design, found that detailed questions about cough characteristics and timing were not useful in determining the cause of cough. Many patients with GERD-related cough may not have esophageal reflux symptoms. Other patients may have symptoms only after the development of cough, suggesting that cough may be the initiating event in the cough reflux cycle [29, 57].

The standard test to diagnose GERD-related cough is 24-hour esophageal pH testing, which has a sensitivity and specificity approaching 100% in the chronic cough population [8, 34]. Ambulatory 24-hour esophageal pH testing also follows correlation of coughs with reflux events. Irwin et al. [39] found that correlation of cough episodes with simultaneous reflux events is more helpful than total esophageal acid contact times, which may be normal in some patients.

In conclusion, all patients with chronic cough should be carefully questioned about GERD symptoms. If GERD symptoms are present, then antireflux therapy should be initiated, as outlined in the previous section. If patients deny reflux symptoms, then 24-hour esophageal pH testing should be performed when cough is unexplained after a detailed evaluation. Esophageal pH testing should also be performed in patients who do not respond clinically to therapy guided by the anatomic diagnostic protocol since cough may be caused by more than one etiology in up to 59% of patients [39]. Correlation of esophageal acid events with coughing should also be examined.

## ASTHMA AND GASTROESOPHAGEAL REFLUX DISEASE

### Prevalence of Gastroesophageal Reflux Disease in Asthmatics

Gastroesophageal reflux also plays a role in asthma [20, 21]. The prevalence of GERD in asthmatics is estimated to be between 34% and 89% [6, 14, 37, 45, 46, 53, 58, 68, 84, 85]. Many asthmatics complain of GERD symptoms. Field et al. [14] examined the prevalence of GERD symptoms using a detailed questionnaire in 109 asthmatics and two control groups (68 patients visiting their family physicians and 67 patients with other medical disorders). Among the asthmatics, 77% experienced heartburn, 55% complained of regurgitation, and 24% experienced swallowing difficulties, higher than in the two control groups [14]. In the week prior to completing the questionnaire, 41% of asthmatics noted reflux-associated respiratory symptoms and 28% used inhalers while experiencing GERD symptoms. As in the chronic cough population, some asthmatics may have significant GERD without classic reflux symptoms. Irwin et al. [37] reported that GERD was clinically silent in 24% of difficult-to-control asthmatics.

There is also a high prevalence of esophageal dysfunction in asthmatics. Kjellen et al. [46] found that 37 of 97 consecutive asthmatics (38%) had evidence of esophageal dysmotility, 26 (27%) had LES hypotension, and 23 (24%) had a positive Bernstein test. Sontag et al. [85] examined 186 consecutive adult asthmatics with endoscopy and esophageal biopsy and found that 79 (43%) had evidence of esophagitis or Barrett's esophagus. The same group evaluated 104 consecutive asthmatics and 44 control subjects with esophageal manometry and 24-hour esophageal pH tests and found that 82% of asthmatics had abnormal amounts of acid reflux [84]. The asthmatics compared to normal controls had significantly lower LES pressure ($p = 0.0001$), more frequent reflux episodes ($p = 0.0001$), and higher esophageal contact times ($p = 0.0001$) [84].

In conclusion, frequency of reflux symptoms, LES hypotension, and esophageal acid contact times are higher in asthmatics compared to normal groups, helping to substantiate the association between GERD and asthma.

## Pathogenesis of Esophageal Acid-induced Bronchoconstriction

There are three proposed mechanisms whereby esophageal acid produces bronchoconstriction, including an esophagobronchial vagal reflex, heightened bronchial reactivity, and microaspiration. These three mechanisms may interact and further augment airway responses. Interestingly, the vagus nerve is involved in all three mechanisms, including microaspiration.

### Vagal Reflex

Airway reflexes may be protective in order to avoid exposure to noxious agents [44]. In a dog model, Mansfield and Stein [55] noted that esophageal acid increased respiratory resistance which was ablated with bilateral vagotomy. They also examined 15 asthmatics with GERD. When symptoms of esophagitis appeared with esophageal acid, there was an increase in total respiratory resistance and a decrease in

airflow at 25% of vital capacity, which returned to baseline after reflux symptoms were relieved with antacids [54]. The same group performed a double-blind, acid infusion study in four subject groups: normal controls, asthmatics with GERD, asthmatics without GERD, and subjects with GERD alone [86]. The asthmatics with a positive Bernstein test group had a 10% increase in total respiratory resistance. The changes in total respiratory resistance were even more pronounced (72% over baseline) in asthmatics with GERD, in whom asthma attacks were associated with reflux symptoms ($p < 0.0001$) [86]. Kjellen et al. [47] found that esophageal acid caused a 0.2 L decrease in vital capacity and an increase in alveolar plateau by 0.9% in asthmatics with GERD. Likewise, Wright et al. [101] studied 136 individuals, measuring airflow and arterial oxygen saturation both before and after esophageal acid infusions, and found significant reductions in airflow and arterial oxygen saturation. Atropine pretreatment abolished these findings, providing more evidence for an acid-induced, vagally mediated esophagobronchial reflex [101].

Because previous studies failed to control for microaspiration, we performed a series of studies utilizing dual esophageal pH testing [22, 23, 77]. Peak expiratory flow rate (PEF) decreased with esophageal acid infusion in normal control subjects, asthmatics with GERD, asthmatics without GERD, and subjects with GERD alone [77]. Esophageal acid clearance improved PEF in all groups except for the asthma with GERD group, which had further deterioration. These effects were not dependent on a positive Bernstein test or evidence of proximal esophageal acid exposure, a prerequisite for microaspiration. The asthma with GERD group also had an increase in specific airway resistance with esophageal acid infusion, which continued to increase despite acid clearance. Subsequently, we infused esophageal acid into subjects in the supine position, and again, esophageal acid decreased PEF and increased specific airway resistance in asthmatics with GERD, which did not improve despite esophageal acid clearance [22]. In a third study, vagolytic doses of intravenous atropine partially ablated the bronchoconstrictive response to esophageal acid, implying the importance of a vagally mediated reflex [23].

To further evaluate the role of the autonomic nervous system in esophageal acid-induced bronchoconstriction, we performed autonomic function testing in 15 asthmatics with GERD, hypothesizing that asthmatics with GERD have exaggerated vagal responsiveness compared to 23 age-matched controls [51]. All asthmatics with GERD had at least one autonomic function test displaying a hypervagal response. Seventy-three percent of asthmatics with GERD had a hypervagal response during the deep-breathing maneuver, 31% had a hypervagal response during the Valsalva maneuver, and 6% had a hypervagal response during the tilt test [51]. The overall response score showed that no asthmatic with GERD had a normal or hyperadrenergic score. These data suggest that asthmatics with GERD have heightened vagal responsiveness, which may be partially responsible for the airway responses to esophageal acid.

However, other reports show conflicting data. Tan et al. [88] studied 15 nocturnal asthmatics with esophageal acid infusions, measuring respiratory flow, tidal volume, and airflow resistance during sleep and found no significant changes in airflow resistance when acid was present in the esophagus.

### Heightened Bronchial Reactivity

Herve et al. [26] examined the effect of esophageal acid on expiratory flow with methacholine challenge testing in asthmatics with and without GERD. The total dose of methacholine required to reduce the forced expiratory volume in 1 second ($FEV_1$) by 20% was significantly lower when esophageal acid was infused versus normal saline [26]. Furthermore, the response to esophageal acid was abolished with atropine pretreatment. They proposed that stimulated esophageal acid-sensitive receptors interact with cholinergic bronchial tone by a vagally mediated reflex, suggesting that GERD aggravates asthma by increasing bronchomotor responsiveness to other stimuli [26].

### Microaspiration

It is well established that mechanical stimulation of the upper airway or instillation of saline into the trachea increases airway resistance [3, 92]. Chernow et al. [2] instilled technetium 99 sulfur colloid into the stomachs of six patients while monitoring overnight esophageal pH. The patients with abnormal lung scans had prolonged episodes of acid reflux. One of the most convincing studies examining the role of microaspiration was performed in a cat model by Tuchman et al. [95]. Instilling 10 mL of acid into the esophagus, they noted a 1.5-fold increase in total lung resistance compared to a nearly a fivefold increase if 0.5 mL of tracheal acid was instilled [95]. Furthermore, the esophageal acid response occurred in only 60% of animals versus 100% of animals given tracheal acid [95]. Interestingly, the effect of tracheal acidification on total lung resistance was abolished

with bilateral cervical vagotomy, so even in the microaspiration model, the vagus nerve plays a role [95]. In a human study, Varkey et al. [99] examined 19 consecutive asthmatics and seven normal controls with dual esophageal pH monitoring and a probe in the pharynx 2 cm above the upper esophageal sphincter. Asthmatics had 31% of reflux episodes associated with a fall in. pH at the proximal esophagus and 5% of episodes associated with a fall in pH at the pharyngeal probe, documenting that microaspiration does exist and is more prevalent in asthmatics than in normal controls [99].

Even more convincing evidence of microaspiration was provided by Jack et al. [40], who monitored simultaneous tracheal and esophageal pH in four patients with severe asthma. Thirty-seven episodes of esophageal reflux lasting more than 5 minutes were observed, and five of these episodes were associated with a fall in tracheal pH. PEF decreased 84 L minute when esophageal acid and tracheal acid were present versus 8 L a minute with esophageal acid alone [40]. Episodes of tracheal microaspiration were associated with significant deterioration in pulmonary function [40].

### Conclusion

Data suggest that all three mechanisms play a role in esophageal acid-induced bronchoconstriction. Both human and animal data show evidence of bronchoconstriction with esophageal acid in the distal esophagus. This bronchoconstriction is modest but present, with PEF decreasing approximately 10 L a minute. Numerous studies have also shown that airway resistance increases with esophageal acid. Atropine inhibits the response to esophageal acid. There is also evidence of heightened bronchial reactivity, with atropine inhibiting this response, so the vagus nerve also plays a role in this model. Microaspiration causes significant alterations in pulmonary mechanics in both human and animal studies. The magnitude of airway responses to tracheal acidification is fivefold over baseline in an animal model, and in a human study, tracheal acidification caused a tenfold worsening in airflow, with PEF decreasing 84 L a minute. The vagus nerve has also been implicated in the microaspiration model. Figure 29–1 shows how all three mechanisms interact through the vagus nerve, leading to airway inflammation.

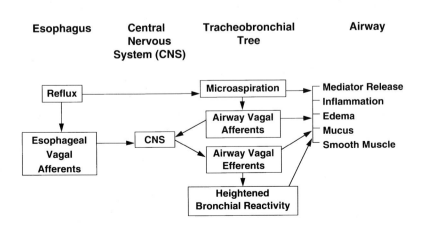

**FIG. 29–1.** Pathophysiologic mechanisms of esophageal acid-induced bronchoconstriction. The three mechanisms include a vagally mediated reflex, heightened bronchial reactivity, and microaspiration, resulting in bronchoconstriction and airway inflammation. The vagus nerve plays a role in all three mechanisms. (Reprinted with permission from ref. 20A.)

**TABLE 29–3.** *Medical therapy trials for gastroesophageal reflux disease-related asthma in adults*

| Study | Study design | Patient number | Intervention | Therapy duration | Document acid suppression | Asthma outcome[a] |
|---|---|---|---|---|---|---|
| Kjellen et al. [48] | Randomized, placebo-controlled | 65 | Antacids, postural therapy | — | No | 54% improved symptoms, no change in PFTs |
| Goodall et al. [19] | Double-blind, placebo-controlled, crossover | 18 | Cimetidine 200 mg q.i.d. | 6 weeks | No | 78% responded, decreased symptom score |
| Harper et al. [25] | Open-label, prepost comparison | 15 | Ranitidine 150 mg b.i.d. | 8 weeks | Endoscopy | Increase in $FEV_1$, decreased symptoms |
| Nagel et al. [67] | Double-blind, placebo-controlled, crossover | 15 | Ranitidine 450 mg/day | 1 week | No | No change |
| Ekstrom et al. [10] | Placebo-controlled, crossover | 48 | Ranitidine 150 b.i.d. | 4 weeks | No | Improvement in night asthma score, no change in PFTs, mild decrease in $\beta_2$ agonist rescue |
| Meier et al. [61] | Placebo-controlled, crossover | 5 | Omeprazole 20 mg b.i.d. | 6 weeks | Endoscopy | 29% increased $FEV_1$ by 20%, only if esophagitis healed |
| Ford et al. [17] | Placebo-controlled, crossover | 11 | Omeprazole 20 mg b.i.d. | 4 weeks | No | No difference |
| Harding et al. [24] | Prospective, pretest, posttest | 30 | Omeprazole 20–60 mg/day for acid suppression | 3 months | pH testing | 73% increased PEF or decreased symptoms by 20% |
| Teichtahl et al. [90] | Placebo-controlled, crossover | 20 | Omeprazole 40 mg | 4 weeks | pH testing but still had acid | Mild improvement in evening PEF |

[a] PFT, Pulmonary function test; $FEV_1$, forced expiratory volume at 1 second; PEF, peak expiratory flow rate.

## Possible Factors Promoting Gastroesophageal Reflux Disease in Asthmatics

There are a number of physiologic factors which may contribute to the development of GERD in asthmatics, including autonomic dysfunction, an increased pressure gradient between the thorax (esophagus) and abdominal cavity (stomach), alterations in crural diaphragm function, and bronchodilators which may promote reflux. We previously discussed the finding that asthmatics show evidence of autonomic dysfunction [51]. Autonomic dysregulation could result in decreased LES pressure and transient relaxations of the LES, major mechanisms of GERD [64].

The pressure gradient between the thorax and the abdomen may be increased in asthmatics with GERD. At the end of expiration, the pressure gradient between the stomach (abdominal cavity) and esophagus (thorax) is 4 to 5 mm Hg [64]. Therefore, a normal LES pressure of 10 to 35 mm Hg at the end of expiration is sufficient to counteract this pressure gradient [64]. With an acute asthma exacerbation, there are wide pressure swings, with a much more negative intrathoracic pressure on inspiration and a more positive abdominal

pressure, increasing the pressure gradient and promoting reflux [27].

Another factor which may be altered in asthmatics with GERD is the crural diaphragm. Multiple investigators have shown that transient relaxation of the LES and the crural diaphragm are responsible for GERD [65, 66]. There is relaxation of the LES associated with an inhibition of the diaphragmatic electromyogram associated with an increase in esophageal pressure, resulting in a reflux episode [66]. Hyperinflation associated with bronchospasm places the diaphragm at a functional disadvantage because of geometric flattening [76]. Flattening and stretching of the diaphragmatic crura may also occur with chronic hyperinflation and airtrapping.

Bronchodilator medications may also promote GERD, especially theophylline and oral beta$_2$-adrenergic agents. Theophylline increases gastric acid secretion and decreases LES pressure; however, there is debate about its clinical importance [12, 41, 87]. In a randomized, double-blind, crossover study, Hubert et al. [28] administered oral theophylline or placebo in asthmatics, finding no difference in the number of reflux episodes or total acid exposure time, while pulmonary function improved. However, Ekstrom et al. [11] examined 25 asthmatics with GERD using 24-hour esophageal pH testing and found that asthmatics with therapeutic theophylline levels had a 24% increase in total esophageal acid exposure and a 170% increase in reflux symptoms. Oral beta$_2$-adrenergic agents may also decrease LES pressure [9]. However, Schindlbeck et al. [79] found no significant difference in GERD parameters or esophageal motility in normal controls taking inhaled albuterol. Likewise, Michoud et al. [63] found that inhaled albuterol had no effect on LES pressure or esophageal function in both normal controls and asthmatics. There are three studies evaluating asthmatics on multiple bronchodilators. Sontag et al. [85] examined the frequency of esophagitis in 186 consecutive asthmatics on versus not on bronchodilators: 38% of asthmatics had esophagitis on bronchodilators versus 39% of asthmatics not on bronchodilators ($p$ = nonsignificant). The same group also evaluated 104 consecutive asthmatics with esophageal manometry and 24-hour esophageal pH testing, finding no significant difference in LES pressure, esophageal acid contact time, or number of reflux episodes in asthmatics on versus not on chronic bronchodilator therapy [84]. Finally, Field et al. [14] examined GERD symptoms in 109 consecutive asthmatics, and no asthma medication was associated with an increased likelihood of having heartburn or regurgitation.

In conclusion, there are physiologic alterations associated with asthma that may promote GERD, which may partially explain the increased prevalence of GERD in asthmatics. There is continued debate about the influence of bronchodilator medications on the severity of GERD.

## Treatment Outcome

If GERD triggers asthma, then adequate control of reflux should improve asthma outcome in selected patients. There have been numerous medical and surgical trials evaluating asthma outcome.

### Medical Therapy

Table 29–3 reviews medical therapy trials in asthmatics with GERD. Many studies have design limitations, including the absence of a control group, small or selected patient populations, inconsistent outcome parameters, and lack of objective evidence of acid suppression. More importantly, many therapeutic trials are too short to assess asthma outcome. Despite these limitations, many studies show modest improvement in asthma symptoms and some show objective improvement in pulmonary function.

More recently, proton pump inhibitors were studied. Meier et al. [61], in a placebo-controlled, crossover trial in 15 asthmatics using omeprazole 20 mg two times a day for 6 weeks, found that 29% had asthma response (FEV$_1$ decreased by 20%). Only subjects without esophagitis had asthma response. Many of the nonresponders still had active esophagitis. This study further emphasizes the need for prolonged therapy before assessing asthma outcome. Ford et al. [17], in a placebo-controlled, crossover trial in 11 asthmatics using omeprazole 20 mg a day for 4 weeks, found no difference in pulmonary outcome; but 4 weeks is not adequate time to assess asthma outcome. Teichtahl et al. [90] also reported a placebo-controlled, crossover trial of 20 nocturnal asthmatics using omeprazole 40 mg a day for 4 weeks and noted a mild improvement in PEF; however, the treatment period was too short. Our laboratory performed a prospective, pretest/posttest evaluation of 30 asthmatics with GERD with 3 months of acid-suppressive therapy (omeprazole 20 to 60 mg per day) [24]. Seventy-three percent of asthmatics with GERD had a 20% increase in PEF and/or a decrease in asthma symptoms by 20% [24]. The asthma responders had improvement in pulmonary function studies, including FEV$_1$ and midexpiratory flow rates. Asthma symptoms required time to improve. After 1 month of acid-suppressive therapy, there was a 30% reduction in asthma symptoms compared to baseline; at 2 months, a 43% reduction; and by 3 months, a 57% reduction (Fig. 29–2). Acid-sup-

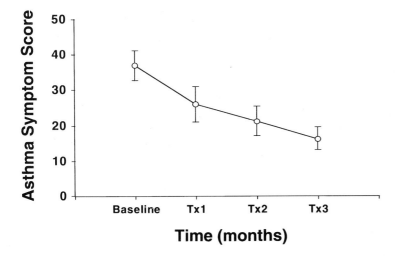

**FIG. 29–2.** Asthma symptom score response to omeprazole over time. Asthma symptom score at baseline, at omeprazole treatment month 1 *(Tx 1)*, treatment month 2 *(Tx 2)*, and treatment month 3 *(Tx 3)* in 22 asthma responders to antireflux therapy. Mean ± standard error shown. Asthma responders had a 30% reduction in asthma symptoms at month 1, a 43% reduction at month 2, and a 57% reduction after 3 months of therapy. (From ref. 24, with permission.)

pressive therapy can improve asthma in nearly 75% of asthmatics with GERD, similar to the reported success rates with antireflux surgery [24].

### Surgical Therapy

Table 29–4 reviews studies that examined outcome in asthmatics with GERD utilizing surgical therapy. Most studies have design flaws, including lack of a control group, poor documentation of airflow obstruction both preoperatively and postoperatively, poor documentation of asthma severity, and no proof that reflux was adequately controlled in the postoperative state. Despite these flaws, combining the results of nine trials [7, 43, 45, 52, 68, 72, 82, 89, 96] showed that there was a total of 297 asthmatics with GERD, of whom 235 (70%) had asthma improvement.

### Combined Medical and Surgical Trials

Two studies examined medical and surgical therapy response in GERD-related asthma using a placebo-controlled design [49, 83]. Unfortunately, proton pump inhibitors were not available when these studies were performed. Larrain et al. [49] examined the effect of cimetidine 300 mg four times a day versus surgery in a placebo-controlled trial in nonallergic asthmatics. After 6 months, there was improvement in $FEV_1$ and PEF in the cimetidine and surgically treated group but not in the placebo group. Medication scores also dropped significantly in both treatment groups compared to placebo. Asthma was considered improved in 36% of the control subjects versus 74% in the medically treated group and 77% in the surgically treated group [49]. Likewise, Sontag et al. [83] performed a placebo-controlled, randomized study comparing ranitidine 150 mg three times a day to surgery (Nissen fundoplication) in 73 asthmatics with GERD. In the surgically treated group, 75% had resolution or improvement in asthma symptoms versus 9% of the ranitidine group and 4% of the control group at 5-year follow-up. They concluded

that surgical treatment of GERD in asthmatics improved pulmonary function and decreased medication usage more often than medical therapy or placebo.

### Conclusion

Aggressive antireflux therapy results in improvement in asthma outcome in approximately 70% of asthmatics with GERD, treated both medically and surgically. Since there are design flaws in many outcome studies performed to date, future studies should be multicentered and placebo-controlled, using acid-suppressive therapy for at least 3 months with documentation of asthma outcome, cost analysis, and quality-of-life assessment.

### Predictors of Asthma Response

Many studies reported predictors of asthma response. Some studies examined subgroups which had excellent asthma response, while others examined predictors using sophisticated statistical analysis. Meier et al. [61] found that only patients with complete endoscopic healing of esophagitis had asthma improvement ($p < 0.01$). Hoarseness, cough, nocturnal reflux symptoms, and asthma duration did not predict asthma improvement [61]. Larrain et al. [49] performed a trial in a subset of nonallergic asthmatics with less than grade 1 esophagitis who had asthma improvement. Another subset with improvement comprised difficult-to-control asthmatics (who require prednisone 10 mg every other day for at least 3 consecutive months per year) [37]. Ekstrom et al. [10] found that a history of reflux-associated respiratory symptoms predicted asthma improvement in 48 moderate to severe asthmatics.

Perrin-Fayolle et al. [72] reported predictors of asthma response in 44 asthmatics with GERD more than 5 years postsurgery. They found that asthmatics who were younger in age and had nocturnal and/or intrinsic asthma had improved outcome. The onset of GERD symptoms before respiratory symptoms, severe GERD, and medical therapy response also predicted asthma improvement [72]. DeMeester

**TABLE 29–4.** *Surgical therapy trials for GERD-related asthma in adults*

| Study | Study design | Patient number | Surgical intervention | Monitoring time | Asthma outcome |
|---|---|---|---|---|---|
| Kennedy et al. [45] | Case series | 15 | Unknown | — | 15 (100%) improved |
| Overholt et al. [68] | Case series | 28 | Transthoracic repair | >6 months | 23 (82%) improved or cured |
| Urschel et al. [96] | Case series | 27 | Unknown | — | 24 (89%) improved |
| Lomasney [52] | Cases series | 129 | Unknown | — | 97 (75%) improved |
| Sontag et al. [82] | Case series | 13 | Nissen fundoplication | 1–5 years | 6/11 (55%) improved |
| Tardif et al. [89] | Case series | 10 | Unknown | 21 months | 5 (50%) improved |
| Perrin-Fayolle et al. [72] | Case series | 44 | Nissen fundoplication | >5 years | 37 (84%) improved |
| DeMeester et al. [7] | Case series of subjects who failed medical therapy | 17 | 14 Nissen fundoplication, Belsey Mark IV | 36–103 months | 14 (82%) improved |
| Johnson et al. [43] | Case series | 14 | Nissen or Belsey fundoplication | 3 years | Group had improvement |

et al. [7] also performed fundoplication in patients who were unresponsive to medical antireflux therapy. Patients with normal esophageal motility and pulmonary symptoms during or within 3 minutes of reflux events or patients who had pulmonary symptoms unrelated to reflux events had a higher success rate than patients who had pulmonary symptoms 3 minutes before reflux events. This study showed that 24-hour esophageal pH monitoring predicted which patients improve with aggressive antireflux therapy [7].

Schnatz et al. [80] also found that esophageal pH testing was able to predict asthma improvement with antireflux therapy. Nine out of 11 (82%) asthmatics with distal only reflux and four out of four (100%) with proximal only reflux events had a favorable response. None of the five patients with normal esophageal acid contact times had asthma improvement.

We examined predictors of asthma response and found that higher amounts of total proximal reflux, higher baseline asthma symptom score, higher baseline reflux symptom score, the presence of regurgitation, asthma exacerbated by upper respiratory tract infection, and asthma exacerbated by allergies showed a trend toward asthma improvement [24]. Forward linear regression analysis found that the presence of regurgitation more than once a week and/or excessive amounts of proximal reflux (i.e., esophageal proximal pH was less than 4 over 1.1% of the time) predicted a greater than 20% improvement in asthma symptoms. These two variables had a 100% sensitivity, a 100% negative predictive value, a specificity of 44%, and a positive predictive value of 79% [24].

In conclusion, there are many possible predictors, as outlined in Table 29–5. These predictors need to be reexamined in an independent study population. This would allow further characterization of which patients to treat aggressively with antireflux therapy.

### Diagnostic and Therapeutic Approach

All asthmatics should be treated in accordance with the Guidelines for the Diagnosis and Management of Asthma, Expert Panel Report 2, supported by the National Institutes of Health [20]. This includes aggressive therapy with bronchodilators and antiinflammatory agents. All asthmatics should be asked about the presence of reflux symptoms. For

**TABLE 29–5.** *Predictors of asthma response*

Healing of esophagitis with antireflux therapy
Asthmatics with < grade 1 esophagitis at study entry
Nonallergic asthma/intrinsic asthma
Difficult-to-control asthma
Reflux-associated respiratory symptoms
Nocturnal asthma
Pulmonary symptoms occur during or within 3 min of a reflux event
Presence of proximal reflux on pH testing
Presence of regurgitation > once a week

patients with symptomatic GERD, conservative lifestyle therapy should be initiated as well as aggressive empiric medical therapy with a proton pump inhibitor for at least 3 months using omeprazole 20 mg b.i.d. or lansoprazole 30 mg b.i.d. During this time, patients should monitor both asthma and GERD symptoms, daily PEF, and asthma medication usage.

In asthmatics with chronic persistent asthma without reflux symptoms, 24-hour esophageal pH testing should be performed to evaluate for the presence of clinically silent GERD. If GERD is present, an aggressive 3-month trial of acid suppression should be initiated. If after the therapeutic trial both GERD and asthma are improved, then GERD is an important asthma trigger. If GERD is improved but asthma is not, then GERD is most likely not a trigger of asthma. If reflux symptoms persist despite antireflux therapy, then 24-hour esophageal pH testing should be performed to see if there is adequate acid suppression on antireflux therapy.

If there is a therapeutic response with aggressive antireflux therapy, then the patient should be placed on chronic maintenance therapy, which may include proton pump inhibitors, a prokinetic agent, or $H_2$ antagonists with or without a prokinetic agent. Surgical therapy should be reserved for patients who are good surgical risks: those without a long esophageal stricture, those with normal esophageal motility, and those with a hypotonic LES pressure. Chronic treatment should be individualized for each patient.

## ROLE OF GASTROESOPHAGEAL REFLUX DISEASE IN OTHER RESPIRATORY DISEASES

GERD may also have an impact on other pulmonary diseases, including aspiration pneumonia, ventilator-associated pneumonia, bronchiectasis, bronchitis, and fibrotic lung diseases including idiopathic pulmonary fibrosis and scleroderma.

Aspiration of esophageal contents has long been recognized as a cause of lung abscess and pneumonia [1]. Diagnosis is usually straightforward because patients often describe regurgitation. Risk factors for aspiration pneumonitis include disruption of normal deglutition and airway protective mechanisms [56]. Pellegrini et al. [71] examined GERD in 48 patients suspected of being aspirators. Eight patients had documented episodes of aspiration during the monitoring period and 75% had esophageal dysmotility. Antireflux surgery improved both aspiration and reflux. Recurrent lung injury in pneumonia from GERD may result from direct contact with caustic reflux gastric contents (acid and pepsin) and possibly aspirated gastric, esophageal, or pharyngeal bacteria [15, 70, 93]. This may be especially true in ventilator-associated pneumonia [18, 93, 98]. Recurrent episodes of aspiration and pneumonitis may lead to bronchiectasis. Although prokinetic agents and acid-secretion inhibitors may decrease regurgitant volume and acid content, selected patients are encouraged to undergo surgical fundoplication for chronic recurring aspiration pneumonia if they are surgical candidates.

There is a small body of data to suggest a relationship between GERD and chronic bronchitis. Crausaz et al. [4] performed scintiscans showing reflux in 27 patients (84%) versus five control subjects (38%). Lung contamination was seen in 24 patients (75%) and two control subjects (15%) ($p < 0.001$) 15 hours after eating a labeled solid meal. Although the two associated phenomena may not be causally related, pulmonary aspiration did correlate with GERD, suggesting that GERD may contribute to chronic bronchial disease [4]. Tibbling [91] further examined the association between GERD with aspiration and bronchitis. She examined 119 patients operated on for hiatal hernia and GERD and compared them with 89 patients treated with omeprazole, examining bronchial symptoms before and after treatment. Patients treated with omeprazole did not have significant relief of bronchial symptoms, whereas patients who underwent fundoplication with crural repair, showed a marked reduction in bronchitis. She concluded that the main reason for chronic bronchitis in patients with GERD is intermittent aspiration due to partial misswallowing [91]. Further research is needed in this area.

GERD has also been implicated in the pathogenesis of interstitial pulmonary fibrosis. Mays et al. [59] examined 48 patients with idiopathic interstitial pulmonary fibrosis and showed that 54% had reflux on barium esophagogram versus 8.5% in a normal control group. This association should probably be ignored because episodes of aspiration are unlikely to be distributed uniformly throughout the lungs (much less to the distal airways) and GERD does not augment our present understanding of idiopathic pulmonary fibrosis.

Esophageal dysfunction and pulmonary interstitial disease are common manifestations of systemic sclerosis (scleroderma). Johnson et al. [42] studied 13 patients with scleroderma and interstitial lung disease with esophageal pH testing and found that 11 had evidence of proximal esophageal reflux. They also found a correlation between proximal acid reflux and a decrease in lung diffusion capacity. Troshinsky et al. [94] examined 39 patients with systemic sclerosis using 24-hour esophageal pH and pulmonary function tests. Patients were grouped into those with and those without abnormal esophageal acid contact times. There was no difference in total lung capacity or diffusion capacity between the two groups. Important measures of lung volume indicative of interstitial lung disease do not appear to be related to abnormal esophageal reflux in patients with systemic sclerosis [94]. Also, lung biopsy findings in patients with systemic sclerosis show interstitial fibrosis without granulomatous inflammation, unlike the biopsy findings of chronic aspiration pneumonitis. Causal links between esophageal reflux and pulmonary fibrosis and scleroderma cannot be made at this time.

In conclusion, GERD should be aggressively sought in patients with chronic persistent cough and asthma. In these two diseases, there is excellent evidence showing that there is an association with gastroesophageal reflux.

## REFERENCES

1. Allen CJ, Newhouse MT. Gastroesophageal reflux and chronic respiratory disease. Clinical commentary. Am Rev Respir Dis 1984;129:645
2. Chernow B, et al. Pulmonary aspiration as a consequence of gastroesophageal reflux: a diagnostic approach. Dig Dis Sci 1979;24:839
3. Colebatch HJH, Halmagyi DFJ. Reflex airway reaction to fluid aspiration. J Appl Physiol 1962;17:787
4. Crausaz FM, Favez G. Aspiration of solid food particles into the lungs of patients with gastroesophageal reflux and chronic bronchial disease. Chest 1988;93:376
5. Cunningham ET Jr, Ravich WJ, Jones B, Donner MW. Vagel reflexes referred from the upper aerodigestive tract: an infrequently recognized cause of common cardiorespiratory responses. Ann Intern Med 1992;116:575
6. Davis MV. Relationship between pulmonary disease, hiatal hernia and gastroesophageal reflux. NY State J Med 1972;72:935
7. DeMeester TR, et al. Chronic respiratory symptoms and occult gastroesophageal reflux: a prospective clinical study and results of surgical therapy. Ann Surg 1990;211:337
8. DeVault KR, Castell DO, for the Practice Parameters Committee of the American College of Gastroenterology. Guidelines for the diagnosis and treatment of gastroesophageal reflux disease. Arch Intern Med 1995;155:2164
9. DiMarino AJ, Cohen S. Effect of an oral beta-2 adrenergic agonist on lower esophageal sphincter pressure in normals and in patients with achalasia. Dig Dis Sci 1982;27:1063
10. Ekstrom T, Lindgren BR, Tibbling L. Effects on ranitidine treatment on patients with asthma and a history of gastroesophageal reflux: a double blind crossover study. Thorax 1989;44:19
11. Ekstrom T, Tibbling L. Influence of theophylline on gastroesophageal reflux and asthma. Eur J Clin Pharmacol 1988;35:353
12. Ekstrom T, Tibbling L. Can mild bronchospasm reduce gastroesophageal reflux? Am Rev Respir Dis 1989;139:52
13. El-Serag HB, Sonnenberg A. Comorbid occurrence of laryngeal or pulmonary disease with esophagitis in United States military veterans. Gastroenterology 1997;113:755
14. Field SK, et al. Prevalence of gastroesophageal reflux symptoms in asthma. Chest 1996;109:316
15. Finegold SM. Aspiration pneumonia. Sem Respir Crit Care Med 1995;16:475
16. Fitzgerald JM, et al. Chronic cough and gastroesophageal reflux. Can Med Assoc J 1989;140:520
17. Ford GA, et al. Omeprazole in the treatment of asthmatics with nocturnal symptoms and gastroesophageal reflux: a placebo-controlled cross-over study. Postgrad Med J 1994;70:350
18. Gavrouste-Orgeas M, et al. Oropharyngeal or gastric colonization and nosocomial pneumonia in adult intensive care unit patients. A prospective study based on genomic DNA analysis. Am J Respir Crit Care Med 1997;156:1647
19. Goodall RJR, et al. Relationship between asthma and gastroesophageal reflux. Thorax 1981;36:116
20. Guidelines for the diagnosis and management of asthma: Expert Panel Report 2. Bethesda MD: National Institutes of Health, publication 97–4051, 1997
20A. Harding SM. Pulmonary abnormalities in gastroesophageal reflux disease. In J.B. Richter, ed. Ambulatory esophageal pH monitoring: Practical approaches and clinical applications. 2nd ed. Baltimore: Williams & Wilkins, 1997, p. 153
21. Harding SM, Richter JE. The role of gastroesophageal reflux in chronic cough and asthma. Chest 1997;111:1389
22. Harding SM, et al. Gastroesophageal reflux-induced bronchoconstriction: is microaspiration a factor? Chest 1995;108:1220
23. Harding SM, et al. Gastroesophageal reflux induced bronchoconstriction: vagolytic doses of atropine diminish airway responses to esophageal acid infusion. Am J Respir Crit Care Med 1995;151:A589 (abstr)
24. Harding SM, et al. Asthma and gastroesophageal reflux: acid suppressive therapy improves asthma outcome. Am J Med 1996;100:395
25. Harper PC, Bergren A, Kaye MD. Anti-reflux treatment in asthma:

improvement in patients with associated gastroesophageal reflux. Arch Intern Med 1987;147:56

26. Herve P, et al. Intraesophageal perfusion of acid increases the bronchomotor response to methacholine and to isocapnic hyperventilation in asthmatic subjects. Am Rev Respir Dis 1986;134:986

27. Holmes PW, Campbell AM, Barter CE. Changes of lung volumes and lung mechanics in asthma and normal subjects. Thorax 1978;33:394

28. Hubert D, et al. Effect of theophylline on gastroesophageal reflux in patients with asthma. J Allergy Clin Immunol 1988;81:1168

29. Ing AJ. Cough and gastroesophageal reflux. Am J Med 1997;103:91S

30. Ing AJ, Ngu MC, Breslin ABX. Chronic persistant cough and gastroesophageal reflux. Thorax 1991;46:479

31. Ing AJ, Ngu MC, Breslin ABX. A randomized double blind placebo controlled cross over study of ranitidine in patients with chronic persistant cough (CPC) associated with gastroesophageal reflux. Am Rev Respir Dis 1992;141;A11 (abstr)

32. Ing AJ, Ngu MC, Breslin ABX. Chronic persistent cough and clearance of esophageal acid. Chest 1992;102:1688

33. Ing AJ, Ngu MC, Breslin ABX. Pathogenesis of chronic persistent cough associated with gastroesophageal reflux. Am J Respir Crit Care Med 1994;149:160

34. Irwin RS. Management of chronic cough. In George R, ed, Pulmonary and Critical Care Update, vol 9. Northbrook, IL: American College of Chest Physicians, 1994:1

35. Irwin RS, Corrao WM, Pratter MR. Chronic persistent cough in the adult: the spectrum and frequency of causes and successful outcome of specific therapy. Am Rev Respir Dis 1981;123:413

36. Irwin RS, Curley FJ, French CL. Chronic cough: the spectrum and frequency of causes, key components of the diagnostic evaluation, and outcome of specific therapy. Am Rev Respir Dis 1990;141:640

37. Irwin RS, Curley FJ, French CL. Difficult-to-control asthma: contributing factors and outcome of a systematic management protocol. Chest 1993;103:1662

38. Irwin RS, et al. Chronic cough as the sole presenting manifestation of gastroesophageal reflux. Am Rev Respir Dis 1989;140:1294

39. Irwin RS, et al. Chronic cough due to gastroesophageal reflux disease. Clinical, diagnostic, and pathogenetic aspects. Chest 1993;104:1511

40. Jack CIA, et al. Simultaneous tracheal and oesophageal pH measurements in asthmatic patients with gastro-esophageal reflux. Thorax 1995;50:201

41. Johannesson N, et al. Relaxation of lower esophageal sphincter and stimulation of gastric secretion and diuresis by antiasthmatic xanthines: role of adenosine antagonism. Am Rev Respir Dis 1985;131

42. Johnson DA, et al. Pulmonary disease in progressive systemic sclerosis. A complication of gastroesophageal reflux and occult aspiration. Arch Intern Med 1989;149:589

43. Johnson WE, et al. Outcome of respiratory symptoms after antireflux surgery on patients with gastroesophageal reflux disease. Arch Surg 1996;131:489

44. Karlsson JA, Sant' Ambrogio G, Widdicombe J. Afferent neural pathways in cough and reflex bronchoconstriction. J App Physiol 1998;65:1007

45. Kennedy JH. "Silent" gastroesophageal reflux. Dis Chest 1962;42:42

46. Kjellen G, et al. Oesophageal function in asthmatics. Eur J Respir Dis 981;62:87

47. Kjellen G, Tibbling L, Wranne B. Bronchial obstruction after esophageal acid perfusion in asthmatics. Clin Physiol 1981;1:285

48. Kjellen G, Tibbling L, Wranne B. Effect of conservative treatment of oesophageal dysfunction on bronchial dysfunction on bronchial asthma. Eur J Respir Dis 1981;62:190

49. Larrain A, et al. Medical and surgical treatment of nonallergic asthma associated with gastroesophageal reflux. Chest 1991;9:1330

50. Locke GR, Talley NJ, Fett SC, Zinmeester AR, Melton ZJ. Prevalence and clinical spectrum of gastroesophageal reflux: a population study in Olmstead County, Minnesota. Gastroenterology 1997;112:1448

51. Lodi U, Harding SM, Coghlan HC, Guzzo MR, Walker LH. Autonomic regulation in asthmatics with gastroesophageal reflux. Chest 1997;111:65

52. Lomasney TL. Hiatus hernia and the respiratory tract. Ann Thorac Surg 1977;24:448

53. Mansfield LE. Gastroesophageal reflux and asthma. Postgrad Med 1989;86:265

54. Mansfield LE, et al. The role of the vagus nerve in airway narrowing caused by intraesophageal hydrochloric acid provocation and esophageal distention. Ann Allergy 1981;76:431

55. Mansfield LE, Stein MR. Gastroesophageal reflux and asthma: a possible reflex mechanism. Ann Allergy 1978;41:224

56. Martin BJW, Robbins JA. Physiology of swallowing: protection of the airway. Semin Respir Crit Care Med 1995;16:448

57. Maukka MA, Cameron AJ, Schei AJ. Gastroesophageal reflux and chronic cough: which comes first? Clin Gastroenterol 1994;19:100

58. Mays EE. Intrinsic asthma in adults: association with gastroesophageal reflux. JAMA 1976;236:2626

59. Mays EE, Dubois JJ, Hamilton GB. Pulmonary fibrosis associated with tracheobronchial aspiration. A study of the frequency of hiatal hernia and gastroesophageal reflux in interstitial pulmonary fibrosis of obscure etiology. Chest 1976;69:512

60. McFadden ER Jr, Gilbert IA. Asthma. N Engl J Med 1992;327:1928

61. Meier JH, et al. Does omeprazole (Prilosec) improve respiratory function in asthmatics with gastroesophageal reflux? A double-blind, placebo-controlled crossover study. Dig Dis Sci 1994;39:2127

62. Mello CJ, Irwin RS, Curley FJ. Predictive values of the character, timing and complications of chronic cough in diagnosing its cause. Arch Intern Med 1996;156:997

63. Michoud MC, et al. Effect of Salbutamol on gastroesophageal reflux in healthy volunteers and patients with asthma. J Allergy Clin Immunol 1991;87:762

64. Mittal RK, Balaban DH. The esophagogastric junction. N Engl J Med 1997;336:924

65. Mittal RK, Holloway RH, Penagiri R, Blackshaw LA, Dent J. Transient lower esophageal sphincter relaxation. Gastroenterology 1995;109:601

66. Mittal RK, Rochester DF, McCallum RW. Electrical and mechanical activity in the human lower esophageal sphincter during diaphragmatic contraction. J Clin Invest 1988;81:1182

67. Nagel RA, et al. Ambulatory pH monitoring of gastro-esophageal reflux in "morning dipper" asthmatics. BMJ 1988;297:1371

68. Overholt RH, Ashraf MM. Esophageal reflux as a trigger in asthma. NY State J Med 1966;66:3030

69. Paterson WG, Murat BW. Combined ambulatory esophageal manometry and dual-probe pH-metry in evaluation of patients with chronic unexplained cough. Dig Dis Sci 1994;39:1117

70. Patti MG, Debas HT, Pellegrini CA. Esophageal manometry and 24-hour pH monitoring in the diagnosis of pulmonary aspiration secondary to gastroesophageal reflux. Am J Surg 1992;163:401

71. Pellegrini CA, DeMeester TR, Johnson LF, Skinner DB. Gastroesophageal reflux and pulmonary aspiration: incidence, functional abnormality, and results of surgical therapy. Surgery 1979;86:110

72. Perrin-Fayolle M, et al. Long-term results of surgical treatment for gastroesophageal reflux in asthmatic patients. Chest 1989;96:40

73. Poe RH, et al. Chronic persistent cough: experience in diagnosis and outcome using an anatomic diagnostic protocol. Chest 1989;95:723

74. Pratter MR, et al. An algorithmic approach to chronic cough. Ann Intern Med 1993;119:977

75. Raiha IJ, et al. Prevalence- and characteristics of symptomatic gastroesophageal reflux disease in the elderly. J Am Geriatr Soc 1992;40:1209

76. Roussos C, Macklem PT. The respiratory muscles. N Engl J Med 1982;307:786

77. Schan CA, et al. Gastroesophageal reflux-induced bronchoconstriction: an intraesophageal acid infusion study using state-of-the-art technology. Chest 1994;106:731

78. Schappert SM. National Ambulatory Medical Care Survey: 1991: Summary. In Vital and Health Statistics 230. Washington DC: US Department of Health and Human Services, March 29, 1993

79. Schindlbeck NE, et al. Effects of albuterol (Salbutamol) on esophageal motility and gastroesophageal reflux in healthy volunteers. JAMA 1988;260:3156

80. Schnatz PF, Castell JA, Castell DO. Pulmonary symptoms associated with gastroesophageal reflux: use of ambulatory pH monitoring to diagnose and to direct therapy. Am J Gastroenterol 1996;91:1715

81. Smyrnios NA, Irwin RS, Curley, FJ. Chronic cough with a history of excessive sputum production. Chest 1995;108:991

82. Sontag S, et al. Is gastroesophageal reflux a factor in some asthmatics? Am J Gastroenterol 1987;82:119

83. Sontag S, et al. Anti-reflux surgery in asthmatics with reflux (GER) improves pulmonary symptoms and function. Gastroenterology 1990;98:A128 (abstr)

84. Sontag SJ, et al. Most asthmatics have gastroesophageal reflux with or without bronchodilator therapy. Gastroenterology 1990;99:613

85. Sontag SJ, et al. Prevalence of oesophagitis in asthmatics. Gut 1992;33:872

86. Spaulding MS Jr, Mansfield LE, Stein MR, Sellner JC, Gremillion DE. Further investigation of the association between gastroesophageal reflux and bronchoconstriction. J Allergy Clin Immunol 1982;69:516

87. Stein MR, et al. The effect of theophylline on the lower esophageal sphincter pressure. Ann Allergy 1980;45:238

88. Tan WC, et al. Effects of spontaneous and stimulated gastroesophageal reflux on sleeping asthmatics. Am Rev Respir Dis 1990;141:1394

89. Tardif C, et al. Surgical treatment of gastroesophageal reflux in 10 patients with severe asthma. Respiration 1989;51:115

90. Teichtahl H, Kronbert IJ, Yeomans ND, Robinson P. Adult asthma and gastroesophageal reflux: the effects of omeprazole therapy on asthma. Aust N Z J Med 1996;26:671

91. Tibbling L. Wrong-way swallowing as a possible cause of bronchitis in patients with gastroesophageal reflux disease. Acta Otolaryngol (Stockh) 1993;113:405

92. Tomori Z, Widdicombe JG. Muscular, bronchomotor and cardiovascular reflexes elicited by mechanical stimulation of the respiratory tract. J Physiol (Lond) 1969;200:25

93. Torres A, et al. Pulmonary aspiration of gastric contents in patients receiving mechanical ventilation: the effect of body position. Ann Intern Med 1992;116:540

94. Troshinsky MB, et al. Pulmonary function and gastroesophageal reflux in systemic sclerosis. Ann Intern Med 1994;121:6

95. Tuchman DN, et al. Comparison of airway responses following tracheal or esophageal acidification in the cat. Gastroenterology 1984;87:872

96. Urschel HC, Paulson DL. Gastroesophageal reflux and hiatal hernia: complications and therapy. J Thorac Cardiovasc Surg 1967;53:21

97. Vaezi MF, Richter JE. Twenty-four hour ambulatory esophageal pH monitoring in the diagnosis of acid reflux-related chronic cough. South Med J 1997;90:305

98. Valles J, Artigas A, Rello J. Continuous aspiration of subglottic secretions in preventing ventilation-associated pneumonia. Ann Intern Med 1995;12:179

99. Varkey B, Pathial K, Shaker R, Dodds WJ, Hogan WJ. Pharyngoesophageal reflux index in asthmatics. Chest 1992;102:152S (abstr)

100. Waring JP, Lacayo L, Hunter J, Katz E, Suwak B. Chronic cough and hoarseness in patients with severe gastroesophageal reflux disease. Diagnosis and response to therapy. Dig Dis Sci 1995;40:1093

101. Wright RA, Miller SA, Corsello BF. Acid-induced esophagobronchial cardiac reflexes in humans. Gastroenterology 1990;99:71

*The Esophagus*, Third Edition,
edited by D. O. Castell and J. E. Richter.
Lippincott Williams & Wilkins, Philadelphia © 1999.

CHAPTER 30

# Regurgitation and Rumination

Steven S. Shay

Physicians commonly evaluate patients with recurrent episodes of regurgitation. Since many disorders present in this manner, a systematic approach is advisable to diagnose the origin of regurgitation in the individual patient with an organic lesion. However, even extensive evaluation may fail to define an underlying disorder. In this situation, consideration of a functional etiology, such as rumination, is warranted. Finally, eating disorders such as bulimia should be considered in the appropriate patient population.

This chapter discusses only the initial approach to patients with chronic regurgitation as the specific disorders are covered in detail elsewhere in this book. Rumination is discussed in detail. The primary eating disorders are not discussed.

## CHRONIC REGURGITATION

### Definition

*Regurgitation* is the sudden, effortless return of small volumes of gastric or esophageal contents into the pharynx and implies cricopharyngeal relaxation or insufficiency. Regurgitation is best differentiated from vomiting by its small volume; predominantly recumbent occurrence; the absence of preceding nausea, retching, or autonomic symptoms; and a lack of abdominal and thoracic muscle contraction.

### Differential Diagnosis

Chronic regurgitation may result from several primary esophageal disorders or gastroesophageal reflux disease (GERD) (Table 30–1). Structural lesions may obstruct the esophagus, or diverticula (midesophageal, epiphrenic) at any level may accumulate food particles and secretions, resulting in regurgitation when the contents are discharged into the esophageal lumen. An esophageal motility disorder [achala-

S. S. Shay: Department of Gastroenterology, The Cleveland Clinic Foundation, Cleveland, Ohio 44195.

sia, hypertensive lower esophageal sphincter (LES), diffuse esophageal spasm] may be responsible. Pseudoregurgitation [i.e., solid or liquid accumulations in the pharynx not resulting from upper esophageal sphincter (UES) relaxation] occurs in several disorders and may be confused with regurgitation. Structural lesions, such as Zenker's diverticula, accumulate food and secretions. In addition, inflammation of the nasal passages (sinuses, pharynx, or hypopharynx) may present with pseudoregurgitation as secretions are perceived as regurgitation by the patient or physician.

Regurgitation can be difficult to distinguish from vomiting, and both symptoms may occur in the same patient. Chronic vomiting is usually of intra-abdominal origin, as in disorders of the pancreas or the hepatobiliary, genitourinary, or gastrointestinal tract; a broad differential encompassing several different organ systems must be considered (Table 30–2).

### Complications

Aspiration is the most feared sequela of chronic regurgitation or pseudoregurgitation. Nocturnal coughing, wheezing, a pillow stained with gastric contents, recurrent pneumonia, and interstitial lung disease are all suggestive of regurgitation. Referred otic pain, globus sensation [33], dental findings [23], and a variety of otolaryngological lesions [14] have been reported in patients with regurgitation caused by gastroesophageal reflux.

### Diagnostic Evaluation

History is valuable in discerning which category of chronic regurgitation may be responsible. Associated symptoms should be sought. Most disorders of esophageal origin can present with dysphagia and, occasionally, odynophagia. Pyrosis suggests GERD, either primary or as a result of gastric retention. Chest pain suggests an esophageal motility disorder or GERD. Regurgitation or vomiting of material eaten many hours previously suggests gastric retention but

**TABLE 30–1.** *Disorders associated with chronic regurgitation and their initial evaluation*

| Disorder | Evaluation |
| --- | --- |
| Esophageal origin | |
|   Structural esophageal lesion | Barium esophagogram, esophagoscopy |
|     Tumor | |
|     Stricture | |
|     Diverticulum | |
|   Esophageal motility disorder | Videoesophagogram, esophageal manometry |
| Gastroesophageal reflux | |
|   LES dysfunction | Esophagoscopy, esophageal manometry, 24-hr pH monitoring |
|     Primary | |
|     Scleroderma | |
|   Gastric retention | UGI series, scintigraphic solid-food gastric emptying |
|     Obstruction | |
|     Gastric atony | |
| Pseudoregurgitation | |
|   Zenker's diverticulum | Videoesophagogram |
|   Nasopharyngeal structural lesion | Nasopharyngoscopy |
|   Sinus disease | Sinus x-ray, CT scan |

LES, lower esophageal sphincter; UGI, upper gastrointestinal; CT, computed tomography.
From ref. 24, with permission.

may also represent material expelled from a diverticulum (esophageal or pharyngeal) or achalasia. Expectoration of small volumes of mucoid or purulent material suggests a nasopharyngeal origin.

The past history can be valuable. Chronic rhinorrhea and coryza, especially seasonal, suggest nasopharyngeal disease. Other examples include a history of peptic ulcer disease (which should lead to suspicion of gastric retention), scleroderma, and Raynaud's disease.

The present and past history should lead one to suspect an esophageal or gastroesophageal source for chronic regurgitation or to suspect pseudoregurgitation. The diagnostic tests available for the evaluation of these disorders are listed in Table 30-1. Occasionally, when the history does not clearly discriminate between the symptoms of regurgitation and vomiting or when they coexist, disorders associated with vomiting must be considered and excluded by appropriate studies. Finally, the patient may have primary rumination or an eating disorder.

## RUMINATION

### Definition

*Rumination* is a diagnosis of exclusion. When there is an absence of organic esophageal or gastric disease, diagnostic

**TABLE 30–2.** *Disorder categories in patients with chronic vomiting*

| | | |
| --- | --- | --- |
| Cerebromedullary | Toxins | Vestibular |
| Intra-abdominal | Drugs | Pregnancy |
|   Intraluminal | Metabolic | Psychogenic |
|   Visceral | | |

criteria recently proposed for the rumination syndrome are as follows: (a) chronic or recurrent regurgitation of recently ingested food into the mouth with subsequent remastication and swallowing present at least 3 months, (b) absence of nausea and vomiting, and (c) rumination usually stopping when the contents become acidic [21]. Regurgitation, remastication, and swallowing may occur as frequently as 20 times after a meal. Finally, in most patients with rumination syndrome, it occurs with most meals.

### Presentations

The rumination syndrome has many different presentations. Voluntary rumination may occur in the mentally retarded. In adults with normal intelligence, presentations can be extremely variable. At one extreme are patients with voluntary rumination performed for a pleasurable or profitable reason. At the other extreme are patients whose rumination is confused with organic disease because the rumination is involuntary and accompanied by other symptoms that mask its diagnosis, such as abdominal pain, weight loss, nausea without vomiting, constipation, and heartburn [19, 27]. This discussion addresses these divergent adult presentations after a review of rumination in animals and the infant rumination syndrome.

### Animal Rumination

Animals such as sheep and cattle have compartmentalized stomachs *(rumens)*. Rumination in cows was first studied by manometry in nineteenth-century experiments. These and later studies employing fluid-filled, nonperfused catheters found two steps in the process [7, 28]. First, a negative intrathoracic pressure ($-40$ mm Hg) occurred during rumen contractions, resulting in gastric contents being delivered to the esophagus. Then, antiperistalsis at a very fast rate (greater than 100 mm per second) was observed delivering ingesta from the esophagus to the mouth. In the cow, this occurs in regular 1-minute cycles. A complex reflex mediated by the brainstem has been proposed since vagal sectioning prevents rumination in cows [6].

Rumination is reported in 79% of captive gorillas. Since they do not have rumens, the mechanism is unknown, although regurgitation typically follows a series of other voluntary motor movements, as in infants and retarded individuals (described later). Interestingly, as in some adults and infants, rumination in gorillas may respond to behavior modification. That is, rumination decreases if time spent eating increases, suggesting that rumination by gorillas in the zoo environment is voluntary and a result of artificially short feeding times in comparison to eating in the wild [11].

### Infant Rumination Syndrome

The typical features of infant rumination syndrome begin at 3 to 8 months of age. It occurs when the baby is awake, quiet, and self-absorbed rather than while asleep or actively interested in objects or surroundings. The act of rumination is typically a stereotyped series of maneuvers. It begins with rhythmic movements of the pharynx, tongue, and abdominal muscles, culminating in regurgitation to the mouth (and usually spilling of regurgitant outside the oral cavity). Then, the regurgitant is masticated and reswallowed. There may be associated self-stimulatory behavior, such as head rolling, hand sucking, etc. The infant often fails to thrive; does not improve with conservative antireflux therapy, formula change, etc.; and, occasionally, exhibits progressive wasting until death [8].

The etiology is thought to be an emotionally distant caregiver, who is unable to sense the baby's needs. Thus, rumination is self-stimulating and satisfies needs ordinarily supplied by the caregiver [8]. Others feel the etiology is behavioral, and rumination persists as a result of the increased attention gained from the caregiver [34].

The key to diagnosis is direct observation of the ruminating activity since rumination can be easily confused with other functional vomiting disorders of infancy (nervous or innocent vomiting [8]. In addition, gastroesophageal diseases, such as pyloric or esophageal obstruction, and especially GERD [29] need to be excluded.

Therapy is behavioral if possible. Increasing social interaction between infant and mother or mother-substitute may stop rumination, especially increased holding during and immediately following meals [18, 32]. If this fails, aversive therapy, such as isolation or placing lemon juice on the tongue after rumination, has been effective [18, 22].

### Voluntary Rumination Syndrome in Adults

Some adults willfully ruminate as a pleasurable experience and may be selective in the food type regurgitated [3, 20]. In this situation, the patient may present out of concern of self-injury or the presence of an underlying disease or if heartburn develops or be presented by a relative who may observe mastication long after meal completion.

Taking advantage economically of their ability to regurgitate on command, some astonishing acts of controlled regurgitation have been described in circus performers. Among the most remarkable was Hadji Ali, an actor, who swallowed a pint of water and a half pint of kerosene, then stood about 6 feet from a candle burning in a box open at the front. The kerosene, being of lower specific gravity, was brought up first in small jets which dramatically burst into flame as they approached the candle. When the kerosene was exhausted, the water was regurgitated in a spraying fashion from his mouth and extinguished the flames [15].

The pathophysiology of voluntary rumination is unknown. However, it is likely to be similar to that in those with involuntary rumination (described later) since observations of professional ruminators describe Valsalva and Müller-like maneuvers preceding or associated with rumination [3, 15, 20]. In addition, upper gastrointestinal (UGI) series in four patients during induced rumination found Müller maneuvers and abdominal contractions simultaneous with rumination [30].

Despite the voluntary nature of rumination in these patients, cessation of rumination behavior should be recommended because of the potential for oropharyngeal, especially dental, complications.

### Voluntary Rumination in Retarded Individuals

Rumination syndrome has been reported to occur in as many as 10% of retarded patients in institutions. It appears to be a voluntary behavior as it is typically repetitive and associated with oropharyngeal movements such as sucking, belching noises, tongue movements, etc. Identifying these stereotyped maneuvers is the key to the correct diagnosis [9]. However, other causes of chronic regurgitation (especially GERD [5]), as well as vomiting (such as poor gastric emptying and hydrocephalus) need to be considered and excluded in the appropriate clinical situation.

Treatment is often necessary due to concern by caregivers about frequent cleaning of the patient and changes of clothing, bedding, etc. A combination of dietary manipulations, such as prescribing peanut butter [12], and behavioral interventions, such as withdrawal of social reinforcement during and after eating [16], should be tried first. If unsuccessful, retarded individuals have been treated successfully with a food-satiation approach [9] or aversive therapy, such as applying Tabasco sauce or lemon juice to the tongue [2, 31].

### Nonvoluntary Rumination Syndrome in Adults

Rumination in some patients is nonvoluntary and not accompanied by other symptoms. This has been termed *simple rumination,* and men predominate in most series [20]. However, in some patients, rumination is accompanied by other symptoms, which may dominate the presentation. For example, *dyspeptic rumination* has been described, where epigastric discomfort, bloating, belching, and regurgitation were present [3, 10]. In a recent report of 16 patients [27], pain (n = 6), nausea (n = 5), constipation (n = 5), and heartburn (n = 1) were present. Weight loss was common. Moreover, 4/16 had been on either total parenteral nutrition or feeding jejunostomy tube. In this report, 10/16 were women.

#### Pathophysiology

Whether rumination in the varied presentations described above has the same pathophysiology and natural history is unknown. Early studies compared human and animal rumination, and separate gastric pouches and antiperistalsis were sought. These were not found. In fact, UGI series in patients not actively ruminating were normal in most cases.

Manometry of the UGI tract has described simultaneous pressure spikes at all monitored sites concomitant with regurgitation and reswallowing (termed an *R wave*) in several reports. Furthermore, simultaneous pH changes have also been described [2, 19, 27]. This manometric finding is characteristic of rumination.

We recorded simultaneous esophageal, gastric, UES, and rectal pressures with esophageal and pharyngeal pH in a 31-year-old patient with rumination and dyspeptic complaints for 20 years. Twenty-five episodes were recorded in the first postprandial hour and revealed the same pathophysiological sequence (Fig. 30–1). First, a spontaneous increase in intraesophageal pressure occurred, with respiratory excursion being the same as intragastric, i.e., a common cavity due to gaseous reflux [4]. A Valsalva maneuver (R wave) documented by sudden increases in intrathoracic and intraabdominal pressures occurred within 1 to 5 seconds of the common cavity and was simultaneous with the esophageal pH change. Relaxation of the UES at the time of the Valsalva maneuver resulted in near simultaneous pH changes in the pharynx and the esophagus. In fact, the calculated velocity of esophagopharyngeal regurgitation was 100 cm per second over the 20-cm distance between the two pH probes. Acid reflux was then cleared from the esophagus and pharynx by primary swallows [25].

In the patient above, rumination was a learned response

to the common cavity phenomenon [25], which is gaseous gastroesophageal reflux. A recent review also postulated that rumination is a learned adaptation of the belch reflex [17]. Another etiology proposed for rumination is voluntary induction of transient LES relaxation after abdominal contractions [26].

### Diagnosis

The rumination syndrome is underdiagnosed and often difficult to diagnose. In a recent study, patients saw a mean of five physicians and had symptoms a mean of 2.8 years before diagnosis [19].

Rumination syndrome is a diagnosis of exclusion. Since any cause of regurgitation can potentially meet the definition of rumination syndrome if the patient chooses (or prefers for social reasons) to reingest the regurgitant, the disorders in Table 30-1 need to be excluded by the studies suggested. Once excluded, if the characteristic history is present, therapy as described below should be prescribed.

If primary GERD is suspected, the pattern of reflux and symptoms recorded during 24-hour pH monitoring can be helpful. That is, predominantly upright postprandial reflux,

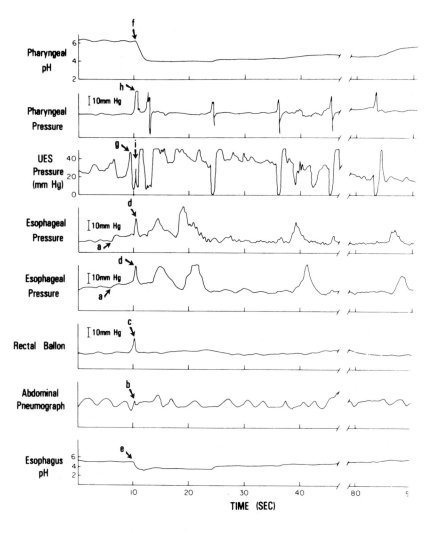

FIG. 30–1. Simultaneous hypopharyngeal and esophageal pH monitoring and manometry during a rumination event (see keys *a–i*). First, a spontaneous increase in intraesophageal pressure occurred (see *Esophageal Pressure, a*) with a respiratory excursion that coincided with that of the intragastric environment, i.e., the common cavity phenomenon. Second, 5 seconds after the onset of the common cavity, a Valsalva maneuver (R wave) occurred, documented by splinting of respiration (see *Abdominal Pneumograph, b*), sudden increase in intraabdominal pressure (see *Rectal Balloon, c*), and spikes in intraesophageal pressure (see *Esophageal Pressure, d*). This sequence was the rumination event, simultaneously documented by the decrease in hypopharyngeal pH (see *Pharyngeal pH, f*) and esophageal pH (see *Esophageal pH, e*). Simultaneous relaxation of the upper esophageal sphincter *(UES)* pressure at the time of the Valsalva maneuver (R wave) appeared to facilitate esophagopharyngeal regurgitation (see *UES Pressure, g*). The velocity of esophagopharyngeal regurgitation was 100 cm per second over the 20-cm distance between the pH probes. Acid reflux was then cleared from both the esophagus and the pharynx by primary peristalsis.

especially when accompanied by symptoms during the reflux events, is characteristic. Finally, if the diagnosis is in question because of accompanying dyspeptic complaints or abdominal pain is present, gastroduodenal manometry can identify the characteristic R waves from abdominal and thoracic contractions and exclude other disorders.

## Therapy

A number of aversive therapies have been attempted in adults, such as alkalies, acids, bitter potions, and gastric lavage [13]. However, no generally accepted and reliable aversive treatment has been reported. We are unaware of reports of prokinetic or antisecretory drugs in rumination.

Nonaversive behavioral therapy employs explanations of the mechanism of rumination and/or behavioral therapy, such as biofeedback, by a behavioral therapist. An eating habit regulation program (six of seven patients), biofeedback and Jacksonian relaxation (two of two patients), and psychotherapy (one of one patient) were associated with improvement or complete cessation of rumination in nine of ten treated patients in one study [1]. My colleagues and I found that biofeedback directed against the abdominal and thoracic contractions stopped rumination, and we documented a decrease in acid exposure and reflux event frequency by 24-hour pH monitoring [25]. Thus, nonaversive behavioral therapy is the modality of choice for rumination in adults of normal intelligence.

## REFERENCES

1. Amarnath RP, Abell TL, Malagelada J. The rumination syndrome in adults. Ann Intern Med 1986;105:513
2. Bright PJ, George GC, Smart DE. Suppression of regurgitation and rumination with aversive events. Mich Ment Health Res Bull 1968;11:17
3. Brockbank EM. Mercyism or rumination in man. BMJ 1907;1:421
4. Butterfield DG, Struthers JE, Showalter BS. A test of gastroesophageal sphincter competence: the common cavity test. Dig Dis Sci 1972;17:415
5. Byrne WJ, Euler AR, Achcraft E, Nash D, Seibert J, Golladay ES. Gastroesophageal reflux in the severely retarded who vomit: criteria for and results of surgical intervention in twenty-two patients. Surgery 1982;91:95
6. Clark C. The nerve control for rumination and reticuloruminal motility. Am J Vet Res 1953;14:376
7. Doughterty RW. Physiology of eructation in ruminants. In Handbook of Physiology, vol 5. Baltimore: Williams & Wilkins, 1968:2695
8. Fleisher DR. Functional vomiting disorders in infancy: innocent vomiting, nervous vomiting, and infant rumination syndrome. J Pediatr 1994;125(suppl):84
9. Foxx RM, Snyder MS, Schroeder F. A food satiation and oral hygiene punishment program to suppress chronic rumination by retarded persons. J Autism Dev Disord 1979;9:399
10. Geffen N. Rumination in man. Am J Dig Dis 1966;11:963
11. Gould E, Bres M. Regurgitation and reingestion in captive gorillas: description and intervention. Zoo Biol 1986;5:241
12. Greene KS, Johnson JM, Rossi M, Rawal A, Winston M, Barron S. Effects of peanut butter on ruminating. Am J Ment Retard 1991;95:631
13. Kanner L. Historical notes on rumination in man. Med Life 1936;43:27
14. Koufman JA. The otolaryngeal manifestations of gastroesophageal reflux disease. Laryngoscope 1991;101(suppl 53):1
15. Long C. Rumination in man. Am J Med Sci 1929;178:814
16. Luiselli JK, Haley S, Smith A. Evaluation of a behavioral medicine consultative treatment for chronic, ruminative vomiting. J Behav Ther Exp Psychiatry 1993;24:27
17. Malcolm A, Thumshirn MB, Camilleri M, Williams DE. Rumination syndrome. Mayo Clin Proc 1997;72:646
18. Murray ME, Keele DK, McCarver JW. Behavioral treatment of rumination. Clin Pediatr 1976;15:591
19. O'Brien MD, Bruce BK, Camilleri M. The rumination syndrome: clinical features rather than manometric diagnosis. Gastroenterology 1995;108:1024
20. Parry-Jones B. Mercyism or rumination disorder: a historical investigation and current assessment. Br J Psychiatry 1994;165:303
21. Richter JE. Functional esophageal disorders. In Drossman DA, ed, Functional Gastrointestinal Disorders, Diagnosis, Pathophysiology and Treatment—A Multinational Consensus. Boston: Little, Brown and Company, 1994:35
22. Sajwaj T, Libet J, Agras S. Lemon juice therapy: the control of life-threatening rumination in a six-month-old infant. J Appl Behav Anal 1974;7:557
23. Schroeder PL, Filler SJ, Ramirez B, Lazarchik DA, Vaezi MF, Richter JE. Dental erosion and acid reflux disease. Ann Intern Med 1995;122:809
24. Shay SS, Johnson LF. Regurgitation, rumination, and disorders of eating. In Castell DO, ed, Esophageal Function in Health and Disease. New York: Elsevier Science, 1983:140
25. Shay SS, et al. Rumination, heartburn, and daytime gastroesophageal reflux: a case study with mechanisms defined and successfully treated with biofeedback therapy. J Clin Gastroenterol 1986;8:115
26. Smout AJ, Breumelhof R. Voluntary induction of transient lower esophageal sphincter relaxations in an adult patient with the rumination syndrome. Am J Gastroenterol 1990;85:1621
27. Soykan I, Chen J, Kendall BJ, McCallum RW. The rumination syndrome: clinical and manometric profile, therapy, and long-term outcome. Dig Dis Sci 1997;42:1866
28. Stevens CE, Sellers AF. Rumination. In Handbook of Physiology, vol 5. Baltimore: Williams & Wilkins, 1968:2699
29. Taminiau JA. Gastro-oesophageal reflux in children. Scand J Gastroenterol 1997;32(suppl 223):18
30. Van Trappen G, Hellemans J. Diseases of the Esophagus. New York: Springer-Verlag, 1974:418
31. White JD, Taylor D. Noxious conditioning as a treatment for rumination. Ment Retard 1967;5:30
32. Whitehead WE, Dresher VM, Corbin EM. Rumination syndrome in children treated by increased holding. Pediatr Gastroenterol Nutr 1985;4:550
33. Wilson JA, et al. Pharyngoesophageal dysmotility in globus sensation. Arch Otol Laryngol Head Neck Surg 1989;115:1086
34. Wolf MM, Birnbrauer J, Lawler J, Williams T. The operant extinction, reinstatement and re-extinction of vomiting behavior in a retarded child. In Ulrich R, Statnik T, Mabry J, eds, Control of Human Behavior, vol 2. Glenview, IL: Scott, Foresman, 1970:146

*The Esophagus*, Third Edition,
edited by D. O. Castell and J. E. Richter.
Lippincott Williams & Wilkins, Philadelphia © 1999.

CHAPTER 31

# Surgical Treatment of Gastroesophageal Reflux Disease

Susan A. Branton, Ronald A. Hinder, Neil R. Floch, Paul J. Klingler, and Matthias H. Seelig

Gastroesophageal reflux disease (GERD) is a very common condition. Gastroesophageal reflux occurs normally postprandially and is usually of no pathologic consequence. About 44% of Americans experience the symptom of heartburn at least once a month, and 18% of these people regularly take some form of nonprescription medication for the problem [26]. Many young people have GERD, with a peak incidence at 30 to 40 years of age. The mean age of patients with severe esophagitis is over 60 years, and more than half of patients presenting with Barrett's esophagus are over 70 years of age [29]. Sex incidence appears to be about equal, with some series reporting more men and others reporting more women [21]. GERD is mainly a disease of the Western world, with a low incidence reported in Africa and Asia.

The vast majority of patients with gastroesophageal reflux can be managed by self-medication or intermittent antireflux medication. In a small number of patients, this may not be adequate and surgery must be considered. The most popular procedure has been the fundoplication, in which the fundus of the stomach is wrapped around the lower esophagus. This procedure was described by Nissen in 1961. Since that time, many patients have undergone this procedure, which has been more frequently performed since 1991, when it was found to be feasible using laparoscopic techniques.

The annual adult mortality rate of GERD is only 0.1 per 100,000 population (from 1957 to 1961) [7]; but complications, such as ulceration, strictures, hemorrhage, Barrett's esophagus, and Barrett's adenocarcinoma, occur relatively commonly. When medical therapy fails to control symptoms or is required continuously, particularly in the presence of complications, surgery may be indicated.

## PATHOPHYSIOLOGY

To understand the rationale for antireflux surgery, it is important to understand the relevant pathophysiology. The luminal environment of the stomach and esophagus is usually totally different, with a low-pH gastric content and neutral pH of the esophagus. Prolonged exposure of the esophageal mucosa to acid and other noxious secretions causes mucosal damage. The severity of the resulting disease depends on the amount of acid refluxed into the esophagus, the length of time that the acid is allowed to remain in contact with the esophageal mucosa, and the susceptibility of the esophageal mucosa to acid. Enzymes such as pepsin and trypsin as well as alkaline secretions from the duodenum and bile acids have also been implicated in esophageal disease.

To prevent reflux of gastric contents into the esophagus, a delicate antireflux mechanism exists at the gastric cardia. The major component of this is the lower esophageal sphincter (LES), which is an imperfect valve that must open to allow for the passage of food, belching, and vomiting. The LES forms the most important part of the physiologic barrier between the esophagus and stomach. The LES is a thickening of the musculature in the lower 5 cm of the esophagus [32]. This is composed of a thickening of the circular muscle layer, particularly on the greater-curvature side of the sphincter. Below this, oblique muscle fibers, named the collar of Helvetius, run from the angle of His toward the lesser curvature of the stomach. The sphincter lies partly within the chest and partly within the abdomen. This area of the esophageal musculature has a higher density of neuronal plexuses than does the esophageal body [45]. Muscle from

S. A. Branton, R. A. Hinder, and N. R. Floch: Department of Surgery, Mayo Clinic Jacksonville, Jacksonville, Florida 32224.

P. J. Klingler: Department of General Surgery, University Hospital of Innsbruck, A-6020 Innsbruck, Austria.

M. H. Seelig: Department of Surgery, General Hospital Ludwigshafen, D-67063 Ludwigshafen/Rhein, Germany.

this region is more responsive to gastrin and has a heightened sensitivity to cholinergic and adrenergic compounds compared with the adjacent smooth muscle.

The LES has a resting pressure that can be measured in the interprandial period by obtaining pressure measurements from within the lumen of the esophagus. Studies of the LES in normal people have shown that the 2.5th percentile of normal is 6 mm Hg pressure, measured at the respiratory inversion point. It has a total length of over 2 cm and an intra-abdominal component measuring more than 1 cm in length. Gastroesophageal reflux is likely to occur if the pressure or length of the sphincter falls below these lower limits of normal. Failure of the LES mechanism can be due to a number of events, including primary weakness of the smooth muscle, short length of the sphincter, defective control mechanisms, an abnormally high number of transient relaxations, and dislocation of the LES into the chest. A combination of several of these events makes reflux more likely to occur. It is not clear whether esophageal mucosal inflammation has a negative influence on LES pressure [4, 15]. An effective way of representing the overall antireflux ability of the LES is the expression of vector volume. This calculation expresses the pressure and length of the sphincter around its circumference as a vector volume. This gives a single value to be compared with a normal range [47]. Not all gastroesophageal reflux events are related to impaired LES resting pressure: Among patients with GERD, a defective sphincter is found in 60% or fewer, and only 18% to 23% of all reflux episodes can be explained by deficient esophageal sphincter pressures [13, 54].

The LES is under various neural and hormonal control mechanisms in addition to the influence of the crura and the surrounding intra-abdominal or intrathoracic pressures. The resting pressure shows large variations and can reach values of about 100 mm Hg. The highest values are seen during phase III of the migrating motor complex in the stomach, which suggests that there is a direct influence of gastric motility on the LES [12]. Hormones that are known to increase the tone in the LES are motilin and gastrin, whereas cholecystokinin, secretin, and vasoactive intestinal peptide cause a decrease in LES tone [15, 16, 17, 53]. Other hormones, such as substance P, are implicated in maintaining LES tone. In patients with GERD, the LES shows a poor response to stimulants such as gastrin and bethanechol [18]. Patients with GERD have significantly lower basal levels of motilin and an impaired postprandial cholecystokinin response [40]. It is not clear whether these are primary or secondary events. Nitric oxide has also been found to play a role in the control of LES pressure.

The resting LES pressure is contributed to by the surrounding crura and the intra-abdominal pressure. If the LES is translocated into the chest, such as occurs with a hiatal hernia, these factors are ineffective, and reflux can occur. The crura play an important part in maintaining LES pressure, with increases in pressure recorded with crural contraction even when the sphincter muscle is relaxed. Intra-abdom-

inal pressure may increase the pressure at the LES by direct pressure on the sphincter or by inducing active contractions in the LES, resulting in pressures much higher than the intra-abdominal pressure.

Dislocation of the LES into the chest can be identified by recording a high-pressure zone at a level located anatomically in the chest. Occasionally, a "double-hump" phenomenon can be identified manometrically with two high-pressure zones in the distal esophagus [28]. The lower high-pressure zone is created by the diaphragmatic crura and the upper by the LES, which has been dislocated into the chest. The pressure that the LES can generate in the chest is lower than normal but is able to prevent reflux under most conditions. Under straining conditions, this can be more easily overcome than when the crura contribute to the pressure [36].

LES relaxation normally occurs with swallowing. So-called transient relaxations of the LES not related to swallowing may play a role in GERD but are probably more significant during normal physiologic events, such as belching. Contradictory evidence exists regarding the number of such relaxations in patients with GERD. Subthreshold swallows may produce them. The clinical importance of transient relaxations of the LES is not known.

## INDICATIONS FOR SURGERY

In the past, there was some reluctance to refer patients for antireflux surgery because of the uncertainty of the outcome and the magnitude of the surgical procedures. In recent years, this has changed due to a better understanding of the mechanisms of reflux and how they can be altered by antireflux surgery. The ability to do these operations using minimally invasive techniques has added to the increase in the rate of surgery. The success of antireflux surgery depends on choosing suitable candidates who can be offered a good chance of cure based on previous experience (Fig. 31–1).

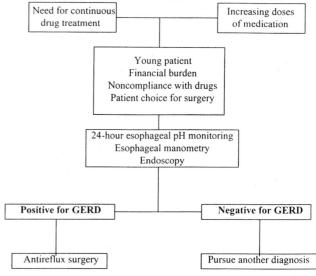

**FIG. 31–1.** Algorithm for identifying appropriate candidates for antireflux surgery.

Excellent medications against reflux are available, but many patients will either fail to obtain relief, develop complications of their disease, or choose not to be dependent on medications for the rest of their lives. Medical treatment of GERD, although intermittent for some, is often a daily, life-long process for others. Patient compliance can be poor, especially for long-term treatment. In addition to the inconvenience of daily treatment, the cost of therapy can be unacceptable to the patient. Cost varies depending on the treatment regimen being used, with proton pump inhibitors (PPIs) being more expensive than histamine receptor antagonists, especially when high-dose therapy is required for relief of symptoms. When continuous therapy is required for several years, the cost and inconvenience can make surgery a viable alternative. In addition, if increasing doses are required to maintain control, surgery may be indicated. Rarely, patients on medical therapy become refractory to their medications and suffer continued symptoms despite increasing doses, making surgery a reasonable alternative.

Complications of GERD characterize another subset of patients for whom surgery is frequently recommended. Patients with severe esophagitis, Barrett's esophagus, ulceration, and esophageal strictures should be considered for surgery.

Severe esophagitis, based on the Savary-Miller classification, is a clear indication for surgery. This is particularly so since these patients are more likely to fail long-term medical therapy [49]. Barrett's esophagus is regarded as a severe form of esophagitis. Barrett's esophagus is diagnosed when a columnar lining of the esophagus is recognized more than 2 to 3 cm above the LES; this is seen in up to 2% of the population. It is now known to be the result of chronic GERD with metaplasia of the normal squamous lining. Reflux is thought to result in destruction and desquamation of the squamous epithelium, with replacement by the inherently more acid-resistant columnar epithelium. Patients with Barrett's esophagus have been found to have a more defective LES than other patients with GERD [25]. These patients also have a decreased amplitude of contractions in the distal esophagus. Increased duodenogastric reflux has been reported in patients with Barrett's esophagus [3]. Treatment of Barrett's esophagus using prolonged therapy against acid may not make sense in a disease that is associated with alkaline exposure of the esophagus. Experiments in rats have indicated that damage to the esophageal mucosa by alkaline reflux is worsened by the addition of acid suppression with omeprazole or by vagotomy. However, in humans, Barrett's patients have increased acid and alkaline exposure of the esophagus and omeprazole decreases the amount of bile in the esophagus [8]. In support of this protective effect, continued medical therapy has not been associated with a significant increase in the level of columnar epithelium in the esophagus. Surgical therapy for Barrett's esophagus is advised in patients who are resistant to medical therapy and in those who develop complications, such as ulceration, stricture, or severe dysplasia. Some have suggested bile diversion procedures for these patients [9]. Antireflux procedures, such as the Nissen fundoplication [37], relieve symptoms and may even prevent extension of the columnar epithelium [6]. It is unclear whether the progression to dysplasia or malignancy is arrested by surgery, but some evidence suggests that dysplastic changes may stop or even reverse it [46]. There are reports of adenocarcinoma developing in Barrett's esophagus after antireflux surgery. Patients with Barrett's, however, should undergo regular surveillance for dysplastic or malignant change even after surgery.

Mucosal ulceration due to severe GERD most commonly occurs at the squamocolumnar junction and is sometimes associated with stricture formation. Ulcers are an indication of severe disease and may heal with stricture formation. Approximately two-thirds of ulcers heal on medical therapy, but this may take weeks to achieve. Barrett's esophagus may also be associated with ulcers which are solitary and usually found in the middle of the columnar epithelium. Surgical therapy can permanently remove the cause of the ulceration and prevent ulcer recurrence and stricture formation from repeated scarring and healing.

GERD patients with strictures are usually older and have a long history of gastroesophageal reflux. They often have significantly reduced LES pressures and may have deranged esophageal body motility. Several conditions can predispose to stricture formation, including scleroderma, Zollinger-Ellison syndrome, ingestion of pills known to cause strictures, and achalasia after myotomy or possibly balloon dilation. Hiatal hernias are associated with strictures. Forty-two percent of reflux patients without endoscopic esophagitis, 63% of those with endoscopic esophagitis, and 85% of those with peptic strictures have hiatal hernias [34]. Strictures can lead to increased risk of food impaction, risk of pulmonary aspiration, and the need for esophageal dilation with the occasional complication of perforation. The disordered body motility experienced by patients with strictures is often very profound and can sometimes occur as complete aperistalsis. More commonly, low-amplitude or failed peristaltic contractions occur. It is unclear whether the peristaltic dysfunction results from esophagitis or reflects a primary motor disorder predisposing to stricture formation. Peptic strictures are found most commonly near the squamocolumnar junction and are usually 1 to 2 cm in length. If longer strictures are found, predisposing conditions such as indwelling nasogastric tubes, pill esophagitis, or Zollinger-Ellison syndrome should be ruled out. Strictures can often be treated successfully with medication and esophageal dilation. Patients who require frequent dilation, have strictures complicated by bleeding or ulceration, or have continued reflux symptoms despite medical therapy should be considered as surgical candidates. We found that the need for dilation was decreased fivefold by surgery and pneumonia was abolished [30].

GERD can also cause several atypical symptoms, which improve with control of reflux. These include chronic cough, reflux-induced asthma, atypical chest pain, recurrent pneu-

**Surgical Goals**

1. Increase resting LES pressure
2. Replace the LES intraabdominally
3. Lengthen the intraabdominal LES
4. Accentuate the angle of His
5. Reduction of hiatal hernia
6. Accelerate gastric emptying

**FIG. 31–2.** Goals of antireflux surgery.

monias, and laryngeal dysfunction. One-third of patients with reflux-induced pulmonary symptoms do not have typical reflux symptoms. Results of antireflux surgery for these conditions are quite variable, and careful evaluation to prove GERD preoperatively, including 24-hour pH monitoring and esophageal manometry, are extremely important.

Reflux disease is quite common in children and can usually be controlled medically. Surgery is again considered only for those experiencing complications of GERD, including stricture, failure to thrive, anemia, and aspiration pneumonia. Esophageal pH monitoring may be normal in infancy as gastric acid production does not reach adult levels until 6 months of age.

## HOW DOES SURGERY PREVENT REFLUX?

Fundoplication causes a rise in LES resting pressure from below 6 mm Hg before surgery to 14 mm Hg, after surgery [22]. There are, however, other important mechanisms responsible for preventing reflux (Fig. 31–2). These involve reduction of the hiatal hernia which replaces the LES in the abdomen and allows it to function better in the positive-pressure abdominal environment with crucal support. The latter also serves to hold the lower esophagus in the abdomen. Other mechanisms are lengthening of the intra-abdominal component of the LES and accentuation of the angle of His with formation of a mucosal rosette at the cardia. Reduction of the volume of the fundus used in the fundoplication results in speeding of gastric emptying [24]. As the stomach fills after a meal, filling of the wrap clasping the lower esophagus prevents shortening and widening of the LES.

## PREOPERATIVE EVALUATION

Meticulous evaluation of the patient preoperatively is the first and most important step in performing antireflux surgery (Fig. 31–3). Performing inappropriate antireflux surgery can have disastrous results. A careful history will elicit the typical symptoms of reflux, as well as atypical symptoms which may require further clinical correlation. Patients with a classic history and those with an atypical presentation should be subjected to clinical testing to confirm the diagnosis and to exclude other causes of their symptoms.

Esophageal manometry is essential because it assesses not only the pressure of the LES but also the esophageal body motility. Manometry can assess the location of the LES, its resting pressure, its ability to relax, its overall length, as well as the length of its intrathoracic and intra-abdominal components. It is important that the LES pressure is measured at the respiratory inversion point, which identifies the junction between the positive abdominal pressure and the negative thoracic pressure with inspiration. This position has been found to be best to avoid interference by either pressure environment. Manometry can also identify the double-hump phenomenon, which is seen in patients with large hiatal hernias. This consists of a distal high-pressure area due to crural pressure and a more proximal LES high-pressure zone. It is also important to establish parameters of esophageal body motility as patients with poor body motility may require a looser wrap at the time of antireflux surgery, to prevent severe and possibly permanent dysphagia after surgery [33]. Deficient body motility is defined as having a mean amplitude of less than 30 mm Hg in response to wet swallows or more than 40% interrupted or simultaneous waves.

Esophagogastroduodenoscopy with biopsies is important in evaluating patients with GERD. This will establish the grade of esophagitis as well as aid in identifying esophageal diverticula, the size of hiatal hernia, strictures, and Barrett's esophagus. Biopsies should be taken to exclude severe dysplasia or malignancy.

Twenty-four-hour esophageal pH testing is useful to confirm the presence of acid reflux. Patients should be tested off of their current therapy, and this requires stopping PPI medication for at least 7 days and histamine blockers for 48 hours prior to the test to ensure that any drug effect is no longer present. Exposure to pH less than 4 for longer than 5% of the time and a positive reflux score are suggestive of abnormal acid exposure. The score is calculated based on the percent of time that the distal esophagus is exposed to pH less than 4 over the total time in the upright and the supine positions, the number of reflux episodes with pH less than 4, the number of episodes lasting longer than 5 minutes, and the length of the longest episode.

A barium esophagram is important to help establish the morphology of the distal esophagus and to rule out malignancy, strictures, and motility disturbances. Hiatal hernia and shortened esophagus can also be identified preoperatively, which may alter the surgical approach.

Evaluation of gastric emptying is sometimes assessed pre-

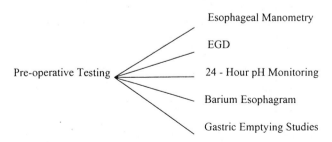

**FIG. 31–3.** Summary suggested preoperative testing.

operatively. Antireflux surgery has been shown to speed gastric emptying and will usually improve delayed emptying, which may be present in some patients preoperatively.

Important conditions to rule out using the above tests are achalasia, scleroderma, and other disorders of the esophageal body, including nutcracker esophagus and diffuse esophageal spasm.

## SURGICAL OPTIONS

Surgery for GERD has been performed since 1956 but has recently undergone a dramatic resurgence of interest with the advent of the option of performing the procedures with laparoscopic techniques. The most popular procedures are the 360-degree Nissen fundoplication, the 270-degree partial Toupet fundoplication, the Hill repair, and the Belsey Mark IV repair. Esophageal lengthening can be achieved using the Collis procedure. The laparoscopic approach offers the advantage of performing antireflux surgery with minimally invasive techniques, which allow for the procedures to be completed either during an overnight stay in the hospital or on an outpatient basis. The laparoscopic approach offers the advantages of decreased pain, a shorter recovery time than is required for most open procedures, and good long-term results. The principle of repair evolved from the Allison repair [2], in which the hiatal hernia was reduced and the esophageal hiatus was narrowed. This procedure did little to restore LES function, and the results were very poor. Nissen fundoplication has a 90% success rate at 10 years and has been demonstrated to be an effective procedure against reflux [11]. The original technique, using the anterior and posterior gastric walls for construction of the wrap, was associated with considerable side effects that have encouraged modifications. Subsequently, a technique of fundoplication was developed that relies on wrapping the greater curve of the fundus around the distal esophagus and fixing it to itself [44]. This technique is considered to allow a more precise formation of the fundic wrap.

The laparoscopic Nissen fundoplication is the standard surgical procedure for GERD. We reserve the partial, or Toupet, fundoplication for those with poor body motility, to avoid postoperative dysphagia. We elect to use laparoscopy in almost all suitable candidates, regardless of the weight of the patient or whether there have been previous abdominal operations. If the esophagus is shortened, the laparoscopic technique is not used, and the repair is carried out by the thoracic approach. This is infrequently required. Shortening of the esophagus is suggested by the combination of a fixed hernia measuring more than 5 cm, poor body motility, severe esophagitis, and deep fibrosis (Fig. 31–4) [43].

## TECHNIQUE OF LAPAROSCOPIC NISSEN FUNDOPLICATION

The patient is positioned in steep reverse Trendelenburg. After establishing the pneumoperitoneum, 10-mm trocars

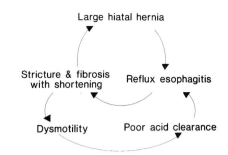

**FIG. 31–4.** Interrelationship of reflux esophagitis, poor acid clearance, dysmotility, stricturing, fibrosis, and hiatal hernia in producing the short esophagus. (From ref. 43, with permission.)

are introduced into the abdominal cavity (Fig. 31–5). To obtain access to the hiatus, the left lobe of the liver is retracted with a liver retractor. Division of the triangular ligament is not recommended because the left liver lobe would drop into the operative field of view.

The next step of the operation is the division of the gastrohepatic omentum superior to the hepatic branches of the

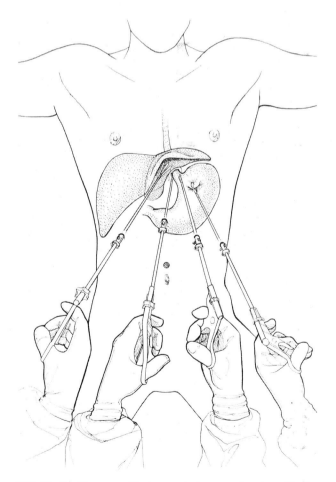

**FIG. 31–5.** Trocar and instrument placement and positioning for laparoscopic Nissen fundoplication. (From *Current techniques in general surgery*. With permission from Miles, Inc., Pharmaceutical Division.)

vagus nerve. These can be seen passing through the omentum in thin patients. Damage to the left gastric artery or an aberrant hepatic artery must be avoided. This is seen in 8% of patients. The anterior edge of the right crus can then be seen and dissected off the right-hand side and front of the esophagus. This should be performed carefully to avoid damage to the esophagus and to fairly large blood vessels in this area. Once the esophagus is identified, the posterior trunk of the vagus nerve can easily be separated from the esophagus. The anterior vagus nerve should be visualized and is usually located within the smooth muscle of the anterior distal esophagus.

Dissection of the crura is continued to establish the point where the left and right crura join anterior to the esophagus. The anterior part of the left crus can usually be separated from the esophagus without difficulty. The posterior portion of the left crus should be mobilized off the left side of the esophagus. To create a window behind the esophagus, it is necessary to elevate the esophagus from its right-hand side and to separate loose tissue behind the esophagus. Dissection too far superiorly should be avoided because it may result in damage to the left pleura. Dissection too far inferiorly may result in muscle fibers of the esophagus or stomach being misidentified as crural fibers, resulting in perforation of these organs. Once this window is established, the crura are approximated behind the esophagus as in the open procedure, with nonabsorbable sutures placed in the crura behind the esophagus (Fig. 31–6). The operation is continued with mobilization of the greater curvature in preparation for the fundoplication. The short gastric vessels can be transected using metallic clips or the harmonic scalpel. The mobilized

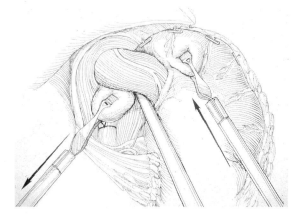

**FIG. 31–7.** The fundus of the stomach being brought around behind the esophagus to form the wrap. (From *Current techniques in general surgery*. With permission from Miles, Inc., Pharmaceutical Division.)

fundus is grasped with a Babcock tissue forceps at a point about 5 to 6 cm from the angle of His measured along the greater curvature and brought behind the esophagus (Fig. 31–7). This is fixed around the esophagus to a more distal part of the fundus so that they snugly approximate. Tightness of the wrap can be assessed by passing a 56F to 60F Maloney bougie into the esophageal lumen. We use visual assessment and no longer use the bougie due to the high incidence of perforation which can occur with its use. For approximation of the left and right fundal wrap around the esophagus, a U-shaped 2-0 Prolene suture is used. This suture also includes the muscle wall of the esophagus to hold the wrap in place and to prevent the stomach from slipping up through the fundoplication. The suture is buttressed using two Teflon felt pledgets, one on each side of the fundic wrap (Fig. 31–8). A second simple suture of silk may be added either above or below this to snug the fundoplication to the desired tension around the esophagus. The wrap is made no longer than 2 cm since any wrap longer than this results in a greater incidence of postoperative dysphagia [10].

There are four essential components of the operation (Fig. 31–9). First, the wrap should be loose. This is achieved by carefully choosing the part of the fundus to be used in the wrap. Furthermore, the wrap should be no longer than 2 cm, to ensure a postoperative dysphagia rate of less than 3%. Second, the gastric fundus must be completely mobilized, to avoid torsion of the esophagus, tension of the wrap, or inclusion of gastric corpus in the wrap, which may lead to incomplete swallowing-induced relaxations of the sphincter with delayed esophageal clearance function [10]. The same effect may occur if a distal portion of the stomach is chosen for the construction of the fundoplication. The ideal point is about 5 to 6 cm distal to the angle of His, measured along the greater curvature. Third, the gastric fundus must be wrapped around the esophagus and not around the upper stomach. This would result in dysphagia and failure to con-

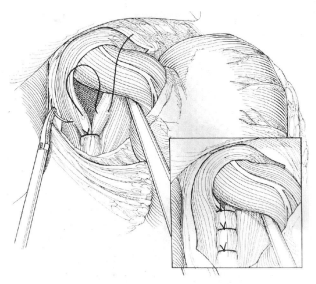

**FIG. 31–6.** Approximation of the crura during laparoscopic Nissen fundoplication. (From *Current techniques in general surgery*. With permission from Miles, Inc., Pharmaceutical Division.)

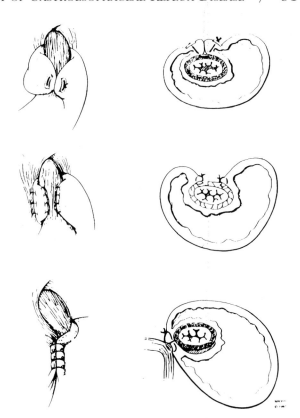

**FIG. 31–10.** Appearance and cross-sectional views of the Nissen fundoplication **(top)**, the Toupet fundoplication **(middle)**, and the Hill repair **(bottom).**

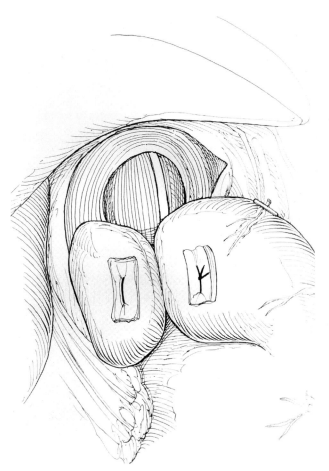

**FIG. 31–8.** The completed laparoscopic Nissen fundoplication. (From *Current techniques in general surgery*. With permission from Miles, Inc., Pharmaceutical Division.)

trol reflux. Finally, the crural repair is important because it helps to hold the fundoplication in the abdomen. Because the diaphragmatic crura are also part of the barrier against reflux, the approximation of the crura supports the effect of the fundal wrap, especially under straining conditions.

## TECHNIQUE OF THE LAPAROSCOPIC TOUPET FUNDOPLICATION

The Toupet fundoplication, which is a 180- to 270-degree wrap, is usually used in patients who are demonstrated to have poor esophageal body motility as these patients are at greater risk for postoperative dysphagia if a complete 360-

1. Loose wrap which is no longer than 2 cm.
2. Complete mobilization of the gastric fungus.
3. Placement of the wrap around the esophagus and not around the upper stomach.
4. Crural repair.

**FIG. 31–9.** Essential components of the proper laparoscopic Nissen fundoplication.

degree fundoplication is performed. (Fig. 31–10). Ineffective esophageal peristalsis is a complication of longstanding gastroesophageal reflux. Others routinely use a partial fundoplication, but the rise in LES pressure is less than after a Nissen fundoplication and reflux control is less. The Toupet fundoplication is performed in a similar manner to the laparoscopic Nissen fundoplication, with the patient in a similar position and using the same placement of five 10-mm trocars. After the pneumoperitoneum is established, division of the gastrohepatic ligament, dissection of the esophagus and hiatal crura, and establishment of a window behind the esophagus are performed as described above for the Nissen procedure. The hiatal hernia, if present, is reduced and the hiatal crura are loosely approximated behind the esophagus using nonabsorbable sutures. The short gastric vessels can be divided within 15 cm of the angle of His along the greater curvature of the stomach. A Babcock grasper is then passed from the right side through the window behind the esophagus, and the gastric fundus is grasped near the short gastric vessels and advanced behind the esophagus, leaving the posterior vagus nerve outside of the fundic wrap. The right side of the wrap is first sutured to the adjacent right crus using three interrupted 2-0 silk sutures and then to the right side of the abdominal esophagus with another three silk sutures. The left limb of the wrap is then sutured to the left side of the abdominal esophagus using three 2-0 silk sutures. A segment of approximately 90 degrees of the anterior esophagus is not covered by the wrap. Suturing is performed using intracorporeal knot tying with two needle holders.

The Dor anterior hemifundoplication can also be performed laparoscopically. This procedure is an anterior hemifundoplication which is performed by suturing the anterior wall of the gastric fundus to the right crus of the diaphragm with interrupted stitches. This procedure is not as effective as a posterior fundoplication and is not generally recommended.

## TECHNIQUE OF HILL REPAIR

This is performed in a similar way to the open Hill repair, which is described below.

## COMPLICATIONS OF LAPAROSCOPIC ANTIREFLUX PROCEDURES

Operative complications consist of perforation, bleeding, pneumothorax, and splenectomy. Perforations occur in about 1% of cases and can be either esophageal or gastric. Perforations do not always require conversion to an open procedure, and if successfully repaired, do not lead to further problems. However, if a perforation occurs, and it is not discovered at operation, the mortality is high. Significant bleeding is uncommon; very few patients require conversion to an open procedure, and even fewer require blood transfusion. Pneumothorax is uncommon and usually does not require chest tube placement as there is rarely any direct parenchymal lung damage but only compromise of the parietal pleura. Splenectomy is much less common with the laparoscopic technique (0.1%) than with the open procedure (3%).

## LATE SEQUELAE AFTER ANTIREFLUX SURGERY

Wound complications are rare after laparoscopic surgery. Delayed perforation of the stomach or esophagus as a result of ischemia or unrecognized iatrogenic injury can occur and usually presents 7 to 10 days after surgery. Postoperative fever and elevated white blood cell counts can be early signs of perforation.

## POSTOPERATIVE MANAGEMENT AFTER LAPAROSCOPIC ANTIREFLUX SURGERY

Patients leave the operating room with no nasogastric tube in place and are allowed clear liquids after the anesthetic has worn off and they can safely swallow. Antireflux medications are discontinued. A meglumine diatrizoate (Gastrografin) videoesophagram is performed only if there is concern prior to allowing the patient to commence a liquid diet. The following morning, the patient is advanced to a pureed diet. He or she ambulates immediately and usually requires only a few doses of intramuscular analgesic injections,

which is then changed to an oral analgesic elixir. The majority of patients are discharged on the first postoperative day. Some young, nonobese patients who have had an uneventful operation may elect to go home on the same day as surgery. If there is any difficulty in advancing the diet or with swallowing, a meglumine diatrizoate swallow can be obtained for clarification. Patients remain on a soft diet for approximately 3 to 4 weeks and are gradually allowed to resume a normal diet by the sixth week.

## OPEN ABDOMINAL APPROACHES

The transabdominal approach for a Nissen fundoplication is through an upper midline laparotomy with exposure of the esophageal hiatus. The gastrohepatic ligament is divided. Care should be taken to avoid damaging the hepatic branches of the vagus nerve, an aberrant left hepatic artery, or the left gastric artery. The incision of the gastrohepatic ligament is then continued over the anterior surface of the esophagus, with division of the parietal peritoneum over the esophagus. The fat pad that usually covers the anterior surface of the cardia and esophagus is removed. Special care must be taken because this tissue contains large blood vessels and the anterior trunk of the vagus nerve, which is adherent to the esophagus. Bleeding in this area leads to poor visualization and difficulty in the identification of anatomic structures. After blunt finger dissection behind the esophagus, the posterior trunk of the vagus is identified, and a sling is passed around the esophagus, excluding the posterior nerve. Retraction on the sling opens the space behind the esophagus, allowing identification of the right and left crura of the esophageal hiatus.

The next step is to mobilize the gastric fundus. Short gastric vessels are divided, starting at a point about 10 cm aboral from the angle of His. It is important to the success of the operation that the gastric fundus is completely mobilized, to allow a tension-free fundoplication around the esophagus without including the gastric corpus. Blood vessels passing from the greater curvature of the stomach to the retroperitoneum should also be divided. These are found mainly on the most superior part of the greater curvature. It is then possible to proceed with the repair. The first step is to approximate the crura using nonabsorbable sutures, followed by the fundoplication. This is established in the same manner as in the laparoscopic method.

The Hill repair depends on fixing the LES in the abdomen and on creating an angulation in the lower esophagus to prevent reflux (Fig. 31–10). Through an upper midline abdominal incision, the liver is retracted in the same way as described for the abdominal approach to the Nissen fundoplication. The gastrohepatic ligament is divided, preserving the hepatic branches of the vagus nerve. The dissection is continued over the anterior surface of the esophagus. The loose fat pad anterior to the esophagus is dissected, taking care not to damage the anterior trunk of the vagus nerve. The right and left diaphragmatic crura are prepared as described for the Nissen procedure. The crura are dissected posteriorly to the point where they decussate over the aorta, and the preaortic fascia is identified and defined. The gastric fundus is mobilized along the greater curve in the same way as for the Nissen fundoplication. After identification of the posterior trunk of the vagus nerve, the esophagus is rotated clockwise when viewed from the abdomen, and both the anterior and posterior bundles of the phrenoesophageal ligament are visualized. The first step of the repair is, as in all other procedures, approximation of the crura. Five sutures are then placed through the anterior and posterior bundles of the phrenoesophageal ligament so that it is plicated at the right-hand side of the esophagus. These sutures also pass through the preaortic fascia. To do this safely, a finger has to be inserted into the hiatus beneath the preaortic fascia. The sutures may be buttressed using Teflon pledgets. These sutures can be tied over a 56F to 60F bougie in the esophagus or, as Hill originally described, by manometric control [20]. Hill ties the upper three sutures with a single throw and measures the sphincter resting pressure, which should be in the range of 35 to 45 mm Hg. If this pressure level is obtained, all sutures are tied completely.

## THORACIC APPROACHES

A transthoracic approach to the Nissen fundoplication can be used. The usual indication for proceeding in this manner is some reason for not operating in the abdomen, such as multiple previous operations or a shortened esophagus. To allow placement of the fundoplication below the diaphragm without tension, maximal mobilization of the esophagus is required. This can best be achieved by the thoracic approach. In addition, it allows for a Collis gastroplasty to be used to gain extra length of the esophagus if the esophagus is still too short after extended mobilization [38]. In patients with a slipped fundoplication located in the chest, the thoracic approach allows for safe dissection, and if necessary, a circumferential incision in the diaphragm can be made, allowing simultaneous dissection from the abdominal side of the diaphragm. Patients with concomitant esophageal spasm or vigorous achalasia who require a long myotomy are best treated using the thoracic approach, as are patients with undefined pulmonary pathology on the left side, which requires operative evaluation.

After a posterolateral left-sided thoracotomy in the sixth intercostal space, mobilization of the esophagus is commenced from the diaphragm up to the aortic arch. In the presence of a previous hiatal hernia repair, thoracotomy can be performed in the seventh intercostal space, which allows for better access to the abdomen through a circumferential incision in the diaphragm. The diaphragmatic incision is made about 3 cm from the chest wall and is about 10 to 15 cm in length. After extensive esophageal mobilization, the hernial sac can be dissected off the diaphragm. This can be achieved through the hiatus or through the circumferential diaphragmatic incision. Care has to be taken not to damage

the thoracic duct or the trunks of the vagus nerve. After division of all attachments, the gastric fundus is pulled into the chest. A few short gastric vessels must be divided. The fat pad on the anterior surface of the distal esophagus and cardia is dissected, taking care to avoid damage to the anterior trunk of the vagus nerve. The posterior vagal trunk must be identified and dissected off the esophagus. The next step is to place the sutures for the approximation of the diaphragmatic crura. Four to six sutures are usually necessary. They are not tied at this time. The fundoplication is then constructed. The fundus is wrapped around the distal esophagus proximal to the angle of His. The U-shaped suture for the fixation of the wrap is placed by the same technique as in the abdominal procedure, except that it is located more posteriorly. Before placing this suture, a 56F to 60F Maloney bougie is passed through the esophagus and into the stomach by the anesthesiologist. The fundoplication is placed in the abdomen. If the tension on the esophagus is not too great, the fundoplication will remain in the abdominal cavity even when the diaphragm is gently manipulated. The crural sutures can then be tied. If the fundoplication tends to slide back into the chest, the esophagus should be further mobilized, which can be accomplished by division of the branches of the posterior vagal trunk to the left pulmonary plexus. If this maneuver fails, a Collis gastroplasty [38] or colon interposition has to be considered. The Collis gastroplasty is performed to provide extra length to the esophagus and can be completed in a cut or uncut fashion. The uncut procedure is the most popular, performed after a 50F dilator is placed in the esophagus. The fundus is elevated superiorly and a stapler applied to the stomach parallel to the dilator at the angle of His. The staple line creates a 3-cm neoesophagus of stomach. This reduces tension as the repair is made over the stomach rather than the distal esophagus (Fig. 31–11). This is necessary only in rare cases, particularly if the wrap is kept short.

Another thoracic procedure to control reflux is the Belsey Mark IV operation, which is quite similar to the transthoracic Nissen fundoplication. The thoracotomy is performed at the same site, and the mobilization of the esophagus is done in the same way. After mobilization of the esophagus, starting from the diaphragm and extending up to the aortic arch, the hernial sac is freed from all its attachments. The posterior trunk of the vagus nerve is protected, and the gastric fundus is pulled into the chest. A few short gastric vessels must be divided. The sutures for approximation of the diaphragmatic crura are placed as described earlier. The fundus is rolled anteriorly onto the esophagus. In this case, the fundus lies at a 90-degree angle to the fundoplication achieved in the transthoracic Nissen fundoplication and comes to lie only around the anterior two-thirds of the distal esophagus. The fundus is fixed to the esophagus with two rows of three nonabsorbable, U-shaped sutures each. The first row is placed about 1.5 cm above the gastroesophageal junction. The sutures grasp the esophageal muscle but do not traverse the entire wall. One of these sutures is placed on the anterior

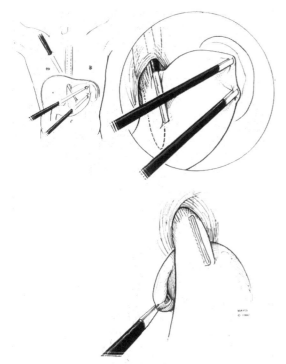

**FIG. 31–11.** The Collis gastroplasty with creation of a neo-esophagus to add esophageal length in the event of a shortened esophagus.

side of the esophagus, the other two on the right and left sides. To place the suture on the right side, the esophagus has to be rotated. It is important that this suture is not placed too far anteriorly, which would result only in an anterolateral fundoplication of lower efficiency. The second row of U-shaped sutures is placed 1 or 2 cm above the first row, and these are carefully tied without strangulating the tissue. The tails of the sutures are not cut off as they are passed through the diaphragm from the abdominal to the thoracic surface about 1.5 cm apart into the edge of the hiatus. These sutures are placed at the 4-, 8-, and 12-o'clock positions. It is important to place the 4-o'clock suture posteriorly so as to avoid the creation of an anterolateral fundoplication. The fundoplication is placed into the abdomen, where it should remain if the esophagus has been correctly mobilized, as described earlier. The three diaphragmatic sutures are tied so that there is close apposition between the fundoplication and the diaphragm. Finally, the crural sutures are tied.

## BILE DIVERSION PROCEDURES

The other type of reflux, which presents occasionally, is duodenogastric reflux, which occurs when duodenal content refluxes into the stomach and, if a defective LES is present, into the esophagus. In the presence of normal gastric acid secretion and normal gastric emptying, these contents are neutralized, diluted, and cleared from the stomach. If the volume of reflux is excessive, gastric acid secretion is diminished, or gastric emptying is delayed, the ability of the stomach to deal with the noxious reflux is exceeded, and esopha-

geal and gastric mucosal injury can occur. Bile acids, activated pancreatic enzymes, and lysolecithin have been implicated as the mediators of damage. The entity of primary duodenogastric reflux, which occurs without a prior gastric operation, has been recognized for some time and has been implicated in many conditions, including Barrett esophagus, esophagitis, and malignant disease of the esophagus and stomach [39]. Duodenogastric reflux is very difficult to diagnose. Patients commonly complain of continuous burning epigastric pain, which is worse after meals and at night. The pain is refractory to antacids. History and physical examination are nonspecific, and often elaborate testing is needed to confirm the diagnosis. Testing should include endoscopy and biopsy, foregut pH monitoring, radionuclide scanning studies, and the Bilitec probe (Synectics Medical, Dallas, TX). Endoscopy may reveal a "bile lake," and biopsy may show foveolar hyperplasia, edema and smooth muscle fibers in the lamina propria, vasodilation and congestion of superficial mucosal capillaries, and a paucity of acute and chronic inflammatory cells. Gastric pH monitoring should be performed 5 cm below the LES, and measurement of the percent of time pH is greater than 3 during fasting periods can differentiate between physiologic and pathologic duodenogastric reflux. A useful test is the measurement of $^{99}$Tc hepatic 2,6-dimethyliminodiacetic acid (HIDA) in the gastric region following its intravenous injection and excretion into the bile. The radionuclide is almost entirely excreted in the bile, allowing for detection of bile reflux. The stomach can be scanned with a gamma camera, and reflux can be detected on serial scans. Gastric aspiration for the measurement of bile acids and pancreatic enzymes has been investigated, but the short duration of these test may be inadequate for detecting significant duodenogastric reflux since this is an intermittent event. A newer option is to measure spectrophotometrically the intraluminal bilirubin concentration using the Bilitec probe. A portable data logger is connected to a fiberoptic probe that is passed transnasally and positioned 5 cm proximal to the LES. The light source is provided by two light-emitting diodes that emit a 460-nm signal light and a 565-nm reference light. The specific wavelength of absorption for bilirubin is 453 nm and is highly reproducible [27].

The management of duodenogastric reflux is very difficult. Multiple forms of drug therapy have been tried, including cholestyramine, aluminum hydroxide-containing antacids, metoclopramide, domperidone, and cisapride. Mucosal protectants such as sucralfate have also been used; all have had little success. A trial of medical therapy is recommended for several months before resorting to surgery.

Bile diversion surgery has been used for treating alkaline gastritis, failed fundoplication with proven duodenogastric reflux, and most recently Barrett's esophagus, with the hope of reversing dysplasia and preventing adenocarcinoma formation. This may take the form of the classic Roux-en-Y or the duodenal switch (Fig. 31–12) [52]. Csendes and co-workers [9] have described a three-armed attack on acid

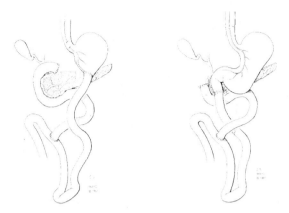

**FIG. 31–12.** The classic Roux-en-Y procedure with partial gastrectomy and vagotomy **(left)** and the duodenal switch **(right)**.

reflux and bile reflux for patients with Barrett's esophagus by combining highly selective vagotomy, an antireflux procedure, and the duodenal switch procedure. They describe clinical improvement as well as disappearance of dysplastic changes in almost 50% of patients. In order to support the widespread application of this procedure, further evidence needs to be collected to ascertain whether current antireflux procedures applied to Barrett's patients are inadequate to prevent further progression of Barrett's esophagus. These data are currently lacking.

## SURGERY FOR PARAESOPHAGEAL HERNIAS

Hiatal hernias occur in approximately 10% of the North American population (Fig. 31–13) [14]. Sliding, or type I, hernias are seven times more common than paraesophageal hernias. Pure paraesophageal, or type II, hernias exist when

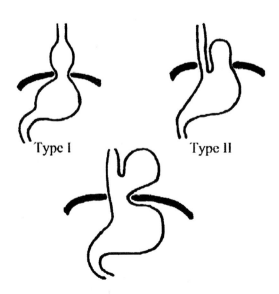

**FIG. 31–13.** Types of hiatal hernia.

the gastric fundus herniates alongside the esophagus into the thorax while the gastroesophageal junction remains in its normal anatomic location. This type is rarely seen. A type II hernia associated with translocation of the LES into the chest is also generally referred to as a paraesophageal hernia. These are called type III, or mixed, hernias. Of the 15% of all hiatal hernias that are paraesophageal, greater than 86% are considered to be type III. For a paraesophageal hernia to occur, the stomach obtains enough mobility to rotate through the diaphragmatic defect. In order for this to occur, there must be some laxity in the gastrocolic and gastrosplenic ligaments which normally secure the stomach in the abdomen [35]. Depending on the relative weakness of these ligaments, two types of volvulus of the stomach may develop. An organoaxial volvulus occurs with movement of the greater curvature of the stomach anterior to the lesser curvature. This results in rotation along its longitudinal axis. The mesentericoaxial volvulus is less common and occurs when the stomach rotates along its transverse axis.

The most common symptoms are regurgitation, heartburn, and dysphagia; but symptoms can vary greatly from this classic triad. Other common symptoms include chest pain, pulmonary problems, nausea, vomiting, bleeding, early satiety, and gastric volvulus. The incidence of iron deficiency anemia has been reported to be as high as 38% [1, 31, 35, 48, 51]. Often, there is no direct evidence of gastrointestinal bleeding. Venous obstruction at the hiatus caused by an incarcerated hernia may result in venous dilation, engorgement, and chronic oozing, which can lead to chronic anemia. Gastric ulcers at the point of constriction of the hernia at the hiatus are termed *Cameron's ulcers.* These ulcers may bleed and lead to chronic anemia. Up to 20% of patients may present as a surgical emergency [50]. Strangulation or perforation can occur, leading to sepsis and shock. Mortality in this situation may be as high as 50% [19]. A contributing factor to the mortality rate is the high incidence of comorbidities in this elderly patient population. This is the reason why elective surgery has previously been recommended in all patients with a paraesophageal hernia.

Diagnosis can be made on upright chest x-ray, esophagram, endoscopy, and manometry. The latter may be difficult to perform because the catheter may not easily advance into the stomach. Esophageal body motility can still be assessed. At least 50% of patients with a paraesophageal hernia have a hypotensive LES [41]. Short intra-abdominal length of the LES may further potentiate reflux [50]. Defective body motility can result in delayed clearance of refluxed acid. These findings lend support to performing an antireflux procedure when repairing the paraesophageal hernia.

Most paraesophageal hernias can be surgically corrected using a laparoscopic approach. Prior to the advent of laparoscopy, paraesophageal hernias were repaired using open techniques. The surgery was performed via either a thoracotomy or a large abdominal incision and was associated with a higher morbidity. Advantages of the laparoscopic technique include smaller incisions, minimal blood loss, and less third spacing of fluid. Recovery is quick, the hospital stay is short, return to normal activities is fast, and patients are satisfied with the cosmetic result. Excellent results and low morbidity and mortality of the laparoscopic approach allow older, more debilitated patients, who could not tolerate open thoracotomy or laparotomy, to have a repair.

When a paraesophageal hernia should be repaired has long been controversial. Some feel that elective surgery is indicated because the low mortality of the elective approach far outweighs the mortality of emergency surgery. In comparison to elective surgery, emergencies result in a 19% mortality [42]. More recent evidence has shown that asymptomatic patients have little risk of complication and that surgery should be recommended for symptomatic patients, with close clinical follow-up of asymptomatic patients [41].

Options for surgical repair are many, ranging from simple repair of the defect to repair of the defect and an antireflux procedure to repairs with gastrostomy or gastropexy. We currently recommend laparoscopic repair of the defect and an antireflux procedure. The technique is very similar to that of the laparoscopic Nissen procedure. Port placement is the same, and division of the gastrohepatic ligament is the first step. Beginning from the inferior, posterior pole of the right crus and working in an anterior direction, the sac is dissected off the right crural edge, followed by clearance of the anterior left crural edge. The entire sac is bluntly peeled from the mediastinal structures into the abdomen using gentle traction with graspers. Surgical emphysema commonly occurs secondary to tracking of air through the mediastinum and into the neck. This is of minimal concern and always resolves. The sac is not excised and is left attached to the front of the stomach because large blood vessels and the vagus nerve may be damaged. Reduction of the sac is necessary to prevent hernia recurrence. Leaving the sac in the chest may also lead to seroma formation. The esophagus must be adequately mobilized in order to facilitate the crural repair. A window behind the esophagus is then created, as described for the Nissen procedure. In patients with paraesophageal hernia, there is almost always great laxity in the gastrosplenic ligament, giving the fundus adequate length for the fundoplication. If the area seems tight, some of the short gastric vessels may need to be divided. Fundoplication is then performed in the usual manner. The fundoplication is tacked to the diaphragm on either side to prevent slippage into the chest.

Recovery is much the same as for a laparoscopic Nissen fundoplication. Similar diet and activity restrictions are instituted, and most patients are released from the hospital the day after surgery.

In our series of 64 patients who had laparoscopic repair of a paraesophageal hernia, two required conversion to an open procedure [41]. Bleeding and pleural entry with a pneumothorax may occur. Vagal injury has been rarely reported. Early reoperation was necessary in 5% of our patients. A slipped Nissen, a small bowel obstruction with wrap disruption, and gastric volvulus were the reasons for reoperation.

The most common early symptom after antireflux surgery is dysphagia, which occurs in 20% of patients according to a review by Perdikis et al. [41]. This decreases to 5.5% in patients who are followed for 6 months after surgery. Other common findings are early satiety (49%), abdominal bloating (36%), diarrhea (20%), nausea (8%), and recurrent reflux symptoms (8%). Approximately 31% of patients are unable to vomit after surgery.

Persistent dysphagia can be successfully treated with dilation in most patients. If persistent symptoms occur, consideration must be given to failure of the wrap due to breakdown, herniation, or if too tight or too loose construction. Evaluation and treatment of these conditions requiring redo surgery are addressed below.

Paraesophageal herniation of the stomach is a rare complication following laparoscopic Nissen fundoplication. In our experience of 760 laparoscopic Nissen fundoplications, seven patients (0.9%) were found to have postoperative paraesophageal hernias requiring reoperation. Early dysphagia after surgery should alert the surgeon to this complication. The correct diagnosis could be confirmed in only four of the seven patients by barium esophagram. Four patients underwent successful laparoscopic repair, two patients required thoracotomy, and one patient had a laparotomy to reduce an intrathoracic gastric volvulus.

## LONG-TERM RESULTS OF ANTIREFLUX SURGERY

When asked how satisfied patients were with their decision to have surgery, satisfaction rates were 87% to 100%. The results of antireflux surgery are good, with a failure rate of approximately 1% per year; 3.2% of patients had recurrent reflux after 3 years and 10% at 10 years. Two-thirds can be controlled on medication and one-third require redo surgery with open or laparoscopic techniques.

## WHO SHOULD DO LAPAROSCOPIC ANTIREFLUX SURGERY?

Laparoscopic antireflux surgery is technically challenging and requires surgeons to be proctored for a number of cases before proficiency is attained. Proctoring should be utilized for 10 to 30 cases. It is sensible that each community should have only a few surgeons who concentrate their efforts on this type of surgery, to ensure that patients are offered optimal expertise associated with low-risk surgery. This allows these surgeons to analyze their results by operating on an adequate number of patients. Gastroenterologists will then be allowed to make appropriate management decisions for their patients. In the case of patients being considered for redo antireflux surgery, it is best to seek a surgeon who has had sufficient experience in performing this procedure.

## REDO SURGERY

### Reasons for Failure of the Primary Operation

The reasons for failure of antireflux surgery are multiple and can vary from a fundoplication that is too tight (Fig. 31–14), too loose, incorrectly positioned, or disrupted. Most

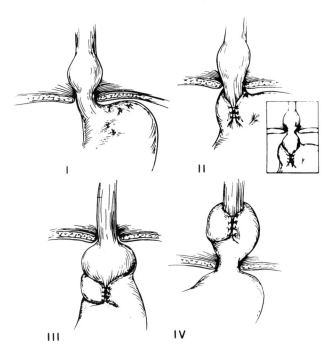

**FIG. 31–14.** Pictorial depiction of surgical failures, types I to IV. (From ref. 3a, with permission.)

descriptions of the failed procedure are classified by their radiologic descriptions. Four types of abnormality exist (Fig. 31–14). Type I represents complete or almost complete disruption of the fundoplication, with recurrence of the hiatal hernia in most cases. This has been called the "missin Nissen." Type II involves slippage of part of the stomach through the fundoplication to lie above the diaphragm. An hourglass defect is created, with part of the stomach above and part below the esophageal hiatus. This is frequently caused by the fundoplication having been incorrectly placed around the upper stomach rather than around the esophagus. Type III is associated with some of the stomach found above the wrap with both the wrap and stomach remaining in the abdomen. This is the so-called slipped Nissen (Fig. 31–15) and may occur as a result of slippage of the stomach through the fundoplication or incorrect placement of the fundoplication around the stomach at the time of surgery. Type IV occurs when the intact fundoplication herniates through the esophageal hiatus into the chest (Fig. 31–14). Other problems include crural disruption with paraesophageal herniation of the stomach into the chest, inadvertent vagotomy, small bowel adhesive obstruction, persistent reflux gastritis, impaired gastric emptying, gas bloat, and problems with an Angelchik prosthesis. Most patients have had a previous open procedure; however, with the increasing number of procedures being performed using the laparoscopic technique, there will be more failed procedures occurring after the laparoscopic technique.

## Evaluation of Symptoms after Surgery

Symptom evaluation after antireflux surgery can be quite complicated. Often, many of the tests which are used to evaluate patients prior to their first procedure can be helpful in eliciting the cause of their postoperative problems. Upper gastrointestinal endoscopy, barium esophagram, esophageal manometry, and 24-hour esophageal pH monitoring are most useful in defining the problem. Gastric acid analysis will indicate if there is excessive gastric acid secretion. In addition, computed tomographic scanning and $^{99}$Tc-HIDA scanning can be of further assistance.

Upper gastrointestinal endoscopy is helpful to evaluate mucosal abnormalities, including esophagitis, gastritis, and mucosal ulceration, as well as to document a residual hiatal hernia or to identify the presence of retained food in the esophagus or stomach. The integrity of the fundoplication can be evaluated. A barium esophagram allows for a functional as well as an anatomic evaluation of the fundoplication. The position of the fundoplication can be assessed, as can the ability and speed with which the barium passes through the fundoplication. The esophagram is also helpful to identify a short esophagus (Plate 51).

Esophageal manometry is essential in evaluating symptomatic patients after fundoplication. Evaluation of the LES pressure can reveal a wrap that is either too tight or too loose. Assessment of body motility can identify motor disturbances such as nutcracker esophagus and diffuse esophageal spasm, which may be the cause of postoperative symptoms and can help to identify misdiagnosed achalasia. Twenty-four-hour pH monitoring can identify the presence of continued reflux after fundoplication and can sometimes suggest the presence of duodenogastric reflux. Often, duodenogastric reflux can best be demonstrated on HIDA scans or by using the Bilitec probe to reveal the presence of bile salts in the esophagus.

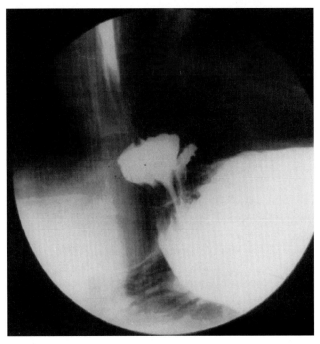

**FIG. 31–15.** The "slipped Nissen" or type III paraesophageal hernia as it appears radiographically.

Gastric emptying studies will determine if gastric emptying is abnormally fast or abnormally slow after surgery. If there is initial rapid emptying of liquids and delayed emptying of solids, the integrity of the vagus nerves needs to be questioned. Confirmation of the completeness of vagotomy can be obtained by measuring the gastric acid response to insulin hypoglycemia or to a sham meal.

### Principles of Redo Surgery

After careful evaluation, a plan for the approach can be made. This may be a simple matter if paraesophageal herniation of the stomach or slippage of the fundoplication has occurred. If a shortened esophagus has been identified, consideration should be given to esophageal lengthening of the Collis type. A Belsy fundoplication is usually added to the lengthening because most patients will have poor body motility and a 360-degree fundoplication would be inappropriate.

The approach may be by laparoscopy, laparotomy, or thoracotomy. Because of scarring, great care must be taken with all of these approaches to avoid perforation of the esophagus or the stomach. Careful identification of the vagus nerves should be undertaken to preserve them intact. This may be quite difficult due to previous scarring and fibrosis. The first step should be to identify the esophageal hiatus and the crura. This is undertaken using the same methods as in first-time antireflux surgery. A relatively well-preserved area in the lower mediastinum can be identified as a starting point, and the esophagus can usually be first isolated here. It is often necessary to take down the previous fundoplication. The greatest risk of perforation occurs at this time. The LES should be placed intra-abdominally, and if this is not possible, consideration should be given to a Collis procedure. In most cases, a partial fundoplication should be undertaken rather than a 360-degree fundoplication, due to the presence of poor esophageal body motility. Occasionally, a Hill repair can be done. The crura should be closed prior to the fundoplication. Careful evaluation using endoscopy at the end of the procedure is the best way to assess for mucosal injury so that the problem can be identified and repaired immediately. Redo antireflux surgery carries a higher mortality than the first procedure. Mortalities of over 10% have been reported, with an average of 2.8% [23].

The success rate of redo surgery is somewhat less than that of primary antireflux surgery. A 79% success rate is quoted by Jamieson and Duranceau [26]. This falls to 66% after a third operation and less than 50% after a fourth operation. Poor outcomes have been shown to be more likely for patients with peptic stricture and poor esophageal body motility.[23] Incorrect choice of technique, inappropriate patient selection, and inexperience of the surgeon are common reasons for failure.

## CONCLUSION

Antireflux surgery is a good alternative to long-term medication in patients with severe reflux disease or in those with complications of their disease. The laparoscopic approach offers patients the advantages of minimally invasive surgery with similar long-term results to open procedures.

## REFERENCES

1. Allen MS, Trastek VF, Deschamps C, Pairolero PC. Intrathoracic stomach. Presentation and results of operation. J Thorac Cardiovasc Surg 1993;105:253
2. Allison PR. Reflux esophagitis, sliding hiatus hernia, and the anatomy of repair. Surg Gynecol Obstet 1951;92:419
3. Attwood SE, DeMeester TR, Bremner CG, Barlow AP, Hinder RA. Alkaline gastroesophageal reflux: implications in the development of complications in Barrett's columnar-lined lower esophagus. Surgery 1989;106:764
4. Biancani P, Barwick K, Selling J, McCallum R. Effects of acute experimental esophagitis on mechanical properties of the lower esophageal sphincter. Gastroenterology 1984;87:8
5. Biancani P, Walsh JH, Behar J. Vasoactive intestinal polypeptide. A neurotransmitter for lower esophageal sphincter relaxation. J Clin Invest 1984;73:963
6. Brand DL, Ylvisaker JT, Gelfand M, Pope CE II. Regression of columnar esophageal (Barrett's) epithelium after anti-reflux surgery. N Engl J Med 1980;302:844
7. Brunner PI, Karmondy AM, Needham CD. Severe peptic oesophagitis. Gut 1969;10:831
8. Champion G, Richter JE, Vaezi MF, Singh S, Alexander R. Duodenogastroesophageal reflux: relationship to pH and importance in Barrett's esophagus. Gastroenterology 1994;107:747
9. Csendes A, Braghetto I, Burdiles P, Diaz JC, Maluenda F, Korn O. A new physiologic approach for the surgical treatment of patients with Barrett's esophagus: technical considerations and results in 65 patients. Ann Surg 1997;226:123
10. DeMeester TR, Bonavina L, Albertucci M. Nissen fundoplication for gastroesophageal reflux disease. Evaluation of primary repair in 100 consecutive patients. Ann Surg 1986;204:9
11. DeMeester TR, Johnson LF, Kent AH. Evaluation of current operations for the prevention of gastroesophageal reflux. Ann Surg 1974;180:511
12. Dent J, Dodds WJ, Sekiguchi T, Hogan WJ, Arndorfer RC. Interdigestive phasic contractions of the human lower esophageal sphincter. Gastroenterology 1983;84:453
13. Dodds WJ, et al. Mechanisms of gastroesophageal reflux in patients with reflux esophagitis. N Engl J Med 1982;307:1547
14. Duranceau A, Jamieson GG. Hiatal hernia and gastroesophageal reflux. In Sabiston DC, Jr, Lyerly HK, eds, Textbook of Surgery: The Biologic Basis of Modern Surgical Practice. Philadelphia: WB Saunders, 1997:767
15. Eastwood GL, Castell DO, Higgs RH. Experimental esophagitis in cats impairs lower esophageal sphincter pressure. Gastroenterology 1975;69:146
16. Goyal RK, McGuigan JE. Is gastrin a major determinant of basal lower esophageal sphincter pressure? A double-blind controlled study using high titer gastrin antiserum. J Clin Invest 1976;57:291
17. Goyal RK, Said SI, Rattan S. Vasoactive intestinal peptides as a possible neurotransmitter of noncholinergic, noradrenergic neurons. Nature 1988;288:378
18. Grossman MI. What is physiological? Gastroenterology 1973;65:994
19. Hill LD. Incarcerated paraesophageal hernia. A surgical emergency. Am J Surg 1973;126:286
20. Hill LD. Intraoperative measurement of lower esophageal sphincter pressure. J Thorac Cardiovasc Surg 1978;75:378
21. Hinder RA. Gastroesophageal reflux disease. In Bell RH, Rikkers LF, Mulholland M, eds, Digestive Tract Surgery: A Text and Atlas. Philadelphia: Lippincott-Raven Publishers, 1996
22. Hinder RA, Filipi CJ, Wetscher G, Neary P, DeMeester TR, Perdikis G. Laparoscopic Nissen fundoplication is an effective treatment for gastroesophageal reflux disease. Ann Surg 1994;220:472
23. Hinder RA, Klingler PJ, Perdikis G, Smith SL. Management of the failed antireflux operation. Surg Clin North Am 1997;77:1083
24. Hinder RA, Stein HJ, Bremner CG, DeMeester TR. Relationship of a satisfactory outcome to normalization of delayed gastric emptying after Nissen fundoplication. Ann Surg 1989;210:458
25. Iascone C, DeMeester TR, Little AG, Skinner DB. Barrett's esophagus.

Functional assessment, proposed pathogenesis, and surgical therapy. Arch Surg 1983;118:543

26. Jamieson GC, Duranceau A. Gastroesophageal Reflux. Philadelphia: WB Saunders, 1988:65

27. Kauer WK, et al. Does duodenal juice reflux into the esophagus of patients with complicated GERD? Evaluation of a fiberoptic sensor for bilirubin. Am J Surg 1995;169:98

28. Kaul BK, et al. The cause of dysphagia in uncomplicated sliding hiatal hernia and its relief by hiatal herniorrhaphy. A roentgenographic, manometric, and clinical study. Ann Surg 1990;211:406

29. Khoury GA, Bolton J. Age: an important factor in Barrett's oesophagus. Ann R Coll Surg Engl 1989;71:50

30. Klingler PJ, et al. Laparoscopic antireflux surgery for treatment of esophageal strictures refractory to medical therapy. Am J Gastroent (in press)

31. Landreneau RJ, Johnson JA, Marshall JB, Hazelrigg SR, Boley TM, Curtis JJ. Clinical spectrum of paraesophageal herniation. Dig Dis Sci 1992;37:537

32. Liebermann-Meffert D, Allgower M, Schmid P, Blum AL. Muscular equivalent of the lower esophageal sphincter. Gastroenterology 1979;76:31

33. Lund R, et al. Laparoscopic Toupet fundoplication for gastroesophageal reflux disease with poor esophageal body motility. J Gastrointest Surg 1997;1:301

34. Marks RD, Richter JE. Peptic strictures of the esophagus. Am J Gastroenterol 1993;88:1160

35. Menguy R. Surgical management of large paraesophageal hernia with complete intrathoracic stomach. World J Surg 1988;12:415

36. Mittal RK, McCallum RW. Characteristics and frequency of transient relaxations of the lower esophageal sphincter in patients with reflux esophagitis. Gastroenterology 1988;95:593

37. Nissen R. Gastropexy and fundoplication in surgical treatment of hiatus hernia. Am J Dig Dis 1961;6:954

38. Pearson FG, Cooer JD, Nelems JM. Gastroplasty and fundoplication in the management of complex reflux problems. J Thorac Cardiovasc Surg 1978;76:665

39. Perdikis G, Hinder RA, Wetscher GJ, Redmond EJ. Duodenogastric reflux and its surgical management. Prog Chir 1994;5:29

40. Perdikis G, et al. Gastroesophageal reflux disease is associated with enteric hormone abnormalities. Am J Surg 1994;167:186

41. Perdikis G, et al. Laparoscopic paraesophageal hernia repair. Arch Surg 1997;132:586

42. Postlewait RW. Hiatal hernia and gastroesophageal reflux. In Postlewait RW, ed, Surgery of the Esophagus. Norwalk CT: Appleton-Century-Crofts, 1986:211

43. Raiser F, et al. Laparoscopic antireflux surgery in complicated gastroesophageal reflux disease. Semin Laparosc Surg 1995;2:46

44. Rossetti M, Hell K. Fundoplication for the treatment of gastroesophageal reflux in hiatal hernia. World J Surg 1977;1:439

45. Sengupta A, Paterson WG, Goyal RK. Atypical localization of myenteric neurons in the opossum lower esophageal sphincter. Am J Anat 1987;180:342

46. Sjogren RW Jr, Johnson LF. Barrett's esophagus: a review. Am J Med 1983;74:313

47. Stein HJ, DeMeester TR, Naspetti R, Jamieson J, Perry RE. Three-dimensional imaging of the lower esophageal sphincter in gastroesophageal reflux disease. Ann Surg 1991;214:374

48. Treacy PJ, Jamieson GG. An approach to the management of paraoesophageal hiatus hernias. Aust N Z J Surg 1987;57:813

49. Vigneri S, et al. A comparison of five maintenance therapies for reflux esophagitis. N Engl J Med 1995;333:1106

50. Walther B, DeMeester TR, Lafontaine E, Courtney JV, Little AG, Skinner DB. Effect of paraesophageal hernia on sphincter function and its implication on surgical therapy. Am J Surg 1984;147:111

51. Wichterman K, Geha AS, Cahow CE, Baue AE. Giant paraesophageal hiatus hernia with intrathoracic stomach and colon: the case for early repair. Surgery 1979;86:497

52. Wilson P, Anselmino M, Hinder RA. The duodenal switch operation for duodenogastric reflux. Probl Gen Surg 1993;10:242

53. Yamashita Y, et al. Neuropeptide release from the isolated, perfused, lower esophageal sphincter region of the rabbit and the effect of vasoactive intestinal peptide on the sphincter. Surgery 1992;112:227

54. Zaninotto G, DeMeester TR, Schwizer W, Johansson KE, Cheng SC. The lower esophageal sphincter in health and disease. Am J Surg 1988;155:104

*The Esophagus*, Third Edition,
edited by D. O. Castell and J. E. Richter.
Published by Lippincott Williams & Wilkins, Philadelphia, 1999.

CHAPTER 32

# Pill-Induced Esophageal Injury

James Walter Kikendall

Medications administered as nonchewable tablets or capsules are intended to pass rapidly through the esophagus and to release their contents in the stomach or more distally. On occasion, these tablets and capsules may lodge in the esophagus and dissolve therein, releasing their undiluted contents directly onto the esophageal mucosa. If the concentrated medication thus released is sufficiently caustic, the esophageal wall may be injured. This process is known as pill-induced esophageal injury [126]. This chapter reviews evidence from 950 cases of pill-induced esophageal injury due to nearly 100 different medications (Tables 32–1 to 32–4).

## CLINICAL PRESENTATION AND DIFFERENTIAL DIAGNOSIS

The typical injured patient has no prior esophageal symptoms but experiences the sudden onset and the progression over 1 to 4 days of retrosternal pain [126]. The pain is almost always exacerbated by swallowing and may be perceived only with swallowing. The pain may remain mild or become so severe as to make swallowing impossible, compromising hydration and alimentation [3, 114, 223, 231]. Symptoms typically resolve in a few days to a few weeks. The sudden onset of odynophagia in a patient taking potentially injurious pills is highly suggestive of pill-induced esophageal injury, the principal differential being infectious esophagitis.

Many patients relate that the tablet or capsule seemed to stick in the esophagus prior to the onset of symptoms. Others admit that they have taken their pills with little or no water. Those patients who have been awakened from sleep by pain may relate that they took their pills immediately prior to going to bed. Many injured patients, however, have taken

their pills entirely properly, and the absence of these predisposing features does not constitute evidence against the diagnosis of pill-induced esophageal injury.

Sometimes symptoms are less clearly defined. A burning quality to the pain may result in confusion with gastroesophageal reflux disease (GERD). Constant pain may suggest a myocardial infarction [12, 84, 158]. Slowly progressive painless dysphagia is uncommon but has been observed, particularly with injury due to quinidine or potassium chloride pills, and may suggest neoplasia. Hemorrhage is unusual, but pill-induced ulcers have indeed penetrated the left atrium and major vessels [56, 98, 156, 227]. Mediastinitis and free esophageal perforation have complicated injuries due to an aspirin–caffeine compound pill [51], sustained-release ferrous sulfate [213], and sustained-release sodium valproate [247].

## DIAGNOSIS, PATHOLOGY, AND COMPLICATIONS

When a patient states that a swallowed pill had become lodged in the chest prior to the onset of rapidly progressive retrosternal pain clearly exacerbated by swallowing, the diagnosis of pill-induced esophagitis is apparent. Such a patient will usually require no diagnostic evaluation other than a history and physical to rule out predisposing factors or complications and to permit the planning of appropriate alternatives to the implicated oral medication.

Endoscopy is indicated when symptoms are gradual rather than acute in onset, atypical, or inordinately persistent, or when the relationship of symptoms to a previously reported potentially injurious pill is unclear. Endoscopy is also indicated in immunocompromised patients or in patients with hemorrhage.

Endoscopy is more sensitive than barium esophagography for subtle pill-induced esophageal lesions. With its biopsy capability, endoscopy is also more likely to provide a definitive alternative diagnosis such as infectious esophagitis, cancer, or GERD. The only apparent advantages of esophagog-

The opinions and assertions contained herein are the personal views of the author and are not to be construed as reflecting the views of the U.S. Department of the Army or Department of Defense. This work was written by a government employee using government resources.

J. W. Kikendall: Gastroenterology Service, Walter Reed Army Medical Center, Washington, D.C. 20307-5001.

raphy over endoscopy are its lower initial cost and its higher sensitivity for extrinsic compression which might lead to a recurrence of injury if undetected. The higher diagnostic yield of endoscopy will make it the most cost-effective procedure if diagnostic testing is reserved for difficult cases as suggested above.

The typical endoscopic appearance of pill-induced esophageal injury is one or more discrete ulcers with normal surrounding mucosa [126]. Discrete ulcers range from pinpoint to several centimeters in size. At times, diffuse inflammation is observed either without ulceration or surrounding the ulcer(s). Remnants of the offending pill may occasionally be identified [2, 28, 51, 105, 146, 179, 209]. Biopsies reveal acute inflammation without evidence for infection or neoplasia.

In contrast to this typical pattern of injury, tenacious exudate and nodularity may be so profuse that neoplasia is suggested, either at endoscopy or on barium swallow [126, 202, 213, 232, 246]. Such inflammatory pseudotumors have been observed in patients injured by sustained-release quinidine [126, 232, 246], sustained-release ferrous sulfate [213], and sustained-release naproxen [202]. Even such flamboyant inflammatory stenoses tend to resolve spontaneously if the offending pill is withdrawn. More ominously, large circumferential ulcers or repetitive injuries may lead to fibrotic strictures requiring dilatation or surgery.

Any area of the esophagus may be injured [126]. The most common site of injury is the junction of the proximal and middle thirds of the esophagus where peristaltic amplitude is relatively low and where the esophagus may be compressed by the aortic arch which passes anteriorly. Patients with left atrial enlargement are susceptible to injury at the site where the esophagus is compressed by the left atrium [42, 45, 242]. The most distal esophagus has uncommonly been reported as the site of injury, perhaps because of the difficulty in differentiating pill-induced injury from GERD in this location.

## THERAPY AND CLINICAL COURSE

The obvious first step in the treatment of pill-induced esophageal injury is withdrawal of the offending pill. Empiric antireflux therapy may be administered to prevent exacerbation of injury by refluxing acid. Swallowing a topical anesthetic will temporarily relieve severe pain. Most patients will become asymptomatic within a few days to a few weeks if the injury is not repeated [126]. Rare patients require parenteral hydration or parenteral alimentation. Complications of esophageal perforation, mediastinitis, hemorrhage, or fibrotic stricture require specific treatment.

## EPIDEMIOLOGY AND PATHOGENESIS

Since the first reported cases of pill-induced esophageal injury in 1970 [115, 130, 179], nearly 1,000 cases have been reported or summarized in the medical literature. These cases represent only the tip of the iceberg. Cases are reported selectively in the literature, usually because of an unusual quality such as a clustering of cases, a newly implicated pill, or a complication. The best estimate of the incidence of pill-induced esophageal injury is derived from 109 cases diagnosed in a region of Sweden during a 4-year period in the 1970s [39], an incidence of 4 cases per 100,000 population per year. The incidence of injury today in the United States is probably higher because of more frequent administration of medications. Still, pill-induced esophageal injury is an uncommon event considering the number of pills consumed each year.

Patients of all ages (3 to 98 years of age) have been injured (Tables 32–1 to 32–4). Women have been injured more frequently than men in a ratio of 2.2:1, largely because more women have been injured by antibiotics, nonsteroidal antiinflammatory drugs (NSAIDs), alendronate (indicated for osteoporosis), and emepronium bromide (indicated for urinary frequency due to bladder irritability).

Most injured patients have normal esophageal structure and function. This is possible because pill transit through the esophagus is commonly interrupted even in normal subjects. When swallowed with water by upright subjects, gelatin capsules were retained in the esophagus longer than 5 minutes by 11 of 18 subjects [31]. Chasing pills with more water makes them more likely to pass rapidly to the stomach but does not guarantee transit [31]. Pills are even more likely to stick in the esophagus if taken without water or while supine, and these predisposing factors are frequently documented in literature case reports. Other factors favoring esophageal retention of pills include advanced patient age, decreased esophageal peristalsis, and extrinsic esophageal compression. Gelatin capsules are more likely to stick in the esophagus than tablets, and large pills are more likely to stick than small ones [101].

When a pill is retained in the esophagus, it may dissolve there and release its contents. If the contents are sufficiently caustic, injury will occur. The pathogenic mechanism for some pills including the tetracyclines, ascorbic acid, and ferrous sulfate may be production of an acid burn. Any of these pills dissolved in 10 ml of water produces a solution with a pH of 3.0 or less [31, 38]. Phenytoin sodium, 100 mg, dissolved in 10 ml of water produced a solution with a pH of 10.4, suggesting that it might produce an alkaline burn [31]. Other dissolved pills produce neutral solutions, so other mechanisms must be invoked. Postulated mechanisms include induction of GERD by anticholinergics and theophylline, production of local hyperosmolarity by potassium chloride [30], and intracellular poisoning after uptake of doxycycline [88], NSAIDs [212], and alprenolol [172, 173] directly from the esophageal lumen into the mucosa.

Several observations suggest that sustained-release medications may be more injurious to the esophagus than standard-release pills of the same medications. First, sustained-release preparations of potassium chloride, quinidine, ferrous sulfate, and alprenolol have caused most of the reported esophageal injuries and most of the reported complicated injuries due to these medications despite the widespread availability and use of standard-release preparations of the latter three medications. Isolated cases of complicated esophageal injury due to other sustained-release pills have also been reported: esophageal hemorrhage and pseudotumor due to slow-release naproxen [202], esophageal perforation due to sustained-release sodium valproate [247], and deep, circumferential esophageal ulceration and hemorrhage due to sustained-release morphine sulfate [104]. Finally, two small prospective clinical trials suggest that sustained-release pamidronate may be more injurious to the esophagus than the standard preparation of this drug [147]. Taken together, these observations demonstrate enhanced causticity for some sustained-release preparations.

## INJURIES DUE TO SPECIFIC PILLS

### Antibiotics and Antiviral Pills

Antibiotics and antivirals have caused 467 of the 950 reported cases of pill-induced esophageal injury (Table 32–1), approximately 50% of the esophageal injuries due to all medicinal pills combined. Doxycycline (most frequently the large-capsule form of this drug) and other tetracyclines have caused over 400 of these cases, but 20 nontetracycline antibiotics and antivirals have also been implicated. Injured patients tend to be younger (mean age 31 years) than those injured by other pills. Predisposing factors other than improper pill-taking behavior have been rare. Almost all injured patients have presented with acute, severe retrosternal

**TABLE 32–1.** *Esophageal injury due to antibiotic and antiviral pills*

| Implicated pill | Cases | Sex M | Sex F | Age (yr) Number for whom reported | Age (yr) Range | Age (yr) Mean | Number of complications Hemorrhage | Number of complications Stricture | Number of complications Death | References |
|---|---|---|---|---|---|---|---|---|---|---|
| Doxycycline | 262 | 43 | 85 | 115 | 10–98 | 30 | 1 | 2 | 1 | a |
| Tetracycline HCl | 42 | 10 | 24 | 23 | 18–72 | 36 | 5 | 1 | — | b |
| Unspecified tetracyclines | 72 | — | — | — | — | — | — | — | — | 40, 171 |
| Oxytetracycline | 10 | 3 | 2 | 5 | 25–32 | 30 | — | — | — | 8, 34, 40, 44, 66, 118 |
| Demethylchlortetracycline | 1 | 1 | — | 1 | — | 24 | — | — | — | 22 |
| Minocycline | 8 | 1 | — | 2 | 16–21 | 18 | — | — | — | 8, 112, 176, 220 |
| Florocycline | 1 | 1 | — | 1 | — | 19 | — | — | — | 152 |
| Metacycline | 1 | — | 1 | 1 | — | 49 | — | — | — | 106 |
| Methylenecycline | 1 | — | 1 | 1 | — | 30 | — | — | — | 178 |
| Pivmecillinam | 32 | 2 | 30 | 32 | — | 35 | — | — | — | 35, 164 |
| Penicillin | 5 | — | 2 | 4 | 18–31 | 23 | — | 1 | — | 32, 35, 39, 91, 226 |
| Ampicillin | 2 | 1 | 1 | 2 | 20–28 | 24 | — | — | — | 190, 197 |
| Pivampicillin | 2 | 1 | — | 1 | — | 35 | — | — | — | 108, 197 |
| Amoxicillin | 2 | 1 | — | 1 | — | 39 | — | — | — | 48, 235 |
| Apocillin | 2 | — | — | — | — | — | — | — | — | 66 |
| Cloxacillin | 1 | — | — | — | — | — | — | — | — | 176 |
| Dicloxacillin + Danzen | 1 | — | — | — | — | — | — | — | — | 176 |
| Trimethoprim-sulfamethoxazole | 2 | 1 | 1 | 2 | 14–63 | 38 | — | — | — | 20, 211 |
| Clindamycin | 5 | 4 | 1 | 4 | 22–35 | 29 | — | — | — | 44, 84, 128, 203, 228 |
| Lincomycin | 1 | — | 1 | 1 | — | 28 | — | — | — | 210 |
| Spiramycine | 1 | 1 | — | 1 | — | 70 | — | — | — | 183 |
| Erythromycin | 1 | — | — | — | — | — | — | — | — | 39 |
| Rifampicin | 1 | — | 1 | 1 | — | 23 | — | — | — | 44 |
| Sulfamethoxypyridazine | 1 | — | — | 1 | — | 24 | — | 1 | — | 239 |
| Tinidazole | 1 | — | — | — | — | — | — | — | — | 39 |
| Grouped antibiotics c | 4 | 3 | 1 | 2 | 33–77 | 55 | 1 | — | — | 169 |
| Unidentified antibiotic | 1 | — | — | — | — | — | — | — | — | 162 |
| Zalcitibine | 1 | 1 | — | 1 | — | 20 | — | — | — | 110 |
| Zidovudine | 3 | 3 | — | 3 | 33–38 | 35 | — | — | — | 70 |
| Totals | 467 | 77 | 151 | 205 | 10–98 | 31 | 7 | 5 | 1 | |

[a] References for doxycycline: 1, 5, 7, 12, 17, 20, 23–25, 29, 31, 32, 39, 40, 44, 46, 47, 53–55, 59, 62–64, 74, 80–82, 85, 87, 88, 90, 95, 99, 100, 106, 112, 114, 117–121, 125, 126, 128, 129, 131, 132, 143, 149–151, 159, 160, 162, 165, 166, 169, 174, 176, 186, 188, 195, 203, 208, 216, 221, 230, 231, 234, 236, 238.

[b] References for tetracycline: 7, 20, 22, 24, 27, 31, 32, 36, 41, 54–56, 66, 67, 89, 112, 123–126, 137, 206, 207.

[c] Erythromycin (two cases), josamycine (one case), clindamycine (one case).

pain and/or odynophagia. Mucosal injury is usually superficial, and symptoms almost always have resolved in a few days to a few weeks. Only 2.5% of reported cases have been complicated, seven by hemorrhage and five by stricture.

### Aspirin and Other Nonsteroidal Anti-inflammatory Drugs

Table 32–2 documents 73 literature case reports of NSAID pill-induced esophageal injury and 81 cases compiled by the U.S. Food and Drug Administration. Considering the cases first reported in the literature, aspirin and other NSAIDs have caused only 73 pill-induced esophageal injuries, less than 10% of the total literature reports, but 22 of these have been complicated by hemorrhage. In contrast, only 25 esophageal injuries due to all other medications com-

bined have been complicated by hemorrhage. NSAIDs are thus strikingly more likely than other pill classes to cause hemorrhage when they injure the esophagus.

Several of these injuries have been devastating. A patient taking indomethacin suffered a fatal esophageal hemorrhage [6], and a patient taking aspirin required surgery for a bleeding, pill-induced esophageal ulcer [209]. Four other patients injured by NSAIDs developed esophageal strictures. Finally, a patient taking pills containing aspirin and caffeine suffered an esophageal perforation [51].

More than half of the cases of NSAID-related esophageal injury documented in Table 32–2 are due to over-the-counter naproxen sodium. These were not reported as literature case reports but were detected by the U.S. Food and Drug Administration's Spontaneous Reporting System [116]. This system is a more sensitive surveillance system than reliance

**TABLE 32–2.** *Esophageal injury due to aspirin and other nonsteroidal anti-inflammatory drug pills*

| Implicated pill | Cases | Sex M | Sex F | Age (yr) Number for whom reported | Age (yr) Range | Age (yr) Mean | Number of complications Hemorrhage | Number of complications Stricture | Number of complications Death | Refs. |
|---|---|---|---|---|---|---|---|---|---|---|
| Aspirin | 19 | 12 | 4 | 10 | 16–89 | 40 | 8 | 2 | — | 31, 32, 39, 110, 126, 130, 194, 209, 243 |
| Aspirin, caffeine | 1 | 1 | — | 1 | — | 26 | — | — | — | 51 |
| Aspirin, phenacetin, caffeine | 1 | 1 | — | 1 | — | 54 | 1 | — | — | 244 |
| Aspirin, Anacin | 1 | — | 1 | 1 | — | 41 | 1 | — | — | 225 |
| Aspirin, ibuprofen | 1 | 1 | — | 1 | — | 20 | 1 | — | — | 225 |
| Doleron[a] | 7 | — | — | — | — | — | — | 1 | — | 39 |
| Decagesic[b] | 1 | 1 | — | 1 | Adolescent | — | — | — | 68 | |
| Paraflex compound[c] | 1 | — | — | — | — | — | — | — | — | 39 |
| Naproxen | | | | | | | | | | |
|    Literature case reports | 3 | 1 | 2 | 3 | 29–87 | 62 | 2 | — | — | 69, 202, 237 |
|    FDA reporting program | 81 | 16 | 65 | — | — | 36 | — | — | — | 116 |
| Indomethacin | 5 | 4 | 1 | 5 | 28–82 | 62 | 2 | — | 1 | 6, 19, 67, 68, 86 |
| Ibuprofen | 5 | 2 | 2 | 4 | 18–63 | 32 | 1 | — | — | 7, 47, 162, 225 |
| Meclofenamate sodium | 2 | — | 2 | 2 | 36–47 | 41 | — | — | — | 161, 204 |
| Mefenamic acid | 1 | 1 | — | 1 | — | 63 | 1 | 1 | — | 60 |
| Phenylbutazone + prednisone | 1 | — | 1 | 1 | — | 75 | 1 | — | — | 115 |
| Tolmetin | 1 | 1 | — | 1 | — | 27 | — | — | — | 57 |
| Sulindac | 1 | 1 | — | 1 | — | 36 | — | — | — | 140 |
| Piroxicam | 4 | 3 | 1 | 4 | 20–27 | 22 | — | — | — | 205 |
| Diclofenac | 1 | — | 1 | 1 | — | 23 | — | — | — | 109 |
| Flurbiprofen | 1 | 1 | — | 1 | — | 26 | — | — | — | 229 |
| Grouped nonsteroidal agents[d] | 6 | 3 | 3 | 2 | 21–75 | 48 | 4 | — | — | 169 |
| Unspecified nonsteroidals | 8 | — | — | — | — | — | — | — | — | 171 |
| Acetaminophen | 1 | — | — | — | — | — | — | — | — | 66 |
| Percogesic[e] | 1 | — | 1 | 1 | — | 31 | — | — | — | 170 |
| Totals | 154 | 49 | 84 | 42 | 16–89 | 43 | 22 | 4 | 1 | |

[a] Components of Doleron: aspirin, dextropropoxyphene, phenothiazine carboxyl-10-hydrochloride, antipyrene, vinbarbital.
[b] Components of Decagesic: aspirin, dexamethasone, aluminum hydroxide gel.
[c] Components of Paraflex compound: aspirin, dextropropoxyphene, chlorzoxazone.
[d] Oxyphenbutazone (three cases), indomethacin (two cases), diclofenac (one case).
[e] Components of Percogesic: acetaminophen, phenyltoloxamine citrate.

**TABLE 32–3.** *Esophageal injury due to other pills available in the United States*

| Implicated pill | Cases | Sex M | Sex F | Number for whom reported | Age (yr) Range | Age (yr) Mean | Hemorrhage | Stricture | Death | References |
|---|---|---|---|---|---|---|---|---|---|---|
| Potassium chloride (KCl) | 33 | 9 | 16 | 23 | 14–77 | 55 | 4 | 17 | 6 | [a] |
| Alendronate | | | | | | | | | | |
|   Literature case reports | 14 | 2 | 12 | 14 | 33–90 | 67 | 1 | 6 | — | 3, 37, 49, 61, 125, 139, 141, 148, 168, 192, 218 |
|   Postmarketing survey | 51 | 2 | 46 | 36 | 23–85 | 65 | 2 | 2 | — | 61 |
| Ferrous sulfate or succinate | 24 | 4 | 10 | 14 | 62–89 | 79 | 4 | 6 | 1 | 2, 39, 132, 213 |
| Quinidine | 13 | 6 | 5 | 11 | 12–76 | 60 | — | 7 | — | 28, 31, 33, 54, 126, 154, 219, 232, 246 |
| Quinidine + KCl | 2 | — | 2 | 2 | 49–73 | 61 | — | 2 | — | 134, 191 |
| Quinidine + indomethacine + multivitamins | 1 | — | 1 | 1 | — | 77 | — | — | — | 67 |
| Mexiletine | 4 | 1 | 2 | 3 | 72–77 | 74 | — | — | — | 4, 169, 181, 200 |
| Captopril | 1 | — | 1 | 1 | — | 84 | 1 | — | — | 11 |
| Nifedipine | 2 | 1 | — | 1 | — | 69 | — | 1 | — | 169, 217 |
| Verapamil (+ zolpidem) | 1 | — | 1 | 1 | — | 50 | — | — | — | 111 |
| Bepridil | 1 | — | — | — | — | — | — | — | — | 169 |
| Unidentified antihypertensive | 1 | — | — | — | — | — | — | — | — | 162 |
| Theophylline/aminophylline | 7 | 2 | 1 | 3 | 28–31 | 30 | — | — | — | 73, 171, 214, 223 |
| Corticosteroids | 6 | 4 | 2 | 3 | 42–81 | 66 | — | — | — | 65, 169 |
| Multivitamin & iron or & minerals | 3 | 2 | — | 3 | 3–62 | 29 | — | — | — | 32, 75, 184 |
| Ascorbic acid | 3 | — | 3 | 3 | 24–61 | 47 | — | 2 | — | 31, 127, 241 |
| 13-*cis*-Retinoate | 3 | 3 | — | 3 | 17–74 | 46 | — | 1 | — | 13, 77 |
| Tryptophan | 1 | — | 1 | 1 | — | 81 | 1 | — | — | 187 |
| Pamidronate[b] | 5 | — | 5 | 5 | 64–74 | 69 | — | — | — | 147 |
| Valproic acid | 1 | 1 | — | 1 | — | 49 | — | — | — | 247 |
| Phenytoin sodium | 1 | 1 | — | 1 | — | 36 | — | 1 | — | 31 |
| Phenytoin + phenobarbital | 1 | — | 1 | 1 | — | 41 | 1 | — | — | 240 |
| Warfarin | 1 | 1 | — | 1 | — | 58 | 1 | — | — | 144 |
| Thioridazine, slow-release | 1 | 1 | — | 1 | — | 22 | — | — | — | 197 |
| Clorazepate | 1 | — | 1 | 1 | — | 25 | — | — | — | 153 |
| Diazepam | 1 | — | 1 | 1 | — | 45 | — | — | — | 99 |
| Morphine sulfate, slow-release | 1 | — | — | — | — | — | 1 | — | — | 104 |
| Glyburide (glibenclamide) | 2 | — | 1 | 1 | — | 82 | — | — | — | 108, 197 |
| Estramustine phosphate | 2 | — | — | — | — | — | — | — | — | 39 |
| Eucalyptus-menthol cough tab | 1 | 1 | — | 1 | — | 9 | — | — | — | 79 |
| Oral contraceptives | 4 | — | 3 | 3 | 19–24 | 21 | — | — | — | 10, 48, 175 |
| Totals | 193 | 41 | 115 | 140 | 3–90 | 60 | 16 | 45 | 7 | |

[a] References for potassium chloride: 15, 16, 31, 33, 39, 45, 72, 98, 105, 136, 145, 146, 156, 162, 169, 171, 179, 185, 199, 201, 227, 230, 242.

[b] Approved only for parenteral use in the United States.

upon review of literature case reports, especially for less serious injuries. Consequently, these 81 cases do not necessarily imply that naproxen is more likely than other NSAIDs to injure the esophagus. None of these 81 patients is known to have suffered a hemorrhage or stricture.

## Potassium Chloride, Quinidine, Ferrous Sulfate or Succinate, and Alprenolol

Many of the 84 patients injured by potassium chloride, quinidine, ferrous sulfate or succinate, and alprenolol (a beta blocker) (Tables 32–3 and 32–4) have presented with progressive dysphagia, often with little or no pain. Esophageal strictures have occurred in 39 (46%) of the patients injured by these four medications, 15 more strictures than have been caused by all other medications combined.

At least 26 of the 33 patients injured by potassium chloride tablets (Table 32–3) have been predisposed to esophageal retention of pills by virtue of extrinsic esophageal compression or esophageal motor dysfunction. At least 21 had previously undergone cardiac surgery, which can result in entrapment of the esophagus between the aorta and vertebral column [242]. When the esophagus is fixed in position by adhesions and neighboring structures, it is especially susceptible to compression by an enlarged left atrium, predisposing these patients to pill retention and injury [242].

Potassium chloride-induced esophageal injuries have often been devastating. Seventeen patients have developed esophageal strictures, four have presented with hemorrhage, and six have died as a result of their injuries. Four patients suffered fatal esophageal hemorrhage, including one patient each with penetration of the aorta [156], the left atrium [227], and a bronchial collateral artery [98]. Another death was due to penetration of the mediastinum [199], and a patient with a potassium chloride-induced esophageal stricture died 1 week after surgical creation of a feeding jejunostomy [242]. All six deaths occurred in patients with cardiomegaly, and four of the six patients had previously undergone cardiac surgery.

Thirteen cases of pill-induced esophageal injury in patients taking no caustic pill other than quinidine have been reported, and seven of the 13 injured patients developed esophageal strictures. In contrast to the situation with regard to potassium chloride, predisposing factors were identified in only two of these subjects.

An unusual feature of quinidine-induced esophageal injury is the occasional presentation with flamboyant exudate that is so thick and tenacious as to suggest neoplasia on barium swallow [126, 232, 246]. This exudate may break up at endoscopy and reveal edematous, ulcerated underlying mucosa. Similar presentations have been documented in injuries due to sustained-release ferrous sulfate [213] and sustained-release naproxen [202]. Although these patients sometimes present with painless dysphagia suggesting a stricture or carcinoma, the lesions and symptoms may resolve without dilatation.

## Alendronate and Pamidronate

Alendronate (Table 32–3) and pamidronate (Table 32–4) are bisphosphonate inhibitors of bone resorption. In the 2 years since the initial marketing of alendronate in late 1995, 14 esophageal injuries due to this medication have been reported as case reports or case series in the medical literature. Six of the injured patients developed esophageal strictures and one presented with hemorrhage. Postmarketing surveillance reports compiled by the manufacturer of alendronate document 51 additional patients with "serious" or "severe" adverse esophageal effects [61]. Two of these patients developed strictures, and two suffered hemorrhage. Most patients injured by alendronate appear to have taken their pills improperly, either failing to remain upright after swallowing the pills or taking the pills with less than the 6 ounces of water recommended by the manufacturer. Nonetheless,

**TABLE 32–4.** *Esophageal injury due to pills not available in the United States*

| Implicated pill | Cases | Sex M | Sex F | Age (yr) Number for whom reported | Age (yr) Range | Age (yr) Mean | Number of complications Hemorrhage | Number of complications Stricture | Number of complications Death | References |
|---|---|---|---|---|---|---|---|---|---|---|
| Emepronium bromide | 90 | 11 | 52 | 67 | 5–89 | 34 | 2 | 2 | — | [a] |
| Alprenolol | 12 | — | 3 | 3 | 32–73 | 59 | — | 7 | — | 39, 171, 222 |
| Pinaverium bromide | 14 | 4 | 7 | 11 | 17–48 | 33 | — | — | — | 14, 135, 169, 196, 224, 234 |
| Thiazinium | 5 | 1 | 3 | 4 | 21–53 | 30 | — | — | — | 169, 180 |
| Naftidrofuryl | 3 | 1 | 2 | 2 | 17–21 | 19 | — | — | — | 157, 158, 195 |
| Pantogar[b] | 1 | — | 1 | 1 | — | 21 | — | — | — | 131 |
| Rhinasal[c] | 3 | 2 | — | 1 | — | 27 | — | — | — | 79, 182, 193 |
| Clomethiazol | 1 | 1 | — | 1 | — | 55 | — | — | — | 197 |
| Diltenate-tetra[d] | 1 | — | — | 1 | — | 75 | — | — | — | 245 |
| Traumanase-cyklin[e] | 1 | — | — | 1 | — | 45 | — | — | — | 245 |
| Acenocoumarol | 1 | — | — | — | — | — | — | — | — | 169 |
| Calcium dobesilate | 1 | — | — | 1 | — | 45 | — | — | — | 78 |
| Pantozyme | 1 | — | — | — | — | — | — | — | — | 176 |
| Minidril | 1 | — | — | — | — | — | — | — | — | 48 |
| Chlormadinone | 1 | — | 1 | 1 | — | 50 | — | — | — | 58 |
| Totals | 136 | 20 | 69 | 94 | 5–89 | 35 | 2 | 9 | — | |

[a] References for emepronium bromide: 18, 21, 39, 43, 50, 52, 71, 76, 83, 92, 93, 96, 97, 102, 103, 106–108, 112, 113, 118, 120, 122, 131, 133, 138, 142, 163, 167, 189, 197, 198, 215, 233.

[b] Components of Pantogar: thiamine HCl, calcium pantothenate, paraaminobenzoic acid, cystin, faex, keratin.

[c] Components of Rhinasal: thiazinium methylsulfate, acetaminophen, norephedrine chlorhydrate.

[d] Components of Diltenate-tetra: tetracycline, theophylline, etafedrine, doxylamine succinate, phenylephrine, guaifenesin.

[e] Components of Traumanase-cyklin: tetracycline, bromelaine.

some patients appear to have been injured despite taking their pills entirely appropriately.

Even though alendronate is a frequent offender compared to other medications, an individual patient taking alendronate properly is at only minimal risk for esophageal injury, considering that only 65 patients are known to have been injured out of more than 500,000 patients for whom prescriptions have been written [61]. In comparing the frequency of esophageal injury induced by alendronate to the frequency of esophageal injury induced by other pills, it is appropriate to compare only the 14 cases reported primarily in the medical literature rather than those compiled by the manufacturer. Even limiting the comparison in this manner, the 14 cases reported as case reports in a 2-year period suggest that alendronate is somewhat more likely than most pills (except, perhaps, for some antibiotics) to injure the esophagus and that the injuries tend to be more serious than injuries resulting from most other pills. Physicians should always caution their patients to take this medication appropriately, in the upright posture with a minimum of 6 ounces of water, and remaining upright for at least 30 minutes after swallowing the pill. The medication should not be prescribed to patients with impaired esophageal transit.

Two controlled clinical trials provide the only documentation of esophageal injury due to oral pamidronate [147]. In these trials, four of 33 subjects taking timed-release pamidronate and one of 33 subjects taking standard pamidronate developed severe chest pain, dysphagia, and vomiting. Endoscopy revealed erosive and exudative distal esophagitis in each. No complications occurred.

Etidronate, a related bisphosphonate, has not been reported in the medical literature to cause esophageal injury, but the manufacturer's packaging literature lists "esophagitis" as a potential adverse reaction.

## PREVENTION OF PILL-INDUCED ESOPHAGEAL INJURY

Pills will not injure the esophagus directly unless they dissolve in the esophagus, so physicians, nurses, and pharmacists should instruct patients in a few simple and prudent steps to enhance esophageal transit of prescribed pills:

1. Patients should drink at least 4 ounces of fluid with any pill, twice this amount with pills that are especially likely to cause injury.
2. Patients should remain upright for at least 10 minutes after taking most pills and for 30 minutes after taking pills likely to cause injury.
3. Pills implicated as causing frequent or severe esophageal injury should be avoided in bedridden patients or patients with esophageal compression, stricture, or dysmotility.

These steps will greatly reduce the frequency of pill-induced esophageal injury but will not completely eliminate injury. A high index of suspicion is required to recognize pill-induced esophageal injury when it occurs, so that repetitive injury may be avoided by prompt withdrawal of the offending pill.

## REFERENCES

1. Aarons B, Bruns BJ. Oesophageal ulceration associated with ingestion of doxycycline. NZ Med J 1980;91:27
2. Abbarah TR, Fredell JE, Ellenz GB. Ulceration by oral ferrous sulfate. JAMA 1976;236:2320
3. Abdelmalek MF, Douglas DD. Alendronate-induced ulcerative esophagitis. Am J Gastroenterol 1996;91:1282
4. Adler JB, Goldberg RI. Mexiletine-induced pill esophagitis. Am J Gastroenterol 1990;85:629
5. Adverse Drug Reactions Advisory Committee. Doxycycline-induced oesophageal ulceration. Med J Aust 1994;161:490
6. Agdal N. Mediciniducerede esophagusskader. Ugeskr Laeger 1979; 141:3019
7. Agha FP, Wilson JAP, Nostrand TT. Medication-induced esophagitis. Gastrointest Radiol 1986;11:7
8. Algayres JP, Valmary J, Chabierski M, Daly JP, Rougier Y. Ulcère oesophagien après prise de minocycline. Presse Med 1989;18:541
9. Allard C. Ulcére iatrogene de l'oesophage. Gastroenterol Clin Biol 1982;6:712
10. Allmendinger G. Esophageal ulcer caused by the "pill." Z Gastroenterol 1985;23:531
11. Al Mahdy H, Boswell GV. Captopril-induced oesophagitis. Eur J Clin Pharmacol 1988;34:95
12. Amendola MA, Spera TD. Doxycycline-induced esophagitis. JAMA 1985;253:1009
13. Amichai B, Grunwald MH, Odes SH, Zirkin H. Acute esophagitis caused by isotretinoin. Int J Dermatol 1996;35,528
14. Andre JM, Voiment YM, Marti RG. Ulcéres oesophagiens après prise de bromure de pinaverium. Acta Endosc 1980;10:289
15. Ashour M, et al. Acute dysphagia induced by bendrofluazide-K. Practitioner 1984;228:524
16. Barbier P, Pringot J, Heimann R, Fiasse R, Jacobs E. Ulcérations digestives induites par le chlorure de potassium. Acta Gastroenterol Belg 1976;39:261
17. Barbier P, Dumont A, Dony A, Toussaint J, Thys O, Engelholm L. Ulcérations oesophagiennes induites par la doxycycline. Acta Gastroenterol Belg 1981;44:424
18. Barrison IG, Trewby PN, Kane SP. Oesophageal ulceration due to emepronium bromide. Endoscopy 1980;12:197
19. Bataille C, Soumagne D, Loly J, Brassinne A. Esophageal ulceration due to indomethacin. Digestion 1982;24:66
20. Bell RL. Tetracycline induced esophagitis. Alabama Med 1986;55: 47
21. Bennett JR. Oesophageal ulceration due to emepronium bromide. Lancet 1977;1:810
22. Berli DE, Salis GB, Chiocca JC. Lesion esofagica por drogas. Acta Gastroent Latin Am 1986;16:109
23. Bezuidenhout DJJ. Iatrogene esofagitis. S Afr Med J 1980;57:1023
24. Biller JA, Flores A, Buie T, Mazor S, Katz A. Tetracycline-induced esophagitis in adolescent patients. J Pediatr 1992;120:144
25. Bissonnette B, Biron P. Ulcère oesophagien causé par la doxycycline. Can Med Assoc J 1984;131:1186
26. Bjarnason I, Bjornsson S. Oesophageal ulcers. Acta Med Scand 1981; 209:431
27. Bliss MR. Tablets and capsules that stick in the oesophagus. J R Coll Gen Pract 1984;34:301
28. Bohane TD, Perrault J, Fowler RS. Oesophagitis and oesophageal obstruction from quinidine tablets in association with left atrial enlargement. Aust Paediatr J 1978;14:191
29. Bokey L, Hugh TB. Oesophageal ulceration associated with doxycycline therapy. Med J Aust 1975;1:236
30. Boley SJ, Allen AC, Schultz L, Schwartz S. Potassium-induced lesions of the small bowel. JAMA 1965;193:997
31. Bonavina L, DeMeester TR, McChesney L, Schwizer W, Albertucci M, Bailey RT. Drug-induced esophageal strictures. Ann Surg 1987; 206:173
32. Bova JG, Dutton NE, Goldstein HM, Hoberman LJ. Medication-induced esophagitis: diagnosis by double-contrast esophagography. Am J Roentgenol 1987;148:731

33. Boyce HW Jr. Dysphagia after open heart surgery. Hosp Pract 1985; 20:40

34. Bretzke G. Tetrazyklin-ulkus der speiserohre. Z Gesamte Inn Med 1982;37:574

35. Brochet E, Croisier G, Grimaldi A, Bosquet F. Stenose oesophagienne liée à la prise de phenoxylmethylpenicilline chez une diabetique insulino-dependante. Presse Med 1984;13:2392

36. Burke EL. Acute oesophageal damage from one brand of tetracycline tablets. Gastroenterology 1975;68:1022

37. Cameron RB. Esophagitis dissecans superficialis and alendronate: case report. Gastrointest Endosc 1997;46:562

38. Carlborg B. Biverkningar vid accidentell losning av lakemedel i esofagus och bronker. Lakartidningen 1976;73:4201

39. Carlborg B, Kumlien A, Olsson H. Medikamentella esofagusstrikturer. Lakartidningen 1978;75:4609

40. Carlborg B, Densert O, Lindqvist C. Tetracycline induced esophageal ulcers. A clinical and experimental study. Laryngoscope 1983;93:184

41. Channer KS, Hollanders D. Tetracycline-induced oesophageal ulceration. BMJ 1981;282:1359

42. Channer KS, Bell J, Virjee JP. Effect of left atrial size on the oesophageal transit of capsules. Br Heart J 1984;52:223

43. Chapman K. Emepronium bromide and the treatment of urge incontinence. Med J Aust 1978;1:103

44. Chen CY, Wang LY, Liu HW, Jan CM, Chien CH. Esophageal ulcers caused by antibiotics. J Formosan Med Assoc 1982;81:618

45. Chesshyre MH, Braimbridge MV. Dysphagia due to left atrial enlargement after mitral Starr valve replacement. Br Heart J 1971;33:799

46. Cleau D. Ulcère oesophagien après prise de doxycycline. Gastroenterol Clin Biol 1982;6:510

47. Coates AG, Nostrant TT, Wilson JAP, Elta GH, Agha FP. Esophagitis caused by nonsteroidal antiinflammatory medication: case reports and review of the literature on pill-induced esophageal injury. South Med J 1986;79:1094

48. Cocheton JJ, Bigot JM, Penalba C. Les avatars du transit oesophagien des medicaments solides. Concours Med 1984;106:3895

49. Colina RA, Smith M, Kikendall JW, Wong RKH. A new, probably increasing cause of esophageal ulceration: alendronate. Am J Gastroenterol 1997;92:704

50. Collins FJ, Matthews HR, Baker SE, Strakova JM. Drug-induced oesophageal injury. BMJ 1979;1:1673

51. Corsi PR, de Aguiar JR, de S Kronfly F, Saad R Jr, Rasslan S. Lesao esofagica provocada por ingestao de pilula. Rev Assoc Med Brasil 1995;41:360

52. Cowan RE, Wright JT, Marsh F. Drug-induced oesophageal injury. BMJ 1979;2:132

53. Craig JM, Giaffer MH, Talbot MD. Drug-induced oesophageal ulceration in a patient with acquired immunodeficiency syndrome. Int J STD AIDS 1996;7:370

54. Creteur V, et al. Drug-induced esophagitis detected by double-contrast radiography. Radiology 1983;147:365

55. Crowson TD, Head LH, Ferrante WA. Esophageal ulcers associated with tetracycline therapy. JAMA 1976;235:2747

56. Cummin ARC, Hangartner JRW. Oesophago-atrial fistual: a side effect of tetracycline? J R Soc Med 1990;83:745

57. Cunningham JT. Induced esophageal ulceration. Gastrointest Endosc 1982;28:49

58. Daghfous R, Hedi Loueslati M, El Aidli S, Srairi S, Lakhal M, Belkahia C. Atteinte inflammatoire du tractus digestif superieur probablement due à un progestatif de synthese. Gastroenterol Clin Biol 1995;19:853

59. Daunt N, Brodribb TR, Dickey JD. Oesophageal ulceration due to doxycycline. Br J Radiol 1985;58:1209

60. de Caestecker JS, Heading RC. Iatrogenic oesophageal ulceration with massive haemorrhage and stricture formation. Br J Clin Pract 1988; 42:212

61. de Groen PC, et al. Esophagitis associated with the use of alendronate. N Engl J Med 1996;335:1016

62. Delpre G. Esophageal ulcers due to tetracycline. Harefuah 1981;101: 281

63. Delpre G, Kadish U. Esophageal ulceration due to enterocoated doxycycline therapy—further considerations. Gastrointest Endosc 1984; 30:44

64. Dent J, et al. Mechanism of gastroesophageal reflux in recumbent asymptomatic human subjects. J Clin Invest 1980;65:256

65. de Witte C, Dony A, Serste JP. Ulcere oesophagien iatrogene. J Belge Radiol 1972;55:655

66. Djupesland G, Rolstad EA. Etsskader i oesophagus forarsaket av medikamenter. Tidsskr Nor Laegeforen 1978;98:696

67. Doman DB, Ginsberg AL. The hazard of drug-induced esophagitis. Hosp Pract 1981;16:17

68. Drug Experience Report. Spontaneous Reporting Program (1969–1980). Rockville, MD: Division of Drug Experience, Food and Drug Administration

69. Ecker GA, Karsh J. Naproxen induced ulcerative esophagitis. J Rheumatol 1992;19:646

70. Edwards P, Turner J, Gold J, Cooper DA. Esophageal ulceration induced by zidovudine. Ann Intern Med 1990;112:65

71. Eichenberger P, Blum AL. Drug-induced esophageal lesions. Acta Endosc 1980;10:273

72. Eng J, Sabanathan S. Drug-induced esophagitis. Am J Gastroenterol 1991;86:1127

73. Enzenauer RW, Bass JW, McDonnell JT. Esophageal ulceration associated with oral theophylline. N Engl J Med 1984;310:261

74. Evenepoel C. Slokdarmzweren door gebruik van doxycycline. Tijdschr Gastroenterol 1977;20:293

75. Ewert B, Ewert G, Glas JE, Thore M. Medikamentell hypofarynxskada. Lakartidningen 1979;76:739

76. Fellows IW, Ogilvie AL, Atkinson M. Oesophageal stricture associated with emepronium bromide therapy. Postgrad Med J 1982;58:43

77. Fennerty B, Sampliner R, Garewal H. Esophageal ulceration associated with 13-cis-retinoic acid therapy in patients with Barrett's esophagus. Gastrointest Endosc 1989;35:442

78. Fernandez Rodriguez C, Moreira V, Boixeda D, Dominguez Rodriguez F, Garcia Plaza A. Ulcera esofagica por dobexilato calcico. Gastroenterol Hepatol 1986;9:102

79. Fiedorek SC, Casteel HB. Pediatric medication-induced focal esophagitis. Clin Pediatr 1988;27:455

80. Florent C, Chagnon JP, Vivet P, Brun JG, Cattan D, Bernier JJ. Accidents oesophagiens associés à la prise orale de doxycycline. Gastroenterol Clin Biol 1980;4:888

81. Foucaud P, Vincent MH, Scart G, Gaudelus J, Nathanson M, Perelman R. Premier cas chez l'enfant d'ulcère aigu oesophagien après pris de doxycycline. Med Infantile 1980;87:233

82. Fraser GM, Odes HS, Krugliak P. Severe localised esophagitis due to doxycycline. Endoscopy 1987;19:86

83. Freysteinsson H, Thorsson AV. Oesophageal ulcerations in two children taking emepronium bromide. Acta Paediatr Scand 1982;70:513

84. Froese EH. Oesophagitis with clindamycin. S Afr Med J 1979;56: 826

85. Garcia Molinero MJ, Vidal Ruiz JV, Garcia Cabezudo J. Ulcera esofagica por doxiciclina. Gastroenterol Hepatol 1981;4:383

86. Gardies A, Gevaudan J, Le Roux C, Cornet C, Warnet-Duboscq J, Viguie R. Ulcére iatrogene de l'oesophage. Nouv Presse Med 1978; 7:1032

87. Geschwind A. Oesophagitis and oesophageal ulceration following ingestion of doxycycline tablets. Med J Aust 1984;1:223

88. Giger M, et al. Das tetracyclin-ulkus der speiserohre. Dtsch Med Wochenschr 1978;103:1038

89. Ginaldi S. Drug-induced esophagitis. Am Fam Physician 1984;30: 169

90. Golindano C, Villalobos MM. Doxycycline esophageal ulcers: are they due to an irritant effect? Gastrointest Endosc 1985;31:408

91. Gould PC, Bartolomeo RS, Sklarek HM. Esophageal ulceration associated with oral penicillin in Marfan's syndrome. NY State J Med 1985;85:199

92. Guignard A, Savary M. L'oesophagite d'origine medicamenteuse. Acta Endosc 1980;10:263

93. Habeshaw T, Bennett JR. Ulceration of mouth due to emepronium bromide. Lancet 1972;2:1422

94. Haefeli W. Der fall aus der praxis. Praxis 1982;71:1396

95. Hatheway GJ. Doxycycline-induced esophagitis. Drug Intell Clin Pharmacy 1982;16:879

96. Hale JE, Barnardo DE. Ulceration of mouth due to emepronium bromide. Lancet 1973;1:493

97. Halter F, Scheurer U. Veratzung des distalen osophagus durch ein anticholinergikum. Z Gastroenterol 1978;16:699

98. Henry JG, Shinner JJ, Martino JH, Cimino LE. Fatal esophageal and bronchial artery ulceration caused by solid potassium chloride. Pediatr Cardiol 1983;4:251

99. Herrerias JM, Bonet M. Esofagitis por diacepam. Med Clin (Barcelona) 1984;83:690

100. Herrerias JM, Bonet M, Jimenez M, Ariza A, Pellicer F. Oesophagite ulcérative et doxycycline. Acta Endosc 1984;14:141

101. Hey H, Jorgensen F, Sorensen K, Hasselbalch H, Wamberg T. Oesophageal transit of six commonly used tablets and capsules. BMJ 1982;285:1717

102. Higson RH. Oesophagitis as a side effect of emepronium. BMJ 1978; 2:201

103. Hillman LC, Scobie BA, Pomare EW, Austad WI. Acute oesophagitis due to emepronium bromide. NZ Med J 1981;94:4

104. Hiraoka T, Okita M, Koganemaru S, Okada H, Sone Y. Hemorrhagic esophageal ulceration associated with slow-release morphine sulfate tablets. Nippon Shokakibyo Gakkai Zasshi 1991;88:1231

105. Howie AD, Strachan RW. Slow release potassium chloride treatment. BMJ 1975;2:176

106. Hugel HE, Schinko H, Bischof HP. Das medikamentos bedingte osophagusulkus. Z Gastroenterol 1982;20:599

107. Hughes R. Drug-induced oesophageal injury. BMJ 1979;2:132

108. Hunert H, Ottenjann R. Drug-induced esophageal ulcers. Gastrointest Endosc 1979;25:41

109. Imada T, Aoyama N, Amano T, Kolzumi H, Goto H. Esophageal ulceration associated with Voltaren therapy. I To Cho 1983;18:227

110. Indorf A, Pegram PS. Esophageal ulceration related to Zalcitabine (ddC). Ann Intern Med 1992;117:133

111. Jacques JP, Llau ME, Mercier JF, Vigreux P, Montastruc JL. Ulcération oesophagienne d'origine medicamenteuse. Therapie 1993;48:513

112. Jeffery PC, Cullis SNR. Drug-induced oesophagitis. S Afr Med J 1983;64:1081

113. Johnsen S, Koefoed-Nielsen B, Tos M. Emepron (Cetiprin) og aetsskader i mund og spiseror. Ugeskr Laeger 1982;144:1477

114. Jost PM. Drug-induced esophagitis. JAMA 1985;254:508

115. Juncosa L. Ulcus peptico yatrogeno del esofago. Rev Esp Enferm Apar Dig 1970;30:457

116. Kahn LH, Chen M, Eaton R. Over-the-counter naproxen sodium and esophageal injury. Ann Intern Med 1997;126:1006

117. Kalar JG, Redwine JN, Persaud MV. Iatrogenic esophagitis. Iowa Med 1988;78:323

118. Kato S, Komatsu K, Harada Y. Medication-induced esophagitis in children. Gastroenterol Jpn 1990;25:485

119. Kato S, Kobayashi M, Sato H, Saito Y, Komatsu K, Harada Y. Doxycycline-induced hemorrhagic esophagitis: a pediatric case. J Pediatr Gastroenterol Nutr 1988;7:762

120. Kavin H. Oesophageal ulceration due to emepronium bromide. Lancet 1977;1:424

121. Keegan AD. Drug-induced oesophageal ulceration. Med J Austr 1990; 152:383

122. Kenwright S, Norris ADC. Oesophageal ulceration due to emepronium bromide. Lancet 1977;1:548

123. Khan SA. Esophageal ulceration related to oral ingestion of tetracycline capsules. Gastrointest Endosc 1983;29:163

124. Khera DC, Herschman BR, Sosa F. Tetracycline-induced esophageal ulcers. Postgrad Med 1980;68:113

125. Kikendall JW. Pill esophagitis. In Brandt LJ, ed, Clinical Practice of Gastroenterology. Philadelphia: Current Medicine 1999:91

126. Kikendall JW, Friedman AC, Oyewole MA, Fleischer D, Johnson LF. Pill-induced esophageal injury: case reports and review of the medical literature. Dig Dis Sci 1983;28:174

127. Kikendall JW, Schmidt M, Graeber GM, Burton NA, Fall SM, Johnson LF. Pill-induced esophageal ulceration and stricture following cardiac surgery. Milit Med 1986;151:539

128. Kimura K, et al. Drug-induced esophageal ulcer. Nippon Shokakibyo Gakkai Zasshi 1978;75:64

129. Klegar KL, Young TL. Pill-induced esophageal injury. J Tenn Med Assoc 1992;85:417

130. Knauer CM, McLaughlin WT, Mark JBD. Esophago-esophageal fistula in a patient with achalasia. Gastroenterology 1970;58:223

131. Kobler E, Buhler H, Nuesch HJ, Deyhle P. Medikamentos induzierte osophagusulzera. Dtsch Med Wochenschr 1978;103:1035

132. Kobler E, Nuesch HJ, Buhler H, Jenny S, Deyhle P. Medikamentos bedingte osophagusulzera. Schweiz Med Wochenschr 1979;109:1180

133. Kunert H. Medikamentos induzierte osophagusulzera. Dtsch Med Wochenschr 1978;103:1278

134. Lambert JR, Newman A. Ulceration and stricture of the esophagus due to oral potassium chloride (slow release tablet) therapy. Am J Gastroenterol 1980;73:508

135. Lamouliatte H, Plane D, Quinton A. Ulcére oesophagien après pris orale de bromure de pinaverium. Gastroenterol Clin Biol 1981;5:812

136. Learmonth I, Weaver PC. Potassium stricture of the upper alimentary tract. Lancet 1976;1:251

137. Lee MG, Hanchard B. Tetracycline-induced proximal oesophagitis. West Ind Med J 1990;39:124

138. Leonard RCF, Adams PC, Parker S, Adams DM. Oesophageal injury associated with emepronium bromide (Ceteprin). Br J Clin Pract 1984; 38:429

139. Levine J, Nelson D. Esophageal stricture associated with alendronate therapy. Am J Med 1997;102:489

140. Levine MS, Rothstein RD, Laufer I. Giant esophageal ulcer due to Clinoril. Am J Roentgenol 1991;156:955

141. Lilley LL, Guanci R. Avoiding alendronate-related esophageal irritation. Am J Nurs 1997;97:12

142. Lind O. Medikamentindusert osofagitt. Tidsskr Nor Laegeforen 1978; 98:742

143. Llanos O, Guzman S, Duarte I. Doxycycline esophageal ulcer. Gastrointest Endosc 1985;31:407

144. Loft DE, Stubington S, Clark C, Rees WDW. Oesophageal ulcer caused by warfarin. Postgrad Med J 1989;65:258

145. Lowry N, Delaney P, O'Malley E. Oesophageal ulceration occurring secondary to slow release potassium tablets. Irish J Med Sci 1975; 144:366

146. Lubbe WF, Cadogan ES, Kannemeyer AHR. Oesophageal ulceration due to slow-release potassium in the presence of left atrial enlargement. NZ Med J 1979;90:377

147. Lufkin EG, et al. Pamidronate: an unrecognized problem in gastrointestinal tolerability. Osteoporosis Int 1994;4:320

148. Maconi G, Bianchi Porro G. Multiple ulcerative esophagitis caused by alendronate. Am J Gastroenterol 1995;90:1889

149. Maffioli C, Segal S, Renard A, Diot J, Segal A. Ulcères oesophagiens à la doxycycline. Nouv Presse Med 1979;8:1264

150. Maffioli C, Segal S, Diot J, Segal A. Oesophagite ulcéreuse a la doxycycline. Acta Endosc 1980;10:285

151. Markin RS, al-Turk M, Zetterman RK. Esophageal ulceration following doxycycline ingestion. Postgrad Med 1992;91:179

152. Maroy B. Ulcère oesophagien après prise de florocycline. Gastroenterol Clin Biol 1983;7:324

153. Maroy B, Moullot P. Esophageal burn due to chlorazepate dipotassium (Tranxene^R). Gastrointest Endosc 1986;32:240

154. Mason SJ, O'Meara TF. Drug-induced esophagitis. J Clin Gastroenterol 1981;3:115

155. Matteo A, Eyssautier B, Rodor F, Gerolami A. Oesophagite ulcérée après prise de Selexid^R. Gastroenterol Clin Biol 1988;12:670

156. McCall AJ. Slow-K ulceration of oesophagus with aneurysmal left atrium. BMJ 1975;3:230

157. McCloy EC, Kane S. Drug-induced oesophageal ulceration. BMJ 1981;282:1703

158. McLean D. Drug-induced oesophageal ulceration. BMJ 1981;282:1975

159. Merino Angulo J, Perez de Diego I, Varas R, Casas JM. Dolor retrosternal y esofagitis inducida por doxiciclina. A proposito de dos observaciones. Rev Clin Esp 1986;179:431

160. Meyboom RHB. Slokdarmbeschadiging door doxycycline en tetracycline. Ned Tijdschr Geneeskd 1977;121:1770

161. Minocha A, Greenbaum DS. Pill-esophagitis caused by nonsteroidal antiinflammatory drugs Am J Gastroenterol 1991;86:1086

162. Mohandas KM, et al. Medication induced esophageal injury. Ind J Gastroenterol 1991;10:20

163. Morck HI, Nielsen VM, Kirkegaard P. Ulcus esophagei forarsaget af emeproniumbromid (Cetiprin). Ugeskr Laeger 1981;143:623

164. Mortimer O, Wiholm BE. Oesophageal injury associated with pivmecillinam tablets. Eur J Clin Pharmacol 1989;37:605

165. Muller, KD. Ulzerose osophitis durch doxycyclin. Z Arztl Fortbild (Jena) 1990;84:659

166. Mur Villacampa M, Guerrero Navarro L, Cabeza Lamban F. Ulcera esofagica por doxiciclina. Rev Esp Enferm Apar Dig 1989;76:67

167. Murray K. Severe dysphagia from emepronium bromide associated with oesophageal diverticulum. Br J Surg 1982;69:439

168. Naylor G, Davies MH. Oesophageal stricture associated with alendronic acid. Lancet 1996;348:1030

169. Netter P, Paille F, Trechot P, Bannwarth B, Royer RJ. Les complica-

tions oesophagiennes d'origine medicamenteuse. Therapie 1988;43: 475

170. Nwakama PE, Jenkins HJ Jr, Bailey RT Jr, Pelligrino J, DeMeester TR, Jones JB. Drug-induced esophageal injury: a case report of Percogesic. Drug Intell Clin Pharmacy 1989;23:227

171. Ollyo JB, et al. L'oesophagite medicamenteuse et ses complications. Schweiz Rundsch Med Prax 1990;79:394

172. Olovson SG, Bjorkman JA, Ek L, Havu N. The ulcerogenic effect on the esophagus of three B-adrenoceptor antagonists, investigated in a new porcine oesophagus test model. Acta Pharmacol Toxicol (Copenh) 1983;53:385

173. Olovson SG, Havu N, Regardh CG, Sandberg A. Oesophageal ulcerations and plasma levels of different alprenolol salts: potential implications for the clinic. Acta Pharmacol Toxicol (Copenh) 1986;58:55

174. O'Meara TF. A new endoscopic finding of tetracycline-induced esophageal ulcers. Gastrointest Endosc 1980;26:106

175. Oren R, Fich A. Oral contraceptive-induced esophageal ulcer. Two cases and literature review. Dig Dis Sci 1991;36:1489

176. Ovartlarnporn B, Kulwichit W, Hiranniramol S. Medication-induced esophageal injury: report of 17 cases with endoscopic documentation. Am J Gastroenterol 1991;86:748

177. Papazian A, Capron JP, Dupas JL. Doxycycline-induced esophageal ulcer. Gastrointest Endosc 1981;27:201

178. Papazian A, Descombes P, Capron JP. Oesophagite ulcérée et mycotique après prise de Physiomycine$^R$. Gastroenterol Clin Biol 1984;8: 389

179. Pemberton J. Oesophageal obstruction and ulceration caused by oral potassium therapy. Br Heart J 1970;32:267

180. Pen J, Van Meerbeeck J, Pelckmans P, Van Maercke Y. Thiazinium-induced oesophageal ulcerations. Acta Clin Belg 1986;41:278

181. Penalba C. Ulcérations oesophagiennes induites par le chlorhydrate de mexiletine. Ann Gastroenterol Hepatol (Paris) 1986;22:267

182. Penalba C, Eugene C. Oesophagite medicamenteuse due au Rhinasal. Presse Med 1983;12:1725

183. Perreard M, Klotz F. Oesophagite ulcérée après prise de spiramycine. Ann Gastroenterol Hepatol (Paris) 1989;25:313

184. Perry PA, Dean BS, Krenelok EP. Drug induced esophageal injury. Clin Toxicol 1989;27:281

185. Peters JL. Benign oesophageal stricture following oral potassium chloride therapy. Br J Surg 1976;63:698

186. Petigny A, Moulinier B. Ulcères oesophagiens après prise de doxycycline. Nouv Presse Med 1979;8:439

187. Piccione PR, Winkler WP, Baer J, Kotler DP. Pill-induced intramural esophageal hematoma. JAMA 1987;257:929

188. Pinos T, Figueras C, Mas R. Doxycycline-induced esophagitis: treatment with liquid sucralphate. Am J Gastroenterol 1990;85:902

189. Puhakka HJ. Drug-induced corrosive injury of the oesophagus. J Laryngol Otol 1978;92:927

190. Rambaud S, Elkharrat D, Gajdos P. Ulcération oesophagienne après prise d'ampicilline. Ann Med Intern (Paris) 1990;141:275

191. Riker J, Swanson M, Schweigert B. Esophageal ulceration caused by wax-matrix potassium chloride. West J Med 1978;128:542

192. Rimmer DE, Rawls DE. Improper alendronate administration and a case of pill esophagitis. Am J Gastroenterol 1996;91:2648

193. Rives JJ, Olives JP, Ghisolfi J. Oesophagite aigue medicamenteuse. Arch Fr Pediatr 1985;42:33

194. Rodino S, Sacca N, De Medici A, Giglio A. Multiple esophageal ulcerations caused by a granular formulation of aspirin. Endoscopy 1994;26:509

195. Rodrigo Moreno M, Pleguezuelo Diaz J, Esteban Carretera J, Martinez Moreno J, Ruiz Cabello Jimenez M. Ulceraciones esofagicas de origen medicamentoso. Aportacion de dos casos y descripcion de un nuevo agente etiologico. Gastroenterol Hepatol 1985;8:311

196. Rodriguez Agullo JL, Vidal Ruiz JV, Benita Leon V. Ulceras esofagicas causadas por una capsula de bromuro de pinaverium. Gastroenterol Hepatol 1983;6:362

197. Rohner HG, Berges W, Wienbeck M. Clomethiazol tablets induce ulcers in the esophagus. Z Gastroenterol 1982;20:469

198. Rose JDR, Tobin GB. Drug-induced oesophageal injury. BMJ 1980; 1:110

199. Rosenthal T, Adar R, Militianu J, Deutsch V. Esophageal ulceration and oral potassium chloride ingestion. Chest 1974;65:463

200. Rudolph R, Seggewiss H, Seckfort H. Oesophagus-ulcus durch Mexiletin. Dtsch Med Wochenschr 1983;108:1018

201. Ryan JR, McMahon FG, Akdamar K, Ertan A, Agrawal N. Mucosal

202. Sacca N, Rodino S, De Medici A, De Siena M, Giglio A. NSAIDS-induced digestive hemorrhage and esophageal pseudotumor: a case report. Endoscopy 1995;27:632

203. Sakai H, Seki H, Yoshida T, Ido K, Kimura K. Radiological study of drug-induced esophageal ulcer. Rinsho Hoshasen 1980;25:27

204. Santalla Pecina F, Gomez Huelgas R, Sanchez Robles C. Sodium meclofenamate-induced esophageal ulcerations. Am J Gastroenterol 1991;86:786

205. Santucci L, Patoia L, Fiorucci S, Farroni del Favero F, Morelli A. Oesophageal lesions during treatment with piroxicam. BMJ 1990;300: 1018

206. Scapa E, Shemesh E, Batt L. Fsophageal ulceration caused by tetracycline. Harefuah 1980;99:373

207. Schmidt-Wilcke HA. Tetracyclin-ulkus der speiserohre. Dtsch Med Wochenschr 1978;103:2053

208. Schneider R. Doxycycline esophageal ulcers. Am J Dig Dis 1977;22: 805

209. Schreiber JB, Covington JA. Aspirin-induced esophageal hemorrhage. JAMA 1988;259:1647

210. Seaman WB. The case of the antibiotic dysphagia. Hosp Pract 1979; 14:206

211. Seibert D, Al-Kawas F. Trimethoprim-sulfamethoxazole, hiccups, and esophageal ulcers. Ann Intern Med 1986;105:976

212. Semble EL, Wu WC, Castell DO. Nonsteroidal antiinflammatory drugs and esophageal injury. Semin Arthritis Rheum 1989;19:99

213. Serck-Hanssen A, Stray N. Jerntablettinduserte oesophaguslesjoner. Tidsskr Nor Laegeforen 1994;114:2129

214. Shaikh YM, Khan AH, Rao N, Rizvi IH, Hameed TA, Rana TA. Phyllocontin (theophylline) induced esophagitis. J Pakistan Med Assoc 1993;43:183

215. Shepperd HWH. Iatrogenic reflux oesophagitis. J Laryngol Otol 1977; 91:171

216. Shiff AD. Doxycycline-induced esophageal ulcers in physicians. JAMA 1986;256:1893

217. Simko V, Joseph D, Michael S. Increased risk in esophageal obstruction with slow-release medications. J Assoc Acad Minority Physicians 1997;8:38

218. Sorrentino D, Trevisi A, Bernardis V, DeBiase F, Labombarda A, Bartoli E. Esophageal ulceration due to alendronate. Endoscopy 1996; 28:529

219. Stanely AJ, Eade OE, Hardwick D. Oesophageal ulceration secondary to potassium tablets. Scot Med J 1994;39:118

220. Stillman AE, Martin RJ. Tetracycline-induced esophageal ulcerations. Arch Dermatol 1979;115:1005

221. Stricker BHCh, van Overmeeren AB, Vegter AW. Doxycycline, tabletten of capsules? Ned Tidschr Geneeskd 1982;126:2200

222. Stiris MG, Oyen D. Oesophagitis caused by oral ingestion of Aptin (alprenolol chloride) Durettes. Eur J Radiol 1982;2:38

223. Stoller JL. Oesophageal ulceration and theophylline. Lancet 1985;2: 328

224. Stricker BHC. Slokdarmbeschadiging door pinaveriumbromide. Ned Tijdschr Geneeskd 1983;127:603

225. Sugawa C, Takekuma Y, Lucas CE, Amamoto H. Bleeding esophageal ulcers caused by NSAIDs. Surg Endosc 1997;11:143

226. Suissa A, Parason M, Lachter J, Eidelman S. Penicillin VK-induced esophageal ulcerations. Am J Gastroenterol 1987;82:482

227. Sumithran E, Lim KH, Chiam HL. Atrio-oesophageal fistula complicating mitral valve disease. BMJ 1979;2:1552

228. Sutton DR, Gosnold JK. Oesophageal ulceration due to clindamycin. BMJ 1977;1:1598

229. Takehana T, et al. A case of drug-induced esophageal ulcer developed at the esophageal constriction due to the right aortic arch. Nippon Kyobu Geka Gakkai Zasshi 1992;40:1131

230. Tanaka S, Yamada A, Yoshida M, Hamano K, Endo M. Drug-induced esophageal ulcer—clinical report of 3 cases. I To Cho 1980;15:255

231. Tankurt IE, Akbaylar H, Yenicerioglu Y, Simsek I, Gonen O. Severe, long-lasting symptoms from doxycycline-induced esophageal injury. Endoscopy 1995;27:626

232. Teplick JG, Teplick SK, Ominsky SH, Haskin ME. Esophagitis caused by oral medication. Radiology 1980;134:23

233. Tobias R, Cullis S, Kottler RE, Goodman H, Marks IN, Hatfield A. Emepronium bromide-induced oesophagitis. S Afr Med J 1982;61: 368

irritant potential of a potassium-sparing diuretic and of wax-matrix potassium chloride. Clin Pharmacol Ther 1984;35:90

234. Tournier C, Lapuelle J, Gerardin A, Canard JM, Pillegand B, Claude R. Ulcères oesophagiens medicamenteux. Rev Med Limoges 1981; 12:160

235. Treille C. Ulcéres de l'oesophage secondaires à la prise d'amoxycilline (1 cas) et de mequitazine (1 cas). Acta Endosc 1985;15:41

236. Tzianetas I, Habal F, Keystone JS. Short report: severe hiccups secondary to doxycycline-induced esophagitis during treatment of malaria. Am J Trop Med Hyg 1996;54:203

237. Vazquez Valdes E, Baptista MA, Barradas Guevara MC. Ulceras esofagicas producidas por medicamentos. Informe de un paciente. Rev Gastroenterol Mex 1987;52:119

238. Viver JM, Bory F, Forne M, Garau J. Ulceraciones esofagicas medicamentosas a proposito de tres casos secundarios a ingestion de doxiciclina. An Med Interna 1986;3:600

239. Voilque G. Oesophagite stenosante apparue au cours d'accidents digestifs graves par intolerance à la sulfamethoxypyridazine. J Fr Otorhinolaryngol 1973;22:923

240. Walsh J, Kneafsey DV. Phenobarbitone induced oesophagitis. Irish Med J 1980;73:399

241. Walta DC, Giddens JD, Johnson LF, Kelley JL, Waugh DF. Localized proximal esophagitis secondary to ascorbic acid ingestion and esophageal motor disorder. Gastroenterology 1976;70:766

242. Whitney B, Croxon R. Dysphagia caused by cardiac enlargement. Clin Radiol 1972;23:147

243. Wilcox CM, Schwartz DA, Clark WS. Esophageal ulceration in human immunodeficiency virus infection. Ann Intern Med 1995;122:143

244. Williams JG. Drug-induced oesophageal injury. BMJ 1979;2:273

245. Winckler K. Tetracycline ulcers of the oesophagus. Endoscopy, histology and roentgenology in two cases, and review of the literature. Endoscopy 1981;13:225

246. Wong RKH, Kikendall JW, Dachman AH. Quinaglute-induced esophagitis mimicking an esophageal mass. Ann Intern Med 1986;105:62

247. Yamaoka K, Takenawa H, Tajiri K, Yamane M, Kadowaki K, Marumo F, Sato C. A case of esophageal perforation due to a pill-induced ulcer successfully treated with conservative measures. Am J Gastroenterol 1996;91:1044

*The Esophagus*, Third Edition,
edited by D. O. Castell and J. E. Richter.
Lippincott Williams & Wilkins, Philadelphia © 1999.

CHAPTER 33

# Esophagitis in the Immunocompromised Host

C. Mel Wilcox

With the continued advancements in and broadening applications of transplantation coupled with the acquired immune deficiency (AIDS) pandemic, esophageal infections continue to be an important clinical problem. Before the 1960s, esophageal infections were uncommon and most often identified at autopsy [172]. The frequency of esophageal infections burgeoned in the 1970s and 1980s as the armamentarium of immunosuppressive therapies expanded, corticosteroids became more widely utilized, and organ transplantation began to flourish. The development of fiberoptic endoscopes coincided with these medical advancements such that the esophagus could now be directly visualized and biopsied. However, more recently, there appears to be a reversal in the growing prevalence of esophageal infections. For example, in patients undergoing transplantation, the prevalence of pathogens as well as incidence of esophagitis have been evolving due to the widespread administration of antimicrobial prophylaxis, which includes the use of strategies to prevent cytomegalovirus (CMV) disease [48, 102]. Likewise, the routine use of antimicrobial prophylaxis for *Pneumocystis carinii* pneumonia has altered the spectrum of infections seen in AIDS [5, 131]. Esophageal infections were a very common complication of AIDS; however, since the release of the protease inhibitors in 1995 and widespread use of effective combination antiretroviral therapies, there has been an overall reduction in opportunistic infections including those involving the esophagus [16].

Given the efficacy of therapies for virtually all esophageal infections, timely and accurate diagnosis is essential. This chapter will focus on esophagitis in the immunocompromised host and review epidemiology, pathology, presentation, diagnosis, and therapy for specific infections. Esophageal infections occurring in the normal host will be briefly discussed. Selected esophageal disorders associated with human immunodeficiency virus (HIV) infection and AIDS will also be reviewed.

## EPIDEMIOLOGY

Given the refinements in immunosuppressive therapy and overall management of the transplant patient as well as the treatment of HIV infection, the epidemiology of esophageal infections is rapidly changing. Much of the early data on the etiology and prevalence of esophageal infections were acquired from retrospective autopsy and radiographic series. Studies performed in the 1970s and 1980s which documented the incidence of esophageal infections following transplantation are now largely outdated because of improvements in management. Similarly, the high incidence of esophageal infections previously documented in patients with AIDS, including those caused by *Candida,* is now inaccurate since the release of the protease inhibitors [16].

Primary esophageal infection is rare in an otherwise *normal person* in whom no permissive factor is present. In this setting, the most common pathogen is herpes simplex virus (HSV) [35, 142], although candidiasis may be observed in elderly patients without any predisposing factors [35]. Almost uniformly, immunocompetent patients who develop esophageal infection have conditions that either weaken esophageal defense mechanisms or alter esophageal flora such as disorders of esophageal emptying (achalasia, diverticula) or treatment with broad-spectrum antimicrobial agents.

Esophageal infection following *solid organ transplantation* is usually due to *Candida* or herpes viruses (CMV, HSV) with an equal frequency of HSV and CMV disease [2, 6]; coinfections have been described. Autopsy series suggest a high prevalence of unsuspected viral-associated esophagitis in transplant patients. The causes of esophageal infection following *bone marrow transplantation* are generally similar to other transplant patients [93, 152]. It is likely that the prevalence of esophageal infection in all transplant patients will continue to decline as immunosuppressive therapy becomes more targeted [49].

C. M. Wilcox: Department of Medicine, University of Alabama at Birmingham, and Division of Gastroenterology, University Hospital, Birmingham, Alabama 35294-0007.

*Candida* is the most common cause of esophageal infection associated with malnutrition, broad-spectrum antibiotics, and corticosteroids, both inhaled and ingested. Patients with *cancer* as well as *lymphoproliferative diseases* are well recognized to develop esophageal infections following chemotherapy, but *Candida* and viral esophagitis may also occur prior to such treatment.

Esophageal infections are common gastrointestinal complications of HIV infection, but as mentioned above, the efficacy of highly active antiretroviral therapy has resulted in an impressive reduction in the incidence of all opportunistic infections including those of the esophagus [16]. Before the development of these antiretroviral regimens and the widespread use of antifungal medications, prospective series of symptomatic patients found that *Candida* esophagitis was the most frequent cause of disease, seen in approximately 50% of patients [14, 31, 166]. Coinfections of *Candida* and viruses are common [157]. In contrast to other immunocompromised hosts, HSV esophagitis is less frequent than CMV esophagitis [162]. Furthermore, HIV-infected patients are susceptible to a number of other unusual pathogens which cause esophagitis, and these patients are commonly affected by the idiopathic esophageal ulcer (see below).

## PREDISPOSING FACTORS

Esophageal infections result from alterations in the normal esophageal flora, or, more commonly, humoral or cellular immune dysfunction. Numerous conditions are associated with immune dysfunction which leads to infections, including diabetes mellitus, alcoholism, malnutrition, malignancies, and advanced age. In diabetes mellitus, hyperglycemia and ketoacidosis impair granulocyte function. Corticosteroids have many deleterious effects on the immune system which result in both lymphocyte and granulocyte dysfunction. Mucosal disruption of the oropharynx and esophagus commonly follows chemotherapy or radiation therapy, providing a portal of entry for pathogens. Depending on the specific type, transplantation predisposes to infection through both qualitative and quantitative effects on B and T cells due to immunosuppressive agents, chemotherapy, and neutropenia. Episodes of rejection in solid organ transplant recipients and graft versus host disease following allogeneic bone marrow transplantation are frequently complicated by infection, because these patients require further immune suppression. Broad-spectrum antibiotics, antiacid therapy, as well as surgical trauma further predispose to esophageal infections in the immunocompromised host.

Infection following solid organ transplantation has a relatively predictable time course [126]. Bacterial and fungal infections are most common during the initial months after transplantation, because it is during this period that granulocyte number and/or function are most compromised. Herpes simplex virus infection also tends to occur early after transplantation due to reactivation of disease, whereas CMV typically presents 2 to 6 months following transplantation at a time when neutropenia is common and T-cell function is most impaired. In HIV-infected patients, opportunistic infections reflect severe immunodeficiency; esophageal infections usually become clinically manifest when the CD4 lymphocyte count falls below 200/mm$^3$, with most occurring below 100/mm$^3$ [5, 9].

## GENERAL CONSIDERATIONS

A number of factors guide the approach to the immunosuppressed patients with suspected esophageal infection. Given the breadth of the potential causes of infection (Table 33–1), the differential diagnosis should be based on the cause, severity and timing of immunodeficiency, character of esophageal complaints, and findings on physical examination, particularly of the oropharynx. In HIV-infected patients, the absolute value of the CD4 lymphocyte count is essential for developing a differential diagnosis. Odynophagia is the most common presenting symptom of esophageal infection, and disorders resulting in esophageal ulceration almost uniformly cause odynophagia. Dysphagia may be observed with esophageal infections, especially *Candida* esophagitis, or may represent esophageal obstruction or dysmotility from some other cause. Bleeding may be the initial manifestation of esophageal ulceration especially when there is an associated coagulopathy. Oropharyngeal candidiasis is commonly associated with esophageal candidiasis [92, 163, 166]. However, the presence of oropharyngeal candidiasis does not prove *Candida* is the only cause of symptoms, nor does the absence of oropharyngeal candidiasis exclude *Candida* esophagitis. Coexistent oropharyngeal ulceration is common in patients with HSV esophagitis but is rarely observed in patients with CMV esophagitis [6, 163]. In patients

**TABLE 33–1.** *Reported etiologies of esophageal infections*[a]

| Fungal | Viral | Bacterial | Mycobacterial | Parasitic |
|---|---|---|---|---|
| *Candida* sp. | CMV | Oral flora | TB | *Cryptosporidia* |
| *Histoplasma* | HSV | *Nocardia* | MAC | *Pneumocystis* |
| *Blastomycosis* | EBV | *Actinomyces* | | *Leishmania* |
| *Mucormycosis* | HPV | *Bartonella* | | *Trympanosoma* |
| *Aspergillus* | Varicella | | | |

[a] CMV, Cytomegalovirus; HSV, herpes simplex virus; EBV, Epstein-Barr virus; HPV, human papilloma virus; TB, tuberculosis; MAC, *Mycobacterium avium* complex.

with AIDS, multiple coexisting esophageal disorders are frequent, which further complicates management.

Documentation of an infectious agent in tissue biopsies is the most specific means of diagnosis. Although barium radiography may suggest infectious esophagitis, rarely will these studies be definitive. Likewise, the clinical presentation may favor an infectious esophagitis, but the specific etiology can rarely be determined by history and physical examination alone.

At the time of endoscopy, the characteristics of the esophageal lesion(s) will provide diagnostic clues. The location, size, and appearance of all endoscopic abnormalities should be documented, because these features form the basis of the differential diagnosis and are useful for comparison on follow-up endoscopic examinations. The differential diagnosis of the lesion will also impact on the methods for acquiring biopsy samples and recommendations for diagnostic testing on the biopsy specimens. Additional stains for pathogens may be required based on the suspected cause clinically, endoscopically, and pathologically, thereby necessitating close collaboration with the pathologist to accurately diagnose these infections. Because most esophageal infections can be diagnosed on tissue biopsy alone, multiple biopsies should be performed of endoscopic abnormalities to increase diagnostic yield. Esophageal brushings with cytologic evaluation may be diagnostically helpful in certain diseases such as those due to Candida and HSV. Viral culture of biopsy specimens may increase the diagnostic yield, although false positives occur. Serologic testing plays no significant role in the diagnosis of acute infectious esophagitis.

## FUNGAL INFECTIONS

### Candida Species

#### Epidemiology

Candida species are the most frequent esophageal pathogens. Although Candida albicans is most common, other reported species include C. dublenis, C. tropicalis, C. parapsilosis, and C. glabrata. Conditions predisposing to Candida esophagitis in the normal host include antibiotics, inhaled or ingested corticosteroids, antiacid therapy or hypochlorhydric states, diabetes mellitus, alcoholism, malnutrition, old age, head and neck radiotherapy, and esophageal motility disturbances. Alterations in cellular immunity lead to candidal colonization and superficial infection, whereas humoral immunity (granulocytes) prevents invasive disease and dissemination. Chronic mucocutaneous candidiasis, a congenital immunodeficiency, may also be complicated by Candida esophagitis. As stated above, the use of immunosuppressive regimens (i.e., cyclosporine) which better target the immune system combined with prophylactic antifungal therapy has reduced the incidence of candidal infections following solid organ and bone marrow transplantation [71, 102, 138]. The incidence of Candida esophagitis in transplant patients administered prophylactic oral nystatin or azole therapy is less than 5% [45].

### Pathology

The gross pathologic appearance of esophageal candidiasis ranges from a few white or yellow plaques on the mucosal surface to a dense, thick plaque coating the mucosa and encroaching on the esophageal lumen. Although occasionally misinterpreted as "ulcer," this plaque material is composed of desquamated squamous epithelial cells, admixed with fungal organisms, inflammatory cells, and bacteria [160]. True ulceration (granulation tissue) is rarely caused by Candida alone, and has been documented most commonly in immunosuppressed patients with profound granulocytopenia or when Candida is a coinfection with another cause of ulceration [38].

### Clinical Manifestations

Although esophageal candidiasis may be an incidental finding in an asymptomatic patient, the usual clinical presentation is odynophagia with dysphagia [92, 166] (Table 33–2). Symptoms are variable in severity ranging from mild difficulty with swallowing to severe pain resulting in an inability to eat and secondary dehydration. When odynophagia is very severe, however, one must always consider causes other than Candida or coinfections, particularly in patients with AIDS.

Physical examination may be helpful in suggesting the diagnosis. Approximately two-thirds of patients with AIDS and esophageal candidiasis have oral candidiasis (thrush) [92, 163]. In other immunocompromised patients, oropharyngeal candidiasis is also commonly associated with esophageal candidiasis [6]. It should be noted, however, that thrush may be absent if antifungal therapy, such as nystatin, is administered. Patients with chronic mucocutaneous candidiasis may have fungal involvement of various mucous membranes, hair, nails, and skin with a history of adrenal or parathyroid dysfunction.

### Complications

Complications from esophageal candidiasis are rare. Hemorrhage may occur when the disease is severe (erosion/ulcer) and there is an associated coagulopathy. Lumenal ob-

**TABLE 33–2.** *Presentations and complications of esophageal infections*

|  | Common | Uncommon |
|---|---|---|
| *Candida* sp. | Dysphagia, odynophagia | Bleeding, chest pain |
| Other fungi | Dysphagia, odynophagia | Fistula |
| Viral | Odynophagia, chest pain | Fever, bleeding |
| Mycobacterial | Odynophagia, dysphagia, fever | Fistula |
| Bacterial | Odynophagia, fever | Dissemination |
| Parasitic | Odynophagia | — |

struction secondary to a mycetoma, fibrosis and stricture formation, and fistulization into the bronchial tree have been described [86, 112, 133], but these lesions probably represent *Candida* colonization of anatomic abnormalities caused by other underlying disorders or unrecognized coinfections.

### Diagnosis

Esophageal candidiasis should be suspected in any patient at risk for esophageal infection, especially the immunocompromised patient, who complains of dysphagia or odynophagia. The presence of thrush further supports this diagnosis, but the absence of thrush does not exclude esophageal disease. Prior to the development of endoscopy, radiographic examination (barium esophagram) was used to evaluate the symptomatic patient. The most characteristic radiographic feature of *Candida* esophagitis is the appearance of diffuse plaquelike lesions usually in a linear configuration. With disease progression, these plaques become confluent causing a ''shaggy'' appearance of the esophagus often described as ulcerations [83, 125, 133] (Fig. 33–1). Additional radio-

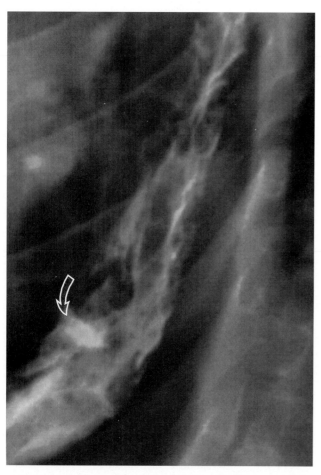

**FIG. 33–1.** *Candida* and cytomegalovirus (CMV) esophagitis. Diffuse irregularity of the proximal esophagus due to extensive candidal plaques in a patient with acquired immune deficiency (AIDS). A well-circumscribed ulcer is present in the distal esophagus (*arrow*), which was caused by coinfection with CMV.

**TABLE 33–3.** *Pathologic findings of esophageal infections[a]*

| | Common | Uncommon |
|---|---|---|
| *Candida* | Plaques | Ulcer (rare) |
| Other fungi | Plaques, ulcer | Fistula |
| Viral | Ulcer | Mass lesions; nodules[b] |
| Mycobacteria | | |
| TB | Ulcer, fistula | Mass lesions |
| MAC | Ulcer | |
| Bacteria | Ulcer, plaques | — |
| Parasites | Plaque, ulcer | — |

[a] TB, *Mycobacterium tuberculosis;* MAC, *Mycobacterium avium* complex.
[b] Human papilloma virus.

graphic findings which have been reported include pseudo-membranes, cobblestoning, polypoid nodules, fungus balls, strictures, esophagopulmonary fistulas, mucosal bridges, or large neoplastic-appearing esophageal ulcers and masses [38, 83, 86, 112, 125, 133]. A large, well-circumscribed ulceration should not be attributed to *Candida.* Importantly, a normal barium esophagram does not exclude esophageal candidiasis. In any patient, the presence of severe odynophagia limits the ability to drink barium, thereby hampering the utility of barium studies.

Cytology brush and balloon devices which do not require endoscopy have been developed for the rapid diagnosis of esophageal infections. These may be placed easily through the nares or mouth, and the material obtained on the brush or balloon after it is withdrawn through the esophagus is then evaluated cytologically and cultured. These devices have been tested primarily in HIV-infected patients, and when compared to endoscopy, they have been found to be sensitive for the diagnosis of *Candida,* less sensitive for the detection of HSV, and unreliable for CMV [15]. Nevertheless, in HIV-infected patients, the frequency of esophageal coinfections and the idiopathic esophageal ulcer (see below) have limited wide acceptance of these techniques.

Endoscopic examination of the esophagus is the most sensitive and specific method of diagnosing esophageal candidiasis (Table 33–3). The gross endoscopic appearance of *Candida* esophagitis is pathognomonic and may be graded according to recently published criteria [160]. During endoscopy, mucosal lesions can be brushed and submitted for cytologic evaluation or biopsied for histologic diagnosis. When ulceration is identified endoscopically, multiple biopsies should be performed of the ulcer to exclude coexisting disorders. The use of periodic acid-Schiff or Gomori methenamine silver stains help highlight the organisms. Cytologic examination of esophageal brushings is more sensitive than histologic examination of biopsy specimens in mild superficial candidiasis (i.e., grades 1 and 2) because organisms may be washed off tissue surfaces during processing of biopsy specimens [59]. Rarely, positive cytology but negative histology indicates colonization rather than infection. Skin testing and serologic tests for candidiasis are not useful for the diagnosis of *Candida* esophagitis.

In patients with AIDS and thrush, the presence of dysphagia and/or odynophagia usually indicates *Candida* esophagitis [30, 166]. Given the prevalence of *Candida* esophagitis in AIDS, in the symptomatic patient with associated thrush an empirical trial of antifungal therapy should be instituted, reserving endoscopy for those patients who fail to respond. Further evaluation should be delayed no longer than 1 week for patients with severe persistent symptoms since the response to antifungal therapy is rapid, with clinical improvement occurring in the majority of patients within days [67, 156, 166]. If patients fail to improve with empirical antifungal therapy, endoscopy should be performed since disorders other than *Candida* are identified in most patients [167]. This empirical strategy has not been critically studied in the transplant setting, yet clinical experience suggests it to be effective.

### Treatment

A number of highly effective oral and intravenous medications are available for the treatment of *Candida* esophagitis (Table 33–4). In general, oral therapies should be initiated first, reserving intravenous treatment for refractory disease or when there are contraindications to orally administered medication. Although candidal species other than *C. albicans* cause esophagitis, speciation is not widely employed, as reliable culturing and sensitivity testing are lacking at most centers and the treatment is the same. For patients with mild disease, minimal immunocompromise, and/or readily reversible immunodeficiency, an abbreviated course of therapy with an oral azole should be given. Immunocompromised transplant patients and AIDS patients with *Candida* esophagitis are best treated with systemically active agents

(azoles). In addition, patients with granulocytopenia are at significant risk for disseminated candidal infection, warranting the use of systemically acting agents. Drug interactions must always be kept in mind particularly in transplant patients.

Orally administered systemically active agents, all of which have efficacy for the treatment of *Candida* esophagitis, include ketoconazole (Nizoral), fluconazole (Diflucan), and itraconazole (Sporanox). These agents, like other azoles, alter fungal cell membrane permeability by cytochrome P-450-dependent interference with ergosterol biosynthesis, resulting in fungal cell injury and death. The newer triazoles (itraconazole and fluconazole) have greater affinity then the imidazoles (miconazole and ketoconazole) for fungal P-450 enzymes [29]. Although other agents such as clotrimazole and nystatin are effective for oral candidiasis and provide prophylaxis against esophageal involvement [117, 134], they are significantly less effective than azoles as primary therapy for esophageal candidiasis.

Ketoconazole therapy (200 to 400 mg per day) requires an acid milieu for optimal absorption, which limits its use in many patients [148]. For example, 10% to 25% of patients with AIDS have reduced gastric acid secretion, which will decrease absorption and thereby impair the efficacy of this agent [12, 78, 155]. Itraconazole absorption is also reduced by an increasing gastric pH [89]. Both ketoconazole and itraconazole are extensively metabolized in the liver and excreted in the bile. The half-life of these two agents is 7 to 10 and 24 to 42 hours, respectively [29]. Dose adjustments are not required for the patient with renal failure.

Randomized studies of patients with AIDS suggest that fluconazole (100 mg per day) has significantly greater efficacy than ketoconazole (200 mg per day) for the treatment of *Candida* esophagitis [77]. A randomized trial of over 2,000 AIDS patients which compared fluconazole to itraconazole

**TABLE 33–4.** *Recommended treatment regimens for esophageal infections[a]*

| Pathogen | Drug | Dosage | Route | Duration | Efficacy (%) |
|---|---|---|---|---|---|
| *Candida* | Ketoconazole | 200–400 mg/d | PO | 7–14 d | <80 |
| | Fluconazole | 100 mg/d | PO/IV | 7–14 d | ~80 |
| | Itraconazole | 200 mg/d | PO | 7–14 d | ~80 |
| | Amphotericin B | 0.5 mg/kg/d | PO/IV | 7 d | >95 |
| *Histoplasma* | Amphotericin B | — | IV | — | >90 |
| | Ketoconazole | | | | |
| Other fungi | Amphotericin B | | | | |
| CMV | Ganciclovir | 5 mg/kg b.i.d. | IV | 2–4 wk | ~75 |
| | Foscarnet | 90 mg/kg b.i.d. | IV | 2–4 wk | ~75 |
| HSV | Acyclovir | 400 mg 5×/d | PO/IV | 14 d | >90 |
| | Valacyclovir | 1 gm t.i.d. | PO | 14 d | >90 |
| | Famciclovir | 500 mg t.i.d. | PO | 14 d | >90 |
| | Foscarnet | 90 mg/kg b.i.d. | IV | 14 d | >95 |
| | Ganciclovir | 5 mg/kg b.i.d. | IV | 14 d | >95 |
| Mycobacteria | Sames as for pulmonary disease | | | | |
| Bacteria | Based on infecting species | | | | |
| Idiopathic ulcer | Prednisone | 40 mg/d taper | PO | 4 wk | >90 |
| | Thalidomide | 200–300 mg/d | PO | 4 wk | >90 |

[a] CMV, Cytomegalovirus; HSV, herpes simplex virus; b.i.d., twice a day; t.i.d., three times a day.

also found fluconazole to be the superior agent [8]. Unlike ketoconazole and itraconazole, fluconazole is highly water soluble, is minimally protein bound or metabolized, and is excreted unchanged in the urine. The half-life of fluconazole is approximately 30 hours if renal function is normal, and the presence of food or hypochlorhydria does not alter absorption. Fluconazole is available in oral and intravenous preparations, and both fluconazole and itraconazole are also now available in oral solutions. These oral solutions are as effective as pills, likely due to an enhanced local effect and/ or improved absorption [76, 169].

Adverse effects of ketoconazole, fluconazole, and itraconazole are primarily dose dependent and include nausea, hepatotoxicity, and inhibition of steroid production and cyclosporine metabolism [29]. Ketoconazole can cause fatal hepatitis, although this is rare with the triazoles [87]. Minor increases in aminotransferases are common with these three agents, but rarely warrant drug discontinuation. Reversible inhibition of gonadal and adrenal steroid synthesis by ketoconazole may occur with doses equal to or greater than 400 mg per day [140], whereas in recommended doses, fluconazole and itraconazole do not affect steroidogenesis. Due to the effects on hepatic microsomal enzymes, all three azoles inhibit the metabolism of cyclosporine, potentially resulting in an increase in cyclosporine blood levels; this effect is most pronounced with ketoconazole [29]. In standard doses, however, fluconazole has no significant effect on cyclosporine metabolism. A number of other important drug interactions have been noted with these agents, although these tend to be more common with ketoconazole.

The other major family of antifungal agents is made up of the polyene antibiotics, represented by amphotericin and nystatin. These agents bind irreversibly to sterols in fungal cell membranes, thereby altering the permeability characteristics of the membrane and causing cell death. Nystatin is effective for treating thrush, but less so for esophageal disease. The efficacy, safety, and ease of administration of azoles have therefore made nystatin a second-line agent. Although amphotericin B (Fungizone) is the most effective agent for systemic mycoses, its severe side effects in conjunction with the availability of azoles have limited its use for the treatment of esophageal candidiasis. When there is resistance to treatment with fluconazole or other azoles, low doses of intravenous amphotericin B (10 to 20 mg daily) are effective. Renal toxicity, which is usually reversible, is the most serious adverse effect of continued use of amphotericin B and can be troublesome in patients receiving cyclosporine. The total dose of amphotericin B for the treatment of esophageal candidiasis is approximately 100 to 200 mg. This agent is also now available in an oral solution for the treatment of thrush.

Flucytosine (Ancobon) is a fluorinated pyrimidine with a narrow spectrum of antifungal activity that acts by interfering with fungal translation of RNA. This oral agent, which is rarely used today, can be combined with amphotericin B, but it should not be used alone because fungi rapidly become resistant. As such, flucytosine monotherapy (50 to 150 mg per kg per day taken every 6 hours) is only modestly effective [7]. Trials evaluating its efficacy in combination with amphotericin B or azole agents are lacking.

### Prophylaxis

The prophylactic use of ketoconazole or nystatin for esophageal candidiasis in cancer and transplant patients has yielded mixed results [71, 93]. Although the frequency of candidal infections is generally reduced, other mycoses still occur, and reductions in mortality have been difficult to establish. The use of azole prophylaxis in transplant patients may also be problematic in those receiving cyclosporine. Low doses of intravenous amphotericin B have been used successfully for prophylaxis in high-risk patients [62]. Although effective [119], primary prophylaxis against oropharyngeal and esophageal candidiasis is not recommended for patients with AIDS [64].

### Drug Resistance

Because of widespread use, azole resistance has become an important clinical problem especially in HIV-infected patients. Both the cumulative dose of azole and severe immunodeficiency have been shown to be highly associated with the development of resistance [94, 124], and clinical resistance correlates with in vitro resistance. Prophylactic fluconazole has similarly been associated with resistance in transplant patients. When resistance occurs, increasing the dose of azole is often helpful. If higher doses fail, switching to another azole or use of an oral solution such as itraconazole [22] may be tried, but higher doses are often necessary because of cross-resistance [21]. Intravenous amphotericin B is usually required when high-dose (greater than 400 mg per day fluconazole) therapy fails, achieving a high response rate. Resistance to amphotericin is rare. With the availability of effective therapy for HIV infection, the current focus in these patients is on improving immune function to treat resistant candidal infections.

## Other Fungi

### Epidemiology

Esophageal involvement with other fungi is rare [27, 28, 44, 53, 55, 95, 96, 90, 100, 104, 105, 107, 174] and results from contiguously infected mediastinal lymph nodes, pulmonary parenchymal infection, primary esophageal disease, or widespread dissemination. Most instances of histoplasmosis and blastomycosis esophagitis represent secondary esophageal involvement from mediastinal lymph nodes rather than primary esophageal infection [53, 96]. Although no particular geographic distribution within the United States has been reported for aspergillosis, blastomycosis, or mucormycosis, histoplasmosis is endemic in the midwestern states and Mississippi Valley. *Aspergillus,* principally a lung pathogen, has been reported to involve the esophagus in patients with leukemia and profound neutropenia [105, 174] and after bone marrow transplantation [28]; contiguous pulmonary disease is usually present. Mucormycosis has been reported to involve the esophagus in a patient with AIDS [107], and only a few cases have been described in other immunocompromised patients [95].

### Pathology, Clinical Manifestations, and Complications

Other than the development of fistula, there are no unique pathologic features for these fungi (Table 33–3). The principal clinical manifestation is usually odynophagia and/or dysphagia, and as such is nonspecific. Pulmonary symptoms may predominate when there is fistula formation to the tracheobronchial tree or coexistent pulmonary involvement. Histoplasmosis and blastomycosis are more likely to cause focal lesions as a consequence of extension from mediastinal lymph nodes, but multiple lesions can occur during the course of dissemination [44]. Other sites of gastrointestinal involvement are common with disseminated histoplasmosis in immunocompromised patients [96]. Massive bleeding can result if there is fistulization to the aorta or heart, or with large ulceration(s) [100, 105]. Invasion of blood vessels is common with mucormycosis [107]. Perforation has been reported with esophageal aspergillosis [174].

### Diagnosis

Histoplasmosis should be considered in the endemic areas or in patients who have previously resided in these regions especially if extraesophageal manifestations such as hilar adenopathy, calcification or atelectasis of adjacent pulmonary tissue, or splenic calcification are present. Esophageal blastomycosis should be considered in patients with skin involvement and dysphagia; pulmonary disease may be present.

Recognition of these fungi depends on appropriate staining of endoscopic biopsy specimens with the identification of the characteristic fungal elements. Barium esophagram or endoscopy may show changes suggestive of *Candida* [104], malignancy [55, 99], extrinsic compression due to lymph nodes usually in the region of the carina, or ulcer with or without fistula. Ulcerative lesions, which may be extensive, are common with all these fungi. Chest radiography may demonstrate acute or chronic pulmonary parenchymal changes which frequently coexist in patients with esophageal histoplasmosis and aspergillosis. Calcification of mediastinal lymph nodes is typical for *Histoplasma.* Endoscopy with biopsies and histologic examination (with cytologic brushings) may establish the diagnosis if the pathologist is able to differentiate the septate hyphae of *Aspergillus* species from the pseudohyphae of *Candida* species. Other fungi can be suggested by their appearance on staining of esophageal biopsies. Culture of biopsy material using fungal media can be diagnostic. Because *Histoplasma capsulatum* does not generally invade the esophageal mucosa and fibrosis is often marked, endoscopic brushings or biopsies are often nondiagnostic, thereby requiring thoractomy or thoracoscopy [96]. Serologic tests are not useful because of the high prevalence of positive results in endemic areas. Recently, a urine antigen test has been developed which is highly specific for disseminated histoplasmosis.

### Treatment

Although in the normal host pulmonary histoplasmosis may spontaneously resolve, therapy is required in those who are immunocompromised or when there is extrapulmonary disease. Ketoconazole, itraconazole, and amphotericin B are effective against histoplasmosis and blastomycosis [29]. Because of the toxicity associated with amphotericin, this agent should probably be reserved for severe infections or in cases of failure of ketoconazole therapy. Systemic aspergillosis should be treated with high-dose amphotericin B, although itraconazole has significant *in vitro* activity. Surgery may be required for drainage of abscesses or excision of fistulas. Amphotericin should be administered with mucormycosis, although surgical debridement may be required.

## VIRAL INFECTIONS

Since the implementation of *Candida* prophylaxis in selected patients undergoing transplantation and the widespread use of oral antifungal therapies in AIDS, viral esophagitis has assumed more etiologic importance. Nevertheless, in the transplant setting, the incidence of clinically apparent viral esophageal disease has been falling. One explanation for the decrease in herpetic esophagitis in the transplant patient is the frequent use of HSV prophylaxis. The incidence of CMV disease has also decreased with the use of CMV-seronegative organs and blood products for seronegative recipients, use of leukocyte-depleted platelets for patients following bone marrow transplantation, and the administration of preemptive ganciclovir for high-risk transplant patients [48, 102]. Without antiviral prophylaxis, viral esophagitis is more common in bone marrow than solid organ transplant recipients because of the greater degree of immunosuppression required for these patients.

### Herpes Simplex Virus

#### Epidemiology

Herpes simplex virus type 1 is one of three herpes viruses that affect the esophagus, the others being CMV and varicella-zoster virus. Herpes simplex virus type 2 rarely involves the esophagus. After *Candida* species, HSV is the next most frequent agent that causes infectious esophagitis. Although well recognized as an esophageal pathogen in otherwise healthy people [10, 35, 63, 113, 142], HSV esophagitis occurs most often in patients with some predisposing factor(s). Following transplantation, HSV and CMV occur with equal frequency as causes of esophagitis [2, 98], whereas in patients with AIDS, HSV esophagitis is relatively uncommon and much less frequent than CMV [162]. In a study of 100 HIV-infected patients with esophageal ulcer, HSV was only found in nine, in four of whom it was a copathogen with CMV (19).

### Pathology

HSV infection is generally limited to squamous mucosa, where the earliest manifestation is a vesicle. As these vesicles enlarge and ulcerate, they coalesce to form larger lesions, and the intervening mucosa between these lesions is often normal [106]. The ulcerative process is uniformly superficial [103, 106]. Microscopic examination of the squamous epithelial cells at the ulcer edge reveals multinucleation, ground-glass nuclei, and eosinophilic Cowdry's type A inclusion bodies that may take up half of the nuclear volume. Over time, these inclusion bodies may be surrounded by haloes, become more basophilic, filling, enlarging, and deforming the nucleus [106, 114].

### Clinical Manifestations and Complications

HSV esophageal infection commonly presents with the sudden onset of severe odynophagia or chest pain. Autopsy studies, however, suggest that esophageal symptoms are absent in many patients [18]. Herpes labialis (i.e., cold sores) and oropharyngeal ulcers may coexist, antedate, or develop during the esophageal infection, whereas skin infection is rare [6, 163]. Low-grade fever or symptoms of an upper respiratory infection may be observed. In untreated immunocompetent persons, spontaneous resolution of HSV esophageal infection occurs within 2 weeks of the onset of symptoms [10, 63, 113, 137]. Complications are rare and include bleeding [19, 123], perforation [32, 136], tracheoesophageal fistula in association with other pathogens [109], or dissemination [18].

### Diagnosis

Esophageal disease caused by HSV appears in barium radiographic studies as focal ulceration on a background of normal mucosa; vesicles are infrequently observed. These ulcers have been described as stellate or volcano-like in appearance often with a thin halo of edema at the margin [84, 137, 173]. There is less propensity to form the longitudinal or linear lesions that are commonly seen in CMV infection [84]. Severe, diffuse herpetic esophagitis may result in a cobblestone or ''shaggy'' mucosal appearance resembling

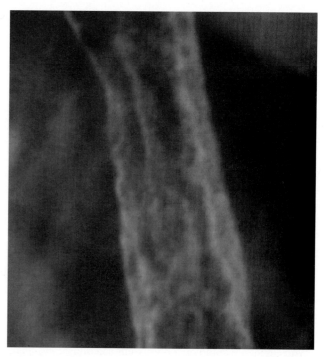

**FIG. 33–2.** Herpes simplex virus esophagitis. Diffuse irregularity of the mucosa in the midesophagus in a patient following renal transplantation.

*Candida* esophagitis [82] (Fig. 32–2). Although the radiographic appearance may be suggestive, definitive diagnosis of herpetic esophagitis requires endoscopic mucosal biopsies. The endoscopic characteristics of herpetic esophagitis reflect the pathologic changes (Table 33–3), appearing as discrete, usually small (less than 2 cm), well-circumscribed shallow ulcers [1, 97], a diffuse erosive esophagitis, or rarely vesicles. Small scattered lesions covered with exudate mimic esophageal candidiasis. Deep ulcers, as seen with CMV, are very rare. Cytologic brushings [88] and endoscopic mucosal biopsies should be taken from the ulcer edge, as the viral cytopathic effect is best identified in epithelial cells rather than granulation tissue in the ulcer bed. Immunohistochemical staining on biopsy samples using specific monoclonal antibodies to HSV will help confirm the diagnosis when the viral cytopathic effect is difficult to appreciate. Viral culture of biopsy specimens helps establish a definitive diagnosis. As with other etiologies of infectious esophagitis, serologic tests play no role in establishing the diagnosis.

### Treatment

A number of uncontrolled trials and vast clinical experience in both immunocompetent and immunodeficient patients suggest the efficacy of acyclovir (Zovirax), a nucleoside analog, for the therapy of esophageal disease. In the largest study, which evaluated 34 patients with AIDS and HSV esophagitis, a clinical response was seen in essentially all treated patients [66]. Although spontaneous resolution of

HSV esophagitis is common in the normal host, acyclovir therapy is usually instituted regardless of immune status because of its safety and efficacy. When oral intake is hampered by severe odynophagia or when there is a question of drug absorption, intravenous administration is required. Side effects of intravenous acyclovir therapy are few and appear limited to irritation of veins used for drug infusion and rash. Although rare, resistance should be suspected when there is clinical failure of acyclovir; in this setting, foscarnet (Table 33–4) is the drug of choice and will lead to clinical cure in most patients [26, 40]. Acyclovir is effective prophylaxis for HSV-antibody-positive patients undergoing transplantation [102]. Long-term secondary prophylaxis should be considered when immunodeficiency persists because the relapse rate is high. More recently, valacyclovir, a prodrug of acyclovir, and famciclovir have been released. The advantage of these agents over acyclovir is that they can be administered three times per day at an equivalent cost. Large studies evaluating the use of these new agents for esophagitis are lacking, but trials in genital disease suggest equivalence to acyclovir [143].

## Cytomegalovirus

### Epidemiology

Until the last several decades, CMV was a rare cause of disease. Currently, CMV is regarded as one of the most common opportunistic infections. In contrast to HSV, CMV esophagitis has very rarely been documented in normal individuals [4, 17, 150]. Studies from developed countries have shown seropositivity rates of 50% or greater, and up to 90% seropositivity has been found in homosexual men, reflecting sexual transmission of the virus [135]. In transplant patients who receive no antiviral prophylaxis, CMV and HSV are equally common esophageal pathogens [2, 98]. As mentioned above, CMV is the most frequent cause of esophageal ulcer in patients with AIDS, comprising greater than 50% of esophageal ulcers in these patients [162].

### Pathology

The histologic hallmark of CMV esophagitis is mucosal ulceration (Table 33–3). Although variable, deep ulcers are very characteristic for disease in AIDS, whereas in other immunocompromised patients, lesions tend to remain more superficial. In contrast to HSV, the viral cytopathic effect of CMV is located in endothelial and mesenchymal cells in the granulation tissue of the ulcer base rather than squamous cells. Inclusions are large (cytomegalo) and often have an eosinophilic appearance which may be located either in the nucleus or cytoplasm [47]. Because these inclusions can appear atypical, especially in patients with AIDS [129], immunohistochemical stains play a valuable role in confirming the presence of CMV and often highlight more infected cells than are appreciated by routine hematoxylin and eosin stain-

ing. As with other esophageal infections, CMV may coexist with HSV or Candida especially in patients with AIDS [157, 162, 166]. The pathogenesis of disease caused by CMV is not well understood. Mucosal ischemia has been hypothesized as the etiologic mechanism given the involvement of endothelial cells [47]. More recently, however, high mucosal concentration of tumor necrosis factor-$\alpha$ has been found in association with CMV esophagitis, which falls after ganciclovir treatment and ulcer healing, suggesting an etiologic role for this proinflammatory cytokine [170].

### Clinical Manifestations and Complications

Odynophagia is almost uniformly present and is typically severe (Table 33–2). Chest pain, weight loss, and fever may be reported. The onset of symptoms is often more subacute than the acute presentation of HSV. A prior or coexistent diagnosis of CMV infection in another organs (e.g., retinitis or colitis) is not infrequent. Although rare in transplant patients, retinitis may be observed in approximately 15% of AIDS patients at the time of diagnosis of gastrointestinal disease [164]. Complications include gastrointestinal bleeding (5% of patients) and rarely strictures, or fistulas to the tracheobronchial tree [24].

### Diagnosis

Like HSV, the radiologic appearance of CMV esophagitis is that of either focal or extensive ulceration, and will depend in large part on the epidemiologic setting. Barium esophagography of CMV esophagitis may reveal only thickening of mucosal folds, but more typically, well-circumscribed ulcers are present which may be vertical, linear with central umbilication, solitary and deep, or occasionally diffuse and superficial [11, 43, 82, 149]. In patients with AIDS, these ulcers are often large and deep, exceeding 2 cm in size (Fig. 33–3). Rarely, the exuberant inflammatory response results in a lesion suggestive of a malignancy [75]. The endoscopic appearance of CMV esophagitis is similarly variable, ranging from multiple shallow ulcers, to solitary giant ulcers, to a diffuse superficial esophagitis [161]. Given the high rate of prior exposure to CMV, serologic testing is not helpful. In addition, some immunosuppressed transplant patients fail to develop a brisk antibody response with acute infection.

Identification of viral cytopathic effect in mucosal biopsies is the best diagnostic method. Multiple biopsies (up to ten) may be required to establish the diagnosis in patients with AIDS and should be taken from the base of the ulcer [168]. Viral culture of mucosal biopsies is less sensitive and specific than histology and can be falsely positive [70]. In contrast to Candida and HSV, cytologic specimens from esophageal lesion have very poor sensitivity for the diagnosis of CMV. Since retinitis may coexist with gastrointestinal disease, and, when present, alters the duration of antiviral therapy, a diagnosis of CMV gastrointestinal disease in any patient with AIDS warrants ophthalmologic examination.

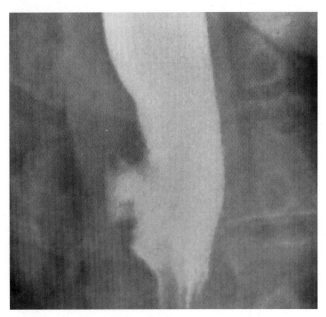

**FIG. 33–3.** CMV esophagitis. Large, deep ulcer in the distal esophagus in a patient with AIDS.

*Therapy*

The therapies available for the treatment of CMV disease require intravenous administration and include ganciclovir, foscarnet, and, more recently, cidofovir. A prospective open-label trial of ganciclovir therapy for CMV esophagitis in 35 AIDS patients documented clinical and endoscopic improvement in 77% of patients [164]. The time course of the clinical response to ganciclovir is variable; 1 week of therapy may be required before there is symptomatic improvement. The total treatment duration should be based on the clinical and endoscopic response, and a 2- to 4-week treatment course is usually adequate. If retinitis is absent and there has been a complete response, the patient may be followed closely without maintenance therapy. Because of low bioavailability (less than 10%), oral ganciclovir is not effective for the treatment of active infections, including those of the gastrointestinal tract [33]. Following acute CMV disease in transplantation patients, treatment with ganciclovir should be given for 1 to 2 months until the immunosuppressive regimen is significantly reduced. Ganciclovir is well tolerated, with its major side effect being myelosuppression, which may be severe when other bone marrow suppressive drugs, such as azidothymidine, are coadministered. Clinical and virologic resistance has been recognized, usually in patients receiving prolonged therapy [39]. Combination therapy with foscarnet has been used to treat refractory disease or when side effects are limiting, as lower doses of each agent may be utilized [34].

Foscarnet inhibits viral DNA polymerase and reverse transcriptase. A randomized trial comparing ganciclovir to foscarnet for AIDS patients with gastrointestinal CMV disease found clinical improvement in over 80% of patients, and there were no significant differences in efficacy between the two agents [13]. There is less information on the use of foscarnet in non-AIDS immunosuppressed patients. Foscarnet has been most frequently utilized when there is clinical resistance to ganciclovir or a major contradiction to ganciclovir use. The major side effect of foscarnet is reversible renal insufficiency [52]. This may be prevented by vigorous saline hydration prior to and during drug administration in combination with dose adjustments based on creatinine clearance. Electrolyte disturbances, which include hypocalcemia and hypophosphatemia, are also common during or shortly after infusion, and slowing the rate of infusion may alleviate the mild cramps induced by these electrolyte shifts. Supplementation of these electrolytes may occasionally be warranted when significant reductions in serum levels are observed. Because of these side effects as well as higher cost, foscarnet remains second-line therapy.

Cidofovir is the newest systemic agent available for the therapy of CMV but has only undergone evaluation for the treatment of retinitis in AIDS [79, 146]. Because of its long half-life, once-weekly administration is adequate, which makes it an ideal agent for selected patients. Like foscarnet, this drug is associated with renal insufficiency.

All drugs for herpes viruses only inhibit viral replication; thus, relapse is frequent when therapy is discontinued. The relapse rate for transplant patients also remains high until immunosuppressive therapy is reduced. In patients with AIDS, the relapse rate of CMV esophagitis is approximately 50%, similar to HSV [13, 66, 164]. With the advent of highly active antiretroviral therapy, treatment for HIV, if associated with improvement in immune function, will serve to prevent relapse, thus negating the need for long-term antiviral therapy for CMV.

*Prophylaxis*

High-dose acyclovir has been used with some success for the prophylaxis of CMV infection in transplant patients, although ganciclovir has been shown to be superior [171]. Because of its cost, potential side effects, and intravenous route of administration, at most transplant centers intravenous ganciclovir prophylaxis is limited to high-risk patients including CMV-seropositive patients, CMV seronegative-recipients who receive CMV-seropositive organs and/or blood products, and patients receiving potent immunosuppression for episodes of rejection [48]. More recently, oral ganciclovir prophylaxis has been shown to decrease CMV disease in high-risk patients after liver transplantation [65]. Oral ganciclovir is effective prophylaxis for CMV retinitis in AIDS patients with a CD4 lymphocyte count less than 200/mm$^3$, but is untested for either primary or secondary prophylaxis of gastrointestinal CMV disease [33]. Fortunately, despite long-term administration, resistance of CMV to ganciclovir and foscarnet is uncommon.

**Other Viruses**

The frequency of esophageal involvement caused by varicella-zoster virus during the course of chicken pox or herpes zoster infections is unknown but clinically uncommon [61, 68]. The esophagitis usually occurs when skin lesions are present rather than antedating the cutaneous disease. Culture of mucosal biopsies is required to differentiate HSV from varicella-zoster virus. The disease is self-limited in the immunocompetent patient. Papilloma virus may infect the esophagus in both normal and immunocompromised patients and characteristically causes small polypoid lesions [111], which may be asymptomatic, or symptomatic ulcers [128]. Esophageal ulcers have been reported due to Epstein-Barr virus in patients with AIDS [58].

## MYCOBACTERIAL INFECTIONS

### Epidemiology

Mycobacterial involvement of the esophagus is rare in both immunocompromised and immunocompetent patients with advanced pulmonary tuberculosis even in countries with high prevalence rates. Previously, *Mycobacterium tuberculosis* (TB) involvement of the esophagus was considered a rare autopsy finding, found in less than 0.15% of necropsies [90]. In developing countries, the rate of TB is much higher, and extrapulmonary manifestations, including esophageal disease, are more common. The upsurge in reported cases of TB linked to the AIDS epidemic has increased the incidence of esophageal infection in developed countries. *Mycobacterium avium* complex (MAC), a pathogen principally restricted to patients with AIDS, is primarily a small bowel pathogen with fewer than ten reported cases of esophageal involvement [36, 37, 73, 145, 153, 173].

### Pathology

Most commonly, TB involves the midesophagus at the level of the carina. Esophageal disease is caused by spread of infection from contiguous TB-infected mediastinal lymph nodes by way of a draining fistula or obstructed lymphatics, resulting in tracheoesophageal fistula. Rarely, TB involves the upper third of the esophagus by direct extension from tuberculous pharyngitis or laryngitis. Primary esophageal TB in the absence of extraesophageal disease is exceedingly rare [130, 147]. Granulomas are often present in ulcer tissue, with bacilli identifiable by mycobacterial staining. Unless multiple biopsies are taken, the diagnosis can be easily missed, especially if there is a significant fibrotic response.

### Clinical Manifestations and Complications

The symptoms of esophageal TB depend on the degree and type of involvement. Dysphagia is the most common presenting symptom. Formation of long strictures or traction diverticula resulting from the fibrotic response or mediastinitus may be the cause of dysphagia [122]. Systemic symptoms of fever and weight loss are common. Pulmonary complaints often predominate due to a fistula to the trachea, bronchus,

or pleural space. Upper gastrointestinal hemorrhage from tuberculous esophageal ulcers [118] and tuberculous arterioesophageal fistulas [23, 110] has been reported. Bleeding caused by extensive mucosal disease has been described in an AIDS patient with esophageal MAC [20].

### Diagnosis

Esophageal TB should be suspected in patients with pulmonary or systemic TB who develop esophageal symptoms. Barium esophagram findings of ulceration and stricture are nonspecific. A sinus tract or fistulous connection to the bronchial tree or mediastinum at the level of the hilum is highly suggestive of TB but is commonly attributed to malignancy, which appears similarly, thus delaying the diagnosis [147]. An ulcerated tuberculous granulomatous mass may also mimic an esophageal neoplasm at endoscopy [74]. When a fistula is present, the diagnosis of TB can be made by sputum staining and culture. Chest radiography is often abnormal and may suggest the diagnosis. Computed tomography of the chest usually demonstrates mediastinal lymphadenopathy, but again, carcinoma may appear similarly. Ulceration is usually present at the site of fistula. Endoscopic biopsies from the edge of the lesions may reveal granulomas and/or acid-fast bacilli, and biopsy material should be cultured for further confirmation of the diagnosis and determination of sensitivities to antimycobacterial agents.

### Treatment

Regardless of the presence of immunodeficiency, a 9-month course of multidrug therapy (in the absence of drug resistance) will often cure esophageal TB and close fistulas. If fistulas do not close with medical therapy alone, surgical intervention will be required. Multidrug-resistant TB is becoming an increasingly complex problem; thus, knowing drug sensitivities to antituberculous therapy is essential to guide therapy.

The most effective agents for the treatment of MAC are clarithromycin and ethambutol [132]. Although a clinical and bacteriologic response is common, long-term therapy for MAC is required if immune function cannot be improved with highly active antiretroviral therapy.

## BACTERIAL INFECTIONS

### Epidemiology

Bacterial esophagitis is a very rare cause of esophageal disease in immunocompromised patients or the normal host [41, 50, 69, 101, 121, 154]. For the most part, this is a polymicrobial infection consisting of oral flora, particularly gram-positive organisms, including *Streptococcus viridans*, staphylococci, and other bacilli. Bacterial esophagitis with these organisms occurs almost exclusively in patients with hematologic malignancies complicated by severe granulocytopenia, but occasionally following bone marrow transplantation [98] or diabetic ketoacidosis [41]. It is likely that these bacteria colonize and then invade mucosa damaged either from reflux disease, radiation therapy, or following chemotherapy, which leads to local infection; dissemination may occur when granulocyte function is poor and/or there is absolute granulocytopenia.

Other bacteria have been reported to involve the esophagus. *Brucella* presenting as a distal submucosal esophageal mass with dysphagia and fever has been noted in a normal host [80]. In patients with AIDS, recent reports have broadened the etiologic spectrum to include *Bartonella hensellae,* the cause of cat scratch disease [25], actinomycoses [108, 116, 141], and *Nocardia* [56].

## Pathology

The gross pathologic appearance of the esophagus in bacterial infection depends on the specific pathogen and ranges from diffuse, shallow ulcerations to ulcers associated with erythema, plaques, pseudomembranes, nodules, or hemorrhage [154]. Microscopic examination reveals pseudomembranes and bacterial invasion that may be superficial and limited to squamous epithelium or may be invasive and transmural with infiltration of blood vessels (i.e., phlegmonous esophagitis). Esophageal actinomycosis is characterized by ulcerative esophagitis sinuses leading from abscess cavities with sulfur granules and filamentous gram-positive branching bacteria seen on tissue biopsies [141]. In the one reported case, *B. hensellae* esophagitis resulted in multiple nodules resulting from a lobulated proliferation of capillary vessels lined by plump endothelial cells [25].

## Clinical Manifestations and Complications

Bacterial esophagitis is usually found in a neutropenic patient with esophageal complaints following chemotherapy for a hematogenous malignancy and rarely in patients with AIDS. Bacterial esophagitis presents with odynophagia and dysphagia typical for any infectious esophagitis. Esophageal infection may serve as a focus for bacteremia and seeding of other organs [154]. Perforation has not been reported.

## Diagnosis

The diagnosis of bacterial esophagitis should be considered in the clinical settings described above. Radiographic findings are nonspecific, and endoscopic biopsy is required to establish this diagnosis. Additional stains including Gram's stain will be necessary to identify the etiologic bacteria. When suspected, bacterial cultures of biopsy material should be submitted. Positive blood cultures will also pinpoint the bacterial pathogen(s) and direct antimicrobial therapy.

## Treatment

Since the infection may be polymicrobial, broad-spectrum antibiotics which effectively treat both Gram-positive and Gram-negative oropharyngeal flora are required for treatment. Treatment of other bacteria found in these patients is similar to infection in other locations.

### *Treponema pallidum*

Although esophageal involvement by *Treponema pallidum* was well recognized many years ago, this disease is unheard of today in developed countries and is primarily of historical interest. The rarity of this esophageal infection has also not been altered by the AIDS epidemic. Tertiary syphilis of the esophagus may present as a submucosal gumma or diffuse inflammatory reaction with fibrosis, which often affects the upper third of the esophagus, and may be associated with mucosal ulcers and structures [51, 144]. Given the rarity of esophageal syphilis, most patients with infectious esophagitis and positive serologic tests for syphilis will have another cause of esophagitis.

## PROTOZOAL INFECTIONS

In developed countries, protozoal infections of the esophagus are very rare, having been reported almost exclusively in AIDS patients. In these patients, reported pathogens include *P. carinii* [72], *Cryptosporidium parvum* [54], and *Leishmania donovani* [151]; coinfections were present in two of these cases [54, 72]. The clinical presentation is similar to other causes of infectious esophagitis. Ulcerations are the most common endoscopic finding and the diagnosis is established by appropriate histologic staining of mucosal biopsies. In normal hosts from endemic areas in South America, however, *Trypanosoma cruzi* may involve the myenteric plexus of the esophagus resulting in Chagas' disease. This disease is indistinguishable clinically, radiographically, manometrically, and endoscopically from idiopathic achalasia. This diagnosis may be established by antibody testing.

## SELECTED HIV-RELATED ESOPHAGEAL DISORDERS

In addition to the infections described above, there are other unique disorders causing esophageal disease in these patients.

### Disorders Associated with Primary HIV Infection

Although primary HIV infection is largely asymptomatic, in some patients, a mononucleosis-like illness occurs around the time of infection consisting of fever, sore throat, and myalgias associated with a maculopapular rash [91, 127]. Spontaneously resolving oropharyngeal and esophageal ulceration or candidal infection may also be observed during this seroconversion illness [46, 91, 115, 120, 127]. Endoscopically, these esophageal ulcerations are multiple, small, and shallow [46, 120]. In some of these patients, electron microscopic examination of biopsy specimens revealed enveloped viruslike particles with morphologic features compatible with retroviruses [120]. Serologic testing is unhelpful, as antibody positivity to HIV is delayed 3 to 18 months after the illness. The diagnosis can be established at the time of presentation by the detection of HIV RNA in serum [127].

## Idiopathic Esophageal Ulcer

### Epidemiology

Large, usually isolated esophageal ulcerations in which no specific etiology could be identified were recognized early in the AIDS epidemic. These ulcers, termed idiopathic esophageal ulcers (IEU) or aphthous ulcers, are very common, comprising approximately 40% of esophageal ulcers in HIV-infected patients [162]. Like other esophageal infections in AIDS, IEU are observed in the later stages of immunodeficiency, when the CD4 lymphocyte count is less than 100/mm³ [162]. These lesions appear to be unique to AIDS.

### Pathology

IEU are variable in size, may be quite large, and are uniformly well circumscribed; a diffuse superficial esophagitis has not been described [60, 158]. Ulcer tissue resembles that in cases of CMV and HSV esophagitis, except that viral cytopathic effect is absent. *Candida* coinfection is common [157]. The presence of a superficial candidal infection overlying a large, well-circumscribed lesion with histopathologic findings of granulation tissue but without viral cytopathic effect should still strongly suggest the diagnosis of IEU rather than *Candida* esophagitis [157]. Since HIV has been observed in ulcer tissue by immunohistochemical staining, it has been suggested that HIV is the direct cause of these lesions [60]. More recently, however, studies have found HIV histopathologically in esophageal biopsies from patients with *Candida*, CMV, and HSV esophagitis [139, 165]. HIV has been uniformly identified in inflammatory cells rather than in squamous epithelial cells, and the infected cells are few in number [139, 165]. In aggregate, these studies suggest that HIV does not cause IEU, at least based on a direct cytopathic mechanism.

### Clinical Manifestations and Complications

IEU present in a fashion indistinguishable from other causes of esophageal ulcer. Coexistent oropharyngeal aphthous ulcers are infrequent [163], whereas thrush is common, especially if the patient has not received empirical antifungal therapy. Complications of IEU include bleeding and fistula to the stomach, but not to the tracheobronchial tree [57, 60]. Esophageal strictures are uncommon.

### Diagnosis

The findings of IEU on barium esophagram are characteristically large, well circumscribed, and often deep ulcers [42,

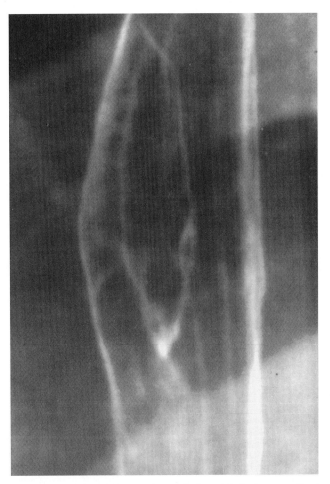

**FIG. 33–4.** Idiopathic esophageal ulcer. Well-circumscribed ulcer in the proximal esophagus in a patient with AIDS. The ulcer had a heaped-up appearance at endoscopy. This type of lesion results in the outline of the ulcer by barium, but without barium in the ulcer crater.

85, 173] (Fig. 33–4). Because of the similarity to CMV esophagitis, a definitive diagnosis cannot be made on the radiographic appearance alone. As IEU is a diagnosis of exclusion, endoscopy with biopsy is required. Endoscopically, these ulcers are variable in size and appearance and larger ulcers are indistinguishable from CMV esophagitis [158, 161]. Pill-induced esophagitis must be excluded by history since the pathologic findings of esophageal biopsies are similar. Likewise, distal esophageal ulcer may suggest gastroesophageal reflux disease, and the histopathologic features cannot distinguish IEU from gastroesophageal reflux disease. However, the clinical history is different, and the endoscopic appearance helps suggest reflux disease.

### Treatment

These ulcers respond rapidly to either prednisone or thalidomide, with clinical and endoscopic cure seen in greater than 90% of cases [3, 159]. The prednisone regimen consists of 40 mg per day tapering 10 mg per week for a 1-month treatment course. Intermittent azole therapy should be coadministered to reduce the likelihood of *Candida* complicating the use of high-dose corticosteroids. Steroid injection into the ulcers has been found to effective, but requires repetitive endoscopy [60]. The relapse rate for IEU is approximately 50%, and retreatment is usually successful. Long-term maintenance therapy may be required for the patient with frequent relapses. Like other opportunistic diseases in AIDS, improvement in immune function with highly active antiretroviral therapy should prevent relapse.

## REFERENCES

1. Agha FP, Horchang HL, Nostrant TT. Herpetic esophagitis: a diagnostic challenge in immunocompromised patients. Am J Gastroenterol 1986;81:246
2. Alexander JA, et al. Infectious esophagitis following liver and renal transplantation. Dig Dis Sci 1988;33:1121
3. Alexander LN, Wilcox CM. A prospective trial of thalidomide for the treatment of HIV-associated idiopathic esophageal ulcers. AIDS Res Hum Retroviruses 1997;13:301
4. Altman C, Bedossa P, Dussaix E, Buffet C. Cytomegalovirus infection of esophagus in immunocompetent adults. Dig Dis Sci 1995;40:606
5. Bacellar H, et al., for the Multicenter AIDS Cohort Study. Incidence of clinical AIDS conditions in a cohort of homosexual men with CD4+ cell counts <100/mm³. J Infect Dis 1994;170:1284
6. Baehr PH, McDonald GB. Esophageal infections: risk factors, presentation, diagnosis, and treatment. Gastroenterology 1994;106:509
7. Barbaro G, Barbarina G, Di Lorenzo G. Fluconazole vs. flucytosine in the treatment of esophageal candidiasis in AIDS patients: A double-blind, placebo-controlled study. Endoscopy 1995;27:377
8. Barbari G, et al. Fluconazole versus itraconazole for *Candida* esophagitis in acquired immunodeficiency syndrome. Gastroenterology 1996;111:1169
9. Bashir RM, Wilcox CM. Symptom-specific use of upper gastrointestinal endoscopy in human immunodeficiency virus-infected patients yields high dividends. J Clin Gastroenterol 1996;23:292
10. Bastian JF, Kaufman IA. Herpes simplex esophagitis in a healthy 10 year old boy. J Pediatr 1982;100:426
11. Balthazar EJ, et al. Cytomegalovirus esophagitis in AIDS: radiographic features in 16 patients. Am J Roentgenol 1987;149:919
12. Belitsos PC, et al. Association of gastric hypoacidity with opportunistic enteric infections in patients with AIDS. J Infect Dis 1992;166:277
13. Blanshard C, Benhamou Y, Dohin E, Lernestedt JO, Gazzard BG, Katlama C. Treatment of AIDS-associated gastrointestinal cytomegalovirus infection with foscarnet and ganciclovir: a randomized comparison. J Infect Dis 1995;172:622
14. Bonacini M, Young T, Laine L. The causes of esophageal symptoms in human immunodeficiency virus infection. Arch Intern Med 1991;151:1567
15. Brandt LJ, et al. Use of a new cytology balloon for diagnosis of esophageal disease in acquired immunodeficiency syndrome. Gastrointest Endosc 1993;4:559
16. Brodt HR, Kamps BS, Gute P, Knupp B, Staszewski S, Helm EB. Changing incidence of AIDS-defining illness in the era of antiretroviral combination therapy. AIDS 1997;11:1731
17. Buckner FS, Pomeroy C. Cytomegalovirus disease of the gastrointestinal tract in patients without AIDS. Clin Infect Dis 1993;17:644
18. Buss DH, Scharyj M. Herpes virus infection of the esophagus and other visceral organs in adults: incidence and clinical significance. Am J Med 1979;66:457
19. Byard RW, Champion MC, Orizaga M. Variability in the clinical presentation and endoscopic findings of herpetic esophagitis. Endoscopy 1987;19:153
20. Cappell MS, Gupta A. Gastrointestinal hemorrhage due to gastrointestinal *Mycobacterium avium intracellulare* of esophageal candidiasis in patients with the acquired immunodeficiency syndrome. Am J Gastroenterol 1992;87:224
21. Cartledge JD, Midgley J, Gazzard BG. Clinically significant azole cross resistance in *Candida* isolates from HIV-positive patients with oral candidiasis. AIDS 1997;11:1839
22. Cartledge JD, Midgley J, Gazzard BG. Itraconazole cyclodextrin solution: the role of *in vitro* susceptibility testing in predicting successful treatment of HIV-related fluconazole-resistant fluconazole-susceptible oral candidosis. AIDS 1997;11:163
23. Catinella FP, Kittle F. Tuberculous esophagitis with aortic aneurysm fistula. Ann Thorac Surg 1988;45:87
24. Chalasani N, Parker KM, Wilcox CM. Bronchoesophageal fistula as a complication of cytomegalovirus esophagitis in AIDS. Endoscopy 1997;29:S28
25. Chang AD, Drachenberg CI, James SP. Bacillary angiomatosis associated with extensive esophageal polyposis: A new mucocutaneous manifestation of acquired immunodeficiency disease (AIDS). Am J Gastroenterol 1996;91:2220
26. Chatis PA, Miller CH, Schrager LE, Crumpacker CS. Successful treatment with foscarnet of an acyclovir-resistant mucocutaneous infection with herpes simplex virus in a patient with acquired immuno-deficiency syndrome. N Engl J Med 1989;320:297
27. Cherniss EI, Waisbren BA. North American blastomycosis: a clinical study of 40 cases. Ann Intern Med 1956;44:105
28. Choi JH, et al. Esophageal aspergillosis after bone marrow transplant. Bone Marrow Transplant 1997;19:293
29. Como JA, Dismukes WE. Oral azole drugs as systemic antifungal therapy. N Engl J Med 1994;330:263
30. Connolly GM, Forbes A, Gleeson JA, Gazzard BG. Investigation of upper gastrointestinal symptoms in patients with AIDS. AIDS 1989;3:453
31. Connolly GM, Hawkins D, Harcourt-Webster JN, Parsons PA, Husain OAN, Gazzard BG. Oesophageal symptoms, their causes, treatment, and prognosis in patients with the acquired immunodeficiency syndrome. Gut 1989;30:1033
32. Cronstedt JL, Bouchama A, Hainau B, Halim M, Khouqeer F, Al Darsouny T. Spontaneous esophageal perforation in herpes simplex esophagitis. Am J Gastroenterol 1992;87:124
33. Crumpacker CS. Ganciclovir. N Engl J Med 1996;335:721
34. Dieterich DT, et al. Concurrent use of ganciclovir and foscarnet to treat cytomegalovirus infection in AIDS patients. J Infect Dis 1993;167:1184
35. Deshmukh M, Shah R, McCallum RW. Experience with herpes esophagitis in otherwise healthy patients. Am J Gastroenterol 1984;79:173
36. de Silva R, Stoopack PM, Raufman JP. Esophageal fistulas associated with mycobacterial infection in patients at risk for AIDS. Radiology 1990;175:449
37. El-Serag HB, Johnston DE. *Mycobacterium avium* complex esophagitis. Am J Gastroenterol 1997;92:1561
38. Eras P, Goldstein MJ, Sherlock P. *Candida* infection of the gastrointestinal tract. Medicine (Balt.) 1972;51:367
39. Erice A, et al. Progressive disease due to ganciclovir-resistant cytomegalovirus in immunocompromised patients. N Engl J Med 1989;320:289
40. Erlich KS, et al. Acyclovir-resistant herpes simplex virus infections in patients with the acquired immunodeficiency syndrome. N Engl J Med 1989;320:293
41. Ezzell JH, Bremer J, Adamec TA. Bacterial esophagitis: an often forgotten cause of odynophagia. Am J Gastroenterol 1990;85:296
42. Frager D, Kotler DP, Baer J. Idiopathic esophageal ulceration in the acquired immunodeficiency syndrome: radiologic reappraisal in 10 patients. Abdom Imaging 1994;19:2
43. Frager DH, et al. Gastrointestinal complications of AIDS: radiologic features. Radiology 1986;158:597
44. Forsmark CE, Wilcox CM, Darragh TM, Cello JP. Disseminated histoplasmosis in AIDS: an unusual case of esophageal involvement and gastrointestinal bleeding. Gastrointest Endosc 1990;36:604
45. Frick T, Fryd DS, Goodale RL, Simmons RL, Sutherland DER, Najarian JS. Incidence and treatment of *Candida* esophagitis in patients undergoing renal transplantation. Data from the Minnesota prospective randomized trial of cyclosporine versus antilymphocyte globulin-azathioprine. Am J Surg 1988;155:311
46. Fusade T, et al. Ulcerative esophagitis during primary HIV infection. Am J Gastroenterol 1992;87:1523
47. Henson D. Cytomegalovirus inclusion bodies in the gastrointestinal tract. Arch Pathol 1972;93:477
48. Hibberd PL, et al. Preemptive ganciclovir therapy to prevent cytomeg-

alovirus disease in cytomegalovirus-positive renal transplant recipients. Ann Intern Med 1995;123:18

49. Hofflin JM, Potasman, I, Baldwin CJ, Oyer PE, Stinson EB, Remington JS. Infectious complications in heart transplant recipients receiving cyclosporine and corticosteroids. Ann Intern Med 1987;106:209

50. Howlett SA. Acute streptococcal esophagitis. Gastrointest Endosc 1979;25:150

51. Hudson TR, Head JR. Syphilis of the esophagus. J Thoracic Surg 1950;20:216

52. Jacobson MA. Review of the toxicities of foscarnet. J Acquir Immune Defic Syndr 1992;5:S11

53. Jenkins DW, Fisk DE, Byrd RB. Mediastinal histoplasmosis with esophageal abscess. Gastroenterology 1976;70:109

54. Kazlow PG, Shah K, Benkov KJ, Dische R, LeLeiko NS. Esophageal cryptosporidiosis in a child with acquired immune deficiency syndrome. Gastroenterology 1986;91:1301

55. Khandekar A, Moser D, Fidler WJ. Blastomycosis of the esophagus. Ann Thorac Surg 1980;30:76

56. Kim J, Minamoto GY, Grieco MH. Nocardial infection as a complication of AIDS: report of six cases and review. Rev Infect Dis 1991; 13:624

57. Kimmel ME, Boylan JJ. Fistulous degeneration of a giant esophageal ulcer in a patient with acquired immunodeficiency syndrome. Am J Gastroenterol 1991;86:890

58. Kitchen VS, et al. Epstein-Barr virus associated oesophageal ulcers in AIDS. Gut 1990;31:1223

59. Kodsi BE, et al. Candida esophagitis. A prospective study of 27 cases. Gastroenterology 1976;71:715

60. Kotler DP, et al. Chronic idiopathic esophageal ulceration in the acquired immunodeficiency syndrome: characterization and treatment with steroids. J Clin Gastroenterol 1992;15:284

61. Kroneke MK, Cuadrado MR. Esophageal stricture following esophagitis in a patient with herpes zoster: case report. Milit Med 1984;149: 479

62. Kruger W, et al. Antimycotic therapy with liposomal amphotericin-b for patients undergoing bone marrow or perpheral blood stem cell transplantation. Leukemia Lymphoma 1997;24:491

63. Galbraith JCT, Shafram SD. Herpes simplex esophagitis in the immunocompetent patient: report of four cases and review. Clin Infect Dis 1992;14:894

64. Gallant JE, Moore RD, Chaisson RE. Prophylaxis for opportunistic infections in patients with HIV infection. Ann Intern Med 1994;120: 932

65. Gane E, Saliba F, Valdecasas GJC, Pescovitz MD, Lyman S, Robtinson CA. Randomised trial of efficacy and safety of oral ganciclovir in the prevention of cytomegalovirus disease in liver transplant recipients. Lancet 1997;350:1729

66. Genereau T, et al. Herpes simplex esophagitis in patients with AIDS: report of 34 cases. Clin Infect Dis 1996;22:926

67. Gil A, et al. Safety and efficacy of fluconazole treatment for Candida oesophagitis in AIDS. Postgrad Med J 1991;67:548

68. Gill RA, et al. Shingles esophagitis: endoscopic diagnosis in two patients. Gastrointest Endosc 1984;30:26

69. Gilver RL. Esophageal lesions in leukemia and lymphoma. Dig Dis Sci 1970;15:31

70. Goodgame RW, Genta RM, Estrada R, Demmler G, Buffone G. Frequency of positive tests for cytomegalovirus in AIDS patients: endoscopic lesions compared with normal mucosa. Am J Gastroenterol 1993;88:338

71. Goodman JL, et al. A controlled trial of fluconazole to prevent fungal infections in patients undergoing bone marrow transplantation. N Engl J Med 1992;326:845

72. Grimes MM, LaPook JD, Bar MH, Wasserman HS, Dwork A. Disseminated Pneumocystis carinii infection in a patient with acquired immunodeficiency syndrome. Hum Pathol 1987;18:307

73. Gray JR, Rabeneck L. Atypical mycobacterial infection of the gastrointestinal tract in AIDS patients. Am J Gastroenterol 1989;89:1521

74. Laajam MA. Primary tuberculosis of the esophagus: pseudotumoral presentation. Am J Gastroenterol 1984;79:839

75. Laguna F, Garcia-Samaniego J, Alonso MJ, Alvarez I, Gonzalez-Lahoz JM. Pseudotumoral appearance of cytomegalovirus esophagitis and gastritis in AIDS patients. Am J Gastroenterol 1993;88:1108

76. Laine L, Rabeneck LR. Prospective study of fluconazole suspension for the treatment of oesophageal candidiasis in patients with AIDS. Aliment Pharmacol Ther 1995;9:553

77. Laine L, et al. Fluconazole compared to ketoconazole for the treatment of Candida esophagitis in AIDS. Ann Intern Med 1992;117:655

78. Lake-Bakaar G, et al. Gastropathy and ketoconazole malabsorption in the acquired immunodeficiency syndrome (AIDS). Ann Intern Med 1988;109:471

79. Lalezari JP, et al. Intravenous cidofovir for peripheral cytomegalovirus retinitis in patients with AIDS. Ann Intern Med 1997;126:257

80. Laso FJ, Cordero M, Giarcia-Sanchez. Esophageal brucelosis: a new location of Brucella infection. Clin Invest 1994;72:393

81. Leotta SMG, Elsborg L. Localized tuberculosis of the esophagus: a rare condition. J Intern Med 1995;238:77

82. Levine MS. Radiology of esophagitis: a pattern approach. Radiology 1991;179:1

83. Levine MS, Macones AJ Jr., Laufer I. Candida esophagitis: accuracy of radiographic diagnosis. Radiology 1985;154:581

84. Levine MS, et al. Herpes esophagitis: sensitivity of double-contrast esophagography. Am J Roentgenol 1988;151:57

85. Levine MS, et al. Giant, human immunodeficiency virus-related ulcers in the esophagus. Radiology 1991;180:323

86. Lewicki AM, Moore JP. Esophageal moniliasis: a review of common and less frequent characteristics. Am J Roentgenol 1975;125:218

87. Lewis JH, Zimmerman HJ, Benson GD, Ishak KG. Hepatic injury associated with ketoconazole therapy. Gastroenterology 1984;86:503

88. Lightdale CJ, Wolf DJ, Marcucci RA, Salyer WR. Herpetic esophagitis in patients with cancer: ante mortem diagnosis by brush cytology. Cancer 1977;39:223

89. Lim SG, Sawyer AM, Hudson M, Sercombe J, Pounder RE. The absorption of fluconazole and itraconazole under conditions of low intragastric acidity. Aliment Pharmacol Ther 1993;7:317

90. Lockard LB. Oesophageal tuberculosis. A critical review. Laryngoscope 1913;23:561

91. Loes S, et al. Symptomatic primary infection due to human immunodeficiency virus type 1: review of 31 cases. Clin Infect Dis 1993;17: 59

92. Lopez-Dulpa M, et al. Clinical, endoscopic, immunologic, and therapeutic aspects of oropharyngeal and esophageal candidiasis in HIV-infected patients: a survey of 114 cases. Am J Gastroenterol 1992; 87:1771

93. Lumbreras C, et al. Randomized trial of fluconazole versus nystatin for the prophylaxis of Candida infection following liver transplantation. J Infect Dis 1996;174:583

94. Maenza JR, Keruly JC, Moore RD, Chaisson RE, Merz WG, Gallant JE. Risk factors for fluconazole-resistant candidiasis in human immunodeficiency virus-infected patients. J Infect Dis 1996;173:219

95. Margolis PS, Epstein A. Mucormycosis esophagitis in a patient with the acquired immunodeficiency syndrome. Am J Gastroenterol 1994; 89:1900

96. Marshall JB, Singh R, Demmy TL, Bickel JT, Everett ED. Mediastinal histoplasmosis presenting with esophageal involvement and dysphagia: case study. Dysphagia 1995;10:53

97. McBane RD, Gross JR Jr. Herpes esophagitis: clinical syndrome, endoscopic appearance, and diagnosis in 23 patients. Gastrointest Endosc 1991;37:600

98. McDonald GB, et al. Esophageal infections in immunosuppressed patients after marrow transplantation. Gastroenterology 1985;88:1111

99. McKenzie R, Khakoo R. Blastomycosis of the esophagus presenting with gastrointestinal bleeding. Gastroenterology 1985;88:1271

100. Meyer RD, Young LS, Armstrong D, Yu B. Aspergillosis complicating neoplastic disease. Am J Med 1973;54:6

101. Miller JT, Slywka SW, Ellis JH. Staphylococcal esophagitis causing giant ulcers. Abdom Imaging 1993;18:225

102. Momin F, Chandrasekaar PH. Antimicrobial prophylaxis in bone marrow transplantation. Ann Intern Med 1995;123:205

103. Moses HL, Cheatham WJ. The frequency and significance of human herpetic esophagitis. Lab Invest 1963;12:663

104. Murata K, Sekigawa T, Sakamoto T, Yamazaki T, Torizuka K. Opportunistic esophagitis caused by Aspergillus fumigatus. Radiat Med 1984;2:24

105. Nakamura S, Vawter G, Sallan S, Chanock S. Fatal esophageal aspergilloma in a leukemic adolescent. Pediatr Infect Dis J 1992;11:245

106. Nash G, Ross JS. Herpetic esophagitis: a common cause of esophageal ulceration. Hum Pathol 1974;5:339

107. Neame P, Rayner D. Mucormycosis. Arch Pathol 1960;70:143

108. Ng FH, Wong SY, Chang CM, Lai ST, Chau KY. Esophageal actinomycosis: a case report. Endoscopy 1997;29:133

109. Obrecht WF Jr, et al. Tracheoesophageal fistula: a serious complication of infectious esophagitis. Gastroenterology 1984;83:1174

110. O'Leary M, Nollet DJ, Blomberg DJ. Rupture of a tuberculous pseudoaneurysm of the innominate artery into the trachea and esophagus: report of a case and review of the literature. Hum Pathol 1977;8:458

111. Orlowska J, Jarosz D, Gugulski A, Pachelwski J, Butruk E. Squamous cell papillomas of the esophagus: report of 20 cases and literature review. Am J Gastroenterol 1994;89:434

112. Ott DJ, Gelfand DW. Esophageal stricture secondary to candidiasis. Gastrointest Radiol 1978;2:323

113. Owensby LC, Stammer JL. Esophagitis associated with herpes simplex infection in an immunocompetent host. Gastroenterology 1978; 74:1305

114. Pearce J, Dagradi A. Acute ulceration of the esophagus with associated intranuclear inclusion bodies. Arch Pathol 1943;35:889

115. Pena M, et al. Esophageal candidiasis associated with acute infection due to human immunodeficiency virus: case report and review. Rev Infect Dis 1991;13:872

116. Poles MA, McMeeking AA, Scholes JV, Dieterich DT. *Actinomyces* infection of a cytomegalovirus esophageal ulcer in two patients with acquired immunodeficiency syndrome. Am J Gastroenterol 1994;89: 1569

117. Pons V, et al. Therapy for oropharyngeal candidiasis in HIV-infected patients: a randomized, prospective multicenter study of oral fluconazole versus clotrimazole troches. J Acquir Immune Defic Syndr 1993; 6:1311

118. Porter JC, Friedland JS, Freedman AR. Tuberculosis bronchoesophageal fistulae in patients infected with the human immunodeficiency virus: three case reports and review. Clin Infect Dis 1994;19:954

119. Powderly WG, et al. A randomized trial comparing fluconazole with clotrimazole troches for the prevention of fungal infections in patients with advanced human immunodeficiency virus infection. N Engl J Med 1995;332:700

120. Rabeneck L, et al. Acute HIV infection presenting with painful swallowing and esophageal ulcers. JAMA 1990;263:2318

121. Radhi JM, Schweiger F. Bacterial oesophagitis in an immunocompromised patient. Postgrad Med J 1994;70:233

122. Ramakantan R, Shah R. Dysphagia due to mediastinal fibrosis in advanced pulmonary tuberculosis. Am J Roentgenol 1990;154:61

123. Rattner HM, Cooper DJ, Zaman MB. Severe bleeding from herpes esophagitis. Am J Gastroenterol 1985;80:523

124. Revankar SG, et al. Detection and significance of fluconazole resistance in oropharyngeal candidiasis in human immunodeficiency virus-infected patients. J Infect Dis 1996;174:821

125. Roberts L Jr, Gibbons R, Gibbons G, Rice RP, Thompson WM. Adult esophageal candidiasis: a radiographic spectrum. Radiographics 1987; 7:289

126. Rubin RR. Infections in the liver and renal transplant patient. In Rubin RH, Young LS, eds, Clinical Approach to Infection in the Compromised Host, 2nd ed. New York: Plenum Publishing, 1988:561

127. Schacker T, Collier AC, Hughes J, Shea T, Corey L. Clinical and epidemiologic features of primary HIV infection. Ann Intern Med 1996;125:257

128. Schechter M, Pannain VLN, de Oliveira AV. Papovavirus-associated esophageal ulceration in a patient with AIDS. AIDS 1991;5:238

129. Schwartz DA, Wilcox CM. Atypical cytomegalovirus inclusions in gastrointestinal biopsy specimens from patients with the acquired immunodeficiency syndrome: diagnostic role of *in situ* nucleic acid hybridization. Hum Pathol 1992;23:1019

130. Seivewright N, Feehally J, Wicks ACB. Primary tuberculosis of the esophagus. Am J Gastroenterol 1984;79:842

131. Selik RM, Chu SY, Ward JW. Trends in infectious diseases and cancers among persons dying of HIV infection in the United States from 1987 to 1992. Ann Intern Med 1995;123:933

132. Shafran SD, et al. A comparison of two regimens for the treatment of *Mycobacterium avium* complex bacteremia in AIDS: rifabutin, ethambutol, and clarithromycin versus rifampin, ethambutol, clofazimine, and ciprofloxacin. N Engl J Med 1996;335:377

133. Sheft DJ, Shrago G. Esophageal moniliasis: the spectrum of the disease. JAMA 1970;231:1859

134. Shepp DH, Klosterman A, Siegel MS. Comparative trial of ketoconazole and nystatin for prevention of fungal infection in neutropenic patients treated in a protective environment. J Infect Dis 1985;152: 1257

135. Shepp DH, Moses JE, Kaplan MH. Seroepidemiology of cytomegalovirus in patients with advanced HIV disease: influence on disease expression and survival. J Acquir Immune Defic Syndr Hum Retroviruses 1996;11:460

136. Shintaku M, Hirai T, Kohno K. Esophageal perforation in association with herpes virus. Report of an autopsy case. Am J Gastroenterol 1992;87:1524

137. Shortsleeve MJ, Levine MS. Herpes esophagitis in otherwise healthy patients: clinical and radiologic findings. Radiology 1992;182:859

138. Slavin MA, et al. Efficacy and safety of fluconazole prophylaxis for fungal infections after marrow transplantation—a prospective, randomized, double-blind study. J Infect Dis 1995;171:1545

139. Smith PD, et al. Esophageal disease in AIDS is associated with pathologic processes rather than mucosal human immunodeficiency virus type 1. J Infect Dis 1993;167:547

140. Sonino N. The use of ketoconazole as an inhibitor of steroid production. N Engl J Med 1987;317:812

141. Spencer GM, Roach D, Skucas J. Actinomycosis of the esophagus in a patient with AIDS: findings on barium esophagograms. Am J Roentgenol 1993;161:795

142. Springer DJ, DaCosta LR, Beck IT. A syndrome of acute self limiting ulcerative esophagitis in young adults probably due to herpes simplex virus. Dig Dis Sci 1979;24:535

143. Spruance SL, Tyring SK, DeGregorio B, Miller C, Meutner K, and the Valaciclovir HSV Study Group. A large-scale, placebo-controlled, dose-ranging trial of peroral valaciclovir for episodic treatment of recurrent herpes genitalis. Arch Intern Med 1996;156:1729

144. Stone J, Friedberg SA. Obstructive syphilitic esophagitis. JAMA 1961;177:7116

145. Stoopack PM, de Silva R, Raufman JP. Inflammatory double-barrelled esophagus in two patients with AIDS. Gastrointest Endosc 1990;36: 394

146. Studies of Ocular Complications of AIDS Research Group. Parenteral cidofovir for cytomegalovirus retinitis in patients with AIDS: The HPMPC peripheral cytomegalovirus retinitis trial. Ann Intern Med 1997;126:264

147. Tassios P, Ladas S, Giannopoulos G, Lariou K, Katsogridakis J, Chalevelakis G. Tuberculous esophagitis. Report of a case and review of modern approaches to diagnosis and treatment. Hepato-Gastroenterol 1995;42:185

148. Tavitian A, et al. Ketoconazole-resistant *Candida* esophagitis in patients with acquired immunodeficiency syndrome. Gastroenterology 1986;90:443

149. Teixidor HS, et al. Cytomegalovirus infection of the alimentary canal: radiologic findings with pathologic correlation. Radiology 1987;163: 317

150. Venkataramani A, Schlueter AJ, Spech TJ, Greenberg E. Cytomegalovirus esophagitis in an immunocompetent host. Gastrointest Endosc 1994;40:392

151. Villanueva JL, et al. *Leishmania* esophagitis in an AIDS patient: An unusual form of visceral leishmaniasis. Am J Gastroenterol 1994;89: 273

152. Vishny ML, Blades EW, Creger RJ, Lazarus HM. Role of upper endoscopy in evaluation of upper gastrointestinal symptoms in patients undergoing bone marrow transplantation. Cancer Invest 1994;12:384

153. Wall SD, et al. Multifocal abnormalities of the gastrointestinal tract in AIDS. Am J Roentgenol 1986;146:1

154. Walsh TJ, Belitsos NJ, Hamilton SR. Bacterial esophagitis in immunocompromised patients. Arch Intern Med 1986;146:1345

155. Welage LS, Carver PL, Revankar S, Pierson C, Kauffman CA. Alterations in gastric acidity in patients infected with human immunodeficiency virus. Clin Infect Dis 1995;21:1431

156. Wilcox CM. Time course of clinical response to fluconazole for *Candida* oesophagitis in AIDS. Aliment Pharmacol Ther 1994;8:347

157. Wilcox CM. Evaluation of a technique to evaluate the underlying mucosa in patients with AIDS and severe *Candida* esophagitis. Gastrointest Endosc 1995;42:360

158. Wilcox CM, Schwartz DA. Endoscopic characterization of idiopathic esophageal ulceration associated with human immunodeficiency virus infection. J Clin Gastroenterol 1993;16:251

159. Wilcox CM, Schwartz DA. Comparison of two corticosteroid regimens for the treatment of idiopathic esophageal ulcerations associated with HIV infection. Am J Gastroenterol 1994;89:2163

160. Wilcox CM, Schwartz DA. Endoscopic-pathologic correlates of *Candida* esophagitis in acquired immunodeficiency syndrome. Dig Dis Sci 1996;41:1337

161. Wilcox CM, Straub RA, Schwartz DA. Prospective endoscopic characterization of cytomegalovirus esophagitis in patients with AIDS. Gastrointest Endosc 1994;40:481

162. Wilcox CM, Schwartz DA, Clark WS. Esophageal ulceration in human immunodeficiency virus infection: causes, diagnosis, and management. Ann Intern Med 1995;123:143

163. Wilcox CM, Straub RF, Clark WS. Prospective evaluation of oropharyngeal findings in human immunodeficiency virus-infected patients with esophageal ulceration. Am J Gastroenterol 1995;90:1938

164. Wilcox CM, Straub RF, Schwartz DA. Cytomegalovirus esophagitis in AIDS: a prospective study of clinical response to ganciclovir therapy, relapse rate, and long-term outcome. Am J Med 1995;98:169

165. Wilcox CM, Zaki SR, Coffield LM, Greer PW, Schwartz DA. Evaluation of idiopathic esophageal ulcer for human immunodeficiency virus. Mod Pathol 1995;8:568

166. Wilcox CM, Alexander LN, Clark WS, Thompson SE. Fluconazole compared with endoscopy for human immunodeficiency virus-infected patients with esophageal symptoms. Gastroenterology 1996;110:1803

167. Wilcox CM, Straub RF, Alexander LN, Clark WS. Etiology of esopha-geal disease in human immunodeficiency virus-infected patients who fail antifungal therapy. Am J Med 1996;101:599

168. Wilcox CM, Straub RF, Schwartz DA. A prospective evaluation of biopsy number for the diagnosis of viral esophagitis in patients with HIV infection and esophageal ulcer. Gastrointest Endosc 1996;44:587

169. Wilcox CM, Darouiche RO, Laine L, Moskovitz BL, Mallegol I, Wu J. A randomized, double-blind comparison of itraconazole oral solution and fluconazole tablets in the treatment of esophageal candidiasis. J Infect Dis 1997;176:227

170. Wilcox CM, et al. High mucosal levels of tumor necrosis factor alpha messenger RNA in AIDS-associated cytomegalovirus-induced esophagitis. Gastroenterology 1998;114:77

171. Winston DJ, Wirin D, Shaked A, Busuttil RW. Randomised comparison of ganciclovir and high-dose acyclovir for long-term cytomegalovirus prophylaxis in liver-transplant recipients. Lancet 1995;346:69

172. Wong TW, Warner NE. Cytomegalic disease in adults. Arch Pathol 1962;74:403

173. Yee J. Wall SD. Infectious esophagitis. Radiat Clin North Am 1994;32:1135

174. Young RC, et al. Aspergillosis: the spectrum of the disease in 98 patients. Medicine (Balt) 1970;49:147

The Esophagus, Third Edition,
edited by D. O. Castell and J. E. Richter.
Lippincott Williams & Wilkins, Philadelphia © 1999.

CHAPTER 34

# Caustic Injuries of the Esophagus

Joseph R. Spiegel and Robert Thayer Sataloff

## INTRODUCTION

The Caustic Substances Labeling Act, passed in 1927, was perhaps the first consumer protection legislation. This law was enacted in large part due to the efforts of Chevalier Jackson, who recognized the hazards of caustic ingestion with the increasing prevalence of caustic substances [47]. Lye, used in soap making, was the original offending agent. In 1967, the introduction of liquid drain cleaners with their much higher alkaline concentrations greatly increased the risk of severe injuries secondary to ingestion. Some control of the problem was achieved as manufacturers reduced the concentration of caustic substances in their products in response to the reports of injuries, and with the Poison Prevention Packaging Act and the Hazardous Substances Act of 1970. In some countries, lye has been outlawed, and the number of caustic ingestions has been reduced greatly, resulting in a trend toward a predominance of acid-induced injuries [62]. However, caustic substances remain ubiquitous and available in the United States and throughout most of the world.

Caustic ingestion can result in a range of injuries from a mild oral burn or sore throat to rapidly progressive life-threatening complications. After recovery from the initial injury, esophageal stricture may develop. Reducing the morbidity of these serious injuries depends on accurate early diagnosis, aggressive treatment of life-threatening complications, and attentive, long-term follow up (Fig. 34–1).

## INCIDENCE

The majority of caustic ingestions occurs in children. The average age of an injured child is under 3 years, and this problem has been reported in a 2-day-old infant [11, 51].

J. R. Spiegel and R. T. Sataloff: Department of Otolaryngology—Head and Neck Surgery, Graduate Hospital, Philadelphia, Pennsylvania 19146, and Department of Otolaryngology—Head and Neck Surgery, Thomas Jefferson University, Philadelphia, Pennsylvania 19107.

It is estimated that there are over 5,000 accidental caustic ingestions each year in the United States [60]. In Denmark, the incidence of pediatric caustic ingestion has been measured at 34.6/100,000 with esophageal burns in 15.8/100,000 [15]. Children are almost always the innocent victims of experimentation with substances found around the home. Even though traditional caustics, such as lye and drain cleaners, are now sold in child-protective containers, they are often transferred to cups or bottles. Other potential caustics, such as dishwasher detergent, denture cleanser, and small batteries, can be found easily by an adventurous toddler. In some cases, toxic ingestions can be part of a pattern of child abuse or child neglect.

Caustic ingestions in adults are less common and almost always associated with suicide attempts. In one study, 92% of 484 adults with caustic swallowing injuries treated in France were found to be suicide attempts [74]. In Denmark, incidence of caustic ingestion in adults has been measured at 1/100,000 with 61% representing suicide attempts. The remaining cases were mostly accidental ingestion by alcoholics [14]. In India, corrosive ingestion is a common mode of poisoning [91].

## PATHOPHYSIOLOGY

### Alkali Ingestion

The sequence of injury in lye burns of the esophagus was first described by Bosher et al. [7]. It includes (a) edema and congestion, principally of the submucosa; (b) inflammation of the submucosa with thrombosis of its vessels; (c) sloughing of the superficial layers; (d) necrosis of the muscularis in varying degrees; (e) organization and fibrosis of the deep layers; and (f) delayed reepithelialization. Superficial mucosal burns often heal without sequelae. Deeper burns into the muscularis can result in delayed healing with fibrosis. Usually only circumferential burns result in strictures. For as long as 2 weeks, inflammation persists, necrotic tissue sloughs, granulation tissue forms, and new collagen is laid

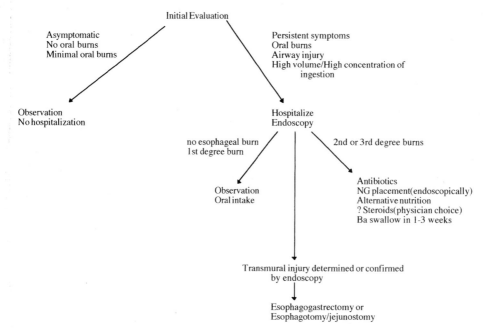

**FIG. 34–1.** Algorithm for care of caustic ingestion.

down. Between 3 and 4 weeks after the initial injury, the collagen begins to contract, and thus, the process of cicatrization begins [82]. When the liquefaction necrosis is transmural, esophageal perforation can result with its attendant high morbidity and mortality rates.

A clinical grading system for esophageal burns has been borrowed from the descriptions of thermal injuries of the skin. First-degree esophageal burns have superficial erythema and edema with only minimal tissue sloughing. Second-degree burns involve the muscularis with ulceration, necrosis, and usually some full-thickness mucosal slough. Third-degree burns are transmural with possible extension to extraesophageal structures [43].

The extent of injury is dependent on two factors: the concentration of the corrosive and the duration of exposure. Esophageal stricture has been induced experimentally with as little as a 0.5% NaOH solution (pH 13) and with an 8.8% ammonia solution (pH 12.5) [50]. However, most serious esophageal injuries result from ingestion of substances with a pH of 14, and the closer the pH to 14, the more likely the patient is to have an injury requiring treatment [81].

A list of common household products with their corrosive components and concentrations can be found in Table 34–1. Even after the safety changes made in the 1970s, all drain cleaners, oven cleaners, and detergents remain sufficiently concentrated to exert their toxic effects at a pH of 14 if swallowed in granular or solid form [52, 80]. Products with less concentrated alkali, such as Clinitests and denture cleaning tablets, can cause severe esophageal injury because their solid form allows them to lodge in the digestive tract and prolong the duration of action [9]. The most common sites of these injuries are at the three natural points of anatomic narrowing in the esophagus: (a) the cricopharyngeus, (b) the aortic arch, and (c) the cardia. Because foreign bodies can lodge at these sites, substances other than traditional caustics can also lead to corrosive injury. A recent report reviewed 679 causes of pill-induced esophageal injuries [48]. Antibiotics were the most common offenders, but anti-inflammatories, potassium chloride, and quinidine led to a high incidence of secondary complications. There is an increased risk of pill-induced injuries in patients with left atrial enlargement, especially after cardiac surgery [48]. Similarly, there have now been many reports of esophageal injury secondary to ingestion of small disk batteries [54]. These batteries are a problem in the pediatric population because they are small, shiny, and nonthreatening in appearance. Over one-third of pediatric disk-battery ingestions have been found in children who wear hearing aids [55]. The injury in disk battery ingestion is secondary to both a caustic burn from leakage of alkali from inside the battery and a thermal burn from electrical discharge of the battery before it dissolves [89]. Because the battery lodges in the esophagus as a foreign body, its effects are concentrated and may lead to esophageal perforation or tracheoesophageal fistula [58, 76].

The liquid bleaches are much less concentrated, but they have also been shown to have the potential to cause esophageal injury in both experimental [84] and clinical settings [53]. It has long been thought that more viscous liquids, such as the liquid drain cleaners, are more dangerous because of their ability to coat the mucosal surface and thus have an increased duration of effect. However, this concept has recently been questioned in a study that found that relative viscosity of offending agents made no difference when their pH was also considered [50]. In recent years, hair relaxers have been involved commonly in caustic ingestions. Hair relaxers are mild alkalis, and although they can cause severe oral burns, they have never been implicated as a source of esophageal or more-distal injury [20].

**TABLE 34–1.** *Common alkaline household corrosives*

| Type of corrosive | Product | Caustic ingredient |
|---|---|---|
| Bleaches | Chlorox | Sodium hypochlorite (5.25%) |
| | Peroxide | Hydrogen peroxide (3%) |
| | Minute mildew remover | Calcium hypochlorite (48%) |
| | Tilex Instant mildew remover | Sodium hypochlorite (5%), sodium hydroxide (1%) |
| Detergents | Oxydol laundry detergent | Sodium tripolyphosphates (25–49%) |
| | Electrasol dishwasher detergent | Sodium tripolyphosphates (20–40%) |
| | Calgonite dishwasher detergent | Sodium phosphates (<50%) |
| | Cascade dishwasher detergent | Phosphates (25–50%) |
| | Comet cleanser | Trisodium phosphate (14.5%) |
| | Polident powder | Sodium tripolyphosphate (<15%) |
| Alkalis | Drano (liquid) | Sodium hydroxide (9.5%) |
| | Drano Professional (liquid) | Sodium hydroxide (32.0%) |
| | Liquid Plummer | Sodium hydroxide (0.5–2%), sodium hypochlorite (5–10%) |
| | Dow oven cleaner (liquid) | Sodium hydroxide (4.0%) |
| | Crystal Drano (granular) | Sodium hydroxide (54.0%) |
| Thermal alkalis | Clinitest tablets | Sodium hydroxide (223 mg) |
| | Efferdent extra-strength tablets | Sodium hydroxide (0.5–1%) |

*Source:* From ref. 60.

## Acid Ingestion

Esophageal injuries secondary to acid ingestion have been reported far less commonly than injuries due to alkaline products. The mechanism of injury differs, with a predominance of coagulation necrosis and the rapid formation of a protective eschar in tissues exposed to acid. This delays the progression of necrosis into the deeper tissues [3]. Additionally, most ingested acids have a rapid transit time in the esophagus, further limiting the opportunity for injury.

Table 34–2 lists the household products involved most often in acid ingestions. Sulfuric acid and hydrochloric acid are the most common offenders by far, but gastric injuries secondary to nitric and trichloroacetic acid, potassium and sodium hydroxide, sodium hypochloride, phenol, zinc chloride, mercurial salts, and formaldehyde have all been reported [36]. Even household vinegar has caused injury in young children [62].

Acid injuries have long been thought to relatively spare the esophagus, although they can cause severe gastric injury [13, 64]. However, a study done in India, where acid ingestion is more common, revealed significant esophageal injury in as many as 85% of patients with gastric or duodenal injuries, and almost one-third of these patients went on to develop esophageal stricture [90]. Thus, patients with acid ingestion require the same rigorous assessment and follow-up as patients with caustic alkaline injuries.

## EVALUATION

### History

Establishing an accurate history of the time of ingestion and the nature of the caustic substance is critical. Since these injuries are common in young children, this often involves sending a parent or guardian back to the home to retrieve a sample of the offending agent, ideally including the labeled bottle. An infant may demonstrate the same level of general distress initially whether a mild or severe corrosive was swallowed, so identifying the substance that was swallowed is often the single most important factor in determining the risk of severe injury. Victims of attempted suicide are often uncooperative historians, and family members or authorities who can investigate the scene of the incident must be interviewed.

### Signs and Symptoms

A wide variety of signs and symptoms are associated with caustic ingestion. Since the earliest investigations, there has been little correlation between the severity of presenting

**TABLE 34–2.** *Common acidic household corrosives*

| Type of corrosive | Products | Caustic ingredient |
|---|---|---|
| Acidic cleaners | Mister Plumber (liquid) | Sulfuric acid (99.5%) |
| | SnoBol toilet cleaner (liquid) | Hydrochloric acid (15%) |
| | Lysol toilet cleaner (liquid) | Hydrochloric acid (8.5%) |
| | Cost Cutter toilet cleaner (liquid) | Hydrochloric acid (9.55%) |
| | Saniflush toilet cleaner (granular) | Sodium bisulfate (75%) |
| | Vanish toilet cleaner (granular) | Sodium bisulfate (75%) |

*Source:* From ref. 60.

**TABLE 34–3.** *Mild to moderate signs and symptoms of caustic ingestion*

| Oral/pharyngeal | Laryngeal | Esophageal | Gastric |
|---|---|---|---|
| Pain | Hoarseness | Dysphagia | Abdominal pain |
| Odynophagia | Aphonia | Odynophagia | Vomiting |
| Mucosal ulceration | Stridor | Chest pain | Hematemesis |
| Drooling | | Back pain | |
| Tongue edema | | | |

symptoms and the extent of the esophageal injury. As many as 10% of patients with significant esophageal injuries may have no early signs or symptoms [21, 28], while up to 70% of patients with oral and oropharyngeal burns will not have any significant distal lesion [38]. However, recent reviews of pediatric patients alone have shown that there is little risk of subsequent problems in children without symptoms appearing within hours following the ingestion [17, 62].

Table 34–3 shows the mild to moderate signs and symptoms of caustic injuries categorized by the anatomic site affected. Oral and pharyngeal findings are established easily by observation and the use of a tongue depressor. Fiberoptic laryngoscopy provides a safe, easy method to complete the laryngeal and pharyngeal examination in almost any setting. Esophageal and gastric examinations must often be repeated to assess findings for signs of complications or long-term sequelae.

Life-threatening complications of airway obstruction, aspiration, or esophagogastric perforation can occur within seconds of the ingestion, or on a delayed basis as inflammation and necrosis progress. Table 34–4 lists the signs and symptoms of the most severe sequelae of caustic ingestions. Death is related to the amount and concentration of caustic substance ingested and has been noted uniformly in patients swallowing more than 6 ml of a concentrated substance, usually alkali [5].

## Endoscopy

Endoscopy is the single most valuable tool in the assessment of caustic trauma of the esophagus. The key is avoiding iatrogenic perforation of the weakened esophageal wall. Fear of endoscopic injury prompted some authors to suggest that endoscopy on patients suspected of having severe burns is contraindicated [90] or that, in children, it be restricted to patients with significant injuries 2 weeks after the ingestion [6]. A review of 115 children evaluated for caustic ingestion

**TABLE 34–4.** *Severe signs and symptoms of caustic ingestion*

| Airway obstruction | Aspiration | Perforation |
|---|---|---|
| Stridor | Cough | Pain |
| Agitation | Hypoxia | Tachycardia |
| Cyanosis | Fever | Fever |
| Hypoxia | Leukocytosis | Leukocytosis |
| | | Shock |

in Denmark has suggested that endoscopy is unnecessary in asymptomatic patients [16]. However, even earlier studies showed large numbers of patients who safely underwent diagnostic esophagoscopy for caustic injuries. Daly [22] reported 105 consecutive patients and Yarrington [88] reported 70 consecutive patients all having rigid esophagoscopy. More recently, Di Costanzo et al. [24] reported 81 consecutive patients and Rappert et al. [66] reported 102 consecutive patients who underwent evaluation for caustic injuries by flexible esophagoscopy, all without complication.

There are two important factors in performing safe esophagoscopy. First, use the procedure for diagnosis only. The procedure should be terminated before passing the scope beyond any area of severe or circumferential burn. Second, perform the endoscopy within 48 hours of the ingestion, while the lumen wall retains its greatest strength. Some authors suggest a more aggressive approach with full esophagogastroscopy in all patients with severe injuries due to the risk of progressively more severe distal lesions that would otherwise be missed [75, 78]. The decision to proceed with endoscopy after encountering a severe circumferential burn must be made by an experienced endoscopist with full regard for the possible risks. With these caveats in mind, esophagoscopy is indicated if the history or any of the signs or symptoms raise the index of suspicion for a distal esophageal injury [32].

Either flexible or rigid instrumentation can be used. The flexible esophagoscope is easier to pass and is better tolerated in an awake patient in most cases. A flexible, fiberoptic system is required to assess fully the cardia and stomach due to the anatomic narrowing and the need to "turn" the scope. However, it can be difficult to maintain visualization with the flexible scope in the presence of bleeding and necrotic tissue, so rigid instrumentation is sometimes necessary. An experienced endoscopist can often perform full rigid esophagoscopy with sedation alone, but general anesthesia with muscle relaxation is usually required. Endoscopic findings in the evaluation of acute caustic injuries are shown in Table 34–5.

## Radiology

A chest x-ray is probably the single most important radiographic study in the earliest stages of severe caustic injuries. Chest x-ray can reveal pulmonary infiltrates secondary to aspiration and signs of esophageal perforation (pneumothorax, pneumomediastinum, subcutaneous emphysema).

**TABLE 34–5.** *Endoscopic findings in esophageal burns*

| | |
|---|---|
| First-degree (superficial) | Nonulcerative esophagitis<br>Mild mucosal erythema and edema |
| Second-degree (transmucosal) | Shallow to deep ulceration with possible extension to muscularis<br>White exudate<br>Severe erythema |
| Third-degree (transmural) | Deep ulceration with possible perforation<br>Dusky or blackened transmural tissue<br>Little remaining mucosa<br>Possible obliteration of lumen |

Contrast swallowing studies appear to be of little use in the early evaluation of caustic esophageal injuries. Findings of atonic dilatation, intramural contrast dissection, and aperistalsis have been reported in severe injuries and have occasionally been precursors of perforation [12, 31]. However, even though the correlation of positive radiologic findings to endoscopic findings is reasonably high in some studies [77], other authors have found very high false-negative rates [56]. In the evaluation of acute injuries, contrast esophagograms are most useful to rule out and localize perforations. Initial examinations are performed with water-soluble contrast medium due to the risk of extravasation [57]. Once perforation is ruled out, studies with barium can proceed.

Contrast swallowing studies are much more important in the evaluation and treatment planning in the later stages of caustic esophageal injury. As patients with moderate to severe injuries are followed, smooth strictures can be noted radiologically as soon as 10 days to 2 weeks after ingestion. Other findings such as diverticulae and aperistaltic segments are not uncommon [32, 77]. Contrast studies can demonstrate functional deficits such as loss of muscle function or coordination, as well as demonstrate all areas of stricture without the risk of endoscopy [63].

## TREATMENT

### Initial Management

All patients who are thought to have suffered a serious caustic ingestion are hospitalized. Intravenous fluids are started, and if hypovolemia is present, central venous access is obtained. Intravenous antibiotics should be given prophylactically in any patient being treated for a presumed caustic ingestion.

Airway injury is not very common in adult caustic ingestions, but it is much more frequent in the pediatric population. Moulin et al. found significant laryngeal lesions in 14 of 33 children assessed after caustic ingestions, and 7 children required intubation [61]. Obstruction may not be present initially but may develop over 24 hours with progressive edema of the tongue and supraglottic larynx. If administered early, intravenous steroids can reduce upper airway swelling. If airway support is necessary, intubation is preferred when adequate visualization is possible. However, "blind" nasotracheal intubation should not be attempted because of the potential presence of necrotic tissue in the upper airway. Emergency tracheotomy is indicated in cases of rapidly progressive upper airway obstruction and when there has been a severe laryngeal burn.

After the patient has been stabilized, esophagoscopy should optimally take place within 24 hours. Treatment is then determined based on the patient's general condition and the endoscopic findings. No treatment is necessary in patients with first-degree injuries. As soon as they are tolerating oral fluids, patients can be discharged from the hospital. A follow-up barium swallow study is performed approximately 3 weeks after the injury. Further study is necessary only if symptoms develop or if the barium study identifies an abnormality. Strictures will rarely, if ever, occur in this group [39, 64].

In more extensive esophageal burns, the risk of severe complications and stricture is higher. Once the patient has been stabilized, there are many therapeutic options that can be considered.

### Nutrition

Most clinicians agree that patients who can swallow should be allowed to take oral nutrition after they are stabilized. Patients unable to swallow should receive total parenteral nutrition (TPN) or have a nasogastric (NG) tube placed under endoscopic guidance, or undergo gastrostomy. If an NG tube is utilized, it should never be placed blindly due to the risk of perforation. It has been suggested that adequate nutrition alone is the most important factor in promoting healing of an esophageal burn [88].

### Steroids

Steroids were originally advocated after they were found to be effective in preventing esophageal stricture in animal models with caustic injury [30, 73, 85]. Infectious complications of perforation and pneumonia were encountered, but were overcome by the addition of antibiotics [37, 72]. Subsequently, many clinical reports have supported the use of steroids to prevent the development of secondary esophageal stricture [10, 18, 21, 38, 63]. A recent review analyzing 13 prior studies (10 retrospective, 3 prospective) found evidence that steroids can prevent strictures in second- and third-degree burns [45]. Summarizing the findings of the studies that support steroid use, the following clinical suggestions are noted: steroids are unnecessary in first-degree superficial burns; steroids are not beneficial and potentially dangerous in third-degree severe burns involving perforation or transmural necrosis; steroids should be given early and in high doses (e.g., prednisone 2 mg per kg per day or its equivalent); and steroids should always be given concomitantly with antibiotics. Last, at least one study suggests that there may be increased effectiveness when steroids are used in conjunction with sucralfate and $H_2$ blockers [68].

Despite both the scientific logic and the clinical support for steroid use, other reports have questioned the effectiveness of this treatment. Ferguson et al. [29] and Kirsh et al. [49] both found no difference in complication rates. Di Costanzo et al. [24] avoided steroid use, advocating "therapeutic nihilism." In this study, 94 patients were treated with supportive care alone, TPN in patients unable to swallow, and oral nutrition in the remaining patients. There were four deaths and five cases of stenosis, four of which required surgery. More recently, Anderson et al. [1] reported a prospective study in which steroids were found to have no affect on stricture rates in patients with moderate and severe circumferential burns.

Thus, there is contradictory evidence regarding the efficacy of steroid use in caustic ingestions. However, if their use is limited to patients with endoscopically confirmed partial thickness injuries, they can be used safely in most cases and may help prevent late sequelae of the injury.

### Stenting

The easiest and simplest stent is an NG tube. The endoscopically placed tube can be used to prevent stricture formation as well as provide nutrition [86, 87]. In patients with deep partial thickness or transmural burns without perforation, a wider intraluminal stent can be considered. This practice was first described in animal models [26, 69] and has subsequently been used successfully in both children and adults [19, 41, 59]. Silicone-rubber or silastic is utilized. The stent can be placed endoscopically, but some surgeons routinely position the tube through a gastrostomy. Steroids and antibiotics have been utilized routinely, but a recent report by Berkovits et al. described excellent results using a custom-made, twin-tube silicone-rubber stent without steroids [4].

### Dilation

At one time, dilation was considered part of the early therapeutic regimen in caustic ingestions. This practice was abandoned due to the risk of perforation. Dilation is now utilized as the initial treatment for secondary esophageal strictures. The stenotic segments can often be managed with antegrade dilation. A rigid or mercury-weighted bougie system can be used. When stenotic segments are multiple, extensive, or involve the esophagogastric junction, retrograde dilation should be considered. The procedure was first popularized by Tucker [79] in the 1920s and involves having the patient swallow a string which is retrieved through a gastrostomy. Serial dilators are then passed over the string and pulled retrograde into the mouth.

All dilations should be gentle with a goal of slow, progressive improvement. Perforation is a hazard with all manipulations of the stenotic lumen. Steroid and antibiotic treatment is not usually necessary in the secondary treatment of strictures. However, one report did describe an advantage with intralesional steroid injections in conjunction with dilations [42].

The development of dysphagia after the initial injury may be multifactorial, rather than due to stricture alone. Dantas and Mamede [23] reported disordered esophageal motility in almost all patients studied 1 to 53 years after their injury. Other investigative studies such as esophageal manometry, gastric emptying studies, and pH monitoring should be considered in these patients.

### Surgery

Surgical treatment is divided into emergency procedures to treat esophagogastric necrosis and perforation, and delayed reconstruction. Widespread necrosis with paraesophageal contamination secondary to a third-degree injury is life-threatening due to the rapid onset of mediastinitis, sepsis, tracheobronchial involvement, and shock. Patients with such severe injuries have routinely responded very poorly to conservative therapy, and thus an aggressive surgical philosophy has been adopted in many institutions [2, 25, 35, 67]. Gastric necrosis with or without esophageal injury is seen in a high percentage of acid ingestions [44]. Often a laparotomy is indicated to diagnose the extent of the intra-abdominal complications. These patients undergo emergency esophagogastrectomy and have reconstruction usually with a colon interposition graft on a delayed basis (at least 4 to 6 weeks later). Esophagectomy can be accomplished "bluntly," sparing the patient a thoracotomy [46, 67], but the esophagus can be left *in situ* if it is minimally burned [70], and it should not be resected when the trachea is involved. This aggressive approach has greatly reduced mortality and morbidity and has also yielded acceptable swallowing rehabilitation [68, 79, 91]. A review of patients severely injured by caustic ingestion has shown excellent results utilizing early cervical esophagostomy and feeding jejunostomy, avoiding esophagectomy in most cases [71].

Reconstruction of the esophagus and pharynx is performed either as a planned second stage after an emergency resection or as an alternative to failed conservative treatment of a secondary stricture. If any swallowing can be preserved with periodic dilation, surgery should be avoided [8]. If esophageal replacement is necessary, the best results are obtained with vascularized grafts from the stomach or bowel. Colon interposition utilizes the right or transverse colon, on a mesenteric pedicle. The bowel is passed through a retrosternal tunnel into the neck for esophagocolonic or pharyngocolonic anastomosis [65]. When the stomach has not been damaged, it can be elongated, passed through the posterior mediastinum, and sutured to the pharynx for total esophageal replacement (a gastric "pullup" procedure) [40].

Over the past decade, the use of microvascular, free jejunal grafts for reconstruction of the pharynx and cervical esophagus has become popular [27, 33]. Although this method is used predominantly after cancer resections, it has also been utilized successfully in patients with caustic strictures [35, 83]. Recent refinements in the procedure may allow free jejunal grafts to be used for total esophageal reconstruction as well [34].

## CONCLUSIONS

Caustic ingestion continues to be a complex clinical challenge. Even though most severe injuries are caused by lye or other solid alkalis, all caustic products have the potential to do harm. Acid ingestion must be evaluated with the same concern for serious complications.

Early, diagnostic esophagoscopy is the crucial component of the initial evaluation. Contrast radiography is the mainstay of diagnosis in secondary strictures.

Superficial burns require no treatment and limited follow-up. Partial thickness injuries are treated with nutritional support and close follow-up. Most clinicians also utilize steroids and antibiotics during the initial treatment interval. Long segments with circumferential burns can be successfully treated with intraluminal stents. Life-threatening perforations and severe, widespread necrosis are best treated by radical surgical resection and delayed reconstruction. Secondary strictures are treated with dilation or esophageal reconstruction.

Although there have been important advances in the diagnosis and treatment of caustic injuries, much remains unknown. Even the use of steroids and antibiotics remains controversial. Study into optimal management of caustic injuries is needly badly, and further refinements in clinical management should be anticipated.

## REFERENCES

1. Anderson KD, Rouse TM, Randolph JG. A controlled trial of corticosteroids in children with corrosive injury of the esophagus. N Engl J Med 1990;323:637
2. Andreoni B, Farina ML, Biffi R, Crosta C. Esophageal perforation and caustic injury: emergency management of caustic ingestion. Dis Esophagus 1997;10:95
3. Ashcraft KW, Padula RT. The effect of dilute corrosives on the stomach. Pediatrics 1974;53:226
4. Berkovits RN, Bos CE, Wijburn FA, Holzki J. Caustic injury of the oesophagus. Sixteen years experience, and introduction of a new model oesophageal stent. J Laryngol Otol 1996;110:1041
5. Berthet B, Castellani P, Brioche MI, Assadourian R, Gauthier A. Early operation for severe corrosive injury of the upper gastrointestinal tract. Eur J Surg 1996;162:951
6. Borja AR, Ransdell HT, Thomas TV, Johnson W. Lye injuries of the esophagus. J Thorac Cardiovasc Surg 1969;57:533
7. Bosher LH, Burford TH, Ackerman L. The pathology of experimentally produced lye burns and strictures of the esophagus. J Thorac Surg 1951; 21:483
8. Braghetto ACI. Surgical management of esophageal strictures. Hepato-Gastroenterology 1992;39:502
9. Burrington JD, Clinitest burns of the esophagus. Ann Thorac Surg 1975;20:400
10. Campbell GS, Burnett HF, Ransom JM, Williams GD. Treatment of corrosive burns of the esophagus. Arch Surg 1977;112:495
11. Casasnovas BA, E Martinez, V Cives. A retrospective analysis of ingestion of caustic substances by children. Eur J Pediatr 1997;156:410
12. Chen YM, Ott DJ, Thompson JN, Gelfand, DW. Progressive roentgenographic appearance of caustic esophagitis. South Med J 1988;81:724
13. Chodak GW, Passaro E. Acid ingestion: need for gastric resection. JAMA 1978;239:225
14. Christesen HB. Caustic ingestion in adults—epidemiology and prevention. J Toxicol 1994;32:557
15. Christesen HB. Epidemiology and prevention of caustic ingestion in children. Acta Paediatr 1994;83:212
16. Christesen HB. Prediction of complications following unintentional caustic ingestion in children. Is endoscopy always necessary? Acta Paediatr 1995;84:1177
17. Clausen JO, Nielsen TL, Fogh A. Admission of Danish hospitals after suspected ingestion of corrosives. A nationwide survey (1984–1988) comprising children aged 0–14 years. Dan Med Bull 1994;41:234
18. Cleveland WW, Chandler JR, Lawson RB. Treatment of caustic burns of the esophagus. JAMA 1963;186:182
19. Coln D, Chang, JHT. Experience with esoophageal stenting for caustic burns in children. J Pediatr Surg 1986;21:588
20. Cox AJ 3rd, Eisenbeis JF. Ingestion of caustic hair relaxer: is endoscopy necessary? Laryngoscope 1997;107:897
21. Crain EF, Gershel JC, Mezey AP. Caustic ingestions: symptoms as predictors of esophageal injury. Am J Dis Child 1984;138:863
22. Daly JF. Corrosive esophagitis. Otolaryngol Clin North Am 1968;1: 119
23. Dantas RO, Mamede RC. Esophageal motility in patients with esophageal caustic injury. Am J Gastroenterol 1996;91:2450
24. Di Costanzo J, Noirclerc M, Jouglard J, Escoffier JM, Cano N, Martin J, Gauthier A. New therapeutic approach to corrosive burns of the upper gastrointestinal tract. Gut 1980;21:370
25. Estrera A, Taylor W, Mills LJ, Platt MR. Corrosive burns of the esophagus and stomach: a recommendation for an aggressive surgical approach. Ann Thorac Surg 1986;41:276
26. Fell SC, Denize A, Becker NH, Hurwitt ES. The effect of intraluminal splinting in the prevention of caustic stricture of the esophagus. J Thorac Cardiovas Surg 1966;52:675
27. Fisher, SR, Cameron R, Hoyt DJ, Cole TB, Seigler HF, Meyers WC. Free jejunal interposition graft for reconstruction of the esophagus. Head Neck Surg 1990;12:126
28. Ferguson MK, Megliore M, Staszak, VM, Little AG. Early evaluation and therapy for caustic esophageal injury. Am J Surg 1989;157:116
29. Ferguson MK, Migliore M, Staszak VM, Little AG. Early evaluation and therapy for caustic esophageal injury. Am J Surg. 1989;157:116
30. Floberg LE, Koch H. The effect of cortisone on the scarification in corrosive lesions of the esophagus. Acta Otolaryngol Suppl 1953;109: 33
31. Franken EA. Caustic damage of the gastrointestinal tract: roentgen features, Am J Radiol 1973;118:77
32. Friedman EM, Lovejoy FH. The emergency management of caustic ingestions, Emerg Med Clin North Am 1984;2:77
33. Gluckman JL, McDonough J, Donegan JO. The role of the free jejunal graft in reconstruction of the pharynx and cervical esophagus. Head Neck Surg 1982;4:360
34. Gorbunov GN, Marinichev VL, Volkov ON, Stolyarov VI. Microvascular reconstruction of the esophagus with pedicled small intestine. Ann Plast Surg 1993;31:439
35. Gossot D, Sarfati E, Celerier M. Early blunt esophagectomy in severe caustic burns of the upper digestive tract. J Thorac Cardiovasc Surg 1987;94:188
36. Gray HK, Holmes CL. Pyloric stenosis caused by ingestion of corrosive substances: report of a case. Surg Clin North Am 1948;28:1041
37. Haller JA, Bachman K. The comparative effect of current therapy on experimental caustic burns of the esophagus. Pediatrics 1964;34:236
38. Haller JA, Andrews G, White JJ, Tamer MA, Cleveland WW. Pathophysiology and management of acute corrosive burns of the esophagus: results of treatment in 285 children. J Pediatr Surg 1971;6:578
39. Hawkins DB, Demeter MJ, Barnett, TE. Caustic ingestion: controversies in management. A review of 214 cases. Laryngoscope 1980;90: 98
40. Heimlich HJ. Esophagoplasty with reversed gastric tube. Am J Surg 1972;123:80
41. Hill JL, Norberg HP, Smith MD, Young JA, Reyes HM. Clinical technique and success of the esophageal stent to prevent corrosive stenosis. J Pediatr Surg 1976;11:443
42. Holder TM, Ashcraft KW, Leape L. The treatment of patients with esophageal strictures by local steroid injections. J Pediatr Surg 1969; 4:646

43. Holinger PH, Management of esophageal lesions caused by chemical burns. Ann Otol Rhinol Laryngol 1968;77:819

44. Horvath OP, Olah T, Zentai G. Emergency esophagogastrectomy for treatment of hydrochloric acid injury. Ann Thorac Surg 1991;52:98

45. Howell JM, Dalsey WC, Hartsell FW, Butzin CA. Steroids for the treatment of corrosive esophageal injury. Am J Emerg Med 1992;10:421

46. Hwang TL, Shen-Chen SM, Chen MF. Nonthoracotomy esophagectomy for corrosive esophagitis with gastric perforation. Surg Gynecol Obstet 1987;164:537

47. Jackson C. Esophageal stenosis following the swallowing of caustic alkalis. JAMA 1921;77:22

48. Kikendall JW, Pill-induced esophageal injury. Gastroenterol Clin North Am 1991;20:835

49. Kirsh MM, Peterson A, Brown JW, Orringer MB, Ritter F, Sloan H. Treatment of caustic injuries of the esophagus: a ten year experience. Ann Surg 1978;188:675

50. Krey H. On treatment of corrosive lesions in the esophagus: experimental study. Acta Otolaryngol Suppl 1952;102:1

51. Kushimo T, Ekanem MM. Acid ingestion in a 2-day old baby. W Afr J Med 1997;16:121

52. Kynaston JA, Patrick, MK, Shepherd RW, Raivadera PV, Cleghorn GJ. The hazards of automatic-dishwasher detergent. Med J Aust 1989;151:5

53. Klein JD. Caustic injury from household bleach too (letter). J Pediatr 1986;108:328

54. Litovitz TL. Button battery ingestions: A review of 56 cases. JAMA 1983;249:2495

55. Litovitz TL. Battery ingestions: product accessability and clinical course. Pediatrics 1985;75:469

56. Mansson I. Diagnosis of acute corrosive lesions of the oesophagus. J Laryngol Otol 1978;92:499

57. Martel WM. Radiologic features of esophagogastritis secondary to extremely caustic agents. Radiology 1972;103:31

58. Maves MD, Carithers JS, Brick HG. Esophageal burns secondary to disc battery ingestion. Ann Otol Rhinol Laryngol 1984;93:364

59. Mills LJ, Estrera AS, Platt MR. Avoidance of esophageal stricture following severe caustic burns by the use of an intraluminal stent. Annals Thoracic Surg 1979;28:60

60. Moore WR. Caustic Ingestions. Clin Pediatr 1986;25:192

61. Moulin D, Bertrand JM, Buts JP, Nyakabasa M, Otte JB. Upper airway lesions in children after accidental ingestion of caustic substances. Pediatrics 1985;106:408

62. Nuutinen M, Uhari M, Karvali T, Kouvalainen K. Consequences of caustic ingestions in children. Acta Paediatr 1997;83:1200

63. Ott DJ, Gelfand DW, Wu WC, Chen YM. Radiologic evaluation of dysphagia. JAMA 1986;256:2718

64. Penner GE. Acid ingestion: toxicology and treatment. Ann Emerg Med 1980;9:374

65. Postlethwait RW, Sealy WC, Dillon ML, Young WG. Colon interposition for esophageal substitution. Ann Thorac Surg 1971;12:89

66. Rappert P, Preier L, Korab W, Neubauer T. Diagnostic and therapeutic management of esophageal and gastric caustic burns in childhood. Eur J Pediatr Surg 1993;3:202

67. Ray JF, Myers WO, Lawton BR, Lee FY, Wenzel FJ, Sautter RD. The natural history of liquid lye ingestion: rationale for an agressive surgical approach. Arch Surg 1974;109:436

68. Reddy AN, Budhraja M. Sucralfate therapy for lye-induced esophagitis. Am J Gastroenterol 1988;83:71

69. Reyes HM, Lin CY, Schlunk FF, Replogle RL. Experimental treatment of corrosive esophageal burns. J Pediatr Surg 1974;9:317

70. Ribet ME. Esophagogastrectomy for acid injury (letter). Ann Thorac Surg 1992;53:738

71. Ribet M, Chambon JP, Pruvot FR. Oesophagectomy for severe corrosive injuries: is it always legitimate? Eur J Card Thor Surg 1990;4:347

72. Rosenberg N, Kunderman PJ, Vroman L, Moolten SE. Prevention of experimental lye strictures of the esophagus by cortisone II. Control of suppurative complications by penicillin. Arch Surg 1953;66:593

73. Rosenberg N, Kunderman PJ, Vroman L, Moolten SE. Prevention of experimental lye strictures of the esophagus by cortisone. Arch Surg 1951;63:147

74. Sarfati E, Gossot D, Assens P, Celerier M. Management of caustic injuries in adults. Br J Surg 1987;74:146

75. Sellars SL, Spence RAJ. Chemical burns of the oesophagus, J Laryngol Otol 1987;101:1211

76. Sigalet D, Lees G. Tracheoesophageal injury secondary to disc battery ingestion. J Pediatr Surg. 1988;23:996

77. Stannard MW. Corrosive esophagitis in children. Am J Dis Child 1978;132:596

78. Thompson J. Corrosive eophageal injuries I. A study of nine cases of concurrent accidental caustic ingestion. Laryngoscope 1987;97:1060

79. Tucker G. Cicatricial stenosis of the esophagus. Ann Otol Rhinol Laryngol 1924;33:1180

80. Vadarikan BA. Ingestion of dishwasher detergent by children. Br J Clin Pediatr 1996;44:35

81. Vancura EM, Clinton JE, Ruize, Krenzelok EP. Toxicity of alkaline solutions. Ann Emerg Med 1980;9:118

82. Waggoner LG. Diagnosis and management of chemical burns of the esophagus. Laryngoscope 1958;68:1790

83. Wang TD, Sun YE, Chen Y. Free jejunal grafts for reconstruction of the pharynx and cervical esophagus. Ann Otol Rhinol Laryngol 1986;95:348

84. Weeks RS, Ravitch MM. The pathology of experimental injury to the cat esophagus by liquid chlorine bleach. Laryngoscope 1971;81:1532

85. Weisskopf A. Effects of cortisone on experimental lye burn of the esophagus. Ann Otol Rhinol Laryngol 1952;61:681

86. Wijburg FA, Beukers MM, Heymans HS, Bartelsman JF, den Hartog Jager FC. Nasogastric intubation as sole treatment of caustic esophageal lesions. Ann Otol Rhinol Laryngol 1985;94:337

87. Wijburg FA, Heymans HS, Urbanus NA. Caustic esophageal lesions in childhood: prevention of stricture formation. J Pediatr Surg 1989;24:171

88. Yarrington C. Steroids, antibiotics and early esophagoscopy in caustic esophageal trauma. NY State J Med 1963;2960

89. Yasui T. Hazardous effects due to alkaline button battery ingestion: an experimental study. Ann Emerg Med 1986;15:901

90. Zargar SA, Kochhar R, Nagi B, Mehta S, Mehta SK. Ingestion of corrosive acids. Gastroenterology 1989;97:702

91. Zargar SA, Kochhar R, Nagi B, Mehta S, Mehta SK. Ingestion of strong corrosive alkalis: spectrum of injury to upper gastrointestinal tract and natural history. Am J Gastroenterol 1992;87:337

*The Esophagus*, Third Edition,
edited by D. O. Castell and J. E. Richter.
Lippincott Williams & Wilkins, Philadelphia © 1999.

CHAPTER 35

# Esophageal Involvement in Other Inflammatory Conditions

David A. Johnson

The esophagus may serve as a mirror for manifestations of systemic disease. As such, it is conceivable that esophageal abnormalities may be the forme fruste presentation of a more widespread disease. Physicians caring for patients with systemic disease therefore need to be attuned to the potential for esophageal involvement in order to direct more appropriately the diagnostic and therapeutic care plan.

Esophageal involvement in systemic disease reflects alteration of either motility or mucosal integrity (esophagitis). There are numerous diseases causing esophageal dysmotility and even a greater number causing esophagitis, particularly with the expanding recognition of esophagitis in the immunocompromised host. These issues are covered in detail in chapters 16 and 32. The focus of this chapter is on disease states, both infectious and noninfectious, that uncommonly have esophageal involvement, particularly esophagitis.

## CROHN'S DISEASE

Crohn's disease of the esophagus is a rare, but definite entity, despite the failure of Marshall [88] to document a single case of esophageal involvement in a series of more than 8,000 cases of regional enteritis. The first case of esophageal involvement in Crohn's disease was reported by Eggers in 1935 [31]. Eighteen years after Crohn's classic paper on ileal disease [20], the first report of a process limited to the esophagus appeared with the description by Franklin and Taylor of three patients with isolated esophageal strictures and a histologic picture of nonspecific granulomatous esophagitis [39]. Subsequently, there have been several reports indicating Crohn's disease involving the esophagus (albeit rarely, with approximately 60 cases described in the world's literature to date) [2, 7, 12, 21, 24, 30, 42–45, 56, 68, 79, 84, 86, 94, 125, 128, 137]. Ulcerative esophagitis has also

been described in a few patients in whom inflammatory bowel disease was categorized as ulcerative colitis [15, 65, 141].

The real incidence of Crohn's disease of the esophagus is not known. Geboes and colleagues [43] retrospectively observed esophageal involvement in 9 of 500 patients (incidence, 1.8%). This figure may be potentially misleading, however, as upper gastrointestinal endoscopy or radiography was not performed on all patients, but rather in the 95 patients with symptoms referable to the upper gastrointestinal tract (19%) and in the 12 patients with stomatitis (2.4%). A more recent, retrospective study of Crohn's disease in 230 children showed that 30% of patients overall had lesions of the esophagus, stomach, and duodenum, with 6.5% having specific esophageal involvement [75]. Tishler and Helman [128], reporting on 140 patients with Crohn's disease of the ileum, colon, or both, noted that 2.8% of patients had esophageal involvement. It appears that when the esophagus is involved in Crohn's disease, these patients almost always have concomitant ileocolic disease, although rare cases of isolated esophageal Crohn's disease have been reported [79].

### Clinical Features

The symptoms of Crohn's esophagitis are nonspecific and depend on the activity and duration of disease. Dyspepsia, dysphagia, chest pain, and weight loss are the more typical presenting complaints [44]. Recognizably, as with any of the extraintestinal manifestations of inflammatory bowel disease, the esophageal symptoms may occasionally precede the clinical manifestations of small- or large-bowel involvement. More commonly, the esophageal involvement is recognized concurrently with or after the diagnosis of granulomatous ileocolitis [12, 128]. As a general rule, those patients with Crohn's esophagitis come to medical attention late in the course of the disease when severe dysphagia, due to strictures or other complications, has developed [51].

D. A. Johnson: Department of Gastroenterology, Eastern Virginia School of Medicine, and Digestive and Liver Disease Specialists, Ltd., Norfolk, Virginia 23502.

Pulmonary symptoms of cough and recurrent infection should strongly suggest esophageal involvement in patients with Crohn's disease, as esophageal-pulmonary fistulization has been described [123]. The symptom of hoarseness—often a protean manifestation of gastroesophageal reflux—is more likely a reflection of involvement of the larynx and bronchial tree [74], as there is no reported increased proclivity for gastroesophageal reflux in patients with Crohn's disease.

## Radiographic Features

The spectrum of radiographic findings resembles the classic features of regional enteritis. Aphthous ulcerations are the earliest manifestation. These appear as punctate, slitlike, or ringlike collections of barium, surrounded by a fine radiolucent halo [24, 76]. These ulcers are usually not numerous (fewer than five) and are sporadically distributed throughout the esophagus, with intervening areas of normal mucosa. As such, these lesions may be quite subtle, and double-contrast radiography will enhance detection. With further involvement, the size and number of these ulcers may increase, producing a localized or diffuse esophagitis. Deep irregular areas of ulceration or a linear serpiginous configuration (reminiscent of the lower colonic involvement) may be seen [12, 21, 24]. Severe esophagitis may be manifest by thickened, nodular, or varicoid folds (Fig. 35–1A), occasionally

associated with pseudomembrane formation or a diffuse cobblestone appearance [12, 21]. In advanced cases, fistula may be evident. Progression of the esophageal fistulization may lead to erosion into adjacent organs and esophagobronchial or esophagomediastinal fistula formation [12, 21]. Progressive scarring and fibrosis eventually may lead to the development of strictures, which are most often found in the distal third of the esophagus and are the most common radiographic finding in the advanced stage of esophageal Crohn's disease (Fig. 35–1B) [12, 30, 79, 134]. These strictures invariably are greater than 1 cm long (unlike uncomplicated peptic strictures) and may involve a considerable segment of the esophagus [56]. They may occasionally be associated with traction-type hiatal hernias due to concomitant scarring and shortening of the esophagus in its longitudinal axis [84]. Rarely, filiform polyposis of the esophagus may develop in advanced esophageal Crohn's disease, analogous to the filiform polyposis of the colon in granulomatous colitis [17].

## Endoscopic Features

The endoscopic appearance of Crohn's disease of the esophagus can be highly variable [3], but two stages have been distinguished [56]. The predominant morphologic changes are more typically localized to the middle or lower esophagus. In stage 1, inflammatory changes predominate,

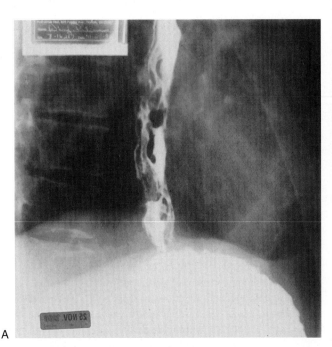

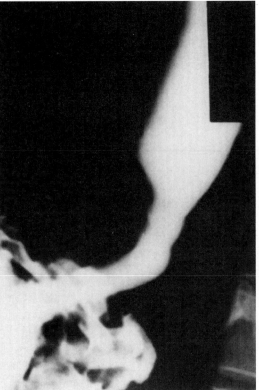

A             B

**FIG. 35–1. A:** Thickened nodular varicoid folds seen with Crohn's involvement of the distal esophagus. **B:** Distal esophageal stricture in a patient with Crohn's disease with concomitant terminal ileal involvement. (Courtesy Dr. James L Buck, Archives of the Department of Radiologic Pathology, Armed Forces Institute of Pathology, Washington, DC.)

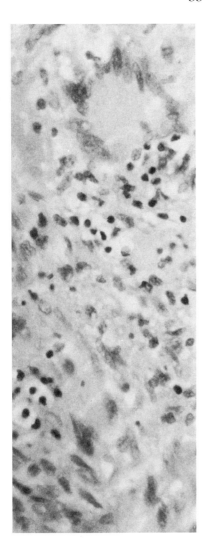

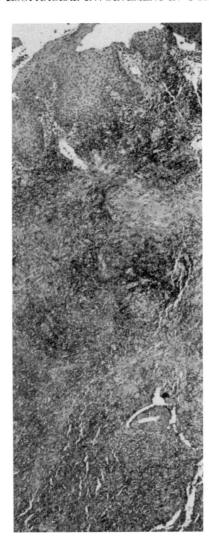

**FIG. 35–2.** Biopsy specimen of an esophageal lesion showing noncaseating granuloma surrounded by polymorphic inflammatory component with diffuse proliferation of the epithelioid histiocytes (hematoxylin and eosin; × 100). Inset (*left*) shows giant cells (× 400).

and the esophagitis is mild or more often erosive and ulcerative. In addition to erosions, shallow, irregular ulcerations with a fibrinous base may be seen, which are surrounded by an erythematous margin and often localized in normal esophageal mucosa (Plate 52). When these changes are more extensive, the macroscopic appearance may be strikingly similar to the colonoscopic features, with flat, extensive ulcerations, polypoid cobblestone-like change, and intervening normal-appearing mucosa (Plate 53A) [40, 56]. Fistulous disease may also be seen (Plate 53B, C). Polypoid or varicoid-like changes may suggest malignancy in some cases and biopsies should be done to exclude dysplasia (Plate 53D).

Stage 2 is categorized by stenosis similar to that from reflux esophagitis or neoplasia [56]. This stenosis is tubular and localized in the middle or lower esophagus. The endoscopic appearance of the stenosis is that of a funnel-like narrowing. Ringlike stenosis has not been described. In some cases, polypoid irregular areas may simulate a malignancy [30, 56, 132]. It has been speculated that a columnar-lined (Barrett's) esophagus might be seen in Crohn's disease in view of the potentially severe inflammatory changes of the

esophagus, and this has been described on rare occasion [51, 72].

### Histopathologic Features

Granulomas are generally accepted as histologic proof of Crohn's disease, provided that other causes of granulomatous involvement of the gastrointestinal tract can be excluded [98, 109]. Such granulomas have been reported, however, in a limited number of cases of esophageal Crohn's disease [42, 43, 79, 93, 108] and only rarely in endoscopic biopsies (Fig. 35–2) [42, 68, 94]. Endoscopic procurement of biopsy material by the use of jumbo forceps, biopsying from the edge of the ulcerated areas, and serial sectioning of the fixed specimens may all augment the yield in discovering granulomatous change [43]. Granulomas are found less often in patients who are treated with steroids [88] and are not essential for the pathologic diagnosis of Crohn's disease [108]. Esophagitis typically shows focal inflammation in the epithelium and lamina propria, with the absence of the other classic epithelial alterations for reflux disease [3, 10, 37].

## Differential Diagnosis

The radiograqphic and endoscopic manifestations of Crohn's esophagitis may pose a diagnostic dilemma if evaluated independently or without clinical correlation. Aphthoid ulcerations can be seen also with peptic, viral, and mycotic esophagitis as well as other inflammatory colitides [15, 65, 77, 141]. Drug-related erosive changes need also to be excluded, as certain drugs, such as doxycycline, quinidine, potassium chloride, ferrous sulfate, and nonsteroidal anti-inflammatory preparations, produce aphthoid ulcerations [64]. Intramural sinus tracts and fistulization to adjacent organs, well-known complications of Crohn's enteritis, may be seen in the esophagus [21, 123], although similar complications have been reported in patients with tuberculosis, actinomycosis, histoplasmosis, and lymphoma [122]. The cicatricial and stenotic phase of esophageal Crohn's disease is suggestive of other differential diagnostic possibilities, including reflux esophagitis, caustic congestion, and infiltrative neoplasia. The distinction from the neoplasia may, at times, be difficult as evidenced by the fact that most cases of Crohn's esophagitis with surgical-pathologic documentation have been operated on with the presumptive diagnosis of esophageal carcinoma.

## Treatment

Corticosteroids have been highly effective in promoting symptomatic relief, within days in some cases [43, 44, 128]. Sulfasalazine has been tried in a few patients, with good subjective results [43]. Clinical activity of the esophageal lesions may parallel the colonic disease [43] and has responded to colectomy in one case [92]. Esophagectomy has been performed in some patients initially believed to have neoplastic disease [21, 56, 79]. It is conceivable that esophagectomy may be required in some cases of extensive Crohn's disease of the esophagus, although there are no reported cases of this primary approach to date.

## TUBERCULOSIS

In immuncompetent patients, tuberculous involvement of the esophagus, be it primary or secondary, is rare [87]. An incidence of 0.14% of macroscopic esophageal tuberculosis was noted in 18,049 autopsies on tuberculosis patients [16, 80]. Primary tuberculosis of the esophagus in patients without demonstrable tuberculous lesions elsewhere is even more rare [70, 106, 107, 111, 117, 121, 129]. It is assumed that infection occurs through ingestion, and the bacilli gain entry into the esophageal wall through a mucosal defect [121].

Secondary esophageal involvement may occur by several mechanisms. It is likely that most cases of reactivation disease are the result of contiguous extension from caseous hilar or mediastinal nodes, tuberculous spondylitis, or adjacent tuberculous lung infections [8, 22, 32]. Infection may also occur by swallowing tuberculous sputum. The rarity of this is striking, despite the large numbers of bacilli swallowed in patients with cavitary tuberculosis. This relative resistance to infection is believed to be due to esophageal mucosal protective factors such as the relatively resistant stratified squamous epithelium and other factors (rapid transit time, tubular structure) that limit prolonged contact of infectious materials [22]. Preexisting esophageal disease such as reflux esophagitis, ulcerative stricture, or carcinoma is believed to be requisite for implantation of the acid-fast bacilli [80, 110]. Caudad extension from pharyngeal or laryngeal involvement may occur in rare instances [22]. Finally, seeding of esophageal tissue during hematogenous spread of disease represents another possible pathogenic mechanism for secondary esophageal involvement [22, 110].

## Clinical Features

Clinical presentations of esophageal tuberculosis are nonspecific and depend on the type and content of pathologic involvement. Three types of the disease have been described—ulcerative, hypertrophic, and granular [34]. Pain is the major presenting symptom in the ulcerative type and is usually manifest as a constant retrosternal pain accompanied by dysphagia for solids and, ultimately, also for liquids. Hypertrophic esophageal tuberculosis involves the middle third of the esophagus and frequently presents with an obstructive stenosis with prominent dysphagia [34]. The granular form of esophageal disease is the least common variety and results from seeding during miliary spread of primary infection. As a result, patients may appear more systemically ill and may not have prominent esophageal complaints [34]. If an esophagobronchial fistula develops, patients may have liquid or particulate expectoration on swallowing, or have minor hematemesis [100]. Massive hematemesis from an aorto-esophageal fistual complicating tuberculosis aortitis has also been reported [54].

## Radiographic Features

The roentgenographic findings are not diagnostic, as the barium swallow may show ulceration, stricture, spasm, disordered motility, or alteration of the mucosal pattern compatible with other disease states [22, 66, 69, 110, 111, 126, 136]. Extraluminal extravasation of barium will be evident if a sinus tract or fistula is present [82, 139] (Fig. 35–3A). Esophageal obstruction may be rarely seen (Fig. 35–3B). If a midesophageal lesion is present in the region of the tracheal bifurcation, a tuberculous basis for this lesion should be considered [69, 78]. With the ulcerative form of esophageal tuberculosis, the ulcer may be solitary or multiple and typically occurs in the proximal third of the esophagus. In the hypertrophic form, a long segment of the esophagus is involved, typically the middle third. The mucosal pattern resembles hypertrophic ileocecal tuberculosis in its appearance and behavior [34]. In the granular form, multiple diffuse ulcerations are present, with typical miliary granuloma evident on chest x-ray.

## Endoscopic Features

The endoscopic appearance is dependent on the pathologic form of the disease [50]. The ulcerative type may demonstrate solitary or multiple ulcers occurring in the proximal

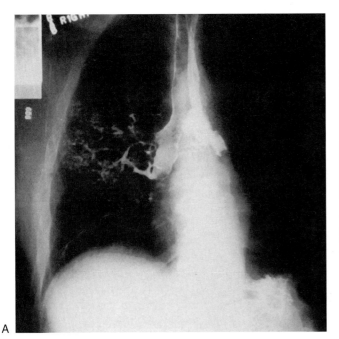
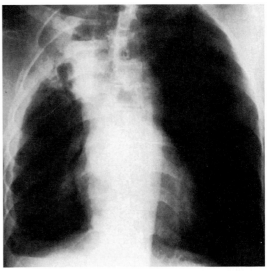

**FIG. 35–3. A:** Barium esophagram demonstrates an esophageal tracheal fistula due to tuberculosis desease. **B:** Air–fluid level seen here to the left of the trachea could be either cavitation or recurrent tuberculosis, a bronchotracheal or bronchoesophageal fistula, but in this case represents a deviated, partially obstructed esophagus secondary to tuberculous involvement. (Courtesy Dr. David J Curtis, Washington, DC.)

third of the esophagus [120] (Plate 54). Tuberculous ulcers in some patients may appear superficial and have a grayish base (Plate 55). Yellow tuberculous nodules may be seen in the surrounding mucosa [109]. Involvement of the carinal nodes may be evident by extrinsic compression or ulcerative change seen 24 to 26 cm from the incisors (Plate 56). Fistulous esophageobronchial communication can develop with progressive disease (Plate 57). The hypertrophic type affects the middle third and typically involves a long segment of the esophagus [121]. The granular form has a velvety appearance and may have yellowish translucent tubercles that are seeded during the miliary spread of primary infection [22, 130]. In general, endoscopy and histologic findings are nonspecific and only occasionally diagnostic in tuberculosis [27] but are more helpful in the exclusion of carcinoma.

## Histopathologic Features

Nonspecific inflammation is the most common finding in proved cases of esophageal tuberculosis. The classic appearance of caseating granulomas is seen in only approximately 50% of cases, and demonstration of acid-fast bacilli occurs in less than 25% of patients [22]. Some of the features, particularly in the hypertrophic form, may suggest Crohn's disease, but fissured ulcers, sinus tracts, and typical nonnecrotic granulomas are absent [121].

## Treatment

The small number of cases of esophageal tuberculosis reported in the literature prohibits vigorous generalizations re-

garding antituberculous chemotherapy regimens. Patients treated with isoniazid and streptomycin plus ethambutol or rifampin were relieved of esophageal symptoms more rapidly and had fewer complications [22]. Successful medical therapy of esophagobronchial fistulas has also been reported [18]. Although the majority of patients have been treated with three-drug regimens, other forms of extrapulmonary tuberculosis have been adequately treated with two-drug regimens, including isoniazid and rifampin [29]. On rare occasions, treatment with antituberculous therapy followed by staged esophageal bypass with gastric interposition and esophagectomy has been done in patients with a severe, long stenosis [121].

## Histoplasmosis

Histoplasmosis is the most common endemic respiratory mycosis in the United States, and most infections are self-limited with a paucity of symptoms. Gastrointestinal involvement with disseminated histoplasmosis has been recognized since Darling's original description of the disease in 1906 [23]. Esophageal involvement has been reported, but is rare [11, 49, 61, 102, 112, 114, 115]. Each of these reported cases represented impingement against or, rarely, erosion into the esophagus by infected mediastinal nodes. Esophageal involvement has also been reported in patients with disseminated histoplasmosis and most likely results from hematogenous spread from a primary pulmonary infection [73]. Histoplasmosis begins, in general, as a pulmonary infection that usually drains into hilar or peritracheal lymph nodes. Only when the posterior mediastinal nodes are affected is there direct esophageal involvement [47]. Esophageal complications from mediastinal histoplasmosis have occurred either during the acute phase of pulmonary infection or as a consequence of healing periadenitis. Occasionally, during acute pulmonary disease, enlarged mediastinal nodes may cause extrinsic esophageal compression. During active infection, inflammatory nodes may attach to the esophagus. During the healing phase, the encapsulated lesions may cause esophageal erosions and dissect into adjacent structures, causing fistulas [20, 25, 47]. During the development of the delayed type of hypersensitivity, intense fibrinogenesis may occur in the process of encapsulation of healing lymphadenitis, resulting in drainage into the esophagus [48].

### Clinical Features

Esophageal symptoms are rare in patients with histoplasmosis. Dysphagia was evident in 1 of 26 patients in one series and 7 of 47 patients in another series of patients with primary histoplasmosis [49]. Sudden onset of odynophagia was reported in one case as a manifestation of esophageal mucosal ulceration [112]. Odynophagia due to an extrinsic lesion will not occur unless the esophageal wall, particularly the muscular layers, is involved in the inflammatory process. Esophageal abscess formation secondary to nodal erosion [61] and fistula formation complicating mediastinal histoplasmosis have also been reported [19, 25, 48].

### Radiologic Features

The chest x-ray may show hilar adenopathy with prominent calcifications and atelectasis in the adjacent parenchyma. Calcification of other visceral organs, in particular the spleen, may be evident on a plain film of the abdomen. Barium studies may show esophageal compression anteriorly at the level of the tracheal bifurcation or carina (Fig. 35–4). The mucosal pattern may be irregular and extravasation evident if a sinus tract is present. Computed tomography

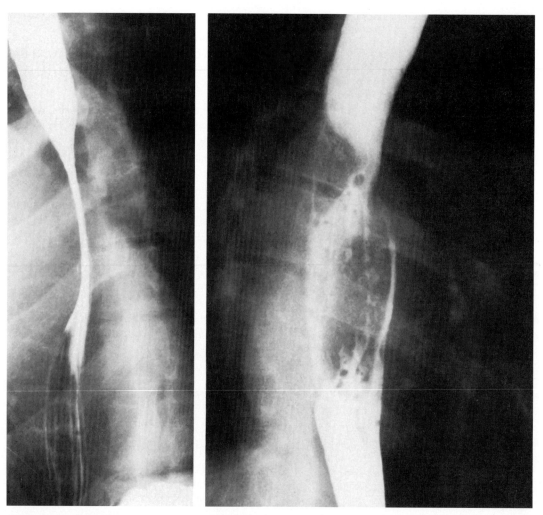

**FIG. 35–4.** Two opposite oblique views of the esophagus demonstrating a long, smooth effacement of the esophageal lumen. This is not a stricture, because the lumen size is different in two views, but rather is a nonspecific mass effect from histoplasmosis adenopathy. (Courtesy Dr. David J Curtis, Washington, DC.)

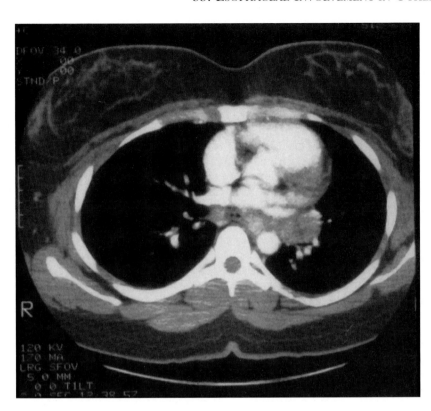

**FIG. 35–5.** A computed tomography of the thorax showing a 4-cm subcarinal mass that is inseparable from the left side of the esophagus and with intraesophageal air, compatible with fistulous communication due to histoplasmosis.

typically shows a perihilar inflammatory process with extension to the esophagus. Air, when seen in the esophagus in this setting, is suggestive of a fistulous communication (Fig. 35–5).

### Endoscopic Features

Endoscopy may reveal luminal narrowing at the level of the carina (24 to 26 cm from the incisors). The submucosal mass effect may be evident, with ulceration present in some cases [112] (Plate 58). In addition, a defect in the mucosal pattern may be appreciated if a sinus tract fistula is present [19] (Plate 59).

### Diagnostic Features

The diagnosis of esophageal disease due to histoplasmosis should be suspected if the appropriate clinical symptoms and radiologic features are present in a patient with exposure to an endemic area. A definite diagnosis is established only by demonstration of the organism in tissue obtained by bronchoscopy, sputum, or surgical means. Highly suggestive evidence of histoplasmosis is a complement fixation titer of 1:32 or more or a fourfold increase in convalescent titers obtained at least 2 weeks later. The histoplasmosis skin test is not diagnostic of active disease, but merely indicates previous infection.

### Treatment

Treatment of esophageal involvement in histoplasmosis has been primarily surgical based on the nature of the involvement [41]. Varying degrees of esophageal compression may be seen in patients with mediastinal granuloma. Mild forms of compression due to associated caseous adenopathy may resolve without treatment [28, 103]. Enucleation of the caseous nodes at the time of thoracotomy resulted in relief in some patients [41]. Mild esophageal compression is commonly seen in patients with fibrosing mediastinitis, although symptoms are rarely present. Tracheobronchial fistula is believed to require immediate intervention [25, 36, 41, 58]. Blind sinus formation has been treated by surgical means [25, 41, 58], although amphotericin B has been used as the sole treatment in a few patients, with excellent response [19, 61]. In general, amphotericin B is usually not recommended because mediastinal involvement is determined by host response to a pulmonary infection and not by activity of infection and because *Histoplasma capsulatum* grows poorly in the mediastinum [48, 112].

## SYPHILIS

Tertiary syphilitic lesions of the esophagus are rare manifestations of the disease. There are fewer than 100 reported cases in the literature, and the validity of many of the reports is lacking, being without autopsy confirmation [1, 6, 52, 57, 99, 101, 122, 138].

The syphilitic process reaches the esophagus by one of two routes [99, 101, 140]: (a) A gumma develops primarily in the wall of the esophagus, usually in the submucosa, or (b) there is direct extension of the syphilitic process from a neighboring organ or tissue such as the aorta, mediastinal lymph nodes, lung parenchyma, or sternum. This latter spread represents the more common of the two pathways for esophageal involvement.

Having involved the esophagus, the syphilitic process may terminate in the esophageal wall in one of three ways [99, 101, 140]. Involution by fatty degeneration may occur, followed by complete healing without ulceration or an appreciable fibrosis. Alternatively, there may be necrosis of tissues and extension to the mucosa without ulceration. As healing takes place, there results a fibrous distortion of the tissue that contracts and produces a rather localized stenosis of the esophageal lumen. A third possibility is that the process is more chronic in its progress and invades the tissues of the esophageal wall in a diffuse manner, encircling the lumen in the greater part of its length. There may be sclerosis and superficial ulceration, as a consequence of which healing results in a very marked esophageal stenosis.

## Clinical Features

Syphilis involving the esophagus occurs equally in men and women. The lesion occurs in adult life during the age period in which syphilis is most commonly acquired and rarely occurs in the congenital form [6]. The esophagus may be involved in the secondary stage and is associated with mucous plaques and ulcerations. Gummas and contractional sclerosis appear in the tertiary type [6].

The symptomatology of this condition is similar in many respects to the other stenosing lesions of the esophagus. There are no early symptoms, though there may be transitory periods of dysphagia in the stage of inflammation, followed by asymptomatic periods. A history of intermittent attacks of mild dysphagia is of significant importance in suggesting the diagnosis. Patients rarely have pain, although there may be some with laryngeal involvement. The onset of dysphagia is gradual, often exceeding a 4- to 12-month duration, and dysphagia increases as the stenosis progresses [140]. Weight loss, anemia, and asthenia occur in the last stage as a function of the malnutrition as well as the syphilitic toxemia [6].

## Radiologic Features

There is no characteristic roentgenographic appearance of diffuse syphilitic esophagitis with stenosis, but there are several features that are more or less peculiar to this condition alone [140]. The walls of the esophagus will be fairly rigid, with little change in the contour or caliber of the barium column as it travels through the esophagus (Fig. 35–6). In addition, as it passes the area of narrowing, the barium will have a finely irregular outline. Dilatation above the lesion is usually not a striking feature. Ulcerations may be evident as a consequence of rupture of a gumma. Extrinsic compression may be evident as lymphatic involvement may be pronounced and demonstrable on x-rays of other organs (Fig. 35–7).

## Endoscopic Features

Esophagoscopy and biopsy studies are essential, particularly to exclude neoplastic disease. Nonspecific esophagitis may be seen, more often involving the midesophagus [124]. In contrast, gummatous ulceration, when present, is usually evident in the upper or lower third of the esophagus [124]. When a gumma is present within the esophageal wall, it may be impossible to make a diagnosis either by roentgenographic or by endoscopic means [101].

## Histopathologic Features

The histologic features are nondiagnostic. In chronic diffuse syphilitic esophagitis, there is a full-thickness inflammatory infiltrate. Parenchymal destruction with an infiltrate of lymphocytes and plasma cells as well as prominent fibrosis are typical features. Lymphocytic infiltration of the small blood vessels with intimal proliferation is a hallmark feature for the syphilitic arteritis that causes tissue devitalization and consequent mucosal and submucosal inflammatory changes [52, 97, 124].

## Diagnosis

Establishing the diagnosis may be difficult. A history of gradual, painless, and intermittent dysphagia is important.

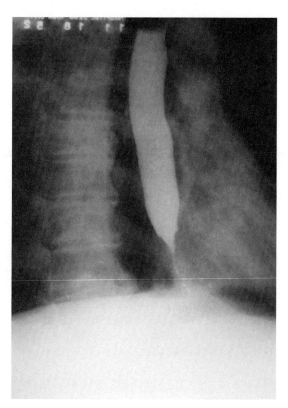

**FIG. 35–6.** Rigid, nondistensible distal esophageal stricture in a patient with tertiary syphilis. (Courtesy Dr. James L Buck, Archives of the Department of Radiologic Pathology, Armed Forces Institute of Pathology, Washington, DC.)

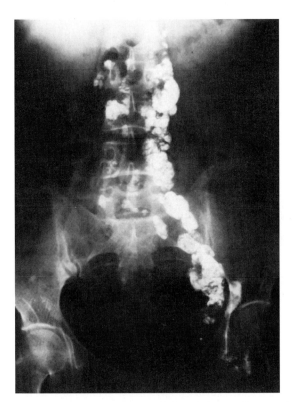

**FIG. 35-7.** Lymphangiogram of the abdomen in a patient with tertiary syphilis demonstrating diffuse, significantly enlarged adenopathy, which can extend into the chest and produce an effect similar to that seen with histoplasmosis. (Courtesy Dr. David J Curtis, Washington, DC.)

The presence of suspicious lesions in adjacent organs or in distant parts of the body may suggest the diagnosis. A positive Wassermann reaction is also important, but a negative reaction does not exclude the diagnosis, any more than a positive reaction establishes it. Radiologic and endoscopic evaluations supplement a careful clinical history and often help exclude other disease states manifesting esophageal involvement.

## Treatment

Treatment of esophageal involvement is directed primarily at the primary infection. Symptomatic response to specific therapy is usually rapid [1, 57, 97, 124]. Esophageal dilatation is required if luminal stricturing is present. As the stenoses are frequently long and may be due to transmural fibrosis, esophageal dilatation should be approached with extreme caution, analogous to the approach of dilating strictures due to radiation or caustic ingestion [111].

## SARCOIDOSIS

Well-documented accounts of esophageal sarcoidosis are exceptionally scarce. Two large necropsy studies of patients with sarcoidosis failed to demonstrate esophageal involve-

ment in any case [59, 81]. To date, from my review, there have been four reported cases in the literature [62, 105, 116, 127].

### Clinical Features

Three of the four reported cases had dysphagia as a primary esophageal complaint [62, 105, 116]. One patient with pulmonary involvement manifested by extensive fibrosis developed dysphasia secondary to moderate stenosis of the distal esophagus [62]. A similar esophagogram was evident in another patient with diffuse sarcoidosis involving the lungs, liver, spleen, and esophagus [81]. The third patient with dysphagia had proximal esophageal involvement of the cricopharyngeus muscle [116]. A fourth patient with esophageal involvement had diffuse gastrointestinal sarcoidosis, but no symptoms referable to the esophagus [127].

Sarcoidosis may cause granulomatous hepatic disease and is a rare cause of portal hypertension. As a consequence, esophageal involvement presenting with variceal hemorrhage may occur [13, 38, 53, 95].

### Radiologic Features

Chest x-rays may demonstrate hilar adenopathy or parenchymal involvement with a nodular or interstitial pattern [60]. Barium esophagography in one case demonstrated distal esophageal irregularity [103]. Regional lymphadenopathy may be evident, demonstrating extrinsic compression on the esophagus (Fig. 35–8). Esophageal varices may also be evident if portal hypertension is present (Fig. 35–9).

### Diagnosis

All patients reported with esophageal involvement demonstrated noncaseating granulomas on biopsy obtained at surgery or autopsy. There have been no reported cases of esophageal sarcoidosis established by endoscopic examination (with or without biopsy). Differentiation from granulomatous infectious diseases may be possible by history, skin testing, and histologic special staining. Serum angiotensin-converting enzyme (ACE) elevations are found almost uniformly in lymph nodes in sarcoidosis and are usually evident in serum as well [53, 119]. Elevated ACE levels may also be found in granulomatous diseases, such as tuberculosis, silicosis, berylliosis, and Gaucher's disease, but not in Crohn's disease, where values are typically lower than normal [120]. Because sarcoidosis rarely causes obstructive diseases elsewhere in the gastrointestinal viscera, differentiation from Crohn's disease may be difficult. The histology of Crohn's disease is characterized by transmural inflammation with lymphoid aggregates in the bowel wall [97], whereas visceral sarcoidosis usually involves only the mucosa. The granulomas are similar in appearance, although deposits of immunoglobulin (Ig) A, IgM, IgG, and IgD have all been demonstrated in granuloma of sarcoidosis, but not in Crohn's

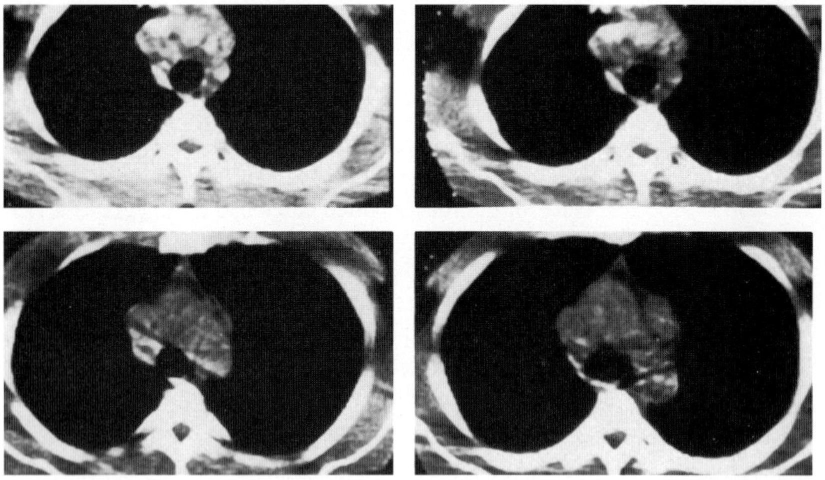

**FIG. 35–8.** Computed tomography demonstrating adenopathy in the region of the esophagus in a patient with sarcoidosis. This would produce the same barium examination as seen in the patient with histoplasmosis (see Fig. 35–4). (Courtesy Dr. David J. Curtis, Washington, DC.)

disease [97]. The presence of Schaumann's bodies has also been used to favor the diagnosis of sarcoidosis [136].

### Treatment

With the paucity of cases in the literature, there is little experience with directed treatment for esophageal sarcoidosis. Palliative dilatation may be required for the symptomatic

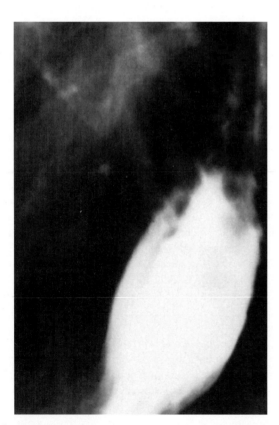

**FIG. 35–9.** Barium esophagogram showing lower esophageal varices caused by portal hypertension in a young woman with far-advanced sarcoidosis. (Courtesy Dr. David J Curtis, Washington, DC.)

relief of obstructive complaints. Resolution of dysphagia was evident in one patient who received steroids and who did not undergo esophageal dilatation [105].

### BLASTOMYCOSIS

North American blastomycosis is a chronic infection by the fungus *Blastomyces dermatitidis,* which predominantly affects the lungs, skin, bone, and genitourinary tract. Gastrointestinal involvement has been exceedingly rare, with review articles and case reports describing esophageal involvement in only eight cases [9, 14, 63, 89, 92, 113, 118, 132, 136].

### Clinical Features

Dysphagia is the primary esophageal symptom and was evident in five of the eight reported cases of esophageal blastomycosis [9, 14, 63, 92, 113, 132]. Dysphagia may be longstanding, and in one case antedated the skin lesions (and diagnosis) by 4 years [14]. Four patients had dysphagia due to disease limited to the esophagus. Fistula formation was evident in two patients, one of whom developed fistula and abscess following bougienage which resulted in an esophageal perforation. Esophageal involvement was part of disseminated infection in three patients, two of whom had no dysphagia, but were found at autopsy to have esophageal involvement. Gastrointestinal bleeding from erosive esophagitis was the presenting symptom in one patient without dysphagia [92].

Pulmonary disease, which is commonly evident in blastomycosis [9, 14], has been present in only four of the eight cases of esophageal blastomycosis reported to date [14, 89, 92, 113, 118]. Two patients had widely disseminated disease [89, 118]. Primary lung involvement with subsequent esophageal fistula formation was found in another patient [14]. Asymptomatic pulmonary disease with positive sputum examinations and chronic interstitial changes on chest x-ray was seen in the fourth patient [92].

### Roentgenographic Features

Barium esophagograms may be suggestive of esophageal carcinoma. Esophageal strictures have been reported involving the proximal esophagus in two patients [113, 118] and the distal esophagus in two patients [63, 92]. The esophageal wall is rigid and may show irregular spicular mucosa [63].

### Endoscopic Features

Esophagogastroscopy results have been reported in only two patients [14, 63]. Distal esophageal stenosis with elevated white mucosa suggestive of neoplasia was seen in one patient [63], whereas erythematous friable mucosa with linear ulcerations was described in the second patient [92].

### Diagnosis

Histopathologic analysis of the esophageal lesion typically shows granuloma formation. Giant cells may contain large, thick-walled yeasts with single buds characteristic of *B. dermatitidis* [63]. In those patients in whom surgical resection has been done to exclude carcinoma, the esophageal wall showed marked thickening due to a pseudoepitheliomatous hyperplasia, granulomatous inflammation, muscular hypertrophy, and fibrosis [63]. Silver staining of the pathologic specimen increases the diagnostic yield. Cultures are typically positive, although fungal serologic findings may be negative [63].

### Treatment

Six of the previously reported cases of esophageal blastomycosis were treated before 1956, the year amphotericin B became available as an antifungal agent. Treatment was invariably ineffective and included iodide, gentian violet, penicillin, stilbamidine, or supportive care. Two patients have been treated with amphotericin B with excellent therapeutic response. One developed a distal esophageal stricture following successful eradication of the organism, but the stricture responded to palliative dilatation [92].

### EOSINOPHILIC ESOPHAGITIS

Eosinophilic esophagitis has rarely been reported as a manifestation of eosinophilic gastroenteritis syndrome, which is characterized by gastrointestinal symptoms, peripheral eosinophilia, and infiltration of the gastrointestinal tissue by mature eosinophils [26, 35, 71, 83, 90, 104, 133]. Approximately one-half of these patients have some allergic manifestation or a specific food intolerance. In patients with idiopathic eosinophilic esophagitis an allergic disorder is frequently present (80%), with the diagnosis based on the history of asthma, allergic rhinitis, allergic urticaria, hay fever, atopic dermatitis, food or medication allergy, and/or a positive response on the radioallergosorbent test or the allergic skin test.

Recently, esophageal eosinophilia without peripheral eosinophilia also was described as a distinct syndrome in a group of patients presenting with dysphagia [5]. Esophageal manometries have shown nonspecific motor disturbance in 14% of these patients and 24-hour esophageal monitoring revealed normal findings in all patients [5]. Manometric abnormalities including diffuse esophageal spasm [133] and vigorous achalasia [71] have been reported in other patients with eosinophilic esophagitis.

### Radiographic Features

A retrospective review of idiopathic eosinophilic gastroenteritis and idiopathic eosinophilic esophagitis demonstrated that a proximal esophageal stricture was the most common esophageal abnormality, seen in approximately 80% of patients [133]. Additionally, both distal esophageal mucosal rings and proximal esophageal webs have been reported [35, 83, 90, 133]. Concomitant changes in the stomach, duodenum, and small bowel are typical in patients with esophageal involvement of eosinophilic gastroenteritis, with luminal narrowing, rigidity, stricture, nodularity, or thickening among the radiographic spectrum of findings.

### Endoscopic Features

Endoscopic identification of a proximal esophageal stricture should suggest eosinophilic esophagitis as a differential concern [83, 90, 133]. The distal esophageal mucosal pattern is typically normal, delineating this from peptic esophagitis. Pseudomembrane formation may be evident proximal to the esophageal stricture [133]. In the syndrome of esophageal eosinophilia with dysphagia in the absence of peripheral eosinophilia, the endoscopic appearance of the esophagus is normal [5].

### Histopathologic Features

Eosinophilic infiltration of the esophageal mucosa and submucosa is evident in all patients with idiopathic eosinophilic esophagitis occurring alone or in conjunction with eosinophilic gastroenteritis [26, 133]. In the syndrome of esophageal eosinophilia with dysphagia in the absence of peripheral eosinophilia, high concentrations of intraepithelial esophageal eosinophils (more than 20 per high-power field) have been used as a diagnostic criterion [5].

### Differential Diagnosis

The radiologic and endoscopic features may suggest neoplasia, esophagitis associated with corrosive agents, pill-induced damage, or radiation injury. Epidermolysis bullosa, and bullous pemphigoid with upper esophageal involvement should also be considered. Nasogastric tube and postoperative strictures are rare complications, but may involve the proximal or distal esophagus. Inflammatory bowel disease (Crohn's-disease-related stricture) is typically found in the midesophagus, in contrast to the more proximal nature for eosinophilic esophagitis [35, 83, 90, 133].

## Treatment

In general, patients with idiopathic eosinophilic esophagitis occurring alone or in conjunction with eosinophilic gastroenteritis do respond to steroids. The subgroup of patients with the esophageal eosinophilia with dysphagia in the absence of peripheral eosinophilia have not been treated with steroids, but this should be considered for patients with incapacitating symptoms [5]. Dilatation of strictures has led to prompt symptomatic improvement, although symptoms may persist due to secondary underlying esophageal motor disorder until the steroid therapy becomes effective [133].

## BACTERIAL ESOPHAGITIS

Bacterial esophagitis is uncommon and has not been well recognized. Difficulty arises in ascertaining whether the bacteria are primary pathogens or coexistent colonization. Walsh and co-workers [135] established strict criteria for this diagnosis. The requisite histopathologic criterion is demonstration of bacterial invasion of esophageal mucosa within deeper layers, with no concomitant fungal, viral, or neoplastic involvement and no previous esophageal surgery. Nonbacteremic, but clinically overt bacterial esophagitis with *Lactobacillus acidophilus* [93] and group A beta-hemolytic streptococci [55] has been documented in two nonimmunocompromised patients. In a radiologic study of 34 patients with opportunistic infections of the upper gastrointestinal tract, two had evidence of *Klebsiella* esophagitis and bacteremia [4]. In an immunocompromised host, bacterial esophagitis may be more common than previously recognized and should be considered a potential source of bacteremia. Bacterial esophagitis has been reported in one patient with human immunodeficiency virus infection [33].

### Clinical Features

Typical features of esophagitis are evident, with dysphagia, odynophagia, and chest pain as prominent manifestations. Fever may be present with invasive disease due to bacteremia. Suspicion should be high for the diagnosis in any immunocompromised host with these clinical findings.

### Radiographic Features

Barium radiography may show diffuse, shaggy, ulcerated mucosa. Esophageal pseudomembrane formation has been described [33, 135].

### Endoscopic Features

A marked exudative inflammatory reaction is the primary endoscopic finding. The presence of a pseudomembrane indicates extensive destruction of the squamous epithelium (Color Plates 60 and 61). Thus, the presence of a pseudomembrane may be a useful endoscopic marker of the severity of the esophageal bacterial infection.

Endoscopic biopsy typically reveals the bacterial organisms. In patients in whom this diagnosis is suspected, a specimen must be sent in nonbacteriostatic saline for appropriate cultures. Special stains for fungal and vital pathogens should also be done.

### Treatment

Treatment is guided initially by the morphologic identification of the organism by Gram's stain. Final identification and sensitivity will be established by appropriate culture results.

### Necrotizing Esophagitis

Noncaustic-related acute esophageal necrosis, also known as acute necrotizing esophagitis or esophageal infarction, has been rarely reported [46, 85, 91, 96]. Acute necrotizing esophagitis seems to occur primarily in critically ill patients and is characterized by a subclinical and rapidly evolving state that may remain undiagnosed or be misdiagnosed as reflux esophagitis. The pathogenesis is unclear, but several facts point to the presence of a potential ischemic mechanism. The histologic lesion is that of a sudden diffuse necrosis with an occasional thrombotic vessel. Recognizably, the blood supply to the distal third of the esophagus is limited. It has been speculated that when the regulatory blood flow is impaired (e.g., critical illness, diabetes, hypoxia), the esophageal mucosa is particularly susceptible, including potentially an abnormal sensitivity to refluxed gastric acid [90]. All patients with necrotizing esophagitis reported to date have had impaired disease status, with hypoxemia, diabetes, and a postoperative state being the more common associated conditions [46, 85, 91, 96].

### Radiologic Features

The radiologic description of acute esophageal necrosis is limited. In one patient, barium x-ray demonstrated a long and extremely narrowed, newly developed stenosis [96].

### Endoscopic Features

The endoscopic picture is striking and shows a diffusely blackened esophagus with or without exudate. The distribution of these findings primarily involves the distal third of the esophagus (Plate 62), ending sharply at the transitional line of the esophagogastric junction. From the endoscopic point of view, the "black esophagus picture" is similar to that of the esophageal necrosis seen after caustic ingestion. Lesser degrees of a blackish or brownish exudate may also be seen as in severe cases of *Candida* esophagitis. Subsequent endoscopies (dependent on the course of the patient with necrotizing esophagitis) have occasionally shown complete resolution, but a time sequence for follow-up endoscopies has not been specified [96]. Interestingly, simultaneous gastric and duodenal damage has been found in the majority of patients, pointing to a common mechanism potentially related to stress. Gastric outlet obstruction was evident in three reported patients [91, 96].

## Histopathology

The histologic picture is one of a diffuse and severe necrosis (without recognizable stratified squamous epithelium) affecting mucosa and submucosa. Diffuse hemorrhage is a constant feature and deranged muscle fibers and scattered thrombosed vessels are frequently evident.

## Treatment

There is no specific treatment apart from support of the patient with efforts to improve perfusion and oxygenation and limit to any concomitant acid reflux-related injury. Obviously, stricture dilatation should be performed if a stricture develops. The use of steroids and antibiotics is of doubtful benefit. Prognosis is usually poor, given the severity of the associated disease process. Esophagectomy has been performed in at least one patient [46]. Acute necrotizing esophagitis, while by itself not necessarily lethal and irreversible, more likely mirrors the severity of the underlying illness.

## ACTINOMYCOSIS

*Actinomyces israelii* was previously considered to be a fungus but is now classified as a bacterium. Morphologically, this organism is a pleomorphic, Gram-positive, rod-shaped bacterium. Involvement of the esophagus may occur as a primary event when the swallowed organism penetrates a traumatized esophagus. More often, the involvement is secondary, developing from contiguous spread from an adjacent structure or from hematogenous spread from a distant site. From the esophagus itself, the infection may spread hematogenously or by direct extension, particularly to the mediastinum.

### Radiographic Features

The radiographic features are nondiagnostic. Nonspecific ulceration and inflammation are typical, and an esophago-bronchial fistula has been demonstrated rarely [131].

### Endoscopic Features

Endoscopic examination in the early stage of esophageal involvement may demonstrate a lesion seen as an abscess or ulceration with irregular, ragged edges [67]. A sinus or fistulous tract opening may be evident, with characteristic yellow "sulfur granules" draining from the site.

### Histopathologic Features

Chronic granulomas are frequently evident [67]. The sulfur granules represent clumps or chains of gram-positive bacteria that have invaded tissue and produced a purulent necrotic debris. Polymorphonuclear leukocytes, plasma cells, histiocytes, and giant cells surround the abscesses and sinuses.

### Diagnosis

The diagnosis may be suggested by endoscopic or histologic examination. In reality, the diagnosis is rarely made until fistulization develops and the sulfur granule drainage is seen. Anaerobic bacterial culture confirms the diagnosis. Skin tests and serologic methods are unreliable [67].

### Treatment

High-dose penicillin is the treatment of choice, using 10 to 20 million units parenterally daily for a minimum of 6 weeks or until the lesions have healed [67]. Tetracycline and clindamycin are less popular alternatives. Surgery may be required if the abscesses, sinuses, or fistulas do not respond to antimicrobial therapy.

## REFERENCES

1. Abel AC. Syphilis of the esophagus. Lancet 1928;2:441
2. Achenbach H, Lynch JP, Dwight RW. Idiopathic ulcerative esophagitis—report of a case. N Engl J Med 1956;225:456
3. Alcantara M, et al. Endoscopic and biopsy findings in the upper gastrointestinal tract in patients with Crohn's disease. Endoscopy 1993;25:282
4. Athey PA, Goldstein HM, Dodd GD. Radiologic spectrum of opportunistic infections of the upper gastrointestinal tract. Am J Respir 1977;129:419
5. Attwood SEA, et al. Esophageal eosinophilia with dysphagia: a distinct clinopathologic syndrome. Dig Dis Sci 1993;38:109
6. Avery PS. Syphilis of the esophagus. Radiology 1936;27:323
7. Bagby RJ, Rogers JV, Hobbs C. Crohn's disease of the esophagus, stomach and duodenum—a review with emphasis on the radiographic findings. South Med J 1972;65:515
8. Bloomberg TJ, Dow CJ. Contemporary mediastinal tuberculosis. Thorax 1980;35:392
9. Busey JF, et al. Blastomycosis: I. A review of 198 collected cases in Veterans Administration Hospitals. Am Rev Respir Dis 1964;89:659
10. Carr DT, Spain DM. Tuberculosis in a carcinoma of the esophagus. Am Rev Tuberculosis 1947;46:346
11. Case records of the Massachusetts General Hospital. N Engl J Med 1976;295:381
12. Chahremani GG, et al. Esophageal manifestations of Crohn's disease. Gastrointest Radiol 1982;7:199
13. Cheitlin MD, et al. Portal hypertension in sarcoidosis. Am J Gastroenterol 1960;38:60
14. Cherniss EI, Waisbren BA. North American blastomycosis: a clinical study of 40 cases. Ann Intern Med 1956;44:105
15. Christopher NL, Watson DW, Faber FW. Relationship of chronic ulcerative esophagitis to ulcerative colitis. Ann Intern Med 1969;70:971

16. Clerf T. Tuberculous pseudoesophageal abscess producing stenosis: report of a case. Ann Otol Rhinol Laryngol 1940;49:793

17. Cockey BM, et al. Filiform polyps of the esophagus with inflammatory bowel disease. AJR 1985;144:1207

18. Conjalka JS, et al. Successful treatment of a tuberculous BE fistula. Mt Sinai J Med 1980;47:283

19. Coss KC, et al. Esophageal fistula formation complicating mediastinal histoplasmosis—response to amphotericin B. Am J Med 1987;83:343

20. Crohn BB, Ginzburg L, Oppenheimer GD. Regional ileitis; a pathological and clinical entity. JAMA 1932;99:1323

21. Cynn W, et al. Crohn's disease of the esophagus. AJR 1975;125:359

22. Damtew B, et al. Esophageal tuberculosis: mimicracy of gastrointestinal malignancy. Rev Infect Dis 1987;9:140

23. Darling ST. A protozoan general infection producing pseudotubercles in the lungs and focal necrosis in the liver, spleen, and lymph nodes. JAMA 1906;46:1283

24. Degryse HR, DeSchepper AM. Aphthoid esophageal ulcers in Crohn's disease of the ileum and colon. Gastrointest Radiol 1984;9(3):197

25. Dines DE, et al. Mediastinal granuloma and fibrosing mediastinitis. Chest 1979;75:320

26. Dobbins JW, Sheahan DG, Beahart J. Eosinophilic gastroenteritis with esophageal involvement. Gastroenterology 1977;72:1312

27. Dow CJ. Esophageal tuberculosis: four cases. Gut 1981;22:234

28. Dukes RJ, et al. Esophageal involvement with mediastinal granuloma. JAMA 1976;80:2313

29. Dutt AK, Moers D, Stead WW. Short-course chemotherapy for extrapulmonary tuberculosis: nine years experience. Ann Intern Med 1986;104:7

30. Dyer NH, Cook PL, Harper RA. Esophageal stricture associated with Crohn's disease. Gut 1969;10:549

31. Eggers C. Resection of thoracic portion of the esophagus for chronic ulcer. Ann Surg 1935;104:940

32. Eng J, Sabanathan S. Tuberculosis of the esophagus, Dig Dis Sci 1991;36:536

33. Ezzell JH, Bremer J, Adamec TA. Bacterial esophagitis: an often forgotten cause of odynophagia. Am J Gastroenterol 1990;95:296

34. Fahmy AR, Guindi R, Fared A. Tuberculosis of the esophagus. Thorax 1969;24:254

35. Feczko PJ, Halpert RD, Martin Z. Radiographic abnormalities in eosinophilic esophagitis. Gastrointest Radiol 1985;10:321

36. Ferguson TB, Burford TH. Mediastinal granuloma: a 15-year experience. Ann Thorac Surg 1965;1:125

37. Fink SM, et al. Reassessment of esophageal histology in normal subjects: a comparison of suction and endoscopic techniques. J Clin Gastroenterol 1983;5:177

38. Fraimow W, Myerson RW. Portal hypertension and bleeding esophageal varices secondary to sarcoidosis of the liver. Am J Med 1957;23:995

39. Franklin RH, Taylor S. Nonspecific granulomatous esophagitis. J Thorac Cardiovasc Surg 1950;19:292

40. Fruhmorgen PW, Rosch P. Endoskopischer aspekt dis morbus crohn in osophagus, magen, duodenum, jejunum, ileum, and kolon. Z Gastroenterol 1974;12:592

41. Garrett HE, Roper CL. Surgical intervention in histoplasmosis. Ann Thorac Surg 1986;42:711

42. Gaucha P, et al. Localisations oesophagiennes de la maladie de Crohn. Nouv Presse Med 1977;6:1369

43. Geboes K, et al. Crohn's disease of the esophagus. J Clin Gastroenterol 1986;8:31

44. Gelfand MD, Krone CL. Dysphagia and esophageal ulceration in Crohn's disease. Gastroenterology 1968;55:510

45. Gohel V, Long BW, Richter G. Aphthous ulcers in the esophagus with Crohn's colitis. AJR 1981;137:872

46. Goldenberg SP, Wain SL, Marignaini P. Acute necrotizing esophagitis. Gastroenterology 1990;98:493

47. Goodwin RA, et al. Disseminated histoplasmosis: clinical and pathologic correlations. Medicine 1980;59:1

48. Goodwin RA, Loyd JE, DesPrez RM. Histoplasmosis in normal hosts. Medicine 1981;60:231

49. Goodwin RA, Nickell JA, DesPrez RM. Mediastinal fibrosis complicating healed primary histoplasmosis and tuberculosis. Medicine 1972;51:227

50. Gordon AH, Marshall JB. Esophageal tuberculosis: definitive diagnosis by endoscopy. Am J Gastroenterol 1990;85:174

51. Gore RM, Ghahremani GG. Crohn's disease of the upper gastrointestinal tract. CRC Crit Rev Diagn Imaging 1986;25(3):305

52. Guyot R. La Syphilis de l'oesophage in particular à point de vue anatomo—pathogique. Ann Otolaryngol 1931;5:505

53. Hagos T, Latour F, Levitt RE. Portal hypertension complicating sarcoid liver disease: case report and review of the literature. Am J Gastroenterol 1984;79:389

54. Hancock BW, Barnett DB. Case of post-pulmonary tuberculosis and massive hematemesis. BMJ 1974;5933:722

55. Howlett SA. Acute streptococcal esophagitis. Gastrointest Endosc 1979;25:150

56. Huchzermeyer H, et al. Endoscopic results in five patients with Crohn's disease of the esophagus. Endoscopy 1976;8:75

57. Hudson TR, Head JR. Syphilis of the esophagus. J Thorac Cardiovasc Surg 1950;20:216

58. Hutchin P, Lindskog GE. Acquired esophagobronchial fistula of infectious origin. J Thorac Cardiovasc Surg 1964;48:1

59. Israel HL, Sones M. Sarcoidosis: clinical observation in one hundred and sixty cases. Arch Intern Med 1958;102:766

60. James DG, et al. Description of sarcoidosis. Report of the Subcommittee on Classification and Definition. In Siltzbach LE, ed, International Conference on Sarcoidosis and Other Granulomatous Disease. New York: Academy of Sciences, 1976:742

61. Jenkins DW, Fisk DE, Byrd RB. Mediastinal histoplasmosis with esophageal abscess. Gastroenterology 1976;70:109

62. Kerley P. Sarcoidosis. In McLaren JW, ed, Modern Trends in Diagnostic Radiology. New York: Hoeber, 1948:150

63. Khaorde Kark A, Moser D, Fidler WJ. Blastomycosis of the esophagus. Ann Thorac Surg 1980;30:76

64. Kikendall JW, et al. Pill induced esophageal injury: case reports and review of the medical literature. Dig Dis Sci 1983;28:174

65. Knudsen KB, Sparberg M. Ulcerative esophagitis and ulcerative colitis. JAMA 1967;201:140

66. Kragh J. Tuberculous diverticula of the esophagus. Acta Otolaryngol (Stockh) 1922;4:49

67. Kramer P, Burakoff R. Infections of the esophagus. In Berk JE, ed, Bakus Gastroenterology. Philadelphia: WB Saunders, 1985:798

68. Kuboi H, et al. Crohn's disease of the esophagus—report of a case. Endoscopy 1988;20:118

69. Kutty CPK, Carstens SA, Funahashi A. Traction diverticula of the esophagus in the middle lobe syndrome. Can Med Assoc J 1981;124:1320

70. Laajam MA. Pulmonary tuberculosis of the esophagus: pseudotumoral presentation. Am J Gastroenterol 1984;79:839

71. Landres RT, Kuster GGR, Strum WB. Eosinophilic esophagitis in a patient with vigorous achalasia. Gastroenterology 1978;74:1298

72. Lee CS, Mangla JC, Lee SS. Crohn's disease in Barrett's esophagus. Am J Gastroenterol 1978;69:646

73. Lee JH, Newman DA, Welsh JD. Disseminated histoplasmosis presenting with esophageal symptomatology. Dig Dis 1977;22:831

74. Lemann M, et al. Crohn's disease with respiratory tract involvement. Gut 1987;28:1669

75. Lenaerts C, et al. High incidence of upper gastrointestinal tract involvement in children with Crohn's disease. Pediatrics 1989;83:771

76. Levine MS. Crohn's disease of the upper gastrointestinal tract. Radiol Clin North Am 1989;25:79

77. Levwohl O, et al. Ulcerative esophagitis and colitis in a pediatric patient with Behcet's syndrome. Am J Gastroenterol 1972;68:550

78. Liv C, Fields WR, Shaw C. Tuberculous mediastinal lymphadenopathy in adults. Radiology 1978;126:369

79. Livolsi VA, Jaretzki A. Granulomatous esophagitis. A case of Crohn's disease limited to the esophagus. Gastroenterology 1973;64:313

80. Lockhard CB. Esophageal tuberculosis, a critical review. Laryngoscope 1913;23:561

81. Longcope WF, Freiman DG. A study of sarcoidosis: based on investigation of 160 cases. Medicine 1952;31:1

82. Lucaya J, et al. Bronchial perforation and bronchoesophageal fistula: tuberculosis origin in children. Am J Radiol 1980;135:525

83. MaCarty RL, Talley JT. Barium studies in diffuse eosinophilic gastroenteritis. Gastrointest Radiol 1990;15:138

84. Madden JL, Ravid JM, Hoddad JR. Regional esophagitis: a specific entity simulating Crohn's disease. Ann Surg 1969;170:351

85. Mangan TF, Colley AT, Wytock DH. Antibiotic associated acute necrotizing esophagitis. Gastroenterology 1990;99:900

86. Mannell A, Hamilton DG. Crohn's disease of the esophagus—a case report. Aust NZ J Surg 1980;50:303

87. Marshall JB. Tuberculosis of the gastrointestinal tract and peritoneum. Am J Gastroenterol 1993;88:989

88. Marshall RH. Granulomatous disease of the intestinal tract (Crohn's disease). Radiology 1975;114:3

89. Martin DS, Smith DT. Blastomycosis: II. A report of thirteen new cases. Arch Intern Med 1939;39:488

90. Matzinger MA, Daneman A. Esophageal involvement in eosinophilic gastroenteritis. Pediatr Radiol 1983;13:35

91. McDonald GB. Acute necrotizing esophagitis. Gastroenterology 1990;99:1193

92. McKenzie R, Khakoo R. Blastomycosis of the esophagus presenting with gastrointestinal bleeding. Gastroenterology 1985;88:1271

93. McManus JPA, Webb JN. A yeast-like infection of the esophagus caused by *Lactobacillus acidophilus*. Gastroenterology 1975;68:583

94. Miller LJ, et al. Crohn's disease involving the esophagus and colon. Mayo Clin Proc 1977;52:35

95. Mino RA, Murphy AI, Livingstone RG. Sarcoidosis producing hypertension. Treatment by splenectomy and splenorenal shunt. Ann Surg 1949;130:951

96. Moreto M, et al. Idiopathic acute esophageal necrosis: not necessarily a terminal event. Endoscopy 1993;25:534

97. Morison BC. Histopathology of Crohn's disease. Proc R Soc Med 1968;61:79

98. Morison BC. Pathology of Crohn's disease. Clin Gastroenterol 1972;1:265

99. Myerson MC. Syphilis of the esophagus. Med Clin North Am 1927;10:919

100. Newman RM, et al. Esophageal tuberculosis: a rare presentation with hematemesis. Am J Gastroenterol 1991;86:751

101. Ole UJ. Syphilis of the esophagus. Am J Med Sci 1914;148:180

102. Orchard JL, Luparello F, Brunskill D. Malabsorption syndrome occurring in the course of disseminated histoplasmosis: case report and review of gastrointestinal histoplasmosis. Am J Med 1979;66:331

103. Peider WR, Woellner RC, Gordon SS. Mediastinal histoplasmosis: report of three cases with dysphagia as the presenting complaint. Dis Chest 1965;47:518

104. Pincus, D, Frank PH. Eosinophilic esophagitis. AJR 1981;136:1001

105. Polockek AA, Matre WJ. Gastrointestinal sarcoidosis: a case involving the esophagus. Am J Dig Dis 1964;4:429

106. Roche JY, et al. Esophageal tuberculosis revealed by massive hemorrhage. Chirurgie 1977;103:177

107. Rosario MT, Raso CL, Comer GM. Esophageal tuberculosis. Dig Dis Sci 1989;34:121

108. Rosch W. Crohn's disease of the upper gastrointestinal tract. Acta Hepatogastroenterol 1973;20:254

109. Rotterdam H, Sommers SC. Biopsy Diagnosis of the Digestive Tract. New York: Raven Press, 1981

110. Rubenstein BM, Pastrana T, Jacobson HG. Tuberculosis of the esophagus. Radiology 1958;70:401

111. Schneider R. Tuberculosis esophagitis. Gastrointest Radiol 1976;1:143

112. Schneider RP, Edwards W. Histoplasmosis presenting as an esophageal tumor. Gastrointest Endosc 1977;23:158

113. Schoenback EB, Miller JM, Long PH. The treatment of systemic blastomycosis with stilbamidine. Ann Intern Med 1952;37:31

114. Schwartz E. Regional roentgen manifestations of histoplasmosis. AJR 1962;87:865

115. Schwartz J, Schaen MD, Picardi JL. Complications of the arrested primary histoplasmic complex. JAMA 1976;236:1157

116. Seigel CI, et al. Dysphagia due to granulomatous myositis of the cricopharyngeal muscle: physiologic and cine radiographic studies prior to and following successful surgical therapy. Trans Am Acad Physicians 1961;74:342

117. Seivewright MB, Freehally J, Wicks ACB. Pulmonary tuberculosis of the esophagus. Am J Gastroenterol 1984;79:842

118. Shepherd FJ, Rhea LI. A fatal case of blastomycosis. J Cutan Dis 1911;29:588

119. Silverstein E, et al. Markedly elevated angiotensin-converting enzyme in lymph nodes containing non-necrotizing granulomas in sarcoidosis. Proc Natl Acad Sci USA 1976;73:2127

120. Silverstein E, et al. Angiotensin-converting enzyme in Crohn's disease and ulcerative colitis. Am J Clin Pathol 1981;75:175

121. Sinha SN, et al. Primary esophageal tuberculosis. Br J Clin Pract 1988;42(9):391

122. Spaulding AR, Burney DP, Richie RE. Acquired benign bronchoesophageal fistula in the adult. Am Thorac Surg 1979;28:378

123. Steel A, Dyer NH, Mathews HR. Cervical Crohn's disease with esophageal-pulmonary fistula. Postgrad Med J 1988;64:706

124. Stone J, Friedberg SA. Obstructive syphilitic esophagus. JAMA 1962;10:711

125. Teruina M, Schamaun M, Waldvogel W. Crohn's disease of the esophagus. German Med Mon 1969;14:49

126. Thoeni RF, Margulis AR. Gastrointestinal tuberculosis. Semin Roentgenol 1979;14:283

127. Tinker MA, et al. Acute appendicitis and pernicious anemia as a complication of gastrointestinal sarcoidosis. Am J Gastroenterol 1984;79:868

128. Tishler JMA, Helman CA. Crohn's disease of the esophagus. J Can Assoc Radiol 1984;35:28

129. Torek F. Tuberculosis of the esophagus. Ann Surg 1981;94:794

130. Tulman AB, Boyce HW. Complications of esophageal dilatation and guidelines for their prevention. Gastrointest Endosc 1981;27:229

131. Vinson P, Sutherland CG. Esophagobronchial fistula resulting from actinomycosis: a report of a case. Radiology 1926;6:63

132. Vinson PP, Broderse AC, Hamilton M, Blastomycosis of the esophagus. Surg Gynecol Obstet 1928;216:255

133. Vitellas KM, et al. Idiopathic eosinophilic esophagitis. Radiology 1993;186:789

134. Vogt-Myko F, Wanke JM. Morbus crohn des terminalen osophagus. Z Gastroenterol 1970;8:163

135. Walsh TJ, Belitsos NJ, Hamilton SR. Bacterial esophagitis in immunocompromised patients. Arch Intern Med 1986;146:1345

136. Watson CJ, et al. Isolated sarcoidosis of the small intestine stimulating non-specific ileojejunitis. Gastroenterology 1945;4:30

137. Werthmer S, et al. Granulomatous esophagitis (Crohn's disease): associated with granulomatous enterocolitis. NY State J Med 1976;76:938

138. Wexels P. Tuberculosis of the esophagus. Acta Tuberc Scand 1954;24:211

139. Wigley FM, et al. Unusual manifestations of tuberculosis: TE fistula. Am J Med 1976;60:310

140. Wilcox LF. Tertiary syphilis of the esophagus. AJR 1934;31:773

141. Zimmerman HM, Rosenblum G, Bank S. Aphthous ulcers of the esophagus in a patient with ulcerative colitis. Gastrointest Endosc 1984;30:298

*The Esophagus*, Third Edition,
edited by D. O. Castell and J. E. Richter.
Lippincott Williams & Wilkins, Philadelphia © 1999.

# CHAPTER 36

# The Esophagus and Noncardiac Chest Pain

Jan Tack and Jozef Janssens

## INTRODUCTION

Anginalike chest pain is an alarming symptom, not only for the patient who is frightened by its cardiac connotations, but also for the physician who has to decide whether or not he or she is dealing with a life-threatening condition. Between 10% and 50% of patients presenting with chest pain sufficiently severe to perform more invasive examinations are reported to have no evidence of coronary artery disease and no evidence of coronary spasm upon provocation [73, 87, 99, 102, 148, 154]. Even after cardiac disease has been ruled out, many patients continue to experience chest pain, anxiety, and compromised lifestyles. Hence, noncardiac chest pain remains a considerable clinical challenge.

## PREVALENCE AND IMPACT OF NONCARDIAC CHEST PAIN

Chest pain of noncardiac origin is a frequent clinical entity in the Western world. On the basis of the number of cardiac catheterizations, it has been estimated that more than 100,000 new cases of noncardiac chest pain are identified yearly in the United States [124]. The clinical relevance of the problem may well be underestimated, because not all patients with chest pain will undergo coronary arteriography. The vital prognosis of patients with anginalike chest pain and normal coronary angiograms is favorable. The incidence of myocardial infarction or death is almost zero in most long-term serial studies of patients with noncardiac chest pain [10, 15, 38, 47, 73, 85, 92, 102, 148]. Myocardial infarction occurs in at most 1% of the cases [105, 151] and cardiac death in 0.6% after follow-up of up to 10 years [20, 74, 108, 151]. In contrast, patients with coronary disease confined to a single vessel had a mortality of 15% at 48 months and 35% at 11 years [43].

Information on the functional disability of noncardiac

J. Tack: Center for Gastrointestinal Research, University of Leuven, and Division of Internal Medicine, University Hospital Gasthuisberg, B-3000 Leuven, Belgium.

J. Janssens: Department of Gastroenterology, University of Leuven, and Department of Gastroenterology, University Hospital Gasthuisberg, B-3000 Leuven, Belgium.

chest pain patients is sparse. However, about three-fourths continue to see a physician, one-half remain or become unemployed, and one-half regard their lives as significantly disabled after having been told that their coronaries were normal [15, 38, 73, 85, 102]. Only about one-third to one-half appear reassured that they do not have a serious cardiac disorder [83, 102]. As many as half of the patients remain on cardiac medications. In 1989, it was estimated that these patients will spend approximately $4,000 per year for medical expenses related to their chest pain syndromes [124].

It has been known for a long time that cardiac and esophageal symptoms can mimic each other. Depending on the criteria used, the esophagus has been implied as a possible source of the chest pain in 20% to 60% of patients characterized as having noncardiac chest pain [21, 37, 42, 48, 73, 77, 102, 126, 154]. A positive diagnosis, establishing the esophageal origin of the noncardiac chest pain, resulted in a significant reduction in the need for medical facilities [102, 128, 139, 147] and increased significantly the number of patients who were able to keep their job [128]. Therefore, a good understanding of the causes of recurrent noncardiac chest pain is of major importance to the quality of life of many patients.

## CLINICAL CHARACTERISTICS OF ESOPHAGEAL CHEST PAIN

The clinical history often does not distinguish between cardiac and esophageal causes of chest pain [99]. Chest pain of esophageal origin is usually located retrosternally and may irradiate to the arms, neck, jaw, or back. The pain is often described as squeezing or burning. It can be triggered by swallowing or ingestion, but it may also be triggered by exercise. The pain may last for minutes up to hours or even be present intermittently for several days. The pain can be sufficiently severe to be accompanied by the patient turning ashen and perspiring.

In patients with noncardiac chest pain, careful evaluation of esophageal symptoms, especially the presence of dysphagia, may increase the likelihood of an underlying motor disorder or gastroesophageal reflux [7]. Unfortunately, as many as 50% of patients with a cardiac cause of chest pain may have one or more symptoms of esophageal pain, such as heartburn, regurgitation, or dysphagia [3]. Furthermore, cardiac and esophageal disease may overlap, and they may interact in the induction of chest pain. Hence, the existence of underlying cardiac or esophageal disease cannot be precluded on the basis of history and clinical presentation alone.

## MECHANISMS OF ESOPHAGEAL CHEST PAIN

The mechanisms underlying chest pain of esophageal origin are incompletely understood. It is well known that patients with achalasia and symptomatic diffuse esophageal spasm may have retrosternal anginalike pain [141, 142] and that some patients with gastroesophageal reflux do not feel typical heartburn, but anginalike chest pain [107, 143]. Thus, chest pain of esophageal origin may arise either from stimulation of acid-sensitive chemoreceptors or from stimulation of mechanoreceptors during abnormal motility. A potential role for thermoreceptors in the induction of esophageal chest pain has received little attention. In addition, hypersensitivity to esophageal balloon distention has been found in a subset of patients with noncardiac chest pain, although studies have shown inconsistent results [55, 120].

### Reflux-related Esophageal Chest Pain

Both acid perfusion tests and ambulatory pH and pressure monitoring in patients with noncardiac chest pain have confirmed that intraesophageal acid may trigger chest pain. The mechanism by which chest pain occurs after exposure of the esophageal mucosa to acid remains largely unknown. Earlier studies suggested that acid perfusion was inducing esophageal motor abnormalities [132]. However, more recent studies have demonstrated that acid-induced pain is usually not accompanied by major changes in esophageal motility [19, 55, 60, 67, 99, 107, 117, 132, 135]. Although structures acting as esophageal chemoreceptors have not formally been identified, it seems likely that intraepithelial free nerve endings may act as acid-sensitive nociceptors [90]. On the other hand, topical anesthetics fail to alter the pain response to acid infusion [63].

It has been shown that intraesophageal acid infusion is able to trigger myocardial ischemia in patients with coronary disease or with microvascular angina [26, 95]. However, there is no convincing evidence that coronary ischemia underlies acid-induced pain in patients with noncardiac chest pain. In these patients, episodes of symptomatic acid reflux are not associated by changes in the electrocardiogram [146].

In gastroesophageal reflux disease, the duration and the minimal pH of reflux episodes seem to be determinant factors in inducing the perception of heartburn [9, 68]. Hypersensitivity to acid seems to be a frequent finding in noncardiac chest pain. In these patients, pain frequently occurs after very brief and less-acidic reflux episodes. Sensitization of nociceptors may play a role in the apparently lower threshold for acid-induced chest pain in these patients. Other factors, such as the acid clearance mechanism, the acid exposure during the period preceding a particular reflux event, and the contribution of other refluxed factors such as pepsin, bile acids, and trypsin may also modulate the occurrence of chest pain during reflux episodes.

### Motility-related Esophageal Chest Pain

It is well known that patients with symptomatic diffuse esophageal spasm may have retrosternal anginalike pain [142]. In many patients with noncardiac chest pain, high-amplitude contractions of prolonged duration and with impaired peristaltic progression can be observed during esophageal manometry. The most frequent findings are nonspecific motor disorders, followed by nutcracker esophagus and diffuse esophageal spasm [16, 29, 55]. Initially, a causal link between these abnormal patterns of contraction and the patient's symptoms seemed obvious.

One popular hypothesis has been that the high pressure occurring during these abnormal contractions would inhibit esophageal blood flow for a sufficiently long time to induce mucosal ischemia. MacKenzie et al. used microthermistors to measure the rewarming time of the chilled esophagus [91]. They observed a longer rewarming time in patients with nutcracker esophagus than in control subjects, suggesting esophageal ischemia as a possible cause of the pain. However, Gustaffson and Tibbling observed that the rewarming times before and after edrophonium administration did not differ between patients with a positive or a negative test [58]. The authors concluded that esophageal chest pain, elicited by intravenous edrophonium, is not caused by a decreased blood flow in the esophageal wall but is directly related to high-amplitude and long-lasting esophageal contractions.

The relationship, however, between the manometric findings and the chest pain has remained complex and incompletely understood. Patients are generally asymptomatic at the time when the motor disorders are identified. It has been assumed that these abnormal contractions might be a marker for even more severe motor disturbances during spontaneous episodes of chest pain. However, prolonged esophageal pressure monitoring studies have demonstrated that this is only rarely the case [55, 107]. Moreover, there is no relationship between the presence of a nutcracker esophagus and the response to provocation tests that stimulate motility [86]. Finally, the reduction of the amplitude of contractions by pharmacotherapy does not correlate with a symptomatic improvement [123]. More recently, it was also demonstrated that the nutcracker esophagus can be associated with gastroesophageal reflux disease [1].

Recent data suggest that psychological factors may contribute to the phenomenon. Psychological stress alone is able to increase the amplitude of esophageal contractions, and this is more marked in patients with a nutcracker esophagus [4].

In a preliminary report, based on 24-hour esophageal pressure, pH, and intraluminal ultrasonograpy monitoring, the majority of episodes of chest pain were accompanied by a transient increase in esophageal muscle thickness on ultrasonography [8]. These increases in esophageal muscle thickness, called sustained esophageal contractions, were not accompanied by sustained increases in intraluminal pressure. In addition, sustained esophageal contractions were associated with chest pain in all patients with a positive edrophonium test. They were not observed in subjects with a negative edrophonium test. These findings suggest that sustained esophageal contractions may be the motor correlate of both spontaneous and induced esophageal chest pain. As they are not detected by esophageal pressure recordings, it has been speculated that sustained esophageal contractions reflect contractions of the longitudinal esophageal muscle layer.

### Visceral Hypersensitivity

Patients with noncardiac chest pain have significantly higher pain sensation scores during intraesophageal balloon distension than healthy control subjects [120]. This abnormal sensory perception appears to be independent of esophageal contractions or esophageal wall tone. Studies by De Caestecker et al. suggest that a stretch receptor linked to the longitudinal muscle of the esophageal wall mediates the sensory response as edrophonium is increasing and atropine is reducing the sensitivity to balloon distension [41].

In contrast to healthy subjects or patients with nonstructural dysphagia, patients with noncardiac chest pain report increasing pain sensation scores during repeated balloon distensions [106]. These data suggest that patients with noncardiac chest pain exhibit a conditioning phenomenon during repeated distensions. The level at which this conditioning occurs is unknown.

### Irritable Esophagus

The irritable-esophagus concept was derived from the observation that some patients with noncardiac chest pain, when studied by 24-hour pH and pressure measurements, sometimes developed pain associated with reflux alone (without motor disorders), and on other occasions during the same study experienced the same pain together with motility disorders alone (without acid reflux) [143]. The esophagus of these patients appears to be hypersensitive to a variety of stimuli. The diagnosis of irritable esophagus is therefore based on the demonstration that the patient's familiar chest pain can be elicited by both mechanical and chemical stimuli. Chest pain induced by mechanical stimuli can be observed during edrophonium provocation or balloon distension, or as motility-related chest pain during ambulatory motoring. Chest pain induced by chemical stimuli can be observed during the Bernstein test or as reflux-related chest pain during ambulatory monitoring.

The mechanism underlying this irritability is unclear. In order to elucidate an interaction between sensitivity to acid and sensitivity to mechanical stimulation, Mehta et al. studied esophageal perception and pain thresholds to balloon distention and electrical stimulation before and after esophageal acid perfusion in patients with noncardiac chest pain and healthy controls [94]. After acid perfusion, balloon perception and pain thresholds decreased in patients with noncardiac chest pain and negative provocation tests and in controls, but did not decrease further in patients who had positive provocation tests. These findings suggest that acid perfusion sensitized stretch-sensitive nociceptors in patients with negative provocation tests and controls. The failure to show such sensitization in patients with positive provocation tests suggests that these nociceptors may already have been sensitized. Mutual sensitization of acid-sensitive and mechanonosensitive mechanisms may contribute to the development of irritability in the esophagus.

### Other Causes of Esophageal Chest Pain

Ingestion of hot or cold liquids can trigger severe chest pain. This does not seem to be caused by accompanying esophageal motor disturbances [96].

A belching disorder may be the mechanism responsible for chest pain in some patients with abnormal sensitivity to intraesophageal balloon distention [56, 69]. Esophageal wall distension, mimicked during balloon distension, may occur spontaneously during eructation against a closed upper esophageal sphincter [56]. A similar mechanism of esophageal distension may underlie chest pain induced by acute food impaction and ingestion of carbonated beverages. However, other factors are likely to be involved, since in patients with noncardiac chest pain, smaller volumes of esophageal balloon distention are required to produce pain than in asymptomatic subjects [56, 120].

Almost 5% of patients taking the serotonin-1D receptor agonist sumatriptan for migraine have chest discomfort. These symptoms are most frequently not associated with changes in cardiac function or enzymes. In healthy subjects, administration of sumatripan in supratherapeutic doses causes small but significant increases in the amplitude and duration of deglutitive contractions, and an increased frequency of repetitive contractions can be observed [64]. These data suggest that sumatriptan might provoke diffuse esophageal spasm in susceptible patients. However, no temporal association has been observed between chest symptoms and abnormal esophageal motility after sumatriptan.

## DIAGNOSTIC TOOLS IN CHEST PAIN OF ESOPHAGEAL ORIGIN

Gastrointestinal endoscopy reveals reflux esophagitis in up to 31% of the patients with noncardiac chest pain [51,

65, 144]. Stationary manometry in patients with noncardiac chest pain is able to demonstrate abnormalities in up to 29% of the patients [16, 29, 55]. As esophageal motor disorders and low-grade reflux esophagitis are a common finding in many patients, the mere presence of these disorders cannot be accepted as proof for the esophageal origin of the chest pain.

Therefore, the best way to accept the esophagus as the likely cause of noncardiac anginalike chest pain is to show a temporal correlation between the occurrence of chest pain and an abnormal esophageal event. To increase the chance of recording a pain episode during esophageal testing, one can use provocation tests, or one can extend the recording period (24-hour intraesophageal pH and pressure recording).

The acid perfusion test (Bernstein), the ergonovine test, the edrophonium test [86, 119], and the esophageal balloon distension test [120] are well known and widely accepted provocation tests. Other tests, such as the use of hot and cold liquids, pentagastrin, vasopressin, solid-food boluses, and bethanechol are less extensively studied, and will not be discussed further.

### The Acid Perfusion Test

The acid perfusion test was first described by Bernstein and Baker [17]. When 0.1 N hydrochloric acid infused into the middle third of the esophagus is able to induce the familiar chest pain, the test is called positive related. When acid induces only a retrosternal burning sensation or another unfamiliar sensation, the test is called positive unrelated and is not accepted as proof that the chest pain has an esophageal origin. Studies in patients with noncardiac chest pain show a wide range of sensitivity in the Bernstein test, probably related to differences in patient selection (Table 36–1). The

**TABLE 36–1.** *Diagnostic accuracy of esophageal provocation tests in patients with noncardiac chest pain*

| Study | Accuracy | | |
|---|---|---|---|
| | Bernstein | Edrophonium | Balloon |
| Vantrappen et al. [143] | 11/33 | 6/12 | — |
| De Caestecker et al. [40] | 21/60 | 12/60 | — |
| Peters et al. [107] | 7/20 | 9/18 | — |
| Soffer et al. [135] | 2/20 | 0/20 | — |
| Hewson et al. [60] | 15/45 | 24/44 | — |
| Ghillebert et al. [55] | 18/50 | 16/50 | 1/20 |
| Humeau et al. [66] | 4/40 | 6/40 | 13/34 |
| Nevens et al. [99] | 14/37 | 7/37 | 3/37 |
| Goudot-Pernot et al. [57] | — | 19/78 | 33/78 |
| Hewson et al. [61] | 18/95 | 15/78 | — |
| Rokkas et al. [111] | 29/110 | 26/110 | — |
| Mehta et al. [94] | 3/25 | 10/25 | — |
| Ghillebert and Janssens [54] | 106/270 | 58/220 | 26/182 |
| Frøbert et al. [52] | 10/63 | 9/63 | — |

Bernstein test is positive related (i.e., reproduces the patient's chest pain) in 10% to 38% of the patients with noncardiac chest pain [29, 40, 55, 60, 107, 111, 135, 143].

### The Ergonovine Test

Intravenous administration of ergonovine is used as a test to provoke coronary artery spasm. If administration of ergonovine causes chest pain in the presence of ischemic ST-T segment changes on the electrocardiogram (ECG), a diagnosis of vasospastic angina (Prinzmetal's angina) is accepted [59]. However, if ergonovine induces chest pain without ST-T segment changes, an esophageal origin of the chest pain is often accepted [88]. As ergonovine is not superior to edrophonium in provoking abnormal motility and chest pain in patients with suspected esophageal pain and as the drug may induce potentially fatal coronary artery spasm, ergonovine no longer has a place in the routine diagnostic work-up of chest pain patients, unless to exclude vasospastic angina.

### The Edrophonium Test

The cholinesterase inhibitor edrophonium has been shown to be the most reliable and safest pharmacologic agent for routine provocative testing in the clinical setting [119]. The test is positive if slow intravenous injection of 80 $\mu$g per kg edrophonium, but not placebo, induces the familiar chest pain within 5 minutes after the administration of the drug. Administration of edrophonium increases esophageal contraction amplitude and the number of repetitive waves after wet swallows in both age-matched control subjects and patients with noncardiac chest pain. The change in duration seems to be significantly higher in patients in whom edrophonium induces chest pain, but there is considerable overlap with patients without chest pain [119]. Hence, only symptoms and no manometric criterion will determine a positive edrophonium test. However, the style of the test administration and the interaction of the tester and the patient may strongly influence the outcome of the provocation test [114]. Hence, inclusion of a placebo intravenous injection when using edrophonium is advisable.

The test has been reported to be positive in 0% to 55% of the patients with noncardiac chest pain (Table 36–1) [29, 40, 55, 60, 107, 135, 143]. Lee et al. proposed the use of a higher dose of 10 mg, but this does not produce a higher response rate, although side effects are more pronounced [36, 86].

### The Balloon Distension Test

In 1955, Bayliss et al., proposed intraesophageal balloon distension as a diagnostic test to distinguish esophageal from cardiac chest pain [12]. In 1986, the test was resurrected as a provocative test in the evaluation of patients with noncardiac chest pain. A small balloon is placed 10 cm above the lower esophageal sphincter and inflated with 1-ml increments to a total volume of 10 ml [120]. The reproducibility of the balloon distension test has been confirmed in healthy subjects [84]. Women have significantly lower pain thresholds to esophageal balloon distention than men [101]. The rate of intraesophageal balloon inflation seems to determine the level of perception. With a rapid inflation rate, the mean volume required to induce perception or discomfort is significantly lower [100]. Sustained inflation seems to induce increasing sensation.

Richter et al. observed that balloon distension with a volume of 8 ml reproduced chest pain in 15 of 30 patients and had no effect in controls [36]. In other studies, the sensitivity of the test has been reported to vary between 5% and 50% [55, 57, 66, 99, 120] (Table 36–1). The reasons for this discrepancy are incompletely understood. It has been shown that acid perfusion is able to decrease the thresholds for perception and pain to balloon distension in patients with noncardiac chest pain and negative provocation tests and in controls, but not in patients who had positive provocation tests [94]. Thus, the examination sequence may explain some of the different results obtained with balloon distension.

Rao et al. [110] used impedance planimetry to perform esophageal balloon distensions. Impedance planimetry provides a way to assess the cross-sectional area of the lumen in a selected plane at a range of distending pressures in an intraesophageal balloon. The authors used this technique in 12 healthy controls and in 24 chest pain patients with negative cardiologic and conventional gastrointestinal studies. The balloon was used to carry out stepwise isobaric distensions of the esophagus, while the cross-sectional area was measured and grades of sensation were reported by the subject. Similar to previous studies, hypersensitivity to esophageal distention was found in the patients who had lower thresholds both for first perception and for pain. Especially at low inflating pressures, patients tended to have a larger cross-sectional area in response to stretching. Paradoxically, however, the reactivity of the esophageal wall to distention was greater in patients who had a higher frequency and amplitude of contractions and a higher motility index than controls. Furthermore, balloon distention normally induces an inhibition of contractions distal to the balloon. In patients, this distal inhibition of the amplitude of pressure waves was attenuated or absent, suggesting neuromuscular dysfunction. The greater reactivity to luminal distention may be partly attributable to the biomechanical properties of the esophageal wall: patients with noncardiac chest pain had a stiffer, less compliant esophageal wall than controls. This study seems to resolve at least partly the inconsistencies of previous studies using balloon distensions to elicit chest pain of esophageal origin [55, 120]. In these studies, increasing balloon volume was used as a stimulus to activate tension receptors in the esophagus, but the variable esophageal diameter in different persons may result in a highly variable tension stimulus. Using isobaric distensions and simultaneously assessing the diameter of the esophagus, as performed in the study by Rao et al., allows one to calculate the wall tension that elicits typical sensations.

## Prolonged Esophageal pH and Pressure Recordings

Ambulatory pH and pressure recordings allow the patient to signal the occurrence of spontaneous chest pain episodes on the record. This allows the demonstration of a temporal relationship between chest pain and the occurrence of an abnormal esophageal event such as reflux or motor abnormalities or both. Several systems for ambulatory pH and pressure recordings are now commercially available. They all record pressure at at least two levels in the esophagus and pH at 5 cm above the lower esophageal sphincter. They have an event marker for the patient to indicate the occurrence of symptoms. Data are collected on tape or on solid-state memory, and are analyzed afterward.

Since the original development of prolonged esophageal pH and pressure recordings [67] several studies have reported the reproducibility of this technique [46, 145]. It has recently been suggested that the esophageal motor abnormalities observed after the onset of chest pain area consequence rather than a cause of the pain. Likewise, episodes of gastroesophageal reflux may be induced by pain. Lam et al. analyzed the occurrence of reflux or esophageal motor abnormalities in a prepain and a postpain window of 2 minutes. During the prepain window, 24.7% of pain episodes were correlated with abnormal motility, compared with only 4.2% in the postpain window. Chest pain was followed by acid reflux in only 3.6% of the events. Therefore, in patients with noncardiac chest pain, gastroesophageal reflux and esophageal motor disorders are infrequently induced by pain [81]. The optimal time window in symptom analysis of 24-hour esophageal pressure and pH data begins at 2 minutes before the onset of the pain and ends at the onset of the pain [80].

The diagnostic accuracy of 24-hour pH and pressure recordings in the diagnosis of an esophageal cause for chest pain ranges from 10% to 56% in several published studies (Table 36–2). These differences likely reflect differences in patient selection, which is also reflected in the variable proportion of patients experiencing chest pain during the recording. An additional problem relates to the many uncertainties that remain in the way 24-hour pH and pressure measurements should be analyzed.

The definition of abnormal motility or abnormal pH used in the analysis of the data is controversial. Abnormal motility can be defined as contraction complexes that significantly exceed in amplitude, duration, or peristaltic disorder the contraction waves that were observed during a control period, consisting of a number of 5-minute periods selected throughout the pain-free periods of the recording [107]. Other authors have used shorter control periods [55] or have used nonparametric statistics based on an automatic analysis of the entire 24-hour recording [19]. The definition of abnormal pH is even less well established. Most authors have used a threshold (pH < 4) to accept a pain episode as pH associated.

**TABLE 36–2.** *Diagnostic accuracy of 24-hour pH and pressure recordings in patients with noncardiac chest pain*

| Study | Number of patients | Number of patients with chest pain related to given factor | | | |
| --- | --- | --- | --- | --- | --- |
| | | Dysmotility | Acid | Both | Global |
| Janssens et al. [67] | 60 | 8 | 4 | 9 | 21 |
| Peters et al. [107] | 24 | 3 | 5 | 5 | 13 |
| Soffer et al. [135] | 20 | 0 | 6 | 4 | 10 |
| Ghillebert et al. [55] | 50 | 4 | 12 | 3 | 19 |
| Hewson et al. [61] | 45 | 6 | 11 | 4 | 21 |
| Breumelhof et al. [19] | 44 | 2 | 2 | 4 | 8 |
| Nevens et al. [99] | 37 | 1 | 4 | 1 | 6 |
| Lam et al. [81] | 41 | 10 | 13 | — | 23 |
| Lux et al. [89] | 30 | 4 | 5 | 1 | 10 |

However, Weusten et al. suggested that optimal pH thresholds varied, ranging from 5.0 to 6.4 in the upright and from 4.5 to 5.7 in the supine position [150]. The most reproducible parameter obtained during pH monitoring is the percentage of time at which the pH is less than [153]. This is often used as a criterion to determine whether or not pathological reflux is present. Esophageal pH monitoring is able to demonstrate pathological gastroesophageal reflux in up to 62% of the patients with noncardiac chest pain [19, 29, 39, 42, 60, 61, 66, 67, 79, 99, 107, 129, 135, 144]. However, even in the absence of pathological reflux, reflux can still be the cause of a patient's symptoms of chest pain. A group of patients have normal acid exposure, but still have a significant temporal relationship between reflux episodes and chest pain events. These patients are considered to have an acid-hypersensitive esophagus [131]. Frøbert et al. performed 24-hour esophageal manometry and pH monitoring and provocative testing with intravenous edrophonium chloride and esophageal acid perfusion in 63 patients with anginalike chest pain, but normal coronary angiograms [52]. Reflux indices and ambulatory recorded esophageal motor function did not differ significantly between patients and healthy controls. On the basis of these observations, the authors question the rationale for routine esophageal investigations in patients with anginalike chest pain, but normal coronary angiograms. However, patients were discussed only as groups, and only the mean time of acid exposure during pH monitoring was taken into account as a marker for reflux disease. Esophageal acid perfusion was positive in 16% of the patients, suggesting that they still might have an acid-sensitive esophagus as a cause of their symptoms.

To quantify a temporal relationship between symptoms and episodes of gastroesophageal reflux, several indices have been developed. The most frequently used is the symptom index, defined as the percentage of reflux-related symptom episodes [152]. However, in contrast to patients with typical heartburn as a predominant symptom, in patients with noncardiac chest pain, receiver-operating-characteristic curve analysis failed to determine a discriminant threshold of the symptom index for use in noncardiac chest pain [134].

In addition, the symptom index does not take into account the total number of reflux episodes.

To overcome these drawbacks, the symptom sensitivity index was defined as the percentage of symptom-associated reflux episodes [18]. However, this index does not take into account the total number of symptoms.

More complex methods have been proposed, such as the binomial symptom index, which is obtained using the values of esophageal acid exposure, total number of symptoms experienced, and number of reflux-related symptoms in a binomial mathematical formula [55]. Emde et al. presented a mathematical approach based on the Kolmogorov–Smirnov test to evaluate the significance of reflux episodes as a cause of pain [45].

The symptom–association probability is a new method to calculate the probability that the observed association between gastroesophageal reflux and symptoms is not caused by chance [149]. The 24-hour signal is divided into consecutive 2-minute periods. These periods are analyzed for the presence of reflux. A contingency table can then be constructed comprising all relevant variables, and the probability can be expressed that the associations of symptoms and events are not caused by chance. However, the method can only be applied to esophageal pH, and not to esophageal pressure events.

### Relationship Between Provocation Tests and 24-Hour pH and Pressure Measurements

The usefulness of the acid perfusion test in predicting symptomatic reflux in patients who had pain during 24-hour pH monitoring is rather low. Ghillebert and Janssens found a sensitivity and specificity for the acid perfusion test of 57% and 62%, respectively [54]. Similar observations were made by Richter et al. Despite an excellent specificity (94%), the Bernstein test was found to be considerably less sensitive than pH monitoring in identifying an acid-sensitive esophagus (32%) [125]. These data suggest that mucosal acid sensitivity and symptomatic reflux should be regarded as separate, although related, aspects of reflux disease [62].

Moreover, a specificity of 62% implies that a positive acid perfusion test will be present in 38% of the patients in whom reflux could not be detected during a spontaneous pain attack. Therefore, acid perfusion is still useful, particularly in patients who have no symptoms during 24-hour pH monitoring.

The sensitivity and specificity of the edrophonium test to find motility-related events during 24-hour recording were 50% and 71% respectively. The sensitivity and specificity of a positive edrophonium test to find reflux-related events during 24-hour recording were 39% and 72% respectively [54]. These data support the idea that a positive edrophonium test mainly suggests the presence of an esophageal origin of chest pain, but often fails to identify the specific pathophysiologic mechanism underlying spontaneous attacks.

### Diagnostic Impact of Provocation Tests versus 24-hour pH and Pressure Measurements

A number of studies performed edrophonium and Bernstein provocation tests and also prolonged ambulatory pH and pressure recording in patients with noncardiac chest pain (Table 36–3). In 50% of the patients, at least one provocation test was positive. Twenty-four-hour recording revealed an esophageal origin in 31% of the patients (Table 36–3).

A combination of the acid perfusion test and the edrophonium test revealed the esophageal origin of the chest pain in 105 patients who did not have painful abnormalities during prolonged monitoring (gain 29%). In contrast, the diagnostic gain of ambulatory pH and pressure monitoring in patients found to have positive provocation tests was only 10%. Hence, it seems logical to perform an acid perfusion test and an edrophonium test first. However, if these provocation tests are negative, the chance to establish the esophageal origin by performing ambulatory pH and pressure monitoring is still 20%.

As discussed above, positive provocation tests are indications that chest pain is of esophageal origin. They often fail to identify the specific pathophysiologic mechanism underlying spontaneous attacks. Prolonged ambulatory pH and pressure recordings are presently the only method to demonstrate the mechanism underlying spontaneous pain attacks.

## DIAGNOSTIC EVALUATION

The existence of coronary artery disease cannot be ruled out on the basis of the history and the clinical presentation only [99]. As this is a potentially life-threatening disorder, evaluation of patients with chest pain should always start with the exclusion of cardiac disease. Furthermore, esophageal disorders have been reported in up to 50% of patients with cardiac disease [89, 112] and their coexistence may induce chest pain via complex interactions. In young patients, an ECG during chest pain as well as a negative exercise stress test may be sufficient. In older patients, in addition to the exercise stress test, a coronary angiogram, possibly with ergonovine provocation, may be mandatory. If the cardiologic work-up is negative, the patient can be considered to have chest pain of noncardiac origin.

Gastrointestinal work-up is aimed at demonstrating symptomatic gastroesophageal reflux, esophageal motor abnormalities, or hypersensitivity of the esophagus to balloon distention. The examination sequence may consist of endoscopy, stationary esophageal manometry, esophageal provocation tests using acid infusion, balloon distention and edrophonium chloride intravenously, and 24-hour ambulatory esophageal pH testing with or without 24-hour ambulatory esophageal manometry. Alternatively, the physician may embark on a therapeutic trial. Endoscopy is the initial examination of choice. If this shows esophagitis or an unusual cause of chest pain such as an ulcer, appropriate treatment can be started. As reflux is the most common esophageal cause of chest pain, an empirical trial of acid suppression with a high dose of a proton pump inhibitor can be considered if the endoscopy was negative. Alternatively, one may proceed to perform stationary esophageal manometry with provocation tests. In case of unrevealing provocative tests, 24-hour ambulatory esophageal pH and pressure monitoring can be performed to try to identify the factors that trigger spontaneously occurring episodes of chest pain. Finally, a psychiatric work-up may identify underlying psychological disorders that require appropriate treatment.

## PSYCHOLOGICAL FACTORS

The perception and verbal report of pain is a complex process modulated by factors such as anxiety, depression,

**TABLE 36–3.** *Diagnostic accuracy of provocation tests compared to 24-hour pH and pressure recordings in patients with noncardiac chest pain*

| Study | Number of patients | Positive provocation tests | Positive 24-hour recording | Positive 24-hour recording and negative provocation | Positive provocation and negative 24-hour recording |
|---|---|---|---|---|---|
| Peters et al. [107] | 18 | 13 | 8 | 3 | 7 |
| Soffer et al. [135] | 20 | 2 | 10 | 8 | 0 |
| Ghillebert et al. [55] | 50 | 24 | 19 | 5 | 11 |
| Hewson et al. [61] | 44 | 30 | 20 | 5 | 15 |
| Nevens et al. [99] | 37 | 17 | 6 | 1 | 6 |
| Ghillebert and Janssens [54] | 190 | 94 | 48 | 14 | 60 |

individual cultural values, and secondary gain. Clouse and Lustman showed that psychiatric illnesses were associated with a specific cluster of esophageal contraction abnormalities (increase in mean wave amplitude, increase in mean wave duration, increased frequency of abnormal motor responses, the presence of triple-peaked waves), suggesting a relationship between emotional disturbances and esophageal motility [30]. The relationship between emotional disturbances and esophageal motility probably also explains why patients with nutcracker esophagus have a more pronounced increase in esophageal contraction amplitude during psychological stress as compared to controls [4].

Patients with noncardiac chest pain and nutcracker esophagus and patients with irritable bowel syndrome have significantly higher scores of gastrointestinal susceptibility and somatic anxiety than controls [121]. Several studies found a high incidence of psychiatric diagnoses, such as panic disorder, generalized anxiety disorder, or depression and somatization disorder in patients with noncardiac chest pain [4, 6, 13, 33, 71, 75]. However, a subset of up to 50% of patients with noncardiac chest pain have no active psychiatric syndrome at the time of evaluation [30, 71]. Sexual or physical abuse seems to be less prevalent in patients with noncardiac chest pain than in patients with irritable bowel syndrome or with gastroesophageal reflux [127].

Anxiety is an important factor that contributes to symptom perception in patients with chest pain. Up to 25% of patients presenting to the emergency department because of chest pain meet the diagnostic criteria for panic disorder [49]. In patients with noncardiac chest pain, hyperventilation can cause altered esophageal motility but is unlikely to cause chest pain through this mechanism [32].

It has been suggested that the psychological features of patients with noncardiac chest pain might be secondary to a long-standing painful medical illness. However, the degree of psychiatric comorbidity seems to be less in groups of patients with chronic organic esophageal or cardiac conditions.

The multiple interactions between psychological factors and chest pain may also explain why patients with contraction abnormalities and symptoms benefit from psychotropic drugs [4, 31] even though the drugs do not influence the manometric parameters. In an uncontrolled study, symptomatic improvement was obtained with benzodiazepine treatment [14]. In addition, a beneficial effect of cognitive-behavioral psychotherapy has been reported [76].

## CARDIAC AND ESOPHAGEAL CHEST PAIN

It has been suggested that gastroesophageal reflux and esophageal motility disorders may elicit myocardial ischemia and chest pain, a phenomenon called *linked angina*. In patients admitted to a coronary care unit for a typical angina episode, ischemic pain episodes provoked by reflux or abnormal esophageal motility are rare [82].

Gastroesophageal reflux disease, a common cause of chest pain, and coronary artery disease are both highly prevalent in the population. Moreover, panic disorder has been reported to be highly prevalent both in patients with coronary artery disease and in patients with noncardiac chest pain. Hence, it seems likely that these disorders may coexist in some patients, thus creating confusion about the origin of chest pain.

Lux et al. compared the frequency of esophageal disturbances in patients with normal coronary angiograms and patients with coronary heart disease [89]. They observed that abnormal esophageal motility or gastroesophageal reflux correlated with chest pain episodes in 33% of patients with normal coronary arteries, but also in 26% of patients with pathologic coronary angiograms. In the latter group, reflux or dysmotility were often accompanied by ST-segment changes. Thus, in patients with coronary artery disease, a significant number of episodes of ST deviation correlates with gastroesophageal reflux or abnormal esophageal motility.

Ros et al. investigated causes of recurrent chest pain at rest in 18 patients with proven coronary artery disease who experienced recurrent rest pain despite appropriate revascularization and absence of ischemic ECG changes (the "problem group") [112]. As a control group, 27 patients who had chest pain with ischemic ST-segment changes in the ECG and who had obstructive coronary artery lesions without prior revascularization procedures were also studied. All patients underwent esophageal manometry, 24-hour pH studies, edrophonium provocation, and a psychiatric diagnostic interview. Based upon these studies, in 44% of the patients in the problem group, the esophagus was considered a likely cause of chest pain, and in 56% a probable cause. In the control group an esophageal cause of chest pain was thought unlikely in 48%, probable in 33%, and likely in only 19%. Panic disorder was diagnosed in 50% of the problem group and in 19% of the control group. The authors conclude that esophageal dysfunction and psychiatric disturbances are common in patients with coronary artery disease presenting with chest pain during rest and may contribute to patients' symptoms. Esophageal investigations may thus be beneficial in many of these patients because they can elucidate treatable causes of chest pain.

Not only may esophageal disorders coexist with coronary artery disease, but it has also been suggested that esophageal stimulation may elicit myocardial ischemia. Esophageal acid infusion reduces the threshold for exercise-induced angina in patients with coronary artery disease, and reduces coronary blood flow in patients with syndrome X and in patients with angiographically proven significant coronary artery disease [3, 26, 28]. In 18 denervated cardiac transplant recipients, coronary blood flow was not affected by esophageal acid infusion. These observations suggest the involvement of a neural cardioesophageal reflex in the pathogenesis of so-called linked angina [28]. The study raises the possibility that patients with coronary artery disease might benefit from acid-suppressive therapy.

## MICROVASCULAR ANGINA

In 1973, Kemp used the term *syndrome X* to denote a group of patients with ischemic-appearing electrocardiograms during exercise, but with normal coronary angiograms during cardiac catheterization [72]. A number of studies have subsequently shown that patients with chest pain and normal coronary angiograms had abnormal coronary flow dynamics during pharmacologically induced vasodilatation, suggestive of an impaired coronary flow reserve [22, 103]. It was hypothesized that the abnormality was due to dysfunction of the coronary microcirculation. Several studies reported that patients with syndrome X had an abnormal endothelial function [44, 98, 109] and an excessive sympathetic responsiveness [5, 53, 113]. Most studies, however, failed to demonstrate metabolic evidence for ischemia [5, 34]. Moreover, even in the presence of some suggestion of ischemia, such as impaired left ventricular functional responses or abnormal exercise thallium scintigraphy, the prognosis of these patients is excellent [70, 97].

A number of groups observed that patients with chest pain and normal coronary angiograms would readily experience chest pain during cardiac catheterization, suggesting that abnormal cardiac pain perception might be present [23, 27, 78, 116, 130]. In patients with atherosclerotic or structural heart disease, chest pain is only rarely elicited during cardiac catheterization. Stimuli causing chest pain are catheter movement in the right atrium, intravenous administration of adenosine, intravenous dipyridamole, injection of saline or contrast medium, and right ventricular pacing. Cannon et al. observed that right ventricular pacing elicited characteristic chest pain in 85% of patients with chest pain and normal coronary angiograms, regardless whether or not they had evidence of microvascular dysfunction [23]. Thus, patients with increased cardiac perception may represent another manifestation of visceral hypersensitivity, present in several functional gastrointestinal disorders. The cause or mechanism underlying this hypersensitivity remains unclear.

The antidepressant drug imipramine is able to improve symptoms in patients with chest pain and normal coronary angiograms [4]. The response to imipramine did not depend on the result of cardiac, esophageal, or psychiatric testing at baseline. It was shown that imipramine was able to improve cardiac sensitivity in this group of patients. Thus, the beneficial effect of imipramine may involve a visceral analgesic effect [4].

## TREATMENT

The medical therapy of anginalike chest pain of esophageal origin remains controversial. Many patients may improve with confident reassurance alone, although it seems important for many patients not only to prove the absence of a cardiac disease or malignancy, but also to establish a definite cause for the symptoms to avoid ongoing concern [102, 140].

Anticholinergics have been suggested for the treatment of chest pain ascribed to underlying motility abnormalities, but there are no controlled studies to justify this therapy. In a single-blind acute study, cimetropium bromide produced a dramatic decrease in esophageal contraction amplitude in patients with nutcracker esophagus, but data about the pain relief were lacking [11]. Nitroglycerin and long-acting nitrates have been shown to be beneficial in patients with symptomatic diffuse esophageal spasm [104, 138], but no data have been published on the effect of these agents in patients with noncardiac chest pain without a manometric picture of diffuse spasm.

Several studies have examined the effect of the calcium channel blocker diltiazem on noncardiac chest pain, but the results are conflicting with regard to symptom relief as well as the effect on esophageal contraction amplitude [50, 122, 136]. Nifedipine was shown to decrease the amplitude of esophageal contractions in patients with nutcracker esophagus, but it was no better than placebo in symptom relief after 6 weeks of treatment [118, 123]. A beneficial effect on symptom relief was obtained with a low dose of the antidepressant trazodone in symptomatic patients with esophageal contraction abnormalities [31].

A thoracic longitudinal myotomy has been reported to give symptomatic relief in some patients with chest pain due to esophageal motor abnormalities. More recently, it was reported that a thoracoscopic esophageal long myotomy is able to provide substantial or complete pain relief in a subset of patients with noncardiac chest pain with diffuse esophageal spasm or symptomatic hypertensive peristalsis [35]. However, we feel that surgical management of esophageal chest pain is extremely rarely indicated.

In patients with noncardiac chest pain and proven gastroesophageal reflux, intensive antireflux therapy with high doses of $H_2$-blockers or with proton pump inhibitors is able to improve symptoms [133, 137]. It is unclear whether acid suppression may improve symptoms in patients with coexisting motor disorders and pathologic acid reflux. Adamek et al. performed prolonged manometric and pH recording in 95 patients with noncardiac chest pain and observed a high rate of coexistence of hypermotility disorders and pathologic acid reflux [2]. When patients with both disorders received omeprazole treatment, improvement in symptoms and reduction of pathologic acid reflux was observed, but the hypermotility disorder persisted, and patients did not become completely symptom-free, suggesting that the motor disorder did not depend on pathologic reflux.

The treatment of patients with an irritable or a hypersensitive esophagus is even more difficult. Acid-blocking agents will at best only partially relieve symptoms, while motor-inhibitory drugs may aggravate reflux. Drugs which interfere with pain perception may well be indicated in these patients. Such a mechanism could explain the beneficial effect on symptom relief obtained with a low dose of the antidepressant trazodone in symptomatic patients with esophageal contraction abnormalities [31]. Imipramine, a tricyclic antidepressant helpful in the management of patients with chronic pain syndromes, was evaluated in the treatment of patients with chest pain and normal coronary angiograms [4]. Imipramine reduced by approximately 50% the number of chest pain episodes, and it also reduced the sensitivity to cardiac pain during electrical stimulation. Esophageal motility testing did not identify patients who were likely to respond to imipramine.

McDonald-Haile et al. evaluated the effect of muscle relaxation training on symptoms reports and esophageal acid exposure in patients with reflux disease [93]. Subjects who received muscle relaxation had lower reflux symptoms and esophageal acid exposure. These data suggest that relaxation might be a useful adjunct to antireflux therapy.

## FOLLOW-UP

More work needs to be done before an efficient treatment scheme for chest pain of esophageal origin can be established. The long-term follow-up of patients with noncardiac chest pain has been inadequately studied. The use of esophageal testing and diagnosis has been controversial. Rose et al. studied prospectively the effect of esophageal testing on patient well-being in subjects with noncardiac chest pain [115]. There was a decline in emergency room visits, and patients tended to resume their normal activities, suggesting that esophageal testing by itself is useful in reassuring the patients of a noncardiac etiology of their symptoms. However, some patients did not fully comprehend the results of esophageal testing, and more than half of the patients who were found to have an esophageal abnormality still did not consider the esophagus as the source of the pain.

## REFERENCES

1. Achem SR, Kolts BE, Wears R, Burton L, Richter JE. Chest pain associated with nutcracker esophagus: a preliminary study of the role of gastroesophageal reflux. Am J Gastroenterol 1993;88:187
2. Adamek RJ, Wegener M, Wienbeck M, Pulte T. Esophageal motility disorders and their coexistence with pathologic acid reflux in patients with non-cardiac chest pain. Scand J Gastroenterol 1995;30:833
3. Alban Davies H, Page Z, Rush EM, Brown EM, Lewis MJ, Petch MC. (1985). Oesophageal stimulation lowers exertional angina threshold. Lancet 1985;1:1011
4. Anderson KO, Dalton CB, Bradley LA, Richter JE. Stress induced alteration of esophageal pressures in healthy volunteers and non-cardiac chest pain patients. Dig Dis Sci 1989;34:89
5. Arbogast R, Bourassa MG. Myocardial function during atrial pacing in patients with angina pectoris and normal coronary arteriograms: comparison with patients having significant coronary artery disease. Am J Cardiol 1973;32:257
6. Ayuso Mateos JL, Bayon Perez C, Santo-Domingo Carrasco J, Olivares D. Atypical chest pain and panic disorder. Psychother Psychosom 1989;52:92
7. Bak YT, Lorang M, Evans PR, Kellow JE, Jones MP, Smith RC. Predictive values of symptoms profiles in patients with suspected esophageal dysmotility. Scand J Gastroenterol 1994;29:392
8. Balaban DH, Yamamoto Y, Liu J, Wisniewski R, Mittal RK. Identification of a unique esophageal motor pattern by probe ultrasonography: a marker of spontaneous and induced esophageal chest pain (abstract). Neurogastroenterol Motil 1998;10:59
9. Baldi F, Ferrarini F, Longanesi A, Ragazzini M, Barbara L. Acid

10. Bass C, Wade C, Hand D, Jackson G. Patients with angina with normal and near normal coronary arteries: clinical and psychosocial state 12 months after angiography. Br Med J 1983;287:1505
11. Bassotti G, et al. Manometric evaluation of cimetropium bromide activity in patients with nutcracker esophagus. Scand J Gastroenterol 1988;23:1079
12. Bayliss JH, Komitz R, Trounce JR. Observation on distension of the lower end of the esophagus. Q J Med 1955;94:143
13. Beitman BD, et al. Panic disorder in patients with chest pain and angiographically normal coronary arteries. Am J Cardiol 1989;63:1399
14. Beitman BD, et al. Pharmacotherapeutic treatment of panic disorder in patients presenting with chest pain. J Fam Pract 1989;28:177
15. Bemiller CR, Pepine CJ, Rogers AK. Long term observation in patients with angina and normal coronary arteries. Circulation 1973;47:36
16. Benjamin SB, Gerhardt DC, Castell DO. High amplitude, peristaltic esophageal contractions associated with chest pain and/or dysphagia. Gastroenterology 1979;77:478
17. Bernstein LM, Baker LA. A clinical test for esophagitis. Gastroenterology 1958;34:760
18. Breumelhof R, Smout AJPM. The symptom sensitivity index: a valuable additional parameter in 24 hour esophageal pH recording. Am J Gastroenterol 1991;86:160
19. Breumelhof R, Nadorp JHSM, Akkermans LMA, Smout AJPM. Analysis of 24-hour esophageal pH and pressure data in unselected patients with noncardiac chest pain. Gastroenterology 1990;99:1257
20. Brushke AVG, Proudfit WL, Sones FM. Clinical course of patients with normal, and slightly or moderately abnormal coronary arteriogram. A follow-up study on 500 patients. Circulation 1973;47:936
21. Cannon RO III, Epstein SE. Microvascular angina as a cause of chest pain with angiographically normal coronary arteries. Am J Cardiol 1988;61:1338
22. Cannon RO, Schenke WH, Leon MB, Rosing DR, Urquhart J, Epstein SE. Limited coronary flow reserve after dipyridamole in patients with ergonovine-induced coronary vasoconstriction. Circulation 1987;75:163
23. Cannon RO, et al. Abnormal cardiac sensitivity in patients with chest pain and normal coronary arteries. J Am Coll Cardiol 1990;16:1359
24. Cannon RO, et al. Imipramine in patients with chest pain despite normal coronary angiograms. N Engl J Med 1994;19:1411
25. Chauhan A, Mullins PA, Taylor G, Petch MC, Schofield PM. Effect of hyperventilation and mental stress on coronary blood flow in syndrome X. Am Heart J 1991;122:458
26. Chauhan A, Petch MC, Schofield PM. Effect of oesophageal acid instillation on coronary blood flow. Lancet 1993;341:1309
27. Chauhan A, Mullins PA, Thuraisingham SI, Taylor G, Petch MC, Schofield PM. Abnormal cardiac pain perception in syndrome X. J Am Coll Cardiol 1994;24:329
28. Chauhan A, Mullins PA, Taylor G, Petch MC, Schofield PM. Cardioesophageal reflex: a mechanism for 'linked angina' in patients with angiographically proven coronary artery disease. J Am Coll Cardiol 1996;27:1621
29. Cherian P, Smith LF, Bardhan DK, Thorpe JAC, Oakley GD, Dawson D. Esophageal tests in the evaluation of non-cardiac chest pain. Dis Esophagus 1995;8:129
30. Clouse RE, Lustman PJ. Psychiatric illnesses and contraction abnormalities of the esophagus. N Engl J Med 1982;309:1337
31. Clouse RE, Lustman PJ, Eckert TC, Ferney DM, Griffith LS. Low dose trazodone for symptomatic patients with esophageal contraction abnormalities. Gastroenterology 1987;92:1027
32. Cooke RA, Anggiansah A, Wang J, Chambers JB, Owen W. Hyperventilation and esophageal dysmotility in patients with non-cardiac chest pain. Am J Gastroenterol 1996;91:480
33. Cornier LE, et al. Chest pain with negative cardiac diagnostic studies. Relationship to psychiatric illness. J Nerv Ment Dis 1988;176:351
34. Crake T, Canepa-Anson R, Shapiro L, Poole-Wilson PA. Continuous recording of coronary sinus oxygen saturation during atrial pacing in patients with coronary artery disease or with syndrome X. Br Heart J 1988;59:31
35. Cuschieri A. Endoscopic esophageal myotomy for specific motility disorders and non-cardiac chest pain. Endosc Surg Allied Technol 1993;1:280

# Color Plates

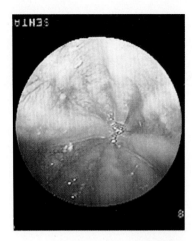

**COLOR PLATE 52.** Endoscopic appearance of punctate aphthoid ulcers.

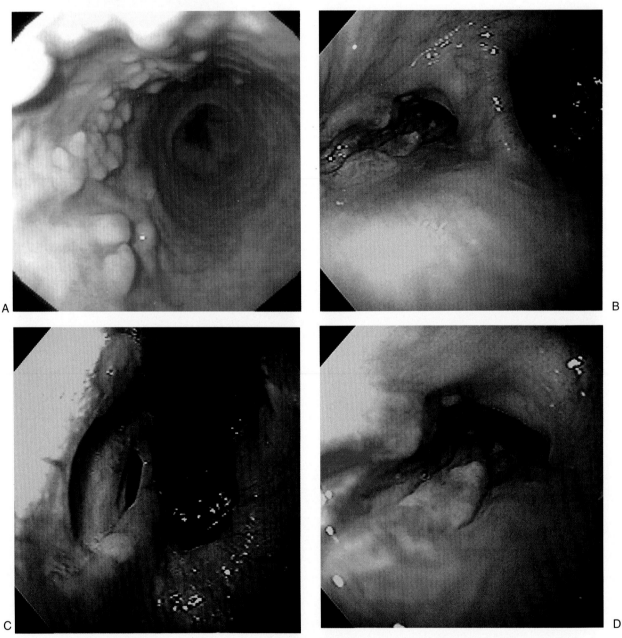

**COLOR PLATE 53. A:** Endoscopic appearance showing extensive polypoid, "cobblestone-like" changes in the distal esophagus in a patient with Crohn's disease. (Courtesy Dr. Kevin Lang, San Antonio, TX.) **B:** Proximal esophageal fistula due to Crohn's disease. **C:** Distal esophageal fistula (seen on retroflexed view) due to Crohn's disease. **D:** Endoscopic view of polypoid/varicoid changes in the mid/distal esophagus corresponding to radiographic changes of Fig. 35-1A.

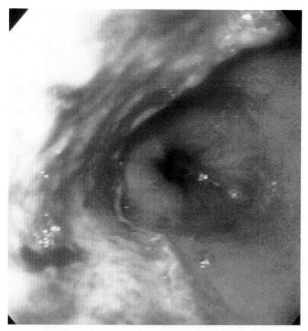

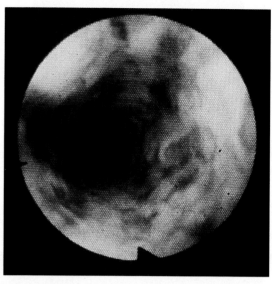

**COLOR PLATE 54.** Focalized esophageal tuberculosis in a 22-year-old man with acquired immunodeficiency syndrome. Ziehl-Nielsen stain showed acid-fast bacilli, and cultures grew *Mycobacterium tuberculosis*. (Courtesy Dr. Benjamin Go, Chicago, IL.)

**COLOR PLATE 55.** Multiple midesophageal superficial ulcerations to *Mycobacterium avium-intracellulare*.

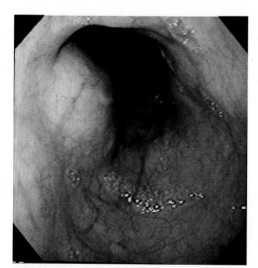

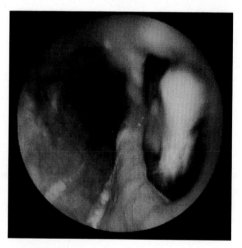

**COLOR PLATE 56.** Esophageal compression due to carinal nodal enlargement in a patient with pulmonary tuberculosis.

**COLOR PLATE 57.** Esophagotracheal fistulous communication (corresponding to the barium esophagram in Fig. 35-3B) due to tuberculosis.

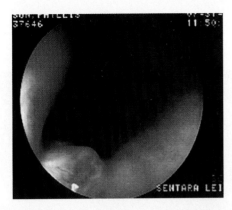

**COLOR PLATE 58.** Endoscopic view of submucosal mass effect in the perihilar area secondary to histoplasmosis.

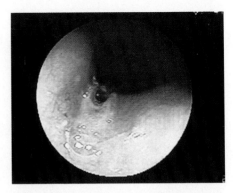

**COLOR PLATE 59.** Endoscopic visualization of the same patient in as Plate 37, now showing mucosal ulceration secondary to sinus tract fistulization from pulmonary histoplasmosis.

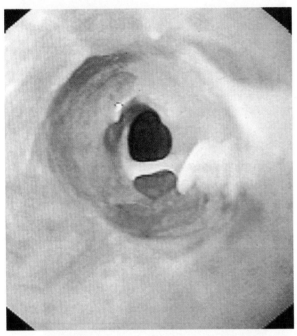

**COLOR PLATE 60.** Esophageal pseudomembrane formation in an immunocompetent patient with *streptococcus viridans* bacteremia. (Courtesy Dr. M. Brian Fennerty, Portland, OR.)

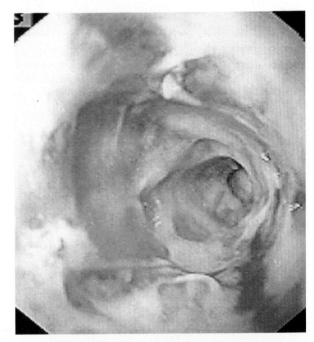

**COLOR PLATE 61.** Endoscopic view of a critically ill patient with *Streptococcus parvus* bacteremia. Extensive pseudomembrane and ulcerative change is evident, shown with the appearance of a pseudodiverticular-like change as a consequence of the plaquelike deposition of the pseudomembrane. (Courtesy Dr. M. Brian Fennerty, Portland, OR.)

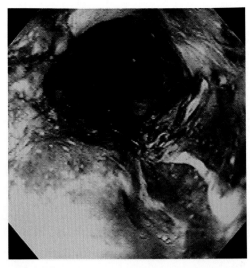

**COLOR PLATE 62.** Diffusely blackened distal esophagus in a critically ill patient.

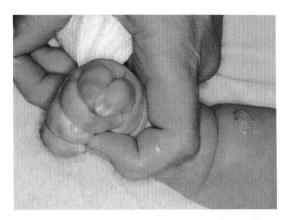

**COLOR PLATE 63.** Epidermolysis bullosa dystrophica. Blisters and erosions on fingers and arms of a newborn infant.

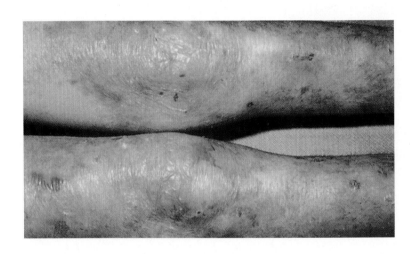

**COLOR PLATE 64.** Epidermolysis bullosa dystrophica. Erosions and scarring in a child.

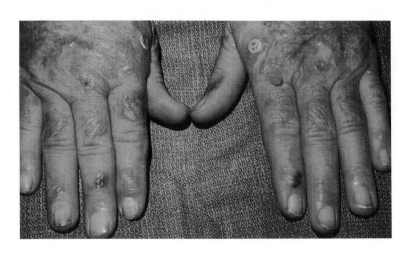

**COLOR PLATE 65.** Epidermolysis bullosa acquisita. Bullous lesions and scarring resemble those seen in porphyria cutanea tarda.

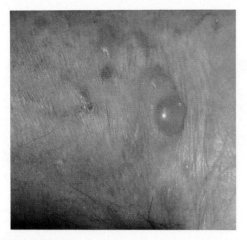

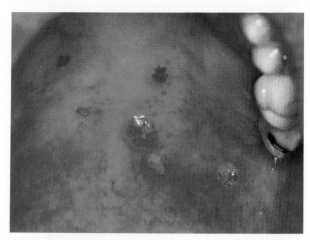

**COLOR PLATE 66.** Bullous pemphigoid. Tense bullae on the wrist.

**COLOR PLATE 67.** Bullous pemphigoid. Bullous lesions on the palate.

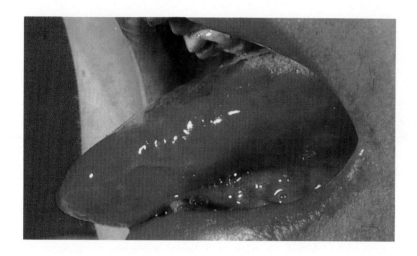

**COLOR PLATE 68.** Cicatricial pemphigoid.

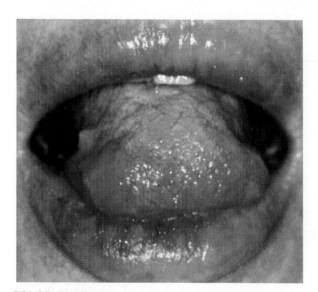

**COLOR PLATE 69.** Pemphigus vulgaris. Oral erosions or desquamative gingivitis may be the presenting sign, prior to cutaneous lesions.

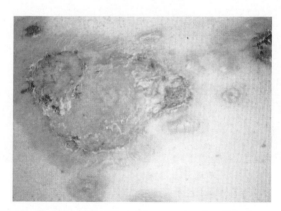

**COLOR PLATE 70.** Pemphigus vulgaris. Erosions and crusting are often more evident than intact blisters.

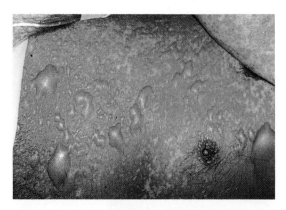

**COLOR PLATE 71.** Toxic epidermal necrolysis. Widespread bullae and erythema, in this case secondary to trimethoprim-sulfamethoxazole.

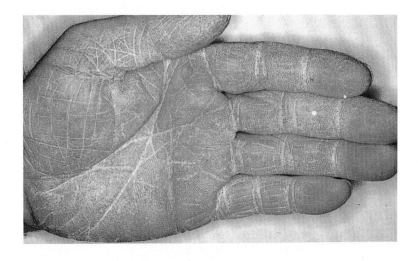

**COLOR PLATE 72.** Tylosis, or acquired palmar keratoderma, in a patient with esophageal carcinoma.

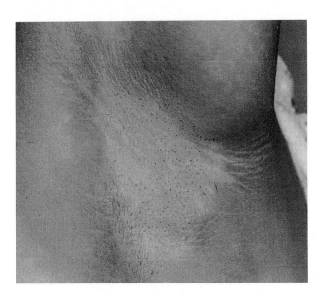

**COLOR PLATE 73.** Acanthosis nigricans. Note brown hyperpigmentation of the axilla.

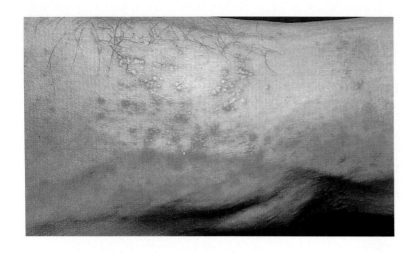

**COLOR PLATE 74.** Lichen planus. Small violaceous papules on the ankle.

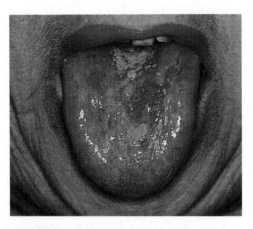

**COLOR PLATE 75.** Lichen planus. Hyperkeratosis and erosion on the tongue. There is also *Candida* infection present.

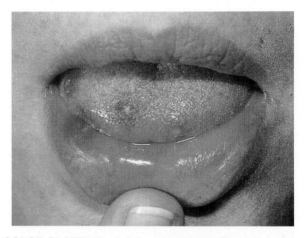

**COLOR PLATE 76.** Aphthous stomatitis. Punctate aphthae of the tongue and lip mucosae.

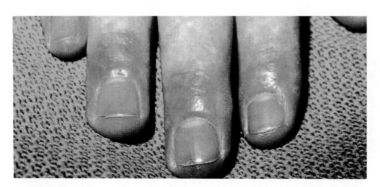

**COLOR PLATE 77.** Dermatomyositis. Note periungual atrophy and telangiectasia.

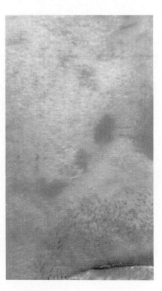

**COLOR PLATE 78.** Scleroderma. Mat telangiectasia and taut skin of the face in a patient with progressive systemic sclerosis.

36. Dalton CB, Hewson EG, Castell DO, Richter JE. Edrophonium provocative test in non-cardiac chest pain. Evaluation of testing techniques. Dig Dis Sci 1990;35:1445

37. Dart AM, Davies AH, Dalal J, Ruttley M, Henderson HH. Angina and normal coronary arteriograms: a follow-up study. Eur Heart J 1980;1:97

38. Day LJ, Sowton E. Clinical features and follow-up of patients with angina and normal coronary arteries. Lancet 1976;ii:334

39. De Caestecker JS, et al. The oesophagus as a cause of recurrent chest pain: which patients should be investigated and which tests should be used? Lancet 1985;2:1143

40. De Caestecker JA, Pryde A, Heading RC. Comparison of intravenous edrophonium and esophageal acid perfusion during esophageal manometry in patients with non-cardiac chest pain. Gut 1988;29:1029

41. De Caestecker JS, et al. Site and mechanism of pain perception with esophageal balloon distension and intravenous edrophonium in patients with esophageal chest pain. Gut 1992;33:580

42. DeMeester TR, O'Sullivan GC, Bermudez G, Midell AI, Cimochowski GE, O'Drobinak J. Esophageal function in patients with angina-type chest pain and normal coronary angiograms. Ann Surg 1982; 196:488

43. Detre KM, Peduzzi P, Takaro T, Hultgren HN, Murphy ML, Kroncke G. The Veterans Administration Coronary Artery Bypass Surgery Cooperative Study Group. Eleven-year survival in the veterans administration randomised trial of coronary bypass surgery for stable angina. N Engl J Med 1984;311:1333

44. Egashira K, et al. Evidence of impaired endothelium-dependent coronary vasodilation in patients with angina pectoris and normal coronary angiograms. N Engl J Med 1993;328:1659

45. Emde C, Armstrong D, Blum AL. Chest pain due to gastroesophageal reflux: presentation of a mathematical procedure to assess its significance. Gastrointest Motil 1990;2:140

46. Emde C, Armstrong D, Castiglione F, Cilluffo T, Riecken EO, Blum AL. Reproducibility of long term ambulatory esophageal combined pH/manometry. Gastroenterology 1990;100:1630

47. Faxon DP, McCabe CH, Kreigel DE, Ryan TJ. Therapeutic and economic value of a normal coronary angiogram. Am J Med 1982;73: 500

48. Ferguson SC, Hodges K, Hersh T, Jinick H. Esophageal manometry in patients with chest pain and normal coronary arteriograms. Am J Gastroenterol 1981;75:124

49. Fleet RP, Dupuis G, Marchand A, Burelle D, Arsenault A, and Beiman BD. Panic disorder in emergency department chest pain patients: prevalence, comorbidity, suicidal ideation and physician recognition. Am J Med 1996;101:371

50. Frachtman RL, Botoman VA, Pope CE. A double blind crossover trial of diltiazem shows no benefit in patients with dysphagia and/or chest pain of esophageal origin. Gastroenterology 1986;90:1420

51. Frobert O, Funch-Jensen P, Jacobsen NO, Kruse A, Bagger JP. Upper endoscopy in patients with angina and normal coronary angiograms. Endoscopy 1995;27:365

52. Frøbert O, Funch-Jensen P, Bagger JP. Diagnostic value of esophageal studies in patients with angina-like chest pain and normal coronary angiograms. Ann Intern Med 1996;124:959

53. Galassi AR, et al. Heart rate response during exercise testing and ambulatory ECG monitoring in patients with syndrome X. Am Heart J 1991;122:458

54. Ghillebert G, Janssens J. Provocation tests versus 24-hour pH and pressure measurements. Eur J Gastroenterol Hepatol 1995;7:1141

55. Ghillebert G, Janssens J, Vantrappen G, Nevens F, Piessens J. Ambulatory 24 hour intraoesophageal pH and pressure recordings vs provocation tests in the diagnosis of chest pain of oesophageal origin. Gut 1990;31:738

56. Gignoux C, et al. Role of upper esophageal reflex and belch reflex dysfunctions in noncardiac chest pain. Dig Dis Sci 1993;38:1909

57. Goudot-Pernot C, Champignuelle B, Bigard MA, Pernot C, Gaucher P. Prospective study comparing the edrophonium test and the intraesophageal balloon distension test in 78 non-cardiac chest pain patients and 12 healthy controls. Ann Gastroenterol Hepatol 1991;27: 41

58. Gustafsson U, Tibbling L. The effect of edrophonium chloride-induced chest pain on esophageal blood flow and motility. Scand J Gastroenterol 1997;32:104

59. Heupler FA, Prandit WL, Razavi M, Shirey EK, Greenstreet R, Sheldon WC. Ergonovine maleate provocation test for coronary artery spasm. Am J Cardiol 1978;41:631

60. Hewson EG, Dalton CB, Richter JE. Comparison of esophageal manometry, provocative testing and ambulatory monitoring in patients with unexplained chest pain. Dig Dis Sci 1990;35:302

61. Hewson EG, Sinclair JW, Dalton CB, Richter JE. Twenty-four-hour esophageal pH monitoring: the most useful test for evaluating noncardiac chest pain. Am J Med 1991;90:576

62. Howard PJ, Maher L, Pryde A, Heading RC. Symptomatic gastroesophageal reflux, abnormal esophageal acid exposure, and mucosal acid sensitivity are three separate, though related aspects of gastroesophageal reflux disease. Gut 1991;32:128

63. Hookman P, Siegel CI, Hendrix TR. Failure of oxethazine to alter acid induced esophageal pain. Am J Dig Dis 1966;11:811

64. Houghton L, Foster JM, Whorwell PJ, Morris J, Fowler P. Is chest pain after sumatriptan esophageal in origin? Lancet 1994;344:985

65. Hsia PC, Maher KA, Lewis JH, Cattau EL, Fleischer DE, Benjamin SB. Utility of upper endoscopy in the evaluation of noncardiac chest pain. Gastrointest Endosc 1991;37:22

66. Humeau B, et al. Angina-like chest pain of esophageal origin. Results of functional tests and value of balloon distension. Gastroenterol Clin Biol 1990;14:334

67. Janssens J, Vantrappen G, Ghillebert G. 24-hour recording of esophageal pressure and pH in patients with non-cardiac chest pain. Gastroenterology 1986;90:1978

68. Janssens J, Vantrappen G, Vos R, Ghillebert G. The acid burden over and extended period preceding a reflux episode is a major determinant in the development of heartburn (abstract). Gastroenterology 1992; 103:A90

69. Kahrilas PJ, Dodds WJ, Hogan WJ. Dysfunction of the belch reflex. A cause of incapacitating chest pain. Gastroenterology 1987;93:818

70. Kaski JC, Rosano GMC, Collins P, Nihoyannopoulos P, Maseri A, Poole-Wilson PA. Cardiac syndrome X: clinical characteristics and left ventricular function. J Am Coll Cardiol 1995;25:807

71. Katon W, et al. Chest pain: relationship of psychiatric illness to coronary arteriography results. Am J Med 1988;84:1

72. Kemp HG. Left ventricular function in patients with the anginal syndrome and normal coronary arteriograms. Am J Cardiol 1973;32:375

73. Kemp HG, Vokonas PS, Cohn PF, Gorlin R. The anginal syndromes associated with normal coronary arteriograms: report of a six year experience. Am J Med 1973;54:735

74. Kemp HG, Kronmal RA, Vlietstra RE, Frye RL. Seven year survival of patients with normal or near normal coronary arteriograms: a CASS registry study. J Am Coll Cardiol 1986;7:479

75. Kisely SR, Creed FH, Cotter L. The course of psychiatric disorder associated with non-specific chest pain. J Psychosom Res 1992;36: 329

76. Klimes I, Mayou RA, Pearce MJ, Coles L, Fagg JR. Psychological treatment for atypical non-cardiac chest pain: a controlled evaluation. Psychol Med 1990;20:605

77. Kubler W, Opherk D. Angina pectoris with normal coronary arteries. Acta Med Scand 1984;694:55

78. Lagerqvist B, Sylven C, Waldenstrom A. Lower threshold for adenosine-induced chest pain in patients with angina and normal coronary angiograms. Br Heart J 1992;68:282

79. Lam HGT, Dekker W, Kan G, Breedijk M, Smout AJPM. Acute noncardiac chest pain in a coronary care unit. Gastroenterology 1992; 102:453

80. Lam HGT, Breumelhof R, Roelofs JMM, Van Berge Henegouwen GP, Smout AJPM. What is the optimal time window in symptom analysis of 24-hour esophageal pressure and pH data? Dig Dis Sci 1994;39:402

81. Lam HGTH, Breumelhof R, Van Berge Henegouwen GP, Smout AJPM. Temporal relationships between episodes of non-cardiac chest pain and abnormal oesophageal function. Gut 1994;35:733

82. Lam HGTH, Dekker W, Kan G, Van Berge Henegouwen GP, Smout AJPM. Esophageal dysfunction as a cause of angina pectoris ("linked angina"): does it exist? Am J Med 1994;96:359

83. Lantinga LJ, Sprafkin RP, McCroskery JH, Baker MT, Warner RA, Hill N. One-year psychosocial follow-up of patients with chest pain and angiographically normal coronary arteries. Am J Cardiol 1988; 62:209

84. Lasch H, DeVault KR, Castell DO. Intra-esophageal balloon distension in the evaluation of sensory thresholds: studies on reproducibility

and comparison of balloon composition. Am J Gastroenterol 1994; 89:1185

85. Lavey EB, Winkle RA. Continuing disability of patients with chest pain and normal coronary arteriograms. J Chron Dis 1979;32:191

86. Lee CA, Reynolds JC, Ouyang A, Baker L, Cohen S. Esophageal chest pain: value of high dose provocative testing with edrophonium chloride in patients with normal esophageal manometries. Dig Dis Sci 1987;32:682

87. Likoff W, Segel BL, Kasparian H. Paradox of normal selective coronary arteriograms in patients considered to have unmistakable coronary heart disease. Engl J Med 1967;276:1063

88. London RL, Ouyang H, Snape WJ Jr, Goldberg S, Hirstfeld JW, Cohen S. Provocation of esophageal pain by ergonovine or edrophonium. Gastroenterology 1981;81:10

89. Lux G, Van Els J, The GS, Bozkurt T, Orth KH, Behrenbeck D. Ambulatory esophageal pressure, pH and ECG recording in patients with normal and pathological coronary angiography and intermittent chest pain. Neurogastroenterol Motil 1995;7:23

90. Lynn RB. Mechanisms of esophageal pain. Am J Med 1992;92:11

91. MacKenzie J, Belch J, Land JD, Park R, KcKillop J. Oesophageal ischemia in motility disorders associated with chest pain. Lancet 1988; ii:529

92. Marchandise B, Bourassa MG, Chaitman BR, Lesperance J. Angiographic evaluation of the natural history of normal coronary arteries and mild coronary atherosclerosis. Am J Cardiol 1978;41:216

93. McDonald-Haile J, Bradley LA, Bailey MA, Schan CA, Richter JE. Relaxation training reduces symptom reports and acid exposure in patients with gastro-esophageal reflux disease. Gastroenterology 1994;107:61

94. Mehta AJ, De Caestecker JS, Camm AJ, Northfield TC. Sensitisation to painful distension and abnormal sensory perception in the esophagus. Gastroenterology 1995;108:311

95. Mellow MH, Simpson AG, Watt L, Schoolmeester L, Haye OL. Oesophageal acid perfusion in coronary artery disease: induction of myocardial ischemia. Gastroenterology 1983;85:306

96. Meyer GW, Castell DO. Human esophageal response during chest pain induced by swallowing cold liquid. JAMA 1981;246:2057

97. Miller TD, Taliercio CP, Zinsmeister AR, Gibbons RJ. Prognosis in patients with an abnormal exercise radionuclide angiogram in the absence of significant coronary artery disease. J Am Coll Cardiol 1988;12:637

98. Motz W, Vogt M, Rabenau P, Scheler S, Luckhoff A, Strauer BE. Evidence of endothelial dysfunction in coronary dysfunction in coronary resistance vessels in patients with angina pectoris and normal coronary angiograms. Am J Cardiol 1991;68:996

99. Nevens F, Janssens J, Piessens J, Ghillebert G, De Geest H, Vantrappen G. Prospective study on the prevalence of esophageal chest pain in patients referred on an elective basis to a cardiac unit for suspected myocardial ischemia. Dig Dis Sci 1991;36:228

100. Nguyen P, Castell DO. Stimulation of esophageal mechanoreceptors is dependent on rate and duration of distension. Am J Physiol 1994; 267:G115

101. Nguyen P, Lee SD, Castell DO. Evidence of gender differences in esophageal pain threshold. Am J Gastroenterol 1995;90:901

102. Ockene IS, Shay MJ, Alpart JA, Weiner BH, Dalen JE. Unexplained chest pain in patients with normal coronary arteriograms. A follow-up study of functional status. N Engl J Med 1980;303:1249

103. Opherk D, et al. Reduced coronary dilatory capacity and ultrastructural changes of the myocardium in patients with angina pectoris but normal coronary arteriograms. Circulation 1981;63:817

104. Orlando RC, Bozymski EM. Clinical and manometric effects of nitroglycerin in diffuse esophageal spasm. N Engl J Med 1973;289:23

105. Pasternak RC, Thibault GE, Savoia M, DeSanctis RW, Hutter AM Jr. Chest pain with angiographically insignificant coronary arterial obstruction. Clinical presentation and long-term follow-up. Am J Med 1980;68:813

106. Patterson WG, Wang H, Vanner SJ. Increasing pain sensation to repeated esophageal balloon distension in patients with chest pain of undetermined etiology. Dig Dis Sci 1995;40:1325

107. Peters L, et al. Spontaneous non-cardiac chest pain. Evaluation by 24-hour ambulatory esophageal motility and pH monitoring. Gastroenterology 1988;94:878

108. Proudfit WL, Bruschke AVG, Sones FM. Clinical course of patients with normal or slightly or moderately abnormal coronary arteriograms. 10 year follow-up of 521 patients. Circulation 1980;62:712

109. Quyyumi AA, Cannon RO, Panza JA, Diodati JG, Epstein SE. Endothelial dysfunction in patients with angina pectoris and normal coronary arteries. Circulation 1992;86:1864

110. Rao SSC, Gregersen H, Hayek B, Summers RW, Christensen J. Unexplained chest pain: the hypersensitive, hyperreactive, and poorly compliant esophagus. Ann Intern Med 1996;124:950

111. Rokkas T, Tanggiansah A, McCullagh M, Owen W. Acid perfusion and edrophonium provocation tests in patients with chest pain of undetermined etiology. Dig Dis Sci 1992;27:1212

112. Ros E, Armengol X, Grande L, Toledo-Pimentel V, Lacima G, Sanz G. Chest pain at rest in patients with coronary artery disease. Myocardial ischemia, esophageal dysfunction, or panic disorder? Dig Dis Sci 1997;42:1344

113. Rosano GMC, et al. Abnormal autonomic control of the cardiovascular system in syndrome X. Am J Cardiol 1994;73:1174

114. Rose S, Achkar E, Falk GW, Flesher B, Revta R. Interaction between patient and test administrator may influence the results of edrophonium provocative testing in patients with non-cardiac chest pain. Am J Gastroenterol 1993;88:20

115. Rose S, Achkar E, Easly KA. Follow-up of patients with non-cardiac chest pain: value of esophageal testing. Dig Dis Sci 1994;39:2069

116. Rosen SD, Uren NG, Kaski JC, Tousoulis D, Davies GJ, Camici PG. Coronary vasodilator reserve, pain perception and sex in patients with syndrome X. Circulation 1994;90:50

117. Richter JE, et al. Are esophageal motility abnormalities produced during the intra-esophageal acid perfusion test? JAMA 1985;253:1914

118. Richter JE, Dalton CB, Castell DO. Nifedipine: a potent inhibitor of esophageal contractions. Is it effective in the treatment of non cardiac chest pain? Dig Dis Sci 1985;30:790

119. Richter JE, Hackshaw BT, Wu WC, Castell DO. Edrophonium: a useful provocative test for esophageal chest pain. Ann Intern Med 1985;103:14

120. Richter JE, Barish CF, Castell DO. Abnormal sensory perception in patients with esophageal chest pain. Gastroenterology 1986;91:845

121. Richter JE, Obrecht WF, Bradley LA, Young LD, Anderson KO. Psychological similarities between patients with the nutcracker esophagus and irritable bowel syndrome. Dig Dis Sci 1986;31:131

122. Richter JE, Spurling TJ, Cordova CM, Castell DO. Effects of oral calcium blocker, diltiazem, on esophageal contractions. Studies in volunteers and patients with nutcracker esophagus. Dig Dis Sci 1984; 29:649

123. Richter JE, Dalton CB, Bradley LA, Castell DO. Oral nifedipine in the treatment of non-cardiac chest pain in patients with the nutcracker esophagus. Gastroenterology 1987;93:21

124. Richter JE, Bradley LA, Castell DO. Esophageal chest pain: current controversies in pathogenesis, diagnosis and therapy. Ann Intern Med 1989;110:66

125. Richter JE, Hewson EG, Sinclair JW, Dalton CB. Acid perfusion test and 24-hour esophageal pH monitoring with symptom index. Comparison of tests for esophageal acid sensitivity. Dig Dis Sci 1991;36:565

126. Sax FL, Cannon SO, Henson L, Epstein SE. Impaired forearm vasodilator reserve in patients with microvascular angina. N Engl J Med 1987;317:1366

127. Scarinci IC, McDonald-Haile J, Bradley LA, Richter JE. Altered pain perception and psychosocial features among women with gastrointestinal disorders and history of abuse: a preliminary report. Am J Med 1994;97:108

128. Schofield PM. Follow-up study of morbidity in patients with angina pectoris and normal coronary angiograms and the value of investigation for esophageal dysfunction. Angiology 1990;41:286

129. Schofield PM, et al. Exertional gastroesophageal reflux: a mechanism for symptoms in patients with angina pectoris and normal coronary angiograms. Br Med J 1987;294:1459

130. Shapiro LM, Crake T, Poole-Wilson PA. Is altered cardiac sensation responsible for chest pain in patients with normal coronary arteries? Clinical observation during cardiac catheterization. Br Med J 1988; 196:170

131. Shi G, Bruley des Varannes S, Scarpignato C, Le Rhun M, Galmiche JP. Reflux-related symptoms in patients with normal oesophageal exposure to acid. The acid hypersensitive oesophagus. Gut 1995;37:457

132. Siegel CI, and Hendrix TR. Esophageal motor abnormalities induced by acid perfusion in patients with heartburn. J Clin Invest 1963;42: 686

133. Singh S, Richter JE, Hewson EG, Sinclair JW, Hackshaw BT. The contribution of gastro-esophageal reflux to chest pain in patients with coronary artery disease. Ann Intern Med 1992;117:824

134. Singh S, Richter JE, Bradley LA, Haile JM. The symptom index. Differential usefulness in suspected acid-related complaints of heartburn and chest pain. Dig Dis Sci 1993;38:1402

135. Soffer EE, Scalabrini P, Wingate DL. Spontaneous non-cardiac chest pain: value of ambulatory esophageal pH and motility monitoring. Dig Dis Sci 1989;24:1651

136. Spuring TJ, Cattau EL, Hirszel R, Richter JE, Chobanian SJ, Castell DL. A double blind crossover study of the efficacy of diltiazem in patients with esophageal motility dysfunction. Gastroenterology 1985;88:1596

137. Stahl WG, Beton R, Johnson CS, Brown CL, Waring JP. Diagnosis and treatment of patients with gastroesophageal reflux and non-cardiac chest pain. South Med J 1994;87:739

138. Swamy N. Esophageal spasm: clinical and manometric responses to nitroglycerine and long acting nitrites. Gastroenterology 1977;72:23

139. Swift GL, Alban-Davies N, McKirdy H, Lowndes R, Lewis D, Rhodes J. A long term clinical review of patients with esophageal pain. Q J Med 1991;295:937

140. Van Dorpe A, Piessens J, Willems JL, De Geest H. Unexplained chest pain with normal coronary arteriograms. A follow-up study. Cardiology 1987;74:436

141. Vantrappen G, Hellemans J, Achalasia. In Vantrappen G, Hellemans J, eds. Diseases of the Oesophagus. Berlin: Springer-Verlag, 1975: 287

142. Vantrappen G, Hellemans J. Diffuse muscle spasm of the oesophagus and hypertensive oesophageal sphincter. Clin Gastroenterol 1976;5:59

143. Vantrappen G, Janssens J, Ghillebert G. The irritable esophagus—a frequent cause of angina-like pain. Lancet 1987;I:1232

144. Voskuil JH, Cramer MJ, Breumelhof R, Timmer R, Smout AJPM. Prevalence of esophageal disorders in patients with chest pain newly referred to the cardiologist. Chest 1996;109:1210

145. Wang H, Beck IT, Paterson WG. Reproducibility and physiological characteristics of 24-hour ambulatory esophageal manometry/pH-metry. Am J Gastroenterol 1996;91:492

146. Wani M, Hishon S. ECG record during changes in oesophageal pH. Gut 1990;31:127

147. Ward B, Wu WC, Richter JE, Hackshaw BT, Castell DO. Long term follow-up of patients with non cardiac chest pain: is diagnosis of esophageal etiology helpful? Am J Gastroenterol 1987;82:215

148. Waxler EB, Kimbiris D, Dreifus LS. The fate of women with normal coronary arteriograms and chest pain resembling angina pectoris. Am J Cardiol 1971;28:25

149. Weusten BLAM, Roelofs JMM, Akkermans LMA, Van Berge Henegouwen OP, Smout AJPM. The symptom association probability: an improved method for symptom analysis of 24 h esophageal pH data. Gastroenterology 1994;107:1741

150. Weusten BLAM, Roelofs JMM, Akkermans LMA, Van Berge Henegouwen, OP, Smout AJPM. Objective determination of pH thresholds in the analysis of 24 hour ambulatory esophageal pH monitoring. Eur J Clin Invest 1996;26:151

151. Wielgosz AT, Fletcher RH, McCants CB, McKinnis RA, Haney TL, Williams RB. Unimproved chest pain in patients with minimal or no coronary disease: a behavioural problem. Am Heart J 1984;108:67

152. Wiener GJ, et al. The symptom index: a clinically important parameter of ambulatory 24-hour esophageal pH monitoring. Am J Gastroenterol 1988;83:358

153. Wiener GJ, Richter JE, Copper JB, Wu WC, Castell DO. Ambulatory 24-hour esophageal pH monitoring: reproducibility and variability of the pH parameters. Dig Dis Sci 1988;33:1127

154. Wilcox RG, Roland JM, Hampton JR. Prognosis of patients with "chest pain? cause." Br Med J 1981;282:431

The Esophagus, Third Edition,
edited by D. O. Castell and J. E. Richter.
Lippincott Williams & Wilkins, Philadelphia © 1999.

CHAPTER 37

# Rupture and Perforation of the Esophagus

Anthony Infantolino and Roland B. Ter

## INTRODUCTION

Approximately 275 years ago, Hermann Boerhaave, a Dutch physician, reported the case of the Grand Admiral of Holland, who died as a result of a ''spontaneous'' rupture of the esophagus [25]. It is doubtful that Boerhaave realized the multitude of people who had suffered or would suffer a similar, almost always fatal demise. However, most additional cases that would be reported would not be classified as ''spontaneous,'' but rather as ''iatrogenic,'' i.e., secondary to either intraluminal or intraoperative injury. Recent improvements in early recognition, initiation of treatment, introduction of antibiotics, and improved surgical technique have lowered the fatality statistics associated with ''spontaneous'' rupture of the esophagus. This chapter will explore adult esophageal rupture and perforation from its etiology, pathophysiology, and clinical presentation through the controversies associated with treatment.

## DEFINITION

In order to clarify many of the different terms in the literature, one must agree on the definition of rupture and perforation. Boerhaave's syndrome has been called *barogenic perforation* and *postemetic perforation* [64]. The term *spontaneous esophageal rupture* will be used interchangeably with *Boerhaave's syndrome*. However, most cases are not truly ''spontaneous,'' since the majority are preceded by intense and prolonged vomiting. Esophageal perforation is similar in its consequence, i.e., full-thickness tear in the wall; most are secondary to manipulation within the esophageal lumen, and the majority have preexisting esophageal pathology. Anastomotic leaks, which have also been called esophageal disruptions [32], often have poor outcomes, are

A. Infantolino: Division of Gastroenterology and Hepatology, Thomas Jefferson Medical College, and Division of Gastroenterology and Hepatology, Thomas Jefferson University Medical Center, Philadelphia, Pennsylvania 19017.
R. B. Ter: Division of Gastroenterology, Graduate Hospital, Philadelphia, Pennsylvania 19146.

postoperative complications, and will not be discussed. A complete list of etiologies is presented in Table 37–1.

## HISTORICAL PROSPECTIVE

In 1946, N. R. Barrett summarized Hermann Boerhaave's description of the case of the Grand Admiral of Holland, Baron Wassenaer [17, 25]. In 1723, Boerhaave was called to the bedside of the admiral, who was complaining of a disagreeable feeling in the stomach. The admiral had overeaten 3 days before and complained of persistent stomach discomfort. He had taken multiple doses of ipecacuanha to induce vomiting as well as almond seed oil. While vomiting violently, he complained of severe pain and exclaimed something had burst, and he was sure he would die. Boerhaave found him doubled over, complaining of constant pain in the chest and epigastric area. Over 16 hours, the admiral became progressively tachycardic, tachypneic, and pale in color; he died shortly thereafter. The autopsy 24 hours later revealed a distended gastrointestinal tract, food and medicine in the chest cavity, and a rupture in the otherwise normal-appearing esophagus.

From 1723 through 1938, there were many reviews of additional, uniformly fatal cases without full explanation. According to Barrett, J. R. Meyer from Berlin in 1858 was the first to recognize this entity prior to death. Barrett described the first early diagnosis and surgical repair in 1946 [17], followed by Olson and Clagett in 1947 [104]. From 1947 through the 1960s, early recognition improved, antibiotics became more widely available, and mortality rates decreased. However, as technology expanded, instrumental perforation became more common and the definitions of rupture, perforation, and esophageal disruption became blurred. In 1979, Cameron et al. reported a 0% mortality in a heterogeneous group of patients who were treated conservatively [32]. In 1983, Larsen et al. [83] reported a 19-year experience on 57 cases (42 iatrogenic, 15 spontaneous) and concluded that early intervention decreased mortality by almost half. Overall, however, there was still a 25% mortality.

**TABLE 37-1.** *Etiology of esophageal perforations*

Iatrogenic
  Instrumentation
    Esophagogastroduodenoscopy
      Flexible, rigid esophagoscopy
    Esophageal dilatation
      Savory, pneumatic, Maloney, Eder-Puestow, through
        the scope (TTS)
    Miscellaneous therapeutic tools
      Nasogastric tube, enteroclysis tube, overtube, band
        ligation/sclerotherapy, Sengstaken-Blakemore
        tube, endoprosthesis, Celestin, expandable metal
        stents, endotracheal tubes, obturator airway, intra-
        cavitary irradiation for esophageal cancer, laser, en-
        doscopic ultrasonography, bicap
    Surgical injury
      Antireflux, Heller myotony, vagotomy, leiomyoma/
        lipoma resection, pneumonectomy, tracheostomy,
        thoracic aneurysm repair, mediatinoscopy, thora-
        costomy tube, cervical spine surgery, thyroid resec-
        tion
Boehaave's syndrome
Trauma
  Blunt, penetrating
Tumor
  Lymphoma, primary esophageal, metastatic
Foreign body
  Meat, bone, pill, Angelchik prosthesis, other
Infection
  Tuberculosis, herpes simplex virus, cytomegalovirus,
    human immunodeficiency virus, syphilis
Acid related
  Barrett's ulcer, Zollinger-Ellison syndrome
Vascular
  Aberrant right subclavian artery, aneurysm, anticardiolipin
    antibody syndrome
Other
  Esophageal diverticulum, radiation therapy, caustic injury

In 1991, Pate et al. [109] retrospectively reviewed 34 cases of spontaneous rupture over 30 years and found an overall mortality of 41%; they concluded that early surgical repair, regardless of the time after onset, appears to be indicated. From Boerhaave's original description in 1724 until the present day, the diagnosis remains difficult, management continues to be controversial, and the diagnosis carries a significant morbidity and mortality.

## IATROGENIC

### Instrumental Perforation

Medical instrumentation in the esophagus is the most common cause of perforation. Flynn and colleagues in their series of 69 patients reported that 48% of ruptures were iatrogenic, 33% were caused by external trauma, and only 8% occurred spontaneously [54]. Diagnostic esophagogastroduodenoscopy is a common procedure worldwide and its risk of perforation extremely low. Flexible esophagoscopy is associated with a lower incidence of perforation (0.03%) compared with rigid endoscopy (0.11%) [42, 75].

The usual location of perforation from endoscopy is at the cricopharyngeus, but when esophageal dilatation is added to the procedure, the location is often proximal to or at the stricture. The risk of perforation is increased tenfold when dilatation is performed at the time of endoscopy and it is dependent on the type of dilator. Cox and Bennett reviewed the literature on esophageal perforation and found that the incidence of perforation related to conventional dilators varies from 0.09% (for Maloney-Hurst-type dilators) to as high as 2.2% (for the Celestin-type dilator) [37]. The American Society of Gastrointestinal Endoscopy Survey estimated that the incidence of esophageal perforation for bougienage and metal-olive dilators was 0.4% and 0.6%, respectively [127]. In a national survey, the incidence of perforation from hydrostatic balloon dilatation was 0.3% [81]. Pneumatic dilatation of the esophagus is a well-established treatment for achalasia, and the most serious complication is perforation. Nair et al. reported a 1.7% risk of perforation [98]. Both higher inflation pressure and previous pneumatic dilatation increase this risk. The risk may increase up to 9.8% when inflation pressure exceeds 11 psi [44, 98].

Endoscopic thermal therapy of gastrointestinal bleeding is associated with 1% to 2% incidence of perforation [52]. Endoscopic variceal sclerotherapy-related perforations, in contrast to other endoscopic complications, occur in a delayed fashion typically 5 to 7 days postprocedure. The incidence of perforation is 1% to 6% and is the result of transmural necroinflammatory injury to the esophagus [35, 85]. Perforation has also been reported as a complication of endoscopic variceal ligation [71, 110]. The injury is due to the pinching of the esophageal mucosa between the endoscope and the overtube [21]. Cotton proposed that the overtube be introduced by riding it over a tapered 45-French Savary or a 44-French Maloney dilator [38].

Palliative endoscopic laser therapy for esophageal tumors is not uncommonly associated with esophageal perforation. It may occur during the procedure or be delayed up to 1 week after treatment. Its incidence is estimated to be about 5% [48]. Photodynamic therapy is currently utilized for palliative treatment of esophageal neoplasm and can be complicated by esophageal perforation. In a multicenter phase III trial of photodynamic therapy, Lightdale and colleagues [86] found a perforation rate of 4.6%. Bipolar electrocoagulation has also been employed to thermally ablate esophageal neoplasm, and the incidence of perforation is similar to laser therapy [72]. Another form of palliative endoscopic therapy is endoprosthesis, which includes expandable metal and plastic stents. Perforation has been reported to occur in 5% to 25% of cases following esophageal stent insertion [139]. The perforation may occur during stent insertion or be delayed secondary to pressure necrosis. Knyrim et al. [79] compared complication rates of expandable metal wall stents and plastic stents. They found that three of 21 patients had perforation during plastic stent insertion, while there was no perforation in the expandable-wall-stent group. A survey of six centers with a large experience in performing endoscopic ultrasound revealed a perforation rate of about 0.1% [11].

Nonendoscopic esophageal instrumentation is rarely responsible for esophageal perforation. These include endotracheal intubation, Sengstaken-Blakemore or Minnesota tubes for tamponading variceal bleeding, and nasogastric tubes. Endotracheal tube intubation can result in perforation of the cervical esophagus, which is usually located in the posterior wall near the cricopharyngeal muscle [148].

**Surgical Perforation**

Esophageal perforation can occur following operations on the esophagus or its contiguous structures. These operations include vagotomy, radical pneumonectomy, Heller myotomy, antireflux surgery, leiomyoma enucleation, thyroid resection, tracheostomy, thoracic aneurysm repair, mediastinoscopy, thoracotomy tube, and anterior cervical spine surgery [148].

## TRAUMATIC PERFORATION

Trauma can cause esophageal perforation and rupture and accounts for 8% to 15.3% of all causes [108, 133]. Trauma-related perforation can be separated into blunt or penetrating. Blunt trauma is an exceedingly rare cause of esophageal perforation, with an incidence of 0.001% [20]. The most common scenario is a high-speed motor vehicle accident with a steering wheel injury where a rapid rise in intraesophageal pressure occurs leading to rupture at the level of the hypopharyngoesophageal junction [20]. Esophageal perforation in the neck can also result from intratracheal disruption, second rib fracture, cervical spine fracture, or improper cervical hyperextension [22].

In contrast, penetrating injuries to the esophagus are more common and most often secondary to knife and gunshot wounds. The incidence of penetrating injury to the esophagus is approximately 11% to 17% [22]. Penetrating injuries of the cervical esophagus are more common than injuries of the thoracic esophagus in surviving patients. Overall mortality remains high (15% to 40%); therefore, early diagnosis with emphasis on location and associated vascular injury is warranted [22].

## TUMOR

Both primary and secondary esophageal cancer can be complicated by perforation. Invasion of the esophagus by contiguous primary or metastatic carcinomas has also been reported.

## FOREIGN BODY

Perforation of the esophagus can occur secondary to foreign-body ingestion and during endoscopic removal. It accounts for 7% to 14% of esophageal perforations [3, 100]. The perforation most often occurs at areas of acute angulation or physiologic narrowing. The level of the cricopha-

ryngeus muscle is the most frequent location. Patients having previous esophageal surgery are at increased risk of perforation [89]. Perforations secondary to foreign bodies occur by a number of pathways. Penetrating injuries from sharp or pointed metallic objects, animal or fish bones, and toothpicks result in high rates of perforation [123, 140]. Pressure necrosis from a blunt foreign body such as a coin can also rarely occur and is more common in children [138]. Clinical manifestation of foreign-body perforation may be seen within 48 hours or as late as 2 weeks with gradual erosion of the impacted foreign body through the esophageal wall.

## CAUSTIC INJURY

Ingestion of caustic substances can result in devastating injuries to the esophagus. Liquefaction necrosis of the esophageal wall following ingestion of lye weakens the wall of the esophagus, leading to rupture. There is a high risk of perforation in the 3- to 5-day postingestion period associated with intense inflammatory response and further vascular thrombosis with ulceration and sloughing of superficial layers of the mucosa. Instrumentation in the esophagus may increase the risk of perforation.

## PILL INDUCED

Pill-induced esophageal injury is common and may occur with a variety of medications. The most common medications are tetracycline preparations, potassium chloride, quinidine, and nonsteroidal antiinflammatory drugs. Sustained-released formulations are more likely to cause injury. Damage caused by prolonged contact of medication with esophageal mucosa may result in perforation [149].

## INFECTION

Infectious esophagitis may occur with pathogens such as *Candida,* herpes simplex virus, or cytomegalovirus, usually in an immunocompromised host. Perforations from esophageal infections are extremely rare. Extensive herpes simplex virus esophagitis and *candida* esophagitis have been reported to cause spontaneous perforations [19, 39]. Adkins et al. [2] reported a case of esophageal erosion and perforation secondary to mediastinal lymph node enlargement from *Mycobacterium* tuberculosis in a human immunodeficiency virus-positive patient.

## OTHERS

Barrett's ulceration and Zollinger-Ellison syndrome with peptic ulcerative esophagitis have also been reported as causal factors in esophageal perforation [89, 140]. Aneurysm and aberrant right subclavian artery have also resulted in esophageal rupture [148]. Cappell et al. [33] reported a case of esophageal necrosis and perforation associated with anticardiolipin antibodies apparently due to thromboemboli and ischemia.

## CLINICAL PRESENTATION

The clinical presentation of esophageal rupture and perforation is largely dependent on location and size of the injury and the time course when the patient is encountered [41]. Although Boerhaave's syndrome is classically postemetic, other entities which can cause a sudden rise in intraesophageal pressure (bursting pressure 3.7 to 5.0 lb/in.²) can result in "spontaneous" rupture [123]. These include weight lifting, laughing, hyperemesis gravidarum, seizures, and others (Table 37–2). Spontaneous rupture almost always occurs on the left side of the esophagus in the distal third [1, 7, 14, 24, 134]. In a review of 184 cases of spontaneous rupture, the vast majority were found to be in the lower third (166 cases), 15 in the middle, and 3 in the upper third of the esophagus [20]. Other large series have confirmed this location distribution [1, 58, 80, 110]. Most tears occur along the longitudinal axis, varying from 0.6 to 8.9 cm in length [6, 7, 73, 80]. Often, the mucosal tear is longer than the muscle tear, which is important surgically. This predilection for the lower left remains unclear, but weakening of the wall by entrance of nerves and vessels, lack of adjacent supporting structures, vertical orientation of the longitudinal muscle bundles, and the anterior angulation of the esophagus have all been considered to contribute [26, 80, 87, 97, 100, 110].

Given the above anatomic considerations, 80% to 100% of cases present with pain [1, 7, 17, 18, 26, 106]. The location is variable, but chest, epigastric, and upper abdominal pain are most common. Mackler's classic triad of vomiting, chest pain, and subcutaneous emphysema is less common than originally thought, and over reliance on this could lead to delayed diagnosis [88] (Table 37–2). Atypical signs and symptoms include back pain [39] and shoulder pain [134], facial swelling, proptosis, dysphonia, polydipsia, and hematemesis [64]. The hematemesis of perforation is usually of small volume relative to the more common Mallory-Weiss tear [13]. Signs include an acutely ill appearing patient with fever, subcutaneous or mediastinal emphysema, tachycardia, tachypnea, cyanosis, and upper abdominal rigidity. Hamman's sign, i.e., mediastinal crunch sound as the heart beats against air-filled tissues, has also been reported [80]. Depending on the time course, shock is not uncommon. Signs consistent with pericardial tamponade secondary to esophagopericardial fistula and food embolism have been reported, but are quite rare [67, 121]. Vomiting, the classic prerupture symptom, occurs in 67% to 100% of cases but is by no means required to suspect the diagnosis [1, 100, 127]. Dyspnea is also common and may be secondary to pleural effusions, pneumothorax, or hydrothorax [1, 7] (Table 37–2). If the perforation is thoracic and instrumental in its etiology, pain, fever, and subcutaneous emphysema predominate [105].

**TABLE 37–2.** *Boerhaave's syndrome: characteristic features*

Classic presentation
  Middle-aged male (35–55 years old), often with a history of dietary and alcohol overindulgence presenting with *chest pain* and *subcutaneous emphysema* after recent *vomiting* or retching (*Mackler's triad*)
Other predisposing factors
  Heavy weightlifting
  Hyperemesis gravidarum
  Excessive coughing
  Inappropriate Heimlich maneuver
  Defecation
  Severe asthma
  Parturition
  Hiccups
  Neurologic disorders (seizures/tumors)
  Idiopathic
Clinical features
  Signs
    Fever
    Tachycardia
    Decreased breath sounds
    Subcutaneous emphysema
    Vascular collapse
    Tachypnea
    Cyanosis
    Abdominal pain
  Symptoms
    Extreme chest/upper abdominal pain
    Vomiting/nausea
    Dysphagia/odynophagia
    Dyspnea
    Palpitations
    Sweats
    Restlessness
    Hematemesis
Histopathology
  Predominantly lower one-third tears
  Longitudinal (0.6–8.9 cm)
  Left greater than right
Radiographic findings
  Chest x-ray
    Subcutaneous/mediastinal emphysema
    Pleural effusions
    Pneumothorax
    Mediastinal widening
    Subdiaphragmatic air
    Pneumomediastinum
    Hydrothorax
    Normal if taken early
  Computed tomography
    Air in soft tissue of mediastinum surrounding the esophagus
    Abscessed cavities in pleural space/mediastinum
    Communication of esophagus with mediastinal fluid collections

Instrumental perforations continue to be predominantly thoracic, but when cervical perforations occur, the pain may initially localize in the neck and may have associated dysphonia, cervical dysphagia, hoarseness, and pain with cervical motion, sternocleidomastoid muscle spasm, and tenderness along with cervical emphysema [105, 112].

## DIAGNOSIS

The diagnosis of spontaneous rupture or perforation most often relies on radiographic findings, but the clinician must first consider the diagnosis. Up to 50% of cases are atypical in nature and lead to diagnostic errors [20, 60]. The diagnoses most often confused with Boerhaave's syndrome are reported in Table 37–3. In terms of instrumental perforation, if the normal anatomic structures are lost during the procedure, a perforation is likely [54, 60]. Patients complaining of pain after endoscopy should always be considered to have a perforation and the burden of proof lies with the physician. Regardless of the etiology of the perforation, the location and the time interval will determine the clinical features. Once suspected, urgent posteroanterior and lateral chest and upright abdominal radiography should be obtained [9]. Experienced radiologists will suspect the diagnosis in 90% of cases [23, 112]. The lateral roentgenogram of the neck is useful in suspected cases of cervical perforation. Some typical chest x-ray findings include pleural effusions, pneumomediastinum, subcutaneous emphysema, hydrothorax, and hydropneumothorax [62, 103, 104] (Table 37–2). If taken early, the chest x-ray can be normal. Soft tissue and mediastinal emphysema can take up to 1 hour to develop. Pleural effusions can take several hours to become evident. Panzini et al. [105] reported that 80% of instrumental perforation patients had abnormal chest x-ray findings. Pneumomediastinum was present in 60%, and 33% had a density adjacent to the descending aorta in the left cardiophrenic angle with a loss of descending aorta contour [104]. The midthoracic esophagus lies next to the right pleura; therefore, perforations in this are associated with right-sided effusions, while distal perforations most often lead to left-sided effusions [62, 82, 105]. Pneumoperitoneum may also be seen secondary to perforation of the intraabdominal esophagus.

Gastrografin and/or barium esophagography should follow plain radiography [29] (Figs. 37–1 and 37–2). If the patient has been sedated, contrast studies should be delayed, pending the return of the gag reflex. Studies should be performed in the upright supine and lateral decubitus position [45]. If a thoracoesophageal fistula or free perforation into the lung is suspected, barium should not be utilized due to the possible risk of mediastinal inflammation. However, if the patient is at high risk for aspiration, barium is the first option due to reported cases of pulmonary edema from gas-

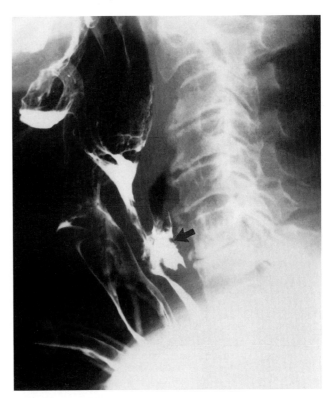

**FIG. 37–1.** Sealed-off perforation of the cervical esophagus by endoscopy. Note the self-contained extraluminal collection of contrast in the prevertebral location (*black arrow*). (Courtesy of Dr. S. Karasick, Thomas Jefferson University Hospital, Philadelphia, PA.)

trografin. Others believe that barium should always be the first study [55]. However, most agree that even if the gastrografin study is negative, it must be repeated with barium [114]. The above technique will detect 60% of cervical and 90% of surgically confirmed perforations, but carries a false-negative rate of 10% to 36% [23, 77, 130]. Esophageal dissections, which are rare, appear radiographically as a double-barreled esophagus [105] (Fig. 37–3). Sawyer et al. [121] stressed the importance of repeating the contrast study after several ours if a clinical scenario suggesting perforation persists, but the initial exam is negative. Spasm, tissue edema, and other factors may contribute to the false negatives [114].

Computed tomography (CT) scanning may also be useful in cases where contrast esophagrams cannot be performed or are difficult to localize or diagnose [13, 51, 69, 131]. CT findings can include air in the soft tissues of the mediastinum surrounding the esophagus, abscess cavities adjacent to the esophagus in either the pleural space or mediastinum, and communication of the air-filled esophagus with adjacent mediastinal or paramediastinal air fluid collection (Fig. 37–4). Left-sided pleural effusion strengthens the suspected diagnosis. CT of the chest may be life-saving in patients with atypical presentations [70]. In patients who do not improve after initial therapy, CT is useful in localizing fluid collections and can assist in their drainage [58]. Whether a CT scan can

**TABLE 37–3.** *Boerhaave's syndrome: misdiagnosis*

| | |
|---|---|
| Pancreatitis | Incarcerated diaphragmatic hernia |
| Tension pneumothorax | |
| Mallory-Weiss tear | Perforated peptic ulcer disease |
| Spontaneous pneumothorax | Myocardial infarction |
| | Pulmonary embolism |
| Gastric volvulus | Aortic dissecting aneurysm |
| Mesenteric thrombosis | Splenic infarction |
| | Pericarditis |
| Pneumonia | Renal colic |

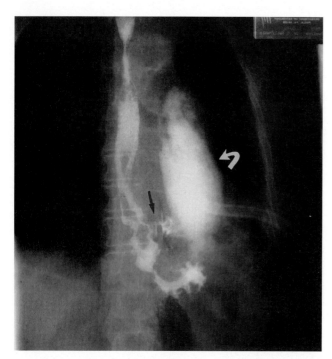

**FIG. 37-2.** Spontaneous esophageal perforation or Boerhaave's syndrome. Water-soluble contrast study shows the presence of a localized perforation of the left lateral wall of the distal esophagus (*black arrow*) communicating with the left pleural cavity (*curved arrow*). (Courtesy of Dr. S. Karasick, Thomas Jefferson University Hospital, Philadelphia, PA.)

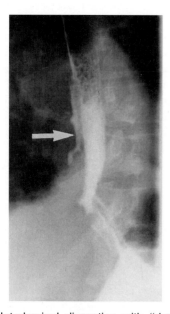

**FIG. 37-3.** Intraluminal dissection with "double-barreled" esophagus. Note the longitudinal intraluminal tract (*arrow*) separated from the esophageal lumen by a radiolucent mucosal stripe. (Courtesy of Dr. S. Karasick, Thomas Jefferson University Hospital, Philadelphia, PA.)

help predict who will benefit from operative versus nonoperative treatment remains to be determined [131].

Endoscopy has been utilized in some studies for diagnosis in difficult cases of perforation and has high accuracy for perforation secondary to external penetrating injuries. However, its role is highly questionable and is not recommended for acute, nonpenetrating perforations [34, 36, 66, 77, 92]. Thoracentesis may aid in diagnosis of perforation. Acidic pH, elevated salivary amylase, purulent foul-smelling material, or the presence of undigested food helps make or confirm the diagnosis [12, 47, 117, 134].

## PATHOPHYSIOLOGY

Lacking a serosal layer, the esophagus is naturally more vulnerable to rupture or perforation. Once a perforation occurs, retained gastric contents, saliva, bile, etc., enter the mediastinum, resulting in a necrotizing mediastinitis [136]. The midesophagus lies adjacent to the right pleura and the distal to the left pleura; therefore, perforations in these locations lead to involvement of their respective pleural cavities. Mediastinal emphysema results and eventually the parietal pleura is compromised, often resulting in hydropneumothorax. The degree of mediastinal contamination and location determines the clinical presentation. Cervical perforation rarely leads to mediastinitis, unless the infection tracks down facial plains or the retroesophageal space into the posterior mediastinum [31]. More commonly, a localized periesophageal abscess is noted [112]. Due to negative intrathoracic pressure, thoracic perforations tend to disseminate mediastinal contamination of fluids and bacteria [18]. Large-volume pleural effusions which contribute to cardiorespiratory difficulty are not uncommon [18]. Within 12 hours, a polymicrobial invasion of bacteria is noted with *Staphylococcus, Pseudomonas, Streptococcus,* and *Bacteroides* leading the way. The natural history of this process is fluid sequestration, sepsis, and death [3]. Perforation of the intraabdominal esophagus rapidly progresses to peritonitis, shock, and death if left unchecked. If the perforation remains localized, signs of sepsis and shock may be absent. This subacute presentation (24 hours to 2 weeks) more often presents with chest pain and dyspnea as the predominant features [77].

## MANAGEMENT

### Medical Management

Esophageal perforation is a lethal condition with a high mortality rate. Therapy depends on the site and size of rupture, the time elapsed between rupture and diagnosis, and the overall health status of the patient. Traditionally, esophageal perforations are treated within 24 hours by surgery with primary closure and external drainage. However, a nonsurgical approach has been advocated by many authors. Medical treatment consists of parenteral nutrition, intravenous antibiotics, and nasogastric suction. In 1965, Mengoli and Klassen

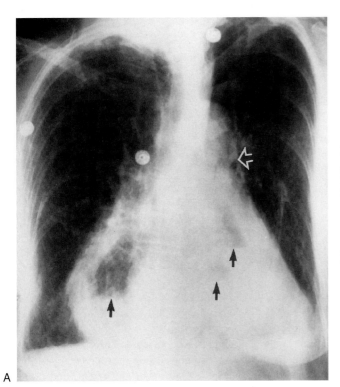

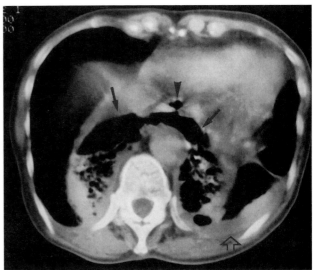

A
B

**FIG. 37–4.** Patient with fever and chest pain 2 weeks following an illness with severe vomiting. Surgical exploration revealed a perforated esophagus. (Courtesy of Dr. A. Salazar, Thomas Jefferson University Hospital, Philadelphia, PA.) **A:** Frontal chest radiograph demonstrates a mediastinal collection which extends on both sides of the midline with multiple air fluid levels (*arrows*). Pneumomediastinum is also present (*open arrow*). **B:** Contrast-enhanced computed tomography at the level of the heart demonstrates a large posterior mediastinal abscess with multiple loculations of fluid and air (*arrows*). There is air within the esophagus (*arrowhead*). There is an accompanying left pleural effusion (*open arrow*).

[92] reported one death among 15 patients treated without operation for instrumental perforation of the thoracic esophagus. They could not duplicate these results for spontaneous rupture of the esophagus, probably secondary to advanced mediastinitis. In 1975, Larriens and Kieffer [84] reported a successful conservative management and care of spontaneous perforation. Wesdorp and colleagues [144] treated 54 patients with instrumental perforation conservatively. They reported no deaths in 19 patients without malignancy and a mortality rate of 8.6% in those with carcinoma who sustained a perforation secondary to palliative intubation. Wesdorp et al. [144] claimed the key to successful conservative management is containment of the contamination of the mediastinum by nasogastric suction and control of local infection by massive doses of intravenous antibiotics.

Criteria to select patients for conservative management were first recommended by Cameron et al. in 1979 [32]. Eight patients with mid- and distal esophageal perforations were managed without operation. The perforations of these patients were well contained with limited soilage. Cameron et al. suggested the following criteria for selection of patients for conservative therapy: absence of clinical sepsis, contained perforation, and drainage of perforation into the esophagus [32]. In 1982, Sarr et al. [120] used these criteria

for patients presenting more than 24 hours after instrumental perforation. They reported that 1 out of 8 patients who were treated medically died, for a mortality of 13%, and concluded that nonoperative management might be entertained in minimally symptomatic patients with late, locally contained perforation and ongoing signs of minimal sepsis. Michel et al. [93] reported similar mortality rate of 12.5% for patients with contained thoracic perforations treated conservatively. Other authors also reported favorable results obtained by conservative treatment for esophageal perforations [28, 48, 54].

In 1992, Shaffer and co-workers [125] reassessed Cameron's criteria by comparing the results in 12 medically treated patients and 13 surgically treated patients. No mortality was seen in the medically treated group, but one surgically treated patient died postoperatively, indicating a nonsurgical approach as treatment for selected patients with esophageal perforation. They concluded that the most relevant of Cameron's criteria was containment of the perforation within the mediastinum and the visceral plane. Patients with pain requiring narcotics, leukocytosis, fever, and the presence of retention or trapping of barium in the mediastinum did not preclude conservative therapy.

From these studies, it is concluded that a nonoperative

approach may apply to specific situations. The guidelines for conservative therapy are (a) patients who are clinically stable with minimal signs of sepsis at the time of presentation and remain so, (b) instrumental perforations in which the patient had been on a regime of nothing by mouth and in which the perforation was detected early or the patient develops "tolerance" for the perforation without need for surgery, and (c) perforation contained within the neck or mediastinum with no extravasation and no signs of crepitus, pneumothorax, or pneumoperitoneum (Table 37–4) [5, 32, 125, 145]. The principles of medical treatment consist of nothing by mouth, parenteral alimentation, nasogastric suction, and broad-spectrum antibiotics covering anaerobes and both Gram-negative and Gram-positive aerobes. The decision to switch over to surgical management should always be considered. Cameron et al. [32] suggested that gastrograffin studies be performed every 3 to 5 days initially until it is evident that the patient is doing well. Deterioration of the patient's condition should prompt either contrast esophagography to look for leakage or a CT scan to detect an abscess. Surgical treatment should be considered early, as a delay in repair alters surgical approach and mortality.

Patients with esophageal cancer or disseminated malignancy who have had instrumental esophageal perforation represent a unique group. Conservative management with the use of endoprosthesis should be considered. Wesdorp and coworkers [144] reported 35 consecutive perforations in such patients, all treated medically with antibiotics, nutritional support, and protection of the perforation site. In 10 of their patients, a prosthesis was inserted to seal the perforated sites. Only one patient developed mediastinitis. In 24 patients, an endoprosthesis was inserted within a week with no mortality. Hine and Atkinson [65] had similar results in 13 patients with disseminated esophageal cancer who underwent endoprosthesis placement for instrumental perforations. Covered self-expanding metal stents were also used in 18 patients with disseminated esophageal cancer with few complications [102, 142].

## Surgical Management

Although conservative management of perforation can be applied successfully, it is only appropriate in a selected group of esophageal perforations. The majority of esophageal perforations are not contained and require operative attention. Indications for surgery include Boerhaave's syndrome, clinically unstable patients with sepsis, respiratory failure or shock, contamination of the mediastinum or

**TABLE 37–4.** *Criteria to select patients for medical management for esophageal perforation*

Clinically stable, minimal sepsis
Elective instrumental perforations
Contained perforation
Absence of crepitus, pneumothorax, and pneumoperitoneum

**TABLE 37–5.** *Criteria to select patients for surgical management for esophageal perforation*

Boerhaave's syndrome
Clinically unstable with sepsis, shock, and respiratory failure
Contaminated mediastinum or pleural space
Perforation with retained foreign bodies
Perforation in esophageal diseases for which elective surgery is considered
Failed medical therapy

pleural space, associated pneumothorax, perforation with retained foreign bodies, and perforation in esophageal diseases for which elective surgery would be considered in the absence of a perforation (e.g., achalasia, stricture, cancer) (Table 37–5) [54, 93, 107, 120, 148]. Perforations caused by forceful vomiting, foreign bodies, and violent trauma are not optimal candidates for medical management because these cases are seldom recognized promptly and may have been grossly contaminated [148]. Failed medical therapy or patients who become clinically unstable while on conservative treatment should be considered for urgent surgery. In general, surgical techniques used for esophageal perforation include drainage alone, drainage and repair, and drainage and diversion.

## Cervical Perforations

Perforations in the hypopharynx and cervical esophagus which are contained can usually be managed conservatively [46, 65, 135]. This usually includes selected patients with small instrumental perforations and perforations that are contained and well tolerated. Selection of the appropriate surgical approach is dependent on location, time period between perforation and diagnosis, and the presence of underlying esophageal disease. When the site of perforation cannot be found due to local inflammation, drainage only with intravenous antibiotics is adequate [82]. An esophageal cervical fistula will close within a few days in the absence of distal obstruction. Some authors recommend primary surgical closure of the perforation with drainage to all perforations without delay, thereby avoiding mortality and reducing morbidity [88, 93, 120]. However, there has been no clear evidence favoring one approach over the other.

## Thoracoabdominal Perforations

In general, thoracic esophageal perforations are more lethal because of direct contamination of the mediastinum and eventually the pleural cavity. Conservative management for selected patients with thoracic perforations has been supported by recent literature [32, 107, 135]. However, for uncontained thoracic esophageal leaks, debridement of necrotic tissue, generous irrigation, and complete mediastinal and pleural drainage are used. As in cervical perforations, care for thoracic perforations varies based on location, underlying disease, and overall condition of the patient. Treatment of choice for intrathoracic perforation within 24 hours is primary closure or reinforced primary closure in the absence of distal obstruction [12, 32, 118]. Bufkin et al. [30] performed primary repair with or without reinforcement in 52% (28 of 54) of the patients with an 82% survival rate. The average time to diagnosis was 20 hours from the onset of perforation. Their success for primary closure was based on early diagnosis, careful intraoperative assessment, and meticulous repair.

The management of perforations diagnosed more than 24 hours later is more complicated and associated with higher mortality and morbidity. Delay in diagnosis results in inflamed and necrotic tissue around the site of the perforation. This tissue holds sutures poorly and results in a high incidence of recurrent leakage after direct closure. Thus, surgeons have included reinforced closure in the operation, even late after the perforation. Pleural flaps, diaphragm, adjacent muscle, and omentum have been employed to reinforce closures of perforations [119, 148]. Bufkin and colleagues [30] suggest that perforations beyond early repair require placement of an esophageal T-tube to divert all secretions and allow time for healing of the surrounding injury. Esophageal resection is performed when a large perforation leads to continued leakage, as it may be the only method of controlling persistent mediastinal and pleural infection [119].

## MORTALITY

The overall mortality of esophageal perforations is 15.5% to 29% [148]. This rate is markedly increased to from 26% to 64% in patients in whom treatment is delayed more than 24 hours [3, 23, 77, 83, 93, 100, 109]. In contrast, patients treated within 24 hours have mortality rates ranging from 0% to 30% [3, 32, 93, 100]. The outcome of esophageal perforation is also dependent on the location and etiology of the perforation. Cervical perforations have a lower mortality rate (0% to 14%) than thoracic perforations (13% to 59%) [54, 75, 77, 83, 145, 148]. The higher mortality rate in thoracic perforations is secondary to direct contamination of the mediastinum and pleural cavity [132]. Boerhaave's syndrome has the highest mortality rate (ranging from 22% to 63%), while instrumental perforations have a lower mortality rate (5% to 26%) [148]. Underlying esophageal disease increases the mortality rate by six times [93].

## CONCLUSION

From Boerhaave's original description in 1724 to the present day, esophageal rupture and perforation remain a diagnostic and therapeutic challenge. Although rare, spontaneous perforation must be considered in any acutely ill patient complaining of respiratory and gastrointestinal symptoms, especially after recent vomiting, and must not be confused with more common diagnoses. Instrumental perforation is far more common and must be suspected in any patient complaining of pain postprocedure. An immediate upright chest

x-ray must be performed. If negative and the clinical presentation continues to suggest perforation, esophagram and/or chest CT should be considered. Thoracic site, delayed diagnosis and treatment are the main factors contributing to poor survival. Selecting patients carefully for conservative versus operative management is important and controversial. If surgery is performed, a 12- to 24-hour window is optimal. Mortality unfortunately remains high (5% to 63%) under the best of circumstances, and therefore continued efforts to improve diagnostic and therapeutic approaches are important.

## REFERENCES

1. Abbott OA, et al. Atraumatic so-called "spontaneous" rupture of the esophagus: a review of 47 personal cases with comments on a new method of surgical therapy. J Thorac Cardiovasc Surg 1970;59:67
2. Adkins MS, Raccuia JS, Acinapura AJ. Esophageal perforation in a patient with acquired immunodeficiency syndrome. Ann Thorac Surg 1990;50:299
3. Ajalat GM, Mulder DG. Esophageal perforations: the need for individualized approach. Arch Surg 1984;119:1318
4. Albin J, et al. Intrathoracic esophageal perforation with the Angelchik antireflux prosthesis: report of a new complication. Gastrointest Radiol 1985;10:330
5. Altorjay A, Kiss J, Voros A, Bohak A. Non-operative management of esophageal perforations. Is it justified? Ann Surg 1997;225:415
6. Anderson RL. Rupture of esophagus. J Thoracic Surg 1952;24:369
7. Anderson RL. Spontaneous rupture of the esophagus. Am J Surg 1957; 93:282
8. Andersson R, Nilsson S. Perforated Barrett's ulcer with esophagopleural fistula: a case report. Acta Chir Scand 1985;151:495
9. Appleton DS, Sandrasagra FA, Flower CDR. Perforated esophagus: review of twenty-eight consecutive cases. Clin Radiol 1979;30:493
10. ASGE Technology Assessment Status Evaluation. Endoscopic band ligation of varices. Gastrointest Endosc 1993;39:877
11. ASGE Technical Assessment Committee. Status evaluation: Endoscopic ultrasound December 1991. Guidelines for training and practice 1997
12. Attar S, et al. Esophageal perforation: a therapeutic challenge. Ann Thorc Surg 1990;50:45
13. Backer CL, et al. Computed tomography in patients with esophageal perforation. Chest 1990;98:1078
14. Baker RW, Spiro AH, Trinka YM. Mallory-Weiss tear complicating upper endoscopy: case reports and review of the literature. Gastroenterology 1982;82:140
15. Banks JG, Bancewicz J. Perforation of the esophagus: experience in a general hospital. Br J Surg 1981;68:580
16. Barber GB, et al. Esophageal foreign body perforation: report of an unusual case and review of the literature. Am J Gastroenterol 1984; 78:509
17. Barrett NR. Spontaneous perforation of the esophagus: review of the literature and report of 3 new cases. Thorax 1946;1:48
18. Barrett NR, Allison PR, Johnstone AS, Bonham-Carter RE. Discussion on unusual aspects of esophageal disease. Proc R Soc Med 1956; 49:529
19. Bauer TM, Dupont V, Zimmerli W. Invasive candidiasis complicating spontaneous esophageal perforation (Boerhaave's syndrome) Am J Gastroenterol 1996;91:1248
20. Beal SL, Pottmeyer EW, Spisso JM. Esophageal perforation following external blunt trauma. J Trauma 1988;28:1425
21. Berkelhammer C, et al. "Pinch" injury during overtube placement in upper endoscopy. Gastrointest Endosc 1993;39:186
22. Bjerke HS. Penetrating and blunt injury of the esophagus. Chest Surgery Clin North Am 1994;4:811
23. Bladergroen MR, Lowe JE, Posthelwaite RW. Diagnosis and recommended management of esophageal perforation and rupture. Ann Thorac Surg 1986;42:235
24. Bobo WO, Billups WA, Hardy JD. Boerhaave's syndrome: review of six cases of spontaneous rupture of the esophagus secondary to vomiting. Ann Surg 1970;172:1034

25. Boerhaave H. *Atrocis, nec descripti pruis, morbi historia: secundum medicae artis leges conscripta.* Lugduni Batavorum, Boutesteniana, 1724 (Summarized by Barrett [17])
26. Borotto E, et al. Risk factors of oesophageal perforation during pneumatic dilatation for achalasia. Gut 1996;39:9
27. Bradley SL, et al. Spontaneous rupture of the esophagus. Arch Surg 1981;116:755
28. Brewer LA III, Carter R, Mulder GA, Stiles QR. Options in the management of perforations of the esophagus. Am J Surg 1986;152:62
29. Brick SH, et al. Esophageal disruption: evaluation with iohexaol esophagography. Radiology 1988;169:141
30. Bufkin BL, Muller JI, Mansour KA. Esophageal perforation: emphasis on management. Ann Thorac Surg 1996;61:1447
31. Burnett CM, Rosemurgy AS, Pfeiffer EA. Life-threatening acute posterior mediastinitis due to esophageal perforation. Ann Thorac Surg 1990;49:979
32. Cameron JL, et al. Selective nonoperative management of contained intrathoracic esophageal disruptions. Ann Thorac Surg 1979;37:404
33. Cappell MS, Sciales C, Biempica L. Esophageal perforation at a Barrett's ulcer. J Clin Gastroenterol 1989;11:663
34. Carter R, Hinshaw DB. Use of the esophagoscope in the diagnosis of rupture of the esophagus. Surg Gynecol Obstet 1965;120:1304–1306
35. Clouse T, et al. Surgical repair of esophageal perforation in cirrhotic patients with varices. Chest 1994;105:1896
36. Coscia MG, Hormuth DA, Huang WL. Back pain secondary to esophageal perforation in an adolescent. Spine 1992;17:1256
37. Cox JGC, Bennett JR. Benign esophageal strictures. In Bennett JR, Hunt RH, eds, Therapeutic Endoscopy and Radiology of the Gut, 2nd ed. Baltimore: Williams & Wilkins, 1990:11
38. Cotton PB. Overtubes (sleeves) for upper gastrointestinal endoscopy. Gut 1983;24:863
39. Cronstedt JL, et al. Esophageal perforation in herpes simplex esophagitis. Am J Gastroenterol 1992;7:124
40. Curci JJ, Horman MJ. Boerhaave's syndrome: the importance of early diagnosis and treatment. Ann Surg 1976;183:401
41. Davis M, et al. Complications from enteroclysis tube insertion. AJR 1995;164:1–274
42. Dawson J, Cockel R. Oesophageal perforation at fibreoptic gastrocopy. Br Med J 1981;283:583
43. Defore WW Jr, et al. Surgical management of penetrating injuries of the esophagus. Am J Surg 1977;134:734
44. Dellipani AW, Hewetson KA. Pneumatic dilation in the management of achalasia: experience with 45 cases. Q J Med 1986;58:253
45. DeMeester TR. Perforation of the esophagus (editorial). Ann Thorac Surg 1986;42:231
46. Dolgia SR, et al. Conservative medical management of traumatic pharyngoesophageal perforations. Ann Otol Rhinol Laryngol 1992;101:209
47. Dubost C, et al. Esophageal perforation during attempted endotracheal intubation. J Thorac Cardiovasc Surg 1979;78:44
48. Ell C, Riemann JF, Lux G, Demling L. Palliative laser treatment of malignant stenoses in the upper gastrointestinal tract. Endoscopy 1986;18(suppl 1):21
49. El-Newihi, Mihas A. Esophageal perforation as a complication of endoscopic overtube insertion. Am J Gastroenterol 1994;89:953
50. Faling LJ, Pugatch RD, Robbins AH. Case report: the diagnosis of unsuspected esophageal perforation by computed tomography. Am J Med Sci 1981;281:31
51. Fennerty B. Esophageal perforation during pneumatic dilatation for achalasia: a possible association with malnutrition. Dysphagia 1990;5:227
52. Fleischer DE. Therapy for gastrointestinal bleeding. In Geenen JE, Fleisher DE, Waye JD, eds, Techniques in Therapeutic Endoscopy, 2nd ed. New York: Gover Medical Publishing, 1992:25
53. Fleischer DF, Kessler F. Endoscopic Nd:YAG laser therapy for carcinoma of the esophagus: a new form of palliative treatment. Gastroenterology 1983;85:600
54. Flynn AE, Verrier ED, Way LW, Thomas AN, Pellegrini CA. Esophageal perforation. Arch Surg 1989;124:1211
55. Foley MJ, Ghahremani GG, Rogers LF. Reappraisal of contrast media used to detect upper gastrointestinal perforations: comparison of ionic water-soluble media with barium sulfate. Radiology 1982;144:231
56. Fulton RL, Garrision RN, Polk HC. The non-operative approach to esophageal perforation due to Celestin tube placement. Arch Surg 1979;114:90
57. Goldschmiedt M, et al. A safety maneuver for placing overtubes during endoscopic variceal ligation. Gastrointest Endosc 1992;38:399
58. Goldstein LA, Thompson WR. Esophageal perforations: a 15 year experience. Am J Surg 1992;143:495
59. Gouge TH, Depan HJ, Spencer FC. Experience with the Grillo pleural wrap procedure in 18 patients with perforation of the thoracic esophagus. Ann Surg 1989;209:612
60. Graeber GM, Niezgoda JA, Burton NA, Collins GJ, Zajtchuk R. A comparison of patients with endoscopic esophageal perforation and patients with the Boerhaave's syndrome. Chest 1987;92:995
61. Hagan WE. Pharyngoesophageal perforations after blunt trauma to the neck. Otolaryngol Head Neck Surg 1983;91:620
62. Han SY, McElvein RB, Aldrete JS, Tishler JM. Perforation of the esophagus: correlation of site and cause with plain film findings. Am J Roentgenol 1985;145:537
63. Haynes DE, Haynes BF, Yong YV. Esophageal rupture complication Heimlich maneuver. Am J Emerg Med 1984;2:507
64. Henderson JA, Ploquin AJ. Boerhaave revisited: spontaneous esophageal perforation as a diagnostic masquerader. Am J Med 1989;86:559
65. Hine KR, Atkinson M. The diagnosis and management of perforations of the esophagus and pharynx sustained during intubation of neoplastic esophageal strictures. Dig Dis Sci 1986;31:571
66. Horwitz B, et al. Endoscopic evaluation of penetrating esophageal injuries. Am J Gastroenterol 1993;88:1249
67. Itabashi HH, Granada LO. Cerebral food embolism secondary to esophageal-cardiac perforation. JAMA 1972;219:373
68. Jackson RH, Payne DK, Bacon BR. Esophageal perforation due to nasogastric intubation. Am J Gastroenterol 1990;85:439
69. Jaffe MH, Fleischer D, Zeman RK, Benjamin SB, Choyke PL, Clark LR. Esophageal malignancy: imaging results and complications of combined endoscopic radiologic palliation. Radiology 1987;164:623
70. Jaworski A, Fischer R, Lippmann M. Boerhaave's syndrome: computed tomographic findings and diagnostic considerations. Arch Intern Med 1988;148:223
71. Johnson P, et al. Complications associated with endoscopic band ligation of esophageal varices. Gastrointest Endosc 1993;39:181
72. Johnston JH, Fleisher D, Pertrini J, Nord HJ. Palliative bipolar electrocoagulation of obstructing esophageal cancer. Gastrointest Endosc 1987;33:349
73. Jones WG, Ginsber RJ. Esophageal perforation: a continuing challenge. Ann Thorac Surg 1992;53:534
74. Justicz AG, Symbas PN. Spontaneous rupture of the esophagus: immediate and late results. Am Surg 1991;57:4
75. Katz D. Morbidity and mortality in standard and flexible gastrointestinal endoscopy. Gastrointest Endosc 1967;14:134
76. Kikendall JW. Pill-induced esophageal injury. Gastroenterol Clin North Am 1991;20:835
77. Kim-Deobald J, Kozarek RA. Esophageal perforation: an 8-year review of a multispeciality clinic's experience. Am J Gastroenterol 1992;87:1112
78. Kirsch HL, et al. Esophageal perforation: an unusual presentation of esophageal lymphoma. Dig Dis Sci 1983;28:371
79. Knyrim K, et al. A controlled trial of an expansile metal stent for palliation of esophageal obstruction due to inoperable cancer. N Engl J Med 1993;329:1302
80. Kossick PR. Spontaneous rupture of the esophagus. S Afr Med J 1973;47:1807
81. Kozarek RA. Hydrostatic balloon dilatation of gastrointestinal stenoses: a national survey. Gastrointest Endosc 1986;23:15
82. Lafontaine E. Instrumentation injury of the oesophagus. In Jaimieson GG, ed, Surgery of the Oesophagus. London: Churchill-Livingstone, 1988:387
83. Larsen K, Skov Jensen B, Axelsen F. Perforation and rupture of the esophagus. Scand J Thorac Cardiovasc Surg 1983;17:311
84. Laurien AJ, Kieffer R. Boerhaave's syndrome: repeat of a case treated nonoperatively. Ann Surg 1975;181:452
85. Lee J, Lieberman D. Complications related to endoscopic hemostasis techniques. Gastrointest Endosc North Am 1996;6:305
86. Lightdale C, et al. A muti-center phase III trial of photodynamic therapy versus Nd YAG laser in the treatment of malignant dysphagia. Gastrointest Endosc 1993;39:283A
87. Loop FD, Groves LK. Esophageal perforations. Ann Thorac Surg 1970;10:571
88. Mackler SA. Spontaneous rupture of the esophagus: experimental and clinical study. Surg Gynecol Obstet 1952;95:345

89. MacManus JE. Perforation of the intestine by ingested foreign body. Am J Surg 1941;53:393

90. McCall AJ. Slow-K ulceration of esophagus with aneurysmal left atrium (letter). Br Med J 1975;3:230

91. McCourtney J, Molloy R, Anderson J. Endoscopic esophageal perforation presenting as surgical emphysema of the scrotum. Gastrointest Endosc 1994;40:121

92. Mengoli LR, Klassen KP. Conservative management of esophageal perforation. Arch Surg 1965;91:238

93. Michel L, Grillo HC, Malt RA. Operative and nonoperative management of esophageal perforations. Ann Surg 1981;194:57

94. Mickisch O, Manegold B. Esophageal perforation in attempted ERCP. Gastroenterology 1992;30:428

95. Moghissi K, Pender D. Instrumental perforations of the esophagus and their management. Thorax 1988;43:642

96. Monnier Ph, Hsieh V, Savary M. Endoscopic treatment of esophageal stenosis using Savary-Gillard bougies: technical innovations. Acta Endosc 1985;15:1

97. Naclerio EA. The V-sign in the diagnosis of spontaneous rupture of the esophagus. Am J Surg 1957;93:291

98. Nair LA, et al. Complications during pneumatic dilatation for achalasia or diffuse esophageal spasm: analysis of risk factors, early clinical characteristics, and outcome. Dig Dis Sci 1993;38:1893

99. Nandi P, Ong GB. Foreign body in the esophagus: review of 2394 cases. Br J Surg 1978;65:5

100. Nesbitt JC, Sawyers JL. Surgical management of esophageal perforation. Am Surg 1987;53:183

101. Newhouse Ke, et al. Esophageal perforation following anterior cervical spine surgery. Spine 1989;14:1051

102. Nicholson AA, et al. Palliation of malignant esophageal perforations and proximal esophageal malignant dysphagia with covered metal stents. Clin Radiol 1995;50:11

103. O'Connell ND. Spontaneous rupture of the esophagus. Am J Roentgenol 1967;99:185

104. Olson AM, Clagett OT. Spontaneous rupture of the esophagus. Report of a case with immediate diagnosis and successful surgical repair. Postgrad Med 1947;2:417

105. Panzini L, Burrell MI, Traube M. Instrumental esophageal perforation: chest film findings. Am J Gastroenterol 1994;89:367

106. Parkin FJS. The radiology of perforated esophagus. Clin Radiol 1973;24:234

107. Pasricha PJ, Fleischer DE, Kalloo AN. Endoscopic perforations of the upper digestive tract: a review of their pathogenesis, prevention, and management. Gastroenterology 1994;106:787

108. Pass LJ, et al. Management of esophageal gunshot wounds. Ann Thorac Surg 1987;44:253

109. Pate JW, et al. Spontaneous rupture of the esophagus: a 30-year experience. Ann Thorac Surg 1989;47:689

110. Perino LE, Gholson CF, Goff JS. Esophageal perforation after fiberoptic variceal sclerotherapy. J Clin Gastroenterol 1987;9:286

111. Pricolo VE, Park CS, Thompson WR. Surgical repair of esophageal perforation due to pneumatic dilatation for achalasia: is myotomy really necessary? Arch Surg 1993;128:540

112. Reeder L, DeFilippi V, Ferguson M. Current results of therapy for esophageal perforation. Am J Surg 1995;169:615

113. Refuel WM, Brioche BS. Esophagi-pleural fistula secondary to perforated esophageal ulcer. Gastrointest Endosc 1972;18:165

114. Richter JE, Castell DO. Balloon dilatation for the treatment of achalasia. In Bennet JR, Hunt RH, eds, Therapeutic Endoscopy and Radiology of the Gut, 2nd ed. Baltimore: Williams & Wilkins, 1990:82

115. Rogers FL, Piug AW, Dooley NB, Cuello L. Diagnostic considerations in mediastinal emphysema: a pathophysiologic roentgenologic approach to Boerhaave's syndrome and spontaneous pneumo-mediastinum. J Surg 1972;115:495

116. Rosch T, et al. Major complications of endoscopic ultrasonography: results of a survey of 42105 cases. Gastrointest Endosc 1993;39:341

117. Roufail WM, Brice BS. Esophago-pleural fistulae secondary to perforated esophageal ulcer. Gastrointest Endosc 1972;18:165

118. Sabanathan S, Eng J, Richardson J. Surgical management of intrathoracic esophageal rupture. Br J Surg 1994;81:863

119. Salo JA, et al. Management of delayed esophageal perforation with mediastinal sepsis: esophagectomy or primary repair? J Thorac Cardiovasc Surg 1993;106:1088

120. Sarr MG, Pemberton JH, Payne WS. Management of instrumental perforations of the esophagus. J Thorac Cardiovasc Surg 1982;84:211

121. Sawyer R, Phillips C, Vakil N. Short and long-term outcome of esophageal perforation. Gastrointest Endsc 1995;41:130

122. Sehkat S, et al. Esophageal moniliasis causing fistula formation and lung abscess. Thorax 1976;31:361

123. Selivanov V, Sheldon GF, Cello JP, Crass RA. management of foreign body ingestion. Ann Surg 1984;199:187

124. Set PA, Flower CD, Stewart S. Delayed presentation of esophageal perforation simulating intrathoracic malignancy. Clin Radiol 1992;46:331

125. Shaffer HA, Valenzuela G, Mittal RK. Esophageal perforation. A reassessment of the criteria for choosing medical or surgical therapy. Arch Intern Med 1992;152:757

126. Sherr HP, et al. Origin of pleural fluid amylase in esophageal rupture. Ann Intern Med 1972;76:985

127. Silvis SE, et al. Endoscopic complications: results of the 1974 American Society for Gastrointestinal Endoscopy Survey. JAMA 1976;235:928

128. Skinner DB, Belsey RHR, Instrumental perforation and mediastinitis. In Management of Esophageal Disease. Philadelphia: WB Saunders, 1988:783

129. Smith JP, et al. The esophageal obturator airway: a review. JAMA 1983;250:1081

130. Snider DM, Crawford DW. Successful treatment of primary aorto-esophageal fistula resulting from aortic aneurysm. J Thorac Cardiovasc Surg 1983;85:457

131. Stephanson SE Jr, Maness G, Scott HW Jr. Esophagopericardial fistula of benign origin. J Thorac Cardiovasc Surg 1958;36:208

132. Sundrasagra FA, English TAH, Milstein BB. The management and prognosis of esophageal perforations. Br J Surg 1978;65:629

133. Symbar PN, et al. Penetrating wounds of the esophagus. Ann Thorac Surg 1972;13:552

134. Tesler MA, Eisenberg MM. Collective review: spontaneous esophageal rupture. Surg Gynecol Obstet Int Abstr Surg 1963;117:1

135. Tilanus HW, et al. Treatment of oesophageal perforation: a multivariate analysis. Br J Surg 1991;78:852

136. Traumatic perforation of esophagus (editorial). Br Med J 1972;2:524

137. Triggiani E, Belsey R. Oesophageal trauma: incidence, diagnosis and management. Thorax 1977;32:241

138. Tucker J, Kim H, Lucas GW. Esophageal perforation caused by coin ingestion. South Med J 1994;87:269

139. Tytgat GN, den Hartos Jager FC, Bartelman JF. Endoscopic prosthesis for advanced esophageal cancer. Endoscopy 1986;18(Suppl 3):32

140. Vizcarrando FJ, Brady PG, Nord HJ. Foreign bodies of the upper gastrointestinal tract. Gastrointest Endosc 1983;29:208

141. Walker WS, Cameron EWJ, Walbaum PR. Diagnosis and management of spontaneous transmural rupture of the oesophagus (Boerhaave's syndrome). Br J Surg 1985;72:204

142. Watkinson A, et al. Plastic covered metallic endoprosthesis in the management of esophageal perforations in patients with esophageal carcinoma. Clin Radiol 1995;50:304

143. Weiss S, Mallory GK. Lesions of the cardiac orifice of the stomach produced by vomiting. JAMA 1932;98:1353

144. Wesdorp IC, et al. Treatment of instrumental esophageal perforation. Gut 1984;25:398

145. White CS, Templeton PA, Attar S. Esophageal perforation: CT findings. Am J Roentgenol 1993;160:767

146. White RK, Morris DM. Diagnosis and management of esophageal perforations. Am Surg 1992;58:112

147. Wichern WA. Perforation of the esophagus. Am J Surg 1970;119:534

148. Williamson WA, Ellis FH. Esophageal perforation. In Taylor MB, Gollan JL, Steer ML, Wolfe MM, eds. Gastrointestinal Emergencies, 2nd ed. Baltimore: Williams & Wilkins, 1997:31

149. Yamaoka K, et al. A case of esophageal perforation due to a pill-induced ulcer successfully treated with conservative measures. Am J Gastroenterol 1996;91:1044

*The Esophagus*, Third Edition,
edited by D. O. Castell and J. E. Richter.
Lippincott Williams & Wilkins, Philadelphia © 1999.

CHAPTER 38

# Cutaneous Diseases and the Esophagus

Michelle L. Bennett, Joseph L. Jorizzo, and Elizabeth F. Sherertz

There are a number of dermatologic diseases with associated esophageal involvement. This may occur because both skin and upper esophagus have stratified squamous epithelium. Table 38–1 summarizes dermatologic diseases that may be associated with dysphagia. The major examples of dermatoses that can also involve the esophageal mucosa are the blistering diseases such as epidermolysis bullosa, bullous pemphigoid, and pemphigus vulgaris. These and other dermatologic diseases that may involve the esophagus are discussed in detail in this chapter.

Mucocutaneous signs may sometimes be helpful in the diagnosis of esophageal disease, such as infections and collagen vascular diseases. These are discussed more thoroughly in other chapters, but the cutaneous features of such diseases are briefly reviewed here.

## GENETIC BULLOUS DERMATOLOGIC DISEASES

### Epidermolysis Bullosa

Epidermolysis bullosa (EB) is a family of inherited mechanobullous diseases with a spectrum of clinical presentations, which have as a major manifestation spontaneous or trauma-induced blisters of the skin (Plates 63 and 64). Mucous membranes are sometimes involved with blisters, erosions, and scarring. In severe dystrophic types, deformities of the extremities may occur.

Classification of EB subtypes is based on inheritance pattern, the level of blistering within the dermal–epidermal junction as determined by immuno- and electron microscopy, and molecular defects [15]. In simplex EB, blistering occurs within the stratum basalis and results from mutations of genes coding for keratins 5 and 14. In junctional EB, the split occurs in the lamina lucida, and molecular defects are seen in the gamma 2-chain gene of laminin 5 (kalinin) coding for anchoring fibrils. In dystrophic EB, the split occurs

M. L. Bennett, J. L. Jorizzo, and E. F. Sherertz: Department of Dermatology, Wake Forest University School of Medicine, Winston-Salem, North Carolina 27157-1071.

below the lamina densa and results from abnormalities in the collagen VII gene coding for anchoring fibrils [48]. Recent studies report another form of EB associated with pyloric atresia and a homozygous mutation in the integrin alpha-6 gene [55, 65].

Onset of gastrointestinal manifestations is often in the first three decades of life [84]. In the esophagus, mechanical passage of food contributes to bullae, with subsequent scarring, stricture, shortening, stenosis, and atony [97]. Dysphagia is the most common complaint. Failure to thrive and nutritional deficiency are also common [4, 52]. Manometric studies of the esophagus in patients with EB have sometimes shown low baseline lower esophageal sphincter pressure even in the absence of strictures.

Treatment of esophageal lesions in EB is symptomatic. Avoidance of solid foods and parenteral nutritional supplementation are used when indicated [85]. Antireflux regimens may help when reflux is present. Systemic corticosteroid or phenytoin therapy improved symptomatic esophageal lesions when employed in recessive dystrophic EB, but the use of either is controversial [37]. Esophageal dilatation may be helpful but should be performed cautiously, particularly in children, since new bullae may be induced by the procedure [82]. In severe cases, when strictured lesions no longer respond to dilatation, surgical treatment is indicated. Colonic interposition is the procedure most often performed, and follow-up indicates successful results [22]. Nutritional support and protection of mucosae and skin from trauma (tape, etc.) must be emphasized to avoid perioperative induction of lesions [82].

Dystrophic (scarring) EB may be inherited in a dominant or recessive fashion, and either type can involve the gastrointestinal tract. Onset of skin lesions occurs at or near the time of birth, and the diagnosis of EB will usually have been made before a patient presents with gastrointestinal symptoms. The major sites of involvement are the oral cavity, anal canal, and esophagus. Esophageal perforation has occurred, requiring esophagectomy in some cases [28]. In the mouth, blistering occurs and leads to scarring, a smooth tongue, and

TABLE 38–1. *Selected dermatologic diseases that may be associated with dysphagia*

Genetic bullous diseases
  Epidermolysis bullosa subtypes
Immunologic bullous diseases
  Epidermolysis bullosa acquisita
  Bullous pemphigoid
  Cicatricial pemphigoid
  Pemphigus vulgaris
Other bullous diseases
  Stevens-Johnson syndrome/toxic epidermal necrolysis (erythema multiforme end of spectrum)
  Hailey-Hailey disease (benign familial pemphigus)
  Darier's disease (keratosis follicularis)
Heritable syndromes
  Cowden's disease (multiple hamartoma syndrome)
  Focal dermal hypoplasia (Goltz's syndrome)
Esophageal carcinomas
  Tylosis/Howel-Evans syndrome
  Paterson-Brown-Kelly syndrome (Plummer-Vinson syndrome)
  Acanthosis nigricans
  Cutaneous metastases
Nonbullous immunologic diseases
  Lichen planus
  Aphthosis and Behçet's disease
  Dermatomyositis
  Scleroderma
  Other collagen vascular diseases
Miscellaneous diseases
  Candidiasis
  Herpes simplex
  Kaposi's sarcoma
  Ehlers-Danlos syndrome
  Osler-Weber-Rendu syndrome

restricted tongue movement and mouth opening, resulting in compromise of chewing, swallowing, and speaking [96]. Dental deformities may also occur [25].

## IMMUNOLOGIC BULLOUS DERMATOLOGIC DISEASES

### Epidermolysis Bullosa Acquisita

Epidermolysis bullosa acquisita (EBA) is an uncommon delayed-onset, immune-mediated blistering disease involving specific immunoglobulins against type VII collagen [90]. It affects both the skin and mucosae. A distinct immunoelectron-microscopic pattern of immunoreactant deposition is observed on skin biopsy specimens from patients with this disorder. Immunoglobulin G deposition has also been shown to occur in the basement membrane zone of the esophagus in EBA [79]. The proximal third of the esophagus is the portion which is involved, with the effect being only seen in stratified squamous epithelium.

Blistering lesions with scarring occur at sites of trauma in EBA (Plate 65). Extensive oral and esophageal scarring may also occur [93]. EBA may rarely be associated with Crohn's disease and may resolve after resection of involved intestine [67, 74]. The relationship between EBA and bullous lupus erythematosus is controversial, as both types of patients may have EBA antibodies in their serum and identical clinical-histologic bullae [51].

### Bullous Pemphigoid and Cicatricial Pemphigoid

Bullous pemphigoid is a vesiculobullous eruption that typically affects older adults. Tense bullae occur on the skin, often with minimal inflammation, but with intense pruritus (Plate 66).

Bullous pemphigoid is an immunologic disease, and skin biopsy specimens reveal a subepidermal blister with variable dermal inflammation [1]. A linear pattern of immunoglobulin G (IgG) and complement deposition in the basement membrane zone is visualized on direct and indirect immunofluorescence microscopy. The bullous pemphigoid antigens BPAG1 (230 kD) and BGAG2 (180 kD) have recently been cloned and mapped to chromosomes 6p12–p11 and 10q24.3, respectively [9].

Mucous membrane involvement occurs, but is less frequent than that seen in cicatricial pemphigoid (Plate 67). Esophageal bullae may occur *de novo* or as a complication of endoscopy and can lead to complete sloughing of the esophageal mucosa, so-called esophagitis dissecans superficialis [95]. Direct immunofluorescence of esophageal biopsy specimens in patients with bullous pemphigoid may show IgG and C3 in the basement membrane zone, even in the absence of macroscopic mucosal lesions [31].

Cicatricial pemphigoid is a disease related to bullous pemphigoid that is characterized by erosive and scarring lesions of the ocular and oral mucosa and possibly of skin (Plate 68). Oral involvement occurs in approximately 33% of patients. Patients most frequently present with desquamative gingivitis [49]. Cicatricial pemphigoid involves the esophagus in about 5% of patients as manifested by cervical esophageal webs, often multiple or complex, and frank strictures [53, 56]. Mucosal biopsy with direct immunofluorescence may be needed to confirm the diagnosis of cicatricial pemphigoid, as cutaneous lesions may be absent [89].

Therapy for bullous pemphigoid and cicatricial pemphigoid is usually initiated with high-dose systemic corticosteroids (e.g., prednisone, 60 to 80 mg per day), with gradual tapering as the disease is controlled. Secondary candidiasis including candidal esophagitis should be sought in patients with persistent erosions who are on this therapy [89]. Corticosteroid-sparing immunosuppressive agents (i.e., methotrexate, azathioprine, or even pulse cyclophosphamide) or sulfone therapy may be used for selected patients. Colon interposition may be required to correct esophageal stenosis [60].

### Pemphigus Vulgaris

Pemphigus vulgaris is another immunologically mediated bullous disease. The autoantigen is desmoglein 3, the gene for which is on chromosome 18q12 [92]. In contrast to bullous pemphigoid, pemphigus is more likely to present with oral mucosal lesions in younger adult individuals, followed by generalized flaccid bullae and erosions on the cutaneous surface (Plates 69 and 70). Skin biopsy specimens reveal acantholysis of epidermal cells, and direct and indirect immunofluorescence microscopic findings include IgG and complement in the intraepidermal space [71]. Symptomatic esophageal involvement in pemphigus vulgaris is not usual, which is surprising given that oral mucosal involvement occurs in more than 85% of patients [18, 21]. It is possible that frequent asymptomatic esophageal disease occurs. A review of ten reported patients with esophageal pemphigus indicates that all patients were middle-aged women in whom dysphagia or odynophagia was the presenting symptom. They experienced bleeding or vomiting of esophageal lining, and none of these patients had skin lesions at the time their esophageal involvement was diagnosed [18]. In two of these patients, esophageal disease was the initial presentation of pemphigus vulgaris, and in some patients, it was the only manifestation [2]. Diagnosis of esophageal pemphigus is suspected with endoscopic demonstration of flaccid bullae and erosions and confirmed with a biopsy specimen showing acantholytic blisters of the esophagus. Positive direct immunofluorescence has been demonstrated in esophageal specimens [31] and was demonstrated in all 12 patients, many of whom lacked gross or histologic evidence of esophageal disease [83].

Although rare reports exist of control of pemphigus using minocycline and nicotinamide [66], more often very high doses of systemic corticosteroids, such as prednisone, 80 to 100 mg per day, are required. In some instances, the addition of a second immunosuppressive agent, such as azathioprine or methotrexate, becomes necessary [58]. Systemic gold therapy is an important alternative or adjunct to therapy in those patients [59]. Patients with a history of pemphigus vulgaris, even those in remission, should be evaluated endoscopically if they present with esophageal symptoms [13].

## OTHER BULLOUS DERMATOLOGIC DISEASES

Stevens-Johnson syndrome is a part of the spectrum of erythema multiforme and is characterized by bullous cutaneous lesions, fever, and mucous membrane lesions (usually ocular and oral). Full epidermal sloughing, with or without prior bullous lesions, is called *toxic epidermal necrolysis* (TEN) (Plate 71). There is a wide range of precipitating factors associated with Stevens-Johnson syndrome or TEN [11]. Drug hypersensitivity reactions and infections are by far the main triggers [70]. Patients infected with human immunodeficiency virus are at higher risk of developing TEN [63]. Hospitalization with supportive care, treatment of septic complications, and burn unit management of severe cases is indicated, and plasmapheresis may be of benefit [8, 98].

Esophageal complications may occur with either Stevens-Johnson syndrome or TEN. Gastrointestinal hemorrhage may occur acutely from erosive involvement of the esophageal mucosa or from focal stress ulceration elsewhere in the gut [44]. An immune-mediated pathogenesis of bullae in the esophagus in drug-induced Stevens-Johnson syndrome has been supported [23]. Complications can include mucosal scarring with esophageal stricture or stenosis and web formation [29, 50].

Other bullous diseases have been associated with blisters, erosions, or stricture of the esophagus. Hailey-Hailey disease (benign familial pemphigus) results from an abnormality on chromosome 3q21–24 [64]. It usually presents with papulovesicular or superficial erosive lesions of intertriginous areas such as the axilla or groin [30]. Biopsy specimens of lesions reveal acantholysis. Esophageal involvement has rarely been reported in these patients. Darier's disease (keratosis follicularis) is an inherited acantholytic disease whose gene abnormality was recently localized to 12q23–24.1 [91]. It presents with pruritic hyperkeratotic papules (rather than bullae) of the neck and upper trunk, with characteristic nail changes, and has also been reported to involve the esophagus [6]. Acantholysis is likely to be seen in esophageal biopsy specimens in each of these diseases, and differentiation from pemphigus would require assessment of clinical and immunopathologic features.

## HERITABLE SYNDROMES WITH CUTANEOUS AND ESOPHAGEAL LESIONS

There are uncommon cutaneous syndromes that may rarely involve an esophageal pathologic process. *Cowden's disease,* also called *multiple hamartoma syndrome,* is an autosomal dominant syndrome resulting from a deletion within the PTEN gene at 10q22–23 [54]. It manifests facial and oral mucosal papules [24]. The oral lesions may have a cobblestone appearance. Histologically, these oral papules are fibromas. Subcutaneous nodules, which are lipomas, hemangiomas, or neuromas, may also occur. The frequency of gastrointestinal involvement is approximately 70% to 85% and usually manifests as benign hamartomatous polyps of the rectum or sigmoid colon. Esophageal lesions have also been seen, and these are papillomas, fibromas, or diffuse glycogenic acanthosis [34]. Recognition of Cowden's disease is important since up to one-third of these patients develop a malignancy, usually of breast or thyroid [45].

*Focal dermal hypoplasia (Goltz's syndrome)* is characterized by skin atrophy and linear areas of hyperpigmentation, localized superficial fat deposits, and perioral and mucosal papillomas [38]. There are also anomalies of the extremities, nails, and teeth [19, 42]. Basement membrane zone disruption suggests abnormal type IV collagen formation, but the underlying chromosome abnormality has not been identified [43]. Almost all reported cases of Goltz's syndrome have been in white women. The mucosal papillomas occur on the lips, tongue, palate, and buccal mucosa, and are similar to papillomatous lesions seen in perianal and genital sites. Very rarely, squamous papillomas have been found in the esophagus in patients with Goltz's syndrome [5, 27]. One patient with chronic gastroesophageal reflux who developed dysphagia was found to have multiple 2- to 3-mm papillomas of the distal esophagus associated with stricture formation [5]. A second patient had laryngeal and esophageal papillomatosis complicating anesthesia administration [27]. In both cases, the diagnosis of focal dermal hypoplasia had already been made.

## CARCINOMA OF THE ESOPHAGUS AND SKIN LESIONS

*Tylosis (palmar and plantar keratoderma)* is a nonspecific presentation of yellow hyperkeratosis of the palms and soles (Plate 72). In patients with long-standing thick palmar and plantar lesions and a strong family history of cancer, the question of gastrointestinal malignancy should be raised when presenting symptoms are suspicious. The strongest association has been with squamous cell carcinoma of the esophagus [14, 3]. This association is known as the Howel-Evans syndrome. It is transmitted in an autosomal dominant fashion, with up to 95% of family members who have palmar and plantar lesions developing esophageal carcinoma by age 65 [47]. The "tylosis–esophageal cancer gene" locus has been mapped to 17q23 by linkage analysis [35]. In such kindreds, regular follow-up with barium swallow and upper endoscopy is warranted (Color Plate 47).

Patients with the *Paterson-Brown-Kelly syndrome (Plummer-Vinson syndrome)* present with spoon-shaped, concave nails (koilonychia), iron deficiency anemia, angular stomatitis, smooth tongue, dysphagia caused by a postcricoid web, and an increased incidence of postcricoid carcinoma [26]. Sjogren's syndrome may occur in association with *Plummer-Vinson syndrome* [10].

*Acanthosis nigricans* presents as a smooth, velvety, dark thickening of skin in the axillae and neck folds, which may become generalized (Plate 73). Palms may be thickened ("tripe palms"), and skin tags (acrochordons) may develop in intertriginous sites [20]. Oral hyperkeratosis may occur in up to 40% of patients with acanthosis nigricans and may be quite verrucous or papillomatous, particularly in the malignant type [86]. Esophageal involvement with acanthosis nigricans can occur and may cause dysphagia due to the thickened, papillated mucosa [40]. Although the strongest association of malignant acanthosis nigricans is with gastric adenocarcinoma, esophageal carcinoma has also been reported [39].

Cutaneous metastases from carcinoma of the esophagus are rare, but present as smooth-surfaced, firm dermal to subcutaneous papules or nodules on the upper trunk [81]. These metastases may rarely be the first manifestation of esophageal malignancy [16]. Of primary dermatologic tumors, malignant melanoma is the type most reported to metastasize to the esophagus. This can occur many years after the cutaneous melanoma is excised and carries a dismal prognosis [68]. Melanoma can arise primarily in the esophagus, but this is extremely rare [78]. *Mycosis fungoides* (cutaneous T-cell lymphoma) or *Kaposi's sarcoma* may rarely involve the esophagus causing hoarseness and dysphagia [62].

## NONBULLOUS CUTANEOUS IMMUNOLOGIC DISEASES

### Lichen Planus

Lichen planus is a disease of uncertain cause that is believed to have an immunologic basis [61]. Skin lesions are violaceous papules, usually acral in distribution (Plate 74). Oral and pharyngeal lesions are not uncommon and range from asymptomatic lacy hyperkeratosis on the buccal mucosa to devastating erosive lesions (Plate 75). Genital, anal, and even gastric mucosal lesions have been well documented [72]. Esophageal involvement with lichen planus has been rarely reported, and patients may present with dysphagia [7]. Endoscopy should be considered in patients with active lichen planus and gastrointestinal manifestations and may reveal erosive changes or stricture [73]. Histologic findings in esophageal lesions may be compatible with lichen planus, but often are not diagnostic. Treatment with systemic corticosteroids has been helpful in reported cases, and regular follow-up is suggested since squamous cell carcinoma is a rare complication of mucosal lichen planus [73].

### Aphthosis and Behçet's Disease

Aphthous stomatitis (canker sores) is a common ulcerative disease of the oral mucosa (Plate 76). *Complex aphthosis* manifests as multiple recurrent aphthae without any systemic manifestations [69]. *Major aphthous stomatitis* (Sutton's disease) has larger ulcerations which can cause severe discomfort, dysphagia, and scarring [41, 75]. In this condition, aphthae have been demonstrated endoscopically to occur in the stomach, esophagus, and at other sites in the gastrointestinal tract.

Behçet's disease is a complex multisystem disease diagnosed clinically by the presence of oral aphthae and at least two of the following clinical criteria: genital aphthae, synovitis, posterior uveitis, cutaneous pustular vasculitis (pathergy), and meningoencephalitis [57]. Perivascular inflammation was the predominant histopathologic finding in a multicenter international analysis [32]. Inflammatory bowel disease must be excluded due to the association of aphthosis with inflammatory bowel disease and confusion with the HLA-B27/enteropathic arthritis spectrum of disease. Esophageal aphthae may also occur in patients with Behçet's disease [36]. This may predispose to the development of candidal esophagitis.

Treatment of Behçet's disease involves a therapeutic "ladder" with aggressive topical and intralesional corticosteroids, colchicine, dapsone, methotrexate, and thalidomide, with systemic corticosteroids and immunosuppressives reserved for severe ocular or severe systemic disease [46].

## Dermatomyositis

Dermatomyositis is characterized by cutaneous poikiloderma (i.e., the presence of telangiectasia, hyperpigmentation and hypopigmentation, and epidermal atrophy), with a violaceous hue affecting the periorbital skin (heliotrope sign), knuckles (Gottron's sign), and other extensor surfaces. Periungual telangiectasias and cuticular dystrophy are also seen (Plate 77). Patients are generally photosensitive. Cricopharyngeal obstruction and distal esophageal dysmotility occur with dermatomyositis; the latter suggests overlap with scleroderma [33]. Frank esophageal rupture attributed to dermatomyositis involvement has been reported in one patient [12].

## Scleroderma

Scleroderma is a cutaneous or multisystem disease of unknown pathogenesis. Variants, which are believed to represent overlapping ends of a spectrum, include a localized cutaneous form (morphea), a milder systemic form called CREST (calcinosis, Raynaud's esophageal dysmotility, sclerodactyly, telangiectasia), and progressive systemic sclerosis [88]. The important esophageal and systemic aspects of this disease are reviewed in chapter 16 and in a recent article by Sjogren [76]. Cutaneous manifestations are variable. Calcinosis cutis occurs as firm papules or nodules, usually located over the joints. A chalky, white discharge may occur. Raynaud's phenomenon often results in trophic (''rat-bite'') lesions on the digits as well as the typical white, blue, and red color changes that occur acutely in association with episodes of vasospasm [94]. Peripheral gangrene is a later sequela. Dermal sclerosis occurs acrally and periorally in the CREST variant of scleroderma, but may be more truncal at the progressive systemic sclerosis end of the spectrum. A salt-and-pepper postinflammatory pigment change may overlie the area of dermal sclerosis in darker skinned patients. Telangiectasias are described as being boxlike or matlike (Plate 78). They occur over the face, neck, hands, oral mucosa, larynx, and esophagus and may bleed spontaneously [87].

## Other Collagen Vascular Diseases

Dysphagia and other esophageal abnormalities are a feature of mixed connective tissue disease and a number of other connective tissue disease overlap syndromes. A discussion of the cutaneous features of systemic lupus erythematosus, mixed connective tissue disease, and other collagen vascular diseases is beyond the scope of this chapter, given the limited primary association with esophageal disease (see Chapter 16).

## MISCELLANEOUS CUTANEOUS DISEASES AND THE ESOPHAGUS

There are other mucocutaneous lesions that may be associated with esophageal disease; however, these are discussed in other chapters. Examples include candidiasis, herpes simplex, and Kaposi's sarcoma (see chapter 33). These entities have particular importance in the setting of human immunodeficiency virus infection. Disorders of connective tissue, such as Ehlers-Danlos syndrome, and syndromes associated with gastrointestinal bleeding, such as Osler-Weber-Rendu disease, may also initially present to a dermatologist due to dermatologic lesions [77].

Treatment of dermatologic diseases may be associated with drug-induced esophageal injury. An example with which most dermatologists are familiar is the use of oral tetracycline antibiotics, which are commonly used for the treatment of inflammatory acne vulgaris [17, 80]. Failure to take the tablets with adequate oral liquids can produce esophageal erosion (see chapter 30). Candidal esophagitis secondary to oral corticosteroids is commonly missed by clinicians and can be prevented with prophylactic clotrimazole troches and intermittent oral fluconazole. It is important that specialists in both dermatology and esophagology be aware of how dermatologic lesions may be associated with esophageal disease for early recognition and optimal management.

## REFERENCES

1. Ahmed AR, Hameed A. Bullous pemphigoid and dermatitis herpetiformis. Clin Dermatol 1993;11:47
2. Amachai B, Grunwald MH, Gasper N, Finkelstein E, Halevy S. A case of pemphigus vulgaris with esophageal involvement. J Dermatol 1996; 23:214
3. Ashworth MT, McDicken IW, Southern SA, Nash JR. Human papillomavirus in squamous cell carcinoma of the oesophagus associated with tylosis. J Clin Pathol 1993;46:573
4. Birge K. Nutrition management of patients with epidermolysis bullosa. J Am Diet Assoc 1995;95:575
5. Brinson RR, Schuman BM, Mills LR, Thigpen S, Freedman S. Multiple squamous papillomas of the esophagus associated with Goltz syndrome. Am J Gastroenterol 1987;82:1177
6. Burge S. Darier's disease—the clinical features and pathogenesis. Clin Exp Dermatol 1994;19:193
7. Celinski K, Krasowska D, Pokora J, Lecewicz-Torun B. Esophageal lichen planus. Endoscopy 1994;26:755
8. Chaidemenos GC, Chrysomallis F, Sombolos K, Mourellou O, Ioannides D, Papakonstantinou M. Plasmapheresis in toxic epidermal necrolysis. Int J Dermatol 1997;36:218
9. Copeland NG, et al. Chromosomal localization of mouse bullous pemphigoid antigens. BPAG1 and BPAG2: identification of a new region of homology between mouse and human chromosomes. Genomics 1993;15:180
10. Dejmkova H, Pavelka K. An unusual clinical manifestation of secondary Sjogren's syndrome and concomitant Paterson-Kelly syndrome. Clin Rheum 1994;13:305
11. Dolan PA, Flowers FP, Shertz EF. Toxic epidermal necrolysis. J Emerg Med 1989;7:65
12. Dougenis D, Papathanasopoulos PG, Paschalis C, Papapetropoulos T. Spontaneous esophageal rupture in adult dermatomyosisis. Eur J Card Thorac Surg 1996;10:1021
13. Eliakim R, Goldin E, Livshin R, Okon E. Esophageal involvement in pemphigus vulgaris. Am J Gastroenterol 1988;83:155
14. Ellis A, et al. Tylosis associated with carcinoma of the oesophagus and oral leukoplakia in a large Liverpool family—a review of six generations. Eur J Cancer 1994;30B:102
15. Eversole LR. Immunopathology of oral mucosal ulcerative, desquamative, and bullous diseases. Selective review of the literature. Oral Surg Oral Med 1994;77:555
16. Farr P, et al. Cutaneous metastasis as the first manifestation of adenocarcinoma in Barrett esophagus. J Belge Radiol 1987;70:329

17. Foster JA, Sylvia LM. Doxycycline-induced esophageal ulceration. Ann Pharmacother 1994;28:1185
18. Goldberg NS, Weiss SS. Pemphigus vulgaris of the esophagus in women. J Am Acad Dermatol 1989;21:1115
19. Goltz RW, Henderson RR, Hitch JM, Ott JE. Focal dermal hypoplasia syndrome. A review of the literature and report of two cases. Arch Dermatol 1970;101:1
20. Gorisek B, Krajnc I, Rems D, Kuhelj J. Malignant acanthosis nigricans and tripe plams in a patient with endometrial adenocarcinoma. Gynecol Oncol 1997;65:539
21. Gorsky M, Raviv M, Raviv E. Pemphigus vulgaris in adolescence. A case presentation and review of the literature. Oral Surg Oral Med 1994;77:620
22. Gryboski JD, Touloukian R, Campanella RA. Gastrointestinal manifestations of epidermolysis bullosa in children. Arch Dermatol 1988;124:746
23. Guitart J. Immunopathology of Stevens-Johnson syndrome. Allerg Proc 1995;16:163
24. Hanssen AM, Fryns JP. Cowden syndrome. J Med Genet 1995;32:117
25. Harel-Raviv M, Bernier S, Raviv E, Gornitsky M. Oral epidermolysis bullosa in adults. Spec Care Dent 1995;15:144
26. Hoffman RM, Jaffe PE. Plummer-Vinson syndrome. A case report and literature review. Arch Int Med 1995;155:2008
27. Holzman RS. Airway involvement and anesthetic management in Goltz's syndrome. J Clin Anesth 1991;3:422
28. Horan TA, Urschel JD, MacEachern NA, Shulman B, Crowson AN, Magro C. Esophageal perforation in recessive dystrophic epidermolysis bullosa. Ann Thorac Surg 1994;57:1027
29. Howell CG, Mansberger JA, Parrish RA. Esophageal stricture secondary to Stevens-Johnson syndrome. J Pediatr Surg 1987;22:994
30. Hunt MJ, Salisbury EL, Painter DM, Lee S. Vesiculobullous Hailey–Hailey disease: successful treatment with oral retinoids. Aust J Dermatol 1996;37:196
31. Jorgensen BG, Pedersen AT, Gjertsen BT. Pemphigus vulgaris and benign cicatrial mucous membrane pemphigoid in the upper respiratory tract and esophagus. Ugeskrift Laeger 1993;155:2126
32. Jorizzo JL, et al. Mucocutaneous criteria for the diagnosis of Behcet's disease: an analysis of clinicopathologic data from multiple international centers. J Acad Dermatol 1995;32:968
33. Kagen LJ, Hochman RB, Strong EW. Cricopharyngeal obstruction in inflammatory myopathy (polymyositis/dermatomyositis): report of three cases and review of the literature. Arth Rheum 1985;28:630
34. Kay PS, Soetikno RM, Mindelzun R, Young HS. Diffuse esophageal glycogenic acanthosis: an endoscopic marker of Cowden's disease. Am J Gastroenterol 1997;92:1038
35. Kelsell DP, et al. Close mapping of the focal non-epidemolytic palmoplantar keratoderma (PPK) locus associated with oesophageal cancer (TOC). Hum Mol Genet 1996;5:857
36. Kemula M, Cabie A, Khuong MA, Chemouilli P, Matherson S, Coulaud JP. Behcet's disease disclosed by recurrent meningitis and esophageal ulcers. Ann Med Int 1995;146:190
37. Kern IB, Eisenberg M, Willis S. Management of oesophageal stenosis in epidermolysis bullosa dystrophica. Arch Dis Child 1989;64:551
38. Kore-Eda S, Yoneda K, Ohtani T, Tachibana T, Furukawa F, Imamura S. Focal dermal hypoplasia (Goltz syndrome) associated with multiple giant papillomas. Br J Dermatol 1995;133:997
39. Koyama S, et al. Transforming growth factor-alpha (TGF alpha) -producing gastric carcinoma with acanthosis nigricans: an endocrine effect of TGF alpha in the pathogenesis of cutaneous paraneoplastic syndrome and epithelial hyperplasia of the esophagus. J Gastroenterol 1997;32:71
40. Kozlowski LM, Nigra TP. Esophageal acanthosis nigricans in association with adenocarcinoma from an unknown primary site. J Am Acad Dermatol 1992;26:348
41. Laccourreye O, Fadlallah JP, Pages JC, Durand H, Brasnu D, Lowenstein W. Sutton's disease (periadenitis mucosa necrotica recurrens). Ann Otol Rhinol Laryngol 1995;104:301
42. Landa N, Oleaga JM, Raton JA, Gardeazabal J, Diaz-Perez JL. Focal dermal hypoplasia (Goltz syndrome) an adult case with multisystemic involvement. J Am Acad Dermatol 1993;28:86
43. Lee IJ, Cha MS, Kim SC, Bang D. Electromicroscopic observation of the basement membrane zone in focal dermal hypoplasia. Pediatr Dermatol 1996;13:5
44. Mahe A, Keita S, Blanc L, Bobin P. Esophageal necrosis in the Stevens-Johnson syndrome. J Am Acad Dermatol 1993;29:103
45. Mallory SB. Cowden syndrome (multiple hamartoma syndrome). Dermatol Clin 1995;13:27
46. Manglesdorf HC, White WL, Jorizzo JL. Behcet's disease. Report of twenty-five patients from the United States with prominent mucocutaneous involvement. J Acad Dermatol 1996;34:745
47. Marger RS, Marger D. Carcinoma of the esophagus and tylosis. A lethal genetic combination. Cancer 1993;72:17
48. Marinkovich MP. The molecular genetics of basement membrane diseases. Arch Dermatol 1993;129:1557
49. Markopoulos AK, Antoniades D, Papanayotou P, Trigonidis G. Desquamative gingivitis: a clinical, histopathologic, and immunologic study. Quintessence Int 1996;27:763
50. Martin Mateos MA, Polemeque A, Pastor X, Munoz Lopez F. Uncommon serious complications in Stevens-Johnson syndrome: a clinical case. J Inv Allerg Clin Immunol 1992;2:278
51. McHenry PM, Dagg JH, Tidman MJ, Lever RS. Epidermolysis bullosa acquisita occurring in association with systemic lupus erythematosus. Clin Exp Dermatol 1993;18:378
52. Meldgaard Lund A, Karlsmark T, Kobayasi T. Protein-losing enteropathy in a child with junctional epidermolysis bullosa and pyloric atresia. Acta Dermato-Venereol 1995;75:59
53. Naylor MF, MacCarty RL, Rogers RS III. Barium studies in esophageal cicatricial pemphigoid. Abdom Imag 1995;20:97
54. Nelen MR, et al. Localization of the gene for Cowden disease to chromosome 10q22–23. Nature Genet 1996;13:114
55. Ng CC, Hung FC, Hsieh CS. Epidermolysis bullosa letalis with pyloric atresia in an infant. J Formosan Med Assoc 1996;95:61
56. Nguyen QD, Foster CS. Cicatricial pemphigoid: diagnosis and treatment. Int Ophthalmol Clin 1996;36:41
57. O'Duffy JD. Behcet's disease. Curr Opin Rheumatol 1994;6:39
58. Paul MA, Jorizzo ML, Fleischer AB Jr, White WL. Low dose methotrexate treatment in elderly patients with bullous pemphigoid. J Acad Dermatol 1994;31:620
59. Penneys NS, Eaglstein WH, Frost P. Management of pemphigus with gold compounds: a long term follow-up report. Arch Dermatol 1976;112:185
60. Popovici Z, Deac M, Rotaru M, Vestemeanu P, Vargatu V. Stenosis of the esophagus in cicatricial pemphigoid resolved by colon interposition: report of a case. Surg Today 1997;27:234
61. Porter SR, Kirby A, Olsen I, Barrett W. Immunologic aspects of dermal and oral lichen planus: a review. Oral Surg Oral Med 1997;83:358
62. Redleaf MI, Moran WJ, Gruber B. Mycosis fungoides involving the cervical esophagus. Arch Otolaryngol Head Neck Surg 1993;119:690
63. Revuz JE, Joujeau JC. Advances in toxic epidermal necrolysis. Semin Cutan Med Surg 1996;15:258
64. Richard G, et al. Hailey-Hailey disease maps to a 5 cM interval on chromosome 3q21–q24. J Inv Dermatol 1995;105:357
65. Ruzzi L, et al. A homozygous mutation in the integrin alpha6 gene in junctional epidermolysis bullosa with pyloric atresia. J Clin Inv 1997;99:2826
66. Sawai T, et al. Pemphigus vegetans with oesophageal involvement: successful treatment with minocycline and nicotinamide. Br J Dermatol 1995;132:668
67. Schattenkirchner S, et al. Localized epidermolysis bullosa acquisita of the esophagus in a patient with Crohn's disease. Am J Gastroenterol 1996;91:1659
68. Schneider A, Martini N, Burt ME. Malignant melanoma metastatic to the esophagus. Ann Thorac Surg 1993;55:516
69. Schreiner DT, Jorizzo JL. Behcet's disease and complex aphthosis. Dermatol Clin 1987;5:769
70. Schwartz RA. Toxic epidermal necrolysis. Cutis 1997;59:123
71. Sciubba JJ. Autoimmune aspects of pemphigus vulgaris and mucosal pemphigoid. Adv Dent Res 1996;10:52
72. Scully G, Et-Kom M. Lichen planus: review and update of pathogenesis. Oral Pathol 1985;14:431
73. Sheehan-Dare RA, Cotterill JA, Simmons AV. Oesophageal lichen planus. Br J Dermatol 1986;115:729
74. Sheridan R, Robbins S, Elston D, Brown C, Quispe G. Resolution of epidermolysis bullosa aquisita with resection of intraabdominal Crohn's disease. Milit Med 1987;152:368
75. Ship JA. Recurrent aphthous stomatitis. An update. Oral Surg Oral Med 1996;81:141
76. Sjogren RW. Gastrointestinal features of scleroderma. Curr Opin Rheumatol 1996;8:569

77. Solomon JA, Abrams L, Lichtenstein GR. GI manifestations of Ehlers-Danlos syndrome. Am J Gastroenterol 1996;91:2282

78. Stranks GJ, Mathai JT, Rowe-Jones DC. Primary malignant melanoma of the oesophagus: case report and review of surgical pathology. Gut 1991;32:828

79. Taniuchi K, Inaoki M, Nishimura Y, Mori T, Takehara K. Nonscarring inflammatory epidermolysis bullosa acquisita with esophageal involvement and linear IgG deposits. J Am Acad Dermatol 1997;36:320

80. Tankurt IE, Akbaylar H, Yenicerioglu Y, Simsek I, Gonen O. Severe, long-lasting symptoms from doxycycline-induced esophageal injury. Endos 1995;27:626

81. Tharakaram S. Metastases to the skin. Int J Dermatol 1988;27:240

82. Touloukian RJ, Schonholz SM, Gryboski JD, Oh TH, McGuire J. Perioperative considerations in esophageal replacement for epidermolysis bullosa: report of two cases successfully treated by colon interposition. Am J Gastroenterol 1988;83:857

83. Trattner A, Lurie R, Leiser A. Esophageal involvement in pemphigus vulgaris: a clinical, histologic, and immunopathologic study. J Am Acad Dermatol 1991;24:223

84. Travis SP, et al. Oral and gastrointestinal manifestations of epidermolysis bullosa. Lancet 1992;340:1505

85. Trotter MM. Tube feeding vs oral intake: nutrition care for patients with epidermolysis bullosa. J Am Diet Assoc 1995;95:1377

86. Tyler MT, Ficarra G, Silverman S Jr, Odom RB, Regezi JA. Malignant acanthosis nigricans with florid papillary oral lesions. Oral Surg Oral Med 1996;81:445

87. Ueda M, et al. Prominent telangiectasia associated with marked bleeding in CREST syndrome. J Dermatol 1993;20:180

88. van den Hoogen FH, de Jong EM. Clinical aspects of systemic and localized scleroderma. Curr Opin Rheumatol 1995;7:546

89. Vincent SD, Lilly GE, Baker KA. Clinical, historic, and therapeutic features of cicatricial pemphigoid. A literature review and open therapeutic trial with corticosteroids. Oral Surg Oral Med 1993;76:453

90. Wakelin SH, et al. Epidermolysis bullosa acquisita associated with epidermal-binding circulating antibodies. Br J Dermatol 1997;136:604

91. Wakem P, et al. Localization of the Darier disease gene to a 2-cM portion of 12q23–24.1. J Inv Dermatol 1996;106:365

92. Wang Y, et al. The human genes for desmogleins (DSG1 and DSG3) are located in a small region on chromosome 18q12. Genomics 1994;20:492

93. Weinman D, Stewart MI, Woodley DT, Garcia G. Epidermolysis bullosa acquisita (EBA) and esophageal webs: a new association. Am J Gastroenterol 1991;86:1518

94. Wigley FM. Raynaud's phenomenon and other features of scleroderma, including pulmonary hypertension. Curr Opin Rheumatol 1996;8:561

95. Witte JT, Icken JN, Lloyd ML. Induction of esophageal bullae by endoscopy in benign mucous membrane pemphigoid. Gastro Endoscopy 1989;35:566

96. Wong WL, Entwisle K, Pemberton J. Gastrointestinal manifestations in the Hallopeau-Siemens variant of recessive dystrophic epidermolysis bullosa. Br J Radiol 1993;66:788

97. Wright JT, Fine JD. Hereditary epidermolysis bullosa. Semin Dermatol 1994;13:102

98. Yarbrough DR III. Experience with toxic epidermal necrolysis treated in a burn center. J Burn Care Rehab 1996;17:30

The Esophagus, Third Edition,
edited by D. O. Castell and J. E. Richter.
Lippincott Williams & Wilkins, Philadelphia © 1999.

CHAPTER 39

# Esophageal Diseases in the Elderly

Lawrence S. Friedman and Donald O. Castell

The aging of the population has become a major social, economic, and political issue, and all aspects of aging have come under close study. Whereas only 13% of the population was age 65 years or older in 1990, it is estimated that 21% of the population will be 65 years or older by 2030. Currently, the elderly account for one-third of total health care expenditures in the United States, and each year persons older than 75 years make six times as many office visits to an internist as do young adults. The elderly are more likely than the young to have multiple chronic and often terminal illnesses [49].

Esophageal diseases are common in all age groups, including the elderly [20]. In a survey in Leiden, Netherlands, 16% of a cohort of residents older than 87 years described symptoms of swallowing dysfunction [12]. Some esophageal diseases are unique to the elderly, including Zenker's diverticulum, cervical osteophytes, and dysphagia aortica. Some disorders may pose special diagnostic considerations in the elderly [159]. For example, in the older patient with achalasia, the possibility of secondary achalasia due to a distal esophageal malignancy is more likely than in a young patient presenting with achalasia. In some cases, diagnosis may be made more complex because of atypical presentations or coexisting illnesses. For example, chest pain due to chronic gastroesophageal reflux may be more difficult to clarify because of associated coronary artery disease or lack of heartburn. Finally, there is a greater potential for the elderly to develop complications of long-standing chronic diseases. For example, the frequencies of Barrett's esophagus and adenocarcinoma of the esophagus increase with the duration of chronic gastroesophageal reflux disease (GERD).

In the elderly patient with esophageal disease, diagnosis is more likely to be delayed compared to younger patients because symptoms are often attributed to underlying cardiac

and pulmonary disorders. Moreover, elderly patients are more likely than younger ones to experience complications resulting from aspiration and malnutrition, which often accompany inadequately treated esophageal diseases [59].

In this chapter, we review changes in pharyngoesophageal function with aging and the unique aspects of esophageal diseases, including clinical presentation, diagnosis, and management, in the elderly.

## CHANGES IN PHARYNGOESOPHAGEAL FUNCTION WITH AGING

### Oropharyngeal Phase

Reduction in lean muscle mass occurs with age. The skeletal muscles involved in the oral and pharyngeal phase of swallowing can thus be affected by aging. In one autopsy study, an age-associated decrease in the number of type 1 (slow-acting) muscle fibers of the pharyngeal constrictor was found [89]. In addition, the standard deviation of fiber diameters was significantly larger in patients older than 50 years than in younger patients; this was associated with a trend toward hypertrophy of individual muscle fibers and decreased fiber density.

These age-related changes may result in functional changes during the oropharyngeal phase of swallowing [111]. Using videofluoroscopy, Ekberg and Feinberg [41] found swallowing to be normal, as defined in young persons, in only 16% of 56 elderly persons without dysphagia or difficulty eating. In one study of 100 asymptomatic individuals older than 65 years, 22 had pharyngeal muscle weakness and abnormal cricopharyngeal relaxation on barium swallow, with pooling of barium in the valleculae and piriform sinuses. Some subjects demonstrated tracheal aspiration of barium [117]. Aging has been reported to affect the coordination of swallowing in some [112], but not other [143] studies.

Upper esophageal sphincter (UES) function is affected by aging. Using a solid-state intraluminal transducer system,

L. S. Friedman: Department of Medicine, Harvard Medical School, and Gastrointestinal Unit (Medical Services), Massachusetts General Hospital, Boston, Massachusetts 02114.

D. O. Castell: Department of Medicine, Graduate Hospital, Philadelphia, Pennsylvania 19146.

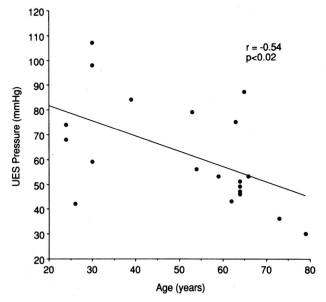

**FIG. 39-1.** Relationship between age and upper esophageal sphincter (UES) pressure. There is a significant trend ($p <$ 0.02) toward diminishing UES pressure with increasing age. (From ref. 50, with permission.)

Fulp and colleagues [50] found that compared to persons younger than 60 years, healthy persons older than 60 years have a lower resting UES pressure (Fig. 39–1) and delayed UES relaxation after swallowing (Fig. 39–2), as confirmed by others [143]. On the other hand, Wilson and coworkers [168] found only marginally lower resting UES pressures, but higher pharyngeal contraction pressures and a reduction in the duration of upper esophageal contractions in older subjects than younger ones. These findings suggest that resistance to flow across the UES is increased because of decreased compliance with age [159]. Indeed, the duration of oropharyngeal swallowing, as measured by videofluoroscopy, is significantly longer in the elderly than in younger persons [131, 143]. A recent study has shown that deglutitive UES opening can be augmented by head-raising exercises with an accompanying decrease in pharyngeal outflow resistance [141], an observation that has implications for therapy. The sensory threshold for initiating a swallow has also been reported to increase with age [9, 140]. It has been suggested that the reported changes in UES function with age reflect an increased frequency of concurrent illnesses in the elderly, rather than age-related physiologic changes per se [45, 48].

## Esophageal Phase

Morphologic changes with age have also been demonstrated in the smooth muscle of the esophagus. Compared to younger persons, elderly individuals show a decrease in the number of myenteric ganglion cells per unit area and thickening of the smooth-muscle layer [6, 39]. As for skeletal muscle, an increased standard deviation of smooth-muscle fiber diameters has been described in the elderly, with a

greater tendency toward hypertrophy than atrophy. Decreases in the number of type 1 muscle fibers and in the density of fibers per unit area have been detected in the distal esophagus [89].

There has long been controversy as to whether aging itself leads to disordered esophageal function. In 1964, Soergel and colleagues [149] found frequent nonpropulsive, tertiary contractions, delayed esophageal emptying, esophageal dilation, decreased lower esophageal sphincter relaxation, and, frequently, the intrathoracic location of the lower esophageal sphincter, in 15 nonagenarians studied with intraluminal manometry and barium radiography. They concluded that these abnormalities represented "presbyesophagus" and resembled diffuse esophageal spasm. In contrast, in 1974, Hollis and Castell [71] were unable to detect an increase in abnormal esophageal motility in a group of men aged 70 to 87 years when compared to a control group of young adults

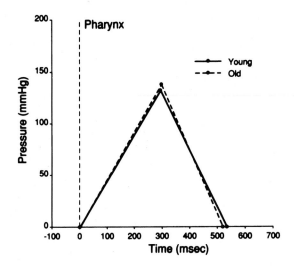

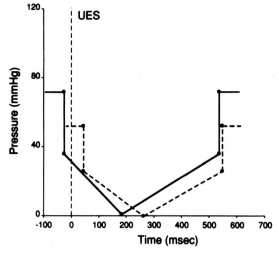

**FIG. 39-2.** A simplified representation of pharyngeal and UES coordination based on computer analysis for pressure dynamics for wet swallows. There is a trend toward delayed UES relaxation in the normal elderly. (From ref. 50, with permission.)

aged 19 to 27 years. However, in a subgroup of 80-year-old men, an age-related reduction in the amplitude of esophageal contractions was noted, implying that the neural system was intact, but that there was weakening of the smooth muscle [56].

In 1977, Ali Khan and colleagues [5] found an increased frequency of abnormal lower esophageal sphincter responses to deglutition, including a reduced amplitude of the aftercontraction, compared to results in a group of healthy persons younger than 40 years. The older persons also showed a reduced amplitude of peristaltic contractions in the upper and lower esophagus, reduced peristaltic velocity, and an increased frequency of simultaneous contractions. Basal lower esophageal sphincter pressures were similar between the two groups. Moreover, a recent study found aperistalsis not otherwise explained by an underlying disease such as achalasia or scleroderma to be much more common in elderly persons with dysphagia than in their younger counterparts [103]. By contrast, Csendes and coworkers [31] found no differences in the amplitude or duration of peristaltic waves in the distal esophagus, but a tendency toward a lower resting lower esophageal sphincter pressure after age 65 years.

In 1987, Richter and colleagues [129], using well-accepted modern manometric techniques, found an increase in distal esophageal amplitude and duration with age until the fifth decade, after which values decreased. In this study, age had no effect on peristaltic velocity, basal lower esophageal sphincter pressure, or the frequency of double- and triple-peaked waveforms.

The clinical significance of the age-related esophageal manometric changes described above is unclear. An increased frequency of radiographic and scintigraphic transit abnormalities in the elderly (e.g., ''tertiary contractions'') has not been shown to correlate with esophageal symptoms [62]. The amount of gastric acid refluxed, as measured by an ambulatory pH system, was shown in one study to increase with age [148]. However, another study found no difference in the frequency of spontaneous gastroesophageal reflux between a group of normal volunteers with a mean age of 49 years and a group with a mean age of 22 years [154]. Moreover, Richter and coworkers [130] found no independent effect of age on ambulatory esophageal pH parameters, although older men experienced a significantly greater number of reflux episodes longer than 5 minutes than did women and younger men. Age-associated changes of the esophageal mucosa have not been studied extensively, but the perception of pain on esophageal distention or infusion of acid has been reported to decline with age [58, 88].

Thus, on the basis of the limited studies available, it appears that in normal healthy individuals, the physiologic function of the esophagus is preserved with increasing age, with the possible exception of the very elderly (older than 80 years), in whom the amplitude of esophageal contractions is decreased. On the other hand, there is evidence to suggest that the perception of pain on distention of the esophagus or infusion of acid declines with age.

## DYSPHAGIA

Dysphagia in the elderly may be caused by any of the diseases that can afflict the young as well as several others unique to the elderly. It is important to note that eating disorders in the elderly may result not only from pharyngoesophageal disease, but also from disturbances not associated with the gastrointestinal tract, including cognitive problems, physical disability of the upper limbs, deterioration of the muscles of mastication, dental disease, and osteoporosis affecting the mandible [64, 155, 166]. Dysphagia occurs in up to 10% of persons over age 50 years [91]. Oropharyngeal dysphagia in particular may occur in up to 50% of nursing home residents [163]. Indeed, irreversible eating and swallowing disturbances in the elderly are associated with a poor prognosis, regardless of the cause. In a study of 240 residents in a skilled nursing facility, persons who could eat without help had a significantly lower mortality rate at 6 months compared to those requiring assistance in eating [144]. Determination of the cause of a patient's inability to maintain adequate nutrition may therefore be of vital prognostic importance.

As in the young, dysphagia in the elderly can be divided into two categories: abnormalities affecting the neuromuscular mechanisms controlling movements of the tongue, pharynx, and UES (oropharyngeal dysphagia), and disorders affecting the esophagus itself (esophageal dysphagia).

### Oropharyngeal Dysphagia

*Oropharyngeal dysphagia* refers to the inability to initiate the act of swallowing, so that food cannot be transferred from the mouth to the upper esophagus. Patients with oropharyngeal dysphagia generally complain of food sticking in the throat, difficulty initiating a swallow, nasal regurgitation, and coughing during swallowing. Because of associated muscle weaknesses, they may also have dysarthria or nasal speech. In fact, oropharyngeal dysphagia is usually one of several manifestations of a local, neurologic, or muscular disease (Table 39–1).

#### Causes of Oropharyngeal Dysphagia

*Central Nervous System Diseases*

Oropharyngeal dysphagia can be caused by any disorder that affects the swallowing center in the brainstem or the nerves that modulate the swallowing process, including the fifth, seventh, ninth, tenth, and twelfth cranial nerves. For example, patients with major strokes often manifest dysphagia as part of their neurologic deficit [57] (Fig. 39–3). In anterior cortical strokes, the motor cortex controlling tongue movement may be affected and thereby result in poor oral

**TABLE 39–1.** *Causes of oropharyngeal dysphagia in the elderly*

Central nervous system disease
  Stroke
    Anterior cortical
    Wallenberg's syndrome
    Pseudobulbar palsy
  Parkinsonism
  Wilson's disease
  Multiple sclerosis
  Neoplasms
Other neuromuscular disorders
  Poliomyelitis and postpolio syndrome
  Myasthenia gravis
  Muscular dystrophies
  Polymyositis and dermatomyositis
  Amyotrophic lateral sclerosis
  Hypothyroidism
  Hyperthyroidism
  Hypercalcemia
  Cricopharyngeal dysfunction
Local structural lesions
  Oropharyngeal tumors
  Abscess
  Web
  Thyromegaly
  Cervical osteoarthritis with vertebral osteophytes
  Stricture
Zenker's diverticulum

control of a food bolus. Dysphagia is more likely with larger cortical strokes than with smaller ones [4]. In cortical strokes, lingual and pharyngeal paresis may be unilateral, thus allowing for a compensatory strategy of turning the head to the paretic side so as to exclude the weakened musculature from the path of the food bolus [57]. Dysphagia may occur in pseudobulbar palsy or in the Wallenberg syndrome, a lesion in the distribution of the posterior inferior cerebellar artery. Brainstem strokes may affect the swallowing center beneath the nucleus of the solitary tract, which coordinates pharyngeal swallowing, or the nucleus ambiguus, which controls the muscles used in swallowing [45]. Rarely, dysphagia has been observed as the sole manifestation of bilateral strokes [24] or an otherwise occult brainstem stroke [19].

Dysphagia may also be seen in patients with parkinsonism, Wilson's disease, multiple sclerosis, amyotrophic lateral sclerosis, and a variety of other congenital and degenerative disorders of the central nervous system. In patients with parkinsonism, oropharyngeal dysphagia may result from tremor of the tongue or hesitancy in swallowing; an abnormality of the pharyngeal phase of swallowing is also likely [94, 145]. Abnormalities may be detected on videofluoroscopy even in the absence of symptoms [11]. In parkinsonism, degenerating dopaminergic neurons in the central nervous system are thought to be replaced by cholinergic neurons, leading to disorganized control of the central swallowing center [16]. Brain stem neoplasms must also be considered in a patient presenting with oropharyngeal dysphagia.

### Other Neuromuscular Disorders

Oropharyngeal dysphagia may also result from disorders affecting the peripheral nervous system or muscles involving the tongue, pharynx, or UES. In the elderly, such disorders include peripheral neuropathy caused by diabetes mellitus, postpolio syndrome, myasthenia gravis, muscular dystrophies, polymyositis and dermatomyositis, hypothyroidism, and hyperthyroidism. In some cases, dysphagia may be the presenting or sole manifestation of the disorder.

Depending on the degree of pharyngeal muscular involvement, polymyositis and dermatomyositis may result in weakness of the muscles controlling pharyngeal function and may lead to nasal regurgitation or aspiration, with abnormal pharyngeal transfer demonstrated on barium swallow [63]. These abnormalities may reverse with treatment of the muscular inflammation. Occasionally, abnormal distal esophageal manometry is also observed [74]. Inflammatory myopathy isolated to the pharynx has also been described [142].

Myasthenia gravis is characterized by increasing muscle weakness on repetitive contractions and typically presents

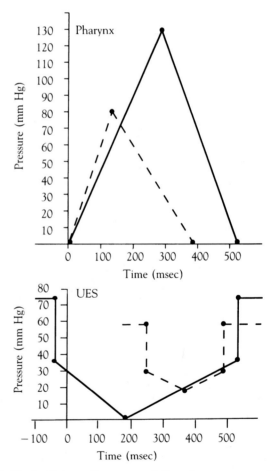

**FIG. 39–3.** Schematic representation of pressures and timings obtained during computed manometry of the pharynx and UES in a normal person (*solid lines*) and in a patient following a stroke (*broken lines*). (From ref. 20, with permission.)

with dysphagia associated with ptosis or diplopia. Although the disease commonly presents in younger women, the onset in men is often after age 70 years, and dysphagia in these cases may not improve with treatment [82]. In advanced myasthenia gravis, dysphagia may be profound.

In amyotrophic lateral sclerosis, oropharyngeal dysphagia is characteristically progressive and severe, resulting in frequent aspiration, which usually signals a preterminal phase of the disease.

In the elderly person with oropharyngeal dysphagia, it is particularly important to consider a diagnosis of hyperthyroidism, since the clinical presentation may otherwise be occult.

### Local Structural Lesions

A variety of lesions may lead to oropharyngeal dysphagia as a result of obstruction. In the elderly, consideration must always be given to the possibility of head and neck tumors. Other obstructing lesions include inflammatory processes, such as an abscess, congenital web, prior surgical resection, an enlarged thyroid gland, and cervical hypertrophic osteoarthropathy. Although cervical osteoarthritis is frequent in the elderly, dysphagia secondary to compression of the esophagus by hypertrophic spurs of the anterior portion of cervical vertebrae is unusual. Patients with this problem complain of difficulty swallowing solid foods, but on occasion, they may also have odynophagia, a foreign body sensation, cough, hoarseness, and an urge to clear the throat. The diagnosis is made by barium swallow with lateral views; endoscopy should be performed to exclude an obstructing neoplasm. Trauma from endotracheal intubation can result in vocal cord weakness, leading to coughing and aspiration with swallowing.

### Upper Esophageal Sphincter Dysfunction

The high-pressure zone of the UES results from contraction of the cricopharyngeus muscle and the adjacent hypopharyngeal musculature [54]. Cricopharyngeal dysfunction may contribute to the development of oropharyngeal dysphagia. As noted above, aging itself has been associated with a decrease in UES tone, although age-related decreases in UES tone do not appear to result in dysphagia [50]. The term *cricopharyngeal achalasia* is often used inappropriately to describe putative cricopharyngeal dysfunction when the cricopharyngeal muscle is actually able to relax. The true abnormality is often an inability of the muscle to function in synchrony with other components of the swallowing mechanism or weakness of the pharyngeal muscles resulting in inability to push the opening of the cricopharyngeus muscle [20]. Other abnormalities in the UES that may result in oropharyngeal dysphagia in the elderly include truly abnormal UES relaxation, a spectrum of disorders that includes oculopharyngeal muscular dystrophy (true cricopharyngeal acha-

lasia), premature closure of the UES, or delayed relaxation of the sphincter, as in familial dysautonomia.

### Zenker's Diverticulum

A Zenker's diverticulum is an outpouching in the posterior pharyngeal wall immediately above the UES (Killian's triangle) and is found almost exclusively in persons over age 50 years. The pathogenesis of Zenker's diverticulum is thought to relate to decreased compliance of the cricopharyngeus muscle, which results in decreased contractility and increased resistance to the passage of a bolus [29, 30]. Intermittent oropharyngeal dysphagia is often the earliest symptom. When the diverticulum becomes large enough to retain food, patients may develop more classic symptoms of cough, fullness and gurgling in the neck, postprandial regurgitation, and aspiration. A Zenker's diverticulum may become large enough to produce a visible mass in the neck or to obstruct the esophagus by compression, thereby contributing to esophageal dysphagia. In some cases, patients learn to perform a variety of maneuvers to empty the diverticulum by applying pressure on the neck and coughing repeatedly. Therapy consists of a diverticulectomy with myotomy. A staged approach (myotomy, diverticulectomy, and cervical esophagostomy, followed later by closure of the esophagostomy) [95] or endoscopic cricopharyngeal myotomy [73] have been advocated in severely debilitated patients.

### Diagnostic Approach to Oropharyngeal Dysphagia

In evaluating the patient with oropharyngeal dysphagia, a careful history and physical examination may provide clues to the diagnosis. For example, evidence of a systemic neurologic disorder should be sought. Careful examination of the head and neck for a neoplasm is also important. The diagnosis of Zenker's diverticulum may be suggested by a typical history. The major diagnostic study in the evaluation of oropharyngeal dysphagia is a barium x-ray of the pharynx and UES with videofluoroscopy. Rapid-sequence pictures must be obtained because bolus transfer from the mouth to the upper esophagus requires only approximately 1 second [37, 38]. Use of thick barium or a solid bolus is particularly helpful in assessing the ability of the patient to transfer food from the mouth to the esophagus [22]. Manometric studies of the pharynx and UES may also be helpful. The development of improved computerized manometric techniques has led to more accurate diagnostic testing, particularly in the evaluation of abnormalities of pharyngeal and UES coordination [22, 50].

### Treatment

Treatment of oropharyngeal dysphagia depends on the underlying cause. Oropharyngeal dysphagia associated with systemic illnesses, such as parkinsonism, myasthenia gravis, polymyositis, and thyroid dysfunction, often improves with treatment of the underlying disorder. Neoplasms require resection and, in some cases, chemotherapy or radiotherapy. Unfortunately, treatment itself may also result in dysphagia, because of the removal or loss of function of structures critical to normal swallowing. Dysphagia following a stroke may respond to techniques aimed at rehabilitation of the physical components of swallowing. Manipulation of the diet and proper positioning of the head may facilitate swallowing in these patients. In some cases, radiographic assessment of swallowing with various types of food (liquids, semisolids, and solids) in different head positions may permit recommendations that lead to improved swallowing. Consultation with a speech pathologist is helpful. There is some encouraging evidence to show that many patients will recover some swallowing function with this approach [57]. For those with permanently impaired swallowing, a feeding gastrostomy or jejunostomy may be the only option.

For patients with cricopharyngeal dysfunction, cricopharyngeal myotomy may be beneficial [86]. In patients with neurologic disorders, including stroke and degenerative conditions, who present with pharyngeal dysphagia due to inadequate pharyngeal contraction or discoordination of the pharynx and UES, myotomy should also be considered, particularly in those with a motility disorder of the pharyngeal phase of swallowing characterized by inadequate pharyngeal contraction pressures, pharyngeal–UES incoordination, or incomplete sphincter relaxation [20]. Studies in small groups of patients with pharyngeal dysphagia have revealed good to excellent results with cricopharyngeal myotomy in patients with strokes, motor neuron disease, head trauma, poliomyelitis, and neoplastic or postsurgical nerve injury [13, 34, 43]. Cineradiographic studies have shown that myotomy produces improvement in the motor function of the entire pharyngoesophageal segment, not just the UES [42]. Injection of botulinum toxin may provide an alternative approach to cricopharyngeal dysfunction, but its exact role in therapy remains to be defined [138]. Passing a large-diameter dilator (18 to 20 mm) may improve dysphagia, particularly in patients in whom manometric studies show high UES pressure or impaired relaxation.

### Esophageal Dysphagia

*Esophageal dysphagia* is characterized by difficulty in the transport of ingested material down the esophagus and can result from a variety of neuromuscular (motility) disorders or mechanically obstructing lesions. A careful history usually allows the physician to place a patient into one of these two main categories of esophageal dysphagia. In approaching the patient with esophageal dysphagia, the three most important questions to answer are (a) Is swallowing liquids or solids associated with dysphagia? (b) Is the dysphagia intermittent or progressive? (c) Is there associated heartburn? The presence of additional associated symptoms, including chest pain, and nocturnal symptomatology may also provide helpful clues to the diagnosis [23]. (See chapter 2 for details.)

**TABLE 39–2.** *Causes of esophageal dysphagia in the elderly*

Motility disorders
  Achalasia
  Diffuse esophageal spasm and related disorders
  Scleroderma
  Diabetes mellitus
  Parkinsonism
Mechanical obstruction
  Neoplasms
  Peptic stricture
  Rings and webs
  Vascular lesions (dysphagia aortica)
  Diverticula
  Medication-induced esophageal injury

The major neuromuscular (motility) disorders to be considered in the elderly include achalasia, diffuse esophageal spasm and related disorders, and scleroderma. As noted above, in some elderly patients with dysphagia, the principal manometric finding is aperistalsis not associated with a classic primary motility disorder [103]. The major mechanical causes of esophageal dysphagia in the elderly include esophageal carcinoma, peptic strictures, rings or webs, vascular lesions, and medication-induced esophageal injury (Table 39–2). In general, motility disorders are characterized by dysphagia for both solids and liquids, whereas mechanical obstructing lesions initially cause dysphagia for solids only.

### Achalasia

Achalasia is characterized by slowly progressive dysphagia for solids and liquids and gradual weight loss (see chapter 10). The onset of achalasia is usually between ages 20 and 40 years, but a second peak occurs in the elderly. In the elderly patient with long-standing achalasia, extreme dilatation and tortuosity of the esophagus as seen on barium x-ray may result in the so-called sigmoid esophagus (Fig. 39–4).

In the elderly patient with apparent achalasia, it is important to perform an upper endoscopy (including a retroflexed view of the gastroesophageal junction) with biopsy of any suspicious area, owing to the possibility of secondary achalasia caused by a cancer that may produce the clinical, radiographic, and manometric abnormalities associated with idiopathic achalasia [20, 164]. Tumors most likely to be associated with secondary achalasia are high gastric cancers and distal esophageal cancers. Occasionally, pancreatic cancer, lung cancer, breast cancer, mesothelioma, hepatocellular carcinoma, sarcoma, and lymphoma can present in this manner [68, 78, 157]. Familial achalasia secondary to diffuse esophageal leiomyomatosis and affecting four generations of a family has also been described [97]. Secondary achalasia should be suspected in a patient with the clinical triad of age greater than 50 years, dysphagia of less than 1 year's duration, and weight loss of greater than 15 lb [164]. However, this triad is not diagnostic and can also be associated with idiopathic achalasia. Moreover, squamous cell carcinoma may develop as a consequence of long-standing achalasia [102]. Certain radiographic changes may be helpful in differentiating primary from secondary achalasia [32], and endoscopic ultrasonography may be particularly sensitive in detecting small neoplasms at the gastroesophageal junction [33].

As in the young patient with achalasia, treatment of the elderly patient can be medical or surgical, and the choice depends on the preference and expertise of the treating physicians, the overall health of the patient, and the patient's preference after being properly apprised of the techniques, risks, and expected outcomes. The principal options are pneumatic dilatation, surgical myotomy, and injection of botulinum toxin. One report has suggested that pneumatic dilatation may be particularly suitable for older patients, in whom improvement in dysphagia is often sustained after pneumatic dilatation and the need for surgical myotomy is infrequent [132]. In fact, in a recent study [40], patients under the age of 40 years had a significantly poorer response to pneumatic dilatation (2-year remission rate of 29%) than did patients older than age 40 years (2-year remission rate of 67%). Myotomy of the abnormal sphincter (Heller procedure) has also been associated with a good outcome in carefully selected elderly patients, although surgery is generally associated with a higher frequency of side effects, including gastroesophageal reflux, compared to pneumatic dilatation [32].

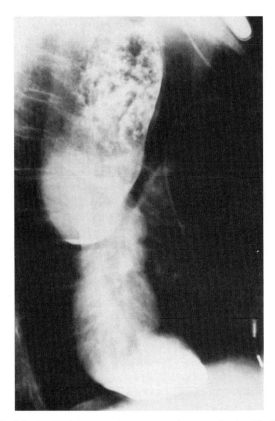

FIG. 39–4. Barium esophagogram from patient with long-standing achalasia showing the marked dilatation and tortuosity of a "sigmoid esophagus."

In the elderly patient with other serious medical problems in whom both pneumatic dilatation and surgery may be associated with a high risk, injection of botulinum toxin into the lower esophageal sphincter provides effective symptomatic relief, at least temporarily [58, 113]. Treatment may need to be repeated when symptoms recur. The noninvasive nature of botulinum toxin injection compared to traditional therapies makes this a particularly attractive first-line approach in the elderly. On the other hand, conservative therapy with smooth-muscle-relaxing agents, such as isosorbide dinitrate or nifedipine given sublingually before meals, has not proven to be very effective in the elderly [55].

### Diffuse Esophageal Spasm and Related Disorders

Diffuse esophageal spasm is characterized by intermittent dysphagia for both solids and liquids, often in association with chest pain. Esophageal manometry shows normal peristalsis interrupted by simultaneous (nonperistaltic) contractions. In fact, diffuse esophageal spasm may be related to a variety of other abnormal motility patterns as part of a spectrum that can progress, on occasion, to frank achalasia. Included in this spectrum are both hypercontractile and hypocontractile abnormalities which which may be associated with chest pain and occasionally with dysphagia (see chapter 11). An increased frequency of psychiatric diagnoses has been reported in patients with spastic esophageal disorders [8].

The aim of treatment of the spastic esophageal disorders is to decrease esophageal pressure or the patient's response to the pain. Agents such as nitrates, calcium antagonists (nifedipine or diltiazem), sedatives, and anticholinergics may be helpful. Occasionally, esophageal dilatation provides relief, and in severe, refractory cases, esophageal myotomy may be considered. Many patients improve after being reassured that their chest pain is esophageal, not cardiac, in origin [21, 125].

### Scleroderma

Esophageal involvement occurs in more than 80% of patients with scleroderma and correlates with the presence of Raynaud's phenomenon [169] (see chapter 16). Patients with scleroderma often experience slowly progressive dysphagia for both solids and liquids, as in achalasia. However, in scleroderma, unlike achalasia, heartburn is a prominent symptom of severe gastroesophageal reflux, and up to 40% of patients with gastroesophageal reflux due to scleroderma develop a peptic esophageal stricture; many develop a Barrett's esophagus [79]. Manometric findings include a low lower esophageal sphincter pressure and decreased peristalsis in the lower esophagus with preserved peristalsis in the upper esophagus. The treatment of esophageal involvement in scleroderma includes measures to treat severe gastroesophageal reflux, as discussed later.

### Esophageal Cancer

In any elderly patient with the new onset of dysphagia, cancer should be the primary initial diagnostic consideration. In esophageal cancer, dysphagia is usually rapidly progressive, initially for solids and then for liquids, and is associated with weight loss. In patients with squamous cell carcinoma of the esophagus, there is often a history of heavy tobacco and alcohol use. The principal risk factor for adenocarcinoma is Barrett's esophagus as a result of long-standing gastroesophageal reflux, and over the past two decades, the incidence of adenocarcinoma of the esophagus (as well as the gastric cardia) has risen faster than that of any other cancer [80, 114]. This increase in incidence may relate to a high frequency of unrecognized "short" segments of specialized columnar epithelium at the gastroesophageal junction [26, 153, 159]. The diagnosis of esophageal cancer may be suggested by a barium x-ray study, but confirmation with tissue diagnosis requires endoscopy with biopsy and cytology, which is safe and well tolerated in the elderly [10].

The treatment of choice for esophageal cancer is surgical resection, which can be performed successfully in selected elderly patients with no or few coexisting medical problems [3, 59, 77, 108, 161]. However, many elderly patients are poor operative risks, and often the disease is unresectable at the time of diagnosis. Computed tomographic scanning and endoscopic ultrasonography are used to determine resectability [33]. In patients who are poor operative risks or who have unresectable disease, palliation with radiotherapy, chemotherapy, or both may be considered. For relief of dysphagia, bougienage or laser photocoagulation of obstructing esophageal lesions, photodynamic therapy, or endoscopic insertion of an expandable mesh stent or Silastic prosthesis are options (see chapter 12). Laser ablation and photodynamic therapy also have shown promise in the treatment of Barrett's esophagus, with or without dysplasia or early cancer [46, 113, 133, 136]. In general, the prognosis of esophageal cancer is poor, with a 5-year survival rate of less than 5%. The prognosis is much better when cancer is detected early as part of endoscopic surveillance in Barrett's esophagus.

### Peptic Stricture

Patients with peptic strictures usually present with progressive dysphagia for solids in the setting of a long history of heartburn and other symptoms of gastroesophageal reflux. Patients with strictures are usually older than patients with gastroesophageal reflux but no stricture, presumably because stricture formation results over a long period of time [96]. Peptic strictures can be demonstrated by barium radiography, but endoscopy is mandatory to exclude carcinoma. The strictures are typically smooth, tapered, and of varying lengths. If they are located above the distal esophagus, Barrett's esophagus may be found.

Most patients with a peptic stricture can be managed with intermittent dilatation using standard Maloney or Savary dilators in combination with aggressive long-term antireflux therapy (see below). Many such patients require proton pump inhibitors or high doses of histamine $H_2$-receptor antagonists. If the stricture does not respond to conservative therapy, surgical antireflux repair (fundoplication) is indicated.

### Rings or Webs

Rings or webs usually present with intermittent dysphagia for solids. Unlike dysphagia associated with esophageal cancer, dysphagia caused by rings or webs is typically nonprogressive. The first episode of dysphagia frequently occurs while the patient is eating steak or bread, so the disorder has been termed the *steakhouse syndrome*. Often the bolus can be forced down by drinking liquids, but occasionally it must be regurgitated, after which the meal can usually be finished without difficulty. The diagnosis is best made by barium swallow with a solid bolus, and endoscopy is indicated if there is any question about the diagnosis.

The most common type of ring is Schatzki's ring, which is composed of invaginated mucosa located at the gastroesophageal mucosal junction [137]. On barium swallow, these rings are seen approximately 3 to 4 cm above the diaphragm. They produce symptoms when the lumen is narrowed to less than 12 or 13 mm. Treatment usually consists of one-time dilatation of the esophagus with a large-caliber bougie. If symptoms occur infrequently, careful chewing of food may suffice. In patients who do not respond to standard bougienage, electrocautery incision of the ring may be successful (see also chapters 3 and 14).

### Vascular Compression

Dysphagia aortica is a disorder of the elderly and results from compression of the esophagus, usually at the gastroesophageal junction, by either a large thoracic aortic aneurysm (Fig. 39–5) or a rigid atherosclerotic aorta posteriorly and the heart or esophageal hiatus anteriorly [158]. Occasionally, the esophagus may be compressed by a markedly enlarged left atrium. Rarely, exsanguinating hemorrhage may result from penetration of an esophageal ulcer into an adjacent major blood vessel [105].

### Medication-Induced Esophageal Injury

Acute esophageal injury may result from ingestion of a variety of medications (see also chapter 32). Resulting symptoms include substernal pain, odynophagia, and dysphagia. The majority of reported cases have been associated with emepronium bromide (an anticholinergic agent used to relax the urinary bladder and not available in the United States), tetracycline derivatives, potassium chloride, quinidine, the bisphosphonate alendronate, and nonsteroidal anti-inflammatory drugs (NSAIDs) [15, 35, 81]. Other medica-

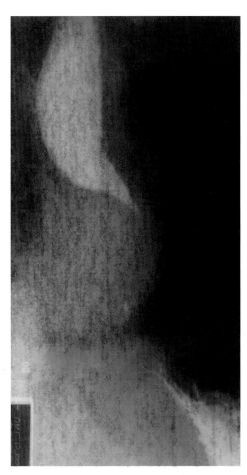

FIG. 39–5. Barium radiograph from a 72-year-old patient with dysphagia aortica from a thoracic aortic aneurysm. Compression of the barium-filled distal esophagus produces a pseudoachalasia appearance.

tions have been implicated less frequently (see tables in chapter 32).

Elderly patients are at particular risk of medication-induced esophageal injury for several reasons: They take more medications than younger patients, are more likely to have anatomic or motility disorders or the esophagus, spend more time in a recumbent position, and may have reduced salivary production. In the elderly, potassium chloride, alendronate, quinidine, and NSAIDs are the drugs most frequently associated with esophageal injury, which often presents with a surprisingly long course [44], whereas in young patients antibiotics are more commonly implicated.

Other factors that predispose to drug-induced esophageal injury include the patient's position at the time the drug is ingested and the volume of fluid ingested with the drug. It has been well established that the likelihood of passage of a pill through the esophagus is reduced when the medication is ingested by a patient in a recumbent position and with less than 15 ml of water [70]. It is thus particularly ill advised to administer medications at bedtime with small sips of water, as is common practice. The majority of patients with

medication-induced esophageal lesions do not have underlying esophageal abnormalities. The site of injury probably relates primarily to anatomic factors, as injury occurs most frequently in the midesophagus at the level of the aortic arch or distally in the area adjacent to the left atrium or above the lower esophageal sphincter.

The diagnosis of medication-induced esophageal injury is usually readily suggested by a history of acute substernal pain, odynophagia, and dysphagia in a patient taking one of the drugs known to cause such injury. A double-contrast barium swallow may identify the lesion and may provide information about possible extrinsic esophageal compression. Endoscopy also may confirm the diagnosis. Lesions vary from an erythematous patch to an ulcer or stricture [13]. Occasional deaths from hemorrhage and perforation have even been reported in patients with potassium chloride-induced esophagitis [15]. However, most medication-induced esophageal lesions heal with discontinuation of the causative agent and short-term therapy with antacids. Occasionally, more aggressive antireflux therapy is required and, in rare instances, resulting strictures must be dilated [14]. Strictures are most likely to occur with esophageal injury from potassium chloride and quinidine preparations, and older age has been shown to be a significant risk factor for the development of such strictures [99].

Recent experience suggests that as many as 20% of patients on NSAID therapy have esophagitis [139]. Whether this is the result of a direct effect of the medications on the esophagus or underlying chronic GERD remains to be determined. In one report [87], evidence of recent aspirin or NSAID use was found in 62% of patients with endoscopically verified esophagitis, compared to 26% of control subjects. It seems prudent to avoid using these agents in any patient with GERD [152].

### Miscellaneous Lesions

Spontaneous intramural hematoma of the esophagus is a rare condition usually affecting middle-aged and elderly women and presenting with acute substernal or epigastric pain and dysphagia or hematemesis. The pathogenesis is uncertain, and symptoms usually resolve with conservative therapy [2]. Spontaneous hemorrhage into a parathyroid adenoma has also been reported to cause acute dysphagia [83]. Intramural esophageal pseudodiverticulosis is another disease associated with dysphagia in persons over age 60 years. The disorder is characterized by multiple small circumferential invaginations of the esophageal wall, either diffusely or focally, presumably as a result of dilatation of the secretory ducts of the submucosal glands [101]. In addition to pseudodiverticulosis, stenoses or areas of reduced distensibility are found, usually in the upper esophagus. The etiology is unknown, but many affected patients have associated *Candida albicans* colonization of the esophageal mucosa. Ischemic infarction due to shock has been described in the elderly [67]. Another entity termed chronic esophagitis dessicans, characterized by chronic dysphagia, shedding of the esophageal mucosa, and localized esophageal strictures, has been described in five older patients with a mean age of 66 years [118].

## GASTROESOPHAGEAL REFLUX DISEASE

It has been estimated that approximately 10% of the U.S. population experiences heartburn every day and that at least one-third of the population has occasional heartburn [110]. Moreover, more than 80% of the over-the-counter antacids sold in the United States are taken for symptoms of gastroesophageal reflux [61]. The questions arise as to whether physiologic antireflux mechanisms deteriorate with age and whether symptoms and complications of GERD are more common in the elderly than in the young.

### Changes in Physiologic Antireflux Mechanisms with Age

Studies of age-related physiologic changes relevant to gastroesophageal reflux have yielded conflicting results. Manometric studies of healthy elderly subjects have not shown a consistent decrease in lower esophageal sphincter pressure with age [71]. However, secondary esophageal peristalsis, an important mechanism to clear refluxed acid, is less consistent in the elderly than in the young [123]. In addition, slight but insignificant decreases in salivary volume and bicarbonate have been found in healthy elderly subjects (mean age, 55 years) compared to younger controls (mean age, 28 years), and the older subjects showed a significantly decreased salivary bicarbonate response to esophageal acid infusion [150].

The acid-peptic injury produced at the esophageal mucosa secondary to chronic gastroesophageal reflux is related, in part, to the acid content of the stomach and the resulting activation of pepsinogen. Although gastric acid secretion does not decrease because of aging per se [72], gastric acid secretion may decline in the large percentage of elderly persons with long-standing *Helicobacter pylori* infection in whom atrophic gastritis develops. (Conversely, eradication of *H. pylori* has been reported to provoke reflux esophagitis, possibly by eliminating gastric ammonia, which is produced by *H. pylori* and may serve to neutralize acid in the esophagus [81].) Thus, in the large majority of elderly persons who are infected with *H. pylori*, refluxed material is often less acidic than in the young [106], an observation that may explain in part a lower frequency of heartburn in elderly patients with GERD compared to young patients (see below) and the underrecognition of GERD in the elderly. Mold and co-workers [107] observed a surprisingly high frequency of distal esophageal alkalinity (more than 30%) among elderly patients undergoing ambulatory esophageal pH testing; such persons had a lower frequency of heartburn, but a higher frequency of pulmonary symptoms compared to those with acid reflux. A role for duodenogastroesophageal reflux in

more severe grades of reflux esophagitis has been suggested [25]. It is also possible that heartburn may be less severe in the elderly than the young because of age-related decreases in pain perception [58, 88].

It has been well documented that the frequency of sliding hiatal hernia increases with age [156]. The presence of a sliding hiatal hernia impairs the diaphragmatic component of the lower esophageal sphincter and may impede the clearance of refluxed acid from the distal esophagus [104, 147, 151]. Therefore, an increased prevalence of hiatal hernia in the elderly could contribute to an increased prevalence of GERD (see below). On the other hand, the rate of gastric emptying does not appear to change with age [51].

Occasional patients over age 60 years are found to have a paraesophageal hernia [98]. Such a hernia may cause little or no symptoms, but can cause considerable morbidity if the stomach becomes mechanically entrapped in the diaphragmatic defect, with resulting hemorrhage, gangrene, and perforation. Because paraesophageal hernias tend to enlarge over time, elective surgical repair is generally advisable before complications ensue.

One factor likely to be important in the elderly is the use of medications known to decrease the lower esophageal sphincter pressure and thereby increase gastroesophageal reflux. Drugs such as theophylline, nitrates, calcium antagonists, benzodiazepines, anticholinergics, antidepressants, lidocaine, and prostaglandins are more likely to be administered to the elderly than to the young and may therefore contribute to gastroesophageal reflux [127]. An increase in body weight with age may also predispose to gastroesophageal reflux [159].

The net effect of the aforementioned reported physiologic changes with age has been difficult to assess. While some investigators have not found a significant increase in the frequency or duration of reflux episodes with age [47, 154], others have observed a longer duration of reflux episodes with age [130, 148], and, in some cases, higher overall esophageal acid exposure [148, 170] (Fig. 39–6). For example, Zhu et al. observed that among patients with symptoms of GERD who underwent prolonged ambulatory esophageal pH monitoring, the mean percent time that the pH was less than 4 was 32.5% among 24 elderly patients with a mean age of 69 years, compared to 12.9% among 147 younger patients with a mean age of 45 years [170].

### Frequency and Presentation of GERD in the Elderly

There is controversy as to whether GERD is more common in the elderly than the young. A Gallup Survey on Heartburn Across America [1] found that 22% of respondents older than 50 years used antacids and other antidyspeptic medications two or more times weekly compared to only 9% of those younger than 50 years. In a Finnish survey of 487 elderly subjects over age 65 years [120], the frequency of daily symptoms suggestive of GERD was 8% in men and 15% in women, and symptoms at least once per month were

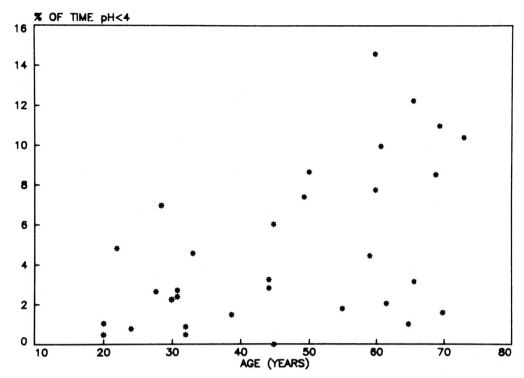

**FIG. 39-6.** Intraesophageal pH data showing increased acid reflux in normal persons with advancing age. (From ref. 148, with permission.)

reported by 54% of men and 66% of women. In an American survey [160], heartburn at least once a week was reported by 22% of persons over age 65 years. On the other hand, among 476 predominantly male veterans who underwent upper endoscopy to evaluate upper gastrointestinal symptoms, the frequency and severity of esophagitis were similar in those over age 65 years and those under age 65 years [161]. Moreover, in a random sample of 2,200 residents aged 25 to 74 years of Olmsted County, Minnesota, the overall prevalence of heartburn or acid regurgitation at least weekly was 20 per 100, and no significant increase in prevalence occurred with age. In fact, the prevalence of heartburn, but not acid regurgitation, declined with age [93].

Compared to younger patients, older patients with GERD are less likely to report heartburn, possibly because of a decline in esophageal sensitivity with age [58, 88]. On the other hand, dysphagia, chest pain, respiratory symptoms, and vomiting are more common [109, 119], and in persons over age 80 years, esophagitis may account for a greater percentage of cases of upper gastrointestinal bleeding than in younger persons [171]. Because the severity of symptoms often does not correlate with the degree of esophagitis, diagnostic endoscopy should be considered in all elderly patients with the new onset of symptoms suggestive of GERD. It may be particularly challenging for the clinician to differentiate chest pain of cardiac origin from that of esophageal origin [17, 21, 126]. Pulmonary and otolaryngologic manifestations of gastroesophageal reflux in the elderly, as in the young, include asthma, bronchitis, aspiration pneumonia,

pulmonary fibrosis, hiccups, and laryngitis [36]. In a study of 195 elderly patients with a mean age of 74 years, Raiha and colleagues [119] found that among those with esophagitis on endoscopy, heartburn was absent in 50% and the presence of heartburn did not correlate with the degree of reflux on ambulatory pH study. On the other hand, respiratory symptoms and dysphagia were common, and vomiting occurred in 25%. On surveying 487 subjects aged 65 years and over, these same investigators also found that typical symptoms of GERD were often associated with abdominal symptoms, chest pain, or respiratory symptoms [120]. Restrictive ventilatory defects [122] and lung parenchymal scars and pleural thickening [121] in particular were more common in elderly patients with abnormalities on 24-hour esophageal pH studies than in those without abnormal results.

Because GERD is a chronic persistent disorder, it seems likely that the frequency of complications associated with gastroesophageal reflux increases with increasing duration of disease and thus with age. In 1969, Brunnen and colleagues [18] reported that in northern Scotland over an 11-year period (1951 to 1962), the incidence of patients referred for surgery for severe esophagitis was 18 per 100,000 in persons aged 60 to 69 years compared to only 1.7 per 100,000 in those aged 40 to 49 years. Despite milder heartburn, older patients may be more likely to have severe esophagitis, strictures, and Barrett's esophagus [125, 170]. The incidence of Barrett's esophagus rises with age. Moreover, elderly patients with Barrett's esophagus are less symptomatic than younger patients with Barrett's esophagus [60, 162]. On the other hand, older patients with GERD seem to need a greater degree of acid suppression to control symptoms and heal esophagitis than younger patients [28, 75].

### Therapy

Therapy of GERD is similar in elderly patients and the young. However, care must be taken in prescribing drugs to elderly patients with GERD, because certain medications are more likely to result in adverse effects in the elderly. In addition, there is a greater frequency of adverse drug interactions in elderly patients, because they are more likely to take a variety of drugs for multiple medical conditions.

### Phase 1 Therapy

Changes in lifestyle can be effective in controlling episodes of heartburn and dyspepsia in the elderly as in the young. In fact, emphasis on phase 1 therapy may be particularly appropriate in the elderly, in whom additional drug therapy may be undesirable [20]. The patient should be instructed to eat three meals per day, with the evening meal taken at least 3 hours before bedtime, in order to avoid recumbency with a full stomach. Obese patients should be advised to lose weight. For patients with nocturnal symptoms, the head of the bed should be elevated at least 6 inches by placing blocks or other elevators under the legs of the bed. Elevation of the head of the bed may be effective in decreasing nocturnal esophageal acid exposure, as assessed by overnight pH monitoring [76]. Alternatively, placing a foam rubber wedge (10 in. high) on top of the mattress and under the patient's head may be as effective as elevating the entire head of the bed [65] and may be more convenient for some elderly patients.

Dietary recommendations include a decrease in the total fat content of the diet, because fat lowers esophageal sphincter pressure and thereby increases gastric acid reflux. Agents that may irritate the esophagus such as citrus juices, tomato products, coffee, and probably alcohol should be restricted. Smoking decreases lower esophageal sphincter pressure and should be discouraged. As noted earlier, medications that may decrease lower esophageal sphincter pressure should be avoided if possible [128].

The intermittent use of antacids, alginic acid, or over-the-counter $H_2$-receptor antagonists completes phase 1 therapy. Antacids must be used with caution because of an increased risk of toxicity in the elderly, including salt overload, constipation, diarrhea, hypercalcemia, and interference with the absorption of other drugs. A major component of phase 1 therapy is the education of the patient about factors that may contribute to gastroesophageal reflux and about beneficial lifestyle changes. In some elderly patients, however, such an interactive approach may not be possible because of physical or mental impairment.

### Phase 2 Therapy

Most patients with GERD require one or more of the available systemic medications. The mainstay of therapy for patients with gastroesophageal reflux has been $H_2$-receptor antagonists. Patients with severe or refractory gastroesophageal reflux or with complications of gastroesophageal disease may require higher than standard doses of $H_2$-receptor antagonists to promote relief of symptoms and heal esophagitis [27]. In the elderly, caution is required in using higher than standard doses of $H_2$-receptor antagonists. Mental status changes have been described in elderly patients, particularly those with renal and liver dysfunction, with both cimetidine and ranitidine [92]. Cimetidine in particular may affect the metabolism of drugs by the hepatic cytochrome $P_{450}$ system, including warfarin sodium (Coumadin), theophylline, and benzodiazepines. The addition of cimetidine to a regimen that already includes such a hepatically metabolized drug requires extreme care and a possible reduction in dose. Famotidine and nizatidine appear to be associated with low rates of side effects in the elderly [27], but in patients with renal insufficiency, the doses of all $H_2$-receptor antagonists may need to be reduced [66].

When an $H_2$-receptor antagonist alone does not result in complete symptomatic and endoscopic improvement, addition of a promotility agent should be considered. However, metoclopramide, a dopamine antagonist that increases lower esophageal sphincter pressure and improves gastric emptying, which is often delayed in patients with gastroesophageal reflux [90], must be used with great caution in the elderly because of side effects in up to one-third of patients, including muscle tremors, spasms, agitation, anxiety, insomnia, drowsiness, and even frank confusion or tardive dyskinesia [165]. Newer peripheral dopamine antagonists such as cisapride and domperidone are preferable in the elderly because of the absence of central nervous system side effects [165]. However, cisapride can cause cardiac arrhythmias and must be used with caution in patients taking other medications that prolong the Q-T interval and those with cardiac disease or renal insufficiency. Cisapride should not be taken with other drugs metabolized by cytochrome $P_{450}$ 3A4, such as fluconazole, itraconazole, ketoconazole, erythromycin, and clarithromycin. Recent studies have reported relief of symptoms and improved healing of esophagitis with cisapride, alone or combined with an $H_2$-receptor antagonist [52], but experience in elderly patients is limited. Bethanecol, which increases resting lower esophageal sphincter pressure, is rarely used and is associated with various side effects, including urinary frequency, abdominal pain, blurred vision, and worsening glaucoma.

### Sulcralfate

Sucralfate has some appeal for the treatment of GERD in elderly patients because of its lack of systemic absorption and a corresponding lack of systemic toxicity. The major side effect is constipation, which is infrequent. However, sucralfate may also bind to other drugs administered by mouth at the same time and, in the elderly patient, it may be challenging to set up an appropriate schedule for the administration of multiple drugs. Moreover, the efficacy of sucralfate in patients with esophagitis has been disappointing [167].

*Proton Pump Inhibitors*

The proton pump inhibitors omeprazole and lansoprazole may be particularly useful in elderly patients with GERD, who seem to require a greater degree of acid suppression than younger patients to heal esophagitis [28, 53, 75]. Analysis of controlled trials has suggested that, as in younger patients, therapy with proton pump inhibitors is more effective than that with $H_2$-receptor antagonists in elderly patients with esophagitis [69, 75, 146]. Whether a greater degree of acid suppression is also required for maintenance treatment is uncertain. Concern has been expressed that maintenance treatment with proton pump inhibitors in *H. pylori*-positive patients with GERD may accelerate progression to atrophic gastritis, a precursor to gastric cancer [84], but the issue is controversial. Although plasma clearance of proton pump inhibitors decreases with age, no reduction in the dose of either omeprazole or lansoprazole is necessary in the elderly [100], even those with impaired renal or hepatic function [53, 100, 146]. Omeprazole and lansoprazole are metabolized by hepatic cytochrome $P_{450}$ and may affect the metabolism of other drugs [53], but the effects are clinically insignificant [7, 116]. Long-term use of a proton pump inhibitor may lead to a reduction in protein-bound vitamin $B_{12}$ absorption [134] but is unlikely to lead to clinically significant fat or carbohydrate malabsorption due to bacterial overgrowth [135].

*Surgery*

Surgery can be performed successfully in selected elderly patients who are reasonable operative risks, but should be avoided in patients with concomitant medical problems that make such surgery hazardous. The role of laparoscopic antireflux surgery in the elderly appears promising, but requires further study [124].

## CONCLUSIONS

In general, the classic symptoms of dysphagia, heartburn, and chest pain are the presenting manifestations of esophageal disorders in the elderly, as in the young. Several unique conditions may occur in the elderly, including Zenker's diverticulum and vascular compression of the esophagus. Certain disorders increase in frequency with age, such as oropharyngeal dysphagia due to neurologic disorders. Treatment approaches are similar in elderly and younger patients,

but the potential for adverse drug effects and drug interactions is greater in the elderly than in the young.

As important as the medical considerations are the special psychosocial, economic, and humanistic aspects of caring for the elderly. Factors that may have an impact on illness in an elderly person include the losses and disability associated with aging, feelings of isolation, a reticence to discuss certain embarrassing problems, and the variety of settings for health care, including nursing homes, home care communities, geriatric units, geropsychiatric units, rehabilitation units, and hospices. The multiplicity of medical problems that often lead to contradictory and mutually exclusive management options and the frequency of multiple-drug use and adverse drug reactions may pose great challenges to treatment of an elderly patient. Clearly, just as children are not "little adults," the elderly are not "big adults," and the delivery of care to the elderly requires special expertise and sensitivity [49].

## REFERENCES

1. A Gallup Survey on Heartburn Across America. Princeton, NJ: Gallup Organization, 1988
2. Ackert JJ, et al. Spontaneous intramural hematoma of the esophagus. Am J Gastroenterol 1989;84:1325
3. Adam DJ, et al. Esophagectomy for carcinoma in the octogenarian. Ann Thorac Surg 1996;61:190
4. Alberts MJ, et al. Aspiration after stroke: lesions analysis by brain MRI. Dysphagia 1992;7:170
5. Ali Khan, et al. Esophageal motility in the elderly. Am J Dig Dis 1977;22:1049
6. Almy TP. Factors leading to digestive disorders in the elderly. Bull NY Acad Med 1981;57:709
7. Andersson J. Pharmacokinetics, metabolism and interactions of acid pump inhibitors. Focus on omeprazole, lansoprazole, and pantoprazole. Clin Pharmacokinet 1996;31:9
8. Anonymous. The oesophagus and chest pain of uncertain cause. Lancet 1992;339:583
9. Aviv JE, et al. Age-related changes in pharyngeal and supraglottic sensation. Ann Otol Rhinol Laryngol 1994;103:749
10. Bannister P, et al. Dysphagia in the elderly: what does it mean to the endoscopist? J R Soc Med 1990;83:552
11. Bird MR, et al. Asymptomatic swallowing disorders in elderly patients with Parkinson's disease: a description of findings on clinical examination and videofluoroscopy in sixteen patients. Age ageing 1994;23:251
12. Bloem BR, et al. Prevalence of subjective dysphagia in community residents aged over 87. Br Med J 1990;300:721
13. Bonavina L, et al. Pharyngoesophageal dysfunctions: the role of cricopharyngeal myopathy. Arch Surg 1985;120:541
14. Bonavina L, et al. Drug-induced esophageal strictures. Ann Surg 1987;206:173
15. Bott S, et al. Medication-induced esophageal injury: survey of the literature. Am J Gastroenterol 1987;82:758
16. Bramble MG, et al. Evidence for a change in neurotransmitter affecting oesophageal motility in Parkinson's disease. J Neurol Neurosurg Psychiatry 1978;41:709
17. Browning TH, et al. Diagnosis of chest pain of esophageal origin: a guideline of the Patient Care Committee of the American Gastroenterological Association. Dig Dis Sci 1990;35:289
18. Brunnen PL, et al. Severe peptic esophagitis. Gut 1969;10:831
19. Buchholz DW, et al. Neurogenic dysphagia: what is the cause when the cause is not obvious? Dysphagia 1994;9:245
20. Castell DO. Esophageal diseases in the elderly. Gastroenterol Clin North Am 1990;19:227
21. Castell DO, ed. Chest pain of undetermined origin. Am J Med 1992;92(5A):2S
22. Castell JA, Castell DO. Upper esophageal sphincter and pharyngeal

function and oropharyngeal (transfer) dysphagia. Gastroenterol Clin North Am 1996;25:35

23. Cattau EL, Castell DO. Symptoms of esophageal dysfunction. Adv Intern Med 1982;27:151

24. Celifarco A, et al. Dysphagia as the sole manifestation of bilateral strokes. Am J Gastroenterol 1990;85:610

25. Champion G, et al. Duodenogastroesophageal reflux: relationship to pH and importance in Barrett's esophagus. Gastroenterology 1994; 107:747

26. Clark GW, et al. Is Barrett's metaplasia the source of adenocarcinomas of the cardia? Arch Surg 1994;129:609

27. Colin-Jones DG. Histamine₂-receptor antagonists in gastroesophageal reflux. Gut 1989;30:1305

28. Collen MJ, et al. Gastroesophageal disease in the elderly: more severe disease that requires aggressive therapy. Am J Gastroenterol 1995; 90:1053

29. Cook IJ, et al. Structural abnormalities of the cricopharyngeus muscle in patients with pharyngeal (Zenker's) diverticulum. J Gastroenterol Hepatol 1992;7:556

30. Cook IJ, et al. Pharyngeal (Zenker's) diverticulum is a disorder of upper esophageal sphincter opening. Gastroenterology 1992;103:1229

31. Csendes A, et al. Relation of gastroesophageal sphincter pressure and esophageal contractile waves to age in man. Scand J Gastroenterol 1978;13:443

32. Csendes A, et al. A prospective randomized study comparing forceful dilatation and esophagomyotomy in patients with achalasia of the esophagus. Gastroenterology 1981;80:789

33. Dancygier H, Classen M. Endoscopic ultrasonography in esophageal diseases. Gastrointest Endosc 1989;35:220

34. David VC. Relief of dysphagia in motor neuron disease with cricopharyngeal myotomy. Ann R Coll Surg Engl 1985;67:229

35. Delpre G, et al. Induction of esophageal injuries by doxycycline and other pills: a frequent but preventable occurrence. Dig Dis Sci 1989; 34:797

36. Deschner WK, Benjamin SB. Extraesophageal manifestations of gastroesophageal reflux disease. Am J Gastroenterol 1989;84:1

37. Dodds WJ, et al. Radiologic assessment of abnormal oral and pharyngeal phases of swallowing. Am J Roentgenol 1990;154:965

38. Dodds WJ, et al. Physiology and radiology of the normal oral and pharyngeal phases of swallowing. Am J Roentgenol 1990;154:953

39. Eckhardt VF, LeCompte PM. Esophageal ganglia and smooth muscle in the elderly. Am J Dig Dis 1978;23:443

40. Eckhardt VF, et al. Predictors of outcome in patients with achalasia treated by pneumatic dilatation. Gastroenterology 1992;103:1732

41. Ekberg O, Feinberg MJ. Altered swallowing function in elderly patients without dysphagia: radiologic findings in 56 cases. Am J Roentgenol 1991;156:1811

42. Ekberg O, Lindgren S. Effect of cricopharyngeal myotomy on pharyngoesophageal function: pre- and postoperative cineradiographic findings. Gastrointest Radiol 1987;12:1

43. Ellis FH, Crozier RE. Cervical esophageal dysphagia. Ann Surg 1981; 194:279

44. Eng J, et al. Drug-induced esophagitis. Am J Gastroenterol 1991;86: 1127

45. Ergun GA, Kahrilas PJ. Oropharyngeal dysphagia in the elderly. Pract Gastroenterol 1993;17:9

46. Ertan A, et al. Esophageal adenocarcinoma associated with Barrett's esophagus: long-term management with laser ablation. Am J Gastroenterol 1995;90:2201

47. Fass R, et al. Age- and gender-related differences in 24-hour esophageal pH monitoring of normal subjects. Dig Dis Sci 1993;38:1926

48. Feinberg MJ, et al. Deglutition in elderly patients with dementia: findings of videographic evaluation and impact on staging and management. Radiology 1992;183:811

49. Friedman LS, ed. Gastrointestinal disorders in the elderly. Gastroenterol Clin North Am 1990;19:227

50. Fulp S, et al. Aging-related alterations in human upper esophageal sphincter function. Am J Gastroenterol 1990;85:1569

51. Gainsborough N, et al. The association of age with gastric emptying. Age Ageing 1993;22:37

52. Galmiche JP, et al. Combined therapy with cisapride and cimetidine in severe reflux oesophagitis. Gut 1988;29:675

53. Garnett WR, Garabedia-Ruffalo SM. Identification, diagnosis, and treatment of acid-related disease in the elderly: implications for long-term care. Pharmacotherapy 1997;17:938

54. Gerhardt DC, et al. Human upper esophageal sphincter. Gastroenterology 1978;75:268

55. Ghosh S, et al. Achalasia of the oesophagus in elderly patients responds poorly to conservative therapy. Age Ageing 1994;23:280

56. Goekas MC, et al. The aging gastrointestinal tract, liver, and pancreas. Clin Geriatr Med 1985;1:177

57. Gordon C, Hewer RL, Wade DT. Dysphagia in acute stroke. Br Med J 1987;295:411

58. Gordon JM, Eaker EY. Prospective study of esophageal botulinum toxin injection in high-risk achalasia patients. Am J Gastroenterol 1997;92:1812

59. Gorman RC, et al. Esophageal disease in the elderly patient. Surg Clin North Am 1994;74:93

60. Grade A, et al. Reduced chemoreceptor sensitivity in patients with Barrett's esophagus may be related to age and not to the presence of Barrett's epithelium. Am J Gastroenterol 1997;92:2040

61. Graham DY, Smith JL, Patterson DJ. Why do apparently healthy people use antacid tablets? Am J Gastroenterol 1983;78:257

62. Grishaw EK, et al. Functional abnormalities of the esophagus: a prospective analysis of radiographic findings relative to age and symptoms. Am J Roentgenol 1996;167:719

63. Grunebaum M, Salinger H. Radiologic findings in polymyositis-dermatomyositis involving the pharynx and upper esophagus. Clin Radiol 1971;22:97

64. Gutmann E. Muscle. In Finch CE, Hayflick L, eds, Handbook of the Biology of Aging. New York: Van Nostrand Reinhold, 1977:709

65. Hamilton J, et al. Sleeping on a wedge diminishes exposure of the esophagus to refluxed acid. Dig Dis Sci 1988;33:581

66. Hatlebakk JG, Berstad A. Pharmacokinetic optimisation in the treatment of gastro-oesophageal reflux. Clin Pharmacokinet 1996;31:386

67. Haviv YS, et al. "Black esophagus": a rare complication of shock. Am J Gastroenterol 1996;91:2432

68. Herrera JL. Case report: esophageal metastasis from breast carcinoma presenting as achalasia. Am J Med Sci 1992;303:321

69. Hetzel DJ, et al. Healing and relapse of severe peptic esophagitis after treatment with omeprazole. Gastroenterology 1988;95:903

70. Hey H, et al. Oesophageal transit of six commonly used tablets and capsules. Br Med J 1982;285:717

71. Hollis JB, Castell DO. Esophageal function in elderly men: a new look at "presbyesophagus." Ann Intern Med 1974;80:371

72. Hurwitz A, et al. Gastric acidity in older adults. JAMA 1997;278:659

73. Ishioka S, et al. Manometric study of the upper esophageal sphincter before and after endoscopic management of Zenker's diverticulum. Hepato-Gastroenterology 1995;42:628

74. Jacob H, et al. The esophageal motility disorder of polymyositis. Arch Intern Med 1983;143:2262

75. James OFW, Parry-Billings KS. Comparison of omeprazole and histamine H₂-receptor antagonists in the treatment of elderly and young patients with reflux esophagitis. Age Ageing 1994;23:121

76. Johnson L, DeMeester T. Evaluation of elevation of the head of the bed, bethanechol, and antacid foam tablets on gastroesophageal reflux. Dig Dis Sci 1981;26:673

77. Jougon JB, et al. Esophagectomy for cancer in the patient aged 70 years and older. Ann Thorac Surg 1997;63:1225

78. Kahrilas PJ, et al. Comparison of pseudoachalasia and achalasia. Am J Med 1987;72:49

79. Katzka D, et al. Barrett's metaplasia and adenocarcinoma of the esophagus in scleroderma. Am J Med 1987;82:46

80. Kelsen D. Multimodality therapy for adenocarcinoma of the esophagus. Gastroenterol Clin North Am 1997;26:635

81. Kikendall JW, et al. Pill-induced esophageal injury: case reports and review of the medical literature. Dig Dis Sci 1983;28:174

82. Kluin KJ, et al. Dysphagia in elderly men with myasthenia gravis. J Neurol Sci 1996;138:49

83. Korkis AM, Miskovitz PF. Acute pharyngoesophageal dysphagia secondary to spontaneous hemorrhage of a parathyroid adenoma. Dysphagia 1993;8:7

84. Kuipers EJ, et al. Atrophic gastritis and Helicobacter pylori infection in patients with reflux esophagitis treated with omeprazole or fundoplication. N Engl J Med 1996;334:1018

85. Labenz J, et al. Curing Helicobacter pylori infection in patients with duodenal ulcer may provoke reflux esophagitis. Gastroenterology 1997;112:1442

86. Lacau ST, et al. Improvement of dysphagia following cricopharyngeal myotomy in a group of elderly patients. Histochemical and biochemi-

cal assessment of the cricopharyngeal muscle. Ann Otol Rhinol Laryngol 1995;104:603

87. Lanas A, Hirschowitz BI. Significant role of aspirin use in patients with esophagitis. J Clin Gastroenterol 1991;13:622

88. Lasch H, Castell DO. Evidence for diminished visceral pain with aging: studies using graded intraesophageal balloon distention. Am J Physiol 1997;272:G1

89. Leese G, Hopwood D. Muscle fibre typing in the human pharyngeal constrictors and oesophagus: the effect of aging. *Acta Anat* (Basel) 1986;127:77

90. Lieberman DA, Keeffe EB. Treatment of severe reflux esophagitis with cimetidine and metoclopramide. Ann Intern Med 1986;104:21

91. Lindgren S, Janzon L. Prevalence of swallowing complaints and clinical findings among 50–79-year-old men and women. Dysphagia 1991; 6:187

92. Lipsy RJ, et al. Clinical review of histamine$_2$-receptor antagonists. Arch Intern Med 1990;150:745

93. Locke III GR, et al. Prevalence and clinical spectrum of gastroesophageal reflux: a population-based study in Olmsted County, Minnesota. Gastroenterology 1997;112:1148

94. Logemann JA, et al. Dysphagia in parkinsonism. JAMA 1975;231: 69

95. Louie HW, Zuckerbraun L. Staged Zenker's diverticulotomy with cervical esophagostomy and secondary esophagostomy closure for treatment of massive diverticulum in severely debilitated patients. Ann Surg 1993;59:842

96. Marks RD, Richter JE. Peptic stricture of the esophagus. Am J Gastroenterol 1993;88:1160

97. Marshall JB, et al. Achalasia due to diffuse esophageal leiomyomatosis and inherited as an autosomal dominant disorder: report of a family study. Gastroenterology 1990;98:1358

98. McArthur KE. Hernias and volvulus of the gastrointestinal tract. In Feldman M, et al., eds, Sleisenger and Fordtran's Gastrointestinal and Liver Disease: Pathophysiology, Diagnosis, Management. Philadelphia: WB Saunders, 1998:317

99. McCord GS, Clouse RE. Pill-induced esophageal strictures: clinical features and risk factors for development. Am J Med 1990;88:512

100. McTavish D, et al. Omeprazole: an updated review of its pharmacology and therapeutic use in acid-related disorders. Drugs 1991;42:138

101. Medeiros LJ, et al. Esophageal intramural pseudodiverticulosis: a report of two cases with analysis of similar, less extensive changes in normal autopsy esophagi. Hum Pathol 1988;19:928

102. Meijssen MAC, et al. Achalasia complicated by oesophageal squamous cell carcinoma: a prospective study of 195 patients. Gut 1992; 33:155

103. Meshinkpour H, et al. Clinical spectrum of esophageal aperistalsis in the elderly. Am J Gastroenterol 1994;89:1480

104. Mittal R, Lange R, McCallum R. Identification and mechanism of delayed esophageal acid clearance in subjects with hiatus hernia. Gastroenterology 1987;92:130

105. Mo KM, et al. Sudden death from perforation of a benign oesophageal ulcer into a major blood vessel. Postgrad Med J 1988;64:687

106. Mold JW, Rankin RA. Symptomatic gastroesophageal reflux in the elderly. J Am Geriatr Soc 1987;35:649

107. Mold JW, et al. Prevalence of gastroesophageal reflux in elderly patients in a primary care setting. Am J Gastroenterol 1991;86:965

108. Muehrcke DD, et al. Oesophagogastrectomy in patients over 70. Thorax 1989;44:141

109. Nano M, et al. Sliding hiatal hernia in the elderly: a clinical entity. J Am Geriatr Soc 1981;29:463

110. Nebel OT, et al. Symptomatic gastroesophageal reflux: incidence and precipitating factors. Am J Dig Dis 1976;21:953

111. Nelson JB, Castell DO. Aging of the gastrointestinal system. In Hazzard WR, et al., eds, Principles of Geriatric Medicine and Gerontology. New York: McGraw-Hill, 1990:593

112. Nilsson H, et al. Quantitative aspects of swallowing in an elderly nondysphagic population. Dysphagia 1996;11:180

113. Overholt BF, Panjehpour M. Barrett's esophagus: photodynamic therapy for ablation of dysplasia, reduction of specialized mucosa, and treatment of superficial esophageal cancer. Gastrointest Endosc 1995; 42:64

114. Pasricha PJ, et al. Botulinum toxin for achalasia: long-term outcome and predictors of response. Gastroenterology 1996;110:1410

115. Pera M, et al. Increasing incidence of adenocarcinoma of the esophagus and esophagogastic junction. Gastroenterology 1993;104:510

116. Petersen KU. Review article: omeprazole and the cytochrome P$_{450}$ system. Aliment Pharmacol Ther 1995;9:1

117. Piaget F, Fouillet J. Le pharynx et l'oesophage seniles: étude clinique radiologique et radiocinématographique. J Med Lyon 1959;40:951

118. Ponsot P, et al. Chronic esophagitis dissecans: an unrecognized clinicopathologic entity? Gastrointest Endosc 1997;45:38

119. Raiha I, et al. Symptoms of gastro-oesophageal reflux disease in elderly people. Age Ageing 1991;20:365

120. Raiha I, et al. Prevalence and characteristics of symptomatic gastroesophageal reflux disease in the elderly. J Am Geriatr Soc 1992;40: 1209

121. Raiha I, et al. Radiographic pulmonary changes of gastro-oesophageal reflux disease in elderly patients. Age Ageing 1992;21:250

122. Raiha I, et al. Pulmonary function in gastro-oesophageal reflux disease of elderly people. Age Ageing 1992;21:368

123. Ren J, et al. Effect of aging on the secondary esophageal peristalsis: presbyesophagus revisited. Am J Physiol 1995;268:G772

124. Richardson WS, et al. Laparoscopic antireflux surgery. Semin Gastrointest Dis 1997;8:100

125. Richter JE. Gastroesophageal reflux disease in the elderly. Geriatr Med Today 1989;8:27

126. Richter JE, Bradley LA. Esophageal chest pain: current controversies in pathogenesis, diagnosis and therapy. Ann Intern Med 1989;110:66

127. Richter JE, Castell DO. Gastroesophageal reflux disease in the Zollinger-Ellison syndrome. Ann Intern Med 1981;95:37

128. Richter JE, Castell DO. Gastroesophageal reflux: pathogenesis, diagnosis, and therapy. Ann Intern Med 1982;97:93

129. Richter JE, et al. Esophageal manometry in 95 healthy adult volunteers: variability of pressures with age and frequency of "abnormal" contractions. Dig Dis Sci 1987;32:583

130. Richter JE, et al. Normal 24-hr ambulatory esophageal pH values: influence of study center, pH electrode, age, and gender. Dig Dis Sci 1992;37:849

131. Robbins J, et al. Oropharyngeal swallowing in normal adults of different ages. Gastroenterology 1992;103:823

132. Robertson CS, et al. Choice of therapy for achalasia in relation to age. Digestion 1988;40:244

133. Salo JA, et al. Treatment of Barrett's esophagus by endoscopic laser ablation and antireflux surgery. Ann Surg 1998;1:40

134. Saltzman JR, et al. Effect of hypochlorhydria due to omeprazole treatment or atrophic gastritis on protein-bound vitamin B$_{12}$ absorption. J Am Coll Nutr 1994;13:584

135. Saltzman JR, et al. Bacterial overgrowth without clinical malabsorption in elderly hypochlorhydric subjects. Gastroenterology 1997;106: 615

136. Sampliner RE. Ablation of Barrett's mucosa. Gastroenterologist 1997; 5:185

137. Schatzki R. The lower esophageal ring. Am J Roentgenol 1963;90: 805

138. Schneider I, et al. Treatment of dysfunction of the cricopharyngeal muscle with botulinum A toxin: introduction of a new, noninvasive method. Ann Otol Rhinol Laryngol 1994;103:31

139. Semble EL, Wu WC, Castell DO. Nonsteroidal anti-inflammatory drugs and esophageal injury. Semin Arthritis Rheum 1989;19:99

140. Shaker R, et al. Effect of aging, position, and temperature on the threshold volume triggering pharyngeal swallows. Gastroenterology 1994;107:396

141. Shaker R, et al. Augmentation of deglutitive upper esophageal sphincter opening in the elderly by exercise. Am J Physiol 1997;272:G1518

142. Shapiro J, et al. Inflammatory myopathy causing pharyngeal dysphagia: a new entity. Ann Otol Rhinol Laryngol 1997;106:357

143. Shaw DW, et al. Influence of normal aging on oral-pharyngeal and upper esophageal sphincter function during swallowing. Am J Physiol 1995;268:G389

144. Siebens H, et al. Correlates and consequences of eating dependency in institutional elderly. J Am Geriatr Soc 1986;34:192

145. Silbiger ML, et al. Neuromuscular disorders affecting the pharynx: cineradiographic analysis. Invest Radiol 1967;2:442

146. Skoutakis VA, et al. Comparative role of omeprazole in the treatment of gastroesophageal reflux disease. Ann Pharmacother 1995;29:1252

147. Sloan S, et al. Determinants of gastroesophageal junction incompetence: hiatal hernia, lower esophageal sphincter, or both? Ann Intern Med 1992;117:977

148. Smout AJPM, et al. Physiological gastroesophageal reflux and esoph-

ageal motor activity studies with a new system for 24-hour recording and automated analysis. Dig Dis Sci 1989;34:372

149. Soergel KH, et al. Presbyesophagus: esophageal motility in nonagenarians. J Clin Invest 1964;43:1472

150. Sonnenberg A, et al. Salivary secretion in reflux esophagitis. Gastroenterology 1982;83:889

151. Sontag S, et al. The importance of hiatal hernia in reflux esophagitis compared with lower esophageal sphincter pressure or smoking. J Clin Gastroenterol 1991;13:628

152. Spechler SJ. Epidemiology and natural history of gastroesophageal reflux disease. Digestion 1992;51(suppl):24

153. Spechler SJ, et al. Prevalence of metaplasia at the gastro-oesophageal junction. Lancet 1994;344:1533

154. Spence RAJ, et al. Does age influence normal gastroesophageal reflux? Gut 1985;26:799

155. Steele CM, et al. Mealtime difficulties in a home for the aged: not just dysphagia. Dysphagia 1997;12:43

156. Stilson W, et al. Hiatal hernia and gastroesophageal reflux. Radiology 1969;93:1323

157. Subramanyam K. Achalasia secondary to malignant mesothelioma of the pleura. J Clin Gastroenterol 1990;12:183

158. Sundaram U, Traube M. Radiologic and manometric study of the gastroesophageal junction in dysphagia aortica. J Clin Gastroenterol 1995;21:275

159. Tack J, Vantrappen G. The aging oesophagus. Gut 1997;41:422

160. Talley NJ, et al. Prevalence of gastrointestinal symptoms in the elderly: a population-based study. Gastroenterology 1992;102:895

161. Thomas P, et al. Esophageal resection in the elderly. Eur J Cardiothorac Surg 1996;10:941

162. Triadafilopoulos G, Sharma R. Features of symptomatic gastroesophageal reflux disease in elderly patients. Am J Gastroenterol 1997;92:2007

163. Trupe EH, et al. Prevalence of feeding and swallowing disorders in a nursing home. Arch Phys Med Rehabil 1984;65:651

164. Tucker HJ, et al. Achalasia secondary to carcinoma: manometric and clinical features. Ann Intern Med 1978;89:315

165. Verlinden M. Review article: a role for gastrointestinal prokinetic agents in the treatment of reflux oesophagitis. Aliment Pharmacol Ther 1989;3:113

166. Wickal KE, Swoope CC. Studies of residual ridge resorption: II. The relationship of dietary calcium and phosphorus to residual ridge resorption. J Prosthet Dent 1974;32:13

167. Williams R, et al. Multicenter trial of sucralfate suspension for the treatment of reflux esophagitis. Am J Med 1987;83(suppl 3B):61

168. Wilson JA, et al. The effects of age, sex, and smoking on normal pharyngoesophageal motility. Am J Gastroenterol 1990;85:686

169. Zamost B, et al. Esophagitis in scleroderma. Gastroenterology 1987;92:421

170. Zhu H, et al. Features of symptomatic gastroesophageal reflux in elderly patients. Scand J Gastroenterol 1993;28:235

171. Zimmerman J, et al. Esophagitis is a major cause of upper gastrointestinal hemorrhage in the elderly. Scand J Gastroenterol 1997;32:906

# Subject Index